The White Cell

A Commonwealth Fund Book

Harvard University Press
Cambridge, Massachusetts, 1975

The White Cell

Martin J. Cline, M.D.

To my wife

This volume is published as part of a long-standing cooperative program between Harvard University Press and the Commonwealth Fund, a philanthropic foundation, to encourage the publication of significant scholarly books in medicine and health.

Preface

At the time I initiated work on *The White Cell*, I did not fully appreciate the problems of critically reviewing and describing the physiology of the normal leukocyte and its abnormal variants. The difficulties in writing a comprehensive summary were soon apparent. The leukocyte is not a single cell type, but three major classes of cells—granulocytes, lymphoid cells, and mononuclear phagocytes. In addition, there are several distinct subpopulations of lymphoid cells and mononuclear phagocytes. Each of these classes and subclasses has a variety of forms at different levels of maturation. Not surprisingly, each normal subclass and each maturational subset has its characteristic morphology, metabolism, and functions. For each of these normal cells there is an abnormal counterpart occurring in various disease states. The consequence is a vast body of literature on normal and abnormal leukocytes.

The problems of selectively summarizing this literature are compounded by the number of fields of basic science embraced by studies of leukocytes: general cell biology, microbiology, immunology, viral oncology, and cell and tissue kinetics. Some of these areas are changing rapidly so that each new issue of the relevant scientific journals brings important new information and sometimes new insight. Consequently, any survey of the white cell that aims at an understanding of cell form and function is destined to be outdated on the day of publication.

The many basic science disciplines related to the white cell present still another challenge—how much material does the reviewer offer in order to clarify cell physiology without writing a textbook of immunology or of cell kinetics? The answer, I would hope, is a compromise between a superficial treatment and a set of encyclopedias.

My purpose in writing this text was to review critically the existing body of knowledge of normal and abnormal leukocyte physiology in order to present the interested reader with a comprehensive bibliography and source book of information on the leukocyte. I have aimed at a sophisticated audience: primarily the medical student, but also the pupil of cell biology and the postgraduate physician concerned with hematology. I have tried to present concepts of leukocyte physiology in a manner that reveals their experimental basis. In pursuing this goal, I have given due consideration to experimentalists who first enunciated certain concepts or made critical observations; for the history of development of a body of scientific information is often as informative as its present status. Consequently, many references to the older as well as the more recent literature have been included. Because the objective was a comprehensive source book of information, over 6,000 articles were reviewed and cited. I have included a number of discussions of immunologic phenomena and general cell biology in order to promote an understanding of leukocyte physiology and function. These areas have been organized for the student of hematology as the principal reader.

To accomplish my objectives, I have arranged the text in the following manner. Three main divisions correspond to the three major types of leukocytes. The interrelationships among these cell types are defined near the beginning of each of these divisions. Each type of leukocyte is discussed in the following sequence. First, *the normal cell:* development and structure, production, life-span and distribution, metabolism, and function; then *the abnormal cell:* abnormalities of morphogenesis, production, metabolism, and function. Finally, disease states illustrating each of these abnormalities are discussed.

Despite the difficulties, writing *The White Cell* has been a rewarding experience. It has offered a unique opportunity to reexamine a body of information and to ascertain that which is firmly based on a solid experimental foundation. For the finished work I am grateful to many: to Dr. T. Hale Ham, who suggested the task and followed

its development with frequent encouragement; to Emma-line Stump, who thoughtfully edited the text; to Gwen Dangerfield for her aid in preparing the manuscript; to Dr. David Golde, Dr. Robert Lehrer, and many other colleagues, who offered specific suggestions and general intellectual stimulation; and to Dr. Maxwell M. Wintrobe, who has long provided a model for dedicated scholarship.

I gratefully acknowledge a grant from the Commonwealth Fund that permitted me to initiate the work, and also support from the United States Public Health Service (Grants CA 11067 and CA 12822), the American Cancer Society (Grant CI-60), and various funds of the Cancer Research Institute of the University of California in San Francisco.

Contents

PART II   Lymphocytes and Plasma Cells

A   THE NORMAL LYMPHOCYTE AND PLASMA CELL

B   THE ABNORMAL LYMPHOCYTE AND PLASMA CELL

PART III   Monocytes and Macrophages

A   THE NORMAL MACROPHAGE

B   THE ABNORMAL MACROPHAGE

The White Cell

Introduction

The Relation of Leukocytes to Other Hematopoietic Cells

The origin of mammalian blood cells can be traced to the blood islands of the fetal yolk sac mesoderm. In the early embryo this organ does not ordinarily contain cells morphologically identifiable as the leukocytes that ultimately circulate in the blood of the adult animal. Rather, it contains progenitor cells capable of giving rise to leukocytes and other hematopoietic cell lines during later embryonic and postnatal development. From the yolk sac, streams of precursor cells migrate to colonize the hematopoietic organs of fetal life: the liver, the spleen, and ultimately the bone marrow. Lymphoid precursors may also migrate from the yolk sac to the epithelial thymic rudiment and thus establish the earliest lymphoid organ. The particular pattern of colonization from the yolk sac differs, of course, among different species.

The migrating hematopoietic progenitors of the early embryo are often referred to as *stem cells*. A hematopoietic stem cell may be defined as a cell with two capabilities: (*a*) the ability to divide and give rise to daughter cells having the same capabilities as the parent; that is, the cell is self-renewing; (*b*) the ability to differentiate into more mature hematologic cells. A stem cell may be either *pluripotent* and capable of giving rise to cells of several hematopoietic lines, or *unipotent* with maturation capabilities along a single line. Both types of stem cells exist in higher animals.

Evidence supporting the existence of pluripotent and unipotent stem cells will be summarized in Chapter 2; however, at the outset it is important to understand that all blood cells are thought to be related in their origins from a pluripotent precursor. The relation between any two types of blood cells may be close or distant, depending upon their point of origin along the branching pathway of potential hematopoietic cell development. This concept is illustrated in Fig. I.1.

The decision for a pluripotent stem cell to develop along one or another potential line appears to be governed directly by local environmental factors operative within a hematopoietic organ, as well as indirectly by specific "cytopoietic" hormones such as erythropoietin. The local microenvironmental factors are poorly understood at present, but almost certainly involve hematopoietic cell interactions that operate over a very short distance. The systemic cytopoietic hormones may be generated by remote organs, which sense the requirements for a given cell line and elaborate a hormonal signal that is distributed systemically.

Leukocyte Functions and Interactions

As indicated earlier, the leukocyte populations of the body are generally considered to be comprised of the granulocytic, lymphoid, and mononuclear phagocyte cell lines. From evidence to be summarized, one can conclude that the origins of granulocytes and monocytes may be more closely related to those of red cells and megakaryocyte precursors than to the origins of lymphoid precursors. For example, certain chromosomal abnormalities may be shared by erythrocyte, megakaryocyte, granulo-

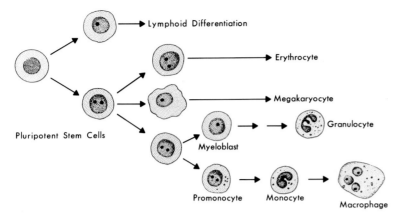

Figure I.1 Schematic representation of the relation of the major hematopoietic cell lines to a pluripotent stem cell. Erthrocytes, megakaryocytes, granulocytes, and macrophages arise from a common pluripotent stem cell different from the stem cell that gives rise to the lymphoid pathway of differentiation. However, both the lymphoid pathway and other hematopoietic cell lines are also linked to a common, more primitive progenitor cell.

cyte, and monocyte-macrophage precursors and are absent in the lymphoid series. Nevertheless, all types of leukocytes seem to have evolved for a common purpose and to function cooperatively in meeting the body's needs. Leukocytes may be regarded as the major defense against foreign invaders. *Foreignness* may be broadly applied to an invading microorganism, a multicellular parasite, an antibody-coated erythrocyte, an exogenously administered protein, or a malignant cell with surface anitgens not native to the host. The multiple aspects of the cooperation of different types of leukocytes in the performance of their defense function will be a recurrent theme in later chapters of this book. At this point, however, an illustration of leukocyte interactions may be helpful.

Let an injection of the facultative intracellular microorganism *Listeria monocytogenes* into an experimental mammal constitute the foreign invasion. Phagocytic neutrophilic granulocytes are the first line of defense, serving to immobilize, phagocytize, and kill a fraction of the inoculated organisms. Should this first line be overwhelmed by proliferating, virulent, intracellular bacteria, mononuclear phagocytes—including monocytes and tissue macrophages—ingest the released organisms and thereby contain their proliferation and spread. With the passage of time, the lymphoid system is also called into play. B lymphocytes and their progeny elaborate immunoglobulin antibody which, together with comple-

ment, "opsonizes" the invaders so that the coated bacteria attach to immunoglobulin and complement receptors on the surface of the phagocytic leukocytes. T and perhaps B lymphocytes elaborate a variety of effector substances that help to activate and direct the distribution of mononuclear phagocytes. Contrariwise, the phagocytes may localize antigen and present it to lymphocytes in a manner that facilitates their immunologic response.

During the course of infection the mononuclear phagocytes and perhaps other leukocytes may release materials that signal the bone marrow to produce more phagocytic cells; that is, the mature cells may be involved in the feedback control of leukopoiesis. Thus monocytes may influence granulopoiesis and mononuclear phagocyte production as part of a prolonged response to a foreign invader.

The leukocyte response to a somatic cell that has undergone malignant transformation appears to be fundamentally similar to the response to a foreign microorganism. The order of appearance of the leukocyte protagonists in the drama and their relative roles may differ, however, in the two situations.

From the above brief sketch it should be apparent that leukocytes possess two major defense mechanisms: phagocytosis and the elaboration of various effector substances, including immunoglobulin. Mature neutrophilic granulocytes and monocytes, and tissue macrophages, are the chief phagocytic cells. Historically, cells in the lymphoid series have been thought to be the major source of effector substances operative in defense reactions. Recently, however, it has become increasingly clear that granulocytes, including eosinophils and basophils, as well as mononuclear phagocytes may release a variety of cellular constituents that operate in defense and inflammatory reactions. These constituents may be beneficial to the host if they localize and destroy foreign invaders, or may sometimes be harmful if the inflammatory response is inappropriate or excessive.

The leukocytes thus may be considered as a widely dispersed organ comprised of three major cell types related in their embryonic origins. Most constituents of this organ are in a state of constant turnover, with cell loss and death being compensated by cell proliferation. Properly functioning, this organ serves its major purpose of defense against external invaders or internal neoplastic change. Abnormalities in organ function, however, may result in serious infection, neoplasia, or excessive inflammatory reactions that are detrimental to the host.

PART I Granulocytes   A The Normal Granulocyte

Chapter 1 Morphology and Morphogenesis of the Granulocytic Series

The granulocytic series encompasses three morphologically distinct cell lines: the neutrophil, the eosinophil, and the basophil. The cells of each series are distinguished by their cytoplasmic granules and certain other morphologic features. Examples of the mature cells of each of these lines are shown in Fig. 1.1. Occasionally the terms *granulocyte* and *neutrophil* are used synonymously. However, granulocyte generally refers to all three of the cell lines and neutrophil to one distinct line.

Controversy exists regarding the cell of origin for the three granulocytic cell lines. The traditional view, evolved at the end of the last century and still held by many hematologists, is that a primitive granule-containing precursor cell, the *promyelocyte*, is common to all three cell lines. The traditionally defined promyelocyte contains a single species of "nonspecific" azurophil granule which, with cellular maturation, differentiates into a "specific" granule characteristic of one of the cell lines. Recent evidence, based on leukocyte fine structure and cytochemical reactions, challenges this view. It suggests that *the earliest cells in which granule development can be detected are already differentiated into a particular series, either neutrophilic, eosinophilic, or basophilic.*

The modern view of granulocyte development, outlined in Fig. 1.2, is that once progenitor cells mature sufficiently to have cytoplasmic granules, they are already committed to one of the three pathways of differentiation. Recent evidence also suggests that the earliest azurophil granules are cytochemically distinct for each cell line and persist in the more mature cells of that line (11, 12, 76, 77, 92, 95). The origins of this modern concept of granulocyte morphogenesis can be found as early as 1918 (41).

Nomenclature and Morphology of Developing Granulocytes

The major morphologic techniques applied to the study of granulocyte differentiation, in order of historical development, are (a) observation of living cells in a transparent suspending medium; (b) staining of fixed or dried specimens of blood or bone marrow; (c) cytochemical methods; and (d) electron microscopy, first of dried or fixed specimens and later of thin sections of cells. These techniques have been refined over a period of time (95). Studies, by light microscopy, of fixed leukocytes stained with Romanovsky dyes have had the greatest influence on the concepts and nomenclature of cellular morphogenesis.

Studies Utilizing Light Microscopy

Since the light microscope is still the most common tool used by the hematologist to study granulocytes, we shall consider the developmental stages of the cell that can be identified with this instrument. The commonly used nomenclature is related to these identifiable stages (34, 43, 62).

Based on morphologic criteria applied to cells stained with Romanovsky dyes, a stepwise series delineating progressively more mature forms of the neutrophilic series

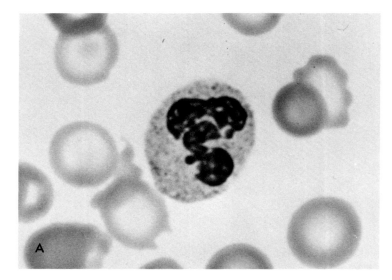

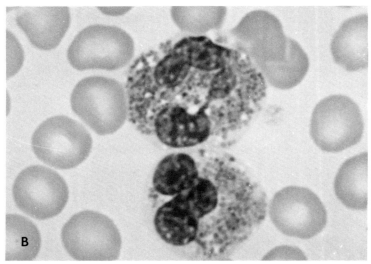

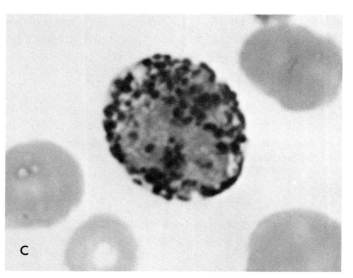

Figure 1.1 Mature granulocytes from human blood; Giemsa stain.

    A. Polymorphonuclear leukocyte
    B. Eosinophil
    C. Basophil

has been identified by means of light microscopy. The maturational process in vivo, however, is continuous rather than stepwise. The clinical hematologist recognized the following sequence of progressively more mature cells, as shown in Fig. 1.3: *myeloblast (granuloblast) → promyelocyte (progranulocyte) → myelocyte → metamyelocyte → band form (stab) → mature neutrophil (polymorphonuclear or PMN leukocyte).* Similar sequences exist for the development of cells in the eosinophilic and basophilic series and will be described in Chapters 6 and 7.

    The general indexes used to identify the different levels of maturation of Romanovsky-stained cells are cell size granule number and appearance, and nuclear morphology.

    From the promyelocyte stage the cell progressively decreases in size as it matures. Large and prominent granules first appear at the promyelocyte stage, becoming less prominent with further maturation. In the myeloblast and promyelocyte the large round or oval nucleus has a relatively loose chromatin structure and the nucleolus, (or nucleoli) is prominent. Nuclear indentation and loss of the nucleoli are characteristics of intermediate-stage cells such as myelocytes and metamyelocytes. Nuclear elongation and lobation and increased condensation (density) define the mature granulocyte.

    Briefly, the characteristics of the cells of this series are as follows.

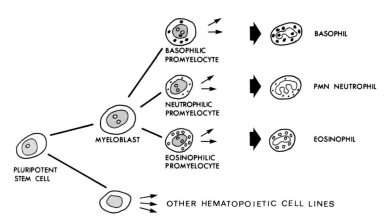

Figure 1.2 Scheme for the development of the three major granulocytic cell lines and other hematopoietic cell lines from a common pluripotent stem cell. Granulocyte differentiation occurs at the promyelocyte stage of development.

MARROW (development, 14 days)

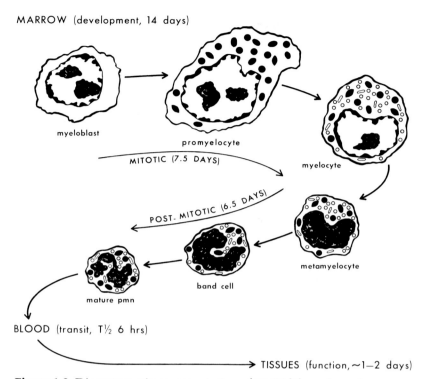

Figure 1.3 Diagrammatic representation of PMN life cycle and stages of PMN maturation. During each of the secretory stages a distinct type of secretory granule is produced: azurophils (*solid black*) are formed only during the promyelocyte stage, and specific granules (*light forms*) are produced during the myelocyte stage. The metamyelocyte and band forms are nonproliferating, nonsecretory stages that develop into the mature PMN. The times indicated for the various compartments were determined by isotope labeling techniques. (From D. F. Bainton, J. L. Ullyot, and M. G. Farquhar, *J. Exp. Med.* 134:907, 1971. Reprinted by permission of authors and publisher.)

Myeloblast (Fig. 1.4): This is a primitive cell normally restricted to the bone marrow. The nucleus, large in relation to the volume of cytoplasm, is round or slightly oval and has one or more prominent nucleoli. The nuclear membrane is smooth without condensation of chromatin. The cytoplasm is deep blue and has no perinuclear clear zone or cytoplasmic inclusions. A foamy appearance is sometimes observed (see Chapter 11). Myeloblasts from patients with leukemia may show considerable variation from the prototype cell.

Promyelocyte (Fig. 1.5): At this stage of maturation, granules ("azurophilic") appear in the cytoplasm and apparently cover the nucleus. Nuclear outline is similar to that of the myeloblast, but the nucleoli may be more difficult to see. The chromatin structure may be more coarse. Cytoplasmic basophilia is still prominent.

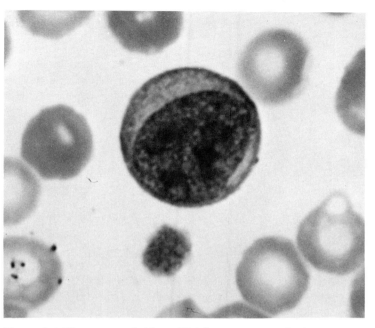

Figure 1.4 Human myeloblast; Wright's stain. Nucleoli are prominent, nuclear chromatin is fine, and cytoplasmic granulation is absent.

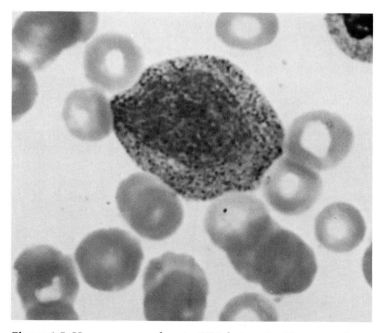

Figure 1.5 Human promyelocyte; Wright's stain. Note prominent nucleoli and cytoplasmic granulation.

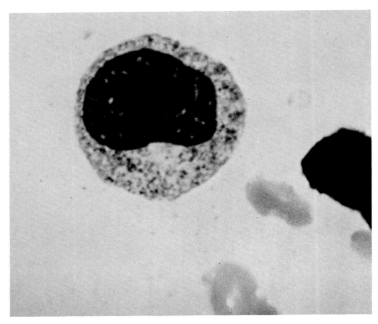

Figure 1.6 Human metamyelocyte (early); Wright's stain. Note dense nuclear chromatin and indented nuclear configuration.

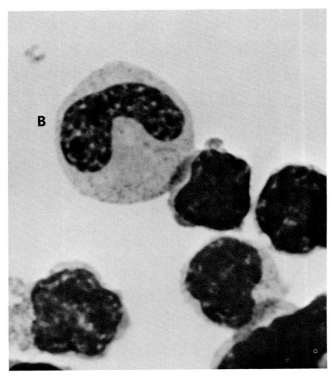

Figure 1.7 Band form (*B*); Wright's stain.

Myelocyte (Fig. 1.6): The nucleus is now oval and may be eccentrically located in the cell. Nucleoli are no longer visible and the nuclear chromatin is more condensed. The cytoplasm loses its basophilia (blue coloring) and becomes acidophilic (light red or pink).

Metamyelocyte (juvenile forms) (Fig. 1.7); The nucleus is dense and elongated with a sausage- or horseshoe-shaped configuration. The nuclear membrane is well defined. The cytoplasm, clearly acidophilic, contains numerous fine granules less coarse and prominent than those of the preceding stages. Some hematologists recognize a further development of this stage of maturation and designate the cells as stab forms or band forms.

Polymorphonuclear neutrophil (Fig. 1.1): This is the final stage of cellular maturation. The nucleus is dense and has assumed its characteristic lobulated appearance. The cytoplasm is pale, acidophilic, and contains fine, uniform pink or violet-pink granules.

Analysis by Electron Microscopy

The study of hematopoietic cell development by light microscopy has many limitations. As a consequence, hematologists and cell physiologists have turned increasingly to electron microscopy for analysis of the fine structure (ultrastructure) of cells.

The most comprehensive studies of the fine structure in developing granulocytes have utilized bone marrow obtained from rabbits (9, 11, 12, 84, 95, 99). A more limited number of comprehensive studies of human marrow is available (5, 26, 63, 74). We shall consider first the fine structure and cytochemistry of the developing rabbit granulocyte; and second, the relatively minor additional features that characterize granulopoiesis in man and other species.

In electron microscopic studies of developing rabbit granulocytes several types of morphologic criteria have been used to identify cells at different levels of maturation. The sequence of events in granulocyte maturation is schematically outlined in Fig. 1.8. As with Romanovsky-strained cells, the important ultrastructural criteria of maturity are nuclear shape, chromatin density, presence of nucleoli, and cytoplasmic organelles. The relative importance of these criteria is indicated in Table 1.1.

Large round or oval nuclei with prominent nucleoli are characteristic of the young myeloblast and early promyelocyte cells. With progressive maturation (15) the large and highly differentiated nucleoli of early cell forms diminish in size and complexity (Fig. 1.3 and 1.8). Maturation involves a progressive increase in the degree of condensation (electron density) of the interphase nuclear chromatin of granulocytes similar to that found in devel-

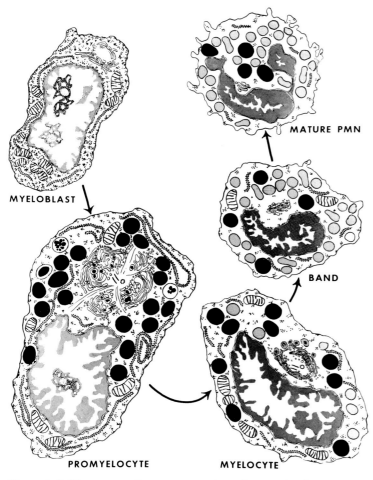

Figure 1.8 Diagrammatic representation of stages in the maturation of PMN leukocytes. Granules are shown 1.5× scale, and only half the average number are shown. The myeoblast lacks granules but contains abundant ribosomes, mitochondria, and a small rudimentary Golgi complex. The promyelocyte (progranulocyte) and myelocyte are stages of intense secretory activity and show elaborate development of cytoplasmic organelles involved in protein synthesis, segregation, and concentration (that is, ribosomes, rough-surface endoplasmic reticulum, and Golgi complex). The larger azurophil granules are formed by condensation of secretory material along the proximal or concave face of the Golgi complex of the progranulocyte. Smaller, less dense specific granules are formed by a similar process occurring along the distal or convex face of the Golgi complex of the myelocyte. The metamyelocyte (not shown) and band cell are nonsecretory stages showing a gradual diminution in most cytoplasmic organelles. The mature PMN has a multilobulated nucleus and a cytoplasm containing primarily glycogen and granules. (From D. F. Bainton and M. G. Farquhar, *J. Cell Biol.* 28:277, 1966. Reprinted by permission of authors and publisher.)

Table 1.1 Morphologic criteria for judging granulocyte maturity.

Reliable nuclear signs	Less reliable nuclear signs	Cytoplasmic signs
Chromatin condensation Nucleolus	Nuclear indentation and lobation Nuclear shape Nuclear size	Organization of granular reticulum Numbers and organization of ribosomes Size and numbers of mitochondria Volume of cytoplasm

oping red cells (80) and thymocytes (70). Progressive nuclear indentation and lobation, although generally concomitant with maturation, are probably the least reliable nuclear signs. Nuclei, immature by other fine structural criteria, sometimes may show indentation. Nuclear shape also may vary considerably in more mature cell forms (23).

The cytoplasmic features useful in determining the maturational level of the cell include: organization of the granular reticulum, amount and organization of ribosomes, size and number of mitochondria, and cytoplasmic volume.

The granular reticulum increases transiently in early cells and decreases during subsequent cell maturation. A parallel increase and succeeding decrease occurs in the numbers of ribosomes attached to the endoplasmic reticulum of the cytoplasm. Presumably this diminution in endoplasmic reticulum and ribosomes reflects a decrease in diversity and capacity of the protein-synthesizing apparatus with cell maturation.

In all the granulocytic lines, and particularly in the neutrophilic series, the size and number of mitochondria decrease as the granulocytes mature (Fig. 1.8). Changes in the aerobic metabolism of these cells reflect this morphologic alteration (see Chapters 3 and 4). Finally, as noted in Romanovsky-stained fixed cells, the volume of the cell cytoplasm at the promyelocyte stage transiently increases and, with further maturation, progressively decreases.

The size, number, and density of cytoplasmic granules are additional guides to cell maturity. They will be considered in detail in subsequent sections of this chapter.

Myeloblast Known also as a granuloblast, the myeloblast is characterized by the following cytologic features (Figs. 1.8 and 1.9): (a) a large round nucleus with a high nucleus/cytoplasm ratio; (b) an "open" or dispersed pattern of nuclear chromatin; (c) large and highly developed nu-

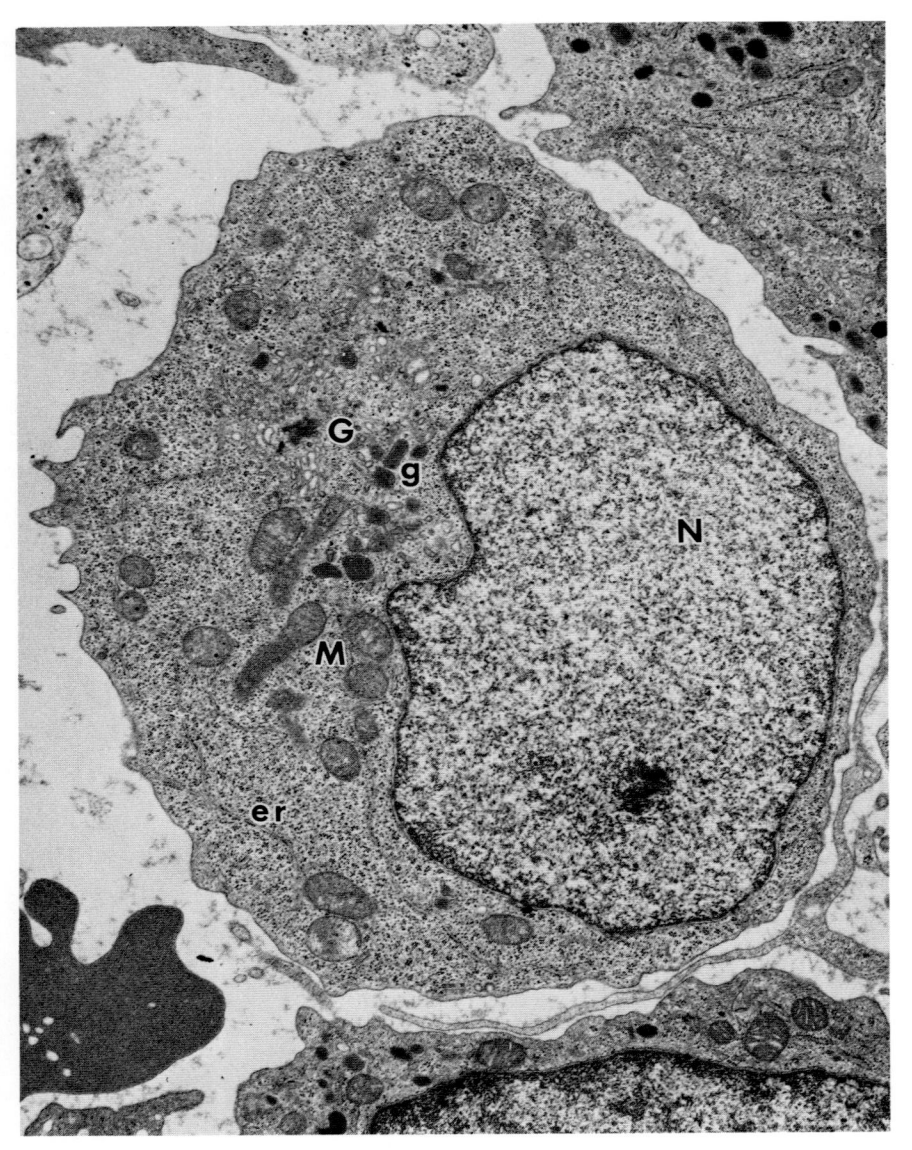

Figure 1.9 Blast cell from a patient with granulocytic hyperplasia. The large, ovoid nucleus (*N*) has finely dispersed chromatin and a prominent nucleolus. The Golgi apparatus (*G*) is well developed. A few dense granules (*g*), mitochondria (*M*), polyribosomes, and some development of endoplasmic reticulum (*er*) are seen in the cytoplasm. (From Y. Tanaka and J. R. Goodman, *Electron Microscopy of Human Blood Cells,* Harper & Row, New York, 1972. Reprinted by permission of authors and publisher.)

cleoli; (*d*) no specific cytoplasmic granules; and (*e*) poorly developed endoplasmic reticulum. The immature cells of patients with acute myelocytic leukemia are often morphologically similar to the myeloblasts of the normal bone marrow (5, 63, 74).

The metabolic correlates of these anatomic structures are (*a*) high levels of synthesis of ribosomal RNA within the nucleoli, and (*b*) the capacity for DNA synthesis (see Chapter 3).

Myeloblasts cannot be distinguished from other primitive hematopoietic cells, such as proerythroblasts and lymphoblasts, on the basis of their fine structure by any wholly reliable morphologic criteria (cf. 70, 73, 80, 88, 95). Both Romanovsky-stained preparations and electron micrographs may show distinctive features in myeloblasts that are absent in erythroblasts or lymphoblasts (41, 89). However, these features are not sufficiently constant to distinguish cell types reliably in the elctron microscope. Instead, one must usually assign a given undifferentiated cell to one of the cell lines on the basis of "the company it keeps"; that is, on the basis of association with more highly differentiated cells of the same series (50, 104). This lack of distinguishing features among the blast cells is not remarkable if there is, in fact, a pluripotent progenitor cell capable of generating several cell lines (see Fig. 1.2 and Chapters 2 and 12).

Neutrophilic Promyelocyte The promyelocyte is the least mature granulated form in the neutrophilic series (Figs. 1.8 and 1.10). The nucleus of this cell is characterized by diffuse chromatin and persistent complex nucleoli. Typically, the nucleus is indented opposite the Golgi zone. The nucleus/cytoplasm ratio is lower than that of the antecedent myeloblast.

Observed within the cytoplasm are occasional mitochondria and lipid droplets, extensive cisternae of granular reticulum, free polyribosomes, and a population of dense granules each about 0.4 micron in diameter (Figs. 1.10 and 1.11). The granules are usually spherical and homogeneously dense after fixation in glutaraldehyde-osmium tetroxide. In the neutrophilic series these granules correspond to the "azurophil granules" of the promyelocyte in Romanovsky-stained preparations and are best designated as *primary granules*, denoting their early appearance in cell maturation (11, 12, 95). In hematologic literature they have been called by a variety of other terms, including type 1, alpha, and A granules. The granules of the neutrophilic leukocyte have many features in common with the lysosomes of other tissues such as the liver and kidney. Lysosomes are membrane-bound substructures containing hydrolases with a low pH optimum activity (32, 33, 71).

In the rabbit neutrophil, primary granules appear as electron-dense spherules on the margins of the Golgi saccules (Fig. 1.12). Individual spherules reach a size of about 0.1 micron. The Golgi saccules fuse and bring the small spherules into contact with one another. The spherules also ultimately fuse, giving rise to the primary granule as the vacuolar space surrounding the granules disappears (cf. 1, 9). Tritium-labeled amino acids are incorporated into the Golgi apparatus (27, 40), which thus appears to be the primary site of production of neutrophil granules.

Cytochemistry of primary granules. The primary granules of the neutrophilic promyelocyte can be shown by cytochemical and biochemical techniques to contain the following enzymes (7, 32):

(a) *Myeloperoxidase*—located exclusively in the primary granules and the best enzymatic marker of this population (8, 11, 12). Peroxidases have been identified in the neutrophil granules of a variety of species, including man and the rabbit (8, 11, 12, 29, 36, 37, 89), the rat (107), the horse (87), and the salamander (69). It occurs in the cat in granules resembling primary granules (3).

(b) *Arginine-rich Basic (Cationic) Proteins*—obtained by a variety of extraction procedures (109) and identified by cytochemical stains, including Fast green (85), Biebrich scarlet (52), and a modified Sakaguchi reaction (11). Approximately one-third of the granule-associated, basic protein *lysozyme* is in the primary granules (8). The bactericidal cationic proteins of the rabbit neutrophils are believed to be localized in the heavy primary granule fraction (110).

(c) *Sulfated Mucopolysaccharides*—contribute to the "azurophilia" of the primary granules and produce a strong metachromasia with the stain azure A (52). These granules also stain with iron diamine, aldehyde, fuchsin, alcian blue, and are PAS positive (49, 52). Chondroitin sulfate and hyaluronic acid have been identified in neutrophil granules (39).

(d) *Acid Phosphatase Activity*—found in the primary granule population of man and the rabbit (8, 11, 12, 53, 97). The situation is somewhat complex, as the precise distribution of acid phosphatase among the granule popu-

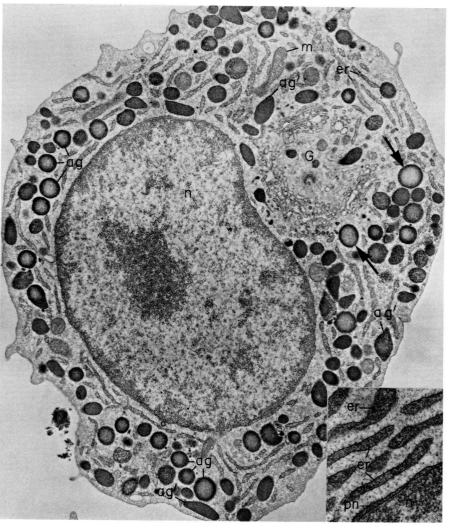

Figure 1.10 PMN promyelocyte, reacted for peroxidase. This cell is the largest (~15 microns) of the neutrophilic series. It has a sizable, slightly indented nucleus (*n*), a prominent Golgi region (*G*), and cytoplasm packed with peroxidase-positive azurophil granules (*ag*). Note the two general shapes of azurophil granules, spherical (*ag*) or ellipsoid (*ag'*). The majority are

spherical, with a homogeneous matrix, but a few ellipsoid forms containing crystalloids (best seen in the three lower rectangles of Fig. 1.11) are also present. Many of the spherical forms (*arrows*) have a dense periphery and a lighter core, presumably owing to incomplete penetration of substrate into the compact centers of mature granules.

Peroxidase reaction product is visible in less concentrated form within all compartments of the secretory apparatus—endoplasmic reticulum (*er*) and perinuclear cisterna (*pn*). No reaction product is seen in the cytoplasmic matrix, mitochondria (*m*), or nucleus (*n*). Magnification ×12,600.

The inset depicts a portion of another promyelocyte at high magnification, showing to better advantage flocculent deposits of peroxidase reaction product in the rough endoplasmic reticulum (*er*) including the perinuclear cisterna (*pn*). Ribosomes do not show up in the section, which has been lightly stained with lead. Magnification ×28,600. (From D. F. Bainton, J. L. Ullyot, and M. G. Farquhar, *J. Exp. Med.* 134:907, 1971. Reprinted by permission of authors and publisher.)

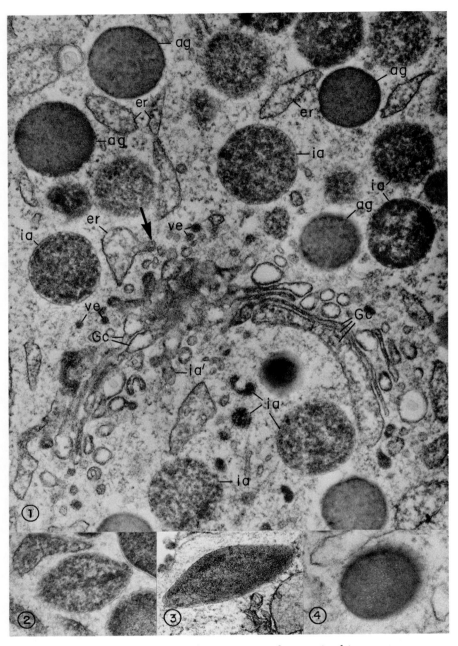

lations depends on the phosphate substrate used in the test system (8, 95). In several other species of mammals acid phosphatase also is found in a granule population that probably corresponds to the primary granules of human and rabbit neutrophil (87, 107). The acid phosphatase marker can be used to trace the origin of the primary granule from the Golgi apparatus (11, 98).

(e) *Other Acid Hydrolases*—a variety of acid hydrolases, including beta-galactosidase, beta-glucuronidase, N-acetyl-beta-glucosaminidase, alpha-mannosidase, arylsulfatase, 5'-nucleotidase, esterase, and naphthylamidase, localize in the primary granules of human and rabbit neutrophils (8, 11, 12, 81).

Differentiation to other cell lines. Differentiation along neutrophilic, eosinophilic, or basophilic lines can first be reliably detected in the late promyelocyte stage of maturation. Available evidence favors production of the characteristic granules of the eosinophils from the Golgi apparatus in a manner similar to that of granulogenesis in the neutrophil (10, 51, 83, 98, 107). Chapters 6 and 7 give details of granulogenesis and the cytochemistry of eosinophils and basophils.

Intermediate Neutrophils: Myelocytes and Metamyelocytes Maturing intermediate neutrophils are characterized by increasing condensation of nuclear chromatin marginated along the inner aspect of the nuclear membrane (77). Nucleoli become less prominent and ultimately disappear. As the nucleus becomes smaller, the nucleus/cytoplasm ratio decreases (Figs. 1.3 and 1.8). Cytoplasm is lost as well, and the cells become progressively smaller from the promyelocyte stage on. The granular endoplasmic reticulum is less developed in intermediate cells than it is in earlier forms; free and bound polyribosomes are less abundant. Mitochondria are small and rela-

Figure 1.11 Golgi region of PMN promyelocyte. At this stage, peroxidase reaction product is present within (1) all cisternae of the rough endoplasmic reticulum (*er*), including transitional elements (*arrow*), and the perinuclear cisterna (not shown here); (2) clusters of smooth vesicles located at the periphery of the Golgi complex (*ve*); (3) all cisternae of the Golgi complex (*Gc*); and (4) all immature (*ia*) and mature azurophil granules (*ag*). Most of the mature granules appear uniformly dense because of the presence of reaction product throughout. Immature granules are larger and their contents less compact. Note that peroxidase is more concentrated in the cisternae along the concave surface of the Golgi complex, suggesting that, as in the case of the rabbit, azurophil granules arise from this Golgi face (see *ia'*). Magnification ×48,000.

Rectangles 2–4: Azurophil granules of promyelocytes occur in two main forms. The majority are spherical, with a dense, homogeneous matrix (*ag*). Others are ellipsoid or football-shaped (rectangles 2 and 3), with a crystalline substructure that may be partially obscured in mature granules by the dense peroxidase reaction product (rectangle 3) but that is clearly visible in the immature ellipsoid (rectangle 2) or in preparations not incubated for peroxidase. Round granule profiles with a central periodicity (rectangle 4) are presumed to represent "footballs" cut perpendicular to the crystal axis. Rectangles 2 and 3, magnification ×54,000; rectangle 4, ×76,500. (From D. F. Bainton, J. L. Ullyot, and M. G. Farquhar, *J. Exp. Med.* 134:907, 1971. Reprinted by permission of authors and publisher.)

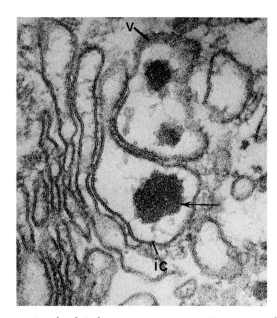

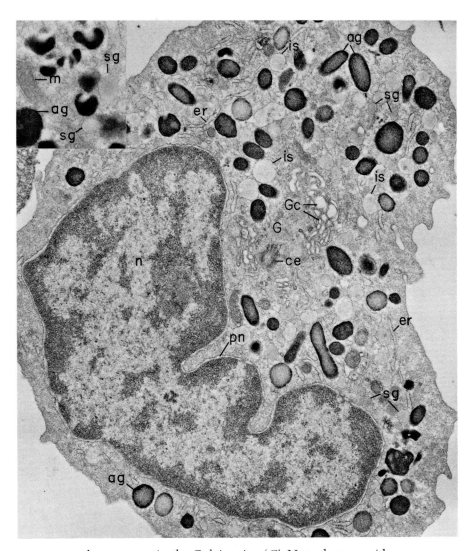

Figure 1.12 Stack of Golgi cisternae in a PMN progranulocyte. The triple-layered structure of the Golgi membranes, which appear nearly symmetrical in this type of preparation, is visible in a number of places. A dense-cored vacuole (*v*), cut in grazing section, is marked. A spherical dense mass (*arrow*), resembling the core material of dense-cored vacuoles, is present within a dilated cisterna (*ic*) along the proximal face of the Golgi complex. Images such as this suggest that dense-cored vacuoles are formed by budding from the ends of the inner one or two Golgi cisternae. Magnification ×100,000. (From D. F. Bainton and M. G. Farquhar, *J. Cell Biol.* 28:277, 1966. Reprinted by permission of authors and publisher.)

tively few in number. These ultrastructural features of intermediate cells correlate with metabolic features of a high level of anaerobic metabolism and rates of RNA and protein synthesis lower than those of younger cell forms (see Chapter 3).

Cytochemistry of secondary granules. In the intermediate neutrophils a second population of granules appears—the secondary (or specific) granules. They are smaller (about 0.3 micron) and less dense than the primary granules (Figs. 1.8 and 1.13). In human neutrophils they may contain crystalloid structures (25, 93).

Two populations of granules are present in the interme-

Figure 1.13 PMN myelocyte. At this stage the cell is smaller (~10 microns) than the promyelocyte (Fig. 1.10), the nucleus is more indented, and the cytoplasm contains two different types of granules: large, peroxidase-positive azurophils (*ag*), and the generally smaller specific granules (*sg*), which do not stain for peroxidase. A number of immature specifics (*is*), which are larger, less compact, and more irregular in contour than mature

granules, are seen in the Golgi region (*G*). Note that peroxidase reaction product is present only in azurophil granules, and is not seen in the rough endoplasmic reticulum (*er*) (which nonetheless has a content of moderate density), perinuclear cisterna (*pn*), or Golgi cisternae (*Gc*) (which appear empty). This is in keeping with the fact that azurophil production has ceased, and only peroxidase-negative specific are produced during the myelocyte stage. Magnification ×16,800.

The inset, a portion of a myelocyte, depicts a cluster of peroxidase-positive granules, most of which are smaller and more pleomorphic than the surrounding specifics (*sg*) and azurophils (*ag*). These are presumed to represent azurophil variants, since they appear during the promyelocyte stage. The presence of such granule variants emphasizes the need for using criteria other than size and shape for identifying PMN granules in the human. Mitochondria (*m*) are also shown. Magnification ×34,400. (From D. F. Bainton, J. L. Ullyot, and M. G. Farquhar, *J. Exp. Med.* 134:907, 1971. Reprinted by permission of authors and publisher.)

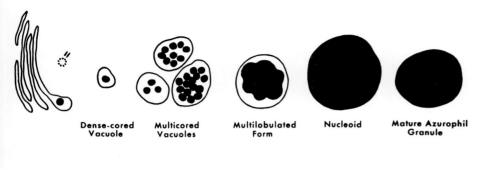

Dense-cored Vacuole   Multicored Vacuoles   Multilobulated Form   Nucleoid   Mature Azurophil Granule

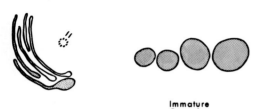 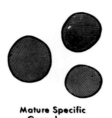

Immature Granules   Mature Specific Granules

Figure 1.14 *Upper diagram:* Diagrammatic representation of azurophil (primary) granule formation in PMN progranulocytes. Dense material condenses within the inner Golgi cisternae and pinches off to form a dense-cored vacuole (~240 millimicrons). Several of the latter merge to form a multicored vacuole. The core material aggregates and becomes a multilobulated mass, which subsequently forms a more compact nucleoid. The finely granular content around the core condenses until it is barely distinguishable from the core material, so that in the mature granule (diameter 600 to 800 millimicrons) the entire content is uniformly dense.

Lower diagram: Diagrammatic representation of specific (secondary) granule formation in PMN myelocytes. Finely granular material condenses within the outer Golgi cisternae. Small granules (~90 millimicrons) bud from the outer Golgi cisternae. Several of these merge to form larger aggregates that further condense to form mature granules, most of which are spherical and measure 300 to 500 millimicrons in diameter. A few dumbbell or smaller forms (not shown) are also present in mature PMN. (From D. F. Bainton and M. G. Farquhar, *J. Cell Biol.* 39:286, 1968. Reprinted by permission of authors and publisher.)

diate neutrophil—the persistent population of primary granules and the new population of secondary granules. Available evidence suggests that at this stage of development the production of primary granules ceases and the neutrophil switches over to production of secondary granules (95). Since manufacture of primary granules is stopped, each cell division reduces the concentration of primary granules as they are parceled out to the daughter cells. As a result of continued synthesis, secondary granules remain numerically high and eventually predominate.

At this intermediate stage of cell development the Golgi apparatus is less developed than in earlier forms

(Figs. 1.10 and 1.13). This organelle appears to be the major site of synthesis of the secondary granules, as it was for primary granules in younger cells. Secondary granules first appear as small structures in the lateral margin of the Golgi saccules and associated small vesicles. Production of secondary granules probably occurs primarily on the convex surface of the Golgi sac, whereas primary granule formation occurs preferentially on the concave face (3, 9). A scheme of granule formation is shown in Fig. 1.14.

By cytochemical techniques the secondary granules can be shown to contain the following components.

(*a*) *Alkaline phosphatase.* This distinctive enzymatic marker appears only in the secondary granules. It was first recognized, relatively early in histochemical studies, that alkaline phosphatase activity is restricted to intermediate or more mature neutrophils and is absent from younger forms (1, 57). Only subsequently was this late emergence of enzymatic activity recognized as corresponding to the appearance of a new granule population (11, 12, 97, 98). Granule fractionation procedures provide evidence consistent with a restriction of alkaline phosphatase activity to the secondary granules (8). Chapter 3 discusses the substrate range and the synthesis of leukocyte alkaline phosphatase.

(*b*) *Lysozyme.* Baggiolini and his co-workers found two-thirds of the cell contents of this basic protein in their "b" granule fraction, which corresponds to the secondary granules of rabbit granulocytes (7, 8). Thus one-third of neutrophil lysozyme is in the primary granules and two-thirds in the secondary granules. This distribution of enzyme is consistent with other primarily morphologic observations (72).

(*c*) *Aminopeptidase.* By biochemical techniques this enzyme appears concomitantly with alkaline phosphatase, relatively late in the development of neutrophils (1, 30). This observation suggests a localization of enzyme in the secondary granule fraction.

The formation and contents of the primary and secondary granules are summarized in Table 1.2.

Late Forms: Bands and Mature Neutrophils The mature forms of the granulocyte are characterized by progressive lobation of the nuclear outline, marked condensation and margination of nuclear chromatin, and absent nucleoli. The endoplasmic reticulum is less developed than in earlier forms; free and bound ribosomes are much less common (Figs. 1.8 and 1.15). These are the fine structural counterparts of the diminished protein and RNA synthetic capacity of the mature cell. Similarly, the Golgi apparatus appears atrophic and granulogenesis has ceased.

Table 1.2 Primary and secondary granules in rabbit neutrophils.

Primary granules	Secondary granules
Formation	*Formation*
Production of primary granules occurs at promyelocyte to intermediate stage of neutrophil development	Production of secondary granules occurs in intermediate neutrophils (myelocytes)
Subsequent cell division reduces concentration of primary granules as they are parceled out to daughter cells	First appear as small structures in lateral margin of Golgi saccules and associated small vesicles
	Production occurs primarily on convex surface of Golgi sac
Contents	Eventually predominate over primary granules
Myeloperoxidase	
Arginine-rich basic (cationic) protein	*Contents*
Sulfated mucopolysaccharides	Alkaline phosphatase
Acid phosphatase	Lysozyme
Other acid hydrolases	Aminopeptidase

The mature cell has a primarily anaerobic metabolism and contains few mitochondria (28). With maturation there is a progressive accumulation of cytoplasmic glycogen.

In addition to the small numbers of primary granules and the large numbers of secondary granules, a third (tertiary) population of granules may exist in the cytoplasm of the mature neutrophil of the rabbit (95). These granules are small, dense, and pleomorphic. They are said to be similar to those observed in lymphocytes and monocytes (98). The identity of this third population of granules is not well established, since their distinctive features are not well preserved in the usual glutaraldehyde-osmium fixative employed to study granulocyte fine structure (95). More recent evidence is against the existence of a distinctive third population of granules.

Summary of Cytologic Features of Maturation

Myeloblasts cannot be definitely distinguished from other immature, nongranulated marrow cells on the basis of their fine structure. When granules appear in early cell forms, their differentiation along neutrophilic, eosinophilic, or basophilic lines is already established. With progressive maturation there is the sequential appearance

Figure 1.15 Mature PMN, reacted for peroxidase. The cytoplasm is filled with granules; the smaller peroxidase-negative specifics (*sg*) are more numerous, the azurophils (*ag*) having

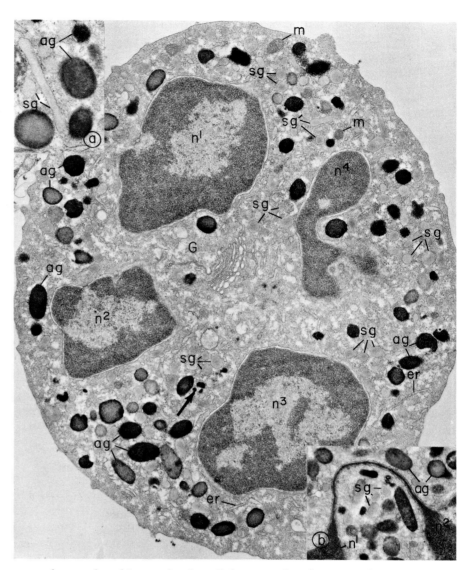

been reduced in number by cell division after the promyelocyte stage. Some small, irregularly shaped azurophil granule variants are also present (*arrow*) (see Fig. 1.13). The nucleus is condensed and lobulated (n^1-n^4), the Golgi region (*G*) is small and lacks forming granules, endoplasmic reticulum (*er*) scanty, and mitochondria (*m*) few. Note that the cytoplasm of this cell has a rather ragged, moth-eaten appearance because the glycogen, which is normally present, has been extracted in this preparation. Magnification ×17,600.

The insets depict portions of the cytoplasm of mature PMN reacted for peroxidase. Inset *a* demonstrates that the peroxidase-positive azurophils (*ag*) can be easily distinguished from the unreactive specifics (*sg*). Note that one of the specifics is quite elongated (~1,000 millimicrons). Inset *b* illustrates the narrow connection between two lobes (n^1-n^2) of the PMN nucleus. Inset *a*, magnification ×30,000; inset *b*, ×11,800. (From D. F. Bainton, J. L. Ullyot, and M. G. Farquhar, *J. Exp. Med.* 134:907, 1971. Reprinted by permission of authors and publisher.)

of two distinct subclasses of granules. The Golgi apparatus is clearly involved in the production of both the primary and the secondary granules (32, 71). As production of the primary granules ceases in intermediate cell forms, cell division dilutes the cellular contents of these granules and the secondary granules come to predominate. The distinctive enzymatic marker of primary granules is peroxidase; of secondary granules, it is alkaline phosphatase. Basic proteins and acid hydrolases are distributed among the different granule populations.

Cytoplasmic features of maturation are a progressive diminution in the size and complexity of the endoplasmic reticulum, and associated polyribosome population that corresponds to a declining protein synthetic capacity. Mitochondria are never abundant in these cells and decrease in numbers with maturity, a change reflected in a diminishing cellular content of mitochondrial enzyme activity. Glycogen accumulates with maturation (105).

Nuclear features of maturation include progressive condensation, margination of interphase chromatin (cf. 90) and, less reliably, a progressive indentation and lobulation of nuclear form.

After the onset of granulation, cells of the eosinophilic and basophilic series develop distinct cytological features; these are considered in subsequent chapters.

Comparative Fine Structure of Mammalian Granulocytes

The basic features of the morphogenesis of human and rabbit neutrophils described in the preceding sections of this chapter appear to be the same for all the mammalian species thus far examined, including the guinea pig (76, 77, 91, 103, 108), the rat (14, 48, 76, 77, 106, 107), the mouse (47, 55, 58), the cat (3), the hamster (86, 96), and the great apes (54). In all these species the earliest granulation detectable in immature cells ostensibly corresponds to the peroxidase-containing primary granules in the early neutrophils of man and the rabbit. Smaller, more dense peroxidase-negative granules appear in the intermediate granulocyte forms of each of these species and probably correspond to secondary granules. Additional granulocyte populations have not been excluded, however, and some clear interspecies differences exist. These differences involve mainly the crystalloid substructures of granules seen in certain species and the enzyme content within a granule class.

Man and the Great Apes

The basic features of granulocyte maturation and differentiation in man are remarkably similar to those of the rabbit. Because of the relative difficulty of obtaining normal human marrow, less is known about the details of granulocyte morphogenesis in man.

The early studies of human granulocyte ultrastructure have been reviewed by Wetzel (96; see also 16, 18, 20, 21, 22, 78). In 1954 Kautz and DeMarsh (59) described the fine structure of human bone marrow. They observed large, dense granules and smaller, less dense granules (probably corresponding to primary and secondary populations). A year later, Bernhard and his colleagues (17) also clearly distinguished granules from other cytoplasmic organelles and discussed their polymorphism. In 1956, Miller (68) documented changes that occur in granulocyte cytoplasmic organelles during maturation.

A number of investigators subsequently distinguished among the various types of human neutrophilic granules (24, 46, 94). The introduction of the glutaraldehyde-osmium tetroxide fixation technique (4, 5) propelled the study of the fine structure of human granulocytes into its modern phase.

The granule populations of human neutrophils are somewhat difficult to classify because they overlap in size distribution, and because they have variable density as a result of susceptibility to extraction during the fixation process. Nevertheless, good evidence supports the existence of two populations of granules. A population of large, dense, "azurophil" primary granules containing peroxidase and mucopolysaccharide is produced in young cells (3, 13, 29, 36, 37, 66, 93). Secondary granules, less dense and generally smaller, seem to originate at the intermediate stage of granulocyte development (36, 37, 93). In addition, there may be a third population of cylindrical granules, large in size and moderately dense, containing filamentous crystalline inclusions (93). These latter granules are usually peroxidase granules and may therefore be related to the primary granule population (cf. 13, 36).

Huser and Webb (54) described large, dense granules and smaller, elongated, less dense granules in the mature neutrophils of gorillas, chimpanzees, and orangutans. Orangutan neutrophils may contain intragranular filamentous crystalloids similar to those described in human cells.

Guinea Pigs, Rats, Mice, and Cats

Developing guinea pig neutrophils closely resemble those of the rabbit with the exception of crystalloids, which occasionally appear in elongate granules (76, 91, 92, 96, 103). No new features of granulocyte morphogenesis have become apparent from studies of this species.

The basic pattern of granulogenesis observed in the developing rat neutrophil is essentially the same as that of the rabbit (48, 76, 103, 106, 107). Rat primary granules are smaller than those of the rabbit. The smaller, less dense granules, which probably correspond to the secondary granules, may be elongate and contain rod-shaped inclusions.

The mouse has no novel granulogenetic features (55, 58). The more mature neutrophils of this species are characterized by a distinctive ring-shaped nucleus. The cat is also unexceptional in its basic pattern of neutrophil morphogenesis. Distinctive features include rod-shaped secondary granules and no histochemically demonstrable acid or alkaline phosphatase (3).

Abnormalities in Disease

Abnormalities of neutrophil morphogenesis in both malignant and nonmalignant conditions are described in detail in Chapters 9, 10, and 11. However, for a better understanding of the development of normal cells a brief consideration of acquired and congenital abnormalities is appropriate at this point.

Inflammatory Diseases

Mature neutrophils accumulating in response to an intense inflammatory stimulus are generally characterized by abundant and prominent primary granules. This phenomenon was appreciated by Horn and his associates (53) in studies of peritoneal exudate granulocytes in the rabbit (cf. 82, 86, 96, 111). The circulating neutrophils of human patients with long-standing infection or intense inflammatory diseases may have prominent azurophilic granulation, often called "toxic granulation." A rather recent study conclusively identifies these "toxic" granules as primary granules (66). Vacuoles containing phagocytized material may also appear as "toxic granules" in Romanovsky-stained preparations when viewed with a light microscope (79, 111, 113).

Other features of toxic neutrophils are an increased alkaline phosphatase activity of the granule fraction (see Chapter 3), decreased nuclear lobation, and persistent granular endoplasmic reticulum (66). These fine structural features suggest that neutrophils in the peripheral blood of patients with chronic inflammatory disease may be less mature than normal. The unusual prominence of the primary granulation suggests that either synthesis of the primary granule persists longer than usual under inflammatory stimuli or that some cell divisions are missed before release of cells into the blood. Examples of "toxic" neutrophils with prominent granulation are shown in Fig. 1.16 (see also Fig. 1.1). Other examples appear in Chapter 9.

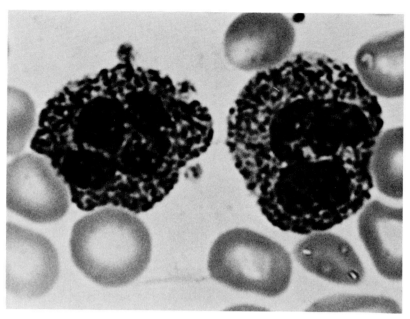

Figure 1.16 Neutrophils with "toxic" cytoplasmic granulation; Giemsa stain.

Myeloproliferative Disorders

Acute Myelocytic Leukemia   Auer rods, possibly unique to the myeloblast and promyelocyte cells of acute myelocytic or myelomonocytic leukemia, may be abnormal developments of the primary granule (see Chapter 11). Along with peroxidase (60), acid phosphatase (45), and esterase (42) activity, the Auer rods are characterized by azurophilia, probably on the basis of mucopolysaccharide content (89). They are structurally distinct from the crystalloid-containing granules of the intermediate and mature human neutrophils described previously (25, 67, 93). Similar structures may be seen in abnormal monocytes as well as in neutrophils (67).

When Romanovsky-stained early granulocytes are viewed by light microscopy, Auer rods appear as needle-shaped, red inclusions 1 to 6 microns in length (Fig. 1.17) (35, 89). Their fine structural detail, revealed in thin sections by electron microscopy, consists of regularly spaced lamellae in the long axis of the rod. Such lamellae occasionally show cross-periodicity at 40 to 60 Å intervals (44, 67, 102). Evidence indicates that the longitudinal substructure consists of small parallel tubules approximately 100A in diameter, in hexagonal array (6, 60).

Asano (6), Bessis (19), and Anderson (5) describe bands of cytoplasmic filaments of 80 to 100A diameter in neutrophils of patients with acute myelocytic leukemia. This is not a uniform finding, however, and similar structures

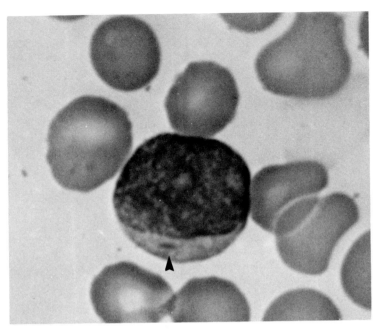

Figure 1.17 A myeloblast with a prominent nucleolus and an Auer body in the cytoplasm (*arrow*).

occasionally have been reported in normal neutrophils (25) and basophils (112).

Chronic Myelocytic Leukemia   Asynchronous nuclear maturation has been observed in the granulocytes of patients with chronic myelocytic leukemia. These granulocytes may demonstrate "mature" nuclear lobation occurring in association with cytoplasmic immaturity (50, 89, 104). A more detailed description of such cells may be found in Chapter 10.

Genetic Defects of Neutrophils

Chediak-Higashi Syndrome and Aleutian Mink Disease
The Chediak-Higashi syndrome is a familial disease char-

acterized by repeated, severe microbial infections and, in patients surviving infection, a tendency to develop early lymphoreticular malignancies (see Chapters 8 and 9). The neutrophils and eosinophils in this disorder contain large cytoplasmic inclusions measuring up to 2 microns in diameter. Such inclusions probably arise from sequestration of white cell cytoplasm in autophagic vesicles (101, cf. 33), although they could also arise from abnormal granulogenesis. The inclusions contain acid phosphatase activity (100, 101, 103).

A similar, but not identical, abnormality has been described in a genetic disease of the Aleutian mink. The neutrophils of affected animals contain a variety of enlarged and irregular secretory storage granules and myelin figures (31, 64, 75). Similar abnormalities have been seen in leukocytes of patients with Niemann-Pick disease (61), in human leukocytes treated with chloroquine (38), and in the beige mouse (65).

May-Heggelin Anomaly and Döhle Bodies   The May-Heggelin anomaly is a familial disorder characterized by giant platelets, thrombocytopenia, bleeding, and abnormal inclusions in granulocytes (56). In Romanovsky stains the inclusions are seen as large, amorphous, basophilic patches resembling so-called Döhle bodies. Döhle bodies are occasionally seen in neutrophils of normal subjects with severe inflammatory diseases, such as massive burns or infections.

Summary
The most important features of granulocytic morphogenesis are (a) the intimate developmental relation between the neutrophilic, eosinophilic, and basophilic cell lines; (b) the morphologic features observed by light and electron microscopy that gauge cellular maturity; (c) the morphologic events in granulogenesis; and (d) the correlation between fine structures and cellular metabolism.

Chapter 1 References

1. Ackerman, G. A. Histochemical differentiation during neutrophil development and maturation, *Ann. N.Y. Acad. Sci.* 113:537, 1964.

2. Ackerman, G. A. Contributions of the nuclear envelope, endoplasmic reticulum, and Golgi to the formation of peroxidase and lysosomal (azurophil) granules during neutrophil granulpoiesis, *Anat. Rec.* 160:304, 1968 (abstract).

3. Ackerman, G. A. Ultrastructure and cytochemistry of the developing neutrophil, *Lab. Invest.* 19:290, 1968.

4. Anderson, D. R. A method of preparing peripheral leukocytes for electron microscopy, *J. Ultrastruct. Res.* 13:263, 1965.

5. Anderson, D. R. Ultrastructure of normal and leukemic leukocytes in human peripheral blood, *J. Ultrastruct. Res.* 9:1, 1966 (suppl.).

6. Asano, M. The use of electron-microscopy in the diagnosis and decision on the therapeutic effect on acute myeloid leukemia, *in* R. Uyeda (ed.), *Electron Microscopy*, vol. 2, p. 711, Maruzen Co., Tokyo, 1966.

7. Baggiolini, M. The enzymes of the granules of polymorphonuclear leukocytes and their functions, *Enzyme* 13:132, 1972.

8. Baggiolini, M., Hirsch, J. G., and DeDuve, C. Resolution of granules from rabbit heterophil leukocytes into distinct populations by zonal sedimentation, *J. Cell Biol.* 40:529, 1969.

9. Bainton, D., and Farquhar, M. G. Origin of granules in polymorphonuclear leukocytes: two types derived from opposite faces of the Golgi complex in developing granulocytes, *J. Cell Biol.* 28:277, 1966.

10. Bainton, D. F., and Farquhar, M. G. Segregation and packaging of granule enzymes in eosinophils, *J. Cell Biol.* 35:6A, 1967 (abstract).

11. Bainton, D. F., and Farquhar, M. G. Differences in enzyme content of azurophil and specific granules of polymorphonuclear leukocytes: I. Histochemical staining of bone marrow smears, *J. Cell Biol.* 39:286, 1968.

12. Bainton, D. F., and Farquhar, M. G. Differences in enzyme content of azurophil and specific granules of polymorphonuclear leukocytes: II. Cytochemistry and electron microscopy of bone marrow cells, *J. Cell Biol.* 39:299, 1968.

13. Bainton, D. F., and Farquhar, M. G. Nature of human neutrophilic leukocyte granules (PMN), *Fed. Proc.* 28:617, 1969 (abstract).

14. Behnke, O. Demonstration of endogenous peroxidase activity in the electron microscope, *J. Histochem. Cytochem.* 17:62, 1969.

15. Bernhard, W., and Granboulan, N. Electron microscopy of the nucleolus in vertebrate cells, *in* A. V. Dalton and J. Haguenau (eds.), Ultrastructure in Biological Systems: The Nucleus, vol. 3, p. 81, Academic Press, New York, 1968.

16. Bernhard, W., Braunsteiner, H., Febvre, H. L., and Harel, J. Les leucocytes du sang humain au microscope électronique, *Presse Med.* 58:472, 1950.

17. Bernhard, W., Haguenau, F., and Leplus, R. Coupes ultrafines d'éléments sanguins et de ganglions lymphatiques étudiées au microscope électronique, *Rev. Hematol.* 10:267, 1955.

18. Bessis, M. Etudes au microscope électronique des leucocytes normaux et leucemiques, *Acta Un. Int. Cancr.* 7:646, 1951.

19. Bessis, M. Cytology of the Blood and Blood-Forming Organs, p. 373, Grune & Stratton, New York, 1956.

20. Bessis, M. Structures cellulaires découvertes par le microscope électronique dans les leucocytes, *Rev. Hematol.* 11:295, 1956.

21. Bessis, M., and Thiery, J-P. Electron microscopy of human white blood cells and their stem cells, *Int. Rev. Cytol.* 12:199, 1961.

22. Bessis, M., Bricka, M., and Gorius, J. Etude du myelogramme au microscope électronique par la method des répliques, *Presse Med.* 60:1076, 1952.

23. Boll, I., and Kühn, A. Granulocytopoiesis in human bone marrow cultures studied by means of kinematography, *Blood* 26:449, 1965.

24. Braunsteiner, H., and Pakesch, F. Elektronenmikroskopische Untersuchungen der Granula menschlicher Leukozyten, *Acta Haematol.* (Basel) 17:136, 1957.

25. Breton-Gorius, J. Structures périodiques dans les granulations eosinophiles et neutrophiles des leucocytes polynucleaires du sang de l'homme, *Nouv. Rev. Fr. Hematol.* 6:195, 1966.

26. Capone, R. J., Weinreb, E. L., and Chapman, G. B. Electron microscope studies on normal human myeloid elements, *Blood* 23:300, 1964.

27. Caro, L. G., and Palade, G. E. Protein synthesis, storage and discharge in the pancreatic exocrine cell: an autoradiographic study, *J. Cell Biol.* 20:473, 1964.

28. Cline, M. J. Metabolism of the circulating leukocyte, *Physiol. Rev.* 45:674, 1965.

29. Daems, W. T., and van der Ploeg, M. On the heterogeneity of human neutrophilic leucocyte granules, *in* R. Uyeda (ed.), Electron Microscopy, vol. 2, p. 83, Maruzen Co., Tokyo, 1966.

30. Dannenberg, A. M., Burstone, M. S., Walter, P. C., and Kinsley, J. W. A histochemical study of phagocytic and enzymatic functions of rabbit mononuclear and polymorphonuclear exudate cells and alveolar macrophages: I. Survey and quantitation of enzymes and states of cellular activation, *J. Cell Biol.* 17:465, 1963.

31. Davis, W. C., Greene, W. B., and Spicer, S. S. Ultrastructure of bone marrow granulocytes in normal and Aleutian mink, *Fed. Proc.* 28:265, 1969 (abstract).

32. DeDuve, C. Lysosomes, a new group of cytoplasmic particles, *in* T. Hiyashi (ed.), Subcellular Particles, p. 128, Ronald Press, New York, 1959.

33. DeDuve, C., and Wattiaux, R. Functions of lysosomes, *Ann. Rev. Physiol.* 28:435, 1966.

34. de Gruchy, G. C. Clinical Haematology in Medical Practice, p. 6, Blackwell Scientific Publications, Oxford, 1964.

35. Downey, H. The myeloblast: its occurrence under normal and pathological conditions, and its relations to lymphocytes and other blood cells, *in* H. Downey (ed.), Handbook of Hematology, vol. 3, p. 1962, Hoeber, New York, 1938.

36. Dunn, W. B., Hardin, J. H., and Spicer, S. S. Ultrastructural localization of myeloperoxidase in

Chapter 2 Production, Destruction, and Distribution of Neutrophilic Granulocytes

Granulocytes are formed in the bone marrow by a series of mitotic divisions that occur in immature cells and cells of intermediate morphologic maturity—myeloblasts, promyelocytes, and myelocytes. The stem cells that are the progenitor of the myeloblasts are not identifiable by morphologic criteria, but from experimental evidence are presumed to exist. Although cytoplasmic and nuclear differentiation continues beyond the myelocyte stage, the cells are no longer capable of division. A variety of overlapping morphologic forms more mature than the myelocyte have been identified (see Chapter 1); for convenience, we have classified the progression as myelocyte → metamyelocyte → band form → segmented neutrophil.

Only mature neutrophils (PMN) and band forms are encountered in the blood of normal man; of these, some are free in the circulation and others adhere to the walls of blood vessels. A variety of stimuli, including infection, endotoxin, burns, and crush injuries, may cause neutrophils, bands, and more primitive forms to be released from the bone marrow granulocyte reserve into the blood stream.

Under both normal and stress conditions, the sojourn of the granulocytes in the circulation is brief and measured in terms of hours. The cells migrate from the blood vessels into the tissues. The short life-span of the mature cell forms is spent primarily outside the circulation and is measured in days. The neutrophils either die in the tissues or are lost from a mucous membrane surface that is in contact with the external world. Once the band or mature neutrophil enters the tissues, it does not normally return to the circulation.

The Stem Cell Concept: Relation between Granulocytes and Other Cell Lines

A hematopoietic stem cell has previously been defined as a dividing cell with the dual capabilities of self-renewal and of differentiating into more mature hematologic cells. A stem cell may be either pluripotent and capable of giving rise to cells of several hematopoietic lines, or unipotent with maturation capabilities along a single line.

Under normal steady-state conditions the stem cell compartment of an animal or man is assumed to be constant in size. Two mechanisms for achieving this constancy are shown in Fig. 2.1. Under a differentiating stimulus, a stem cell could divide asymmetrically, one offspring remaining within the stem cell compartment while the other leaves and provides progeny (Fig. 2.1A). These progeny mature along one or more hematopoietic cell lines depending upon the nature of the stimulus—whether it be hormonal or the microenvironment in which the cell finds itself (cf. 60, 95, 146). In an alternative scheme, a stem cell leaves a compartment under a differentiating stimulus and is replaced by the progeny of another stem cell (Fig. 2.1B).

Evidence for Pluripotent Stem Cells in Man

Patients with chronic myelocytic leukemia have elevated peripheral blood neutrophil counts. In addition, the

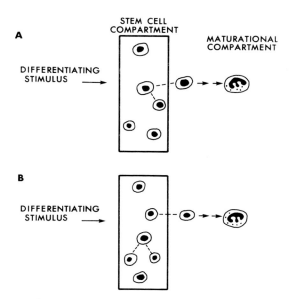

Figure 2.1 Schematic representation of the major alternatives for renewal of the proliferating stem cell compartment. In *A*, a stem cell divides and one of the daughters leaves the compartment to differentiate into more mature hematopoietic elements. In *B*, a stem cell leaves the compartment in order to differentiate, its place being taken by the progeny of another dividing stem cell.

number of circulating basophils and platelets, and occasionally eosinophils, is often increased (Chapter 10). The abnormal chromosome characteristic of this disorder is found in neutrophilic granulocytes, erythroid and platelet precursors (153), and eosinophils (76); but it is not present in fibroblasts or lymphocytes. These observations strongly suggest that in chronic myelocytic leukemia the erythroid, megakaryocytic, neutrophilic, and eosinophilic cell lines are derived from a single stem cell bearing the chromosomal abnormality. Similar evidence has been adduced from the distribution of 6-phosphogluconate dehydrogenase phenotypes among cell lines (55). The membrane defect observed in platelets, granulocytes, and erythrocytes of patients with paroxysmal nocturnal hemoglobinuria also supports the idea of a stem cell common to several hematopoietic cell lines (2).

Animal Models for the Study of Stem Cells

If a lethally irradiated mouse is transfused promptly with a sufficient number of syngeneic bone marrow or spleen cells, death is prevented. Hematopoietic cells proliferate within the marrow cavity, and macroscopic nodules of circumscribed hematopoietic tissue appear on the surface of the spleen. A linear relation exists between the numbers of administered cells and the numbers of spleen

colonies that develop (145). Studies utilizing radiation-induced chromosome markers have clearly demonstrated the clonal nature of the great majority of these colonies; that is, they are the progeny resulting from the proliferation of a single cell (11). Since some of the colonies contain a mixture of erythrocytes, neutrophils, eosinophils, and megakaryocytes, it has been inferred that these cell lines may arise, as in humans, from a common single precursor—a pluripotent stem cell. Since chromosome defects common to the hematopoietic lines were not observed in lymphoid tissues, it was inferred that lymphoid cells do not share the same stem cell as the other hematopoietic cell lines. However, in more recent studies utilizing heavily irradiated donors, the same chromosomal defect has been found in lymphoid cells and in certain spleen colony cells (110, 155). These last observations indicate that, under certain conditions, a pluripotent stem cell is capable of giving rise to lymphoid as well as nonlymphoid hematopoietic cell lines. This concept is illustrated in Fig. I. 1 of the Introduction.

The existence of unipotent, more mature stem cells has also been investigated and documented (12, 13, 19, 79, 123, 137).

Characteristics of the Pluripotent Stem Cell

The pluripotent hematopoietic stem cell has not been morphologically identified with certainty, although candidates have been proposed (149). However, several of its characteristics are known. For example, evidence shows that under normal conditions the pluripotent stem cell capable of producing spleen colonies is resting rather than in active cycle. Bruce and his collaborators (35, 148) examined this question utilizing the spleen colony assay (145). If a donor animal is treated with chemotherapeutic drugs, which act only during the DNA synthetic phase (S phase) of the cell cycle (42), the ability of its marrow cells to establish spleen colonies in an irradiated recipient is only marginally affected. These observations suggest the pluripotent stem cells are usually not in active DNA synthesis.

The exact size of the compartment containing colony-forming cells is not known. The marrow is the richest source of the colony-forming cells and is probably the major site of the stem cell compartment in normal animals (25, 44, 142). The spleen is also a rich source of colony-forming cells in the mouse, but is not so important quantitatively as the bone marrow. Colony-forming cells are also demonstrable in the circulating blood, the peritoneal cavity, and the fetal liver of the mouse. Both adult liver and lymphoid organs, including lymph nodes and thymus, have either very low levels or no detectable spleen colony-forming cells (19). The detection of colony-forming cells in the blood implies that, under normal circumstances, pluripotent stem cells may circulate.

The numbers and behavior of the colony-forming cell may be influenced by the age of the animal (92) and also by a wide variety of agents including foreign plasma, endotoxin, mumps vaccine, phytohemagglutinin, erythropoietin, and testosterone (19, 93). Hypertransfusion of irradiated marrow recipients results in suppression of erythropoietic colonies in the spleen—an observation suggesting that colony-forming cells are susceptible to normal hormonal control of differentiation (93, 111). They are also susceptible to ionizing irradiation (38, 92).

A depleted stem cell compartment cannot meet competing demands for two cell lines simultaneously, as suggested in studies of competition for granulopoiesis and erythropoiesis (19, 70). Two types of genetic disease of hematopoiesis in mice have been identified: in one type the stem cell compartment is abnormal (37, 87), and in the other the environment for proliferation of stem cells is abnormal (88). The W/W^v mouse is genetically anemic and has reduced numbers of bone marrow megakaryocytes and neutrophils. W/W^v mouse bone marrow given to an irradiated normal recipient forms abnormally small spleen colonies. Normal marrow given to an irradiated W/W^v mouse behaves normally. These observations suggest a stem cell defect in the W/W^v mouse that leads to pancytopenia (12, 37, 60, 87).

Genetic and acquired diseases affecting the stem cell compartment of man probably exist, but have not yet been defined with certainty. Examples may be myeloproliferative syndromes and certain hypoplastic anemias.

Methods of Studying Granulopoiesis and Granulocyte Kinetics

In this and subsequent sections of this chapter the terms *neutrophil* and *granulocyte* are used interchangeably. Most of the data cited refer to neutrophils rather than other types of granulocytes. In Table 2.1 a number of terms are listed that are used frequently in the field of cell and tissue kinetics.

Various techniques have been applied to the study of granulocyte kinetics and granulopoiesis. The major ones are (a) granulocyte depletion or destruction to determine the size and rate of mobilization of reserves and the rate of granulopoiesis; (b) radioisotopic and other labels of granulocytes to study distribution, production rates, and survival times; (c) study of mitotic indexes, under a variety of conditions, of cells obtained from bone marrow, blood, or tissues; (d) induced inflammatory lesions to

Table 2.1 Definitions relating to cell and tissue kinetics.

Generation time — time interval between successive mitoses (cell cycle time)

Doubling time — time for entire cell population to go through one division and double in number

Turnover time — time to replace cells of a replicating pool (population renewal time)

Growth fraction — ratio of cells in active cycle to total number of cells in pool. When generation time = doubling time, growth fraction is 1.

Labeling index — number of cells labeled after pulse of ^{3}H-thymidine per 100 cells

Pool — population of cells having at least one characteristic in common

Compartment — subdivision of pool

study the type and rate of cell movement into tissue sites under a variety of conditions; (e) administration of various cell populations to irradiated syngeneic animals depleted of granulocyte precursors (this enables a study of the type of cell capable of granulocyte repopulation); and (f) in vitro culture of granulocyte precursors.

Repopulation of irradiated animals was discussed in the preceding section, and in vitro study of granulopoiesis will be considered at the end of this chapter. A brief description of the other methods follows.

Granulocyte Depletion Techniques

Techniques for this method, all of which remove or destroy large numbers of granulocytes, involve either (a) extensive leukapheresis (14, 46, 47), (b) cross-circulation of a donor with a leukopenic recipient (143), or (c) cytotoxic agents or antileukocyte antibodies (24, 83, 115). Such techniques permit, with certain limitations, examination of the size of granulocyte reserves, their rate of mobilization and resynthesis, and the rate of repopulation of a depleted compartment, such as the circulation or marrow granulocyte reserve.

Labeling Techniques

These techniques have, in recent times, generally used isotopic labels; but the administration of stable, morphologically identifiable variants of granulocytes (Pelger-Huët anomaly) to a normal recipient has also been used. The distribution and survival of cells can be observed by this latter method (133).

The first radioisotopic labels used were incorporated into the DNA of dividing early granulocyte forms; that is, cells up to the myelocyte stage of development. The distribution and fate of the label could then be followed. The first such label to be used was [32]P (47, 112, 151). This label suffers the disadvantage of being incorporated into a variety of cell constituents other than DNA, including phospholipids and phosphoproteins. It labels cells of all ages, not just dividing cells. Furthermore, reutilization of the isotope after cell destruction causes it to label fresh cells for long periods of time. For these reasons a superior DNA label, tritiated thymidine (41, 72), has largely replaced [32]P. This ^{3}H-thymidine has the advantages of selective DNA labeling, rapid degradation of unincorporated material, nonreutilization of label, and a weak beta particle emission which is ideal for radioautography (41).

The major use of DNA markers in the study of neutrophil kinetics is to label S-phase cells (cells in DNA synthesis) in the pool of mitotically active cells. The subsequent movement of labeled cells can then be followed as they progress through sequentially more mature compartments.

Another label, diisopropylfluorophosphate (DFP), containing either ^{32}P or tritium, was introduced as a granulocyte marker in the late 1950s (4, 6, 94). This radioactively labeled chemical binds exclusively to the granulocytic series and not to other types of leukocytes. DFP may be used as either an in vivo or an in vitro label and may be used in nonsteady-state conditions of granulopoiesis (134). It does not elute (leak off) significantly from a labeled cell and is not reutilized. Because the DFP label can be applied in vitro, the radiolabeled cells can be used to determine the total blood granulocyte pool by the isotope dilution method (4, 94). Intravenously administered DFP permits measurement of marrow transit times, granulocyte reserves, and marrow myelocyte turnover rate (80).

More recently, [51]chromium has been introduced as a leukocyte label (53, 85, 89, 116). Although it has the advantage that its radioactive decay permits surface monitoring of distribution of label, it also has disadvantages in that the large majority of labeled cells never circulate and label probably elutes from the cell.

Other Techniques

Detailed explanations of the use of mitotic indexes and other methods of measuring granulocyte kinetics are presented in the excellent reviews of LoBue (84; see also 48, 72, 77, 82).

Several techniques have been used to study the type of cell migrating from the circulation into areas of inflammation and the rate of that migration. The technique of Rebuck and Crowley, utilizing the adherence of leukocytes to sterile cover slips overlying areas of superficially abraded skin, was introduced in 1955 (125). Since this

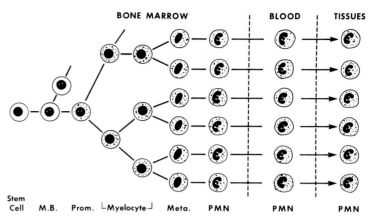

Figure 2.2 The major compartments for granulocyte proliferation and distribution: bone marrow, blood, and tissues. The bone marrow compartment is made up of the proliferating compartment (stem cells through myelocytes) and the maturation and storage compartment (metamyelocytes and mature polymorphonuclear neutrophils). Under normal conditions, there is no return of cells from the tissue compartment to the blood or bone marrow.

method is qualitative rather than quantitative and, in addition, nonadherent cells are missed altogether, attempts have been made to introduce more quantitative techniques. Examples are skin blisters (20) and skin chambers (138). None of these methods is, however, wholly satisfactory.

Granulocyte Kinetics

In most analyses of granulopoiesis and granulocyte kinetics, the granulocyte movement between a number of interconnected compartments has had the greatest consideration. These compartments appear to be arranged in three major groups: the bone marrow phase, the blood phase, and the tissue phase (Fig. 2.2). Each of these phases may have several subcompartments. For example, the marrow

Table 2.2 Definitions and calculations relating to neutrophil kinetics.

Circulating granulocyte pool (CGP) = blood neutrophil concentration × blood volume

Total blood granulocyte pool (TBGP) = all granulocytes in the circulation

Marginal granulocyte pool (MGP) = total blood granulocyte pool less circulating granulocyte pool (MGP = TBGP − CGP)

Blood clearance half-time ($T_{1/2}$) = half disappearance time of labeled granulocytes from the circulation

Granulocyte turnover rate (GTR) = $\dfrac{0.693 \times \text{TBGP}}{T_{1/2}}$

Table 2.3 Data for neutrophil kinetics in normal man.

Pool	Mean pool size × 10⁻⁷/kg	95% limits	References
TBGP	70	14–160	3
CGP	31	11–46	3
MGP	39	0–85	3

Rate	Mean value	95% limits	References
Blood clearance $T_{1/2}$	6.7 hours	4–10 hours	5, 85, 89
GTR	163×10^7/kg/day	$50–340 \times 10^7$/kg/day	3, 5, 62

phase is comprised of the mitotic compartment (pool) and the marrow maturation and storage (reserve) compartment; the blood phase is comprised of the circulating and marginal granulocyte pools (compartments). Presumably the tissue phase could also be divided into subcompartments; for example, a compartment to which neutrophils have free access and egress, and compartments in which egress is restricted. An abscess cavity might be an example of the latter.

Some of the terms used in granulocyte kinetics are defined in Table 2.2 and values found in normal man are in Table 2.3.

The Blood Phase

Pool Size The total blood granulocyte pool encompasses all granulocytes in the vascular space. Some of the cells in this pool do not circulate freely, presumably because they are temporarily sequestered in small blood vessels or adhere to the walls of larger vessels (150). In any event, these marginated cells are not ordinarily sampled when one inserts a needle into a brachial vein; only freely circulating cells are sampled.

Precise quantitative analysis of the size and distribution of the blood neutrophil mass was first provided by studies with the ³²P-DFP label (94). When labeled cells are injected into a series of normal subjects, a mean of 44 percent of the cells can be accounted for in the circulating granulocyte pool (CGP). The circulating granulocyte pool is always less than the total blood granulocyte pool (TBGP). The difference between these pools is the compartment known as the marginal granulocyte pool (MGP); its size is calculated as follows: MGP = TBGP − CGP.

Turnover Rates When the rate of granulocyte disappearance from the circulation is measured in normal subjects

in a steady state, the mean half disappearance time $(T_{1/2})$ of labeled granulocytes is 6.7 hours (5, 85, 89) (Table 2.3). In other words, granulocyte-associated radioactivity in the blood compartment has fallen to one-half its initial value by 6.7 hours. The slope of the disappearance curve (a single exponential curve) indicates that the labeled granulocytes leave the blood in random fashion, and do not follow a "first-in, first-out" pattern in the circulation (3, 57, 113). This is in contrast to the disappearance of labeled red cells, which in the normal subject have a finite life-span and do leave the blood in a first-in, first-out pattern.

The possibility of a minor component of age-dependent neutrophil loss from the circulation, rather than a completely random loss, has been suggested by the ³H-thymidine studies of Fliedner and his associates (56). These investigators proposed that two curves should be considered for human neutrophils: (a) an exponential (age-independent) loss with a half-time of 6 to 7 hours, and (b) a senescent (age-dependent) loss that commences at about 30 hours for a given cohort of cells. No evidence for senescent loss has ever been obtained from DFP-labeling studies (18).

Provided the assumption of random neutrophil loss from the bloodstream is correct, one can calculate the granulocyte turnover rate (GTR) from the data for the total blood granulocyte pool and half disappearance time:

$$GTR = \frac{0.693 \times TBGP}{T_{1/2}}.$$

The values for granulocyte turnover rate of normal human subjects are given in Table 2.3 (3, 5, 62); they have also been reported for the dog (124).

If the subject under study is in a steady state, *the granulocyte turnover rate is the measure of the rate of effective granulopoiesis.* The higher the granulocyte turnover rate, the greater the rate of granulocyte production.

Abnormalities in Disease States Abnormalities of granulocyte production and granulocyte kinetics are considered in detail in Chapter 9. For a better understanding of normal granulocyte physiology, a brief description of these abnormalities is included here.

Neutrophilia refers to conditions in which the blood neutrophil count is higher than normal; neutropenia refers to conditions in which it is lower than normal.

A good correlation between the total blood granulocyte pool and the blood neutrophil count is generally characteristic of patients with neutropenia or neutrophila (5–8).

However, a transient (3) and perhaps sustained (135) "shift neutrophilia" may occasionally be observed. In this condition the total blood granulocyte pool is not increased, but neutrophils are shifted from the marginal into the circulating granulocyte pools. Similarly, "shift neutropenia" sometimes may be noted when the marginal granulocyte pool is increased at the expense of the circulating granulocyte pool. This shift results in a diminished circulating granulocyte concentration (3).

In patients with polycythemia vera and myelofibrosis (see Chapter 10) the marginal granulocyte pool often expands more than the circulating granulocyte pool. In such patients the circulating neutrophil concentration underestimates the actual increase in intravascular mass of granulocytes (8).

Boggs described an entity of "masked" granulocytosis wherein the total blood granulocyte pool is slightly increased, although the neutrophil count is normal. This phenomenon was observed in some patients with mild skin inflammation (23).

In neutrophilia resulting from a variety of causes, including chronic myelocytic leukemia, polycythemia vera, and chronic inflammation, the granulocyte turnover rate (that is, effective granulopoiesis) is usually increased to a variable extent and may be as much as twelve times normal (7, 8). An exception to this rule of increased granulocyte turnover rate in association with blood granulocytosis is the neutrophilia associated with adrenocorticosteroids. In this case the granulocyte turnover rate is generally normal (5, 6, 20).

In disease states such as chronic myelogenous leukemia and myeloid metaplasia, where immature neutrophils circulate in the blood, the half disappearance time for cells leaving the blood is generally prolonged—up to 90 hours as compared to the normal $T_{1/2}$ of 6 to 7 hours. In conditions where the neutrophilia comprises mainly mature cells, the prolongation of the $T_{1/2}$ is less striking (mean, 18 hours). It is not certain whether the prolonged clearance time associated with cellular immaturity is the result of a delayed egress from the blood or a recirculation of immature cells through the marrow and spleen (9, 61, 116, 117, 119).

In acute inflammatory conditions neutrophils are mobilized from the blood to the inflammatory sites within hours (20, 68). In dogs given an intrabronchial injection of pneumococci, the total blood granulocyte pool increases within 4 hours as a consequence of release of cells from the marrow reserve. Thereafter the granulocyte turnover rate increases until the infection is brought under control (91). If the infection is massive, however, peripheral blood

neutropenia may result from the excessive demand for granulocytes in the tissues.

In neutropenic states with impaired granulocyte production and a resultant decrease in granulocyte turnover rate, the blood half clearance time is generally normal (15, 135). In patients with neutropenia as a consequence of hypersplenism and excessive cell destruction, the $T_{1/2}$ is shortened as cells rapidly leave the blood stream (126, 136) (see Chapter 9). The $T_{1/2}$ and total blood granulocyte pool may return to normal following splenectomy.

The Marrow Phase

The bone marrow phase of granulopoiesis is often considered as two interlocking compartments: the proliferating or mitotic compartment and the nonproliferating or maturation and storage compartment. The stem cell pool is often considered as a subunit of the proliferating compartment (see Figs. 2.2 and 2.3).

The Mitotic Compartment As shown in Fig. 2.2, this compartment consists of mitotically active cells of the granulocytic series: myeloblasts, promyelocytes, and myelocytes (27, 28, 114). Although the precursor stem cells are also mitotically active, they are not morphologically identifiable and the techniques of DNA labeling and radioautography cannot be applied directly to assess their behavior.

The maturing cells are thought to progress in the direction of: myeloblasts→promyelocytes→myelocytes. The number of cell divisions between each stage is unknown, although the studies of Warner and Athens suggest that at least three divisions occur at the myelocyte stage (152). The major increase in granulocyte numbers most likely occurs at the myelocyte stage, since the myelocyte pool is at least four times the size of the preceding promyelocyte pool (see Fig. 2.2). Several models of granulopoiesis within

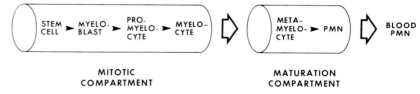

Figure 2.3 The bone marrow compartment is usually divided into the mitotic, or proliferating, compartment and the maturation and storage compartment. The mitotic compartment consists of granulocytes through the myelocyte stage of development; the maturation and storage compartment consists of metamyelocytes and mature polymorphonuclear neutrophils.

the mitotic compartment have been described (22), but no one model has been ascertained as definitive.

In the dog, the mean transit time from labeling of a myelocyte to appearance of a labeled mature neutrophil in the peripheral blood is about 102 hours (90).

Whether the production of cells in the mitotic compartment exactly balances the granulocyte turnover rate or whether ineffective granulopoiesis occurs—that is, death of some immature cells in the marrow—is not known. Patt and Maloney have presented evidence of some ineffective granulopoiesis in the dog (114), but firm evidence of ineffective granulopoiesis in man is not available. The difficulties involved in the measurement of total intramarrow granulocyte production are reviewed well by Athens (3) and by Killmann and his associates (78).

Marrow Granulocyte Reserve　Initial demonstrations of the existence of a granulocyte reserve compartment in the bone marrow of man and the dog involved removal of large quantities of granulocytes by leukapheresis (14, 47). In these studies the number of granulocytes, neutrophils, band forms, and metamyelocytes mobilized into the blood was several times larger than the circulating granulocyte pool.

Evidence from radioautographic studies with ^{3}H-thymidine supports the notion of an orderly progression from metamyelocytes to band to neutrophil within the reserve compartment, and suggests a first-in, first-out pattern for cells leaving the reserve compartment and entering the peripheral blood (90).

Kinetic studies of the appearance of labeled cells after a pulse of ^{32}P or tritiated thymidine permit estimates of the time required for cells to do the following: finish division within the mitotic compartment, enter and traverse the reserve (storage) compartment, and then enter the circulation. The peak of labeled cells generally occurs 6 to 8 days after a radioisotope pulse, with 4 to 6 days usually the minimal transit time. Thus at the normal rate of utilization the marrow reserve represents 4 to 8 days' supply of neutrophils, or a marrow granulocyte reserve of between 6.5 and 13×10^9 cells/kg in normal man (3). A similar figure for marrow granulocyte reserve is provided by a ^{59}iron labeling technique (52), but longer transit times and larger bone marrow reserves have been calculated from ^{32}P-DFP labeling studies (152).

A summary of the size of the marrow granulocyte reserve, calculated by a variety of techniques, is given in Table 2.4. Reasons for the discrepancy in results obtained by different methods of calculation are not entirely clear but may reflect different populations and subjects studied.

The size of the marrow granulocyte reserve and the

Table 2.4　Characteristics of the marrow granulocyte reserve.

Size (cells × 10⁹/kg)	Transit time (days)	Method of determination	References
6.5–13	4–8	^{3}H-thymidine, in vitro ^{32}P-DFP	3
3–23	8–14	In vivo and in vitro ^{32}P-DFP	152
8.8	—	^{59}Fe	52

time required for cell transit through the compartment may be abnormal in disease states. For example, the transit time is often greatly shortened in inflammatory processes (22, 56, 78, 118, 151). Fliedner and his colleagues (56) observed a marrow myelocyte-to-blood transit time of only 48 hours in a patient with severe infection, as compared with normal transit times of 96 to 144 hours. Others have made similar observations (22, 118, 151). It appears, then, that under certain stress conditions (*a*) maturation may be accelerated, (*b*) divisions may be skipped, or (*c*) release into the blood may occur at an earlier than normal stage.

Clinically, the bone marrow reserve is often tested by the ability of administered endotoxin to mobilize granulocytes into the peripheral blood (49).

The Stem Cell Compartment　As indicated earlier in this chapter, the concept of a pluripotential bone marrow stem cell capable of generating progeny that can, in turn, differentiate into granulocytic, erythrocytic, or megakaryocytic cell lines has a long history in hematology. The modern basis for this concept rests on two lines of evidence. First, when syngeneic bone marrow is injected into lethally irradiated mice, the hematopoietic colonies that develop in the spleen almost certainly arise from a single progenitor stem cell (11). These colonies sometimes contain a mixture of granulocytic, erythrocytic, and megakaryocytic cell elements (145). A second line of evidence comes from the observations of the cellular distribution of the Philadelphia (Ph¹) chromosome abnormality in chronic myelogenous leukemia. This chromosomal abnormality is found in nucleated erythroid, granulocytic, and megakaryocytic precursors, but not in lymphocytes or fibroblasts (153). The simplest interpretation of this observation is that the chromosomal abnormality exists in a pluripotential stem cell that is a precursor of erythrocytes, granulocytes, and megakaryocytes.

As yet, the morphologic and physical characteristics of the stem cell have not been identified with certainty. Some progress has been made in studies that use two types of assay systems for detecting stem cells. The system developed first assayed stem cells by their ability to form hematopoietic colonies in the spleens of lethally irradiated mice (145). The second assay system measured the ability of cells, presumed to be related to stem cells, to form hematopoietic colonies in a semisolid agar-containing medium in vitro (34). In these assay systems some cells resembling lymphocytes may have properties of stem cells (149). Progress has been made in separating stem cells from other types of hematologic cells on the basis of physical properties such as size and density (109). Techniques used to separate the stem cells are still new and the technical difficulties involved in identifying a few stem cells among a vast multitude of more differentiated nucleated cells are great. As a result, the characteristics of stem cells are relatively unknown. One feature of the bone marrow stem cell compartment generally agreed upon is its self-renewing abilities under normal conditions That is, the stem cell must give rise to other stem cells as well as cells capable of differentiating along erythroid, granulocytic, and megakaryocytic lines.

Control of Granulopoiesis and Granulocyte Distribution

The concentration of circulating neutrophils is very nearly constant in normal subjects and returns to the normal steady state after various perturbations of the normal state such as acute inflammation. This observation suggests that the neutrophil level is under some sort of control mechanism (cf. 66). Several such mechanisms can be envisaged: they may control (a) the rate of granulopoiesis from the stem cell compartment, (b) the rate of entry of cells from the marrow reserve compartment into the peripheral blood, (c) the distribution of granulocytes between marginal and circulating pools, (d) the rate of egress of cells from the blood into the tissues, and (e) the life-span of the mature cells. Of these possibilities, the first two are probably critical in controlling the numbers of neutrophils in the circulation (Fig. 2.4).

Several substances have been suggested as possible hormonal control factors in the regulation of granulokinetics. Gordon and his co-workers (67) perfused rat femurs with fluid and measured the rate of granulocyte release. When the perfusate had a low leukocyte content, the rate of cells released from the marrow stores was high. As leukocytes accumulated in the recycled perfusate, the rate of release from the marrow decreased. Based on these observations, the investigators suggested a negative feedback control system of release of granulocytes from the marrow mediated by the mature granulocyte (see Fig. 2.4).

In 1965 Delmonte and Liebelt (50) demonstrated a neutrophil-releasing factor in an extract of a mouse mammary

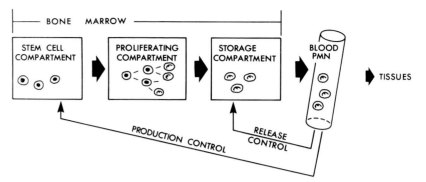

Figure 2.4 Two types of controls on the level of circulating polymorphonuclear neutrophils (as indicated by present evidence): (a) control at the level of production by the stem cell compartment, and (b) control of release from the bone marrow storage compartment.

tumor. The following year Boggs and his colleagues (24) demonstrated a neutrophil-releasing factor in the plasma of dogs rendered leukopenic by either nitrogen mustard or vinblastine, or injection with endotoxin. An apparently similar factor was later demonstrated in the plasma of man after endotoxin injection (26). Relatively little progress has been made in purifying the putative neutrophil-releasing factor. Clearly, ubiquitous endotoxin must always be excluded as an active contaminant of any preparation under study for neutrophil-releasing properties (17).

Some control of neutrophil kinetics may possibly occur at sites of granulocyte egress from the vascular space and from the tissues. Boggs (18) suggested the existence of channels of neutrophil loss that in some manner "sense" the numbers of granulocytes leaving the circulation and appropriately signal for more cell release from the bone marrow. No concrete facts are available, however, to support such a concept.

Indirect evidence suggests that the rate of granulocyte production may be under some feedback control (17, 18, 21, 129); however, the nature of the control mechanisms operative in vivo remains unknown. Recently, in an attempt to identify stem cells and the control mechanisms influencing their differentiation along granulocytic lines, attention has been directed to techniques for growth of bone marrow colonies in vitro where variables can be manipulated more readily than in vivo.

In Vitro Studies of Granulopoiesis

The Agar Culture Technique

A technique for the culture of hematopoietic cells was developed independently by Pluznik and Sachs (121) and by Bradley and Metcalf (30). Basically the technique involves the culture of single-cell suspensions in a mixture of tissue culture medium, serum, and semisolid agar or methyl cellulose (30, 33, 99, 121). Usually some source of colony-stimulating factor (CSF) is incorporated directly into the medium, or CSF is incorporated in an underlayer (feeder layer) of more solid agar. When an appropriate stimulus is provided, the bone marrow cells begin proliferation and form discrete colonies of cells. Colonies arise from single cells and grow progressively over a 7-to 14-day period. After 7 to 10 days of culture, colonies may contain anywhere from 100 to 4,000 cells. This technique of bone marrow culture has been applied with success to a number of strains of mice (102), rats (31), rabbits, guinea pigs, and hamsters (102), and to human bone marrow (63, 65, 139).

Two types of cells may be recognized in in vitro bone marrow colonies: (a) granulocytic lines that mature progressively from myeloblasts to metamyelocytes and sometimes to mature neutrophils (102, 104) (Fig. 2.5), and (b) a mononuclear (macrophage) cell line whose earliest identifiable precursor is the promonocyte and whose most mature element is the macrophage (43, 73, 104, 139). The mature neutrophils develop the appropriate complement of lysosomal enzymes (cf. 54, 71). The mononuclear cells are actively phagocytic for a variety of particles (43) and have the ultrastructural characteristics of macro-

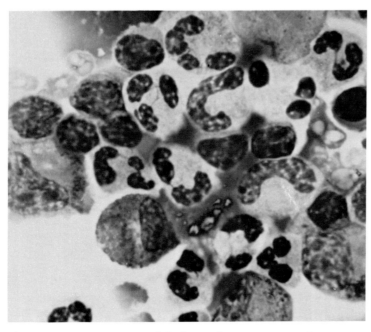

Figure 2.5 Mature neutrophils from a bone marrow colony growing in agar culture; Giemsa stain.

phages (81). Similar cells are seen when the bone marrow is cultured in liquid suspension (154). Initially the cells in culture demonstrate active division, but they cease dividing as the growth of the colonies begins to slow after 7 to 10 days.

It seems likely that the granulocyte colonies originate from a single cell. The question of the single-cell or dual-cell origin of mixed granulocytic-mononuclear colonies is presently unresolved; recent evidence suggests that both cell lines may share a common progenitor (103). Studies in the intact animal also suggest that granulocytes and monocyte-macrophages may share a common progenitor cell (see reference 45 and Chapter 23).

When bone marrow colonies grow in the presence of some form of colony-stimulating factor, the granulocytic elements begin to disappear by the sixth to seventh day of culture. This phenomenon appears to follow progressive cellular differentiation and death. No concomitant replenishment of the proliferating progenitor cell pool is evident. By the seventh to tenth day of culture most of the granulocytic elements have disappeared, although the rate of disappearance depends on such factors as the stimulating factor and feeder layers (102). At this time the mononuclear cells predominate in the colonies.

The Colony-forming Cell

In the mouse embryo, colony-forming cells first make their appearance in the yolk sac at day 8 (108). By day 10 of fetal life, colony-forming cells are detectable in the liver and, subsequently, in the spleen. The yolk sac also has been demonstrated to be the source of erythroid and lymphoid cells, as well as colony-forming cells (107, 147). Interestingly, granulopoiesis, first observed in the fetal liver, is never seen in the yolk sac. The microenvironment of the yolk sac is perhaps unsuitable for development of granulocytic differentiation of the pluripotent stem cell. Such differentiation must await the spread of these precursor cells to other embryonic hematopoietic organs such as the liver.

In the adult mouse, cells capable of giving rise to hematopoietic colonies in vitro are found in the bone marrow, blood, and spleen, but not in the thymus or lymph nodes (34, 102). The bone marrow is most efficient in this regard and generally gives rise, under "basal conditions," to one colony for every 500 to 1,000 nucleated cells plated. It requires 20,000 to 50,000 spleen cells and approximately 500,000 peripheral blood cells to generate one colony in vitro. The efficiency of colony formation can be increased as much as ten-fold by introducing a variety of stimulatory agents into the culture system. Such stimuli include thiol-containing compounds.

Bone marrow colonies from any of the adult sources demonstrate considerable heterogeneity in size and pattern of differentiation (99, 102, 104). This suggests a heterogeneity within the colony-forming population. Heterogeneity in response to colony-stimulating factor is also evident (34, 102, 104, 130).

Numerous attempts have been made to isolate colony-forming cells in the bone marrow (1, 75, 106, 109). These techniques have been partially successful in providing sufficiently enriched cell populations with a high plating efficiency. In primate marrow the colony-forming cell is of low density (less than 1.062); it is sticky in the sense that it adheres to nylon fiber columns. Although the morphology of the colony-forming cell has not been securely identified, the "transitional" lymphocyte has been suggested as a candidate (51, 109, 149). However, early colonies comprised of two to four cells in these studies always contained primitive cells in the granulocytic series, suggesting that the colony-forming cell may also be an undifferentiated blast cell or a morphologically identifiable primitive cell of the granulocytic series.

The number of colony-forming cells in adult mouse bone marrow varies with the erythropoietic status (33, 96). Marrow from mice rendered polycythemic by blood transfusion, with subsequent decreased erythropoiesis, has a greater than normal proportion of colony-forming cells in the marrow. Anemic mice have a smaller than normal portion of colony-forming cells among the nucleated marrow cells.

Whole-body X-irradiation produces a progressive fall in the number of colony-forming cells (105, 131). The relation between the dose of X ray and the fraction of surviving colony-forming cells is linear, with a shoulder at the lower doses. The D_0 value is approximately 85 rads, which compares to that for mouse marrow cells X-irradiated either in vitro or in vivo and assayed by the in vivo spleen colony technique (86, 145). This level represents a high degree of radiosensitivity in colony-forming cells in relation to the level of sensitivity found in blood and blast cells.

Barnes and Loutit (10) demonstrated that treatment of mice with pertussis vaccine results in an increase of the number of spleen colony-forming cells in the peripheral blood (145). An analogous phenomenon occurs when the number of colony-forming cells is assayed by the in vitro soft agar technique (34). A similar relation between the in vitro colony-forming cell and the in vivo colony-forming cell is suggested by the work of Wu and his associates (156). Other studies, however, have suggested that, in fact, the in vivo and in vitro colony-forming cells are not identical (13, 34). At the present time, most of the available evidence supports nonidentity of these two pluripotent colony-forming cells.

Colony-stimulating Factor

Colony formation by bone marrow cells in agar cultures is wholly dependent on the addition of a variety of substances collectively called "colony-stimulating factor" (CSF). This may be a misnomer in the sense that a single substance has not been sufficiently purified and characterized. It is not clear, for example, that a number of substances may be involved in stimulating colony formation. Although "colony-stimulating activity" may be a more appropriate term, we shall at this point retain the original designation of colony-stimulating factor.

In the absence of factor, in vitro colony formation does not occur and only isolated single cells are seen to survive after two to ten days of culture. Colony-stimulating factor is not only required for initiation of colony formation, but also must be continuously present in order that progressive colony growth may occur (100). A number of sources of colony-stimulating factor have been described, including a variety of tissue feeder layers and conditioned media, sera from various species, human urine, and human white blood cells (34, 102).

In the early studies of bone marrow culture techniques, an underlayer of intact or irradiated cells was included as a feeder layer (29, 30, 73, 121). A number of tissues served as an adequate feeder layer for the growth of mouse bone marrow colonies (Table 2.5); of these, newborn kidney cells generally proved to be the best. Since direct contact between feeder layer cells and the developing mouse colonies is not required, a diffusable factor is likely to be operative. There is some degree of species specificity of feeder layers, although mouse kidney cells will stimulate the growth of human bone marrow cells (139).

In cells incubated in vitro in liquid medium for a period

Table 2.5 Sources of colony-stimulating factor for growth of mouse bone marrow in soft agar.

Feeder layer cells	Conditioned media
Whole mouse embryo	Whole mouse embryo
Embryonic skeletal muscle and gastrointestinal tract	Embryonic skeletal muscle
Newborn kidney	Newborn kidney
Newborn thymus	Newborn spleen
Adult kidney	
Adult thymus	
Leukemic thymus	
Spleen cells	

of time the supernatant medium, when removed and rendered cell free by centrifugation, is said to be "conditioned." Some of this conditioned medium may substitute for feeder layers as a source of colony-stimulating factor (Table 2.5) (32, 102, 122). Of the various tissues tested, whole embryo cells or neonatal kidney cells proved the best source of stimulatory conditioned medium for mouse bone marrow. Viable cells are required for production of colony-stimulating factor. The medium thus formed is active for long periods of time when stored at 4° C and resists heat inactivation at 60° for 30 minutes. Dialysis of the conditioned medium against distilled water results in a slight increase in activity (32, 34, 102).

After the initial observation that the sera of some AKR mice with lymphoid leukemia possessed strong colony-stimulating activity (33, 130), a proportion of sera from normal mice of a variety of strains also was shown to have stimulatory activity. The frequency and potency of the stimulatory activity of leukemic or preleukemic mouse sera are generally higher than those of normal sera (99, 100, 102, 105, 130, 141).

Studies of mouse serum colony-stimulating activity have demonstrated that no clear relation exists between that activity and the blood neutrophil concentration (69, 102). Activity levels in serum may be increased by endotoxin and antigen administration (97). Another observation with significance as yet unclear is that administration of a filterable agent from the serum of normal or leukemic Swiss mice is associated with a sharp rise in serum colony-stimulating factor activity (59). Mouse serum activity is quite complex, and inhibitory, as well as stimulatory, substances have been identified (141).

Colony-stimulating activity for mouse bone marrow has been observed in human sera also. Activity is more commonly observed in sera from patients with neoplastic hematologic disease and with infectious mononucleosis than in normal sera (58, 101). Inhibitory, as well as stimulatory, substances have been identified in human serum (36).

In addition to its production by certain cells in tissue culture and its observation in mouse and human sera, colony-stimulating activity has been identified in dialyzed human urine. Levels of factor tend to be higher in the urine of patients with chronic granulocytic leukemia and of some patients with acute leukemia than in that of normal subjects (127, 132).

Physical Properties A preliminary study of the physical characteristics of CSF from serum was reported several years ago (140); but attention has shifted to the material present in human urine because of its greater availability for study. This factor is stable to storage at −20° for long periods, is resistant to heat inactivation at 60° for 30 minutes, but is inactivated at higher temperatures. It is stable in the pH range 2–12. The activity is precipitated by 40–48 percent ethanol and 50–70 percent ammonium sulfate. It is resistant to ether, periodate, DNAase and RNAase, and may be separated by electrophoresis (moving in the postalbumin region on starch at pH 8.2) on DEAE cellulose and Sephadex G 100 (102). Activity sediments in sucrose gradients at S 3–3.6. Estimates of molecular weight vary between 50,000 and 100,000.

The physical properties of colony-stimulating factor in human and mouse serum and serum-free conditioned medium are similar to those described for human urine except that the factor in conditioned medium is not electrophoretically homogeneous.

Sera from rabbits immunized with active concentrates of human urine do not show colony-stimulating activity in assays with bone marrow and, when preincubated with active material, inhibit colony-stimulating activity (102).

The existing evidence on the physical characteristics of CSF suggests a protein containing an active carbohydrate moiety of molecular weight 50,000 (140).

In Vivo Action Only preliminary work has been described on the in vivo action of urine concentrates or conditioned medium containing high levels of colony-stimulating activity (34). Animals injected with such materials develop moderate granulocytosis and splenic enlargement without change in other formed elements of the blood. The numbers of colony-forming cells in such animals increase in the blood and spleen.

At the present time the role of colony-stimulating factor either as a specific growth-promoting substance or as an essential metabolite for in vitro bone marrow colony growth is not well defined. Notwithstanding, the agar colony technique and the identification of growth-promoting factors represent a novel and promising approach to the study of granulopoiesis.

Production of CSF by Human Leukocytes As noted earlier, clonal growth of bone marrow cells in soft gel culture is largely dependent on the availability of stimulating substances. Since CSF stimulates and supports the growth of bone marrow granulocytes and macrophages in semisolid culture, it has been postulated that CSF may be a humoral mediator of leukopoiesis in vivo as well (98).

Several lines of evidence indicate that human white blood cells themselves may provide an important source of CSF. The stimulation of colony formation by feeder layers of peripheral white cells and conditioned media

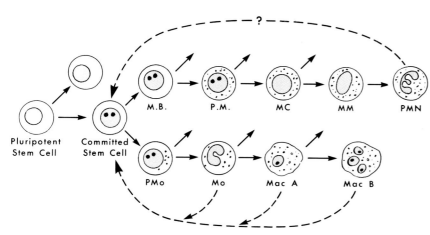

Figure 2.6 A hypothetical scheme for control of granulopoiesis and mononuclear phagocyte (monocyte-macrophage) proliferation. Neutrophils and monocytes arise from a common committed stem cell. Monocytes and macrophages produce colony-stimulating factor, which may have a physiologic role in the control of leukopoiesis. The production of colony-stimulating factor by mature neutrophils is less certain. *PMo* = promonocyte; *Mo* = monocyte; *Mac A* = immature macrophage capable of proliferation; *Mac B* = mature nonproliferating macrophage; *M.B.* = myeloblast; *P.M.* = promyelocyte; *MC* = myelocyte; *MM* = metamyelocyte; *PMN* = polymorphonuclear neutrophil.

from leukocyte cultures suggests that leukocytes produce a factor or factors that influence granulocyte and macrophage proliferation in vitro (39, 74, 120, 128).

These observations have led to a hypothesis about feedback control of granulopoiesis by peripheral blood leukocytes (129). Human blood monocytes and tissue macrophages have been shown to be the source of leukocyte colony-stimulating activity (40, 63, 65). Recently my own laboratory has shown that activated lymphocytes also produce CSF. Since monocytes and granulocytes arise

from a common progenitor cell, autoregulation of granulopoiesis may still be a valid theory. The concept of feedback control of the production of granulocytes and mononuclear phagocytes by CSF produced from monocytes and macrophages is illustrated in Fig. 2.6.

Other In Vitro Culture Methods

Recently techniques for growing human (64) and murine (143) bone marrow in liquid suspension cultures have been described. The liquid culture techniques have the advantage that the proliferative and functional capabilities of cells at various stages of differentiation can easily be studied, whereas in agar culture the growing cells are not easily retrieved. The liquid system, however, does not permit estimation of the number of colony-forming units in a given cell population.

Summary

Neutrophilic granulocytes arise from hematopoietic stem cells under microenvironmental and hormonal influences. Cell production occurs in the proliferative compartment of the bone marrow, comprising stem cells, myeloblasts, promyelocytes, and myelocytes. The myelocytes then enter the maturation and storage compartment of the marrow as they differentiate into myelocytes and PMN leukocytes. The mature cells leave the marrow to enter the blood and within a few hours enter the tissues, where they complete their life-span of a few days. Normally there is no return from the tissues to the blood or marrow compartments. The major controls of the level of circulating neutrophils are exerted on the proliferating compartment and at the point of departure from the marrow storage compartment into the blood. In vitro techniques of bone marrow culture have begun to provide insights about the proliferating cell and the hormonal factors influencing its proliferation and differentiation.

Chapter 2 References

1. Amato, D., Dowan, D. H., and McCulloch, E. A. Separation of immunocompetent cells from human and mouse hemopoietic cell suspensions by velocity sedimentation, *Blood* 39:472, 1972.
2. Aster, R. H., and Enright, S. E. A platelet and granulocyte membrane defect in paroxysmal nocturnal hemoglobinuria: usefulness for the detection of platelet antibodies, *J. Clin. Invest.* 48:1199, 1969.
3. Athens, J. W. Neutrophilic granulocyte kinetics and granulocytopoiesis, *in* A. S. Gordon (ed.), Regulation of Hematopoiesis, p. 1143, Appleton-Century-Crofts, New York, 1970.
4. Athens, J. W., Mauer, A. M., Ashenbrucker, H., and Cartwright, G. E. Leukokinetic studies: I. A method for labeling leukocytes with diisopropylfluorophosphate (DFP³²), *Blood* 14:303, 1959.
5. Athens, J. W., Haab, O. P., Raab, S. O., Mauer, A. M., Ashenbrucker, H., Cartwright, G. E., and Wintrobe, M. M. Leukokinetic studies: IV. The total blood, circulating and marginal granulocyte pools and the granulocyte turnover rate in normal subjects, *J. Clin. Invest.* 40:989, 1961.
6. Athens, J. W., Raab, S. O., Haab, O. P., Mauer, A. M., Ashenbrucker, H., Cartwright, G. E., and Wintrobe, M. M. Leukokinetic studies: III. The distribution of granulocytes in the blood of normal subjects, *J. Clin. Invest.* 40:159, 1961.
7. Athens, J. W., Raab, S. O., Haab, O. P., Boggs, D. R., Ashenbrucker, H., Cartwright, G. E., and Wintrobe, M. M. Leukokinetic studies: X. Blood granulocyte kinetics in chronic myelocytic leukemia, *J. Clin. Invest.* 44:765, 1965.
8. Athens, J. W., Haab, O. P., Raab, S. O., Boggs, D. R., Ashenbrucker, H., Cartwright, G. E., and Wintrobe, M. M. Leukokinetic studies: XI. Blood granulocyte kinetics in polycythemia vera, infection, and myelofibrosis, *J. Clin. Invest.* 44:778, 1965.
9. Athens, J. W., Bishop, C. R., and Cartwright, G. E. The kinetics of neutrophilic granulocytes in chronic myelocytic leukemia—a review, *in* C. J. D. Zarafonetis (ed.), Proceedings of the International Conference on Leukemia-Lymphoma, p. 219, Lea & Febiger, Philadelphia, 1968.
10. Barnes, D. W. H., and Loutit, J. F. Haemopoietic stem cells in the peripheral blood, *Lancet* 2:1138, 1967.
11. Becher, A. J., McCulloch, E. A., and Till, J. E. Cytologic demonstration of the clonal nature of spleen colonies derived from transplanted mouse marrow cells, *Nature* 197:452, 1963.
12. Bennett, M., and Cudkowicz, G. Hemopoietic progenitor cells with limited potential for differentiation: erythropoietic function of mouse marrow "lymphocytes," *J. Cell. Physiol.* 72:129, 1968.
13. Bennett, M., Cudkowicz, G., Foster, R. S., and Metcalf, D. Hemopoietic progenitor cells, of W anemic mice studied *in vivo* and *in vitro*, *J. Cell. Physiol.* 71:211, 1968.
14. Bierman, H. R., Kelly, K. H., Byron, R. L., Jr., and Marshall, G. J. Leucopheresis in man: I. Hematological observations following leucocyte withdrawal in patients with non-hematological disorders, *Br. J. Haematol.* 7:51, 1961.
15. Bishop, C. R., and Athens, J. W. A study of leukokinetic parameters in neutropenic dogs treated with melphalan and busulfan, *in* Proceedings of the XII Congress International Society of Hematology, F-X:36, New York, 1968.
16. Bloom, W., and Fawcett, D. W. A Textbook of Histology, p. 190, W. B. Saunders, Philadelphia, 1968.
17. Boggs, D. R. Homeostatic regulatory mechanisms of hematopoiesis, *Ann. Rev. Physiol.* 28:39, 1966.
18. Boggs, D. R. The kinetics of neutrophilic leukocytes in health and disease, *Semin. Hematol.* 4:359, 1967.
19. Boggs, D. R., and Chervenick, P. A. Hematopoietic stem cells, *in* T. J. Greenwalt and G. A. Jamieson (eds.), Formation and Destruction of Blood Cells, p. 240, J. B. Lippincott Co., Philadelphia, 1970.
20. Boggs, D. R., Athens, J. W., Cartwright, G. E., and Wintrobe, M. M. The effect of adrenal glucocorticosteroids upon the cellular composition of inflammatory exudates, *Am. J. Pathol.* 44:763, 1964.
21. Boggs, D. R., Athens, J. W., Haab, O. P., Cancilla, P. A., Raab, S. O., Cartwright, G. E., and Wintrobe, M. M. Leukokinetic studies: VII. Morphology of the bone marrow and blood of dogs given vinblastine sulfate, *Blood* 23:53, 1964.
22. Boggs, D. R., Athens, J. W., Cartwright, G. E., and Wintrobe, M. M. Leukokinetic studies: IX. Experimental evaluation of a model of granulopoiesis, *J. Clin. Invest.* 44:643, 1965.
23. Boggs, D. R., Athens, J. W., Cartwright, G. E., and Wintrobe, M. M. "Masked" granulocytosis, *Proc. Soc. Exp. Biol. Med.* 118:753, 1965.
24. Boggs, D. R., Athens, J. W., Cartwright, G. E., and Wintrobe, M. M. The different effects of vinblastine sulfate and nitrogen mustard upon neutrophil kinetics in the dog, *Proc. Soc. Exp. Biol. Med.* 121:1085, 1966.
25. Boggs, D. R., Marsh, J. C., Chervenick, P. A., Cartwright, G. E., and Wintrobe, M. M. Factors influencing hematopoietic spleen colony formation in irradiated mice. V. Effect of foreign plasma upon colony forming cell kinetics, *J. Cell. Physiol.* 71:227, 1968.
26. Boggs, D. R., Marsh, J. C., Chervenick, P. A., Cartwright, G. E., and Wintrobe, M. M. Neutrophil releasing activity in plasma of normal human subjects injected with endotoxin, *Proc. Soc. Exp. Biol. Med.* 127:689, 1968.
27. Boll, I., and Kühn, A. Granulocytopoiesis in human bone marrow cultures studied by means of kinematography, *Blood* 26:449, 1965.
28. Bond, V. P., Fliedner, T. M., Cronkite, E. P., Rubini, J. R., and Robertson, J. S. Cell turnover in blood and blood forming tissues studied with tritiated thymidine, *in* F. Stohlman, Jr. (ed.), The Kinetics of Cellular Proliferation, p. 188, Grune & Stratton, New York, 1959.
29. Bradley, T. R. Aspects of stimulation of bone marrow colony growth *in vitro*, *Aust. J. Exp. Biol. Med.* 46:335, 1968.
30. Bradley, T. R., and Metcalf, D. The

growth of mouse bone marrow cells *in vitro, Aust. J. Exp. Biol. Med.* 44:287, 1966.

31. Bradley, T. R., and Siemienowicz, R. Colony growth of rat bone marrow cells *in vitro, Aust. J. Exp. Biol. Med.* 46:595, 1968.

32. Bradley, T. R., and Sumner, M. A. Stimulation of mouse bone marrow colony growth *in vitro* by conditioned medium, *Aust. J. Exp. Biol. Med.* 46:607, 1968.

33. Bradley, T. R., Robinson, W., and Metcalf, D. Colony production *in vitro* by normal polycythaemic and anaemic bone marrow, *Nature* 214:511, 1967.

34. Bradley, T. R., Metcalf, D., Sumner, M., and Stanley, R. *in* P. A. Farnes (ed.), Hemic Cells in Vitro, vol. 4, Williams & Wilkins Co., Baltimore, 1969.

35. Bruce, W. R., Meeker, B. E., and Valeriote, F. A. Comparison of the sensitivity of normal hematopoietic and transplanted lymphoma colony-forming cells to chemotherapeutic agents administered *in vivo, J. Natl. Cancer Inst.* 37:233, 1966.

36. Chan, S. H., Metcalf, D., and Stanley, E. R. Stimulation and inhibition by normal human serum of colony formation *in vitro* by bone marrow cells, *Br. J. Haematol.* 20:329, 1971.

37. Chervenick, P. A., and Boggs, D. R. Decreased neutrophils and megakaryocytes in anemic mice of genotype W/W^v, *J. Cell. Physiol.* 73:25, 1969.

38. Chervenick, P. A., and Boggs, D. R. A kinetic model of hematopoietic stem cell repopulation and differentiation, *J. Clin. Invest.* 48:15a, 1969.

39. Chervenick, P. A., and Boggs, D. R. Bone marrow colonies: stimulation *in vitro* by supernatant from incubated human blood cells, *Science* 169:691, 1970.

40. Chervenick, P. A., and LoBuglio, A. F. Human blood monocytes: stimulators of granulocyte and mononuclear colony formation *in vitro, Science* 178:164, 1972.

41. Cleaver, J. E. Thymidine Metabolism and Cell Kinetics, John Wiley and Sons, New York, 1967.

42. Cline, M. J. Cancer Chemotherapy, W. B. Saunders, Philadelphia, 1971.

43. Cline, M. J., Warner, N. L., and Metcalf, D. Identification of the bone marrow colony mononuclear phagocytes as a macrophage, *Blood* 39:326, 1972.

44. Cole, L. J., and Maki, S. E. Hemopoietic colony-forming cells in mouse blood: effect of pertussis vaccine injection and of thymectomy-irradiation, *Exp. Hematol.* 15:82, 1968.

45. Craddock, C. G. Kinetics of lymphoreticular tissue with particular emphasis on the lymphatic system, *Semin. Hematol.* 4:387, 1967.

46. Craddock, C. G., Adams, W. S., Perry, S., Skoog, W. A., and Lawrence, J. S. Studies of leukopoiesis: the technique of leukapheresis and the response of myeloid tissue in normal and irradiated dogs, *J. Lab. Clin. Med.* 45:881, 1955.

47. Craddock, C. G., Perry, S., and Lawrence, J. S. The dynamics of leukopoiesis and leukocytosis as studied by leukapheresis and isotopic techniques, *J. Clin. Invest.* 35:285, 1956.

48. Cronkite, E. P., and Fliedner, T. M. Granulocytopoiesis, *N. Engl. J. Med.* 270:1347, 1964.

49. DeConti, R. C., Kaplan, S. R., and Calabresi, P. Endotoxin stimulation in patients with lymphoma: correlation with the myelosuppressive effects of alkylating agents, *Blood* 39:602, 1972.

50. Delmonte, L., and Liebelt, R. A. Granulocytosis-promoting extract of mouse tumor tissue: partial purification, *Science* 148:521, 1965.

51. Dicke, K. A., Van Noord, M. J., Maat, B., *et al.* Identification of cells in primate bone marrow resembling the hemopoietic stem cell in the mouse, *Blood* 42:195, 1973.

52. Donohue, D. M., Reiff, R. H., Hanson, M. L., Betson, Y., and Finch, C. A. Quantitative measurement of the erythrocytic and granulocytic cells of the marrow and blood, *J. Clin. Invest.* 37:1571, 1958.

53. Dresch, C., and Najean, Y. Étude de la cinetique des polynucleaires après marquage "in vitro" par le radiochrome, *Nouv. Rev. Fr. Hematol.* 7:27, 1967.

54. Farquhar, M. G., Bainton, D. F., Baggiolini, M., and DeDuve, C. Cytochemical localization of acid phosphatase activity in granule fractions from rabbit polymorphonuclear leukocytes, *J. Cell Biol.* 54:141, 1972.

55. Fialkow, P. J., Lisker, R., Detter, J., Giblett, E. R., Zavala, G. C. 6-phosphogluconate dehydrogenase: hemizygous manifestation in a patient with leukemia, *Science* 163:194, 1969.

56. Fliedner, T. M., Cronkite, E. P., and Robertson, J. S. Granulocytopoiesis: I. Senescence and random loss of neutrophilic granulocytes in human beings, *Blood* 24:402, 1964.

57. Fliedner, T. M., Cronkite, E. P., Killmann, S. A., and Bond, V. P. Emergence and pattern of labeling neutrophilic granulocytes in humans, *Blood* 24:683, 1964.

58. Foster, R., Metcalf, D., Robinson, W. A., and Bradley, T. R. Bone marrow colony stimulating activity in human sera. Results of two independent surveys in Buffalo and Melbourne, *Br. J. Haematol.* 15:147, 1968.

59. Foster, R., Metcalf, D., and Kirchmyer, R. Induction of bone marrow colony stimulating activity by a filterable agent in leukemic and normal mouse serum, *J. Exp. Med.* 127:853, 1968.

60. Fowler, J. H., Till, J. E., McCulloch, E. A., and Siminovitch, L. The cellular basis for the defect in haemopoiesis in flexed-tailed mice. II. The specificity of the defect for erythropoiesis, *Br. J. Haematol.* 13:256, 1967.

61. Galbraith, P. R.: Studies on the longevity, sequestration and release of the leukocytes in chronic myelogenous leukemia, *Can. Med. Assoc. J.* 95:511, 1966.

62. Galbraith, P. R., Valberg, L. S., and Brown, M. Patterns of granulocyte kinetics in health, infection and in carcinoma, *Blood* 25:683, 1965.

63. Golde, D. W., and Cline, M. J. Identification of the colony-stimulating cell in human peripheral blood, *J. Clin. Invest.* 51:2981, 1972.

64. Golde, D. W., and Cline, M. J. Growth of human bone marrow in liquid culture, *Blood* 41:45, 1973.

65. Golde, D. W., Finley, T. N., and Cline, M. J. Production of colony-

stimulating factor by human macrophages, *Lancet* 2:1397, 1972.

66. Goldscheider, A., and Jacob, P. Ueber die Variationen der Leukocytose, *Z. Klin. Med.* 25:373, 1894.

67. Gordon, A. S., Handler, E. S., Siegel, C. D., Dornfest, B. S., and LoBue, J. Plasma factors influencing leukocyte release in rats, *Ann. N.Y. Acad. Sci.* 113:766, 1964.

68. Grant, L. The sticking and emigration of white blood cells in inflammation, in B. W. Zweifach, L. Grant, and R. J. McCluskey (eds.), The Inflammatory Process, p. 197, Academic Press, New York, 1965.

69. Hall, B. M. The effects of whole body irradiation on serum colony stimulating factor and *in vitro* colony-forming cells in the bone marrow, *Br. J. Haematol.* 17:553, 1969.

70. Hellman, S., and Grate, H. E. Enhanced erythropoiesis with concomitant diminished granulopoiesis in preirradiated recipient mice. Evidence for a common stem cell, *J. Exp. Med.* 127:605, 1968.

71. Horn, R. G., Wetzel, B. K., and Spicer, S. S. Fine-structural localization of nonspecific acid and alkaline phosphatases in rabbit myeloid elements, *J. Appl. Physics* 34:2517, 1963 (abstract).

72. Hughes, W. L., Bond, V. P., Brecher, G., Cronkite, E. P., Painter, R. B., Quastler, H., and Sherman, F. G. Cellular proliferation in the mouse as revealed by autoradiography with tritiated thymidine, *Proc. Natl. Acad. Sci. U.S.A.* 44:476, 1958.

73. Ichikawa, Y., Pluznik, D. H., and Sachs, L. *In vitro* control of the development of macrophage and granulocyte colonies, *Proc. Natl. Acad. Sci. U.S.A.* 56:488, 1966.

74. Iscove, N. N., Senn, J. S., Till, J. E., and McCulloch, E. A. Colony formation by normal and leukemic human marrow cells in culture: effect of conditioned medium from human leukocytes, *Blood* 37:1, 1971.

75. Janoshwitz, H., Moore, M. A. S., and Metcalf, D. Density gradient segregation of bone marrow cells with the capacity to form granulocytic and macrophage colonies *in vitro*, *Exp. Cell Res.* 68:220, 1971.

76. Kauer, G. L., Jr., and Engle, R. L.,

Jr. Eosinophilic leukaemia with Ph 1-positive cells, *Lancet* 2:1340, 1964.

77. Killmann, S. A., Cronkite, E. P., Fliedner, T. M., and Bond, V. P. Mitotic indices of human bone marrow cells: I. Number and cytologic distribution of mitoses, *Blood* 19:743, 1962.

78. Killmann, S. A., Cronkite, E. P., Fliedner, T. M., Bond, V. P., and Brecher, G. Mitotic indices of human bone marrow cells: II. The use of mitotic indices for estimation of time parameters of proliferation in serially connected multiplicative cellular compartments, *Blood* 21:141, 1963.

79. Kubanek, B., Ferrari, L., Tyler, W. S., Howard, D., Jay, S., and Stohlman, F. Regulation of erythropoiesis. 23. Dissociation between stem cell and erythroid response to hypoxia, *Blood* 32:586, 1968.

80. Kurth, D., Athens, J. W., Cronkite, E. P., Cartwright, G. E., and Wintrobe, M. M. Leukokinetic studies: V. Uptake of tritiated diisopropylfluorophosphate by leukocytes, *Proc. Soc. Exp. Biol. Med.* 107:422, 1961.

81. Lagunoff, D., Pluznik, D. H., and Sachs, L. The cloning of macrophages in agar. Identification of the cells by electron microscopy, *J. Cell. Physiol.* 68:385, 1966.

82. Lala, P. K., Maloney, M. A., and Patt, H. M. A comparison of two markers of cell proliferation in bone marrow, *Acta Haematol.* 31:1, 1964.

83. Lawrence, J. S., Craddock, C. G., Jr., and Campbell, T. N. Antineutrophilic serum, its use in studies of white blood cell dynamics, *J. Lab. Clin. Med.* 69:88, 1967.

84. LoBue, J. Analysis of normal granulocyte production and release, in A. S. Gordon (ed.), Regulation of Hematopoiesis, p. 1167, Appelton-Century-Crofts, New York, 1970.

85. McCall, M. S., Sutherland, D. A., Eisentraut, A. M., and Lanz, H. The tagging of leukemic leukocytes with radioactive chromium and measurement of the *in vivo* cell survival, *J. Lab. Clin. Med.* 45:717, 1955.

86. McCulloch, E. A., and Till, J. E. The sensitivity of cells from

normal mouse bone marrow to gamma radiation *in vitro* and *in vivo*, *Radiat. Res.* 16:822, 1962.

87. McCulloch, E. A., Siminovitch, L., and Till, J. E.: Spleen-colony formation in anemic mice of genotype W/W, *Science* 144:844, 1964.

88. McCulloch, E. A., Siminovitch, L., Till, J. E., Russel, E. J., and Bernstein, S. E. The cellular basis of the genetically determined hemopoietic defect in anemic mice of genotype S1-S1d, *Blood* 26:399, 1965.

89. McMillan, R., Scott, J. L., and Marino, J. V. Survival of Cr51-labeled leukocytes, *Clin. Res.* 15:133, 1967.

90. Maloney, M. A., and Patt, H. M. Granulocyte transit from bone marrow to blood, *Blood* 31:195, 1968.

91. Marsh, J. C., Boggs, D. R., Cartwright, G. E., and Wintrobe, M. M. Neutrophil kinetics in acute infection, *J. Clin. Invest.* 46:1943, 1967.

92. Marsh, J. C., Boggs, D. R., Bishop, C. R., Chervenick, P. A., Cartwright, G. E., and Wintrobe, M. M. Factors influencing hematopoietic spleen colony formation in irradiated mice. I. The normal pattern of endogenous colony formation, *J. Exp. Med.* 126:833, 1967.

93. Marsh, J. C., Boggs, D. R., Chervenick, P. A., Cartwright, G. E., and Wintrobe, M. M. Factors influencing hematopoietic spleen colony formation in irradiated mice: IV. The effect of erythropoietic stimuli, *J. Cell. Physiol.* 71:65, 1968.

94. Mauer, A. M., Athens, H. W., Ashenbrucker, H., Cartwright, G. E., and Wintrobe, M. M. Leukokinetic studies: II. A method for labeling granulocytes *in vitro* with radioactive diisopropylfluorophosphate (DFP32), *J. Clin. Invest.* 39:1481, 1960.

95. Metcalf, D. Potentiation of bone marrow colony growth *in vitro* by the addition of lymphoid or bone marrow cells, *J. Cell. Physiol.* 72:9, 1968.

96. Metcalf, D. The effect of bleeding on the number of *in vitro* colony-forming cells in the bone marrow, *Br. J. Haematol.* 16:397, 1969.

97. Metcalf, D. Acute antigen-induced elevation of serum colony stimu-

lating factor (CSF) levels, *Immunology* 21:427, 1971.

98. Metcalf, D. The nature of leukemia: neoplasm or disorder of hemopoietic regulation? *Med. J. Aust.* 2:739, 1971.

99. Metcalf, D., and Foster, R. Bone marrow colony-stimulating activity of serum from mice with virus-induced leukemia, *J. Natl. Cancer Inst.* 39:1235, 1967.

100. Metcalf, D., and Foster, R. Behavior on transfer of serum stimulated bone marrow colonies, *Proc. Soc. Exp. Biol. Med.* 126:758, 1967.

101. Metcalf, D., and Wahren, B. Bone marrow colony-stimulating activity of sera in infectious mononucleosis, *Br. Med. J.* 3:99, 1968.

102. Metcalf, D., and Bradley, T. R. Factors regulating *in vitro* colony formation by hematopoietic cells, *in* A. S. Gordon (ed.), Regulation of Hematopoiesis, p. 187, Appleton-Century-Crofts, New York, 1970.

103. Metcalf, D., and Moore, M. A. S. Haemopoietic Cells, North-Holland Publishing Co., Amsterdam, 1971.

104. Metcalf, D., Bradley, T. R., and Robinson, W. Analysis of colonies developing *in vitro* from mouse bone marrow cells stimulated by kidney feeder layers or leukemic serum, *J. Cell. Physiol.* 69:93, 1967.

105. Metcalf, D., Foster, R., and Pollard, M. Colony stimulating activity of serum from germfree normal and leukemic mice, *J. Cell. Physiol.* 70:131, 1967.

106. Metcalf, D., Moore, M. A. S., and Shortman, K. Adherence column and buoyant density separation of bone marrow stem cells and more differentiated cells, *J. Cell. Physiol.* 78:441, 1971.

107. Moore, M. A. S., and Owen, J. J. T. Chromosome marker studies in the irradiated chick embryo, *Nature* 215:1081, 1967.

108. Moore, M. A. S., and Metcalf, D. Ontogeny of the haemopoietic system: Yolk sac origin of *in vivo* and *in vitro* colony forming cells in the developing mouse embryo, *Br. J. Haematol.* 18:279, 1970.

109. Moore, M. A. S., Williams, N., and Metcalf, D. Purification and characterization of the *in vitro* colony forming cell in monkey hemo-

poietic tissue, *J. Cell. Physiol.* 79:283, 1972.

110. Nowell, P. C., and Cole, L. J. Clonal repopulation in reticular tissues of x-irradiated mice: effect of dose and limb-shielding, *J. Cell. Physiol.* 70:37, 1967.

111. O'Grady, L. F., Lewis, J. P., Lange, R. D., Trobaugh, F. E., Jr. Effect of erythropoietin on transplanted hematopoietic tissue, *Am. J. Physiol.* 215:176, 1968.

112. Ottesen, J. On the age of human white cells in peripheral blood, *Acta Physiol. Scand.* 32:75, 1954.

113. Patt, H. M. Discussion of data obtained with DFP[32]-labeled granulocytes, *in* F. Stohlman, Jr. (ed.), The Kinetics of Cellular Proliferation, p. 241, Grune & Stratton, New York, 1959.

114. Patt, H. M., and Maloney, M. A. Kinetics of neutrophil balance in the kinetics of cellular proliferation, *in* F. Stohlman, Jr. (ed.), The Kinetics of Cellular Proliferation, p. 201, Grune & Stratton, New York, 1959.

115. Patt, H. M., Maloney, M. A., and Jackson, E. M. Recovery of blood neutrophils after acute peripheral depletion, *Am. J. Physiol.* 188:585, 1957.

116. Perry, S. Leukocyte kinetics in leukemia, *in* C. J. D. Zarafonetis (ed.), Proceedings of the International Conference on Leukemia-Lymphoma, p. 299, Lea & Febiger, Philadelphia, 1968.

117. Perry, S., and Moxley, J. H., III. Investigations of leukocyte kinetics in normal and leukaemic individuals by means of scintillation counting, *Nature* 209:882, 1966.

118. Perry, S., Craddock, C. G., Jr., and Lawrence, J. S. Rates of appearance and disappearance of white blood cells in normal and in various disease states, *J. Lab. Clin. Med.* 51:501, 1958.

119. Perry, S., Moxley, J. H., III, Weiss, G. H., and Zelen, M. Studies of leukocyte kinetics by liquid scintillation counting in normal individuals and in patients with chronic myelocytic leukemia, *J. Clin. Invest.* 45:1388, 1966.

120. Pike, B. L., and Robinson, W. A. Human bone marrow growth in

agar-gel, *J. Cell. Physiol.* 76:77, 1970.

121. Pluznik, D. H., and Sachs, L. The cloning of normal "mast" cells in tissue culture, *J. Cell. Physiol.* 66:319, 1965.

122. Pluznik, D. H., and Sachs, L. The induction of clones of normal "mast" cells by a substance from conditioned medium, *Exp. Cell Res.* 43:553, 1966.

123. Porteous, D. D., and Lajtha, L. J. On stem-cell recovery after irradiation, *Br. J. Haematol.* 12:177, 1966.

124. Raab, S. O., Athens, J. W., Haab, O. P., Boggs, D. R., Ashenbrucker, H., Cartwright, G. E., and Wintrobe, M. M. Granulokinetics in normal dogs, *Am. J. Physiol.* 206:83, 1964.

125. Rebuck, J. W., and Crowley, J. H. A method of studying leukocytic functions *in vivo*, *Ann. N.Y. Acad. Sci.* 59:757, 1955.

126. Reed, I. L., Barry, P., Wong, H., and Greenberg, M. S. Disappearance rates of circulating granulocytes in cirrhosis. XI Congress International Society of Hematology, Abstracts of Papers, AC4:26, 1966.

127. Robinson, W. A., and Pike, B. L. Leukopoietic activity in human urine, *N. Engl. J. Med.* 282:1291, 1970.

128. Robinson, W. A., and Otsuka, A. Production of granulocyte colony stimulating activity by human WBC and subcellular localization, *in* D. W. van Bekkum and K. A. Dicke (eds.), In Vitro Culture of Hemopoietic Cells, p. 266, Radiobiological Institute TNO, Rijswijk, 1972.

129. Robinson, W. A., and Mangalik, A. Regulation of granulopoiesis: positive feed-back, *Lancet* 2:742, 1972.

130. Robinson, W. A., Metcalf, D., and Bradley, T. R. Stimulation by normal and leukemic mouse sera of colony formation *in vitro* by mouse bone marrow cells, *J. Cell. Physiol.* 69:83, 1967.

131. Robinson, W. A., Bradley, T. R., and Metcalf, D. Effect of whole body irradiation on colony production by bone marrow cells *in vitro*, *Proc. Soc. Exp. Biol. Med.* 125:388, 1967.

132. Robinson, W. A., Stanley, E. R., and Metcalf, D. Stimulation of bone

38   Part I   Granulocytes

marrow colony growth *in vitro* by human urine, *Blood* 33:396, 1969.

133. Rosse, W. F., and Gurney, C. W. The Pelger-Huët anomaly in three families and its use in determining the disappearance of transfused neutrophils from the peripheral blood, *Blood* 14:170, 1959.

134. Rothstein, G., Bishop, C. R., Athens, J. W., and Ashenbrucker, H. E. A method for leukokinetic study in the nonsteady state, *Blood* 38:302, 1971.

135. Sacchetti, C., and Boccacio, P. Riconoscimento del sequestro di granulociti nella mitza, *Minerva Nucl.* 9:207, 1965.

136. Sacchetti, C., Boccacio, P., Ponassi, A., and Morra, L. Neutrophilic leukocyte reserve of the bone marrow, *Minerva Nucl.* 1, 1964.

137. Schooley, J. C., Hayes, J. M., Cantor, L. N., and Havens, V. W. Studies on the behavior of erythropoietin-sensitive cells in the mouse during recovery from 200 roentgens of whole-body irradiation, *Radiat. Res.* 32:875, 1967.

138. Senn, H. J., and Holland, J. F. Kinetics of localized leukocyte mobilization (LLM) in health and hematologic neoplasia. XII Congress International Society of Hematology, Abstract of Papers, F-16:40, 1968.

139. Senn, J. S., McCulloch, E. A., and Till, J. E. Comparison of colony-forming ability of normal and leukaemic human marrow in tissue culture, *Lancet* 2:597, 1967.

140. Stanley, E. R., and Metcalf, D. Partial purification and some properties of the factors in normal and leu-

kaemic urine stimulating bone marrow colony growth *in vitro*, *Aust. J. Exp. Biol. Med.* 47:467, 1969.

141. Stanley, E. R., Robinson, W. A., and Ada, G. L. Properties of the colony stimulating factor in leukaemic and normal mouse serum, *Aust. J. Exp. Biol. Med.* 46:715, 1968.

142. Storb, R., Epstein, R. B., and Thomas, E. D. Marrow repopulating ability of peripheral blood cells compared to thoracic duct cells, *Blood* 32:662, 1968.

143. Sumner, M. A., Bradley, T. R., Hodgson, G. S., Cline, M. J., Fry, P. A., and Sutherland, L. The growth of bone marrow cells in liquid culture, *Br. J. Haematol.* 23:221, 1972.

144. Thomas, E. D., Plain, G. L., and Thomas, D. Leukocyte kinetics in the dog studied by cross-circulation, *J. Lab. Clin. Med.* 66:64, 1965.

145. Till, J. E., and McCulloch, E. A. A direct measurement of radiation sensitivity of normal mouse bone marrow cells, *Radiat. Res.* 14:213, 1961.

146. Trentin, J. J. Determination of bone marrow stem cell differentiation by stromal hemopoietic inductive microenvironments (HIM), *Am. J. Pathol.* 65:621, 1971.

147. Tyan, M. L. Studies on the ontogeny of the mouse immune system. I. Cell bound immunity, *J. Immunol.* 100:535, 1968.

148. Valeriote, F. A., Bruce, W. R., and Meeker, B. E. Comparison of the sensitivity of normal hematopoietic and transplanted lymphoma colony-forming cells of mice to

vinblastine administered *in vivo*, *J. Natl. Cancer Inst.* 36:21, 1966.

149. van Bekkum, D. W., van Noord, M. J., Maat, B., and Dicke, K. A. Attempts at identification of hemopoietic stem cell in mouse, *Blood* 38:547, 1971.

150. Vejlens, G. The distribution of leukocytes in the vascular system, *Acta Pathol. Microbiol. Scand.* 33:1, 1938 (suppl.).

151. Walker, R. I., Herion, J. C., Herring, W. B., and Palmer, J. G. Leukocyte kinetics in hematologic disorders studied by DNA phosphorus labeling, *Blood* 23:795, 1964.

152. Warner, H. R., and Athens, J. W. An analysis of granulocyte kinetics in blood and bone marrow, *Ann. N.Y. Acad. Sci.* 113:523, 1964.

153. Whang, J., Frei, E. III, Tjio, J. H., Carbone, P. P., and Brecher, G. The distribution of the Philadelphia chromosome in patients with chronic myelogenous leukemia, *Blood* 22:664, 1963.

154. Woodliff, H. J. Blood and Bone Marrow Cell Culture, Eyre and Spottiswoode, London, 1964.

155. Wu, A. M., Till, J. E., Siminovitch, L., and McCulloch, E. A. Cytological evidence for a relationship between normal hematopoietic colony-forming cells and cells of the lymphoid system, *J. Exp. Med.* 127:455, 1968.

156. Wu, A. M., Siminovitch, L., Till, J. E., and McCulloch, E. A. Evidence for a relationship between mouse hemopoietic stem cells and cells forming colonies in culture, *Proc. Natl. Acad. Sci. U.S.A.* 59:1209, 1968.

Chapter 3   Neutrophil Metabolism and Composition

A considerable number of reviews interpreting single and multiple aspects of white cell metabolism were published between 1939 and 1970 (2, 3, 23, 25, 33, 52, 72, 90, 96, 97, 104, 147, 259, 275, 276, 282, 424, 487, 515–518, 540). A unified description of granulocyte biochemistry and metabolism has been difficult to achieve, however, as granulocytes are not a single type. The several varieties of circulating granulocytes (neutrophils, basophils, and eosinophils) may be even further subdivided into different stages of maturity and differentiation. The problem of achieving a unified description is additionally complicated by the neoplastic leukocyte which, at a given stage of development, is not necessarily biochemically identical to its normal counterpart. Furthermore, leukocytes are extremely sensitive to the mechanical trauma of isolation procedures and in vitro study conditions (212, 346, 547). Consequently, studies of granulocyte metabolism often have been merely studies of procedural artifacts. In most metabolic studies of white cells reported prior to 1960, few attempts were made to fractionate leukocyte populations into their component elements, so that the contribution of the granulocytic elements in these studies is difficult to analyze. Our knowledge of granulocyte metabolism is still only fragmentary. However, application of improved methods of white cell isolation (89, 175, 297, 507, 557), separation of subtypes (85, 251, 264, 268, 372, 416, 533), and new, sophisticated biochemical techniques have added greatly to our understanding in the past few years.

Respiration

In 1911 Grafe demonstrated the presence of oxidative metabolism in leukemic human leukocytes (227). White cells and platelets subsequently were shown to account for the bulk of the oxygen consumption of whole blood. In human and guinea pig leukocytes, the following appears to be the order of decreasing oxygen consumption per cell: alveolar macrophage, monocyte, polymorphonuclear leukocyte, and lymphocyte (275, 276, 486, 488, 531).

The size and numbers of mitochondria decrease with the progressive maturation of granulocytes. A reasonable inference is that the mature neutrophil derives much of its energy from anaerobic metabolism and is not critically dependent upon available oxygen. Key neutrophil functions, such as movement and phagocytosis, continue perfectly well in the absence of oxygen; and neutrophils demonstrate, even under aerobic conditions, a high level of glycolysis. These observations make teleological sense for a cell that must often function at low partial pressures of oxygen as, for example, in an abscess cavity. In neutrophils the only two important cellular processes known to be dependent on molecular oxygen are the killing of certain ingested microorganisms (466) and the generation of certain vasoactive peptides (354, 355).

Neutrophil oxygen consumption increases markedly with particle ingestion, 10- or even 20-fold. Stimulation of respiration is proportional to the load of particles ingested within a finite range (22, 34, 111, 208, 261, 275–277, 312,

342, 379, 453, 488, 497). The same pattern of enhanced consumption with phagocytosis can be observed in primitive amoebae and in human eosinophils, monocytes, and granulocytes (98, 99, 312).

An outstanding feature of this "respiratory burst," which occurs with phagocytosis, is that it is not poisoned by cyanide (276). This means the enhanced oxygen consumption is not mediated via the usual cyanide-sensitive mitochondrial pathway. The precise mechanisms of the increased oxygen intake are not known, although NADH- and NADPH-oxidase may be instrumental in effecting the process (15, 254, 262, 600) (see Chapter 4). These enzymes are also relatively insensitive to poisoning by cyanide (170, 171, 276). However, they have not been identified in all mammalian leukocytes. Human and guinea pig granulocytes also contain D-amino acid oxidase (100), which may be important in oxygen utilization when D-amino-acid-containing bacteria are ingested. This oxidase cannot, however, account for the respiratory burst that follows the phagocytosis of inert particles.

Guinea pig leukocyte respiration is relatively insensitive to cyanide and antimycin, but is sensitive to amobarbital, an inhibitor of flavoproteins. Based on this evidence, extramitochondrial NADPH-dependent reactions (possibly a malic-malic dehydrogenase system) could be one of the main pathways of reoxidation of reduced pyridine nucleotides (441, 599). Decidedly, insufficient data are available and one cannot make a firm statement about which of these various pathways is critical to the enhanced oxygen consumption accompanying phagocytosis.

Despite these complexities, the granulocytic oxygen burst that follows particle ingestion is clearly utilized in part for generation of hydrogen peroxide (261). Other features of the interesting respiratory phenomenon characteristic of phagocytosis are considered in more detail in the next chapter.

The oxygen consumption of the granulocyte is influenced by certain hormones, a variety of chemicals, biological materials, and the trauma of cell isolation procedures (90). Oxygen utilization may be rapidly altered by the administration of triiodothyronine (8, 50). In human white cells, enzymes active at physiologic pH are capable of de-iodinating thyroxin (305). Respiration is also affected by the partial pressure of carbon dioxide (49, 441), concentration of glucose (169, 331, 423), homologous serum (275, 333, 342, 470, 559), bacterial pyrogens (101), and antigen-antibody complexes (497). White cell respiration is depressed by saponin (410), thiouracil (558), chloramphenicol (193), cyanide, fluoroacetate, malonate, and P-chloromercuribenzoate (331, 342, 346); whereas ascorbic

Table 3.1 Features of granulocyte oxygen metabolism.

There are few mitochondria and low levels of mitochondrial enzymes.

Movement and phagocytosis, key neutrophil functions, do not require oxygen.

Phagocytosis causes increased oxygen consumption by a mitochondria-independent pathway.

Postphagocytic oxygen consumption is utilized for H_2O_2 generation.

Bacterial killing and vasoactive peptide generation require oxygen.

acid (348) and dinitrophenol (331, 346) increase oxygen consumption.

Specific elements of the cytochrome system (87) and oxidative phosphorylation (139, 197) have been identified in mammalian leukocytes. The principal features of granulocyte oxygen metabolism are summarized in Table 3.1.

Carbohydrate Metabolism

Important features of the carbohydrate metabolism of the mature granulocyte are (a) a high level of anaerobic glycolysis utilizing either exogenous sugars or endogenous glycogen stores, (b) dependence upon glycolysis for production of the energy for phagocytosis, and (c) greatly enhanced glucose oxidation via the hexose monophosphate shunt during particle ingestion.

Glycolysis

In 1912 Levene and Meyer demonstrated the conversion of glucose and other monosaccharides to lactic acid by leukocytes prepared from sterile exudates (319, 320). In 1927 Fleischmann and Kubowitz (190) described glycolysis in white cells of goose blood. In 1939 Kempner, reviewing earlier studies, noted that most investigators found the glycolytic rate of normal white cells to be high in comparison with oxidative metabolism, and lactic acid to be formed anaerobically (282). Considerable subsequent evidence has demonstrated that the chief pathway of leukocyte glucose metabolism is to lactate via pyruvate and that leukocytes from normal individuals of several species and from patients with chronic myelocytic leukemia have a high level of aerobic glycolysis (21, 27, 28, 31–33, 205, 207, 276, 281, 282, 310, 329, 331, 332, 427, 548, 549).

Numerous analogies have been drawn between white cell carbohydrate metabolism and the high rate of aerobic glycolysis found in certain neoplastic cells (554). However, this type of metabolic pattern is observed also in certain nonneoplastic cells with a high mitotic rate, such as embryonic tissues (212, 465).

The hexokinase reaction is thought to be the rate-limiting step in the glycolytic sequence in both normal and malignant white cells (27, cf. 28, 249, 362, 518, 550). A variety of factors influences the rate of granulocyte glycolysis: the concentration of glucose and, to a lesser extent, of fructose (331, 342, 423); the presence of insulin (346, 347); cell integrity (331); and viral infection (185, 186). Some bacterial pyrogens stimulate glycolysis (112), but other bacterial products inhibit the process (590). Human leukocytes bind cortisol (285), a hormone capable of inhibiting neutrophil glycolysis without affecting respiration (331, 423). The glycolytic rate is higher in the white cells of infants than in those of older children and adults (456). Granulocytes found in tissue exudates have a higher level of glycolytic activity than do circulating cells (239, 240). The lactic acid thus produced may be instrumental in inducing a cycle of inflammation in the tissues (338) (see Chapter 5).

Possible carbohydrate sources for glycolysis in normal granulocytes are glucose, glycogen, galactose, or fructose (270, 314, 342, 346, 496, 561, 562).

The striking feature of the glycolytic metabolism of mammalian granulocytes, including those of man, is the enhancement of glycolysis by phagocytosis under both aerobic and anaerobic conditions (111, 208, 276, 453). The energy for phagocytosis results from glycolysis (34, 37, 111, 186, 223, 261, 277, 453, 470). Most investigators have found that compounds interfering with glycolysis have a profound inhibitory effect on phagocytosis, whereas inhibitors of cell respiration have little effect except at very high concentrations (230, 427).

Degradation of ingested bacteria occurs after phagocytosis and the subsequent degranulation of neutrophils. Inhibitors of glycolysis and respiration have no effect on this degradation (110). These data suggest that once the degradative enzymes contained in the neutrophilic granules (108, 109, 261) are released, destruction of ingested microorganisms does not require the expenditure of chemical energy.

Table 3.2 Features of granulocyte glycolytic metabolism.

Phagocytosis depends on glycolytic energy production.
High levels of aerobic glycolysis occur in the intact cell.
The hexokinase reaction is the rate-limiting step in glycolysis.
Glycolytic rate is influenced by the concentration of glucose and, to a lesser extent, of fructose, presence of insulin, hormonal factors, some viral infections, and particle ingestion.

Morphologically separable types of leukocytes vary in their range of lactate production. In man the order of decreasing rate of glycolysis per cell is monocyte, neutrophil, lymphocyte (24, 207, 456, 486, 531).

The important features of granulocytic glycolytic metabolism are summarized in Table 3.2.

The Tricarboxylic Acid Cycle

Mature granulocytes have few mitochondria. Consequently, a metabolism based on oxygen-dependent carbohydrate utilization is only poorly developed. Data on the tricarboxylic acid cycle intermediates are scanty. However, the tricarboxylic acid cycle enzymes of the leukocyte, including malic dehydrogenase, fumarase, isocitric dehydrogenase, and aconitase, have been defined (55).

Although only pyruvate of the various Krebs-cycle intermediates stimulates oxygen consumption in intact granulocytes, several intermediates—of which succinate is the most active—stimulate respiration in white cell homogenates (32, 331, 342, 346).

Hexose Monophosphate Shunt

In 1956 Coxon and Robinson demonstrated the existence of a glucose-6-phosphate (phosphogluconate) oxidation pathway in the circulating leukocytes of several mammalian species (120). The reaction sequence of this pathway is summarized in Fig. 3.1. The 5-carbon intermediates interact to form a heptose and a triose and then a hexose

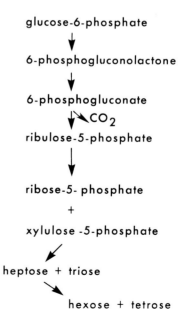

Figure 3.1 Outline of the hexose monophosphate shunt pathway.

and a tetrose, which may then reenter the glycolytic pathway.

Glucose-6-phosphate dehydrogenase (53, 54, 269) is the first enzyme in the direct glucose oxidation pathway. In Caucasians, where the erythrocyte activity of this enzyme is decreased, the granulocyte (422) enzyme activity is 10 to 20 percent of the normal level. Only 10 percent, or less, of total granulocyte glucose is normally metabolized via the hexose monophosphate shunt (27–29, 276, 279, 497).

Most authors stress the role of oxidized NADP in regulating the activity of the direct oxidative pathway from glucose in granulocytes (194). This regulatory mechanism exists in other tissues as well as in white cells (74, 415). Substances such as methylene blue, phenazine methosulfate, and certain quinones, which act as electron acceptors for NADPH, increase the activity of the shunt pathway in white cells (172, 263). Systems for glucose oxidation via the hexose monophosphate shunt are present in the nonparticulate cytoplasmic fraction of the leukocyte. The distribution is similar to that in other mammalian tissues (219, 220, 261).

The most striking feature of the hexose monophosphate shunt pathway in mammalian granulocytes is its great augmentation during the phagocytic process (94, 261, 276, 277, 453). Changes in glucose oxidation by monocytes, macrophages, and eosinophils are similar to those associated with phagocytosis in neutrophils (98, 99, 573). If the availability of NADP controls the rate of glucose oxidation during phagocytosis as well as at rest, it is logical to ask what factors influence the availability of NADP. Some researchers propose that the increase in available NADP with phagocytosis is mediated via an NADP-linked lactic dehydrogenase (172, 276). Iyer and his coworkers suggest that the oxidation of reduced phosphopyridine nucleotides by molecular oxygen is flavine catalyzed and results in the formation of hydrogen peroxide (261, 262, 436). A variety of NADPH and NADH oxidases have been described in the cytoplasm and granules of neutrophils (171, 261, 262, 276, 600) (see Chapter 4). Despite these observations, the mechanism of enhancement of shunt metabolism by phagocytosis of the granulocyte is uncertain at present.

A new analysis of the significance of the pentose phosphate cycle has recently been reported (579).

Glycogen Synthesis and Degradation

On the basis of chemical and histochemical evidence, several authors identify granulocytes as the principal source of glycogen in mixed leukocyte populations. Small amounts of glycogen are present in normal erythrocytes and lymphocytes (276, 313, 429, 522). Human granulocyte glycogen content is comparable to that of the liver and muscle, normally comprising 1 to 2 percent of the wet weight of the tissue.

The quantitative analyses of Wagner, and histochemical observations, suggest that glycogen first appears in granulocytes at the myelocyte stage of development and increases with cell maturation. In electron micrographs of mature neutrophils, glycogen appears in cytoplasmic granules approximately 20 millimicrons in diameter (463). Myeloid blast cells are either glycogen free or have a very low glycogen content (429, 539, 544, 546). The unit cell glycogen is low in chronic granulocytic leukemia, although its synthetic capacity is unimpaired (530). It is high in infectious granulocytosis and polycythemia vera with leukocytosis (520, 522, 546), and decreased in uncontrolled diabetics who are not receiving insulin (168, 522).

The assembly of glycogen from 2- and 3-carbon substrates has been defined in the granulocytes of several mammalian species (170, 315, 323, 381–383, 494–496).

Studies of individuals with inborn errors of glycogen metabolism indicate that liver and white cells utilize similar mechanisms of glycogen degradation, which are distinct from those of muscle (499, 576). Wagner was among the first to demonstrate increased granulocyte glycogen content in glycogen storage disease (545). Leukocyte phosphorylase activity is reduced only in the hepatic phosphorylase-deficient glycogen disease, and not in other hepatic glycogen-storage diseases or in muscle phosphorylase deficiency (256, 576–578). Although leukocyte- and hepatic-debranching enzyme activities are abnormally low in type III glycogenosis, white cell debranching enzyme levels are normal in other forms of hepatic glycogen-storage disease (578). Leukocytes can be used to demonstrate the enzyme defects of types II, III, IV, and VI glycogen-storage disease (75, 490).

The macromolecular state of glycogen in granulocytes and characteristics of its synthesis and turnover have been reviewed in detail by Scott and Still (462, 463). These authors found the glycogen content of the normal adult's granulocyte to be 7.36 ± 2.05 mg/10^9 cells. They also demonstrated that the glycogen portion of the "glycogen organelle" is in a state of constant turnover, although the enzymes of glycogen synthesis and degradation are relatively stable.

Glyoxalase

Glyoxalases utilize glutathione as cofactor in the conversion of methyl glyoxal to lactate (211, 419). As far back as 1913 Dakin and Dudley described glyoxalase activity in formed elements of whole blood (129) and, in the same year, Levene and Meyer observed glyoxalase activity in leukocytes prepared from sterile exudates in dogs (321). Methyl glyoxal is synthesized from glucose and hexose diphosphate by both human and canine leukocytes (330, 332).

Substantial glyoxalase activity is observed in immature leukocytes, but the highest levels are found in disorders characterized by predominantly mature granulocytes (329, 332, 481). McKinney and others (340, 346) have suggested that the white cell glyoxalase system has sufficient capacity to account for the bulk of the cells' anaerobic lactate production. However, the conventional glycolytic pathway is presently favored as the principal source of white cell lactate production. The role of granulocyte glyoxalase is still unknown.

Lipid Composition and Metabolism

Composition

The lipid content, and composition, of normal and abnormal mammalian leukocytes was studied extensively by Boyd and his colleagues approximately 40 years ago (65–69), and more recently by other investigators (286–288). Lipid accounts for between 3 and 5 percent of the total neutrophil mass (66, 82, 225, 226). The total lipid of human neutrophilic leukocytes is subdivided approximately as follows: neutral fat, 30 percent; phospholipid, 35 percent; cholesterol, 10 percent. Fatty acid accounts for about 65 percent of the total lipid (66, 225, 226). Glycolipid, predominantly ceramide dihexoside, may constitute one-sixth of total lipid weight (364). Phosphatidylethanolamine and -choline make up the bulk of the phospholipid fraction of the granulocyte (182, 226, 278).

The phospholipid and free cholesterol contents of a mixed population of leukocytes are roughly proportional to the fraction of granulocytes (51, 67–69). Lymphocytes and myeloblasts do not stain with sudan black; but granulocytes beyond the myelocyte stage do take up lipid stain (51, 167, 308, 429). These histochemical observations agree with quantitative biochemical data, suggesting that granulocytes beyond the myelocyte stage of development are the principal sources of leukocyte lipid.

Miras and his collaborators provided data on the isolation and partial characterization of the glycolipids of normal human leukocytes (364). The best general summary of the lipid composition of leukocytes is found in the 1972 review by Gottfried (226).

Metabolism

The important features of granulocyte lipid metabolism are summarized in Table 3.3 and are discussed below.

Table 3.3 Features of granulocyte lipid metabolism.

The mature granulocyte is incapable of de novo fatty acid synthesis, but is capable of chain elongation reactions.
Significant exchange occurs between granulocyte lipids and plasma lipids.
Neutrophils can utilize lipids as an energy source.
Lipid, especially phospholipid, turnover rates are increased during phagocytosis.

Neutral Lipids and Fatty Acids Reports from many investigators indicate that leukocytes are incapable of de novo fatty acid synthesis, but are capable of chain elongation reactions (78, 337, 344, 363, 448). Normal mature leukocytes lack acetyl CoA carboxylase, the first enzyme unique to the fatty acid synthesis pathway (337).

Leukocytes are some 100 to 1,000 times more active than mature erythrocytes in the incorporation of acetate-1-C^{14} into lipid, principally triglyceride and phospholipid (78, 265, 287, 318, 343, 387, 396, 397, 448). Incorporation proceeds under anaerobic conditions (396). Kidson found a high rate of white cell lipid synthesis with an abnormal partition in acute myeloid leukemia and a low or normal rate of synthesis in polycythemia vera (286, 288). A correlation between leukocyte maturity and lipid synthesis exists in the granulocyte series (287). Rabbit neutrophils, for instance, apparently can incorporate free fatty acid, but not phospholipid or triglyceride, into cellular lipid. The fatty acids are rapidly esterified, probably at the cell surface, in a reaction that is glycolysis dependent (155). The pattern of glycerol labeling in the rabbit neutrophil suggests glycerol synthesis from hexose via aldolase, triophosphate isomerase, and glycerol dehydrogenase (496).

Phospholipids If ^{32}P is administered in vivo, it principally labels leukocyte phosphatidyl ethanolamine, -choline, -serine, and phosphoinositide. In vitro, the isotope principally labels phosphoinositol and a component believed to be phosphatidic acid (182, 446). The incorporation of ^{32}P into phospholipids, especially into phosphatidic acid, phosphatidyl inositol, and -serine, is increased during phagocytosis (see below) (278, 454) and may also be stimulated by staphylococcal leucocidin (591).

Interaction with Plasma Elsbach (154) suggested that leukocyte fatty acid composition depends both upon synthesis and upon transport from the plasma. He studied the uptake of palmitic, stearic, oleic, and linoleic acids by neutrophils (156). Significant exchange occurs between white cell and plasma lipids (78, 182, 265, 326, 344). Triglycerides exchange the most rapidly, but there is also significant exchange of phospholipid and cholesterol. Only a portion of the total cellular phospholipid is involved in these exchange reactions (447).

Lipid Degradation   Neutrophils can degrade many lipids (156, 157, 173) and, not surprisingly, they have a number of lipolytic activities. Esterase activity, found in both granulocytes and mononuclear cells, can be released by surface-active agents (55, 207, 432, 442). The many leukocyte long-chain fatty acid ester hydrolases that have been identified (55, 71, 162, 237) include a neutrophil lipolytic activity capable of using human chylomicrons as substrate. This lipolytic activity is abundant in the neutrophil granules (158, 161).

Effect of Phagocytosis   The phagocytizing neutrophil has a much higher rate of lipid turnover and biosynthesis than does the resting cell. Radioactively labeled carbons of glucose, acetate, and ^{32}P are all incorporated to a greater extent in lipids after particle ingestion than in resting cells (153, 278, 454). Recently, Elsbach (159) demonstrated that neutrophils can synthesize cellular lecithin by acetylation of plasma lysolecithin. Lecithin is a constituent of membrane phospholipid, and its synthesis is greatly augmented during the phagocytic process. Karnovsky (276) suggested that the increased lipid turnover in phagocytic neutrophils reflects new membrane lipid synthesis that occurs when portions of the membrane envelop phagocytized particles. The "signal" for the initiation of new membrane synthesis is not known.

Glycolipids   The hydrolysis of glucocerebroside and sphingomyelin is catalyzed by enzymes found in human granulocytes. The activity level of these enzymes is reduced in white cells as well as in other tissues taken from patients with Gaucher's disease and Niemann-Pick disease (271). Leukocyte activity is normal in other sphingolipodystrophies. Higher activity levels of glucocerbroside-cleaving enzymes are demonstrable in leukocytes taken from patients with acute and chronic myelocytic leukemia (272).

Amino Acid and Protein Composition and Metabolism

Amino Acid Composition and Metabolism

The concentration of amino acid in leukocytes, with the exception of arginine, is much higher than the concentration in plasma or erythrocytes (334, 390)—it is approximately the magnitude found in most other mammalian tissues (334, 404, 503). The leukocyte/plasma ratio of most amino acids ranges from 4.8 to 14.5, and the ratio for glutamic acid, ornithine, and glycine + serine is in excess of 20 (334). The low concentration of leukocyte arginine is probably attributable to the high levels of arginase in mature neutrophils (57, 428, 504).

Amino acids have been isolated from leukocyte nuclei and chromosomes (515, 595). A pattern exists of readily extractable amino acids characteristic for each white cell element, including granulocytes, and for each species. This coincides with the observation that in a particular species each tissue has a characteristic pattern of easily extractable ninhydrin-reactive constituents (435, 445).

Changes in the content of three amino acids are said to be characteristic of leukemic leukocytes. These changes are increased levels of glutamic acid and proline, and decreased levels of ornithine (260, 335, 384). Leukemic granulocytes usually have higher than normal rates of amino acid incorporation (20, 145, 201, 216, 377, 567, 588). These data indicate that the rate of amino acid incorporation into white cells, and presumably of concomitant protein synthesis, is highest in the myeloblast, lowest in the mature granulocyte, and intermediate in white cells of intermediate degrees of maturity.

Interest in leukocyte sulphur-containing amino acids resulted from observations that L-cysteine, and to a lesser extent homocysteine and glutathione, modifies the leukopenia induced by nitrogen mustard (565–567). L-cystine and L-methionine are incorporated independently of each other (201, 568). In decreasing the influx and incorporation of ^{35}S-L-cystine into leukemic white cells, L-cysteine and selenium cystine, but not D-cysteine, homocysteine, or isocysteine, are effective (564, 569).

Increased levels of glutamic acid dehydrogenase occur in white cells isolated from patients with acute leukemia and chronic myelocytic leukemia (55, 551, 552).

Despite earlier reports to the contrary (298), granulocytes from normal subjects and patients with chronic myelocytic leukemia undoubtedly possess significant arginase activity (57, 428, 504). Evidence demonstrating that neutrophils contribute most of the buffy coat arginase activity also shows that there is little of this enzyme activity in lymphocytes or blast cells (56, 57, 428, 504). The role of this enzyme in granulocyte economy is not known.

Histamine   Histidine and its metabolic product, histamine, are of special interest in leukocyte metabolism (102, 103, 241). The basophil is the principal carrier of blood histamine (150, 202, 228, 229, 517, 525) and thus resembles the tissue mast cell (431, 432). However, significant quantities of histamine may exist in other granulocytes, including neutrophils and eosinophils (228). Histamine appears to be associated with the granule fraction of leukocytes (413, 414). Leukocytes may have cell surface receptors which selectively bind histamine. Their significance is unknown (352).

Blood histamine concentration may be strikingly increased in disorders such as chronic myelocytic leukemia, which has large numbers of circulating basophils (103, 509, 517). Lesser elevations of blood histamine are found in polycythemia vera (520). An attempt has been made, in patients with myeloproliferative disorders (218), to correlate the symptoms of itching and blood histamine concentration.

Genetic Abnormalities   Inherited abnormalities of amino acid metabolism may be evident in leukocytes, including granulocytes. These cells provide a convenient tissue for biopsy. Enzymes for the oxidative decarboxylation of branched-chain keto acids of leucine, isoleucine, and valine are widely distributed in tissues (131, 133). In maple-syrup urine disease there appears to be a biochemical defect in the oxidative decarboxylation of these keto acids. The defect is also apparent in the leukocytes isolated from patients with this disorder, and these cells can be used to establish the diagnosis (130–132). Similarly, in patients with isovaleric acidemia—a genetic defect of leucine metabolism—the leukocytes are subnormal in their oxidation of radioactive isovaleric acid. The genetic defect appears to be the enzyme isovaleryl-CoA dehydrogenase (80).

The concentration of free cystine is 80 times greater than normal in leukocytes of homozygous patients with cystinosis and six times greater in heterozygotes with cystinosis. Three-fourths of the cystine is recovered in the granule fraction of neutrophils (349). No defect in the transport of dibasic amino acids or cystine was found in leukocytes from cystinuric patients (371, 438). Occasional cystine crystals can be seen in leukocytes in the blood of patients with cystinosis (349).

Protein Synthesis

The molecular mechanisms of protein synthesis have been studied extensively in bacterial systems and in a limited number of mammalian systems. Except for the lymphocyte (see Chapter 14), the molecular mechanisms of protein assembly have been minimally studied in mammalian leukocytes. Major reasons for this paucity of data are the technical difficulties associated with high levels of protease activity in phagocytic leukocytes and the great diversity of proteins made by these cells.

Although the bulk of amino acid activating enzyme activity in whole blood hemolysates is derived from erythrocytes, the specific activity of these enzymes on either a cell basis or per milligram of protein is higher in leukocytes than in red cells (263). Whether this enzymatic activity derives from granulocytes or lymphocytes is not known. On the basis of fine structural observations of the mature granulocyte, which indicate a paucity of protein-synthesizing apparatus, one would predict little protein synthesis in this cell.

A logical question to ask is whether important granulocyte functions, such as phagocytosis, affect protein synthesis. If mature granulocytes "rearm" themselves by replacing, through synthesis, enzymes lost into the phagocytic vacuoles during particle ingestion, one would anticipate a burst of protein synthesis or at least new enzyme synthesis. However, this seems not to take place. Incorporation of L-leucine into protein by guinea pig granulocytes is unaffected by phagocytosis (454). In human granulocytes, protein synthesis is not enhanced during the phagocytic process (93, 94), and granule enzymes are not replaced (96). These observations suggest that the mature granulocyte is a "one-shot cell" and does not replace a depleted arsenal.

Nucleic Acid Metabolism

Nucleic Acid Content

Human white cells, as well as other human diploid cells, contain about 0.7×10^{-12} gm of DNA phosphorus per cell (138, 317). Occasional observations of increased DNA content per cell in acute leukemia may be attributable to polyploidy (138, 233, 403, 426, 452, 573). Although no differences in the DNA composition of normal and leukemic leukocytes have been observed (152, 291), variations in the physical-chemical properties of DNA isolated from these two sources have been reported. The molecular weight and other physical properties of DNA isolated from chronic myelocytic leukemic cells differ from those of isolated normal white cells (144, 408, 409, 472).

Although DNA content per cell is approximately the same in different white cell populations of a given species, RNA content varies significantly (55, 138, 233, 339, 357, 358, 431, 432, 573). It usually is greatest in immature white cells of all cell lines, and decreases with cellular maturation. The RNA/DNA ratio is highest in the white cells of acute leukemia (138, 431, 573).

Levels of adenosine phosphates in leukocytes of human

and guinea pig blood have been determined by several groups of investigators (205, 206, 208, 324, 581).

Pyrimidine Metabolism

The pathways of pyrimidine synthesis and interconversions in mammalian cells have been determined (125, 137) (Fig. 3.2). Enzymes for de novo pyrimidine synthesis—aspartate carbamyl transferase, dihydro-orotase, dihydro-orotic-dehydrogenase, and orotidylic decarboxylase—exist in the leukocyte (412, 482–484). The activity level of these enzymes ordinarily parallels the degree of immaturity of the white cells. High levels are found in the immature leukocytes of patients with leukemia and infectious leukocytosis. The mature granulocyte has low or undetectable enzyme activity. Decreased levels of orotidylic decarboxylase are found, after treatment with the antimetabolite, 6-azauridine (176), and in the leukocytes of patients with congenital orotic aciduria (485).

End product inhibition, by cytidylate and uridylate, of aspartate carbamyl transferase—the first enzyme unique to the pathway—has been observed in bacteria, but not in human leukocytes (412, 483, 596). The mechanism of control of pyrimidine biosynthesis in mammalian leukocytes remains undefined.

Thymidylate synthetase catalyzes the conversion of dUMP to TMP and may be a key enzyme in the control of pyrimidine production for DNA synthesis. Activity of this enzyme has been detected in extracts of leukocytes from patients with chronic myelocytic leukemia and acute leukemia. Since normal mature granulocytes have little or no capacity for DNA synthesis, it is not surprising that thymidylate synthetase has not been detected in these cells (461, 475, 571). Thymidylate kinases, which catalyze the conversion of TMP to the triphosphate, are present in immature leukocytes (46, 47); the capacity for generating TTP for DNA synthesis therefore exists in these cells.

The feedback control of dCMP deaminase, the first enzyme in a biosynthetic sequence of pyrimidine deoxy-

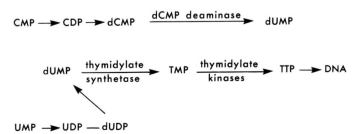

Figure 3.2 Schematic outline of interconversion of pyrimidine nucleotides.

ribonucleotide interconversions, has been demonstrated in normal and leukemic human leukocytes (473).

A salvage pathway for utilization of exogenous thymidine via thymidine kinases also exists. The quantitative contribution of this pathway for normal DNA synthesis is uncertain (46, 345, 449); however, we do know that at least some exogenous thymidine can be used for DNA synthesis. Cooper and his colleagues (117) showed that exogenous thymidine, added to leukocytes of patients with chronic myelocytic leukemia, competes with TTP synthesized de novo for incorporation into DNA. The DNA-thymidine derived from exogenous thymidine increases from 13 percent to 87 percent over a 0.3 to 300 μm range of exogenous thymidine concentrations. Detailed studies of thymidine incorporation into nucleotide pools of normal and chronic myelocytic leukocytes have been reported (117, 118). Bresnick and Karjala (73) have demonstrated end product inhibition of thymidine kinase activity in normal and leukemic leukocytes.

The relatively low levels of thymidine kinase combined with leukocyte thymidine phosphorylase, which degrades the riboside to the base and deoxyribose phosphate (345, 402), may explain the low levels of tritiated thymidine incorporation sometimes observed in leukocytes cultured in vitro or labeled in vivo (174, 214, 215). Enzymes for catabolizing thymine are found in normal and leukemic leukocytes (455).

The incorporation of labeled pyrimidine deoxyribonucleosides, especially tritiated thymidine, has been used extensively in radioautographic studies of leukocytes (121, 123, 124, 214, 215) and more recently in biochemical studies (417). Myeloblasts have enzyme systems for methylating the purine and pyrimidine bases of DNA (471). Membrane systems for transporting purine and pyrimidine nucleosides have been identified in rabbit polymorphonuclear leukocytes (508).

Nucleoside Phosphorylase Guinea pig neutrophils have nucleoside phosphorylase activity which, on a per-cell basis, is eight to ten times greater than that of the erythrocyte (304). This enzymatic activity, the bulk of which can be isolated from the soluble 30,000 × g supernatant, has not been found in nuclei and mitochondria.

Thymidine Phosphorylase Normal and leukemic human leukocyte extracts possess thymidine phosphorylase activity (345, 402). Normal cells have a higher specific activity of this enzyme on both a per-cell basis and a per-milligram-of-cell-protein basis than do leukemic leukocytes (345).

Purine Metabolism

Purines are synthesized from small precursors, including glycine, 5-phosphoribosylpyrophosphate, formate, and the amide nitrogen of glutamine (79). Apparently human leukocytes either cannot perform the early steps in purine biosynthesis or have only a limited capacity for de novo synthesis (461, 481, 571). Leukocytes can utilize either purine intermediates, preformed bases, or nucleosides and nucleotides derived from exogenous sources (307, 401, 593). Presumably, preformed purine bases can be converted to nucleotides by enzymes similar to those described in yeast and liver and in circulating normal and leukemic leukocytes (136, 300, 580).

Purine nucleotides are incorporated only after dephosphorylation to the nucleosides (461). Cleavage of purine-ribosyl bonds occurs when nucleosides and nucleotides are used as precursors (574). When ^{14}C-labeled adenine or guanine is used as a nucleic acid precursor in normal and leukemic leukocytes, a significant intracellular interconversion of the purine bases also occurs (461, 468, 574, 575).

Resistance to 6-mercaptopurine by the leukemic cells of certain mammalian species may result from their inability to utilize exogenous purine (135, 461). This does not appear to be the situation in human 6-mercaptopurine-resistant leukemia (136).

It is generally accepted that in mammals purines are catabolized by xanthine oxidase via the pathway purine → hypoxanthine → xanthine → uric acid (35, 301). A minor pathway may involve the intermediate formation of 8-hydroxy xanthine and 2, 8-dihydroxy purine (266). Normal mouse leukocytes are reported to contain xanthine oxidase, which converts xanthine to uric acid. Activity of this enzyme is greater in granulocytes than in splenic lymphocytes (513).

Nucleic Acid Synthesis

In the last decade the major features of RNA synthesis in mammalian cells have been delineated, although much remains to be learned. Knowledge of DNA replication in mammalian cells is less complete, although there has been considerable recent progress. Investigation of the nucleic acid synthesis mechanisms in leukocytes has similarly advanced, but less rapidly than the progress in knowledge of other mammalian systems. Part of the difficulty lies in the structural makeup of granulocytes and monocytes. Their high levels of nuclease activity interfere both with procedures designed to isolate intact nucleic acid and with studies of polymerase activity.

The major features of RNA synthesis in mammalian cells can be summarized briefly (cf. 398). Under the influence of RNA polymerase, ribonucleotide triphosphates are polymerized into a polyribonucleotide strand. This strand is a transcription of one of the twin strands of DNA. Apparently, only certain regions of the chromosomal DNA are transcribed—those corresponding to the euchromatin (209). Ribosomal RNA synthesis occurs in the nucleolus. The principal species of RNA made by the cell are a low-molecular-weight RNA (4S), which is principally transfer RNA; a high-molecular-weight RNA, which undergoes rearrangement and yields two ribosomal RNA moieties, 28 and 18S (555); 5S RNA; messenger RNA; and several other "minor" RNA species (563). Interestingly, kinetic evidence suggests that the turnover rate of nuclear RNA is very high and a considerable short-lived fraction never reaches the cytoplasm (556).

Although these basic features of RNA metabolism are presumably true also for human leukocytes, including granulocyte precursors and lymphocytes (92, 93, 116, 247, 477, 479), we are still uncertain about the sites within these cells where different events in RNA metabolism take place. Myeloblasts and lymphocytes predictably have the highest rates of RNA synthesis (92, 477, 478); however, granulocytes also have significant levels of RNA synthesis despite an absence of the fine structural features usually indicative of RNA and protein synthesis (see Chapter 1).

RNA synthesis and turnover are increased in human granulocytes after particle ingestion (91). Blocking of RNA synthesis with actinomycin-D has no effect on the other metabolic changes accompanying phagocytosis (94). Particle ingestion by human monocytes appears unaffected by inhibition of RNA synthesis, and only slightly affected by inhibition of protein synthesis (99).

No direct measurements of the stability or turnover rate of messenger RNA in mammalian leukocytes have been made. All measurements have been indirect and based on the rate of decay of protein synthesis after inhibition of RNA synthesis with actinomycin-D. Such measurements have shown a fall in the rate of protein synthesis, with a half-life of 30 to 60 minutes in populations of granulocytes and myeloblasts (92, 95). This rate is slower than that found in bacteria, but faster than that characteristic of liver and immature red cells; however, in none of these biological systems does the rate of decay of protein synthesis necessarily reflect the turnover rate of messenger RNA.

Just as protein synthesis is sensitive to interruption of RNA synthesis, the converse is also true. In leukemic human leukocytes RNA and DNA synthesis is inhibited when protein synthesis is inhibited (96). The precise mechanism is not clear; however, the phenomenon is similar to that in microorganisms and mammalian cells in tissue culture (166).

Kiss and his co-workers (290) and Silber and his colleagues (477) presented data concerning the composition of RNA and acid-soluble nucleotide pools of normal and leukemic human leukocytes.

The principal features of granulocyte purine, pyrimidine, and RNA metabolism are summarized below:

(a) Enzymes for de novo pyrimidine synthesis are found only in immature normal and malignant granulocytes.

(b) Thymidylate synthetase and thymidine kinases are found only in immature granulocytes.

(c) Competition exists between de novo thymidine synthesis and the "salvage pathway" in immature granulocytes.

(d) Little or no de novo purine biosynthesis occurs in immature leukocytes; exogenous sources are utilized.

(e) RNA turnover in mature granulocytes is increased by phagocytosis.

Water and Electrolyte Metabolism

The water and mineral contents of both normal and malignant white cells of several species have been extensively documented (163, 165, 180, 189, 203, 244–246, 309, 340, 415, 430, 432, 560, 583–585). In general, a high intracellular sodium/potassium ratio exists in animal and human leukocytes relative to that in red cells, brain, and muscle. Rigas (430) analyzed the changes that occur with maturation in the composition of leukemic white cells. He reported that as granulocytes age, water, potassium, and sodium remain unaltered, magnesium decreases, and total solids, nitrogen, and calcium increase.

In 1902 Hamburger and van der Schroeff, using suspensions of pus cells from septic abscesses, demonstrated the permeability of leukocytes to several anions (234). In 1929 Fleischmann (189) extended these observations, and in 1937 Shapiro and Parpart (469) measured the permeability of rabbit and human white blood cells to water. Subsequently, several investigators examined permeability and ion transport processes in leukocytes (244–246, 415, 585). Although concentration gradients are maintained for sodium and potassium, intracellular chloride varies with the concentration of the ion in the suspending medium (585). When metabolic activity is depressed at 0°C, rabbit neutrophils lose potassium and gain sodium. Restoration to 37°C permits concentration of intracellular potassium against the gradient (246). Separate transport mechanisms may exist for sodium and potassium (163).

Karnovsky and Sbarra made the interesting suggestion that during phagocytosis solutes normally excluded from the cell may enter along with the ingested particle (276, 277), a phenomenon called "piggyback phagocytosis." This situation has a biological analogy in the increased uptake of glucose by phagocytizing amoebas (88).

Recent studies suggest that the osmotic fragility of leukemic leukocytes may be different from normal (380).

One metal of particular interest is zinc. White cells account for approximately 3 percent of the zinc in whole blood (526, 527). The individual leukocyte is extremely rich in zinc, containing about 25 times more of this metal per cell than the erythrocyte (440, 527, 537, 589). Zinc is rapidly incorporated from plasma into white cells in vivo and in vitro. Once taken up, it is firmly bound (142, 143, 440). A protein containing about 0.3 percent zinc and accounting for up to 80 percent of the total white cell content of the cation has been extracted from leukocytes (244, 253, 529). This protein has no enzymic activity, and no correlation has been established between leukocyte zinc content and the activity of any zinc metaloenzyme (203, 526). However, like swine kidney alkaline phosphatase (350), leukocyte alkaline phosphatase appears to be a zinc metaloenzyme (511), and other leukocyte zinc metaloenzymes have been described (191).

Low zinc levels have been reported in the white cells of patients with leukemia, myeloid metaplasia, and cirrhosis (141, 142, 203, 204, 217, 589). High levels have been described in some cases of refractory anemia (528).

Vitamins and Coenzymes

Folic Acid

Folic acid coenzymes are involved in the synthesis of key precursors of nucleic acids and proteins. They act generally as carriers of one-carbon units although, in some instances, they may also participate in oxido-reduction of the one-carbon units (210).

In 1943 Daft and Sebrell presented evidence that folic acid is essential for murine leukocyte maturation (128). Levels of folinic acid active material are considerably higher in acute leukemic than in normal leukocytes (151, 500). Most of this citrovorum factor activity is present in a form not freely extractable in phosphate buffers of pH 6.6 to 6.8 (386).

The activities of N^5, N^{10}-methylene tetrahydrofolate dehydrogenase, formate-activating enzyme, dihydrofolate reductase, and of several folic acid coenzyme-dependent enzymes are elevated in the white cells of acute leukemia (38, 42–44, 365, 582). Formate-activating enzyme and dihydrofolate reductase activities are also increased in leukocytes of patients with chronic myelocytic leukemia, but not chronic lymphocytic leukemia (44, 365, 582). These enzymes appear to have the same physical properties in leukemic cells as in normal white cells (41, 43). Dihydrofolate reductase is inhibited by folic acid antagonists such as amethopterin (39, 41–43). During therapy with a folic acid antagonist, significant increases in white cell dihydrofolate reductase activity are observed and may in part account for the resistance to these drugs (40, 41, 43, 45, 183, 366). Transport of drugs into the cell may also be important in drug resistance or sensitivity (184). The biochemistry and pharmacology of folic acid antagonists have been reviewed (36).

Vitamin C

In 1936 Stephens and Hawley (491) and in 1940 Butler and Cushman (83) observed high concentrations of ascorbic-acid–like reducing substances in the white cell fraction of blood. These reducing substances are normally found in significantly higher concentration in the buffy coat than in the plasma or red cell layers (83, 113, 122, 242, 328, 491). The level of vitamin C material in the white cell layer is a function of the adequacy of the ascorbic acid intake and is a good measure of total body ascorbic acid (83, 113, 122, 327, 361, 421, 489). Ascorbic acid can be transferred from serum or plasma to white cells, but not in the reverse direction (242, 243, 420, 421). Leukocytes isolated from scorbutic animals are reported to be excessively fragile and to demonstrate impaired phagocytic activity (119, 385).

Riboflavin

Significant amounts of riboflavin are found in white cells (81, 213). The levels of leukocyte riboflavin in several mammalian species are remarkably similar (213). In rats fed a riboflavin-deficient diet the level of the vitamin in white cells falls (81). Low riboflavin levels have also been reported in whole leukocytes and isolated nuclei of patients with lymphocytic leukemia (411).

Thiamine

Fujita and Yamadori reported leukocyte thiamine levels in several mammalian species (213). The vitamin B_1 content of white cells and platelets is approximately ten times that of erythrocytes (224). The leukocyte thiamine content reflects the state of body thiamine stores (224). Higher than normal levels of the vitamin have been reported in whole blood and leukocytes of chronic myelocytic leukemia (1, 222).

Pyridoxine

The leukocyte levels of vitamin B_6 in normal humans are comparable to the levels in liver, muscle, and nervous system (64). White cell vitamin B_6 levels are affected by the intake of the vitamin, and the level tends to be low in women at term and higher in the white cells of cord blood than in the maternal leukocytes (64, 541, 543). Low levels of vitamin B_6 have been reported in both mature and immature leukemic white cells (542). Donald and Ferguson have described a micromethod for determination of leukocyte pyridoxal phosphate that utilizes the enzyme apotryptophanase (148).

Vitamin B_{12}

In 1952 Harris demonstrated that human leukocytes carry significant amounts of vitamin B_{12} (238). In patients with chronic myelocytic leukemia (CML) in relapse and in some individuals with polycythemia vera, the serum-vitamin B_{12} binding capacity is markedly increased above normal (359, 369, 418) (see Chapter 10). In 1955 Mollin and Ross reported that the breakdown products of granulocytes from patients with CML were capable of binding vitamin B_{12} in vitro (369). In 1956 Thomas and Anderson reported a study of leukocyte vitamin B_{12} content and binding capacity in a variety of acute and chronic leukemias (510). Except for one individual with CML, the white cells of leukemic patients had approximately the same B_{12} binding capacity as those of normal subjects. The vitamin B_{12} content of normal leukocytes and white cells from cases of CML were essentially the same. Meyer and his colleagues (360) reported that mature neutrophilic leukocytes show the highest Co^{60}-vitamin B_{12} binding capacity and that immature granulocytes and eosinophils have only a limited binding capacity. Meyer and his co-workers suggested that the disintegration products of mature neutrophils are important in the increased vitamin B_{12} binding capacity of serum in patients with CML and polycythemia vera (see also 369).

Pyridine Nucleotides

There is a marked increase in the NAD content of leukemic cells and, in particular, those of acute leukemia (474). The levels of NADH, NADP, and NADPH are about the same in normal and leukemic white cells except in the case of chronic lymphocytic leukemia, where the nucleotide levels per cell tend to be low (474). Striking increases in pyridine nucleotide transhydrogenases have been reported in leukemic leukocytes (476), but the significance of these observations is unknown.

Granule Constituents: Hydrolases and Oxygenases

Lysosomes are membrane-bound cytoplasmic organelles containing a variety of hydrolytic enzymes (16, 105–107, 140, 250, 570). Destruction of the lysosome is required to demonstrate maximal enzyme activity, a phenomenon termed "structure-linked latency." Classic descriptions of these organelles resulted from studies of liver and kidney cells (140). Clearly, however, certain granules of phagocytic leukocytes closely resemble the lysosomes of liver and kidney tissues, and for practical purposes they may be taken as analogous. The enzymatic content of these organelles is considered in detail in Chapters 1 and 24 and in a recent review by Baggiolini (16).

For convenience, the constituents of leukocyte granules may be classified as acid hydrolases, neutral and alkaline hydrolases, oxygenases, and nonenzymatic constituents. The last category includes substances that have biological activity but no identifiable enzymatic activity. The hydrolases—neutral, acid, and alkaline—are probably concerned mainly with the digestion of phagocytized particles. The oxygenases are probably concerned mainly with the killing of ingested microorganisms (Chapter 4). The nonenzymatic cationic protein may also be microbicidal in function.

In the following paragraphs are detailed considerations of a few of these constituents (see also Table 3.4).

Alkaline and Acid Phosphatases

In 1929 Kay (280) suggested that human white cells may contain phosphatase activity, and in 1931 Roche (437) succeeded in demonstrating alkaline phosphatase activity in preparations of mammalian leukocytes. Subsequently, especially in the past 15 years, leukocyte phosphatases

Table 3.4 Enzymatic constituents of leukocyte granules.

Hydrolases:

α and β-glucosidases	Naphthylamidase	Lipase
α and β-galactosidases	N-acetyl-beta	Phospholipase A, B
α-mannosidase	glucosaminidase	Lecithinase A
Alkaline phosphatase	Arylsulfatase	Lysolecithinase
Lysozyme	Phosphodiesterase	α-amylase
Acid ribonuclease	5′-nucleotidase	Dextranase
Acid deoxy-	Proteases (several)	Prolidase
ribonuclease	Peptides (several)	Elastase
Acid phosphatase	Esterases (several)	Collagenase
γ-glucuronidase		

Oxygenase:
Myeloperoxidase

have been demonstrated histochemically (221, 274, 538, 592) and by quantitative biochemical techniques (179, 232, 283, 519, 598). Investigators have distinguished between alkaline phosphatase with a pH optimum near 10 and acid phosphatase with a pH optimum near 5. The most commonly employed substrate for both histochemical and biochemical studies has been β-glycerophosphate. Occasionally, however, the hydrolysis of other substrates including mono- and diphosphoesters of 3-, 4-, 5-, 6-, and 7-carbon sugars and purine and pyrimidine riboside mono-, di-, and triphosphates has been examined (196, 437, 501, 511, 512). Follette and his colleagues (196) compared leukocyte alkaline phosphatase activities with 5′-AMP, glucose-1-phosphate, and β-glycerophosphate as substrates. On the basis of the distribution of the enzyme in different white cell populations and the lack of an additive effect of multiple substrates, they concluded that leukocyte alkaline phosphatase is probably a single phosphomonoesterase or a group of similar monoesterases. Trubowitz and his colleagues (512) extended these observations. They achieved a 250-fold purification of leukocyte alkaline phosphatase and demonstrated that the specific activity of the enzyme preparation for five different phosphoester-containing substrates rose proportionally during enzyme purification. They also have presented evidence that the white cell enzyme is a zinc metaloenzyme (511, 512). More recent studies suggest that there are isozymes which are zinc-containing and others which are magnesium-containing (439). These observations indicate that white cell alkaline phosphatase is probably a single enzyme or a group of very similar enzymes. They do not exclude the possibility that there may be, in addition, phosphomonoesterases with more limited specificities.

There are marked species differences in the levels and cellular distribution of leukocyte alkaline phosphatase (232, 370, 407, 518, 538). In man the enzyme is restricted to the neutrophilic leukocyte. Activity is first detectable at the myelocyte stage and increases with increasing cellular maturity (232, 274, 407, 480, 518, 586). In normal individuals, but not in patients with chronic myelocytic leukemia, the leukocyte alkaline phosphatase activity may be strikingly increased by the administration of ACTH or adrenal corticosteroids (523, 524). In subjects with a variety of nonneoplastic "stress" conditions, including pyogenic infection, myocardial infarction, and surgery, alkaline phosphatase activity of neutrophilic white cells is elevated (283, 316, 514, 519, 521, 523). In the light of these observations, it has been suggested that leukocyte alkaline phosphatase activity is responsive to changes in pituitary-adrenal activity in normal persons, but not in individuals with CML (518, 521, 524). Moloney, in experiments with adrenalectomized rats, has presented evidence that in this species increased levels of neutrophil alkaline phosphatase are not necessarily mediated via the adrenal gland (370).

Interest in leukocyte alkaline phosphatase as a diagnostic clinical tool has been stimulated by observations that circulating white cells of patients with CML usually have low levels of enzyme activity (299, 316, 407, 519, 520, 538, 586) as well as a chromosomal abnormality (231). Histochemical evidence suggests that this is true even in the mature granulocytes of this disorder (283, 538, 586). In contrast, the mature granulocytes of patients with acute monocytic and lymphocytic leukemia may have normal or elevated levels of alkaline phosphatase activity (399). In leukocyte populations, comparable in maturity to those of CML but isolated from patients with polycythemia vera and certain cases of myeloid metaplasia, the level of alkaline phosphatase tends to be higher than normal (30, 283, 299, 316, 367, 520, 586). These data suggest that the low levels of enzymatic activity in the white cells of patients with CML are a function of the neoplastic process rather than of immaturity per se.

Low levels of leukocyte alkaline phosphatase are not restricted to chronic myelocytic leukemia and have been reported in patients with paroxysmal nocturnal hemoglobinuria, idiopathic thrombocytopenic purpura, infectious mononucleosis, pernicious anemia, aplastic anemia, and in occasional cases of myeloid metaplasia, sarcoidosis, and granulocytopenia (30, 127, 306, 368, 480, 506, 604). In patients with hypophosphatasia, an inborn error of metabolism, alkaline phosphatase levels are also markedly decreased or absent in the white cells as well as in the bones, liver, and kidney (303).

The functions of leukocyte acid and alkaline phosphatase in the economy of the cell are not known. In view of the diverse substrates acted upon by these enzymes, they may be involved in carbohydrate, phospholipid, and nucleic acid metabolism. The association with other hydrolases in the granules of neutrophilic leukocytes suggests that they may be especially important in the white cell defense and digestive functions. A familial deficiency of lysosomal acid phosphatase has been described (376).

Peroxidase

Peroxidases and catalases are ferric iron-porphyrin-containing enzymes that catalyze reactions in which hydrogen peroxide is the electron acceptor. The type of reaction catalyzed by peroxidases may be written:

$AH_2 + H_2O_2 \rightarrow A + 2H_2O$, where AH_2 is an electron donor such as cytochrome c, ascorbic acid, or redox indicators. Catalase decomposes hydrogen peroxide according to the equation $2H_2O_2 \rightarrow 2H_2O + O_2$.

Catalases and peroxidases may be quite similar in their mode of action and may belong to a single group of enzymes termed "hydroperoxidases." In some instances, catalases and peroxidases may exhibit differences in specificity for the electron donor (86, 211). Leukocytes are rich in peroxidase activity and the enzymes involved have been variously designated myeloperoxidase and verdoperoxidase. The latter term arose because the green color of chloroleukemic infiltrates was attributed to the peroxidase content (4). The published reports have not always distinguished clearly between leukocyte catalase and peroxidase activities. However, Vercauteren has stated that these enzymic activities are distinguishable and are associated with different intracellular particles (534). They can be separated by ammonium sulfate fractionation procedures (436) and are differentially inhibited by 3-amino-1,2,4,-triazole (425).

Klebs in 1868 (295) and Struve in 1872 (498) demonstrated that tincture of guaiac became blue in the presence of pus cells. In 1907 Winkler (587) demonstrated Nadi reaction-positive granules in myelocytic, but not lymphocytic, leukocytes. Dating from that time, histochemical peroxidatic reactions have been widely used in the morphological classification of white blood cells. In 1943 Agner isolated myeloperoxidase from tuberculous empyema fluid; he found little associated catalase activity (5). Other investigators have demonstrated myeloperoxidase or catalase activity in nontuberculous empyema and in isolated leukocytes (87, 198, 492, 535). It has been estimated that myeloperoxidase constitutes between 1 and 5 percent (4, 459) of the dry weight of mammalian white blood cells. An experimental leukemic tumor of rats has been an especially rich source of myeloperoxidase (457).

Rabbit neutrophil myeloperoxidase is demonstrable only in the primary granules by histochemical (18), cytochemical (19), and biochemical (17) techniques. It is absent from other granule populations.

Peroxidase plays a role in the defense reactions of mammalian granulocytes against microorganisms (Chapter 4) (292–294, 348). Agner suggested that an additional role for myeloperoxidase may be the destruction of bacterial toxins (6, 7). He also suggested that myeloperoxidase may function as a respiratory pigment in white cells (4), but Chance (87) subsequently presented evidence against this hypothesis. Canellakis and his co-workers demonstrated that in the presence of hydrogen peroxide myeloperoxidase was capable of degrading uric acid to urea and allantoin (84).

Investigation of a patient with a genetic lack of neutrophil myeloperoxidase demonstrated that the peroxidase enzymes of the neutrophil and eosinophil are different (312, 451). These observations confirmed earlier suggestions that these two types of cells have distinct peroxidases (13). Schultz and his associates (458, 460) purified and characterized neutrophil peroxidase.

Lysozyme

Lysozyme is a low-molecular-weight protein capable of depolymerizing certain bacterial mucopolysaccharides. Cohn and his colleagues demonstrated that bacteria with cell walls susceptible to lysozyme were more readily broken down to acid-soluble fragments than were nonsusceptible bacteria (110). Lysozyme-like activity, which has been extracted from white cells from several species (9, 23), is associated with granulocytes and monocytes rather than lymphocytes (23, 188, 248). The major portion of lysozyme is found in the secondary granules of rabbit neutrophils (the "B" fraction of Baggiolini and his colleagues) (17, 602) and probably of other species as well (55, 108, 252, 389).

In 1966 Osserman and Lawlor (393) demonstrated that some patients with acute monocytic and myelomonocytic leukemia have elevated levels of serum and urinary lysozyme (see Chapter 27). This finding aroused interest in the lysosomal enzyme as a possible diagnostic marker for these diseases (400). Lysozyme also may be used indirectly in the study of neutrophil kinetics (181).

Nucleases

Ribonucleases and deoxyribonucleases have been described in rabbit polymorphonuclear leukocytes (23, 58, 149). Evidence indicates that these enzymatic activities may be localized in the granule fraction (108). Several nucleosideases and nucleotideases have been described in human leukemic white cells and rabbit neutrophils (23, 108, 501). A phosphodiesterase present in mouse leukocytes resembles snake venom phosphodiesterase, but differs in its substrate requirements (10). The 5'-nucleotidase appears to be localized in the primary granules of rabbit neutrophils (19).

Proteases and Peptidases

Numerous leukocyte proteases and peptidases are described in early biochemical and medical literature (23, 115, 257, 267, 296, 325, 356, 374, 375, 388, 391, 392). Leukocyte proteolytic enzymes of several species subsequently have been described and characterized in more

detail, and a number of proteases, both acid and neutral, have been identified (55, 191, 192, 199, 200, 373, 394, 493, 597). Extracts prepared from human white cells are also capable of degrading chondromucoprotein; the active agents appear to be endopeptidases (603). Macrophages contain an aminopeptidase (594), and human granulocytes have collagenase activity (311). Baggiolini (16) has recently reviewed the literature on leukocyte proteases.

Esterases

Esterases and lipases have been demonstrated repeatedly in white cells of several species. "Esterases" are defined as those enzymes hydrolyzing esters of short-chain fatty acids. In 1949 Rossiter and Wong reviewed previous reports of leukocyte esterases and described an aliesterase capable of hydrolyzing tributyrin and methobutyrate (442). Esterase activity, present in both granulocytes and mononuclear cells (55, 207), is reported to be decreased in the white cells of patients with chronic myelocytic leukemia (237). Significant lipase activity is also demonstrable in both normal and abnormal leukocytes (49, 162, 237, 378). Esterases histochemically demonstrable in human leukocytes are probably localized in the primary granules (134, 592).

Other Granule Hydrolytic Enzymes

In addition to the enzymes already discussed, the following enzyme activities have been identified in the granules of mammalian neutrophils.

Beta-glucuronidase has been found in the white cells of several species, including man (3, 11, 55, 108, 187, 252, 443, 444). The function of this enzyme in leukocytes is not definitely known (194, 195, 443). It is found mainly in neutrophils, but some activity has been noted in lymphocytes (12, 194, 195, 597).

Alpha-galactosidase is found in neutrophil granules. The activity of this enzyme is reduced in patients with Fabry's disease (289).

Leukocyte arylsulfatase activity has been reported by Tanaka and his colleagues, and by others (70, 505, 507). In the myeloid series, eosinophils are especially rich in arylsulfatase activity (14).

Other enzymes described in neutrophil granules include naphthylamidase (450), N-acetyl-beta-glucosaminidase, beta-galactosidase, alpha-mannosidase (17), and kininase (353, 354).

Nonenzymatic Constituents

Granule fractions from exudate neutrophils contain acid mucopolysaccharides that resemble chondroitin sulfate and hyaluronic acid (177, 284). These sulfated mucopolysaccharides probably account for the labeling of newly formed primary granules by radiosulfate (255).

An arginine-rich basic protein with bactericidal activity can be extracted from the granules of guinea pig and rabbit neutrophils (601, 602).

Cyclic AMP

The following observations suggest that cyclic 3',5'-adenosine monophosphate (cyclic AMP) may mediate hormonal effects as a "second messenger" in granulocytes and perhaps in lymphocytes (59): (a) glucagon activates human leukocyte phosphorylase in vitro; the mechanism of activation is probably similar to that of liver phosphorylase (576); (b) in most tissues containing a cyclic AMP system, epinephrine enhances adenyl cyclase (the enzyme involved in cyclic AMP generation) and methyl xanthines inhibit the phosphodiesterase that destroys cyclic AMP; in leukocytes, methyl xanthines potentiate epinephrine's inhibitory effect on the release of histamine by antigen-antibody complexes (322); (c) epinephrine and prostaglandin E_1 stimulate accumulation of cyclic AMP in human leukocytes (464); (d) adenyl cyclase and phosphodiesterase exist in human leukocytes; granulocytes have much more of these activities than do lymphocytes (60); (e) accumulation of intracellular cyclic AMP is increased by compounds that activate adenyl cyclase and is potentiated by methyl xanthine inhibition of phosphodiesterase (60).

The adenyl cyclase of human leukocytes may be activated by beta-adrenergic compounds and certain prostaglandins. Separate cell surface receptors may exist for these two classes of agents (62).

The precise role of cyclic AMP in mammalian granulocytes is not known. Phagocytosis has little effect on the cyclic AMP concentration of human granulocytes (341, 467). Conflicting lines of evidence are available on the effect of cyclic AMP on phagocytosis-induced degranulation (60, 351). Maneuvers that increase intracellular cyclic AMP clearly may interfere with neutrophil microbicidal activity (60) and may block allergic histamine release

from leukocytes (61, 63) or the release of enzymes from isolated granules (258).

Miscellaneous Constituents

Guinea pig neutrophils are rich in sialic acid (26).

Leukemic blast cells can convert porphobilinogen to porphyrin (126, 207, 532). Homogenates prepared from normal white cells and leukocytes from patients with chronic leukemia fail to synthesize heme from iron and protoporphyrin. Similar homogenates of leukocytes from patients with acute myeloblastic and lymphoblastic leukemia do synthesize heme (553). Normal mature granulocytes lack ALA synthetases, whereas this activity is present in immature cells (502).

In 1931 Platt first reported the presence of glutathione in white cells (406). The glutathione content of leukocytes is approximately seven times that of red cells (236). Many types of leukemic leukocytes contain greater than normal amounts of glutathione (48, 114, 164, 405, 406). Most investigators have reported significant increases in leukocyte glutathione in chronic myelocytic leukemia, but differ in their findings for acute leukemia (114, 236) and other hematologic abnormalities (236, 273, 395). The glutamine-glutathione transpeptidation system described in the kidney and pancreas has been demonstrated in the white cell also (235, 445).

Summary

The principal features of granulocyte metabolism are the following: (a) immature cells have a well-developed mitochondrial system, while mature cells derive their energy primarily from glycolysis; (b) oxygen consumed by phagocytizing granulocytes is used in part for hydrogen peroxide generation by nonmitochondrial pathways; (c) nucleic acid synthesis, active in immature cells, diminishes with maturation; and (d) granulocytes have a well-developed lysosomal system.

Clearly, much of the metabolism of mature neutrophils is directed at fulfillment of the primary functions of these cells—the phagocytosis and killing of microorganisms.

Chapter 3 References

1. Abels, J. C., Gorham, A. T., Craver, L., and Rhoads, C. P. The measurement and metabolism of thiamin and of a pyrimidine stimulating yeast fermentation found in the blood cells and urine of patients with leukemia, *J. Clin. Invest.* 21:177, 1942.

2. Ackerman, G. A. Cytochemical properties of the blood basophilic granulocyte, *Ann. N.Y. Acad. Sci.* 103:376, 1963.

3. Ackerman, G. A. Histochemical differentiation during neutrophil development and maturation, *Ann. N.Y. Acad. Sci.* 113:537, 1964.

4. Agner, K. Verdoperoxidase. A ferment isolated from leucocytes, *Acta Physiol. Scand.* 8:1, 1941 (suppl.).

5. Agner, K. Verdoperoxidase, *Adv. Enzymol.* 3:137, 1943.

6. Agner, K. Detoxifying effect of verdoperoxidase on toxins, *Nature* 159:271, 1947.

7. Agner, K. Studies on peroxidative detoxification of purified diphtheria toxin, *J. Exp. Med.* 92:337, 1950.

8. Alexander, W. D., and Bisset, S. K. The correlation of thyroid function with the rate of O_2 uptake of human leukocytes, *Q. J. Exp. Physiol.* 46:46, 1961.

9. Amano, T., Inai, S., Seki, Y., Kashiba, S., Fujikawa, K., and Nishimura, S. Studies on the immune bacteriolysis. I. Accelerating effect on the immune bacteriolysis by lysozyme-like substance of leucocytes and egg-white lysozome, *Med. J. Osaka Univ.* 4:401, 1954.

10. Anderson, E. P., and Heppel, L. A. Purification and properties of a leukemic cell phosphodiesterase, *Biochim. Biophys. Acta* 43:79, 1960.

11. Anlyan, A. J., and Fishman, W. H. β-glucuronidase activity in human neoplastic tissues and in certain body fluids and secretions, *Bull. Am. Coll. Surg.* 32:262, 1947.

12. Anlyan, A. J., Gamble, J., and Hoster, H. A. Beta-glucuronidase activity of the white blood cells in human leukemias and Hodgkin's disease, *Cancer* 3:116, 1950.

13. Archer, G. T., Jackas, M., and Morell, D. B. Studies on rat eosinophil peroxidase, *Biochim. Biophys. Acta* 99:96, 1965.

14. Austin, J. H., and Bischel, M. A histochemical method for sulfatase activity in hemic cells and organ imprints, *Blood* 17:216, 1961.

15. Baehner, R. L., and Karnovsky, M. L. Deficiency of reduced nicotinamide-adenine dinucleotide oxidase in chronic granulomatous disease, *Science* 162:1277, 1968.

16. Baggiolini, M. The enzymes of the granules of polymorphonuclear leukocytes and their functions, *Enzyme* 13:132, 1972.

17. Baggiolini, M., Hirsch, J. G., and DeDuve, C. Resolution of granules from rabbit heterophil leukocytes into distinct populations by zonal sedimentation, *J. Cell Biol.* 40:529, 1969.

18. Bainton, D. F., and Farquhar, M. G. Differences in enzyme content of azurophil and specific granules of polymorphonuclear leukocytes: I. Histochemical staining of bone marrow smears, *J. Cell Biol.* 39:286, 1968.

19. Bainton, D. F., and Farquhar, M. G. Differences in enzyme content of azurophil and specific granules of polymorphonuclear leukocytes: II. Cytochemistry and electron microscopy of bone marrow cells, *J. Cell Biol.* 39:299, 1968.

20. Baker, W. H., Zamecnik, P. C., and Stephenson, M. L. *In vitro* incorporation of C^{14}-DL-leucine into normal and leukemic white cells, *Blood* 12:822, 1957.

21. Bakker, A. Einige Ubereinstimmungen im Stoffwechsel der Carcinomzellen und Exudatleukocyten, *Klin. Wochenschr.* 6:252, 1927.

22. Baldridge, C. W., and Gerard, R. W. The extra respiration of phagocytosis, *Am. J. Physiol.* 103:235, 1933.

23. Barnes, J. M. The enzymes of lymphocytes and polymorphonuclear leucocytes, *Br. J. Exp. Pathol.* 21:261, 1940.

24. Barron, E. S. G., and Harrop, G. A., Jr. Studies on blood cell metabolism. V. The metabolism of leucocytes, *J. Biol. Chem.* 84:89, 1929.

25. Bazin, S., and Delaunay, A. Biochimie des polynucleaires neutrophiles, *Rev. Fr. Etudes Clin. Biol.* 1:1019, 1956.

26. Bazin, S., and Delaunay, A. Teneur en acide sialique de polynucléaires inflammatoires prélevés chez le cobaye, *Rev. Fr. Etudes Clin. Biol.* 8:592, 1963.

27. Beck, W. S. Leukocyte glycolysis: an investigation of the factors controlling the rate behavior in multienzyme systems, *Ann. N.Y. Acad. Sci.* 75:4, 1958.

28. Beck, W. S. The control of leukocyte glycolysis, *J. Biol. Chem.* 232:251, 1958.

29. Beck, W. S. Occurrence and control of the phosphogluconate oxidation pathway in normal and leukemic leukocytes, *J. Biol. Chem.* 232:271, 1958.

30. Beck, W. S., and Valentine, W. N. Biochemical studies on leukocytes. II. Phosphatase activity in chronic lymphatic leucemia, acute leucemia and miscellaneous hematologic conditions, *J. Lab. Clin. Med.* 38:245, 1951.

31. Beck, W. S., and Valentine, W. N. The aerobic carbohydrate metabolism of leukocytes in health and leukemia. I. Glycolysis and respiration, *Cancer Res.* 12:818, 1952.

32. Beck, W. S., and Valentine, W. N. The aerobic carbohydrate metabolism of leukocytes in health and leukemia. II. The effect of various substrates and coenzymes on glycolysis and respiration, *Cancer Res.* 12:823, 1952.

33. Beck, W. S., and Valentine, W. N. The carbohydrate metabolism of leukocytes: a review, *Cancer Res.* 13:309, 1953.

34. Becker, H., Munder, G., and Fischer, H. Über den Leukocytenstoffwechsel bei der Phagocytose, *Z. Physiol. Chem.* 313:266, 1958.

35. Bergmann, F., and Dikstein, S. Studies on uric acid and related compounds. III. Observations on the specificity of mammalian xanthine oxidases, *J. Biol. Chem.* 223:765, 1956.

36. Berlin, N. I., Rall, D., Mead, J. A. R., Freireich, E. J., Van Scott, E., Hertz, R., and Lipsett, M. B. Folic acid antagonists, *Ann. Intern. Med.* 59:931, 1963.

37. Berry, L. J., and Derbyshire, J. E. Effect of Malonate on selected body defenses, *Proc. Soc. Exp. Biol. Med.* 92:315, 1956.

38. Bertino, J. R., Alenty, A., Gabrio, B. W., and Huennekens, F. M. Folic acid coenzymes and one-carbon metabolism in leukocytes, *Clin. Res.* 8:206, 1960.

39. Bertino, J. R., Booth, B. A., Bieber, A. L., Cashmore, A., and Sartorelli, A. C. Studies on the inhibition of dihydrofolate reductase by the folate antagonists, *J. Biol. Chem.* 239:479, 1964.

40. Bertino, J. R., Donohue, D. M., Gabrio, B. W., Silber, R., Alenty, A., Meyer, M., and Huennekens, F. M. Increased level of dihydrofolic reductase in leucocytes of patients treated with amethopterin, *Nature* 193:140, 1962.

41. Bertino, J. R., Donohue, D. M., Simmons, B., Gabrio, B. W., Silber, R., and Huennekens, F. M. The "induction" of dihydrofolic reductase in leucocytes and erythrocytes of patients treated with amethopterin, *J. Clin. Invest.* 42:466, 1963.

42. Bertino, J. R., Gabrio, B. W., and Huennekens, F. M. Dihydrofolic reductase in human leukemic leukocytes, *Biochem. Biophys. Res. Commun.* 3:461, 1960.

43. Bertino, J. R., Gabrio, B. W., and Huennekens, F. M. Increased activity of leukocyte dihydrofolic reductase in amethopterin-treated patients, *Clin. Res.* 9:103, 1961.

44. Bertino, J. R., Silber, R., Freeman, M., Alenty, A., Albrecht, M., Gabrio, B. W., and Huennekens, F. M. Studies on normal and leukemic leukocytes. IV. Tetrahydrofolate-dependent enzyme systems and dihydrofolate reductase, *J. Clin. Invest.* 42:1899, 1963.

45. Bertino, J. R., Simmons, B. M., and Donohue, D. M. Studies on the mechanism of resistance to the folic acid antagonists, *Clin. Res.* 9:157, 1961.

46. Bianchi, P. A. Thymidine phosphorylation and deoxyribonucleic acid synthesis in human leukaemic cells, *Biochim. Biophys. Acta* 55:547, 1962.

47. Bianchi, P. A., Farina, M. B., and Polli, E. Phosphorylation of thymidine diphosphate in resting and proliferating mammalian cells, *Biochim. Biophys. Acta* 91:322, 1964.

48. Bichel, J. Blood glutathione in leucoses, *J. Acta Med. Scand.* 124:160, 1946.

49. Bicz, W. The influence of carbon dioxide tension on the respiration of normal and leukemic human leukocytes. I. Influence on endogenous respiration, *Cancer Res.* 20:184, 1960.

50. Bisset, S. K., and Alexander, W. D. The effect of intravenous injections of triiodothyroacetic acid and *l*-triiodothyronine on the oxygen consumption of circulating human leucocytes, *Q. J. Exp. Physiol.* 46:50, 1961.

51. Bloom, M. L., and Wislocki, G. B. The localization of lipids in human blood and bone marrow cells, *Blood* 5:79, 1950.

52. Bodansky, O. Blood enzymes in cancer and other diseases, *Adv. Cancer Res.* 6:1, 1961.

53. Bonsignore, A., Fornaini, G., Fantoni, A., and Leoncini, G. Purification and properties of the glucose-6-phosphate dehydrogenase from the human erythrocytes and leukocytes, *Ital. J. Biochem.* 14:217, 1965.

54. Bonsignore, A., Fornaini, G., Leoncini, G., Fantoni, A., and Segni, P. Characterization of leukocyte glucose-6-phosphate dehydrogenase in Sardinian mutants, *J. Clin. Invest.* 45:1865, 1966.

55. Borel, C., Frei, J., Horvath, G., Montri, S., and Vannotti, A. Etude comparée du métabolisme du polynucléaire et de la cellule mononucléé chez l'homme, *Helv. Med. Acta* 26:785, 1959.

56. Borghetti, A., and Scarpioni, L. Sull'attivita arginasica nei leucociti, *Rass. Fisiopat. Clin. Ter.* 27:941, 1955.

57. Borghetti, A., and Scarpioni, L. Attivita arginasica nei leucociti umani, *Enzymologia* 17:338, 1956.

58. Bornstein, D. L., Weinberg, A. N., and Swartz, M. N. A deoxyribonuclease from rabbit leukocytes, *Proc. Soc. Exp. Biol. Med.* 121:677, 1966.

59. Bourne, H. R. Leukocyte cyclic AMP: pharmacologic regulation and possible physiologic implications, *in* P. Ramwell and B. B. Pharriss (eds.), Prostaglandins in Cellular Biology, p. 111, Plenum Press, New York, 1972.

60. Bourne, H. R., Lehrer, R. I., Cline, M. J., and Melmon, K. L. Cyclic 3',5'-adenosine monophosphate in the human leukocyte: synthesis, degradation, and effects on neutrophil candidacidal activity, *J. Clin. Invest.* 50:920, 1971.

61. Bourne, H. R., Lichtenstein, L. M., and Melmon, K. L. Pharmacologic control of allergic histamine release *in vitro*: evidence for an inhibitory role of 3',5'-adenosine monophosphate in human leukocytes, *J. Immunol.* 108:695, 1972.

62. Bourne, H. R., and Melmon, K. L. Adenyl cyclase in human leukocytes: evidence for activation by separate *beta* adrenergic and prostaglandin receptors, *J. Pharmacol. Exp. Ther.* 178:1, 1971.

63. Bourne, H. R., Melmon, K. L., and Lichtenstein, L. M. Histamine augments leukocyte adenosine 3',5'-monophosphate and blocks antigenic histamine release, *Science* 173:743, 1971.

64. Boxer, G. E., Pruss, M. P., and Goodhart, R. S. Pyridoxal-5-phosphoric acid in whole blood and isolated leukocytes of man and animals, *J. Nutr.* 63:623, 1957.

65. Boyd, E. M. Low phospholipid in dog plasma, *J. Biol. Chem.* 91:1, 1931.

66. Boyd, E. M. The lipid content of the white blood cells in normal young women, *J. Biol. Chem.* 101:623, 1933.

67. Boyd, E. M. The lipid composition of the white blood cells in leukemia, *Arch. Pathol.* 21:739, 1936.

68. Boyd, E. M., and Stephens, D. J. A comparison of lipid composition with differential count of the white blood cells, *Proc. Soc. Exp. Biol. Med.* 33:558, 1936.

69. Boyd, E. M., and Wilson, K. M. The exchange of lipids in the umbilical circulation at birth, *J. Clin. Invest.* 14:7, 1935.

70. Boysen, G. An evaluation of aryl sulphatose activity in leukaemic

cells, *Scand. J. Haematol.* 6:246, 1969.

71. Braunsteiner, H., Dienstl, F., Sailer, S., and Sandhofer, F. Lipase activity in leukocytes and macrophages, *Blood* 24:607, 1964.

72. Braunsteiner, H., and Zucker-Franklin, D. The Physiology and Pathology of Leukocytes, p. 574, Grune & Stratton, New York, 1962.

73. Bresnick, E., and Kariala, R. J. End-product inhibition of thymidine kinase activity in normal and leukemic human leukocytes, *Cancer Res.* 24:841, 1964.

74. Brin, M., and Yonemoto, R. H. Stimulation of the glucose oxidative pathway in human erythrocytes by methylene blue, *J. Biol. Chem.* 230:307, 1958.

75. Brown, B. I., and Brown, D. H. Lack of a^{-1}, 4-glucan: a^{-1}, 4-glucan 6 glycosyl tranferase in a case of Type IV glycogenosis, *Proc. Natl. Acad. Sci. U.S.A.* 56:725, 1966.

76. Bryant, B. J. Reutilization of leukocyte DNA by cells of regenerating liver, *Exp. Cell Res.* 27:70, 1962.

77. Bryant, B. J. Reutilization of lymphocyte DNA by cells of intestinal crypts and regenerating liver, *J. Cell Biol.* 18:515, 1963.

78. Buchanan, A. A. Lipid synthesis by human leucocytes *in vitro*, *Biochem. J.* 75:315, 1960.

79. Buchanan, J. M. Biosynthesis of purine nucleotides, *in* E. Chargaff and J. N. Davidson (eds.), The Nucleic Acids, vol. 3, p. 304, Academic Press, New York, 1960.

80. Budd, M. A., Tanaka, K., Holmes, L. B., Efron, M. L., Crawford, J. D., and Isselbacher, K. J. Isovaleric acidemia, *N. Engl. J. Med.* 277:321, 1967.

81. Burch, H. B., Bessey, O. A., and Lowry, O. H. Fluorometric measurements of riboflavin and its natural derivatives in small quantities of blood serum and cells, *J. Biol. Chem.* 175:457, 1948.

82. Burt, N. S., and Rossiter, R. J. Lipids of rabbit blood cells. Data for red cells and polymorphonuclear leucocytes, *Biochem. J.* 46:569, 1950.

83. Butler, A. M., and Cushman, M. Distribution of ascorbic acid in the blood and its nutritional significance, *J. Clin. Invest.* 19:459, 1940.

84. Canellakis, E. S., Tuttle, A. L., and Cohen, P. P. A comparative study of the end-products of uric acid oxidation by peroxidases, *J. Biol. Chem.* 213:397, 1955.

85. Cassen, B., Hitt, J., and Hays, E. F. The efficient separation of lymphocytes from normal human blood, *J. Lab. Clin. Med.* 52:778, 1958.

86. Chance, B. On the reaction of catalase peroxides with acceptors, *J. Biol. Chem.* 182:649, 1950.

87. Chance, B. The cytochromes of respiring cells, *in* J. L. Tullis (ed.), Blood Cells and Plasma Proteins, p. 306, Academic Press, New York, 1953.

88. Chapman-Andersen, C., and Holter, H. Studies on the ingestion of C^{14}-glucose by pinocytosis in the amoeba, *Chaos chaos, Exp. Cell Res.* 3:52, 1955 (suppl.).

89. Christlieb, A. R., Sbarra, A. J., and Bardawil, W. A. Isolation of highly purified leukocytes from blood, *Am. J. Clin. Pathol.* 37:257, 1962.

90. Cline, M. J. Metabolism of the circulating leukocyte, *Physiol. Rev.* 45:674, 1965.

91. Cline, M. J. Ribonucleic acid biosynthesis in human leukocytes: the effects of phagocytosis on RNA metabolism, *Blood* 28:188, 1966.

92. Cline, M. J. Ribonucleic acid biosynthesis in human leukocytes: the fate of rapidly labeled RNA in normal and abnormal leukocytes, *Blood* 28:650, 1966.

93. Cline, M. J. Isolation and characterization of RNA from human leukocytes, *J. Lab. Clin. Med.* 68:33, 1966.

94. Cline, M. J. Phagocytosis and synthesis of ribonucleic acid in human granulocytes, *Nature* 212:1431, 1966.

95. Cline, M. J. Effect of vincristine on synthesis of ribonucleic acid and protein in leukaemic leukocytes, *Br. J. Haematol.* 41:17, 1968.

96. Cline, M. J. Leukocyte metabolism, *in* A. S. Gordon (ed.), Regulation of Hematopoiesis, p. 1045, Appleton-Century-Crofts, New York, 1970.

97. Cline, M. J. Leukocyte function in inflammation: the ingestion, killing, and digestion of microorganisms, *Ser. Haematol.* III:3, 1970.

98. Cline, M. J. Hanifin, J., and Lehrer, R. I. Phagocytosis by human eosinophils, *Blood* 32:922, 1968.

99. Cline, M. J., and Lehrer, R. I. Phagocytosis by human monocytes, *Blood* 32:423, 1968.

100. Cline, M. J., and Lehrer, R. I. D-amino acid oxidase in leukocytes: a possible D-amino-acid-linked antimicrobial system, *Proc. Natl. Acad. Sci. U.S.A.* 62:756, 1969.

101. Cline, M. J., Melmon, K. L., Davis, W. C., and Williams, H. E. Mechanism of endotoxin interaction with human leukocytes, *Br. J. Haematol.* 15:539, 1968.

102. Code, C. F. The source in blood of the histamine-like constituents, *J. Physiol. (Lond.)* 90:349, 1937.

103. Code, C. F. The histamine-like activity of white blood cells, *J. Physiol. (Lond.)* 90:485, 1937.

104. Cohn, Z. A. The structure and function of monocytes and macrophages, *Adv. Immunol.* 9:163, 1968

105. Cohn, Z. A., and Benson, B. The differentiation of mononuclear phagocytes: morphology, cytochemistry and biochemistry, *J. Exp. Med.* 121:153, 1965.

106. Cohn, Z. A., and Benson, B. The *in vitro* differentiation of mononuclear phagocytes: I. The influence of inhibitors and the results of autoradiography, *J. Exp. Med.* 121:279, 1965.

107. Cohn, Z. A., and Benson, B. The *in vitro* differentiation of mononuclear phagocytes: III. The reversibility of granule and hydrolytic enzyme formation and the turnover of granule constituents, *J. Exp. Med.* 122:455, 1965.

108. Cohn, Z. A., and Hirsch, J. G. The isolation and properties of the specific cytoplasmic granules of rabbit polymorphonuclear leucocytes, *J. Exp. Med.* 112:983, 1960.

109. Cohn, Z. A., and Hirsch, J. G. The influence of phagocytosis on the intracellular distribution of granule-associated components of polymorphonuclear leucocytes, *J. Exp. Med.* 112:1015, 1960.

110. Cohn, Z. A., Hirsch, J. G., and Wiener, E. Lysosomes and endocytosis. The cytoplasmic granules of phagocytic cells and the degradation of bacteria, *in* A. V. S. de

Reuck and M. P. Cameron (eds.), Ciba Foundation Symposium on Lysosomes, p. 126, Little, Brown and Co., Boston, 1963.

111. Cohn, Z. A., and Morse, S. I. Functional and metabolic properties of polymorphonuclear leucocytes. I. Observations on the requirements and consequences of particle ingestion, *J. Exp. Med.* 111:667, 1960.

112. Cohn, Z. A., and Morse, S. I. Functional and metabolic properties of polymorphonuclear leucocytes. II. The influence of a lipopolysaccharide endotoxin, *J. Exp. Med.* 111:689, 1960.

113. Constantinides, P. Estimation of vitamin C in leucocytes by the hydrazine method, *Lancet* 1:750, 1947.

114. Contopoulos, A. N., and Anderson, H. H. Sulfhydryl content of blood cells in dyscrasias, *J. Lab. Clin. Med.* 36:929, 1950.

115. Cooke, J. V. Proteolytic leukocytic enzyme in leukemia, *Arch. Intern. Med.* 49:836, 1932.

116. Cooper, H. L. Ribonucleic acid metabolism in lymphocytes stimulated by phytohemagglutinin, *J. Biol. Chem.* 243:34, 1968.

117. Cooper, H. L., Perry, S., and Breitman, T. R. Pyrimidine metabolism in human leukocytes: I. Contribution of exogenous thymidine to DNA-thymine and its effect on thymine nucleotide synthesis in leukemic leukocytes, *Cancer Res.* 26:2267, 1966.

118. Cooper, H. L., Perry, S., and Breitman, T. R. Pyrimidine metabolism in human leukocytes: II. Metabolism of the thymine nucleotide pools in normal and leukemic leukocytes, *Cancer Res.* 26:2276, 1966.

119. Cottingham, E., and Mills, C. A. Influence of environmental temperature and vitamin-deficiency upon phagocytic functions, *J. Immunol.* 47:493, 1943.

120. Coxon, R. V., and Robinson, R. J. Carbohydrate metabolism in blood cells studied by means of isotopic carbon, *Proc. R. Soc. Lond. (Biol.)* 145:232, 1956.

121. Craddock, C. G., and Nakal, G. S. Leukemic cell proliferation as determined by *in vitro* desox-

yribonucleic acid synthesis, *J. Clin. Invest.* 41:360, 1962.

122. Crandon, T. H., Lund, C. C., and Dill, D. B. Experimental human scurvy, *N. Engl. J. Med.* 223:353, 1940.

123. Cronkite, E. P., Bond, V. P., Fliedner, T. M., and Killmann, S. A. The use of tritiated thymidine in the study of haemopoietic cell proliferation, *in* G. E. W. Wolstenholme and M. O'Connor (eds.), Ciba Foundation Symposium on Haemopoiesis, p. 70, Churchill, London, 1960.

124. Cronkite, E. P., Bond, V. P., Fliedner, T. M., and Rubini, J. R. The use of tritiated thymidine in the study of DNA synthesis and cell turnover in hemopoietic tissues, *Lab. Invest.* 8:263, 1959.

125. Crosbie, G. W. Biosynthesis of pyrimidine nucleotides, *in* E. Chargaff and J. N. Davidson (eds.), The Nucleic Acids, vol. 3, p. 323, Academic Press, New York, 1960.

126. Cullity, B., and Vannotti, A. Porphyrin biosynthesis in the leucocyte, *Nature* 185:187, 1960.

127. Dacie, J. V., Smith, M. D., White, J. C., and Mollin, D. L. Refractory normoblastic anaemia: clinical and haematological study of seven cases, *Br. J. Haematol.* 5:56, 1959.

128. Daft, F. S., and Sebrell, W. H. The successful treatment of granulocytopenia and leukopenia in rats with crystalline folic acid, *Public Health Rep.* 58:1542, 1943.

129. Dakin, D. H., and Dudley, H. W. On glyoxalase, *J. Biol. Chem.* 14:423, 1913.

130. Dancis, J., Hutzler, J., and Levitz, M. Metabolism of the white blood cell in maple-syrup-urine disease, *Biochim. Biophys. Acta* 43:342, 1960.

131. Dancis, J., Hutzler, J., and Levitz, M. The diagnosis of maple-syrup-urine disease by the *in vitro* study of peripheral leukocytes, *Pediatrics* 32:234, 1963.

132. Dancis, J., Hutzler, J., and Rokkones, T. Intermittent branched-chain ketonuria, *N. Engl. J. Med.* 276:84, 1967.

133. Dancis, J., Levitz, M., and Westall, R. G. Maple-syrup-urine disease: branched-chain ketoaciduria, *Pediatrics* 25:72, 1960.

134. Dannenberg, A. M., Burstone, M. S., Walter, P. C., and Kinsley, J. W. A histochemical study of phagocytic and enzymatic functions of rabbit mononuclear and polymorphonuclear exudate cells and alveolar macrophages: I. Survey and quantitation of enzymes and states of cellular activation, *J. Cell Biol.* 17:465, 1963.

135. Davidson, J. D. Studies on the mechanism of action of 6-mercaptopurine in sensitive and resistant L_{1210} leukemia *in vitro, Cancer Res.* 20:225, 1960.

136. Davidson, J. D., and Winter, T. S. Purine nucleotide pyrophosphorylase in 6-mercaptopurine-sensitive and -resistant human leukemias, *Cancer Res.* 24:261, 1964.

137. Davidson, J. N. The Biochemistry of the Nucleic Acids, Methuen and Co., London, 1960.

138. Davidson, J. N., Leslie, J., and White, J. C. Quantitative studies on the content of nucleic acids in normal and leukemic cells from blood and bone marrow, *J. Pathol. Bacteriol.* 63:471, 1951.

139. Davis, V. E., Wilson, W. L., and Spurr, C. L. The efficiency of oxidative phosphorylation by normal and leukemic human leukocytes, *Blood* 13:367, 1958.

140. De Duve, C., and Wattiaux, R. Functions of lysosomes, *Ann. Rev. Physiol.* 28:435, 1966.

141. Dennes, E., Tupper, R., and Wormall, A. Zinc content of erythrocytes and leucocytes of blood of normal and leukaemic subjects, *Nature* 187:302, 1960.

142. Dennes, E., Tupper, R., and Wormall, A. The zinc content of erythrocytes and leucocytes of blood from normal and leukaemic subjects, *Biochem. J.* 78:578, 1961.

143. Dennes, E., Tupper, R., and Wormall, A. Studies on zinc in blood. Transport of zinc and incorporation of zinc in leucocytes, *Biochem. J.* 82:466, 1962.

144. DiMajorca, G., Rosenkranz, H. S., Polli, E. E., Korngold, G. C., and Bendich, A. A chromatographic study of the deoxyribonucleic acids from normal and leukemic human tissues, *J. Natl. Cancer Inst.* 24:1309, 1960.

145. Dimitrov, N. V., Hansz, J., Toth,

M. A., and Bartolotta, B. Serine and aspartic acid metabolism in leukemic leukocytes: correlation to effectiveness of therapy, *Blood* 38:638, 1971.

146. Dioguardi, N., Agostoni, A., and Fiorelli, G. Characterization of lactic dehydrogenase in cells of myeloid leukemia, *Enzymol. Biol. Clin.* 2:116, 1962–63.

147. Doan, C. A. The white blood cells in health and disease, *Bull. N.Y. Acad. Med.* 30:415, 1954.

148. Donald, E. A., and Ferguson, R. F. A micro method for determination of pyridoxal phosphate in leukocytes and liver, *Ann. Biochem.* 7:335, 1964.

149. Dubos, R. J., and MacLeod, C. M. The effect of a tissue enzyme upon pneumococci, *J. Exp. Med.* 67:791, 1938.

150. Ehrich, W. E. Histamine in mast cells, *Science* 118:603, 1953.

151. Ellison, R. R., and Hutchison, D. J. Metabolism of folic acid and citrovorum factor in leukemic cells, *in* J. W. Rebuck, F. H. Bethell, and R. W. Monto (eds.), The Leukemias, p. 467, Academic Press, New York, 1957.

152. Elmes, P. C., Smith, J. D., and White, J. C. The composition of human deoxyribonucleic acid isolated from haemopoietic and other tissues. II. Congrès International de Biochimie, Résumé des Communications, pp. 7–8, 1952.

153. Elsbach, P. Composition and synthesis of lipids in resting and phagocytizing leukocytes, *J. Exp. Med.* 110:969, 1959.

154. Elsbach, P. Preferential and active transport of linoleic acid by polymorphonuclear leukocytes, *J. Clin. Invest.* 39:983, 1960.

155. Elsbach, P. Role of phagocytosis in the uptake of lipid by a phagocytic cell, *Nature* 195:383, 1962.

156. Elsbach, P. Comparison of uptake of palmitic, stearic, oleic and linoleic acid by polymorphonuclear leukocytes, *Biochim. Biophys. Acta Previews* 3:Nov., 1963.

157. Elsbach, P. Incorporation of (1-^{14}C) linoleic acid into lipids of polymorphonuclear leukocytes, *Biochim. Biophys. Acta* 70:157, 1963.

158. Elsbach, P. Uptake of fat by phagocytic cells—an examination of the role of phagocytosis: I. Rabbit polymorphonuclear leukocytes, *Biochim. Biophys. Acta* 98:402, 1965.

159. Elsbach, P. Stimulation of lecithin synthesis from medium lysolecithin during phagocytosis, *J. Clin. Invest.* 46:1052, 1967 (abstract).

160. Elsbach, P. Increased synthesis of phospholipid during phagocytosis, *J. Clin. Invest.* 47:2217, 1968.

161. Elsbach, P., and Kayden, H. J. Chylomicron-lipid-splitting activity in homogenates of rabbit polymorphonuclear leukocytes, *Am. J. Physiol.* 209:765, 1965.

162. Elsbach, P., and Rizack, M. A. Acid lipase and phospholipase activity in homogenates of rabbit polymorphonuclear leukocytes, *Am. J. Physiol.* 205:1154, 1963.

163. Elsbach, P., and Schwartz, I. L. Studies on the sodium and potassium transport in rabbit polymorphonuclear leukocytes, *J. Gen. Physiol.* 42:883, 1959.

164. Émile-Weil, P., Ashkenasy, A., and Capron, L. Le glutathion sanguin dans les polyglobuiles, les leucémies et les érythroblastoses chroniques, *Sang* 13:705, 1939.

165. Endres, G., and Herget, L. Mineralzusammensetzung der Bluplättchen und weissen Blutkörperchen, *Z. Biol.* 88:451, 1929.

166. Ennis, H. L. Synthesis of ribonucleic acid in L cells during inhibition of protein synthesis by cycloheximide, *Mol. Pharmacol.* 2:543, 1966.

167. Eränkö, O. Demonstration of glycogen and lipids in the cytoplasm of human neutrophilic leucocytes, *Nature* 165:116, 1950.

168. Esman, V. The glycogen content of leukocytes from diabetic and nondiabetic subjects, *Scand. J. Clin. Lab. Invest.* 13:134, 1961.

169. Estes, F. L., Austin, N. S., and Gast, J. H. Metabolic characterization of polymorphonuclear leukocytes, *Clin. Chem.* 6:501, 1960.

170. Evans, W. H., and Karnovsky, M. L. Metabolic pathways associated with phagocytosis, *Fed. Proc.* 19:42, 1960.

171. Evans, W. H., and Karnovsky, M. L. A possible mechanism for the stimulation of some metabolic functions during phagocytosis, *J. Biol. Chem.* 236:PC30:1961.

172. Evans, W. H., and Karnovsky, M. L. The biochemical basis of phagocytosis. IV. Some aspects of carbohydrate metabolism during phagocytosis, *Biochem.* 1:159, 1962.

173. Evans, W. H., and Mueller, P. S. Effects of palmitate on the metabolism of leukocytes from guinea pig exudate, *J. Lipid Res.* 4:39, 1963.

174. Everett, N. B., Reinhardt, W. O., and Yoffey, J. M. The appearance of labeled cells in the thoracic duct lymph of the guinea pig after the administration of tritiated thymidine, *Blood* 15:82, 1960.

175. Fallon, M. J., Frei, E., III, Davidson, J. D., Trier, J. S., and Burke, D. Leukocyte preparations from human blood: evaluation of their morphologic and metabolic state, *J. Lab. Clin. Med.* 59:779, 1962.

176. Fallon, H. J., Lotz, M., and Smith, L. H., Jr. Congenital orotic aciduria: demonstration of an enzyme defect in leukocytes and comparison with drug induced orotic aciduria, *Blood* 20:700, 1962.

177. Fedorko, M. E., and Morse, S. I. Isolation, characterization and distribution of acid mucopolysaccharides in rabbit leucocytes, *J. Exp. Med.* 121:39, 1965.

178. Feinendegen, L. E., Bond, V. P., and Hughes, W. L. Physiological thymidine reutilization in rat bone marrow, *Proc. Soc. Exp. Biol. Med.* 122:448, 1966.

179. Feissinger, N., and Boyer, F. Les phosphatases des leucocytes, *Enzymologia* 1:172, 1936.

180. Fenninger, L. D., Waterhouse, C., and Keutmann, E. H. The interrelationship of nitrogen and phosphorus in patients with certain neoplastic diseases, *Cancer* 6:930, 1953.

181. Finch. S. C., Lamphere, J. P., and Jablon, S. The relationship of serum lysozyme to leukocytes and other constitutional factors, *Yale J. Biol. Med.* 36:350, 1964.

182. Forkin, B. G., and Williams, W. J. The incorporation of radioactive phosphorus into the phospholipids of human leukemic leukocytes and platelets, *J. Clin. Invest.* 40:423, 1961.

183. Fischer, G. A. Increased levels of folic reductase as a mechanism of resistance to amethopterin in

mouse leukemia cells, *Proc. Am. Cancer Res.* 3:111, 1960.

184. Fischer, G. A., Bertino, J. R., Calabresi, P., Clement, D. H., Zanes, R. P., Lyman, M. S., Burchenal, J. H., and Welch, A. D. Uptake of tritium-labeled methotrexate by human leukemic leukocytes, *Blood* 22:819, 1963.

185. Fisher, T. N., and Ginsberg, H. S. Reactions of influenza viruses with guinea pig polymorphonuclear leucocytes. II. The reduction of white blood cell glycolysis by influenza viruses and receptor-destroying enzyme (RDE), *Virology* 2:637, 1956.

186. Fisher, T. N., and Ginsberg, H. S. The reaction of influenza virus with guinea pig polymorphonuclear leucocytes. III. Studies on the mechanism by which influenza viruses inhibit phagocytosis, *Virology* 2:656, 1956.

187. Fishman, W. H., Springer, B., and Brunetti, R. Application of an improved glucuronidase assay method for the study of human blood β-glucuronidase, *J. Biol. Chem.* 173:449, 1948.

188. Flanagan, P., and Lionetti, F. Lysozyme distribution in blood, *Blood* 10:497, 1955.

189. Fleischmann, W. Über die Permabilität der Leukocyten für Ionen, *Pflüger's Arch. Ges. Physiol.* 223:47, 1929.

190. Fleischmann, W., and Kubowitz, G. Über den Stoffwechsel der Leucocyten, *Biochem. Z.* 181:395, 1927.

191. Fleisher, G. A. Peptidases in human blood. IV. The hydrolysis of glycyl-L-leucine and other dipeptides by leucocytes, *Arch. Biochem. Biophys.* 61:119, 1956.

192. Folds, J. D., Welsh, I. R. H., and Spitznagel, J. K. Neutral proteases confined to one class of lysosomes of human polymorphonuclear leukocytes, *Proc. Soc. Exp. Biol. Med.* 139:461, 1972.

193. Follette, J. H., Shugarman, P. M., Reynolds, J., Valentine, W. M., and Lawrence, J. S. The effect of choramphenicol and other antibiotics on leukocyte respiration, *Blood* 11:234, 1956.

194. Follette, J. H., Valentine, W. N., Hardin, E. B., and Lawrence, J. S. Studies on the glucuronic acid content of human leukocytes in health

and in disease, *J. Lab. Clin. Med.* 43:134, 1954.

195. Follette, J. H., Valentine, W. N., and Lawrence, J. S. The beta-glucuronidase content of human leukocytes in health and in disease, *J. Lab. Clin. Med.* 40:825, 1952.

196. Follette, J. H., Valentine, W. N., and Reynolds, J. A comparison of human leucocyte phosphatase activity toward sodium β-glycerophosphate, adenosine 5'-phosphate and glucose 1-phosphate, *Blood* 14:415, 1959.

197. Foster, J. M., and Terry, M. L. Studies on the energy metabolism: I. Oxidative phosphorylation by human leukocyte mitochondria, *Blood* 30:168, 1967.

198. Foulkes, E. C., Lemberg, R., and Purdom, P. Verdohaem and Verdoglobins, *Proc. R. Soc. Lond. (Biol.)* 138:386, 1951.

199. Fraenkel-Conrat, J., and Chew, W. B. Catheptic activity of leukocytes in normal and leukemic subjects, *Blood* 16:1447, 1960.

200. Fraenkel-Conrat, J., Chew, W. B., Pitlick, F., and Barber, S. Certain properties of leukocytic cathepsins in health and disease, *Cancer* 19:1393, 1966.

201. Frantz, I. D., Jr., and Zamecnik, P. C. Use of C14-labeled amino acids in the study of peptide bond synthesis, *in* J. B. Youmans (ed.), Symposia on Nutrition, vol. 2, Plasma Proteins, p. 94, Charles C Thomas, Springfield, Ill., 1950.

202. Fredricks, R. E., and Moloney, W. C. The basophilic granulocyte, *Blood* 14:571, 1959.

203. Fredricks, R. E., Tanaka, K. R., and Valentine, W. N. Zinc in human blood cells: normal values and abnormalities associated with liver disease, *J. Clin. Invest.* 39:1651, 1960.

204. Fredricks, R. E., Tanaka, K. R., and Valentine, W. N. Variations of human blood cell zinc in disease, *J. Clin. Invest.* 43:304, 1964.

205. Frei, J. Energy levels in the human circulating leucocyte, *in* G. E. W. Wolstenholme and M. O'Connor (eds.), Ciba Foundation Study Group 10; Biological Activity of the Leucocyte, p. 86, Little, Brown and Co., Boston, 1961.

206. Frei, J. Métabolisme énergétique du

leucocyte, *Enzymol. Biol. Clin.* 2:175, 1962–63.

207. Frei, J., Borel, C., Horvath, G., Cullity, B., and Vannotti, A. Enzymatic studies in the different types of normal and leukemic human white cells, *Blood* 18:317, 1961.

208. Frei, J., Borel, C., and Vannotti, A. Modification métabolitique au niveau du leucocyte humain pendant la phagocytose, *Enzymol. Biol. Clin.* 1:149, 1961–62.

209. Frenster, J. H., Allfrey, V. G., and Mirsky, A. E. Repressed and active chromatin isolated from interphase lymphocytes, *Proc. Natl. Acad. Sci. U.S.A.* 50:1026, 1963.

210. Friedkin, M. Enzymatic aspects of folic acid, *Ann. Rev. Biochem.* 32:185, 1963.

211. Fruton, J. S., and Simmonds, S. General Biochemistry, p. 479, John Wiley & Sons, Inc., New York, 1958.

212. Fujita, A. Über den Stoffwechsel der weissen Blutzellen, *Klin. Wochenschr.* 7:897, 1928.

213. Fujita, A., and Yamadori, M. Distribution of thiamine and riboflavin in components of blood, *Arch. Biochem. Biophys.* 28:94, 1950.

214. Gavosto, F., Maraini, G., and Pileri, A. Nucleic acids and protein metabolism in acute leukemia cells, *Blood* 16:1555, 1960.

215. Gavosto, F., Maraini, G., and Pileri, A. Proliferative capacity of acute leukaemia cells, *Nature* 187:611, 1960.

216. Gavosto, F., Pileri, A., and Maraini, G. Protein metabolism in bone marrow and peripheral blood cells: evaluation of H3-DL-leucine uptake by high resolution autoradiographic technique, VII European Congr. Haematol., London, pt. 2, p. 380, 1959.

217. Gibson, J. G., II, Vallee, B. L., Fluharty, R. G., and Nelson, J. E. Studies on the zinc content of the leucocytes in myelogenous leukemia, *Un. Int. Clin. contra Cancr. Acta* 6:1102, 1950.

218. Gilbert, H. S., Warner, R. R., and Wasserman, L. R. A study of histamine in myeloproliferative disease, *Blood* 28:795, 1966.

219. Glock, G. E., and McLean, P. Further studies on the properties and assay of glucose-6-phosphate dehy-

drogenase and 6-phosphogluconate dehydrogenase of rat liver, *Biochem. J.* 55:400, 1953.

220. Glock, G. E., and McLean, P. Levels of enzymes of the direct oxidative pathway of carbohydrate metabolism in mammalian tissues and tumours, *Biochem. J.* 56:171, 1954.

221. Gomori, G. Microchemical demonstration of phosphatase in tissue sections, *Proc. Soc. Exp. Biol. Med.* 42:23, 1939.

222. Goodheart, R. S., and Sinclair, H. M. Cocarboxylase (vitamin B_1 diphosphate) in blood, *J. Physiol.* (*Lond.*) 95:57P, 1939.

223. Gordon, G. B., and King, D. W. Phagocytosis, *Am. J. Pathol.* 37:279, 1960.

224. Gorham, A. T., Abels, J. C., Robins, A. L., and Rhoads, C. P. The measurement and metabolism of thiamin and of a pyrimidine stimulating yeast fermentation found in the blood cells and urine of normal individuals, *J. Clin. Invest.* 21:161, 1942.

225. Gottfried, E. L. Lipids of human leukocytes: relation to cell type, *J. Lipid Res.* 8:321, 1967.

226. Gottfried, E. L. Lipid patterns of leukocytes in health and disease, *Semin. Hematol.* 9:241, 1972.

227. Grafe, E. Die Steigerung des Stoffwechsels bei chronischer Leukaemic und ihre Ursachen, *Dtsch. Arch. Klin.* 102:406, 1911.

228. Graham, H. T., Lowry, O. H., Wheelwright, F., Lenz, M. A., and Parish, H. H., Jr. Distribution of histamine among leukocytes and platelets, *Blood* 10:467, 1955.

229. Graham, H. T., Wheelwright, F., Parish, H. H., Jr., Marks, A. R., and Lowry, O. H. Distribution of histamine among blood elements, *Fed. Proc.* 11:350, 1952.

230. Greendyke, R. M., Brierty, R. E., and Swisher, S. N. *In vitro* studies on erythrophagocytosis, *Blood* 22:295, 1963.

231. Gunz, F. W., and Fitzgerald, P. H. Chromosomes and leukemia, *Blood* 23:394, 1964.

232. Haight, W. F., and Rossiter, R. J. Acid and alkaline phosphatase in white cells. Data for the lymphocyte and the polymorphonuclear leukocyte of man and the rabbit, *Blood* 5:267, 1950.

233. Hale, A. J., and Wilson, S. J. The deoxyribonucleic acid content of the nuclei of leukemia leukocytes, *Lancet* 1:577, 1960.

234. Hamburger, H. J., and van der Schroeff, H. J. Die Permeabilität von Leukocyten und Lymphdrusenzellen für die Anionen von Natriumsalzen, *Arch. Anat. Physiol., Physiol. Abt.* 119, 1902 (suppl.).

235. Hanes, C. S., Hird, F. J. R., and Isherwood, F. A. Synthesis of peptides in enzymatic reactions involving glutathione, *Nature* 166:288, 1950.

236. Hardin, E. B., Valentine, W. N., Follette, J. H., and Lawrence, J. S. Studies on the sulfhydryl content of human leukocytes and erythrocytes, *Am. J. Med. Sci.* 228:73, 1954.

237. Hardin, E. B., Valentine, W. N., Follette, J. H., and Lawrence, J. S. Esterase and lipase activity of leukocytes and erythrocytes in health and disease, *Am. J. Med. Sci.* 229:397, 1955.

238. Harris, J. W. Vitamin B_{12} levels in pernicious anaemia, *Lancet* 2:285, 1952.

239. Hartman, J., and Reidenberg, M. Comparison of the glycolytic activity of blood and exudate leucocytes, *J. Appl. Physiol.* 12:477, 1958.

240. Hartman, J. D., and Goretsky, D. M. Changes in the glycolytic activity of blood and exudate leukocytes during an inflammatory reaction, *Anat. Rec.* 138:149, 1960.

241. Hartman, W. J., Clark, W. G., and Cyr, S. D. Histidine decarboxylase activity of basophils from chronic myelogenous leukemic patients. Origin of blood histamine, *Proc. Soc. Exp. Biol. Med.* 107:123, 1961.

242. Heinemann, M. Distribution of ascorbic acid between cells and serum of human blood, *J. Clin. Invest.* 20:39, 1941.

243. Heinemann, M. The influences of erythrocytes and of leukocytes on stability and transfer of ascorbic acid in human blood, *J. Clin. Invest.* 20:467, 1941.

244. Hempling, H. G. K and Na content in dogfish leukocytes, *Biol. Bull.* 103:303, 1952.

245. Hempling, H. G. Potassium loss in rabbit leukocytes in response to mechanical agitation, *J. Cellular Comp. Physiol.* 40:161, 1952.

246. Hempling, H. G. Potassium and sodium movements in rabbit polymorphonuclear leukocytes, *J. Cellular Comp. Physiol.* 44:87, 1954.

247. Henry, P., Reich, P., Karon, M., and Weissman, S. M. Characteristics of RNA synthesized in vitro by lymphocytes of chronic lymphocytic leukemia, *J. Lab. Clin. Med.* 69:47, 1967.

248. Hiatt, R. B., Engle, C., Flood, C., and Karush, A. The role of the granulocyte as a source of lysozyme in ulcerative colitis, *J. Clin. Invest.* 31:721, 1952.

249. Hieber, F. R., Boyer, P. D., and Hagen, P. S. The nature of glucose 6-phosphate inhibition of hexokinase from normal and leukemic leukocytes, *Clin. Res.* 9:161, 1961.

250. Hirsch, J. G., and Cohn, Z. A. Digestive and autolytic functions of lysosomes in phagocytic cells, *Fed. Proc.* 23:1023, 1964.

251. Hirschhorn, R., Hirschhorn, K., and Weissmann, G. Appearance of hydrolase-rich granules in human lymphocytes induced by phytohemagglutinin and antigens, *Blood* 30:84, 1967.

252. Hirschhorn, R., and Weissmann, G. Isolation and properties of human leukocyte lysosomes *in vitro*, *Proc. Soc. Exp. Biol. Med.* 119:36, 1965.

253. Hoch, F. L., and Vallee, B. L. Extraction of zinc-containing protein from human leucocytes, *J. Biol. Chem.* 195:531, 1952.

254. Holmes, B., Page, A. R., and Good, R. A. Studies of the metabolic activity of leukocytes from patients with a genetic abnormality of phagocytic function, *J. Clin. Invest.* 46:1422, 1967.

255. Horn, R. G., and Spicer, S. S. Sulfated mucopolysaccharide and basic protein in certain granules of rabbit leucocytes, *Lab. Invest.* 13:1, 1964.

256. Hülsman, W. C., Oei, T. L., and van Creveld, S. Phosphorylase activity in leukocytes from patients with glycogen storage disease, *Lancet* ii:581, 1961.

257. Husfeldt, E. Proteolytische Enzyme in den Leukocyten des Menschen, *Z. Physiol. Chem.* 194:137, 1931.

258. Ignarro, L. J., and Colombo, C. Enzyme release from polymorphonuclear leukocyte lysosomes: regulation by autonomic drugs and cyclic

nucleotides, *Science* 180:1181, 1973.

259. Introzzi, P., Notario, A., and Nespoli, M. Su alcune particularitá biochemiche del leucocita leucemico, *Haematol. Arch.* 46:401, 1961.

260. Iyer, G. Y. N. Free amino acids in leukocytes from normal and leukemic subjects, *J. Lab. Clin. Med.* 54:229, 1959.

261. Iyer, G. Y. N., Islam, M. F., and Quastel, J. H. Biochemical aspects of phagocytosis, *Nature* 192:535, 1961.

262. Iyer, G. Y. N., and Quastel, J. H. NADPH and NADH oxidation by guinea pig polymorphonuclear leucocytes, *Can. J. Biochem. Physiol.* 41:427, 1963.

263. Izak, G., Wilner, T., and Mager, J. Amino acid activating enzymes in red blood cells of normal, anemic and polycythemic subjects, *J. Clin. Invest.* 39:1763, 1960.

264. Jago, M. A simple method for the separation of living lymphocytes from human blood, *Br. J. Haematol.* 2:439, 1956.

265. James, A. T., Lovelock, J. E., and Webb, J. P. W. The lipids of whole blood. I. Lipid biosynthesis in human blood *in vitro*, *Biochem. J.* 73:106, 1959.

266. Jamison, C. E., and Gordon, M. P. The formation of 8-hydroxypurine from purine by rat liver extracts, *Biochim. Biophys. Acta* 72:106, 1963.

267. Jobling, J. W., and Stronse, S. Studies in ferment action. II. The extent of leucocytic proteolysis, *J. Exp. Med.* 16:269, 1912.

268. Johnson, J. M., and Garvin, J. E. Separation of lymphocytes in human blood by means of glass wool columns, *Proc. Soc. Exp. Biol. Med.* 102:333, 1959.

269. Justice, P., Shih, L., Gordon, J., Grossman, A., and Hsia, D. Y. Characterization of leukocyte glucose-6-phosphate dehydrogenase in normal and mutant human subjects, *J. Lab. Clin. Med.* 68:552, 1966.

270. Kalant, H., and Schucher, R. Concentration of galactose by leucocytes, *Can. J. Biochem. Physiol.* 41:849, 1963.

271. Kampine, J. P., Brady, R. O., Kanfer, J. N., Feld, M., and Shapiro, D. Diag-

nosis of Gaucher's disease and Niemann-Pick disease with small samples of venous blood, *Science* 155:86, 1967.

272. Kampine, J. P., Brady, R. O., Yankee, R. A., Kanfer, J. N., Shapiro, D., and Gal, A. E. Sphingolipid metabolism in leukemic leukocytes, *Cancer Res.* 27:1312, 1967.

273. Kandel, E. V., and LeRoy, G. V. The blood gluthathione in hematologic diseases, *J. Lab. Clin. Med.* 24:669, 1939.

274. Kaplow, L. S. A histochemical procedure for localizing and evaluating leukocyte alkaline phosphatase activity in smears of blood and marrow, *Blood* 10:1023, 1955.

275. Karnovsky, M. L. Metabolic shifts in leucocytes during the phagocytic event, *in* G. E. W. Wolstenholme and M. O'Connor (eds.), Ciba Foundation Study Group 10, Biological Activity of the Leucocyte, p. 60, Little, Brown and Co., Boston, 1961.

276. Karnovsky, M. L. Metabolic basis of phagocytic activity, *Physiol. Rev.* 42:143, 1962.

277. Karnovsky, M. L., and Sbarra, A. J. Metabolic changes accompanying the ingestion of particulate matter by cells, *Am. J. Clin. Nutr.* 8:147, 1960.

278. Karnovsky, M. L., and Wallach, D. F. H. The metabolic basis of phagocytosis. III. Incorporation of inorganic phosphate into various classes of phosphatides during phagocytosis, *J. Biol. Chem.* 236:1895, 1961.

279. Katz, J., and Wood, H. G. The use of glucose-C^{14} for the evaluation of the pathways of glucose metabolism, *J. Biol. Chem.* 235:2165, 1960.

280. Kay, H. D. Plasma-phosphatase in osteitis deformans and in other diseases of bone, *Br. J. Exp. Pathol.* 10:253, 1929.

281. Keibl, E., and Spitzy, K. H. Zum Problem des Leukozytenstoffwechsels, *Arch. Exp. Pathol. Pharmakol.* 213:162, 1951.

282. Kempner, W. The nature of leukemic blood cells as determined by their metabolism, *J. Clin. Invest.* 18:291, 1939.

283. Kenny, J. J., and Moloney, W. C. Leukocytic alkaline phosphatase. Behavior during prolonged incuba-

tion and infection in normal and leukemic leukocytes, *Blood* 12:295, 1957.

284. Kerby, G. P. The occurrence of acid mucopolysaccharides in human leukocytes, *J. Clin. Invest.* 34:944, 1955.

285. Ketchel, M. M. Physiological and radio-isotopic evidence for the binding of hydrocortisone by human leucocytes *in vitro*, *Endocrinology* 69:60, 1961.

286. Kidson, C. Lipid synthesis in human leucocytes in acute leukaemia, *Australas. Ann. Med.* 10:282, 1961.

287. Kidson, C. Relation of leucocyte lipid metabolism to cell age: studies in infective leucocytosis, *Br. J. Exp. Pathol.* 42:597, 1961.

288. Kidson, C. Leucocyte lipid metabolism in myeloproliferative states, *Australas. Ann. Med.* 11:50, 1962.

289. Kint, J. A. Fabry's disease: alphagalactosidase deficiency, *Science* 167:1268, 1970.

290. Kiss, K., Astaldi, G., and Airo, R. The RNA nucleotide composition in human leukocytes from normal and leukemic cases, *Blood* 30:707, 1967.

291. Kit, S. The nucleic acids of normal tissues and tumors, *in* John T. Edsall (ed.), Amino Acids, Proteins and Cancer Biochemistry, p. 147, Academic Press, New York, 1960.

292. Klebanoff, S. J. A peroxidasemediated antimicrobial system in leukocytes, *J. Clin. Invest.* 46:1078, 1967 (abstract).

293. Klebanoff, S. J. Iodination of bacteria: A bactericidal mechanism, *J. Exp. Med.* 126:1063, 1967.

294. Klebanoff, S. J., Clem, W. H., and Luebke, R. G. The peroxidasethiocyanate-hydrogen peroxide antimicrobial system, *Biochim. Biophys. Acta* 117:63, 1966.

295. Klebs, E. Die pyrogene Substanz, *Zentralbl. Med. Wiss.* 6:417, 1868.

296. Kleinmann, H., and Scharr, G. Untersuchungen über tierische Gewebsproteasen. VIII. Über proteolytische Fermente in der weissen Blutkörperschen verscheidener Tieraten, *Biochem. Z.* 251:275, 1932.

297. Kline, D. L. A modification of Ottsen's method for the separation of granulocytes from lymphocytes, *J. Lab. Clin. Med.* 46:781, 1955.

298. Kochakian, C. D., Keutmann, E. H., and Garber, E. E. Studies on blood arginase, *Conf. Metabol. Aspects Convalescence, Tr.* 17:187, 1948.

299. Koler, R. D., Seaman, A. J., Osgood, E. E., and Vanbellinghen, P. Myeloproliferative diseases. Diagnostic value of the leukocyte alkaline phosphatase test, *Am. J. Clin. Pathol.* 30:295, 1958.

300. Kornberg, A., Lieberman, I., and Simms, E. S. Enzymatic synthesis of purine nucleotides, *J. Biol. Chem.* 215:417, 1955.

301. Krebs, H. A., and Orström, A. Microdetermination of hypoxanthine and xanthine, *Biochem. J.* 33:984, 1939.

302. Kresse, H. Mucopolysaccharidosis IIIA (San Filippo A disease): deficiency of heparin sulfamidase in skin fibroblasts and leucocytes, *Biochem. Biophys. Res. Commun.* 54:1111, 1973.

303. Kretchmer, N., Stone, M., and Bauer, C. Hereditary enzymatic effects as illustrated by hypophosphatasia, *Ann. N.Y. Acad. Sci.* 75:279, 1958.

304. Kržalic, Lj., Mandic, V., and Mihailović, Lj. Nucleoside phosphorylase activity in guinea pig polymorphonuclear leukocytes, *Experientia* 18:369, 1962.

305. Kurland, G. S., Krotkov, M. V., and Friedburg, A. S. Oxygen consumption and thyroxine deiodination by human leukocytes, *J. Clin. Endocrinol.* 20:35, 1960.

306. Lacher, M. J., and Ley, A. B. The value of leukocyte alkaline phosphatase determinations in the malignant lymphomas, *Cancer* 17:402, 1964.

307. Lajtha, L. G., and Vane, J. R. Dependence of bone marrow cells on the liver for purine supply, *Nature* 182:191, 1958.

308. Lambers, K., and Eggstein, M. Der Fettgehalt der Granulocyten und ihrer Vorstufen unter normalen und pathologischen Bedingungen, *Verh. Dtsch. Ges. Inn. Med.* 65:191, 1959.

309. Larizza, P. Beitrag zur Kenntnis der chemischen Zusammensetzung der weissen Blutzellen des menschlichen Blutes, *Z. Ges. Exp. Med.* 101:615, 1937.

310. Laszlo, J. Energy metabolism of human leukemic lymphocytes and granulocytes, *Blood* 30:151, 1967.

311. Lazarus, G., Brown, R. S., Daniels, J. R., and Fullmer, H. M. Human granulocyte collagenase, *Science* 159:1483, 1968.

312. Lehrer, R. I., and Cline, M. J. Leukocyte myeloperoxidase deficiency and disseminated candidiasis: the role of myeloperoxidase in resistance to candida infection, *J. Clin. Invest.* 48:1478, 1969.

313. Leikin, S. L. Glycogen content of normal lymphocytes, *Proc. Soc. Exp. Biol. Med.* 106:286, 1961.

314. Leloir, L. F. The metabolism of hexosephosphates, *in* W. D. McElroy and B. Glass (eds.), Phosphorus Metabolism, p. 67, Johns Hopkins University Press, Baltimore, 1951.

315. Leloir, L. F., Olavarria, J. M., Goldemberg, S. H., and Carminatti, H. Biosynthesis of glycogen from uridine diphosphate glucose, *Arch. Biochem. Biophys.* 81:508, 1959.

316. Leonard, B. J., Israels, M. C. G., and Wilkinson, J. F. Alkaline phosphatase in the white cells in leukaemia and leukaemoid reaction, *Lancet* 1:289, 1958.

317. Leslie, I. The nucleic acid content of tissues and cells, *in* E. Chargaff and J. N. Davidson (eds.), The Nucleic Acids, vol. 2, p. 1, Academic Press, New York, 1955.

318. Leupold, F., and Kremer, G. Zur Biosynthese der Polyenfettsäuren in menschlichen Vollblut, *Z. Physiol. Chem.* 324:226, 1961.

319. Levene, P. A., and Meyer, G. M. The action of leukocytes on glucose, *J. Biol. Chem.* 11:361, 1912.

320. Levene, P. A., and Meyer, G. M. On the action of leukocytes on glucose, *J. Biol. Chem.* 12:265, 1912.

321. Levene, P. A., and Meyer, G. M. On the action of leukocytes on hexoses, IV. On the mechanism of lactic acid formation, *J. Biol. Chem.* 14:551, 1913.

322. Lichtenstein, L. M., and Margolis, S. Histamine release *in vitro*: inhibition by catecholamines and methylxanthines, *Science* 161:902, 1968.

323. Ljungdahl, L., Wood, H. G., Racker, E., and Couri, D. Formation of unequally labeled fructose 6-phosphate by an exchange reaction catalyzed by transaldolase, *J. Biol. Chem.* 236:1622, 1961.

324. Löhr, G. W., and Waller, H. D. Zellstoffwechsel und Zellalterung, *Klin. Wochenschr.* 37:833, 1959.

325. Longcope, W. T., and Donhauser, J. L. A study of the proteolytic ferments of the large lymphocytes in a case of acute leukemia, *J. Exp. Med.* 10:618, 1908.

326. Lovelock, J. E., James, A. T., and Rowe, C. E. The lipids of whole blood II. The exchange of lipids between the cellular constituents and the lipoproteins of human blood, *Biochem. J.* 74:137, 1960.

327. Lowry, O. H., Bessey, O. A., Brock, M. J., and Lopez, J. A. The interrelationship of dietary serum, white blood cell and total body ascorbic acid, *J. Biol. Chem.* 166:111, 1946.

328. Lubschez, R. Studies in ascorbic acid with especial reference to the white layer. I. Description of method and comparison of ascorbic acid levels in whole blood, plasma, red cells and white layer, *J. Clin. Invest.* 24:573, 1945.

329. McKinney, G. R. Glyoxalase activity in human leukocytes, *Arch. Biochem. Biophys.* 46:246, 1953.

330. McKinney, G. R., and Gocke, D. J. Determination of glyoxalase activity, *J. Biol. Chem.* 219:605, 1956.

331. McKinney, G. R., Martin, S. P., Rundles, R. W., and Green, R. Respiration and glycolytic activities of human leukocytes in vitro, *J. Appl. Physiol.* 5:335, 1953.

332. McKinney, G. R., and Rundles, R. W. Lactate formation and glyoxalase activity in normal and leukemic leukocytes *in vitro, Cancer Res.* 16:67, 1956.

333. MacLeod, J., and Rhoads, C. Metabolism of leucocytes in Ringer-phosphate and in serum, *Proc. Soc. Exp. Biol. Med.* 41:268, 1939.

334. McMenamy, R. H., Lund, C. C., Neville, G. J., and Wallach, D. F. H. Studies of unbound amino acid distribution in plasma, erythrocytes, leukocytes and urine of normal human subjects, *J. Clin. Invest.* 39:1675, 1960.

335. McMenamy, R. H., Lund, C. C., and Wallach, D. F. H. Unbound amino acid concentrations in plasma, erythrocytes, leukocytes and urine

of patients with leukemia, *J. Clin. Invest.* 39:1688, 1960.

336. McRipley, R. J., and Sbarra, A. J. Role of the phagocyte in host-parasite interactions: XI. Relationship between stimulated oxidative metabolism and hydrogen peroxide formation, and intracellular killing, *J. Bacteriol.* 94:1417, 1967.

337. Majerus, P. W., and Lastra, R. R. Fatty acid biosynthesis in human leukocytes, *J. Clin. Invest.* 46:1596, 1967.

338. Malawista, S. E. The action of colchicine in acute gout, *Arthritis Rheum.* 8:752, 1965.

339. Mandel, P., and Métais, P. Sur la constance de l'acide désoxypentose-nucléique des leukocytes chez l'homme, *Bull. Acad. Natl. Med. (Paris)* 134:449, 1950.

340. Manery, J. F., Fisher, K. C., Gourley, D. R. H., Wilson, D. L., and Taylor, M. F. J. The influence of carbohydrate and insulin on the potassium content of leucocytes and muscle, *Biol. Bull.* 99:312, 1950.

341. Manganiello, V., Evans, W. H., Stossel, T. P., Mason, R. J., and Vaughn, M. The effect of polystyrene beads on cyclic 3',5'-adenosine monophosphate concentration in leukocytes, *J. Clin. Invest.* 50:2741, 1971.

342. Marinelarena, R. The effects of various chemical substances and bacteria on the glycolytic and respiratory activities of leukocytes (Ph.D. dissertation), University of Michigan, 1950.

343. Marks, P. A., and Gellhorn, A. Lipid synthesis in human leukocytes and erythrocytes *in vitro*, *Fed. Proc.* 18:281, 1959.

344. Marks, P. A., Gellhorn, A., and Kidson, C. Lipid synthesis in human leukocytes, platelets and erythrocytes, *J. Biol. Chem.* 235:2579, 1960.

345. Marsh, J. C., and Perry, S. Thymidine catabolism by normal and leukemic human leukocytes, *J. Clin. Invest.* 43:267, 1964.

346. Martin, S. P., McKinney, G. R., and Green, R. The metabolism of human polymorphonuclear leukocytes, *Ann. N.Y. Acad. Sci.* 59:996, 1955.

347. Martin, S. P., McKinney, G. R., Green, R., and Becker, C. Effect of glucose, fructose and insulin on the leukocytes of diabetes, *J. Clin. Invest.* 32:1171, 1953.

348. Massa, V. Acide ascorbique et metabolisme respiratoire des leukocytes, *Bull. Soc. Chim. Biol.* 29:732, 1947.

349. Mateles, R. I., Baruah, J. N., and Tannenbaum, S. R. Increased cystine in leukocytes from individuals homozygous and heterozygous for cystinosis, *Science* 157:1321, 1967.

350. Mathies, J. C. Preparation and properties of highly purified alkaline phosphatase from swine kidneys, *J. Biol. Chem.* 233:1121, 1958.

351. May, C. D., Levine, B. B., and Weissmann, G. Effects of compounds which inhibit antigenic release of histamine and phagocytic release of lysosomal enzyme on glucose utilization by leukocytes in humans, *Proc. Soc. Exp. Biol. Med.* 133:758, 1970.

352. Melmon, K. L., Bourne, H. R., Weinstein, J., and Sela, M. Receptors for histamine can be detected on the surface of selected leukocytes, *Science* 177:707, 1972.

353. Melmon, K. L., and Cline, M. J. Interaction of plasma kinins and granulocytes, *Nature* 213:90, 1967.

354. Melmon, K. L., and Cline, M. J. The interaction of leukocytes and the kinin system, *Biochem. Pharmacol.* 271, 1968 (suppl.).

355. Melmon, K. L., Cline, M. J., Hughes, T., and Nies, A. S. Kinins: possible mediators of neonatal circulatory changes in man, *J. Clin. Invest.* 47:1295, 1968.

356. Merten, R., and Winschuh, M. L- and D-Dipeptidasen in den Formelementen des menschlichen Blutes, *Z. Vitamin-Hormon-Ferment-Forsch.* 1:351, 1947.

357. Métais, P., Cuny, S., and Mandel, P. La teneur en acide pentose-nucléique des leucocytes chez diverses espéces de mammifères et en particulier chez l'homme, *C. R. Soc. Biol. (Paris)* 145:1235, 1951.

358. Métais, P., and Mandel, P. La teneur en acide désoxypentose-nucléique des leucocytes chez l'homme normal et à l'état pathologique, *C. R. Soc. Biol. (Paris)* 144:277, 1950.

359. Meyer, L. M., Bertcher, R. W., and Cronkite, E. P. Serum Co^{60} vitamin B$_{12}$ binding capacity in some haematologic disorders, *Proc. Soc. Exp. Biol. Med.* 96:360, 1957.

360. Meyer, L. M., Cronkite, E. P., Miller, I. F., Mulzoc, C. W., and Jones, I. Co^{60} vitamin B$_{12}$ binding capacity of human leukocytes, *Blood* 19:229, 1962.

361. Milne, J. S., Lonergan, M. E., Williamson, E. M., Moore, F. M. L., McMaster, R., and Percy, N. Leukocyte ascorbic acid levels and vitamin C intake in older people, *Br. Med. J.* 4:383, 1971.

362. Minakami, S. Studies on leukocyte metabolism: I. Glycolytic intermediates and nucleotides in guinea pig exudate granulocytes, *J. Biochem. Japan* 63:83, 1968.

363. Miras, C. J., Mantzos, J. D., and Levis, G. M. Fatty acid synthesis in human leukocytes, *Biochem. Biophys. Res. Commun.* 19:79, 1965.

364. Miras, C. J., Mantzos, J. D., and Levis, G. M. The isolation and partial characterization of glycolipids of normal human leukocytes, *Biochem. J.* 98:782, 1966.

365. Misra, D. K. A direct assay for dihydrofolate reductase in human leukocytes, *Blood* 23:572, 1964.

366. Misra, D. K., Humphreys, S. R., Friedkin, M., Goldin, A., and Crawford, E. J. Dihydrofolate reductase activities in tissues of mice with antifolate-sensitive and antifolate-resistant leukemia, *Fed. Proc.* 19:398, 1960.

367. Mitus, W. J., Mednicoff, I. B., and Dameshek, W. Alkaline phosphatase of mature neutrophils in various "polycythemias," *N. Engl. J. Med.* 260:1131, 1959.

368. Mohler, D. N., and Leavell, B. S. Aplastic anemia: an analysis of 50 cases, *Ann. Intern. Med.* 49:326, 1958.

369. Mollin, D. L., and Ross, G. I. M. Serum vitamin B$_{12}$ concentrations in leukaemia and in some other haematological conditions, *Br. J. Haematol.* 1:155, 1955.

370. Moloney, W. C. Leukocyte alkaline phosphatase activity in the rat, *Ann. N.Y. Acad. Sci.* 75:31, 1958.

371. Moore, W. T., Rodarte, J., and Smith, L. H., Jr. Urea synthesis by hemic cells, *Clin. Chem.* 10:1059, 1964.

372. Morrison, J. H. Separation of lymphocytes of rat bone marrow by combined glass-wool filtration and dextran-gradient centrifugation, *Br. J. Haematol.* 13:229, 1967.

373. Mounter, L. A., and Atiyeh, W. Proteases of human leukocytes, *Blood* 15:52, 1960.

374. Müller, E., and Jochmann, G. Über eine einfache Methode zum Nachweis proteolytischer Fermentwirkungen, *Munch. Med. Wochenschr.* 53:1394, 1906.

375. Müller, E., and Jochmann, G. Über proteolytische Fermentwirkungen der Leukozyten, *Munch. Med. Wochenschr.* 53:1507, 1906.

376. Nadler, H. L., and Egan, T. J. Deficiency of lysosomal acid phosphatase, *N. Engl. J. Med.* 282:302, 1970.

377. Nadler, S. B., Hansen, H. J., Sprague, C. C., and Sherman, H. The effect of 6-mercaptopurine on the incorporation of labeled amino acids into cellular protein of chronic granulocytic leukemia leukocytes, *Blood* 18:336, 1961.

378. Nees, F. Über die lipolytische Fähigkeit der weissen Blutkorperchen, *Biochem. Z.* 124:156, 1921.

379. Nelson, R. A., Jr., and Lebrun, J. The requirement for antibody and complement for *in vitro* phagocytosis of starch granules, *J. Hyg.* 54:8, 1956.

380. Nir, E., Efrati, P., and Danon, D. The osmotic fragility of human leucocytes in normal and in some pathological conditions, *Br. J. Haematol.* 18:237, 1970.

381. Noble, E. P., Stjernholm, R. L., and Ljungdahl, L. Carbohydrate metabolism in leukocytes. III. Carbon dioxide incorporation in the rabbit polymorphonuclear leukocyte, *Biochim. Biophys. Acta* 49:593, 1961.

382. Noble, E. P., Stjernholm, R. L., and Weisberger, A. S. Carbohydrate metabolism in the leukocyte. I. The pathway of two- and three-carbon compounds in the rabbit polymorphonuclear leukocyte, *J. Biol. Chem.* 235:1261, 1960.

383. Noble, E. P., Stjernholm, R. L., and Weisberger, A. S. Carbohydrate metabolism in lymphocytic leukemia leukocytes, *Blood* 17:361, 1961.

384. Nour-Eldin, F., and Wilkinson, J. F. Amino acid content of white blood cells in human leukaemias, *Br. J. Haematol.* 1:358, 1955.

385. Nungester, W. J., and Ames, A. M. The relationship between ascorbic acid and phagocytic activity, *J. Infect. Dis.* 83:50, 1948.

386. O'Brien, J. S., and Walsh, J. R. Folinic acid activity in leukocytes, *Proc. Soc. Exp. Biol. Med.* 109:843, 1962.

387. O'Donnell, V. J., Ottolenghi, P., Malkin, A., Denstedt, O. F., and Heard, R. D. H. The biosynthesis from acetate-1-C[14] of fatty acids and cholesterol in formed blood elements, *Can. J. Biochem. Physiol.* 36:1125, 1958.

388. Oelkers, H. A. Untersuchungen über Fermente der Lymphocyten, *Arch. Exp. Pathol. Pharmakol.* 161:344, 1931.

389. Ohta, H. A biochemical study on the neutrophilic granules isolated in a pure state from leukocyte homogenate, *Acta Haematol. Jap.* 27:555, 1964.

390. Okada, S., and Hayashi, T. Studies on the amino-acid nitrogen content of the blood, *J. Biol. Chem.* 51:121, 1922.

391. Opie, E. L. Enzymes and anti-enzymes of inflammatory exudates, *J. Exp. Med.* 7:316, 1905.

392. Opie, E. L. Intracellular digestion. The enzymes and anti-enzymes concerned, *Physiol. Rev.* 2:552, 1922.

393. Osserman, E. F., and Lawlor, D. P. Serum and urinary lysozyme (muramidase) in monocytic and monomyelocytic leukemia, *J. Exp. Med.* 124:921, 1966.

394. Pantlitschko, M., and Stattmann, K. Die proteolytischen Enzyme der weissen Blutkörperchen, *Biochem. Z.* 326:252, 1955.

395. Parker, E. P., and Kracke, R. R. Further studies on experimental granulopenia with particular reference to sulfhydryl (glutathione) metabolism in blood dyscrasias, *Am. J. Clin. Pathol.* 6:41, 1936.

396. Pastore, E. J., and Lionetti, F. J. Incorporation of acetate into lipids of human leukocytes, *Fed. Proc.* 17:287, 1958.

397. Pastore, E. J., and Lionetti, F. J. Biosynthesis of long-chain fatty acids from acetate-1-C[14] by a cell-free system from human leukocytes, *Fed. Proc.* 18:299, 1959.

398. Penman, S. Ribonucleic acid metabolism in mammalian cells, *N. Engl. J. Med.* 276:502, 1967.

399. Perillie, P. E., and Finch, S. C. Leukocyte alkaline phosphatase activity in acute leukemia, *Clin. Res.* 9:164 1961.

400. Perillie, P. E., Kaplan, S. S., Lefkowitz, E., Rogaway, W., and Finch, S. C. Studies of muramidase (lysozyme) in leukemia, *J.A.M.A.* 203:317, 1968.

401. Perretta, M., and Pieber-Perretta, M. Evidence for a species difference in the pattern of C[14]-formate incorporation into marrow nucleic acids *in vitro*, *Biochim. Biophys. Acta* 61:828, 1962.

402. Perry, S., and Marsh, J. C. The effect of normal and leukemic human leukocytes on the uptake of thymidine by leukemic cells, *Blood* 22:821, 1963.

403. Petrakis, N. L. Microspectrophotometric estimation of the desoxyribonucleic acid (DNA) content of individual normal and leukemic human lymphocytes, *Blood* 8:905, 1953.

404. Piez, K. A., and Eagle, H. The free amino acid pool of cultured human cells, *J. Biol. Chem.* 231:533, 1958.

405. Pisciotta, A. V., and Daly, M. The reduced glutathione (GSH) content of leukocytes in various hematologic diseases, *Blood* 15:421, 1960.

406. Platt, R. The blood glutathione in disease, *Br. J. Exp. Pathol.* 12:139, 1931.

407. Plum, C. M. Die alkalische Phosphatase in den Zellen des normalen und pathologischen Knochemarkes und des peripheren Blutes, *Acta Haemctol.* 4:73, 1950.

408. Polli, E. E., Rosoff, M., DiMajorca, G., and Cavalieri, L. F. Physicochemical characterization of deoxyribonucleic acids from human leukemic leukocytes, *Cancer Res.* 19:159, 1959.

409. Polli, E. E., and Shooter, K. V. The sedimentation characteristics of deoxyribonucleic acid from normal and diseased human tissues, *Biochem. J.* 69:398, 1958.

410. Ponder, E., and MacLeod, J. The effect of hemolytic substances on

white cell respiration, *J. Gen. Physiol.* 20:267, 1936.

411. Prager, M. D., Malicky, M., Goerner, M., and Hill, H. M. Riboflavin activity in normal and leukemic human leukocytes and nuclei, *J. Lab. Clin. Med.* 53:926, 1959.

412. Prager, M. D., Young, J. E., and Atkins, I. C. A study of the possible role of feedback inhibition of aspartate transcarbamylase in regulation of pyrimidine synthesis in human leukocytes, *J. Lab. Clin. Med.* 70:768, 1967.

413. Pruzansky, J. J., and Patterson, R. Stability of human leukocyte granules which contain histamine, *J. Immunol.* 100:1165, 1968.

414. Pruzansky, J. J., and Patterson, R. Histamine in human leukocytes, *Int. Arch. Allergy Appl. Immunol.* 37:98, 1970.

415. Pulver, R., and Verzar, F. Kalium- und Kohlhydrat-Stoffwechsel der Leukocyten, *Helv. Chim. Acta* 24:272, 1941.

416. Rabinowitz, Y. Separation of lymphocytes, polymorphonuclear leukocytes, and monocytes on glass columns, including tissue culture observations, *Blood* 23:811, 1964.

417. Rabinowitz, Y., Farmer, R., and Czebotar, V. Deoxycytidine pathway in separated normal and leukemic leukocytes with effects of cell culture, *Blood* 38:312, 1971.

418. Raccuglia, G., and Sacks, M. S. Vitamin B_{12} binding capacity of normal and leukemic sera, *J. Lab. Clin. Med.* 50:69, 1957.

419. Racker, E. Glutathione as a coenzyme in intermediary metabolism, *in* S. Colowick (ed.), Glutathione, p. 165, Academic Press, New York, 1954.

420. Ralli, E. P., and Sherry, S. The effect of insulin on the metabolism of vitamin C, *Am. J. Physiol.* 133:418, 1941.

421. Ralli, E. P., and Sherry, S. Adult scurvy and metabolism of vitamin C, *Medicine* 20:251, 1941.

422. Ramot, B., Fisher, S., Szeinberg, A., Adam, A., Sheba, C., and Gafni, D. A study of subjects with erythrocyte glucose-6-phosphate dehydrogenase deficiency. II. Investigation of leukocyte enzymes. *J. Clin. Invest.* 38:2234, 1959.

423. Rauch, H. C., Loomis, M. E., Johnson, M. E., and Favour, C. B. *In vitro* suppression of polymorphonuclear leukocyte and lymphocyte glycolysis by cortisol, *Endocrinology* 68:375, 1961.

424. Rebuck, J. W. The functions of the white blood cells, *Am. J. Clin. Pathol.* 17:614, 1947.

425. Rechcigl, M., Jr., and Evans, W. H. Role of catalase and peroxidase in the metabolism of leucocytes, *Nature* 199:1001, 1963.

426. Reisman, L. E., Mitani, M., and Zuelzer, W. W. Chromosome studies in leukemia. I. Evidence for the origin of leukemic stem lines from aneuploid mutants, *N. Engl. J. Med.* 270:591, 1964.

427. Remmele, V. W. Atmung und Glykolyse der Leukocyten, *Acta Haematol.* 13:103, 1955.

428. Reynolds, J., Follette, J. H., and Valentine, W. N. The arginase activity of erythrocytes and leukocytes with particular reference to pernicious anemia and thalassemia major, *J. Lab. Clin. Med.* 50:78, 1957.

429. Rheingold, J. J., and Wislocki, G. B. Histochemical methods applied to hematology, *Blood* 3:641, 1948.

430. Rigas, D. A. Electrolyte, nitrogen and water content of human leukemic leukocytes: relation to cell maturity, *J. Lab. Clin. Med.* 58:234, 1961.

431. Rigas, D., Duerst, M. L., Jump, M. E., and Osgood, E. E. The nucleic acids and other phosphorus compounds of human leukemic leukocytes: relation to cell maturity, *J. Lab. Clin. Med.* 48:356, 1956.

432. Rigas, D. A., and Osgood, E. E. Phosphorus compounds of human leukemic leucocytes: relation to cell maturity, *Fed. Proc.* 14:269, 1955.

433. Riley, J. F. Histamine in tissue mast cells, *Science* 118:332, 1953.

434. Riley, J. F. Functional significance of histamine and heparin in tissue mast cells, *Ann. N.Y. Acad. Sci.* 103:151, 1963.

435. Roberts, E., and Frankel, S. Free amino acids in normal and neoplastic tissues of mice as studied by paper chromatography, *Cancer Res.* 9:645, 1949.

436. Roberts, J., and Quastel, J. H. Oxidation of reduced triphosphopyri-

dine nucleotide by guinea pig polymorphonuclear leucocytes, *Nature* 202:85, 1964.

437. Roche, J. Blood-phosphatases, *Biochem. J.* 25:1724, 1931.

438. Rosenberg, L. E., and Downing, S. Transport of neutral and dibasic amino acids by human leukocytes: absence of a defect in cystinuria, *J. Clin. Invest.* 44:1382, 1965.

439. Rosner, F., and Lee, S. L. Zinc and magnesium content of leukocyte alkaline phosphatase isoenzymes, *J. Lab. Clin. Med.* 79:228, 1972.

440. Ross, J. F., Ebaugh, F. G., Jr., and Talbot, T. R., Jr. Radioisotopic studies of zinc metabolism in human subjects, *Trans. Assoc. Am. Physicians* 71:322, 1958.

441. Rossi, F., and Zatti, M. Pathway of glucose oxidation in leukocytes, *Exp. Cell Res.* 25:182, 1961.

442. Rossiter, R. J., and Wong, E. Esterase of rabbit polymorphonuclear leucocytes, *J. Biol. Chem.* 180:933, 1949.

443. Rossiter, R. J., and Wong, E. β-glucuronidase of human white blood cells, *Blood* 5:864, 1950.

444. Rossiter, R. J., and Wong, E. β-glucuronidase of rabbit polymorphonuclear leukocytes, *Can. J. Res.* 28:69, 1950.

445. Rouser, G. Free or easily extractable amino acids in blood cells and body fluids, *in* J. W. Rebuck, F. H. Bethell, and R. W. Monto (eds.), The Leukemias, p. 361, Academic Press, New York, 1957.

446. Rowe, C. E. The biosynthesis of phospholipids by human blood cells, *Biochem. J.* 73:438, 1959.

447. Rowe, C. E. The phospholipids of human blood plasma and their exchange with the cells, *Biochem. J.* 76:471, 1960.

448. Rowe, C. E., Allison, A. C., and Lovelock, J. E. Lipid biosynthesis in human blood. The incorporation of acetate into lipids by different types of human-blood cells, *Biochem. J.* 74:26P, 1960.

449. Rubini, J. R., Westcott, E., and Keller, S. *In vitro* DNA labeling of bone marrow and leukemic blood leukocytes with tritiated thymidine: II. H^3 thymidine biochemistry *in vitro*, *J. Lab. Clin. Med.* 68:566, 1966.

450. Rutenberg, A. M., and Rosales, C. L.

A histochemical method for the demonstration of leucocyte naphthylamidase using two substrates: alanyl- and methionyl-4-methoxy-2-naphthylamide, *Br. J. Haematol.* 12:595, 1966.

451. Salmon, S. E., Cline, M. J., Schultz, J., and Lehrer, R. I. Myeloperoxidase deficiency: immunologic study of a genetic leukocyte defect, *N. Engl. J. Med.* 282:250, 1970.

452. Sandberg, A. A., Koepf, G. F., Crosswhite, L. H., and Hauschka, T. S. Chromosome constitution of human marrow in various developmental and blood disorders, *Am. J. Hum. Genet.* 12:231, 1960.

453. Sbarra, A. J., and Karnovsky, M. L. The biochemical basis of phagocytosis. I. Metabolic changes during the ingestion of particles by polymorphonuclear leukocytes, *J. Biol. Chem.* 234:1355, 1959.

454. Sbarra, A. J., and Karnovsky, M. L. The biochemical basis of phagocytosis. II. Incorporation of C[14]-labeled building blocks into lipid, protein, and glycogen of leukocytes during phagocytosis, *J. Biol. Chem.* 235:2224, 1960.

455. Schandl, E. K. Thymine 7-hydroxylase activity in normal and leukemic leukocytes, *Biochem. Biophys. Res. Commun.* 52:524, 1973.

456. Schuler, D., Kiss, S., and Siegler, J. About the glycolysis of lymphocytes and granulocytes in infancy and childhood, *Ann. Paediatr.* 198:279, 1962.

457. Schultz, J. Myeloperoxidase, *Ann. N.Y. Acad. Sci.* 75:22, 1958.

458. Schultz, J., Corlin, R., Oddi, F., Kaminker, K., and Jones, W. Myeloperoxidase of the leucocyte of normal human blood: III. Isolation of the peroxidase granule, *Arch. Biochem. Biophys.* 111:73, 1965.

459. Schultz, J., and Kaminker, K. Myeloperoxidase of leucocytes of normal human blood. I. Content and localization, *Arch. Biochem. Biophys.* 96:465, 1962.

460. Schultz, J., and Schmuckler, H. W. Myeloperoxidase of the leucocyte of normal human blood: II. Isolation, spectroscopy and amino acid analysis, *Biochemistry* 3:1234, 1964.

461. Scott, J. L. Human leukocyte metabolism *in vitro*. I. Incorporation of adenine-8-C[14] and formate C-14 into the nucleic acids of leukemic leukocytes, *J. Clin. Invest.* 41:67, 1962.

462. Scott, R. B. Glycogen in peripheral blood leukocytes: I. Characteristics of the synthesis and turnover of glycogen *in vitro*, *J. Clin. Invest.* 47:344, 1968.

463. Scott, R. B., and Still, W. J. S. Glycogen in human peripheral blood leukocytes: II. The macromolecular state of leukocyte glycogen, *J. Clin. Invest.* 47:353, 1968.

464. Scott, R. E. Effects of prostaglandins, epinephrine and NaF on human leukocyte, platelet and liver adenyl cyclase, *Blood* 35:514, 1970.

465. Seelich, F. The metabolism of normal and abnormal leukocytes, in H. Braunsteiner and D. Zucker-Franklin (eds.), The Physiology and Pathology of Leukocytes, p. 152, Grune & Stratton, New York, 1962.

466. Selvaraj, R. J., and Sbarra, A. J. Relationship of glycolytic and oxidative metabolism to particle entry and destruction in phagocytosing cells, *Nature* 211:1272, 1966.

467. Seyberth, H. W., Schmidt-Gayk, H., Jakobs, K. H., and Hackenthal, E. Cyclic adenosine monophosphate in phagocytizing granulocytes and alveolar macrophages, *J. Cell Biol.* 57:567, 1973.

468. Shapira, J., Bornstein, I., Wells, W., and Winzler, R. J. Metabolism of human leukocytes *in vitro*. IV. Incorporation and interconversion of adenine and guanine, *Cancer Res.* 21:265, 1961.

469. Shapiro, H., and Parpart, A. K. The osmotic properties of rabbit and human leucocytes, *J. Cellular Comp. Physiol.* 10:147, 1937.

470. Sherstneva, O. S. Dependence of phagocytic activity of leucocytes on respiratory phosphorylation, *Bull. Exp. Med. Biol.* 50:705, 1961.

471. Shirakawa, S., and Saunders, G. F. *In vivo* methylation of DNA in human leukocytes, *Proc. Soc. Exp. Biol. Med.* 138:369, 1971.

472. Shooter, K. V. The sedimentation characteristics of DNA from human leucocytes and spleen, Proc. VII Intern. Congr. Hematol., Rome, p. 28, Grune & Stratton, New York, 1958.

473. Silber, R. Regulatory mechanisms in the human leukocyte: I. The feedback control of deoxycytidylate deaminase, *Blood* 29:896, 1967.

474. Silber, R., Gabrio, B. W., and Huennekens, F. M. Studies on normal and leukemic leukocytes. III. Pyridine nucleotides, *J. Clin. Invest.* 41:230, 1962.

475. Silber, R., Gabrio, B. W., and Huennekens, F. M. Studies on normal and leukemic leukocytes. VI. Thymidylate synthetase and deoxycytidylate deaminase, *J. Clin. Invest.* 42:1913, 1964.

476. Silber, R., Huennekens, F. M., and Gabrio, B. W. Studies on normal and leukemic leukocytes. V. Pyridine nucleotide transhydrogenases, *J. Clin. Invest.* 42:1908, 1963.

477. Silber, R., Unger, K. W., and Ellman, L. RNA metabolism in normal and leukaemic leucocytes: further studies on RNA synthesis, *Br. J. Haematol.* 14:261, 1968.

478. Silber, R., Unger, K. W., and Grooms, R. RNA synthesis in normal leucocytes, leukaemia and macroglobulinemia, *Nature* 205:1211, 1965.

479. Sinks, L. F., and Hayhoe, F. G. J. Unstable rapidly labeled RNA in chronic lymphocytic leukaemic cells, *Nature* 213:1140, 1967.

480. Sirola, I., and Sirola, K. Histochemical study of alkaline phosphatase in leukocytes of blood and bone marrow in various diseases, *Acta Haematol.* 18:313, 1957.

481. Smellie, R. M. S., Thomson, R. Y., and Davidson, J. N. The nucleic acid metabolism of animal cells *in vitro*. I. The incorporation of C[14]-formate, *Biochim. Biophys. Acta* 29:59, 1958.

482. Smith, L. H., Jr., and Baker, F. A. Pyrimidine metabolism in man. I. The biosynthesis of orotic acid, *J. Clin. Invest.* 38:798, 1959.

483. Smith, L. H., Jr., and Baker, F. A. Pyrimidine metabolism in man. III. Studies on leukocytes and erythrocytes in pernicious anemia, *J. Clin. Invest.* 39:15, 1960.

484. Smith, L. H., Jr., Baker, F. A., and Sullivan, M. Pyrimidine metabolism in man. II. Studies of leukemic cells, *Blood* 15:360, 1960.

485. Smith, L. H., Jr., Sullivan, M., and Huguley, C. M., Jr. IV. The enzymatic defects in orotic aciduria, *J. Clin. Invest.* 40:656, 1961.

486. Soffer, L. J., and Wintrobe, M. M. The metabolism of leukocytes from normal and leukemic blood, *J. Clin. Invest.* 11:661, 1932.

487. Spiers, R. S. Physiological approaches to an understanding of the function of eosinophils and basophils, *Ann. N.Y. Acad. Sci.* 59:706, 1955.

488. Stähelin, H., Suter, E., and Karnovsky, M. L. Studies on the interaction between phagocytes and tubercle bacilli. I. Observations on the metabolism of guinea pig leucocytes and the influence of phagocytosis, *J. Exp. Med.* 104:121, 1956.

489. Steele, B. F., Liner, R., Pierce, Z. H., and Williams, H. H. Content of ascorbic acid in the white cells of human subjects receiving controlled low intakes of the vitamin, *Fed. Proc.* 12:430, 1953.

490. Steinitz, K. Laboratory diagnosis of glycogen storage diseases, *Adv. Clin. Chem.* 9:227, 1967.

491. Stephens, D. J., and Hawley, E. E. The partition of reduced ascorbic acid in blood, *J. Biol. Chem.* 115:653, 1936.

492. Stern, G. H. Über die Katalase fabloser Blutzellen, *Z. Physiol. Chem.* 204:259, 1932.

493. Stern, K., Birmingham, M. K., Cullen, A., and Richter, R. Peptidase activity in leukocytes, erythrocytes and plasma of young adult and senile subjects, *J. Clin. Invest.* 30:84, 1951.

494. Stjernholm, R. L., and Noble, E. P. Glucose and galactose metabolism in rabbit polymorphonuclear leukocytes, *Fed. Proc.* 19:82, 1960.

495. Stjernholm, R. L., and Noble, E. P. Carbohydrate metabolism in leukocytes. II. The pathway of ribose and xylose metabolism in the rabbit polymorphonuclear leukocyte, *J. Biol. Chem.* 236:614, 1961.

496. Stjernholm, R. L., and Noble, E. P. Carbohydrate metabolism in leukocytes. IV. The metabolism of glucose and galactose in polymorphonuclear leukocytes from rabbits, *J. Biol. Chem.* 236:3093, 1961.

497. Strauss, B. S., and Stetson, C. A., Jr. Studies on the effect of certain macromolecular substances on the respiratory activity of the leucocytes of peripheral blood, *J. Exp. Med.* 112:653, 1960.

498. Struve, H. Ueber die Einwerkung des activen Sauerstoffs auf Pyrogallussäure, *Justus Liebigs Ann. Chem.* 163:160, 1872.

499. Sutherland, E. W. The effect of epinephrine and hyperglycemic factor on liver and muscle metabolism *in vitro,* in W. D. McElroy and B. Glass (eds.), Phosphorus Metabolism, a Symposium, vol. 2, p. 577, Johns Hopkins University Press, Baltimore, 1952.

500. Swendseid, M. E., Bethell, F. H., and Bird, O. D. The concentration of folic acid in leukocytes. Observations on normal subjects and persons with leukemia, *Cancer Res.* 11:864, 1951.

501. Swendseid, M. E., Wright, P. D., and Bethell, F. H. Variations in nucleotidase activity of leukocytes. Studies with leukemia patients, *J. Lab. Clin. Med.* 40:515, 1952.

502. Takaku, F., Wada, O., Sassa, S., and Kakao, K. Heme synthesis in normal and leukemic leukocytes, *Cancer Res.* 28:1250, 1968.

503. Tallan, H. H., Moore, S., and Stein, W. H. Studies on the free amino acids and related compounds in the tissues of the cat, *J. Biol. Chem.* 211:927, 1954.

504. Tanaka, K. R., and Valentine, W. N. The arginase activity of human leukocytes, *J. Lab. Clin. Med.* 56:754, 1960.

505. Tanaka, K. R., Valentine, W. N., and Fredricks, R. E. Arylsulfatase activity of human leukocytes: distinctive pattern in eosinophils, *J. Clin. Invest.* 39:1034, 1960.

506. Tanaka, K. R., Valentine, W. N., and Fredricks, R. E. Diseases or clinical conditions associated with low leucocyte alkaline phosphatase, *N. Engl. J. Med.* 262:912, 1960.

507. Tanaka, K. R., Valentine, W. N., and Fredricks, R. E. Human leucocyte arylsulphatase activity, *Br. J. Haematol.* 8:86, 1962.

508. Taube, R. A., and Berlin, R. D. Membrane transport of nucleosides in rabbit polymorphonuclear leukocytes, *Biochim. Biophys. Acta* 255:6, 1972.

509. Thiersch, J. B. Histamine and histaminase in chronic myeloid leukemia of man, *Aust. J. Exp. Biol. Med. Sci.* 25:73, 1947.

510. Thomas, J. W., and Anderson, B. B. Vitamin B_{12} content of normal and leukaemic leucocytes, *Br. J. Haematol.* 2:41, 1956.

511. Trubowitz, S. Isolation, purification properties of alkaline phosphatase from human leukocytes, *Blood* 15:419, 1960.

512. Trubowitz, D., Feldman, D., Morgenstern, S. W., and Hunt, V. M. The isolation, purification and properties of the alkaline phosphatase of human leucocytes, *Biochem. J.* 80:369, 1961.

513. Ultmann, J. E., and Feigelson, P. Cellular xanthine oxidase and uricase levels in leukemic and normal mouse leukocytes, *Blood* 15:418, 1960.

514. Vaccari, F., Sabotto, B., and Manzini, E. Alkaline phosphatase activity of leukocytes in shock, *Blood* 10:730, 1955.

515. Valentine, W. N. Quantitative biochemical studies on leukocytes in man: a review, *Blood* 6:845, 1951.

516. Valentine, W. N. The leukocytes and leukopathies, *Ann. Rev. Med.* 6:77, 1955.

517. Valentine, W. N. The biochemistry and enzymatic activities of leukocytes in health and disease, in L. M. Tocantins (ed.), Progress in Hematology, vol. 1, p. 293, Grune & Stratton, New York, 1956.

518. Valentine, W. N. The metabolism of the leukemic leukocyte, *Am. J. Med.* 28:699, 1960.

519. Valentine, W. N., and Beck, W. S. Biochemical studies on leucocytes. I. Phosphatase activity in health, leucocytosis and myelocytic leucemia, *J. Lab. Clin. Med.* 38:39, 1951.

520. Valentine, W. N., Beck, W. S., Follette, J. H., Mills, H., and Lawrence, J. S. Biochemical studies in chronic myelocytic leukemia, polycythemia vera and other idiopathic myeloproliferative disorders, *Blood* 7:959, 1952.

521. Valentine, W. N., Follette, J. H., Hardin, E. B., Beck, W. S., and Lawrence, J. S. Studies on leucocyte alkaline phosphatase activity: relation to "stress" and pituitary-

adrenal activity, *J. Lab. Clin. Med.* 44:219, 1954.

522. Valentine, W. N., Follette, J. H., and Lawrence, J. S. The glycogen content of human leukocytes in health and various disease states, *J. Clin. Invest.* 32:251, 1953.

523. Valentine, W. N., Follette, J. H., Solomon, D. H., and Reynolds, J. The relationship of leukocyte alkaline phosphatase to "stress," to ACTH, and to adrenal 17-OH-corticosteroids, *J. Lab. Clin. Med.* 49:723, 1957.

524. Valentine, W. N., Follette, J. H., Solomon, D. H., and Reynolds, J. Biochemical and enzymatic characteristics of normal and leukemic leukocytes (with particular reference to leukocyte alkaline phosphatase), *in* J. W. Rebuck, F. H. Bethell, and R. W. Monto (eds.), The Leukemias, p. 457, Academic Press, New York, 1957.

525. Valentine, W. N., Lawrence, J. S., Pearce, M. L., and Beck, W. S. The relationship of the basophil to blood histamine in man, *Blood* 10:154, 1955.

526. Vallee, B. L. Biochemistry, physiology and pathology of zinc, *Physiol. Rev.* 39:443, 1959.

527. Vallee, B. L., and Gibson, J. G. The zinc content of normal human whole blood, plasma, leucocytes and erythrocytes, *J. Biol. Chem.* 176:445, 1948.

528. Vallee, B. L., and Gibson, J. G. The zinc content of whole blood plasma, leukocytes and erythrocytes in the anemias, *Blood* 4:455, 1949.

529. Vallee, B. L., Hoch, F. L., and Hughes, W. L., Jr. Studies on metalloproteins: soluble zinc-containing protein extracted from human leucocytes, *Arch. Biochem. Biophys.* 48:347, 1954.

530. VanderWende, C., Miller, W. L., and Glass, S. A. Glycogen metabolism of normal and leukemic leukocytes, *Life Sci.* 3:223, 1964.

531. Vannotti, A. Metabolic pattern of leucocytes within the circulation and outside it, *in* G. E. W. Wolstenholme and M. O'Connor (eds.), Ciba Foundation Study Group 10, Biological Activity of the Leucocyte, p. 79, Little, Brown and Co., Boston, 1961.

532. Vannotti, A., and Cullity, B. Biosynthèse du système phorphyrique dans le leucocyte humain, *Schweiz. Med. Wochenschr.* 90:955, 1960.

533. Venetzke, L. E., Perry, S., and Crepaldi, G. A practical method for separation of lymphocytes from granulocytes, *J. Lab. Clin. Med.* 53:318, 1959.

534. Vercauteren, R. E. Oxidoreductases of leucocytes. II. Evidence for particulate bound catalase and peroxidase in leukocyte homogenates, *Enzymologia* 24:37, 1962.

535. Vercauteren, R. E., and Gillis-van-Maele, A. The oxidoreductases of leucocytes. I. Ultramicroassays for peroxidase, catalase, succinate dehydrogenase and protein in small amounts of leucocyte homogenates. Preparation of particulate hydroperoxidases, *Enzymologia* 24:25, 1962.

536. Vetter, Von K. Über das Verhalten von Fermenten in normalen und pathologischen menschlichen Leukozyten, *Acta Haematol.* 26:344, 1961.

537. Vikbladh, I. Studies on zinc in blood, *Scand. J. Clin. Lab. Invest.* 2:1, 1951 (suppl.).

538. Wachstein, M. Alkaline phosphatase activity in normal and abnormal human blood and bone marrow cells, *J. Lab. Clin. Med.* 31:1, 1946.

539. Wachstein, M. The distribution of histochemically demonstrable glycogen in human blood and bone marrow cells, *Blood* 4:54, 1949.

540. Wachstein, M. Histochemistry of leukocytes, *Ann. N.Y. Acad. Sci.* 59:1052, 1955.

541. Wachstein, M., Kellner, J. D., and Ortiz, J. M. Pyridoxal phosphate in plasma and leukocytes of normal and pregnant subjects following B6 load tests, *Proc. Soc. Exp. Biol. Med.* 103:350, 1960.

542. Wachstein, M., Kellner, J. D., and Ortiz, J. M. Pyridoxal phosphate in plasma and leukocytes in patients with leukemia and other diseases, *Proc. Soc. Exp. Biol. Med.* 105:563, 1960.

543. Wachstein, M., Moore, C., and Graffeo, L. W. Pyridoxal phosphate (B6-al-PO₄) levels of circulating leukocytes in maternal and cord blood,

Proc. Soc. Exp. Biol. Med. 96:326, 1957.

544. Wagner, R. The estimation of glycogen in whole blood and white blood cells, *Arch. Biochem.* 11:249, 1946.

545. Wagner, R. Glycogen content of isolated white blood cells in glycogen storage disease, *Am. J. Dis. Child.* 73:559, 1947.

546. Wagner, R. Studies on the physiology of the white blood cell: the glycogen content of leukocytes in leukemia and polycythemia, *Blood* 2:235, 1947.

547. Wagner, R., Meyerriecks, N., and Sparaco, R. Enzyme studies on white blood cells and platelets. V. Dehydrogenase activity, *Arch. Biochem.* 61:278, 1956.

548. Wagner, R., and Reinstein, S. Enzyme studies on white blood cells. II. Phosphorylating glycogenolysis. Accumulation of an intermediary reducing substance and formation of lactic acid, *Arch. Biochem.* 29:260, 1950.

549. Wagner, R., and Yourke, A. Enzyme studies on white blood cells. III. Phosphorylating glycogenolysis and phosphorylated intermediates, *Arch. Biochem.* 39:174, 1952.

550. Wagner, R., and Yourke, A. Enzyme studies on white blood cells. IV. Glycolysis of added glucose. Hexokinase and adenylpyrophosphatase activity, *Arch. Biochem.* 44:415, 1953.

551. Waisman, H. A. Some aspects of amino acid metabolism in leukemia, *in* J. W. Rebuck, F. H. Bethell, and R. W. Monto (eds.), The Leukemias, p. 339, Academic Press, New York, 1957.

552. Waisman, H. A., Monder, C., and Williams, J. N., Jr. Glutamic acid dehydrogenase and transaminase of leucemic and nonleucemic leucocytes, *Fed. Proc.* 14:299, 1955.

553. Walters, T. R., Gribble, T. J., and Schwartz, H. C. Synthesis of haem in normal and leukaemic leucocytes, *Nature* 197:1213, 1963.

554. Warburg, O., Posener, K., and Negelein, R. Über den Stoffwechsel der Carcinomzelle, *Biochem. Z.* 152:309, 1924.

555. Warner, J. R. Species of RNA in the HeLa cell, *in* L. Goldstein (ed.), The Control of Nuclear Activity, p. 79,

Prentice-Hall, Englewood Cliffs, N.J., 1967.

556. Warner, J. R. An evaluation of studies of RNA synthesis by animal cells, *in* Exploitable Molecular Mechanisms of Neoplasia, 22nd Annual Symposium on Fundamental Cancer Research, M. D. Anderson Hospital, Houston, Texas, 1968.

557. Warren, B., Wenk, E. J., and Roath, S. A simple method for the collection of leucocytes from rat blood, *Experientia* 23:1, 1967.

558. Warren, C. O. The effect of thiouracil on the respiration of bone marrow and leukocytes *in vitro*, *Science* 102:175, 1945.

559. Warren, C. O. Fractionation of serum with respect to its action in enhancing tissue respiration, *J. Biol. Chem.* 167:543, 1947.

560. Waterhouse, C., Terepka, A., and Sherman, C. D., Jr. The gross electrolyte composition of certain human malignant tissues, *Cancer Res.* 15:544, 1955.

561. Weinberg, A. Detection of congenital galactosemia and the carrier state using galactose-C^{14} and blood cells, *Metabolism* 10:728, 1961.

562. Weinberg, A. N., and Segal, S. Effect of galactose-1-phosphate on glucose oxidation by normal and galactosemic leukocytes, *Science* 132:1015, 1960.

563. Weinberg, R. A., Loening, U., Willems, M., and Penman, S. Acrylamide gel electrophoresis of HeLa cell nucleolar RNA, *Proc. Natl. Acad. Sci. U.S.A.* 58:1088, 1967.

564. Weisberger, A. S. Studies on cysteine metabolism in leukemia, *in* J. W. Rebuck, F. H. Bethell, and R. W. Monto (eds.), The Leukemias, p. 423, Academic Press, New York, 1957.

565. Weisberger, A. S., and Heinle, R. W. The protective effect of cysteine on leukopenia induced by nitrogen mustard, *J. Lab. Clin. Med.* 36:872, 1950.

566. Weisberger, A. S., Heinle, R. W., and Levine, B. Some structural requirements for the prevention of leukopenia induced by nitrogen mustard, *J. Clin. Invest.* 31:217, 1952.

567. Weisberger, A. S., and Levine, B. Incorporation of radioactive L-cys-

tine by normal and leukemic leukocytes *in vivo*, *Blood* 9:1082, 1954.

568. Weisberger, A. S., Suhrland, L. G., and Griggs, R. C. Incorporation of radioactive L-cystine and L-methionine by leukemic leukocytes *in vivo*, *Blood* 9:1095, 1954.

569. Weisberger, A. S., Suhrland, L. G., and Seifter, J. Studies on analogues of L-cysteine and L-cystine. I. Some structural requirements for inhibiting the incorporation of radioactive L-cystine by leukemic leukocytes, *Blood* 11:1, 1956.

570. Weissmann, G. The role of lysosomes in inflammation and disease, *Ann. Rev. Med.* 18:97, 1967.

571. Wells, W., and Winzler, R. J. Metabolism of human leukocytes *in vitro*. III. Incorporation of formate-C^{14} into cellular components of leukemic human leukocytes, *Cancer Res.* 19:1086, 1959.

572. West, J., Morton, D. J., Esmann, V., and Stjernholm, R. L. Carbohydrate metabolism in leukocytes: VIII. Metabolic activities of the macrophage, *Arch. Biochem. Biophys.* 124:85, 1968.

573. Will, J. J., Glazer, H. S., and Vilter, R. W. Nucleic acids, nucleases and nuclease inhibitors in leukemia, *in* J. W. Rebuck, F. H. Bethell, and R. W. Monto (eds.), The Leukemias, p. 417, Academic Press, New York, 1957.

574. Williams, A. M. Nucleic acid metabolism in leukemic human leukocytes. I. In vitro incorporation by leukocytes from chronic granulocytic leukemia, *Cancer Res.* 22:314, 1962.

575. Williams, A. M., and Schilling, R. F. The *in vitro* incorporation of nucleic acid precursors into leukemic human leukocytes. I. Methodology and effects of therapy on incorporation *in vitro*, *J. Lab. Clin. Med.* 58:76, 1961.

576. Williams, H. E., and Field, J. B. Low leukocyte phosphorylase in hepatic phosphorylase-deficient glycogen storage disease, *J. Clin. Invest.* 40:1841, 1961.

577. Williams, H. E., and Field, J. B. Further studies on leukocyte phosphorylase in glycogen storage disease, *Metabolism* 12:464, 1963.

578. Williams, H. E., Kendig, E. M., and

Field, J. B. Leukocyte debranching enzyme in glycogen storage disease, *J. Clin. Invest.* 42:656, 1963.

579. Williams, J. F., and Clark, M. G. An error in metabolism: the pentose phosphate cycle, *Search* 2:80, 1971.

580. Williams, W. J., and Buchanan, J. M. Biosynthesis of the purines. V. The conversion of hypoxanthine to inosinic acid by liver enzymes, *J. Biol. Chem.* 203:583, 1953.

581. Willoughby, W. H., and Waisman, H. A. Nucleic acid precursors and nucleotides in normal and leukemic blood. I. Comparison of formic acid chromatograms, *Cancer Res.* 17:942, 1957.

582. Wilmanns, W. Bestimmung, Eigenschaften und Bedeutung der Dihydrofolsäure-Reduktase in den weissen Blutzellen bein Leukämien, *Klin. Wochenschr.* 40:533, 1962.

583. Wilson, D. L. Direct effects of adrenal cortical steroids on the electrolyte content of rabbit leucocytes, *Am. J. Physiol.* 190:104, 1957.

584. Wilson, D. L., and Manery, J. F. Permeability of rabbit leucocytes to sodium and potassium, *Fed. Proc.* 8:168, 1949.

585. Wilson, D. L., and Manery, J. F. The permeability of rabbit leucocytes to sodium, potassium and chloride, *J. Cell. Comp. Physiol.* 34:493, 1949.

586. Wiltshaw, E., and Moloney, W. C. Histochemical and biochemical studies on leukocyte alkaline phosphatase activity, *Blood* 10:1120, 1955.

587. Winkler, F. Der Nachweis von Oxydase in den Leukozytenmittels der Dimethylparaphenylendiamin-Alphanaphtol-Reaktion, *Folia Haematol.* 4:323, 1907.

588. Winzler, R. J., Wells, W., Shapira, J., Williams, A. D., Bornstein, I., Burr, M. J., and Best, W. R. Metabolism of human leukocytes *in vitro*. II. The effect of several agents on the incorporation of radioactive formate and glycine, *Cancer Res.* 19:377, 1959.

589. Wolff, H. P. Untersuchungen zur Pathophysiologie des Zinkstoffwechsels, *Klin. Wochenschr.* 34:409, 1956.

590. Woodin, A. M. The effect of staph-

ylococcal leucocidin on the leucocyte, *Biochem. J.* 80:562, 1961.

591. Woodin, A. M. The extrusion of protein from the rabbit polymorphonuclear leucocyte treated with staphylococcal leucocidin, *Biochem. J.* 82:9, 1961.

592. Wulff, H. R. Histochemical studies of leukocytes from an inflammatory exudate: V. Alkaline and acid phosphatases and esterases, *Acta Haematol. (Basel)* 30:159, 1963.

593. Yamada, E. W. The phosphorolysis of nucleosides by rabbit bone marrow, *J. Biol. Chem.* 236:3043, 1961.

594. Yarborough, D. J., Meyer, O. T., Dannenberg, A. M., Jr., and Pearson, B. Histochemistry of macrophage hydrolases: III. Studies on β-galactosidase, β-glucuronidase and aminopeptidase with indolyl and naphthyl substrates, *J. Reticuloendothel. Soc.* 4:390, 1967.

595. Yasuzumi, G., and Miyao, G. Amino acid constituents of poly-chromosomes isolated from blood cells of various animals, *Science* 114:38, 1951.

596. Yates, R. A., and Pardee, A. B. Control of pyrimidine biosynthesis in Escherichia coli by a feed-back mechanism, *J. Biol. Chem.* 221:757, 1956.

597. Young, J. E., and Prager, M. D. Some hydrolytic enzymes in normal and leukemic human leukocytes, *J. Lab. Clin. Med.* 60:385, 1962.

598. Yu, B. P., Kummerow, F. A., and Nishida, T. Acid phosphatases of rat polymorphonuclear leucocytes, *Proc. Soc. Exp. Biol. Med.* 122:1045, 1966.

599. Zatti, M., and Perona, G. Leukocyte physio-pathology. Some metabolic properties of exudate polynuclears, *G. Biochim.* 6:342, 1957.

600. Zatti, M. and Rossi, F. Mechanism of the respiratory stimulation in phagocytzing leukocytes: the KCN-insensitive oxidation of NADPH, *Experientia* 22:758, 1966.

601. Zeya, H. I., and Spitznagel, J. K. Antibacterial and enzyme basic proteins from leukocyte lysosomes: separation and identification, *Science* 142:1085, 1963.

602. Zeya, H. I., and Spitznagel, J. K. Cationic protein-bearing granules of polymorphonuclear leucocytes: separation from enzyme-rich granules, *Science* 163:1069, 1969.

603. Ziff, M., Gribetz, H. J., and Lospalluto, J. Effect of leukocyte and synovial membrane extracts on cartilage mucoprotein, *J. Clin. Invest.* 39:405, 1960.

604. Zuelzer, W. W. "Myelokathexis"—a new form of chronic granulocytopenia: report of a case, *N. Engl. J. Med.* 270:699, 1964.

Chapter 4 Chemotaxis, Phagocytosis, and Microbial Killing

The primary role of neutrophils in the economy of the body is localization and removal of microorganisms. Several integrated functions are necessary for the achievement of these goals. First, the neutrophils must reach the site of infection (chemotaxis), then they must ingest or otherwise immobilize the organism (phagocytosis), and finally they must kill or inhibit the replication of the invaders (microbial killing). The mechanisms by which neutrophils achieve these goals will be considered sequentially.

Chemotaxis

Methods of Study

In Vivo The traditional method of studying leukocyte migration into areas of inflammation is by the examination of stained sections of fixed tissue in the light microscope. By this method one can assess relative numbers of the different types of leukocytes and the relation of leukocytes to blood vessels at various times after a given stimulus (79). The examination of thin sections of tissue with the electron microscope can provide additional evidence about the route of leukocyte migration (113). The obvious limitation of these methods is that they provide no insights into the kinetics of a dynamically changing situation.

Several methods are effective in the study of leukocyte migration in tissues of intact animals or man. Insertion of a transparent chamber into the ear of a rabbit enables one to view the vasculature and perivascular tissues and the movement of white cells (26, 54). A method widely used in studies of human leukocytes is the "skin window" technique of Rebuck and Crowley (137). This method entails placing a sterile cover slip over a superficial skin abrasion and fixing and staining the leukocytes that migrate into the area of inflammation and adhere to the cover slip (Fig. 4.1).

The major disadvantage of all these techniques is that they are qualitative, rather than quantitative. Other techniques have had to be devised in order to determine the numbers of leukocytes migrating over a given period of time; for example, differential counts of cells entering exudates in the pleural or peritoneal cavity. Skin blisters (13) and skin chambers (156, 162) have also been used for similar purposes. These techniques are, again, not wholly satisfactory for providing quantitative data on the numbers and types of cells migrating under various conditions.

In Vitro Various techniques have been used to study leukocyte movement and chemotaxis in vitro. These were reviewed by Harris in 1954 (67). The technique most widely used today was devised by Boyden in 1962 (15) and consists in a plastic chamber divided into two parts by a millipore filter of known pore size. A leukocyte suspension is introduced into one half of the chamber, while fluid containing a substance with chemotactic activity awaiting evaluation is introduced into the other. After a variable interval the filter membrane is removed and stained, and the number of leukocytes that have migrated

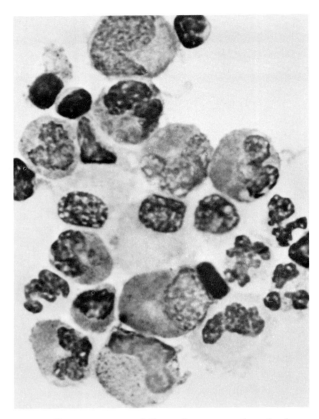

Figure 4.1 Adherent neutrophils and mononuclear leukocytes from a Rebuck "skin window." The sterile cover slip is placed over an area of abraded skin; after several hours it is removed, fixed, and stained with Giemsa.

through the small pores in response to the chemotactic stimulus is determined. A fairly good correlation can be established between chemotaxis measured by this technique and by in vivo methods (143). However, this method has numerous technical problems. For example, migrating cells do not necessarily adhere to the membrane but may pass directly through.

High magnification cinemicrography has also been used in studying chemotaxis (135).

Random Movement and Directional Responses

In studies of living tissues, leukocytes appear to move in random fashion (1), but respond to an appropriate stimulus with nonrandom movement. Harris summarized evidence showing that leukocytes move in nearly straight lines when responding to chemotactic stimuli (67). He discriminated between "true" chemotaxis on the one hand, and accelerated random movement with subsequent leukocyte immobilization on the other. The latter phenomenon may operate in vivo under certain circumstances, simulating chemotaxis, and lead to leukocyte ac-

cumulation. Chemotaxis has, in fact, been suggested as accelerated random movement within a concentration gradient of chemotactic influence. Under such conditions one would expect responding cells to accumulate at the highest point of the gradient unless prevented from doing so by either the toxic effects resulting from very high concentrations of the influential substance, or by overcrowding of the responding cells (94, 143, 163). Chemotaxis does not involve a change in the speed of the leukocytes, merely in their directional movement (135, 136). Movement in leukocytes, like that in amoeba, may be mediated by contractile protein (131).

Locomotion by human neutrophils is temperature dependent but is independent of pH between 6.5 and 7.5 (124). Cytoplasmic flow is continuous in moving cells and occurs throughout the entire width of the cell. "Lamellipodia" are randomly produced; however, chemotactic movement is associated with preferential flow of cellular contents into lamellipodia on the side of the cell nearest the attractant (135, 136).

Some Chemotactic Substances

Many substances, such as those listed below, have been shown to have chemotactic activity for mammalian leukocytes:

Certain bacterial products
Leukocyte components
Damaged tissues
Lymph node permeability factor
Complement components

Bacteria Credit for the first observation that many bacteria are chemotactic for leukocytes probably goes to Gabritchevsky in 1890 (62). Further studies have attempted to recognize and characterize the specific bacterial constituents that exert a chemotactic influence (93, 117, 176). On the basis of studies with *Escherichia coli* and *Staphylococcus albus*, Keller and Sorkin (93) concluded that at least two chemotactic mechanisms were involved. The first depended on a dialyzable factor operating independently of serum. The second involved the induction of chemotactic activity from fresh serum by bacterial products. Ward and his colleagues (176) also concluded that a low-molecular-weight bacterial product was chemotactically active in the absence of serum and appeared in culture filtrates of some, but not all, bacterial species.

Leukocytes In 1961 Hurley and Spector (79) observed that saline extracts of leukocytes are in themselves chemotactic for other viable leukocytes in vivo. Chemotactic activity was enhanced by the presence of serum. Whether this phenomenon results from the induction of a cycle of cell injury by the lysosomal leukocyte enzymes present in the leukocyte extract is not known (see Chapter 5).

Damaged Tissue   Various tissues, when incubated in sterile saline, produce chemotactically active substances; activity is enhanced if serum is included in the incubation mixture (77, 79, 143). Perhaps the most extensively studied of these factors is a permeability factor extracted from lymph node cells (LNPF) that induces leukocyte migration in vivo (181) and is capable of attracting leukocytes in vitro (163). A plasma protein constituent is closely linked to the active fraction of LNPF (116).

Yoshida and his colleagues (183) have described the extraction of a protein-like material from tissue sites of the Arthus reaction, a reaction that is chemotactic for leukocytes and in which there is considerable tissue necrosis.

Other Factors   Prostaglandin E₁ recently has been shown to have chemotactic activity in vitro for rabbit neutrophils (85). This is one of the few chemically defined agents known both to have leukotactic activity and to mediate acute inflammatory reactions.

The Role of Complement and Other Serum Factors

In 1962 Boyden reported that antigen-antibody complexes were chemotactic for neutrophils if a heat-labile serum factor was present (15). Ward and his colleagues (170, 172, 174, 175) subsequently demonstrated that the trimolecular complement complex C'5-C'6-C'7 is exceedingly active chemotactically, although earlier complement components are inactive. Chemotactic response to this complex is blocked by hydrocortisone and chloroquine (170). These observations have not been universally confirmed (167).

In addition to the chemotactic activity of the trimolecular complex C'5-C'6-C'7, evidence exists that the action of plasmin or tissue proteases on C'3 releases a low-molecular-weight, heat-labile substance also capable of exerting chemotactic activity (69, 171). The action of trypsin and of endotoxin-treated serum on C'5 also releases a chemotactically active fragment (160, 161, 177).

In complement-depleted animals neutrophil accumulation does not occur at the site of an Arthus reaction (108, 129, 170), an observation suggesting that complement components are indeed the active chemotactic factors in antigen-antibody-complex–induced acute inflammatory reactions. Keller and Sorkin considered the possibility of chemotactic factors in serum, in addition to complement, since initiation of chemotactic activity and fixation of complement may occur independently (91, 92, 94).

Relatively little information is available on the mechanism responsible for the influence of complement and other serum chemotactic factors on granulocyte movement, although cellular serine esterases have been implicated as possible important factors (9, 173). Chemotactic interaction of complement with the neutrophil may depend upon cell surface receptors for complement (103). Interestingly, phagocytosis seems to interfere with the subsequent migration of neutrophil (19, 180).

In 1968 Keller and Sorkin reviewed the recent work on neutrophil chemotaxis (95).

Phagocytosis

Phagocytosis, illustrated schematically in Fig. 4.2, means the ingestion of a particle by a cell. In this process the mature granulocyte makes contact with a particle of the appropriate size. Firm contact may be mediated by surface receptors on the leukocyte that recognize immunoglobulins coating the particle, or the particle may be trapped between the cell and an unyielding surface. The surface membrane of the leukocyte invaginates, encompassing the particle. The invagination is ultimately pinched off, enclosing the particle within the granulocyte cytoplasm in a vacuole. Phagocytosis is an active process requiring the expenditure of chemical energy by the cell.

For several decades after the classical descriptions of

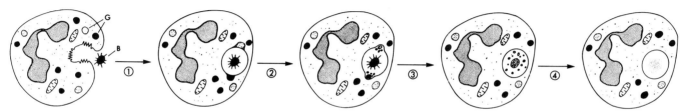

Figure 4.2 Schematic representation of the phagocytic process. An opsonized particle, such as a bacterium (*B*), is recognized by IgG and complement receptors on the neutrophil surface. The neutrophil membrane invaginates, and the particle is enclosed in a phagocytic vacuole. Some of the granules (*G*) of the neutrophil fuse with the vacuole, and the enzymatic contents of the granules are discharged into the vacuole. The bacterium is killed and ultimately digested.

phagocytosis by Metchnikoff (118, 119), physiologists, and later immunologists, were concerned mainly with techniques allowing quantitation of the process and with the study of extrinsic factors modifying particle ingestion. In the 1920s and 1930s the leading students of phagocytosis believed the process to be passive, requiring no energy expenditure, and governed by physical forces at the surface of the cell (56, 123, 132). This concept so dominated the thinking of the day that the report of Baldridge and Gerard (8) in 1933 was scarcely noted. Their analysis first documented the greatly increased oxygen uptake following ingestion of bacteria by granulocytes.

Important contributions to the study of the metabolism of phagocytosis were made early in the 1950s (114), but the field did not gain momentum until the late fifties and early sixties (10, 41, 88, 146, 165, 166). At the time that biochemical data relating to phagocytosis were accumulating, Cohn, Hirsch, and their collaborators made important morphologic and chemical observations (36, 37, 40) identifying the correlation between physical events and biochemical phenomena and placing the entire subject in perspective.

What is the current concept of phagocytosis? The answer to this question must necessarily be divided into component parts: requirements for the mobilization of chemical energy for particle ingestion; the complex morphologic and metabolic events that are initiated when the particle first makes contact with the cell membrane; the requirements for extracellular factors such as opsonins and the proper ionic environment; the chemical events leading to killing of an ingested viable organism; and finally the enzymatic digestion of phagocytized organic material. This sequence of events will be considered in subsequent sections of this chapter.

Measurement of Phagocytosis

Since the first description of phagocytosis by Haeckel in 1862 (65), a number of methods have been devised for measuring the degree or amount of phagocytosis. Most have been based on visual counts of the particles ingested (11, 28, 29, 39, 66, 88, 123). More recently, the use of particles labeled with radioactive material has been introduced (14, 21, 121). In addition, radioactively labeled proteins have been added to the suspending medium. These are swept into the phagocytic vacuole along with the particle being ingested. The cell-associated radioactivity then may be used to measure the extent of phagocytosis (23).

Morphologic Events during Phagocytosis

While Ehrlich studied the specific granules of the neutrophil in 1879 (48), not until eighty years later—when De

Duve (44) described the lysosome structures in liver cells—was the possible significance of the leukocyte granules made clear. Shortly thereafter Cohn and Hirsch (36, 37) demonstrated a close similarity in physical properties and enzyme content between some neutrophil granules and hepatic lysosomes. These and earlier investigators (140) demonstrated the following sequence of events of the phagocytic process (Fig. 4.2): (a) the surface membrane of the neutrophil invaginates to surround the particle being phagocytized (Fig. 4.3), (b) the membrane enclosing the particle gradually pinches off from the surface membrane and is internalized within the cell, forming a phagocytic vacuole (Fig. 4.4), (c) some of the granules of the leukocyte come into apposition with the phagocytic vacuole, and the membranes of granule and vacuole fuse, and (d) the granules rupture, discharging their enzyme-rich contents into the vacuole, where they come into contact with the ingested particle (Figs. 4.5 and 4.6). With extensive degranulation some of the digestive enzymes leak from the vacuole into the cytoplasm and ultimately reach the suspending medium (43). This process of degranulation occurs within five to thirty minutes of particle ingestion. By light microscopy the vacuoles are not apparent and the organisms appear to be lying free in the cytoplasm (Fig. 4.7). The electron microscope is necessary to demonstrate the phagocytic vacuole.

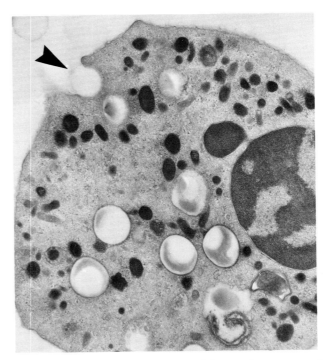

Figure 4.3 Invagination of the neutrophil membrane around a particle (polystyrene bead, *arrow*) to form a phagocytic vacuole. Other polystyrene particles are seen within vacuoles.

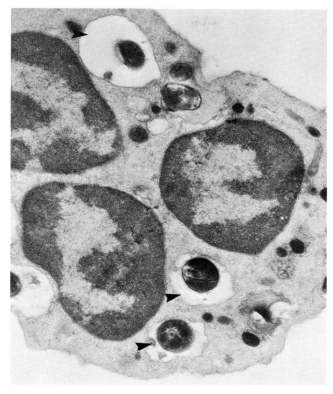

Figure 4.4 Bacteria contained within phagocytic vacuoles (*arrows*) of a human polymorphonuclear leukocyte.

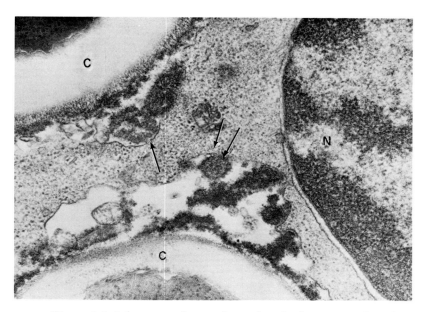

Figure 4.6 A human polymorphonuclear leukocyte incubated for 30 minutes with *Candida albicans*. The thick-walled *Candida* (*C*) are within phagocytic vacuoles containing electron-opaque material derived from the leukocyte granules. The arrows indicate lysosomal granule material entering the vacuole. The nucleus (*N*) is at the right. Magnification ×51,300.

The population of granules containing alkaline phosphatase and lysozyme (secondary granules) probably ruptures into the vacuole before the population that contains the acid hydrolases (primary granules). The mechanisms involved in granule fusions and lysis are unknown. Lysis may be facilitated by a fall in pH within the phagocytic vacuole (36), by leukocyte lysolecithin (50, 53, 179), by protein-phospholipid interactions (68), or by lipid peroxidation (3,22). Whatever the mechanism, the extent of degranulation is dependent upon the amount of material phagocytized. These observations were made by numerous investigators using a variety of phagocytizable particles (88, 140, 145, 164). The similarity between the events of phagocytosis by granulocytes and those associated with particle ingestion by certain unicellular organisms, such as amoebae, is striking. As Metchnikoff first noted, phagocytosis is a very primitive and ancient phenomenon.

An interesting facet of the phagocytic process is that some of the external medium is carried into the cell along with the phagocytized particle. Substances in the medium that normally are excluded from the cell thereby may gain entry into the interior. This phenomenon is called "piggyback phagocytosis" (89) and is directly analogous to a similar process in phagocytizing amoebae (24). The amount of medium carried in by this process is relatively small,

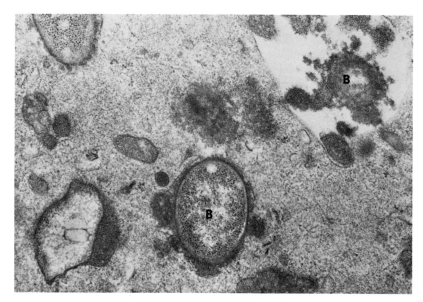

Figure 4.5 Phagocytized bacteria (*B*) within phagocytic vacuoles of a human polymorphonuclear leukocyte. Lysosomal granules, which are electron opaque, are seen adjacent to and within phagocytic vacuoles. Magnification ×42,500.

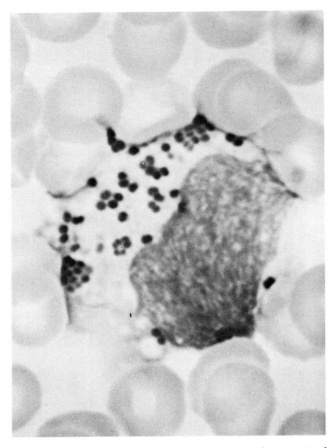

Figure 4.7 An immature neutrophil containing phagocytized *Staphylococcus aureus*; Giemsa stain.

however, since there is a tight fit of the vacuole around the phagocytized particle.

Requirement for Extracellular Factors

In addition to a source of energy, phagocytosis by neutrophils has complex requirements for osmolality. High concentrations of salt and glucose (for example, those found in the renal medulla of man in certain diseases) may significantly impair leukocyte phagocytosis and aggregation (102). Thus a disease such as diabetes mellitus may render the kidney and other tissues more susceptible to bacterial infection by increasing osmolality and reducing leukocyte effectiveness (25). Renal failure per se does not affect phagocyte function (18), although urine itself appears to be detrimental to neutrophil function (20).

The cation requirements for granulocyte adhesion and phagocytosis are not completely understood. Human granulocytes may require magnesium ions for attachment to a charged surface (19). In this requirement the phenomena of phagocytosis and glass adhesiveness may be related (17, 57, 58, 101, 134).

The serum protein components necessary for particle ingestion are equally complex. Since the turn of the century serum factors, including both specific antibodies and nonspecific serum components, have been known to play a role in the phagocytosis of microorganisms. The nonspecific components include complement factors (64, 84, 96), but are not necessarily limited to them. The existence of receptors for complement on the surface membranes of neutrophils has been inferred (103), as have receptors for immunoglobulin G (see Figs. 4.8 and 8.1).

Immunoglobulin G (IgG) opsonins are the main classes of antibody involved in the phagocytosis of infecting microorganisms in human subacute bacterial endocarditis (133). Various observations indicate that the Fc fragment of the IgG antibody molecule is critical in enabling human phagocytic leukocytes, including neutrophils, to ingest certain classes of microorganisms. Components of the cell wall of certain microorganisms, such as protein A of *Staphylococcus aureus*, may interact nonspecifically with this Fc component and thereby inhibit phagocytosis (46). Similarly, although not necessarily by the same mechanism, virulent pneumococci may resist phagocytosis by virtue of their polysaccharide capsule. Their shedding of soluble polysaccharides into the medium protects avirulent organisms against phagocytosis (157).

Studies of yeast and bacteria indicate that absorbed complement or other heat-labile factors are important for ingestion of yeast (84, 105). Once the organisms are internalized within the leukocyte, the next phase of killing is not influenced by the absorbed complement or other heat-labile factors (105). Similar findings have been reported for the staphylocidal ability of human neutrophils

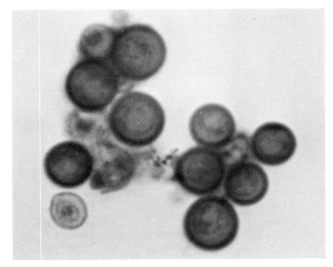

Figure 4.8 *Cryptococcus neoformans* coated with IgG globulin, forming rosettes around human neutrophils.

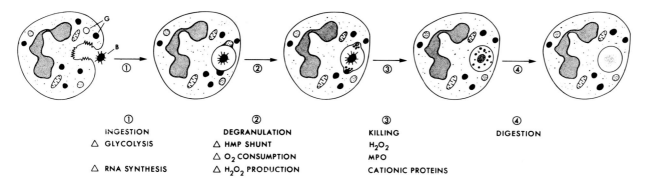

<table>
<tr><td>①</td><td>②</td><td>③</td><td>④</td></tr>
<tr><td>INGESTION</td><td>DEGRANULATION</td><td>KILLING</td><td>DIGESTION</td></tr>
<tr><td>△ GLYCOLYSIS</td><td>△ HMP SHUNT</td><td>H_2O_2</td><td></td></tr>
<tr><td></td><td>△ O_2 CONSUMPTION</td><td>MPO</td><td></td></tr>
<tr><td>△ RNA SYNTHESIS</td><td>△ H_2O_2 PRODUCTION</td><td>CATIONIC PROTEINS</td><td></td></tr>
</table>

Figure 4.9 Events of phagocytosis. The morphologic events are as illustrated in Fig. 4.2; some of the biochemical changes are listed in this figure.

(42). *Complement components thus appear to be necessary for phagocytosis, but not for the subsequent killing of the ingested organism* (122). Recently described familial defects in neutrophil phagocytosis appear related to abnormalities of serum factors, rather than to intrinsic defects in the neutrophil. These familial defects will be discussed in detail in Chapter 8. The constituents of the cell surface that are necessary for phagocytosis are poorly understood. Sialic acid does not seem to be crucial (126).

Metabolic Events

As the leukocyte membrane invaginates to encompass and internalize a microorganism, a series of biochemical changes is initiated in the neutrophil (27, 32, 71, 88, 128, 148). Table 4.1 and Fig. 4.9 summarize these events, which include increased glycolysis, a burst of increased oxygen consumption, increased hexose monophosphate shunt activity, increased lipid synthesis, and RNA turnover.

Glycolysis A moderate increase in the glucose consumption, glycogen breakdown, and lactic acid production occurs during neutrophil phagocytosis (27, 40, 60, 61, 88, 146). Clearly, the energy for particle ingestion derives principally from glycolysis, despite the modest increase in

Table 4.1 Metabolic events during phagocytosis.

Increased glycolysis
Increased hexose monophosphate shunt activity
Increased oxygen utilization
Increased H_2O_2 generation
Increased lipid synthesis
Increased RNA synthesis and degradation
Fall in pH in the phagocytic vacuole
Activation of acid-active enzymes

anaerobic glucose utilization. Evidence for this statement rests on observations demonstrating that particle ingestion is not significantly affected by the poisons of oxidative metabolism (dinitrophenol, cyanide, antimycin A) or by anaerobiosis, but is reduced by glycolytic poisons such as sodium fluoride (10, 40, 88, 146) or certain virus infections (59). Some phagocytosis occurs when glycolysis is suppressed, probably by utilization of preformed adenosine triphosphate (ATP) (12). The absence of available oxygen does not affect the ability of the neutrophil to function and to ingest particles. The neutrophil thus differs from the alveolar macrophage in that it is not dependent upon an adequate oxygen supply for phagocytosis (see Chapter 24).

The mechanism coupling the physical process of particle ingestion to glycolytic energy production is not understood. Senda (154, 155) has suggested that pseudopod formation is necessary for phagocytosis and that the formation of pseudopods is linked to an ATP-dependent "actomysin-like" contractile protein. A somewhat similar thesis has been suggested by North (125). The ATP is rapidly consumed during phagocytosis (12) and is reformed mainly through glycolysis (82).

The suppression of phagocytosis by glycolytic inhibitors can be reversed by supplying certain metabolic intermediates that occur beyond the inhibitor block (149).

Oxygen Consumption and the Hexose Monophosphate Shunt The increase in oxygen consumption and the stimulation of the hexose monophosphate shunt pathway by phagocytosis is dramatic and, under certain conditions, can be observed within a minute following particle ingestion (8, 27, 88, 146). Oxygen consumption and shunt activity may increase 3- to 20-fold with particle engulfment (Fig. 4.10). These phenomena occur in human as well as other mammalian neutrophils (28, 106, 150, 153). Clearly, the oxygen burst can take place at concentrations of cyanide poisonous to mitochondrial enzymes; therefore the "extra respiration" occurs by an extramitochondrial

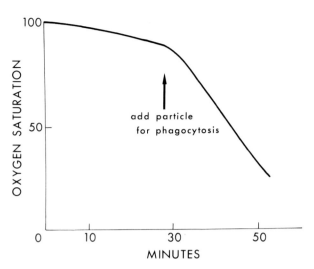

Figure 4.10 Effect of phagocytosis on oxygen consumption by human neutrophils. The oxygen saturation of a solution containing suspended neutrophils falls abruptly as the cells utilize oxygen with particle ingestion.

pathway. Several explanations, given below, have been put forward to explain this unusual phenomenon.

Evans and Karnovsky (55) suggested that the increase in lactic acid production occurring with phagocytosis results in a decreased intracellular pH, which in turn produces a release or activation of a granular enzyme NADH oxidase. Conversion of NADH to NAD by the oxidase would diminish the supply of NADH necessary for the reduction of pyruvate by lactic dehydrogenase. Under this circumstance, NADPH could substitute for NADH, with a resultant generation of large quantities of NADP. Since NADP limits the hexose monophosphate shunt, the increased supply of NADP would activate the shunt pathway, with consequent enhanced oxygen utilization. In this explanation, pyruvate is the oxidant. However, this complex and interesting hypothesis is probably not an accurate explanation of postphagocytic events in the neutrophil. For example, molecular oxygen is considerably more effective at stimulating the shunt pathway than is pyruvate (80).

Iyer and Quastel (81) described a leukocyte enzyme system utilizing oxygen for the conversion of NADPH to NADP (NADPH oxidase, Fig. 4.11); the enzyme system also had some activity in oxidizing NADH to NAD. The NADPH oxidase appears to be activated or released during phagocytosis and stimulated by the presence of manganous ions, which could explain the enhanced oxygen utilization of phagocytic granulocytes.

Zatti, Rossi, and their collaborators (141, 184-186) and more recently Hohn and Lehrer (73) described a somewhat similar system. They found increased NADPH and

NADH oxidase activity in granules from phagocytizing cells and observed that increased oxygen uptake and shunt activity occurred before detection of degranulation. This increased oxidase activity may be related to the swollen, but not disrupted, granules observed in phagocytic leukocytes. Addition of NADPH or NADH to granule fractions of phagocytic cells (but not granule fractions of resting cells) results in a striking increase in cyanide-insensitive oxygen uptake.

Granulocyte oxygen metabolism can be stimulated, under certain conditions, by using sodium fluoride in place of phagocytizable particles (152). This observation indicates that enhanced glycolysis is not critical for the enhanced respiration and stimulation of the hexose monophosphate shunt. The respiratory burst may be inhibited by high concentrations of chloramphenicol (87) and influenced by colchicine (111).

One other enzyme system involved in the conversion of NADPH to NADP should be mentioned: the glutathione peroxidase system (168). As shown in Fig. 4.11, glutathione peroxidase oxidizes GSH to GSSG in the presence of H_2O_2. The cycle is complete when GSSG is reduced to

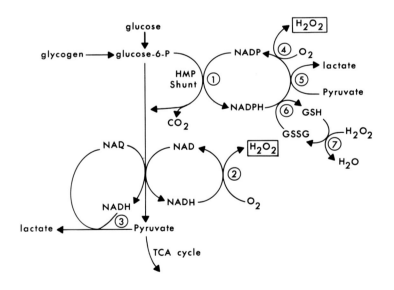

KEY ENZYMES
1. glucose 6-phosphate dehydrogenase
2. NADH oxidase
3. NADH-linked lactic dehydrogenase
4. NADPH oxidase
5. NADPH-linked lactic dehydrogenase
6. GSSG reductase
7. GSH peroxidase

Figure 4.11 Pathways of oxygen utilization by human neutrophils.

GSH and NADPH is concomitantly oxidized to NADP. Indirect evidence suggests that this is one mechanism by which NADP is made available to stimulate the hexose shunt with phagocytosis (138, 139). Human leukocytes contain GSSG reductase (4, 75), and GSH peroxidase has been detected by some investigators (16, 76) but not others (4).

Hydrogen Peroxide and Superoxide Generation Concomitant with enhanced oxidative metabolism, H_2O_2 and superoxide (O_2^-) are generated in the phagocytic leukocyte. Phagocytizing cells contain two to four times more hydrogen peroxide than resting neutrophils (130). The generation of H_2O_2 is ultimately linked to molecular oxygen and does not occur under anaerobic conditions. Iyer, Islam, and Quastel (80) showed that oxidation of exogenously added formate increases during phagocytosis and that this oxidation is linked to H_2O_2 formation from reduced phosphopyridine nucleotides and molecular oxygen.

Another possible means of generating hydrogen peroxide is via oxidation of the D-amino acid found in the bacterial cell wall by the leukocyte enzyme, D-amino acid oxidase (35). Although such a mechanism would provide H_2O_2 as a consequence of D-amino acids that occur naturally in bacteria but not in mammalian tissue, it is unlikely that this is a critical system for generating hydrogen peroxide. The respiratory burst and enhanced hydrogen peroxide generation occurs with nonbacterial and inert materials such as polystyrene. No matter what its mechanism or origin, the hydrogen peroxide generated apparently is important in certain microbicidal mechanisms of the phagocyte (see below). A scheme for the complex changes in oxidative metabolism occurring with phagocytosis is outlined in Fig. 4.11.

In addition to H_2O_2, metabolically stimulated phagocytizing neutrophils produce superoxide, O_2^-. The levels of superoxide produced may be influenced by the intracellular concentration of cyclic nucleotides (2, 3).

Lipid Synthesis The phagocytic neutrophil has a higher rate of lipid turnover and synthesis than does the resting cell. Radioactive carbons of glucose and acetate are more extensively incorporated into lipids after particle ingestion than in the resting cell (49, 88, 90, 146). Incorporation of ^{32}P into phospholipid, and especially into phosphatidic acid, phosphatidyl-inositol, and phosphatidyl-serine, is increased during phagocytosis. The increased lipid turnover may reflect synthesis of new membrane lipids. This synthesis occurs after portions of the membrane enter the cytoplasm associated with a phagocytic vacuole (53). Elsbach has recently reviewed the extensive alterations in leukocyte lipid metabolism occurring with particle engulfment (51).

RNA Turnover Neutrophil phagocytosis is associated with an increased rate of entry of ribonucleotides into cellular acid-soluble pools and an increased turnover rate of RNA (28–30). The enhanced RNA synthesis is not associated with increased protein synthesis (30, 147) and no evidence indicates that neutrophils replace the enzymes lost from the granule fraction during the phagocytic process by new protein synthesis (31). The increased RNA synthesis associated with phagocytosis is not critical for particle ingestion, or for the accompanying changes in oxidative metabolism, or for the subsequent killing of ingested microorganisms (105). These events continue even though RNA synthesis is blocked with actinomycin D. Similarly, high doses of irradiation have relatively little effect on the phagocytic process (150).

pH A critical metabolic effect occurring with particle ingestion is a fall in pH within the phagocytic vacuole (83, 112, 120, 142). Within eight to ten minutes the pH may fall as low as 4.0 to 4.5 (83). This concentration of hydrogen ions is necessary for activation of the acid hydrolases discharged into the vacuole from the granules and for the activation of myeloperoxidase.

Several mechanisms have been proposed to explain the fall in pH within the vacuole, including production of lactic acid, discharge of acid mucopolysaccharides with change in the Donnan equilibrium, and the working of an ATP-dependent proton pump. The human neutrophil may utilize the enzyme carbonic anhydrase for acidification of the phagocytic vacuole. The acidification process may thus resemble the mechanisms used by the stomach and kidney to reduce extracellular pH. A hypothetical scheme for acidification of the phagocytic vacuole is illustrated in Fig. 4.12.

Microbial Killing

The mechanisms by which neutrophils kill microorganisms are as yet ill defined. Multiple interlocking mechanisms probably exist within the cell, some of which are likely to be effective against only a specific class of microorganisms. For example, the mechanisms for killing *Candida* species may be different from those utilized in the killing of *Serratia marcescens*, which in turn may differ from the method of disposal of *Streptococci*. The microbicidal killing mechanisms comprise two broad categories: oxidative and nonoxidative mechanisms. Recent evidence suggests that during fetal life, the phagocytic capacity of leukocytes reaches full development before the bactericidal capacity (74).

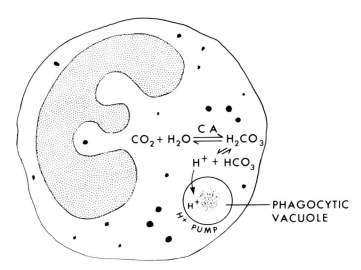

Figure 4.12 Schematic representation of one of the hypothetical mechanisms of acidification of the neutrophil phagocytic vacuole. In the presence of carbonic anhydrase (*CA*), carbon dioxide is hydrated to form carbonic acid. A proton pump restricts the hydrogen ion thus generated to the phagocytic vacuole.

Measurement of microbial killing generally depends upon reduction of bacterial numbers by phagocytic leukocytes (Fig. 4.13) (72) or upon a technique in which inhibition of intracellular bacterial replication is measured by incorporation of thymidine-^{3}H and autoradiography (Figs. 4.14 and 4.15) (33, 34).

Oxidative Mechanisms

The microbicidal function of neutrophils has been studied more extensively than that of any other type of white cell. Any hypothesis pertaining to the killing of microorganisms by this type of leukocyte must take into account the following observations (see Chapter 8): (*a*) for some microbial species bactericidal activity is reduced under anaerobic conditions and in the presence of cyanide, although phagocytosis is unaffected; (*b*) bacterial and fungal killing is reduced as the result of a genetic defect of leukocyte function characterized by impairment of postphagocytic oxygen consumption, hexose monophosphate activity, and hydrogen peroxide generation (182); (*c*) killing of *Candida* is absent or greatly reduced, and bactericidal activity is diminished, in a genetic deficiency of leukocyte myeloperoxidase (106, 107). These observed requirements for microbial killing may be summarized as follows:

Available oxygen
Intact hydrogen peroxide generation
Myeloperoxidase

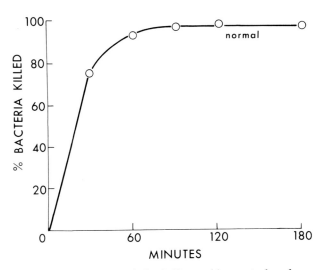

Figure 4.13 Time course of the killing of bacteria by phagocytic human neutrophils. Within 60 minutes essentially all extracellular bacteria are phagocytized and killed.

Reduced killing under anaerobic conditions affects some, but not all, microorganisms tested. Therefore not all organisms are equally sensitive to aerobic neutrophil-killing mechanisms. Susceptible organisms are killed when hydrogen peroxide is added, under anaerobic conditions, to neutrophils (109). This observation, as well as the others cited below, suggests that hydrogen peroxide is an important component of the aerobic killing mechanism.

Much of our knowledge of normal leukocyte function has come from studies of genetic defects in leukocyte metabolism. The most extensively studied of these "experiments of nature" is chronic granulomatous disease of childhood, a disorder considered in more detail in Chapter 8. The important point to understand at this juncture is that in chronic granulomatous disease a rather complete defect of microbicidal activity is associated with abnormal neutrophil oxidative metabolism. This defect in oxidative metabolism is reflected in the absence of the postphagocytic respiratory burst, stimulation of the hexose monophosphate shunt, and hydrogen peroxide generation (75, 86). Similarly, a genetic defect of the neutrophil enzyme, myeloperoxidase, is associated with a partial killing defect for certain bacteria and a complete defect for certain fungi (106, 107). The enhanced oxygen consumption, hexose monophosphate shunt activity, and H_2O_2 generation of phagocytosis are undoubtedly linked to bacterial killing. Studies suggest that, in the presence of H_2O_2, the granule enzyme myeloperoxidase oxidizes intracellular halide, which results in production of a compound lethal to ingested bacteria (97, 98, 100, 110). This

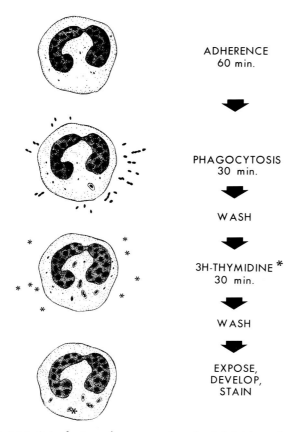

Figure 4.14 A technique for measuring the inhibition of replication of phagocytized bacteria by human neutrophils. The neutrophils are permitted to adhere to a glass surface for 60 minutes. Bacteria are then added, and 30 minutes is allowed for phagocytosis. Extracellular bacteria are removed by washing; tritiated thymidine is added to label any intracellular microorganisms that continue to replicate. Replicating organisms can be identified by radioautography.

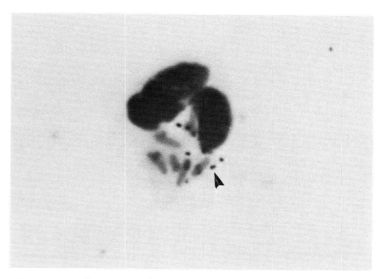

Figure 4.15 Phagocytized *Escherichia coli* labeled with tritiated thymidine. Silver grains are seen adjacent to the *E. coli* (*arrow*). The neutrophil is from a patient with acute myelocytic leukemia and is defective in its ability to kill ingested bacteria. Organisms have been phagocytized and exposed to tritiated thymidine as outlined in Fig. 4.14.

hypothesis has been tested in a patient with a genetic lack of myeloperoxidase in his neutrophils and monocytes (106, 107). An alternative mechanism by which oxygen may be microbicidal is in the production of superoxide, O_2^- (2, 3).

From available data it seems reasonable to postulate the following sequence of events in the *oxidative* killing of phagocytized microorganisms: (a) glycolytic activity supplies the energy necessary for particle engulfment and increases in phagocytizing cells; (b) intracellular phosphopyridine nucleotide oxidases (probably NADPH oxidase in particular) are "activated"; (c) under the catalytic activity of these oxidases, hydrogen peroxide is generated from reduced NADPH, NADH, and molecular oxygen; (d) the hexose monophosphate shunt is probably stimulated by the increased availability of NADP; the shunt pathway in turn generates more NADPH as substrate for NADPH oxidase, with resultant enhanced hydrogen peroxide generation; and (e) hydrogen peroxide interacts with myeloperoxidase, and perhaps intracellular halide, to effect microbial killing.

The putative role of hydrogen peroxide in labilizing leukocyte granules (178) cannot yet be evaluated. Aberrations in this pathway resulting from either genetic disease or acquired abnormality will be discussed in Chapter 8.

Nonoxidative Bactericidal Mechanisms

The fall in pH within the phagocytic vacuole may be sufficient to inhibit the replication of some sensitive bacterial species such as pneumococci. Clearly, however, mechanisms in addition to acid are involved in microbial killing.

A number of compounds possessing a broad range of antibacterial activity have been extracted from phagocytic leukocytes. In 1956 Skarnes and Watson isolated an antibacterial cationic protein from autolysed neutrophils (158, 159). They labeled the protein *leukin* and thought it was derived from nucleohistone. In the same year Hirsch (70) reported the extraction, by citric acid, of an antimicrobial substance from leukocytes. He termed the substance *phagocytin* and subsequently demonstrated it to be extractable from the granule fraction of neutrophils (36, 37). Phagocytin is probably a conglomerate of antibacterial substances. Zeya and Spitznagel (187) found that the rabbit neutrophil granules contain several basic proteins, distinct from nucleohistones, which have antibacterial activity. They demonstrated that separable cationic proteins differ substantially in their composition and antibacterial specificity. Subsequently these authors identified cationic protein-bearing granules in rabbit neutrophils. These distinctive granules were separable from the enzyme-rich granules (188). No particles containing cationic proteins were found in macrophages.

Lactoferrin is an iron-binding protein present in the secondary granules of neutrophils (5). It is bacteriostatic when not fully saturated with iron, presumably by reducing the iron available for growing microorganisms (115, 128). It may represent another antimicrobial substance present in neutrophils.

The role of these various protein fractions in bacterial killing is still problematical. It is not known whether they are enzymes or act by nonenzymatic mechanisms. Furthermore, the function of this group of antibacterial substances in human neutrophils is not yet certain, although there is inferential evidence for their existence (104). As stated in an editorial in the *New England Journal of Medicine* (47):

Most of the basic information on the metabolic and functional behavior of leukocytes has come from studies on guinea pigs and rabbits. There has been perhaps a rather expansive attitude on the part of clinical investigators in translating data from those two species to the situation in man. A clearer recognition of the differences between the behavior of cells of different species during phagocytosis, rather than too bland an acceptance of similarities, would help unravel some of the questions that presently puzzle us.

Digestion of Microorganisms

Once particle ingestion and the subsequent degranulation of neutrophils has taken place, inhibitors of glycolysis and respiration are without effect on the degradation of the killed microorganisms (38). This observation suggests that once the degradative enzymes contained within granules are released into the phagocytic vacuole, destruction of ingested organisms does not require the expenditure of chemical energy. Mammalian leukocytes are rich in acid hydrolytic enzymes (45), which may digest bacterial cell walls (169); Their compartmentalization has been studied by histochemical techniques (7) and cell separation techniques (5, 6). As noted earlier, activation of these enzymes is dependent upon a fall in pH within the phagocytic vacuole.

Summary

To achieve its mission of localizing and destroying microorganisms, the neutrophil must be capable of directed movement, of particle ingestion, and ultimately of killing of the ingested organism. Movement and phagocytosis require energy derived primarily from anaerobic glycolysis and mediated through ATP. The mechanisms of microbial killing are diverse. Some organisms are killed by oxidative mechanisms that probably involve interaction of the enzyme myeloperoxidase with hydrogen peroxide, which is generated from the respiratory burst that accompanies phagocytosis. Another leukocyte microbicidal system is independent of oxygen and comprises several cationic proteins that are lethal for specific species of organisms. Activation of myeloperoxidase and of acid hydrolases requires a low pH within the phagocytic vacuole. These hydrolases ultimately degrade the killed microorganism.

Chapter 4 References

1. Allison, F., Jr., Smith, M. R., and Wood, W. B., Jr. Studies on the pathogenesis of acute inflammation: I. The inflammatory reaction to thermal injury as observed in the rabbit ear chamber, *J. Exp. Med.* 102:655, 1955.

2. Babior, B. M., Curnutte, J. T., and Kipnes, R. S. The influence of cyclic nucleotides on granulocyte superoxide production, Progr. 66th Ann. Mtg. Am. Soc. Clin. Invest., p. 3a, 1974.

3. Babior, B. M., Kipnes, R. S., and Curnutte, J. T. Biological defense mechanisms. The production by leukocytes of superoxide, a potential bactericidal agent, *J. Clin. Invest.* 52:741, 1973.

4. Baehner, R. L., Gilman, N., and Karnovsky, M. L. Respiration and glucose oxidation in human and guinea pig leukocytes: comparative studies, *J. Clin. Invest.* 49:692, 1970.

5. Baggiolini, M., De Duve, C., Masson, P. L., and Heremans, J. F. Association of lactoferrin with specific granules in rabbit heterophil leukocytes, *J. Exp. Med.* 131:559, 1970.

6. Baggiolini, M., Hirsch, J. G., and De Duve, C. Resolution of granules from rabbit heterophil leukocytes into distinct populations by zonal sedimentation, *J. Cell Biol.* 40:529, 1969.

7. Bainton, D. F., and Farquhar, M. G. Differences in enzyme content of azurophil and specific granules of polymorphonuclear leukocytes. I. Histochemical staining of bone marrow smears, *J. Cell Biol.* 39:286, 1968.

8. Baldridge, C. W., and Gerard, R. W. The extra respiration of phagocytosis, *Am. J. Physiol.* 103:235, 1933.

9. Becker, E. L., and Ward, P. A. Esterases of the polymorphonuclear leukocyte capable of hydrolyzing acetyl DL-phenylalanine β-naphthyl ester, *J. Exp. Med.* 129:569, 1969.

10. Becker, H. J., Munder, G, and Fischer, H. Über den Leukocytenstoffwechsel bei der Phagocytose, *Hoppe Seylers Z. Physiol. Chem.* 313:266, 1958.

11. Berry, L. J., and Spies, T. D. Phagocytosis, *Medicine* 28:239, 1949.

12. Bodel, P., and Malawista, S. E. Phagocytosis by human blood leukocytes during suppression of glycolysis, *Exp. Cell Res.* 56:15, 1969.

13. Boggs, D. R., Athens, J. W., Cartwright, G. E., and Wintrobe, M. M. The effect of adrenal glucocorticosteroids upon the cellular composition of inflammatory exudates, *Am. J. Pathol.* 44:763, 1964.

14. Bourne, H. R., Lehrer, R. I., Cline, M. J., and Melmon, K. L. Cyclic 3′, 5′-adenosine monophosphate in the human leukocyte: synthesis, degradation, and effects on neutrophil candidacidal activity, *J. Clin. Invest.* 50:920, 1971.

15. Boyden, S. The chemotactic effect of mixtures of antibody and antigen on polymorphonuclear leucocytes, *J. Exp. Med.* 115:453, 1962.

16. Bracci, R., Calabri, G; Bettini, F., and Princi, R. Glutathione peroxidase in human leukocytes, *Clin. Chim. Acta* 29:345, 1970.

17. Brandt, L. Adhesiveness to glass and phagocytic activity of neutrophilic leukocytes in myeloproliferative diseases, *Scand. J. Haematol.* 2:126, 1965.

18. Brogan, T. D. Phagocytosis by polymorphonuclear leucocytes from patients with renal failure, *Br. Med. J.* 3:596, 1967.

19. Bryant, R. E., DesPrez, R. M., VanWay, M. H., and Rogers, D. E. Studies on human leukocyte motility: I. Effects of alterations in pH, electrolyte concentration and phagocytosis on leukocyte migration, adhesiveness and aggregation, *J. Exp. Med.* 124:483, 1966.

20. Bryant, R. E., Sutcliffe, M. C., and McGee, A. Z. Human polymorphonuclear leukocyte function in urine, *Yale J. Biol. Med.* 46:113, 1973.

21. Brzuchowska, W. Use of radioactive isotopes in studies on phagocytosis *in vitro, Nature* 212:210, 1966.

22. Buckley, R., Hochstein, P., and Sidbury, J. B., Jr. A study of the defect in septic granulomatosis, *J. Reticuloendothel. Soc.* 4:430, 1967.

23. Chang, Y-H. Studies on phagocytosis, *Exp. Cell Res.* 54:42, 1969.

24. Chapman-Andresen, C., and Holter, H. Studies on the ingestion of ^{14}C glucose by pinocytosis in the amoeba *chaos chaos, Exp. Cell Res.* 3:52, 1955 (suppl.).

25. Chernew, I., and Braude, A. I. Depression of phagocytosis by solutes in concentrations found in the kidney and urine, *J. Clin. Invest.* 41:1945, 1962.

26. Cliff, W. J. The acute inflammatory reaction in the rabbit ear chamber with particular reference to the phenomenon of leukocyte migration, *J. Exp. Med.* 124:543, 1966.

27. Cline, M. J. Metabolism of the circulating leukocyte, *Physiol. Rev.* 45:674, 1965.

28. Cline, M. J. Ribonucleic acid biosynthesis in human leukocytes: effects of phagocytosis on RNA metabolism, *Blood* 28:188, 1966.

29. Cline, M. J. Isolation and characterization of RNA from human leukocytes, *J. Lab. Clin. Med.* 68:33, 1966.

30. Cline, M. J. Phagocytosis and synthesis of ribonucleic acid in human granulocytes, *Nature* 212:1431, 1966.

31. Cline, M. J. Leukocyte metabolism, *in* A. S. Gordon (ed.), Regulation of Hematopoiesis, p. 1045, Appleton-Century-Crofts, New York, 1970.

32. Cline, M. J. Leukocyte function in inflammation: the ingestion, killing, and digestion of microorganisms, *Ser. Haematol.* 3:3, 1970.

33. Cline, M. J. Microbicidal activity of human eosinophils, *J. Reticuloendothel. Soc.* 12:332, 1972.

34. Cline, M. J. A test of individual phagocyte function in a mixed population of leukocytes. Identification of a neutrophil in acute myelocytic leukemia, *J. Lab. Clin. Med.* 81:311, 1973.

35. Cline, M. J., and Lehrer, R. I. D-amino acid oxidase in leukocytes: a possible D-amino-acid-linked antimicrobial system, *Proc. Natl. Acad. Sci. U.S.A.* 62:756, 1969.

36. Cohn, Z. A., and Hirsch, J. G. The isolation and properties of the specific cytoplasmic granules of rabbit polymorphonuclear leucocytes, *J. Exp. Med.* 112:983, 1960.

37. Cohn, Z. A., and Hirsch, J. G. The influence of phagocytosis on the intracellular distribution of granule-associated components of polymorphonuclear leucocytes, *J. Exp. Med.* 112:1015, 1960.

38. Cohn, Z. A., Hirsch, J. G., and

Wiener, E. Lysosomes and endocytosis. The cytoplasmic granules of phagocytic cells and the degradation of bacteria, *in* A. V. S. de Reuck and M. P. Cameron (eds.), Ciba Foundation Symposium on Lysosomes, p. 126, Little, Brown and Co., Boston, 1963.

39. Cohn, Z. A., and Morse, S. I. Interactions between rabbit polymorphonuclear leucocytes and staphylococci, *J. Exp. Med.* 110:419, 1959.

40. Cohn, Z. A., and Morse, S. I. Functional and metabolic properties of polymorphonuclear leucocytes: I. Observations on the requirements and consequences of particle ingestion, *J. Exp. Med.* 111:667, 1960.

41. Coxon, R. V., and Robinson, R. J. Carbohydrate metabolism in blood cells studied by means of isotopic carbon, *Proc. R. Soc. Lond. (Biol.)* 145:232, 1956.

42. Craig, C. P., and Suter, E. Extracellular factors influencing staphylocidal capacity of human polymorphonuclear leukocytes, *J. Immunol.* 97:287, 1966.

43. Crowder, J. G., Martin, R. R., and White, A. Release of histamine and lysosomal enzymes by human leukocytes during phagocytosis of staphylococci, *J. Lab. Clin. Med.* 74:436, 1969.

44. De Duve, C. Lysosomes, a new group of cytoplasmic particles, *in* T. Hayashi (ed.), Subcellular Particles, p. 128, Ronald Press, New York, 1958.

45. De Duve, C., and Wattiaux, R. Functions of lysosomes, *Ann. Rev. Physiol.* 28:435, 1966.

46. Dossett, J. H., Kronvall, G., Williams, R. C., Jr., and Quie, P. G. Protein A: An antiphagocytic factor of staphylococcus aureus, *J. Clin. Invest.* 48:21a, 1969.

47. Editorial. Phagocytes and the "bench-bedside interface," *N. Engl. J. Med.* 278:1014, 1968.

48. Ehrlich, P. Über die spezifischen Granulationen des Blutes, *Arch. Physiol., Leipzig*, 571, 1879.

49. Elsbach, P. Composition and synthesis of lipids in resting and phagocytizing leukocytes, *J. Exp. Med.* 110:969, 1959.

50. Elsbach, P. Increased synthesis of phospholipid during phagocytosis, *J. Clin. Invest.* 47:2217, 1968.

51. Elsbach, P. Lipid metabolism by phagocytes, *Semin. Hematol.* 9:227, 1972.

52. Elsbach, P., Patriarca, P., Pettis, P., Stossel, T. P., Mason, R. J., and Vaughn, M. The appearance of lecithin -^{32}P synthesized from lysolecithin -^{32}P in phagosomes of polymorphonuclear leukocytes, *J. Clin. Invest.* 51:1910, 1972.

53. Elsbach, P., and Rizack, M. A. Acid lipase and phospholipase activity in homogenates of rabbit polymorphonuclear leukocytes, *Am. J. Physiol.* 205:1154, 1963.

54. Elsert, R. H. *In vivo* observations on the effect of cortisone on experimental tuberculosis using the rabbit ear chamber technique, *Ann. Rev. Tuberc.* 65:64, 1952.

55. Evans, W. H., and Karnovsky, M. L. The biochemical basis of phagocytosis. IV. Some aspects of carbohydrate metabolism during phagocytosis, *Biochemistry* 1:159, 1962.

56. Fenn, W. O. The theoretical response of living cells to contact with solid bodies, *J. Gen. Physiol.* 4:373, 1921-22.

57. Fenn, W. O. The adhesiveness of leucocytes to solid surfaces, *J. Gen. Physiol.* 5:143, 1923.

58. Fenn, W. O. Effect of the hydrogen ion concentration on the phagocytosis and adhesiveness of leucocytes, *J. Gen. Physiol.* 5:169, 1923.

59. Fisher, T. N., and Ginsberg, H. S. The reaction of influenza viruses with guinea pig polymorphonuclear leucocytes: II. The reduction of white blood cell glycolysis by influenza viruses and receptor-destroying enzyme (RDE), *Virology* 2:637, 1956.

60. Frei, J., Borel, C., Horvath, G., Cullity, B., and Vannotti, A. Enzymatic studies in the different types of normal and leukemic white cells, *Blood* 18:317, 1961.

61. Frei, J., Borel, C., and Vannotti, A. Modification métabolique au niveau du leucocyte humain pendant la phagocytose, *Enzymol. Biol. Clin.* 1:149, 1961.

62. Gabritchevsky, G. Sur les propriétés chimiotactiques des leucocytes, *Ann. Inst. Pasteur* 4:346, 1890.

63. Gewurz, H., Page, A. R., Pickering, R. J., and Good, R. A. Complement activity and inflammatory neutrophil exudation in man: studies in patients with glomerulonephritis, essential hypocomplementemia and agammaglobulinemia, *Int. Arch. Allergy* 32:64, 1967.

64. Gigli, I., and Nelson, R. A., Jr. Complement dependent immune phagocytosis, *Exp. Cell Res.* 51:45, 1968.

65. Haeckel, E. Die Radiolarien, p. 104, Georg Reimer, Berlin, 1862.

66. Hanks, J. H. Quantitative aspects of phagocytosis as influenced by the number of bacteria and leucocytes, *J. Immunol.* 38:159, 1940.

67. Harris, H. Role of chemotaxis in inflammation, *Physiol. Rev.* 34:529, 1954.

68. Hawiger, J., Horn, R. G., Koenig, M. G., and Collins, R. D. Activation and release of lysosomal enzymes from isolated leukocytic granules by liposomes. A proposed model for degranulation in polymorphonuclear leukocytes, *Yale J. Biol. Med.* 42:57, 1969.

69. Hill, J. H., and Ward, P. A. C3 leukotactic factors produced by a tissue protease, *J. Exp. Med.* 130:505, 1969.

70. Hirsch, J. G. Phagocytin: a bactericidal substance from polymorphonuclear leukocytes, *J. Exp. Med.* 103:589, 1956.

71. Hirsch, J. G. Neutrophil and eosinophil leukocytes, *in* B. W. Zweifach, L. Grant, and R. T. McCluskey (eds.), The Inflammatory Process, p. 245, Academic Press, New York, 1965.

72. Hirsch, J. G., and Strauss, B. Studies on heat labile opsonin in rabbit serum, *J. Immunol.* 92:145, 1964.

73. Hohn, D. C., and Lehrer, R. I. Identification of the defect in X-linked chronic granulomatous disease, *Clin. Res.* 22:394A, 1974.

74. Holmes, B., Day, N., Haseman, J., and Good, R. A. Development of bactericidal capacity and phagocytosis-associated metabolism of fetal pig leukocytes, *Infect. Immunol.* 5:232, 1972.

75. Holmes, B., Page, A. R., and Good, R. A. Studies of the metabolic activity of leukocytes from patients with a genetic abnormality of phagocytic function, *J. Clin. Invest.* 46:1422, 1967.

76. Holmes, B., Park, B. H., Malawista, S. E., Quie, P. G., Nelson, D. L.,

and Good, R. A. Chronic granulomatous disease in females. A deficiency of leukocyte glutathione peroxidase, *N. Engl. J. Med.* 283:217, 1970.

77. Hurley, J. V. Substances promoting leukocyte emigration, *Ann. N.Y. Acad. Sci.* 116:918, 1964.

78. Hurley, J. V., Ryan, G. B., and Friedman, A. The mononuclear response to intrapleural injection in the rat, *J. Pathol. Bacteriol.* 91:575, 1966.

79. Hurley, J. V., and Spector, W. G. Delayed leucocytic emigration after intradermal injections and thermal injury, *J. Pathol. Bacteriol.* 82:421, 1961.

80. Iyer, G. Y. N., Islam, M. F., and Quastel, J. H. Biochemical aspects of phagocytosis, *Nature* 192:535, 1961.

81. Iyer, G. Y. N., and Quastel, J. H. NADPH and NADH oxidation by guinea pig polymorphonuclear leucocytes, *Can. J. Biochem. Physiol.* 41:427, 1963.

82. Jemelin, M., and Frei, J. Leukocyte energy metabolism. III. Anaerobic and aerobic ATP production and related enzymes, *Enzymol. Biol. Clin.* (Basel) 11:289, 1970.

83. Jensen, M. S., and Bainton, D. F. Temporal changes in pH within the phagocytic vacuole of the polymorphonuclear neutrophilic leukocyte, *J. Cell Biol.* 56:379, 1973.

84. Johnston, R. B., Jr., Klemperer, M. R., Alper, C. A., and Rosen, F. S. The enhancement of bacterial phagocytosis by serum, *J. Exp. Med.* 129:1275, 1969.

85. Kaley, G., and Weiner, R. Effect of prostaglandin E$_1$ on leukocyte migration, *Nature* (*New Biol.*) 234:114, 1971.

86. Kaplan, E. L., Laxdal, T., and Quie, P. G. Studies of polymorphonuclear leukocytes from patients with chronic granulomatous disease of childhood: bactericidal capacity for streptococci, *Pediatrics* 41:591, 1968.

87. Kaplan, S. S. The effect of chloramphenicol on human leukocyte phagocytosis and respiration, *Proc. Soc. Exp. Biol. Med.* 130:839, 1969.

88. Karnovsky, M. L. Metabolic basis of phagocytic activity, *Physiol. Rev.* 42:143, 1962.

89. Karnovsky, M. L., and Sbarra, A. J. Metabolic changes accompanying the ingestion of particulate matter by cells, *Am. J. Clin. Nutr.* 8:147, 1960.

90. Karnovsky, M. L., and Wallach, D. F. H. The metabolic basis of phagocytosis: III. Incorporation of inorganic phosphate into various classes of phosphatides during phagocytosis, *J. Biol. Chem.* 236:1895, 1961.

91. Keller, H. U., and Sorkin, E. Studies on chemotaxis: I. On the chemotactic and complement-fixing activity of α-globulins, *Immunology* 9:241, 1965.

92. Keller, H. U., and Sorkin, E. Studies on chemotaxis: II. The significance of normal sera for chemotaxis induced by various agents, *Immunology* 9:441, 1965.

93. Keller, H. U., and Sorkin, E. Studies on chemotaxis: V. On the chemotactic effect of bacteria, *Int. Arch. Allergy* 31:505, 1967.

94. Keller, H. U., and Sorkin, E. Studies on chemotaxis: VII. Cytotaxins in rabbit serum, *Experientia* 23:549, 1967.

95. Keller, H. U., and Sorkin, E. Chemotaxis of leucocytes, *Experientia* 24:641, 1968.

96. Kindmark, C. O. Stimulating effect of C-reactive protein on phagocytosis of various species of pathogenic bacteria, *Clin. Exp. Immunol.* 8:941, 1971.

97. Klebanoff, S. J. Iodination of bacteria: a bactericidal mechanism, *J. Exp. Med.* 126:1063, 1967.

98. Klebanoff, S. J. Myeloperoxidase-halide-hydrogen peroxide antibacterial system, *J. Bacteriol.* 95:2131, 1968.

99. Klebanoff, S. J., Clem, W. H., and Luebke, R. G. The peroxidase-thiocyanate-hydrogen peroxide antimicrobial system, *Biochim. Biophys. Acta* 117:63, 1966.

100. Klebanoff, S. J., and Hamon, C. B. Role of myeloperoxidase-mediated antimicrobial systems in intact leukocytes, *J. Reticuloendothel. Soc.* 12:170, 1972.

101. Kvarstein, B. A methodological study of human leukocyte adhesiveness to glass beads, *Scand. J. Clin. Lab. Invest.* 23:259, 1969.

102. Lancaster, M. G., and Allison, F., Jr. Studies on the pathogenesis of inflammation, *Am. J. Pathol.* 49:1185, 1966.

103. Lay, W., and Nussenzweig, V. Complement dependent receptor sites for antigen-antibody complexes on macrophages, polymorphonuclear leukocytes and lymphocytes, *Fed. Proc.* 27:621, 1968 (abstract).

104. Lehrer, R. I. Functional aspects of a second mechanism of candidacidal activity by human neutrophils, *J. Clin. Invest.* 51:2566, 1972.

105. Lehrer, R. I., and Cline, M. J. Interaction of candida albicans with human leukocytes and serum, *J. Bacteriol.* 98:996, 1969.

106. Lehrer, R. I., and Cline, M. J. Leukocyte myeloperoxidase deficiency and disseminated candidiasis: the role of myeloperoxidase in resistance to candida infection, *J. Clin. Invest.* 48:1478, 1969.

107. Lehrer, R. I., Hanifin, J., and Cline, M. J. Defective bactericidal activity in myeloperoxidase-deficient human neutrophils, *Nature* 223:78, 1969.

108. Linscott, W. D., and Cochrane, C. G. Guinea pig B1c-globulin: its relationship to the third component of complement and its alteration following interaction with immune complexes, *J. Immunol.* 93:972, 1964.

109. McRipley, R. J., and Sbarra, A. J. Role of the phagocyte in host-parasite interactions: XI. Relationship between stimulated oxidative metabolism and hydrogen peroxide formation and intracellular killing, *J. Bacteriol.* 94:1417, 1967.

110. McRipley, R. J., and Sbarra, A. J. Role of the phagocyte in host-parasite interactions: XII. Hydrogen peroxide-myeloperoxidase bactericidal system in the phagocyte, *J. Bacteriol.* 94:1425, 1967.

111. Malawista, S. E., and Bodel, P. T. The dissociation by colchicine of phagocytosis from increased oxygen consumption in human leukocytes, *J. Clin. Invest.* 46:786, 1967.

112. Mandell, G. L. Intraphagosomal pH of human polymorphonuclear neutrophils, *Proc. Soc. Exp. Biol. Med.* 134:447, 1970.

113. Marchesi, V. T., and Florey, H. W. Electron micrographic observations on the emigration of leucocytes, *Q. J. Exp. Physiol.* 45:343, 1960.

114. Marinelarena, R. The effect of various chemical substances and bacteria on the glycolytic and respiratory activities of leukocytes, Ph.D. thesis, University of Michigan, Ann Arbor, 1950.

115. Masson, P. L., Heremans, J. F., and Schonne, E. Lactoferrin, an iron-binding protein in neutrophilic leukocytes, *J. Exp. Med.* 130:643, 1969.

116. Meacock, S. C. R., and Willoughby, D. A. Purification of serum proteins from lymph node cell extracts with permeability activity characteristic of the lymph node permeability factor, *Immunology* 15:101, 1968.

117. Meier, R., and Schär, B. Vorkommen leukocytotaktischer Polysaccharide in bakteriellem, pflanzlichem und tierischem Ausgangsmaterial, *Hoppe Seylers Z. Physiol. Chem.* 307:103, 1957.

118. Metchnikoff, E. Lectures on the Comparative Pathology of Inflammation (Kegan Paul, London); quoted in J. Hirsch, in Phagocytosis: *Ann. Rev. Microbiol.* 19:339, 1893.

119. Metchnikoff, E. L'immunité dans les maladies infectieuses, Masson et Cie, Paris (Eng. trans. F. G. Binnie, Cambridge University Press), 1901.

120. Metchnikoff, E. Immunity in Infective Diseases (reprint of 1905 ed.), Johnson Reprint Corp., New York, 1968.

121. Michell, R. H., Pancake, S. J., Noseworthy, J., and Karnovsky, M. L. Measurement of rates of phagocytosis, *J. Cell Biol.* 40:216, 1969.

122. Morelli, R., and Rosenberg, L. T. The role of complement in the phagocytosis of *Candida albicans* by mouse peripheral blood leukocytes, *J. Immunol.* 107:476, 1971.

123. Mudd, S., McCutcheon, M., and Lucké, B. Phagocytosis, *Physiol. Rev.* 14:210, 1934.

124. Nahas, G. G., Tannieres, M. L., and Lennon, J. F. Direct measurement of leukocyte motility: effects of pH and temperature, *Proc. Soc. Exp. Biol. Med.* 138:350, 1971.

125. North, R. J. The uptake of particulate antigen, *J. Reticuloendothel. Soc.* 5:203, 1968.

126. Noseworthy, J., Korchak, H., and Karnovsky, M. L. Phagocytosis and the sialic acid of the surface of polymorphonuclear leukocytes, *J. Cell. Physiol.* 79:91, 1972.

127. Ohta, H. Metabolic responsiveness of human leukemic leukocytes to phagocytic stimulation, *Acta Hematol.* 33:28, 1965.

128. Oran, J. D., and Reiter, B. Inhibition of bacteria by lactoferrin and other iron-chelating agents, *Biochim. Biophys. Acta* 170:351, 1968.

129. Page, A. R., Gewurz, H., Pickering, R. J., and Good, R. A. The role of complement in the acute inflammatory response, *in* P. A. Miescher and P. Grabor (eds.), Immunopathology: Vth International Symposium, p. 221, Schwabe and Co., Basel, 1968.

130. Paul, B., and Sbarra, A. J. The role of the phagocyte in host-parasite interactions: XIII. The direct quantitative estimation of H_2O_2 in phagocytizing cells, *Biochim. Biophys. Acta* 156:168, 1968.

131. Pollard, T. D., and Korn, E. D. Filaments of amoeba proteins. II. Binding of heavy meromyosin by thin filaments in motile cytoplasmic extracts, *J. Cell Biol.* 48:216, 1971.

132. Ponder, E. The influence of surface charge and of cytoplasmic viscosity on the phagocytosis of a particle, *J. Gen. Physiol.* 11:757, 1928.

133. Quie, P. G., Messner, R. P., and Williams, R. C., Jr. Phagocytosis in subacute bacterial endocarditis. Localization of the primary opsonic site to Fc fragment, *J. Exp. Med.* 128:553, 1968.

134. Rabinowitz, Y. Separation of lymphocytes, polymorphonuclear leukocytes and monocytes on glass columns, including tissue culture observations, *Blood* 23:811, 1964.

135. Ramsey, W. S. Analysis of individual leucocyte behavior during chemotaxis, *Exp. Cell Res.* 70:129, 1972.

136. Ramsey, W. S. Locomotion of human polymorphonuclear leucocytes, *Exp. Cell Res.* 72:489, 1972.

137. Rebuck, J. W., and Crowley, J. H. A method of studying leukocytic functions *in vivo*, *Ann. N.Y. Acad. Sci.* 59:757, 1955.

138. Reed, P. W. Glutathione and the hexose monophosphate shunt in phagocytizing and hydrogen peroxide-treated rat leukocytes, *J. Biol. Chem.* 244:2459, 1969.

139. Reed, P. W., and Tepperman, J. Phagocytosis-associated metabolism and enzymes in the rat polymorphonuclear leukocyte, *Am. J. Physiol.* 216:223, 1969.

140. Robineaux, J., and Frederic, J. Contribution a l'étude des granulations neutrophiles des polynucléaires par le microcinématographic en contraste de phase, *C. R. Soc. Biol.* 149:486, 1955.

141. Rossi, F., and Zatti, M. Biochemical aspects of phagocytosis in polymorphonuclear leucocytes: NADH and NADPH oxidation by the granules of resting and phagocytizing cells, *Experientia* 20:21, 1964.

142. Rous, P. The relative reaction within living mammalian tissues. II. On the mobilization of acid material within cells, and the reaction as influenced by the cell state, *J. Exp. Med.* 41:399, 1925.

143. Ryan, G. B., and Hurley, J. V. The chemotaxis of polymorphonuclear leucocytes towards damaged tissues, *Br. J. Exp. Pathol.* 47:530, 1966.

144. Salton, M. R. J. The Bacterial Cell Wall, Elsevier Publishing Co., Amsterdam, 1964.

145. Sbarra, A. J., Bardawil, W. A., Shirley, W., and Gilfillan, R. F. Degranulation of guinea pig leukocytes accompanying phagocytosis, *Exp. Cell Res.* 24:609, 1961.

146. Sbarra, A. J., and Karnovsky, M. L. The biochemical basis of phagocytosis: I. Metabolic changes during the ingestion of particles by polymorphonuclear leukocytes, *J. Biol. Chem.* 234:1355, 1959.

147. Sbarra, A. J., and Karnovsky, M. L. The biochemical basis of phagocytosis: II. Incorporation of C^{14}-labeled building blocks into lipid, protein, and glycogen of leukocytes during phagocytosis, *J. Biol. Chem.* 235:2224, 1960.

148. Sbarra, A. J., Paul, B., Strauss, R., and Mitchell, G. W., Jr. Metabolic and bactericidal activities of phagocytizing leukocytes, *in* A. S. Gordon (ed.), Regulation of Hematopoiesis, p. 1081, Appleton-Century-Crofts, New York, 1970.

149. Sbarra, A. J., and Shirley, W. Phago-cytosis inhibition and reversal: I. Effect of glycolytic intermediates and nucleotides on particle uptake, *J. Bacteriol.* 86:259, 1963.

150. Selvaraj, R. J., McRipley, R. J., and Sbarra, A. J. The effect of phagocy-tosis and x-irradiation on human leukocyte metabolism, *Cancer Res.* 27:2280, 1967.

151. Selvaraj, R. J., and Sbarra, A. J. Phagocytosis inhibition and re-versal: II. Possible role of pyruvate as an alternative source of energy for particle uptake by guinea pig leukocytes, *Biochim. Biophys. Acta* 127:159, 1966.

152. Selvaraj, R. J., and Sbarra, A. J. Re-lationship of glycolytic and oxida-tive metabolism to particle entry and destruction in phagocytizing cells, *Nature* 211:1272, 1966.

153. Selvaraj, R. J., and Sbarra, A. J. The role of the phagocyte in host-parasite interactions: VII. Di- and tri-phosphopyridine nucleotide kinetics during phagocytosis, *Biochim. Biophys. Acta* 141:243, 1967.

154. Senda, N. The phagocytosis of leu-kocytes, Proc. VIII Int. Congr. He-matol., Tokyo, p. 702, 1960.

155. Senda, N. The phagocytosis of leu-kocytes, *Tohoku J. Exp. Med.* 76:119, 1962.

156. Senn, H. J., and Holland, J. F. Plastic skin chamber technique for comparative studies on localized leukocyte mobilization in man, *Rev. Fr. Etudes Clin. Biol.* 14:373, 1969.

157. Sia, R. H. P. Studies on pneumo-coccus growth inhibition. VI. The specific effect of pneumococcus sol-uble substance on the growth of pneumococci in normal serum-leucocyte mixtures, *J. Exp. Med.* 43:633, 1926.

158. Skarnes, R. C. Leukin, a bac-tericidal agent from rabbit polymor-phonuclear leukocytes, *Nature* 216:806, 1967.

159. Skarnes, R. C., and Watson, D. W. Characterization of leukin: an an-tibacterial factor from leucocytes active against gram-positive path-ogens, *J. Exp. Med.* 104:829, 1956.

160. Snyderman, R., Phillips, J. K., and Mergenhagen, S. E. Biological activ-ity of complement *in vivo, J. Exp. Med.* 134:1131, 1971.

161. Snyderman, R., Shin, H. S., Phillips, J. K., Gewurz, H., and Mergenhagen, S. E. A neutrophil chemotactic factor derived from C'5 upon interaction of guinea pig serum with endotoxin, *J. Immunol.* 103:413, 1969.

162. Southam, C. M., and Levin, A. G. A quantitative Rebuck technic, *Blood* 27:734, 1966.

163. Spector, W. G., and Willoughby, D. A. Mechanisms of leukocyte emi-gration in inflammation, *in* A. S. Gordon (ed.), Regulation of Hema-topoiesis, p. 959, Appleton-Century-Crofts, New York, 1970.

164. Spicer, S. S., and Hardin, J. H. Ul-trastructure, cytochemistry, and function of neutrophil leukocyte granules, *Lab. Invest.* 20:488, 1969.

165. Stähelin, H., Karnovsky, M. L., and Suter, E. Studies on the interaction between phagocytes and tubercle bacilli: II. The action of phagocytes upon C14-labeled tubercle bacilli, *J. Exp. Med.* 104:137, 1956.

166. Stähelin, H., Suter, E., and Kar-novsky, M. L. Studies on the in-teraction between phagocytes and tubercle bacilli: I. Observations on the metabolism of guinea pig leu-kocytes and the influence of phago-cytosis, *J. Exp. Med.* 104:121, 1956.

167. Stecher, V. J., and Sorkin, E. Studies on chemotaxis, *Im-munology* 16:231, 1969.

168. Strauss, R. R., Paul, B. B., Jacobs, A. A., and Sbarra, A. J. The role of the phagocyte in host-parasite interac-tions. XIX. Leukocytic glutathione reductase and its involvement in phagocytosis, *Arch. Biochem. Biophys.* 135:265, 1969.

169. Strominger, J. L., and Ghuysen, J-M. Cell walls of bacteria are solu-bilized by action of either specific carbohydrases or specific pep-tidases, *Science* 156:213, 1967.

170. Ward, P. A. The chemosuppression of chemotaxis, *J. Exp. Med.* 124:209, 1966.

171. Ward, P. A. A plasmin-split frag-ment of C'3 as a new chemotactic factor, *J. Exp. Med.* 126:189, 1967.

172. Ward, P. A. Complement-derived leukotactic factors in pathological fluids, *J. Exp. Med.* 134:109s, 1971.

173. Ward, P. A., and Becker, E. L. Mechanisms of the inhibition of chemotaxis by phosphonate esters, *J. Exp. Med.* 125:1001, 1967.

174. Ward, P. A., and Cochrane, C. G. Bound complement and im-munologic injury of blood vessels, *J. Exp. Med.* 121:215, 1965.

175. Ward, P. A., Cochrane, C. G., and Müller-Eberhard, H. J. The role of serum complement in chemotaxis of leukocytes *in vitro, J. Exp. Med.* 122:327, 1965.

176. Ward, P. A., Lepow, I. H., and Newman, L. J. Bacterial factors chemotactic for polymorphonuclear leukocytes, *Am. J. Pathol.* 52:725, 1968.

177. Ward, P. A., and Newman, L. J. A neutrophil chemotactic factor from human C'5, *J. Immunol.* 102:93, 1969.

178. Weissmann, G. The role of lyso-somes in inflammation and disease, *Ann. Rev. Med.* 18:97, 1967.

179. Weissmann, G., Becher, B., and Thomas, L. Studies on lysosomes. V. The effects of streptolysins and other hemolytic agents on isolated leucocyte granules, *J. Cell Biol.* 22:115, 1964.

180. Williams, K. E., and Walters, M. N-i. Inhibitions of leucocytic emi-gration after phagocytosis, *J. Pathol. Bacteriol.* 95:167, 1968.

181. Willoughby, D. A., and Spector, W. G. The lymph node permeability factor: a possible mediator of the delayed hypersensitivity reaction, *Ann. N.Y. Acad. Sci.* 116:874, 1964.

182. Windhorst, D. B., Page, A. R., Holmes, B., Quie, P. G., and Good, R. A. The pattern of genetic trans-mission of the leukocyte defect in fatal granulomatous disease of childhood, *J. Clin. Invest.* 47:1026, 1968.

183. Yoshida, K., Yoshinaga, M., and Hayashi, H. Leukoegresin: a factor from rabbit skin associated with leucocytic emigration in the Arthus reaction, *Nature* 218:977, 1968.

184. Zatti, M, and Rossi, F. Early changes of hexose monophosphate pathway activity and of NADPH oxidation in phagocytizing leuco-cytes, *Biochim. Biophys. Acta* 99:557, 1965.

185. Zatti, M., and Rossi, F. Mechanism of the respiratory stimulation in phagocytizing leukocytes: the KCN-insensitive oxidation of NADPH, *Experientia* 22:758, 1966.

186. Zatti, M., Rossi, F., and Meneghelli, V. Metabolic and morphological changes of polymorphonuclear leucocytes during phagocytosis, *Br. J. Exp. Pathol.* 46:227, 1965.

187. Zeya, H. I., and Spitznagel, J. K. Arginine-rich proteins of polymorphonuclear leukocyte lysosomes. Antimicrobial specificity and biochemical heterogeneity, *J. Exp. Med.* 127:927, 1968.

188. Zeya, H. I., and Spitznagel, J. K. Cationic protein-bearing granules of polymorphonuclear leukocytes: separation from enzyme-rich granules, *Science* 163:1069, 1969.

Chapter 5 Neutrophils and the Inflammatory Process

Because of their active motility, phagocytic activity, and complex microbicidal systems, neutrophilic granulocytes constitute one of the body's most important defense systems against microbial pathogens. They are also a key participant in acute, and some forms of chronic, inflammation. Inflammatory reactions in which neutrophils are active may be incited by a variety of agents: microbial, chemical, thermal, or immunologic. Components of the leukocyte that are important in normal defense functions may also participate in the inflammatory process. For example, the numerous hydrolytic substances of the neutrophil are important in their normal function of degradation and disposal of microorganisms, immune complexes, and injured cells. When these hydrolytic substances escape extracellularly in high concentrations, they augment the inflammatory process. As a result, in certain pathological conditions normal tissues may be injured by leukocyte products. The precarious balance between the normal function of neutrophils and their potential for damage in an inflammatory process was probably first recognized by Metchnikoff in the late nineteenth century (93). Excellent reviews of the role of leukocytes in the inflammatory process and in tissue damage can be found in articles by Hirsch (59), Janoff (65), Thomas (130), and Henson (57).

Mediators of Inflammation in Granulocytes

In 1955 De Duve and his colleagues (37) drew attention to a cellular cytoplasmic organelle containing acid-active hydrolases capable of digesting proteins, carbohydrates, lipids, and nucleic acids. These structures, called *lysosomes,* subsequently were found to contain a multiplicity of enzymatic and nonenzymatic constituents (Table 5.1). In Chapter 1 we traced the development of the neutrophil granules, some of which resemble lysosomes. In Chapter 3 we considered some of the enzyme systems and nonenzymatic constituents of granules, and in Chapter 4 we discussed the interaction of these constituents with ingested microorganisms.

Normally, the granule constituents are isolated within the granule itself or within the phagosome (Chapter 4). This membrane-bound isolation, and the fact that many of the enzymes are not active except at low pH, serves to protect the granulocyte and surrounding cells from the destructive action of these enzymes (38). When the leukocyte is overwhelmed by its phagocytic burden or injured by other mechanisms, the granule constituents may be released and subsequently injure the neutrophilic cell and other cells in its vicinity. Clearly, lysosomal disrupting agents injected in vivo induce a marked inflammatory response, and lysosmal stabilizing agents may inhibit the development of inflammatory reactions (138).

The Role of Neutrophil Proteolytic Enzymes in Tissue Injury

Burke (23), Uriuhara (132), and their colleagues injected extracts of neutrophils into rabbit skin and observed a subsequent increased vascular permeability and hemorrhagic reaction. Vascular permeability was decreased when the extracts were treated with inhibitors of proteases, whereas hemorrhage was not affected (30). Therefore, in-

Table 5.1 Enzymes and nonenzymatic substances associated with neutrophil granules. Some of the substances listed as nonenzymatic may well have enzyme activity when tested with an appropriate substrate.

Enzymes:	Hyaluronidase
Acid phosphatase	Lysozyme
Acid ribonuclease	Collagenase
Acid deoxyribonuclease	Elastase
Cathepsins	Aryl sulfatases
Neutral protease	Phospholipase
Acid lipase	Myeloperoxidase
Phosphoprotein phosphatase	Kininogenase
Phosphatidic acid phosphatase	*Nonenzymatic substances:*
Organophosphate-resistant esterases	Phagocytin and related bactericidal proteins
β-glucuronidase	? Endogenous pyrogen
β-galactosidase	Plasminogen activator
β-N-acetylglucosaminidase	Mucopolysaccharides and glycoproteins
α-L-fucosidase	Histamine
α-1,4-glucosidase	Cationic proteins: bactericidal proteins, histamine-liberating agent, histamine-independent permeability factors
α-mannosidase	
α-N-acetylglucosaminidase	
α-N-acetylgalactosaminidase	

SOURCE: Adapted from reference 140.

creased vascular permeability and hemorrhage induced by granulocyte components are probably independent phenomena.

Neutrophils are involved in the injury to vascular and glomerular basement membranes induced by immune complexes (29). Consequently, Cochrane and Aikin (30) incubated glomerular basement membranes of rabbit kidney with neutrophil granules. Membrane fragments and peptides were released from the membranes at acid pH, indicating proteolytic digestion by the granules. Subsequent purification showed the leukocyte proteases to be cathepsin D and E with low pH optima of 3.4 and 2.5 respectively (74).

Whether or not proteases activated at these very low pH's can induce tissue injury in vivo is not known; however, neutrophils probably can reduce the pH of their phagocytic vacuoles to the very low levels necessary for activation of acid cathepsin (122). Phagocytic neutrophils can also produce lactic acid at a rate sufficient to reduce the pH in their immediate environment (80). It may be unnecessary, however, to invoke acid-activated proteases in tissue injuries. Human neutrophils also contain proteases that may degrade isolated basement membranes at neutral pH (64, 75). These proteases may produce inflammatory reactions at physiologic hydrogen ion concentrations.

Enzymes Hydrolyzing Protein Polysaccharides (Collagenase)

Extracts of leukocytes can degrade crude protein polysaccharides obtained from cartilage (5, 144, 153). The activity, extractable from the leukocyte granules, is expressed at neutral pH and may be inhibited by epsilon-aminocaproic acid (144). Collagenase activity is associated with the secondary (specific) granules containing alkaline phosphatase activity (119).

The neutral proteases of neutrophils can degrade large glycoproteins and cartilage matrix (36, 144). They may therefore be involved in inflammatory degeneration of joint cartilage and also in the lysis of vascular membranes that occurs at physiologic pH and leads to hemorrhagic vasculitis (75, 76, 140).

Elastinolytic Activity

Granules from human leukocytes contain enzymes capable of degrading elastin (68). This activity is distinguishable from the collagenase activity present in these cells and has different properties from pancreatic elastase. The leukocyte enzyme is active at pH 6 to 7 and is resistant to serum elastase inhibitor. This white cell enzyme may be involved in acute arteritis. For example, the elastica staining of human arterial vessels is reduced after incubation of tissue with leukocyte granules.

Fibrinolytic and Fibrin-precipitating Systems

Neutrophils are capable of phagocytizing fibrin, fibrinogen, and their breakdown products (6). Exudate cells from the inflamed joints of patients with rheumatoid arthritis may have phagosomes filled with fibrin-like material. Leukocyte preparations rich in eosinophils can degrade fibrinogen (7). A lysosomal protein fraction from rabbit neutrophils can form an insoluble precipitate of soluble fibrin monomers (55). Therefore, granulocytes possibly are involved in both fibrinogen deposition and resorption.

The Role of Basic Proteins

A number of activities have been ascribed to basic proteins extractable from mammalian granulocytes. These include bacterial killing (see Chapter 4), mast cell membrane activation (25), and increased vascular permeability. A number of investigators have partially purified neutrophilic basic (cationic) proteins and demonstrated that they have the property of inducing vascular permeability (50, 65, 67, 69). Janoff and his colleagues (67) found that neutrophil cationic proteins induced degranulation of rat mast cells. Whether these proteins are the same ones that possess the potent antibacterial activity described in Chapter 4 is unknown.

A variety of basic proteins is undoubtedly involved in these reactions. Chromatography on DEAE cellulose and Sephadex followed by electrophcresis on polyacrylamide has been used to identify at least four distinct vasoactive proteins (30, 116). Some of these appear to increase vascular permeability directly; others work through mast cell degranulation and histamine release. Most have a relatively low molecular weight—2,000 to 12,000 (29). The ability of some of these molecules to degranulate mast cells probably depends in part on their strong positive charge (66). Similar basic proteins have been found in granulocytes of several species (117, 124).

Leukocytes and the Plasma Kinin System

The plasma kinin system consists of several polypeptides of low molecular weight (kinins) that are released from an inactive plasma alpha globulin substrate (kininogen) by a number of enzymes. These enzymes can be isolated from the plasma and certain tissues (45). The basic polypeptide *bradykinin* is the prototype of this group. Bradykinin, an extremely potent constrictor of nonvascular smooth muscle, possesses the properties of inducing vasodilatation, increasing capillary permeability, and causing pain. In intact animals it can produce all the major manifestations of the inflammatory process. In addition, bradykinin has been isolated from inflammatory fluids, including those induced by thermal injury and experimental arthritis. Considerable circumstantial evidence therefore implicates these polypeptides in the inflammatory processes.

The polypeptides of this class have an extremely brief

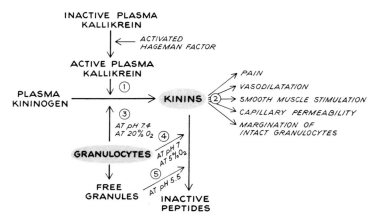

Figure 5.1 Interaction of leukocytes and the plasma kinin system. Granulocytes are a source of kininogen-activating enzymes resulting in the production of kinins from plasma kininogen. Granulocytes also contain enzymes (kininases) capable of degrading kinins to inactive peptides.

life-span in the blood and are inactivated within seconds or minutes by a series of kininases found in the plasma and in certain tissues. Kinin-generating and kininase enzyme activities have been identified in human and animal leukocytes (53, 88–90). These activities are associated with both mature and immature cells of the granulocytic series and with mature eosinophils; they have not been identified in either normal or malignant lymphocytes. The kinin-generating system of the human granulocytes is found in the extragranular portion of the cytoplasm, is most active at pH 7.4, and requires oxygen. Kinin-generating activity is inhibited at concentrations of glucocorticoids achieved by clinical therapy (26). The distribution of kininase activity within the granulocyte is less certain, but a significant proportion—perhaps most—of the activity is found in the granule fraction. This enzyme activity is most potent at pH 6 to 7 and does not require molecular oxygen.

The interaction of leukocytes and kinins in the inflammatory process is illustrated in Fig. 5.1.

Neutrophils and Slow-reacting Substance

Slow-reacting substance (SRS-A) is a poorly characterized vasoactive material found in certain inflammatory exudates. It is released during anaphylactic shock in certain species of animals (105). In rats depleted of neutrophils by antiserum or by alkylating agents, the release of slow-reacting substance induced by immunologic reactions is almost completely abolished (106, 107). When the number of neutrophils in the peritoneal cavity is increased, the release of slow-reacting substance is also increased. The logical conclusion from these observations is that the generation of this vasoactive material is linked in some way to the presence of granulocytes.

Histamine and Histamine-releasing Substances

The exact cellular distribution of histamine, long presumed to be a key mediator in many acute inflammatory reactions, is uncertain. Certainly the bulk of leukocyte histamine is contained within basophils; however, investigators have suggested that small amounts can be localized within neutrophils as well, and specifically within their granule fraction (52, 108, 112).

When basophils and neutrophils disintegrate, they may release histamine. In addition, these cells may release histamine via another mechanism involving cationic protein. A lysosomal cationic protein extracted from rabbit heterophile leukocytes has the property of inducing mast cell degranulation and histamine release with an attendant increase in vascular permeability (67, 69, 127). Simi-

Table 5.2 Molecules and macromolecules hydrolyzed by leukocyte enzymes.

Substrate	Leukocyte enzyme
Collagen	Collagenase
Protein polysaccharides	Neutral protease
C'1	Neutral protease
C'3 and C'5	Neutral protease
Elastic-tissue arterial walls	Elastase
Basement membrane proteins	Cathepsins D, E
Kininogen	Kinin-generating enzymes
Kinin	Kininase
Fibrin	Acid peptidase

lar substances have been obtained from granulocytes of several mammalian species (65).

Although basophils are the major source of histamine in the blood, mast cells are the principal repository of this vasoactive amine in the tissues. The mechanisms of histamine release from basophils and mast cells are discussed in detail in Chapter 7.

Miscellaneous Mediators

In addition to histamine and histamine-releasing factors, permeability factors that are histamine independent have been identified among the cationic proteins of rabbit neutrophil granules (117).

In various types of inflammation and tissue damage the concentration of certain "acute phase" proteins increases in the serum. Examples of these acute phase proteins are C-reactive protein in man and the alpha-2 acute phase globulin of the rat. Studies indicate that most of these are manufactured in the liver in response to some circulating factor (51, 123). Darcy (35) demonstrated that the alpha-2 acute phase serum protein of the rat increases when the animal is injected with disrupted neutrophils or microsomal fractions from such cells.

In addition to the various mediators of inflammation identified in mammalian granulocytes, other cellular and humoral components of the inflammatory process interact in a complex way with neutrophils. These components include mast cells, platelets, anaphylotoxin, and complement.

Some of the identified substrates of granulocyte enzyme systems are listed in Table 5.2.

Release of Granulocyte Mediators

In the preceding paragraphs we have established that neutrophils contain a variety of substances that are in themselves either inflammatory or capable of interacting with external mediators to incite inflammation. Normally,

neutrophils circulate without inducing such reactions. It is logical therefore to question the mechanisms by which neutrophil-mediated inflammatory reactions are triggered.

When neutrophils are irreparably damaged and the integrity of the cell membrane is disrupted, macromolecules, including soluble mediators of inflammation, leak into the surrounding fluid. This mechanism of release of hydrolytic "ferments" was first proposed by Metchnikoff (94). In an alternative mechanism, the neutrophils may remain morphologically intact (at least by light microscopy) and yet leak hydrolases. An example of the latter phenomenon is observed when granulocytes phagocytize a large load of particles, particularly poorly digestible particles. Under such circumstances, lysosomal enzymes may be observed both in the neutrophil cytoplasm and in

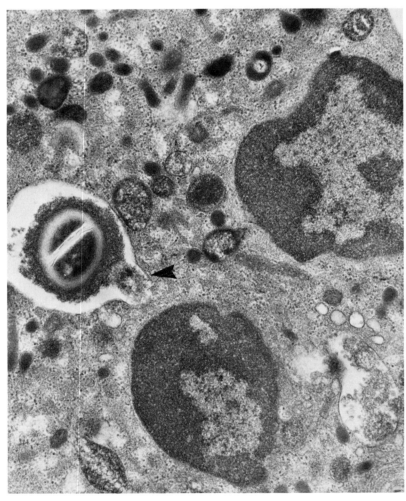

Figure 5.2 An electron micrograph of a polymorphonuclear neutrophil demonstrating fusion of a granule with a phagocytic vacuole. Granule contents, which are electron opaque, are discharged into the vacuole (*arrow*).

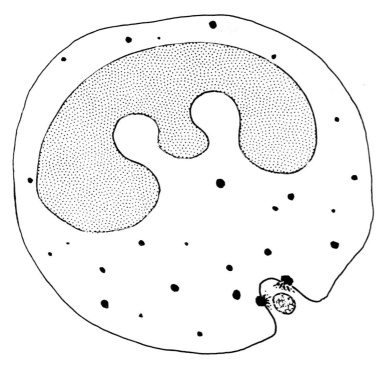

Figure 5.3 Schematic representation of the discharge of leukocyte granules into the external medium as a phagocytic vacuole is being formed around a particle destined for phagocytosis.

the extracellular fluid (19, 151). This mechanism, which has been called "regurgitation during feeding," probably results from the fusion of lysosomes with phagosomes still open at the external surface of the cell (155). The phenomenon is illustrated in Figs. 5.2 and 5.3.

A number of agents are known to alter the stability of lysosomal membranes and may influence the release of inflammatory substances. Table 5.3 summarizes some of the agents thought to influence the degranulation process. Although many of these substances may exert an effect on lysosomal integrity in the test tube, one cannot necessarily extrapolate this observation to explain their in vivo effects. Furthermore, some agents, such as antibody to a lysosomal enzyme, may have multiple effects, depending on experimental conditions (109).

Agents that may disrupt neutrophil lysosomes can be grouped in several categories: (a) bacterial products, (b) immune complexes, (c) poorly soluble crystalline particles, and (d) lipid-soluble compounds interacting directly with the granule membrane. The general phenomenon of release is illustrated in Fig. 5.4.

Bacterial Products

Some interesting examples of leukocyte lysosome disruption by bacterial products have been recorded. For ex-

Table 5.3 Agents influencing the stability of lysosomal membranes or lysosomal enzyme release in vitro. These agents may not necessarily exert their primary effect in vivo by influencing lysosomal integrity.

Agents that may make the membrane more labile
Streptolysin-O	Endotoxin
Streptolysin-S	Antibodies to membranes
Etiocholanolone	Polyene antibiotics
Progesterone	
Vitamin A	

Agents that may stabilize the membranes or prevent enzyme release
Glucocorticoids	Phenylbutazone
Colchicine	Acetylsalicylic acid
Chloroquine	Stilbamidines
Vinblastine	Cyclic AMP
	Prostaglandin E

SOURCE: Adapted from references 138–140.

ample, streptolysin-O and streptolysin-S are known to lyse isolated neutrophil granules (141). When streptolysin-O is added to intact rabbit granulocytes, the granules lyse within minutes, leaving a clear cytoplasm (60, 146, 154). When injected into the joint space of rabbits, streptolysin-S induces a neutrophil accumulation and, subsequently, a mononuclear cell accumulation. Repeated injections result in chronic arthritis and the appearance of antibodies to lysosomal membranes (29, 142).

Streptococcal M-proteins also cause granulocyte lysis, as well as platelet aggregation and lysis (8). Protein antigen-A of *Staphylococci* will release histamine from mixed leukocyte suspensions.

Bacterial infection in man may produce a number of changes in granulocytes resulting in "the toxic neutrophil" (73, 78). These include (a) "toxic" granules that are more prominent than normal granules; (b) light blue,

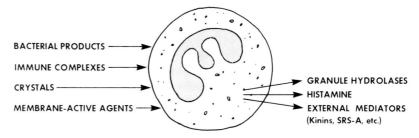

Figure 5.4 Release of granulocyte mediators of inflammation. Bacterial products, immune complexes, certain crystals, and membrane-active agents can cause granulocytes to discharge their hydrolytic enzymes, histamine, and other mediators of inflammation into the external environment.

amorphous inclusions called Döhle bodies (43) (see Chapter 1); (c) cytoplasmic vacuoles (152); and (d) lysosomal lability (78).

A variety of bacterial products may induce release of inflammatory constituents of the leukocyte, although the mechanism by which they accomplish this is not always apparent. Bacterial exotoxins may enter leukocytes by pinocytosis (91). Endotoxin, the product of gram-negative bacteria, has a complex interaction with granulocytes. This interaction is considered in a later section of this chapter.

Immune Complexes

Neutrophils ingest complexes of antigen-antibody and complement during the development of the vasculitis of the Arthus reaction (29, 34, 99, 133). Phagocytosis of such complexes causes degranulation with release of proteases into the surrounding fluid (100, 147). Antibody and complement fixed to a nonphagocytizable surface will also cause neutrophils to release granule constituents (56). The relation of granulocytes to the immunologic tissue injury is considered in detail later in this chapter.

Crystal Ingestion: Pathogenesis of Gouty Arthritis

In studying the mechanism of gouty arthritis, McCarty and his colleagues (80, 110) infused uric crystals into the joint spaces of dogs. The resultant inflammatory exudate contained primarily neutrophils. Small crystals were phagocytized by the cells, large crystals were surrounded by cellular aggregates (79). When crystals were injected into neutropenic animals, inflammation was minimal. The inference is that neutrophils are necessary for the induction of joint inflammation by urate crystals. One postulated mechanism (Fig. 5.5) is that following phagocytosis of the insoluble crystals, a fall in intra- and extracellular pH occurs, and hydrolytic enzymes leak out from the neutrophil granules. The low pH and the acid-active hydrolases induce an inflammatory reaction. Activation of the kinin system by leukocytes may contribute to this reaction. Furthermore, activation of certain complement components by neutrophil proteases from the granules may chemotactically attract more neutrophils, thus augmenting the inflammatory cycle (136).

Colchicine and corticosteroids may function as antiinflammatory agents by interfering with release of lysosomal enzymes. Colchicine may inhibit degranulation following phagocytosis (83) and may also interfere with the chemotactic activity of neutrophils (24). Glucocorticoids may stabilize lysosomes (138) and inhibit neutrophil migration to the site of inflammation. Other antiinflamma-

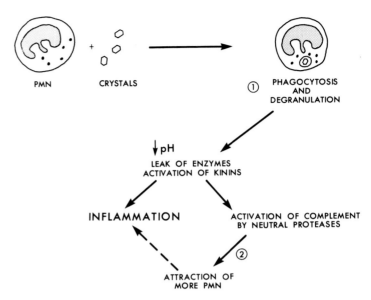

Figure 5.5 Schematic representation of one possible mechanism of the induction of inflammation by the interaction of urate crystals with polymorphonuclear leukocytes. Crystals are phagocytized, resulting in degranulation with a leak of hydrolytic enzymes. Attendant phenomena are a fall in extracellular pH and activation of the kinin system and of complement by neutrophil proteases. A cycle of inflammation is induced with the chemotactic attraction of more neutrophils.

tory agents, such as indomethacin, are also thought to inhibit neutrophil migration (110, 111). Inflammation induced by other phagocytizable crystals (such as silica) may follow a similar pathway, although macrophages, rather than neutrophils, probably are the chief protagonists in these reactions (1).

This model of crystal-induced arthritis leaves several unanswered questions. Whether the disrupting lysosomes come from neutrophils or synovial lining cells and macrophages is uncertain. What first brings the neutrophils into the joint space and why the inflammatory reaction is self-limited are also unknown.

Membrane-active Agents

When polyene antibiotics, which interact with lysosomal membrane, are injected into joint spaces they produce an arthritis reminiscent of that induced by urate (143). The inflammatory reaction may be inhibited by intra-articular cortisone. These antibiotics disrupt membranes by reacting with certain lipid components—phospholipids and/or cholesterol. Again, whether synovial lining cells or neutrophils make the greater contribution to the release of hydrolases is problematical.

Granulocytes and Immunologic Tissue Injury

The injury induced by antigen-antibody complexes is determined largely by the extent of their localization in a given tissue. These complexes seem to localize in a particular site for anatomic reasons rather than because of immunologic specificity. Small complexes may be retained in the circulation for long periods of time; they escape deposition and do not produce tissue injury. High concentrations of large aggregates, such as those seen in serum sickness, may rapidly clear from the circulation, localize in tissues, and induce an exudative granulocyte response and tissue necrosis. Complexes intermediate in size and concentration may circulate for weeks and months and slowly deposit, thereby inducing chronic inflammatory lesions of the vessel walls (42). As will be discussed, the lesions induced by immune complexes often involve neutrophils as one of the mediators of the inflammatory response. In his excellent reviews of this subject, Cochrane (28, 29, 31) describes three experimental models of neutrophil-mediated immunologic tissue injury: the vasculitis of the Arthus phenomenon, immune-complex–induced arteritis in serum sickness, and the acute glomerulonephritis of nephrotoxic nephritis. Since certain diseases of man closely resemble these experimental models, the role of neutrophils in these systems is of more than casual interest. *The critical series of events in all these models is (a) the formation and tissue localization of immune complexes, (b) the fixation of complement components, (c) the attraction of neutrophils, and (d) the release of inflammatory mediators from the leukocytes.*

The Arthus Phenomenon as a Model

The Arthus reaction is one of the simplest and best-understood models of immune complex disease (2, 29, 31). It is induced by local injection of antigen that reacts with circulating antibodies, or local injection of antibody that reacts with circulating antigen. Pathologically it is a localized, acute, necrotizing vasculitis associated with the deposition of large amounts of antigen-antibody precipitates in the walls of the blood vessels (33). These antigen-antibody complexes fix complement, which chemotactically attracts neutrophils (134). The leukocytes phagocytize the complexes and may degrade them (34). This sequence of events is illustrated in Fig. 5.6. By eight hours, mononuclear cells are present in the lesions; later, eosinophils and then histiocytes and plasma cells appear.

Depletion of circulating neutrophils by cytotoxic agents inhibits development of the Arthus lesion and prevents disruption of vascular structures and increased vascular

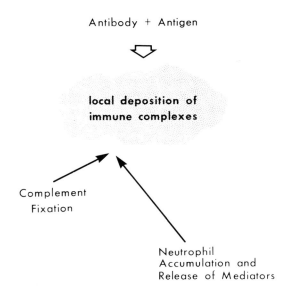

Figure 5.6 Schematic representation of events in the Arthus reaction. Antibody and antigen interact, resulting in local deposition of immune complexes. These fix complement and attract neutrophils that initiate an inflammatory cycle.

permeability (34). The inference that neutrophils are critical to the pathogenesis of this immune complex model is apparent.

Serum Sickness and Nephrotoxic Nephritis

The human disorder of serum sickness is closely mimicked when an experimental animal is given a single dose of foreign serum or serum protein. The course of the disease is outlined in Fig. 5.7. During the first 6 to 8 days after administration, the amount of antigen in the circulation slowly falls as the antigen is catabolized by nonimmune mechanisms. About day 9 to 11 the rate of antigen disappearance is abruptly accelerated.

As can be seen in Fig. 5.7, complexes of antigen and antibody first become evident in the circulation about day 6 or 7. Because these complexes are first seen under conditions of antigen excess, they are small and tend to remain in the circulation. Later, as more antibody is formed, the complexes become larger and are cleared rapidly. Union of antigen and antibody activates the complement sequence, and immune complexes bind complement. Serum hemolytic complement may be low during this phase of clinical symptomatology. As immune complexes are deposited in the tissues, clinical manifestations are seen in the kidney, joint, and heart (29, 31). The vascular lesions in these organs are characterized by increased permeability, endothelial proliferation, and neutrophil infiltration. Im-

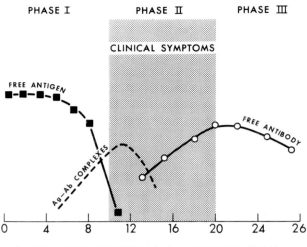

PHASE I   PHASE II   PHASE III

CLINICAL SYMPTOMS

FREE ANTIGEN

FREE ANTIBODY

Ag-Ab COMPLEXES

| | | | | | | | |
0   4   8   12   16   20   24   26

DAYS AFTER INJECTION OF FOREIGN SERUM

Figure 5.7 Schematic representation of the time course of events in the reaction to foreign serum. As antibody to the foreign protein is formed, free antigen is cleared from the serum, and antigen-antibody complexes make their appearance. Such complexes are deposited in the tissues and initiate a cycle of inflammation that is manifested in clinical symptoms. When all antigen is cleared from the circulation, free antibody persists for a period of time. (Modified from C. G. Cochrane and D. F. Dixon, *Calif. Med.* 111:99, 1969.)

munofluorescent techniques reveal immunoglobulin and complement in the lesions (10, 29, 81).

When neutrophils are depleted in rabbits immediately preceding development of the vascular lesions, the usual necrotizing arteritis with fibrinoid necrosis and disruption of the arterial lamina elastica does not occur (71). Again, the inference is that neutrophils are necessary for the full development of the inflammatory lesions of serum sickness.

In nephrotoxic nephritis, intravenous injection of antibody against kidney is followed within a few hours by accumulation of neutrophils in this organ (32). In studies of glomerulitis induced by nephrotoxic antiserum in the rat, Cochrane and his colleagues concluded that two immune mechanisms of injury were operative. The first required small amounts of complement-fixing antibody and was neutrophil dependent; the second required large amounts of antibody and did not require leukocytes (29, 32).

In both the Arthus reaction and acute nephrotoxic nephritis, there is a correlation between the ability of antibody to fix complement and the accumulation of neutrophils at the site of antigen-antibody deposition (29, 32, 134). Complement probably has a dual function: (a) release of factors chemotactic for neutrophils (see Chapter

4) (17, 20, 135, 137); and (b) immune adherence, a phenomenon in which neutrophils and macrophages bind immune complexes containing certain complement components.

Based on accumulated evidence, neutrophil hydrolases are probably critical in the development of these acute immune complex disorders as well as in more chronic varieties of serum sickness (29). The sites of attack for these hydrolases are the internal elastic lamina of arteries and the vascular basement membrane.

Glomerulonephritis

Glomerular lesions induced by circulating immune complexes in animals are very similar to those observed in human acute and chronic glomerulonephritis, and in the renal lesions of Henoch-Schonlein purpura and systemic lupus erythematosus (41, 42, 46, 47, 126). Neutrophil infiltration is seen both in the experimental models and in the human diseases. These observations suggest an immunologic mechanism that is associated with neutrophil accumulation in the pathogenesis of these disorders. Hydrolytic enzymes released from neutrophils by various tissue-injurious agents at sites remote from the kidneys may also induce renal damage (84).

Rheumatoid Arthritis

The joint lesions of rheumatoid arthritis are characterized by infiltration with leukocytes and their accumulation in synovial fluid, as well as by hyperplasia and hypertrophy of the synovial lining cells. Similar lesions can be induced in experimental animals by the intra-articular injection of isolated lysosomes (145).

The following is a hypothetical mechanism for the induction of tissue injury in rheumatoid arthritis. Rheumatoid factor forms immune complexes with altered immunoglobulin G. Such complexes may activate the complement sequence (156), some of whose components are chemotactic for neutrophils. The granulocytes that infiltrate the synovial cavity ingest the immune complexes. These cells, filled with engulfed complexes, have been called "RA cells" or "ragocytes." Since phagocytosis of immune complexes by neutrophils is known to result in degranulation, such cells have been presumed to release hydrolases into the synovial cavity (155). Although this hypothetical mechanism is quite attractive, it is by no means certain that it is the actual mechanism operative in vivo. The induction of inflammation in rheumatoid arthritis may be quite complex, and recent evidence suggests that high concentrations of rheumatoid factor may inhibit complement-mediated phagocytosis by granulocytes (82).

Granulocytes and Endotoxin

The interactions of endotoxin (21) with the intact animal or the human patient are so complex that one must of necessity focus on restricted aspects. Here we shall consider primarily the mechanism of endotoxin interaction with granulocytes of man and primates.

Bacterial endotoxin has complex effects on the formed elements of the blood. These effects appear to be a function of three variables: the dose of endotoxin, the species under investigation, and the presence or absence of immunologic memory of previous exposure to endotoxin. In rabbits, thrombocytopenia is the principal hematologic effect of endotoxin (39). In man and other primates, the granulocyte appears to be the principal target cell in the blood. Endotoxin injected intravenously produces a decrease in the numbers of circulating neutrophils followed, after a variable period of time, by "rebound" granulocytosis (16, 150). The granulocytopenic phase is presumed to result from vascular margination and sequestration of circulating leukocytes (101). The magnitude of the granulocytopenia varies with the amount of endotoxin administered (87). At low doses, sequestration of granulocytes in the pulmonary capillary bed occurs (61). At high concentrations of endotoxin, granulocyte destruction may occur.

The granulocytic phase of the endotoxin response in man has been used as a test of bone marrow reserve capacity (85). Granulocytes may be important in modulating

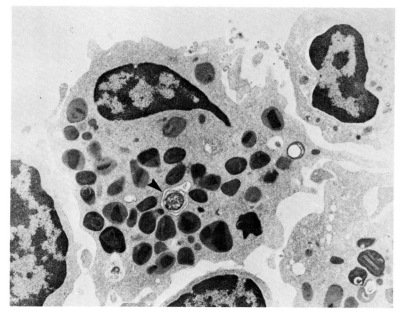

Figure 5.8 Electron micrograph of particulate endotoxin (a fragment of a gram-negative bacterium) within a phagocytic vacuole (*arrow*) of a human eosinophil.

the response of the whole animal to endotoxin, since cardiovascular changes and fever induced by bacterial lipopolysaccharide are modified in leukopenic animals (49).

Endotoxin has a number of effects on human granulocytes in vitro. It stimulates cellular glycolysis, the hexose monophosphate shunt, and RNA turnover; it induces loss of lysosomal enzymes from the granules into the external medium (27); it decreases neutrophil motility and induces cellular aggregation (22); and it stimulates thromboplastic activity (77, 103). These effects closely resemble those accompanying phagocytosis of particulate matter. By electron microscopy (Fig. 5.8) and autoradiographic studies with radioactive endotoxin, the bacterial lipopolysaccharide can be shown to enter the granulocyte (27, 91, 92). If similar events occur in vivo after endotoxemia, one might anticipate release of lysosomal hydrolases and activation of the kinin system in areas of leukocyte sequestration.

Endotoxin may occur in the form of aggregates of high molecular weight (1 to 24×10^6) (125) and is therefore in the range where uptake by phagocytic cells may be expected. Phagocytosis of endotoxin by platelets may occur also and result in dramatic cellular and biochemical changes in these cells (39).

A "naturally occurring" antibody to endotoxin, usually IgM, is present in the sera of many species of animals (95). Such antibodies are presumed to arise from repeated exposure to gram-negative bacteria and usually are not found in the blood of neonatal or germ-free animals. They occur at high concentrations after gram-negative bacterial infection. The requirement for such antibody in the interaction of endotoxin with granulocytes is not certain and may vary in different species. Very young animals lacking antibody are relatively resistant to certain of the effects of endotoxin (96, 128). In contrast, there is no demonstrable requirement for antibody for the in vitro effects of endotoxin on human granulocytes, whereas complement components appeared to be necessary (27).

The generalized Shwartzman reaction is an experimental model in which endotoxin induces widespread intravascular clotting and lesions in many organs, including the lungs and kidneys. Granulocytes appear to have an important function in the pathogenesis of this syndrome. Granulocytopenic rabbits with marrow depression induced by nitrogen mustard are not susceptible to the generalized reaction; infusion of granulocytes renders them susceptible (61, 131). Infusion of disrupted granulocytes into endotoxin-treated rabbits produces pulmonary artery thrombosis in most animals and glomerular thrombosis in some (61). These observations suggest a granulocyte clot-promoting factor operative in the pathogenesis of the generalized Shwartzman reaction. In addition, fragments of granulocytes may be observed in the pulmonary capillaries (62).

Leukocyte Pyrogen

Granulocytes and monocytes derived from either peripheral blood or inflammatory exudates of several mammalian species produce, upon appropriate stimulation, a pyrogenic substance designated *leukocyte pyrogen*. This material, a protein (72, 114), produces a characteristic febrile response when injected into rabbits (4, 9, 11, 12, 15, 18, 54).

Abundant evidence indicates that leukocyte pyrogen from peripheral blood cells is synthesized de novo after stimulation rather than released as a preformed cellular product (70, 120). Intact energy production and new RNA and protein synthesis appear to be necessary for its production (97, 98, 104). The pyrogenic proteins produced by granulocytes and mononuclear phagocytes are physically different (40).

Stimuli for release of leukocyte pyrogen include phagocytosis (11, 120), endotoxin (102, 120, 129), tuberculin (for mononuclear cells) (3), pyrogenic steroids such as etiocholanolone (13, 14, 149), and perhaps antigen-antibody com-plexes (121). Granulocyte pyrogens provoked by many different stimuli are physically identical (98), suggesting that only one leukocyte product is involved.

Endotoxin may also exert a pyrogenic effect on the central nervous system that is independent of the granulocyte mechanism (44).

In general, a latent phase occurs between the application of stimulus and the first detectable release of pyrogen.

Conclusion

The neutrophil serves a critical defense function against infectious microorganisms, utilizing its phagocytic activities and intracellular microbicidal systems. Under certain circumstances, it is important in localization and removal of immune complexes and damaged cells. Neutrophil substances involved in intracellular killing and digestion sometimes are released extracellularly. Tissue damage results when such extracellular release exceeds the ability of host inhibitors (for example, protease inhibitors) to neutralize the effects of these hydrolytic substances. The phenomenon appears to be particularly prominent with the ingestion of certain immune complexes and nondigestible crystals. Under such circumstances the action of neutrophils is detrimental to the host.

Chapter 5 References

1. Allison, A. C., Harington, J. S., and Birbeck, M. An examination of the cytotoxic effects of silica on macrophages, *J. Exp. Med.* 124:141, 1968.
2. Arthus, M. Injections répétées de sérum de chez le lapin, *C. R. Soc. Biol. (Paris)* 55:817, 1903.
3. Atkins, E., Bodel, P., and Francis, L. Release of an endogenous pyrogen *in vitro* from rabbit mononuclear cells, *J. Exp. Med.* 126:357, 1967.
4. Atkins, E., and Snell, E. S. Fever, *in* B. W. Zweifach, L. Grant, and R. T. McCluskey (eds.), The Inflammatory Process, p. 495, Academic Press, New York, 1965.
5. Barland, P., Janis, R., and Sandson, J. Immunofluorescent studies of human articular cartilage, *Ann. Rheum. Dis.* 25:156, 1966.
6. Barnhart, M. I. Importance of neutrophilic leukocytes in the resolution of fibrin, *Fed. Proc.* 24:846, 1965.
7. Barnhart, M. I. Proteases in inflammation, *Ann. N.Y. Acad. Sci.* 146:527, 1968.
8. Beachey, E. H., and Stollerman, G. H. Toxic effects of streptococcal M protein on platelets and polymorphonuclear leukocytes in human blood, *J. Exp. Med.* 134:351, 1971.
9. Beeson, P. B. Temperature-elevating effect of a substance obtained from polymorphonuclear leukocytes, *J. Clin. Invest.* 27:524, 1948.
10. Benacerraf, B., Potter, J. L., McCluskey, R. T., and Miller, F. The pathologic effects of intravenously administered soluble antigen-antibody complexes. II. Acute glomerulonephritis in rats, *J. Exp. Med.* 111:195, 1960.
11. Bodel, P., and Atkins, E. Human leukocyte pyrogen producing fever in rabbits, *Proc. Soc. Exp. Biol. Med.* 121:943, 1966.
12. Bodel, P., and Atkins, E. Release of endogenous pyrogen by human monocytes, *N. Engl. J. Med.* 276:1002, 1967.
13. Bodel, P., and Dillard, M. Studies on steroid fever. I. Production of leukocyte pyrogen *in vitro* by etiocholanolone, *J. Clin. Invest.* 47:107, 1968.
14. Bodel, P., Dillard, M., and Bondy, P. K. The mechanism of steroid in-

15. Bodel, P., and Hollingsworth, J. W. Pyrogen release from human synovial exudate cells, *Br. J. Exp. Pathol.* 49:11, 1968.
16. Boggs, D. R., Marsh, J. C., Chervenick, P. A., Cartwright, G. E., and Wintrobe, M. M. Neutrophil releasing activity in plasma of normal human subjects injected with endotoxin, *Proc. Soc. Exp. Biol. Med.* 127:689, 1968.
17. Bokisch, V. A., Müller-Eberhard, H. J., and Cochrane, C. G. Isolation of a fragment (C3a) of the third component of human complement containing anaphylatoxin and chemotactic activity and description of an anaphylatoxin inactivator of human serum, *J. Exp. Med.* 129:1109, 1969.
18. Bornstein, D. L., and Woods, J. W. Species specificity of leukocytic pyrogens, *J. Exp. Med.* 130:707, 1969.
19. Bourne, H., Lehrer, R. I., Cline, M. J., and Melmon, K. L. Cyclic 3′, 5′-adenosine monophosphate in the human leukocyte: synthesis, degradation and effects on neutrophil candidacidal activity, *J. Clin. Invest.* 50:920, 1971.
20. Boyden, S. The chemotactic effect of mixtures of antibody and antigen on polymorphonuclear leukocytes, *J. Exp. Med.* 115:453, 1962.
21. Braude, A. I. Bacterial endotoxins, *Sci. Am.* 210:36, 1964.
22. Bryant, R. E., Des Prez, R. M., and Rogers, D. E. Studies on human leukocyte motility. II. Effects of bacterial endotoxin on leukocyte migration, adhesiveness and aggregation, *Yale J. Biol. Med.* 40:192, 1967.
23. Burke, J. S., Uriuhara, T., MacMorine, D. R. L., and Movat, H. Z. A permeability factor released from phagocytosing PMN-leukocytes and its inhibition by protease inhibitors, *Life Sci.* 3:1505, 1964.
24. Caner, J. E. Z. Colchicine inhibition of chemotaxis, *Arthritis Rheum.* 8:757, 1965.
25. Clark, J. M., and Higginbotham, R. D. Significance of the mast cell response to a lysosomal protein, *J. Immunol.* 101:488, 1968.
26. Cline, M. J., and Melmon, K. L. Plasma kinins and cortisol: a pos-

sible explanation of the anti-inflammatory action of cortisol, *Science* 153:1135, 1966.
27. Cline, M. J., Melmon, K. L., Davis, W. C., and Williams, H. E. Mechanism of endotoxin interaction with human leucocytes, *Br. J. Haematol.* 15:539, 1968.
28. Cochrane, C. G. The role of immune complexes and complement in tissue injury, *J. Allergy* 42:113, 1968.
29. Cochrane, C. G. Immunologic tissue injury mediated by neutrophilic leukocytes, *Adv. Immunol.* 9:97, 1968.
30. Cochrane, C. G., and Aikin, B. S. Polymorphonuclear leukocytes in immunologic reactions. The destruction of vascular basement membrane *in vivo* and *in vitro*, *J. Exp. Med.* 124:733, 1966.
31. Cochrane, C. G., and Dixon, F. J. Cell and tissue damage through antigen-antibody complexes, *Calif. Med.* 111:99, 1969.
32. Cochrane, C. G., Unanue, E. R., and Dixon, F. J. A role of polymorphonuclear leukocytes and complement in nephrotoxic nephritis, *J. Exp. Med.* 122:99, 1965.
33. Cochrane, C. G., and Weigle, W. O. The cutaneous reaction to soluble antigen-antibody complexes. A comparison with the Arthus phenomenon, *J. Exp. Med.* 108:591, 1958.
34. Cochrane, C. G., Weigle, W. O., and Dixon, F. J. The role of polymorphonuclear leukocytes in the initiation and cessation of the Arthus vasculitis, *J. Exp. Med.* 110:481, 1959.
35. Darcy, D. A. Polymorphonuclear cell fractions which stimulate increase of an acute phase protein in the rat, *Br. J. Exp. Pathol.* 49:525, 1968.
36. Davies, P., Krakauer, K., and Weissmann, G. Subcellular distribution of neutral protease and peptidases in rabbit polymorphonuclear leucocytes, *Nature* 228:761, 1970.
37. De Duve, C., Pressman, B. C., Gianetto, R., Wattiaux, R., and Appelmans, F. Intracellular distribution patterns of enzymes in rat-liver tissue, *Biochem. J.* 60:604, 1955.
38. De Duve, C., and Wattiaux, R.

Functions of lysosomes, *Ann. Rev. Physiol.* 28:435, 1966.

39. Des Prez, R. M., and Bryant, R. E. Effects on bacterial endotoxin on rabbit platelets. IV. The divalent ion requirements of endotoxin-induced and immunologically induced platelet injury, *J. Exp. Med.* 124:971, 1966.

40. Dinarello, C. A., and Wolff, S. M. A new human endogenous pyrogen. Prog. 66th Ann. Mtg. Am. Soc. Clin. Invest., p. 20a, 1974.

41. Dixon, F. J. The pathogenesis of glomerulonephritis, *Am. J. Med.* 44:493, 1968.

42. Dixon, F. J., Feldman, J. D., and Vazquez, J. J. Experimental glomerulonephritis. The pathogenesis of a laboratory model resembling the spectrum of glomerulonephritis, *J. Exp. Med.* 113:899, 1961.

43. Döhle, H. Leukocyteneinschlusse bei Scharlach, *Z. Bakteriol. Parasitenk. Infektionskr. Abt. Orig.* 61:63, 1911.

44. DuBuy, B. Role of the granulocyte in the pyrogenic response to intracisternal endotoxin, *Proc. Soc. Exp. Biol. Med.* 123:606, 1966.

45. Erdös, E. G. Hypotensive peptides: bradykinin, kallidin and eledoisin, *Adv. Pharmacol.* 4:1, 1966.

46. Farquhar, M. G., Vernier, R. L., and Good, R. A. An electron microscope study of the glomerulus in nephrosis, glomerulonephritis and lupus erythematosus, *J. Exp. Med.* 106:649, 1957.

47. Feldman, J. D. Pathogenesis of ultrastructural glomerular changes induced by immunologic means, *in* P. Grabar and P. Miescher (eds.), Immunopathology III, p. 263, Benno Schwabe, Basel, 1963.

48. Fraser, J. R. E., and Clarris, B. J. On the reactions of human synovial cells exposed to homologous leucocytes *in vitro*, *Clin. Exp. Immunol.* 6:211, 1970.

49. Gillman, S. M., Bornstein, D. L., and Wood, W. B., Jr. Studies on the pathogenesis of fever. VIII. Further observations on the role of endogenous pyrogen in endotoxin fever, *J. Exp. Med.* 114:729, 1961.

50. Golub, E. S., and Spitznagel, J. K. The role of lysosomes in hypersensitivity reactions: tissue damage by polymorphonuclear neutrophil lysosomes, *J. Immunol.* 95:1060, 1965.

51. Gordon, A. H., and Darcy, D. A. Production of α_1-globulins by the perfused rat liver, *Br. J. Exp. Pathol.* 48:81, 1967.

52. Graham, H. T., Lowry, O. H., Wheelwright, F., Lenz, M. A., and Parish, H. H., Jr. Distribution of histamine among leukocytes and platelets, *Blood* 10:467, 1955.

53. Greenbaum, L. M., and Kim. K. S. The kinin-forming and kininase activities of rabbit polymorphonuclear leukocytes, *Br. J. Pharmacol. Chemother.* 29:238, 1967.

54. Hahn, H. H., Char, D. C., Postel, W. B., and Wood, W. B., Jr. Studies on the pathogenesis of fever. XV. The production of endogenous pyrogen by peritoneal macrophages, *J. Exp. Med.* 126:385, 1967.

55. Hawiger, J., Collins, R. D., and Horn, R. G. Precipitation of soluble fibrin monomer complexes by lysosomal protein fraction of polymorphonuclear leukocytes, *Proc. Soc. Exp. Biol. Med.* 131:349, 1969.

56. Henson, P. M. Immunologic release of constituents from neutrophil leukocytes, *J. Immunol.* 107:1535, 1971.

57. Henson, P. M. Pathologic mechanisms in neutrophil-mediated injury, *Am. J. Pathol.* 68:593, 1972.

58. Herion, J. C., Spitznagel, J. K., Walker, R. I., and Zeya, H. I. Pyrogenicity of granulocyte lysosomes, *Am. J. Physiol.* 211:693, 1966.

59. Hirsch, J. G. Neutrophil and eosinophil leucocytes, *in* B. W. Zweifach, L. Grant, and R. T. McCluskey (eds.), The Inflammatory Process, p. 245, Academic Press, New York, 1965.

60. Hirsch, J. G., Bernheimer, A. W., and Weissmann, G. Motion picture study of the toxic action of streptolysins on leucocytes, *J. Exp. Med.* 118:223, 1963.

61. Horn, R. G., and Collins, R. D. Studies on the pathogenesis of the generalized Shwartzman reaction, *Lab. Invest.* 18:101, 1968.

62. Horn, R. G., and Collins, R. D. Fragmentation of granulocytes in pulmonary capillaries during development of the generalized Shwartz-

man reaction, *Lab. Invest.* 19:451, 1968.

63. Janoff, A. Effect of an antihistamine on the increased vascular permeability induced by leucocyte lysosome fractions, *Nature* 212:1605, 1966.

64. Janoff, A. Destruction of vascular basement membrane at neutral pH by human leukocyte granules, *Fed. Proc.* 27:250, 1968.

65. Janoff, A. Mediators of tissue damage in human polymorphonuclear neutrophils, *Ser. Haematol.* 3:96, 1970.

66. Janoff, A., and Schaefer, S. Mediators of acute inflammation in leucocyte lysosomes, *Nature* 213:144, 1967.

67. Janoff, A., Schaefer, S., Scherer, J., and Bean, M. A. Mediators of inflammation in leukocyte lysosomes. II. Mechanism of action of lysosomal cationic protein upon vascular permeability in the rat, *J. Exp. Med.* 122:841, 1965.

68. Janoff, A., and Scherer, J. Mediators of inflammation in leukocyte lysosomes. IX. Elastinolytic activity in granules of human polymorphonuclear leukocytes, *J. Exp. Med.* 128:1137, 1968.

69. Janoff, A., and Zweifach, B. W. Production of inflammatory changes in the microcirculation by cationic proteins extracted from lysosomes, *J. Exp. Med.* 120:747, 1964.

70. Kaiser, H. K., and Wood, W. B., Jr. Studies on the pathogenesis of fever. IX. Production of endogenous pyrogen by polymorphonuclear leukocytes, *J. Exp. Med.* 115:27, 1962.

71. Kniker, W. T., and Cochrane, C. G. Pathogenic factors in vascular lesions of experimental serum sickness, *J. Exp. Med.* 122:83, 1965.

72. Kozak, M. S., Hahn, H. H., Lennarz, W. J., and Wood, W. B., Jr. Studies on the pathogenesis of fever. XVI. Purification and further chemical characterization of granulocytic pyrogen, *J. Exp. Med.* 127:341, 1968.

73. Kugel, M. A., and Rosenthal, N. Pathologic changes occurring in polymorphonuclear leukocytes during the progress of infections, *Am. J. Med. Sci.* 183:657, 1932.

74. Lapresle, C., and Webb, T. The purification and properties of a pro-

teolytic enzyme, rabbit cathepsin E, and further studies on rabbit cathepsin D, *Biochem. J.* 84:455, 1962.

75. Lazarus, G. S., Brown, R. S., Daniels, J. R., and Fullmer, H. M. Human granulocyte collagenase, *Science* 159:1483, 1968.

76. Lazarus, G. S., Daniels, J. R., Brown, R. S., Bladen, H. A., and Fullmer, H. M. Degradation of collagen by a human granulocyte collagenolytic system, *J. Clin. Invest.* 47:2622, 1968.

77. Lerner, R. G., Goldstein, R., and Cummings, G. Stimulation of human leukocyte thromboplastic activity by endotoxin, *Proc. Soc. Exp. Biol. Med.* 138:145, 1971.

78. McCall, C. E., Katayama, I., Cotran, R. S., and Finlan, M. Lysosomal and ultrastructural changes in human "toxic" neutrophils during bacterial infection, *J. Exp. Med.* 129:267, 1969.

79. McCarty, D. J., Jr. Phagocytosis of urate crystals in gouty synovial fluid, *Am. J. Med. Sci.* 243:288, 1966.

80. McCarty, D. J., Phelps, P., and Pyenson, J. Crystal-induced inflammation in canine joints. I. An experimental model with quantification of the host response, *J. Exp. Med.* 124:99, 1966.

81. McCluskey, R. T., Benacerraf, B., Potter, J. L., and Miller, F. The pathologic effects of intravenously administered soluble antigen-antibody complexes. I. Passive serum sickness in mice, *J. Exp. Med.* 111:181, 1960.

82. McDuffie, F. C., and Brumfield, H. W. Effect of rheumatoid factor on complement-mediated phagocytosis, *J. Clin. Invest.* 51:3007, 1972.

83. Malawista, S. E., and Bodel, P. Dissociation by colchicine of phagocytosis per se from increased oxygen consumption in human leukocytes, *J. Clin. Invest.* 45:1044, 1966.

84. Manaligod, J. R. Glomerular changes induced by extrarenal foci of inflammation and by polymorphonuclear cell lysates, *Am. J. Pathol.* 56:533, 1969.

85. Marsh, J. C., and Perry, S. The granulocyte response to endotoxin in patients with hematologic disorders, *Blood* 23:581, 1964.

86. Martin, R. R., and White, A. The *in*

vitro release of leukocyte histamine by staphylococcal antigens, *J. Immunol.* 102:437, 1969.

87. Mechanic, R. C., Frei, E., III, Landy, M., and Smith, W. W. Quantitative studies of human leukocytic and febrile response to single and repeated doses of purified bacterial endotoxin, *J. Clin. Invest.* 41:162, 1962.

88. Melmon, K. L., and Cline, M. J. Kinins (editorial), *Am. J. Med.* 43:153, 1967.

89. Melmon, K. L., and Cline, M. J. Interaction of plasma kinins and granulocytes, *Nature* 213:90, 1967.

90. Melmon, K. L., and Cline, M. J. The interaction of leukocytes and the kinin system, *Biochem. Pharmacol.* 271, 1968 (suppl.).

91. Mesrobeanu, I., Bona, C., Ioanid, L., and Mesrobeanu, L. Pinocytosis of some exotoxins by leucocytes, *Exp. Cell Res.* 42:490, 1966.

92. Mesrobeanu, I., Mesrobeanu, L., and Bona, C. La pinocytose des neurotoxines par les leucocytes, *Arch. Roum. Pathol. Exp. Microbiol.* 24:301, 1965.

93. Metchnikoff, E. Sur la lutte des cellules de l'organisme contre l'invasion des microbes, *Ann. Inst. Pasteur* 1:321, 1887.

94. Metchnikoff, E. Immunity in Infective Diseases (reprint of 1905 ed.), Johnson Reprint Corp., New York, 1968.

95. Michael, J. G., and Rosen, F. S. Association of "natural" antibodies to gram-negative bacteria with the α_1-macroglobulins, *J. Exp. Med.* 118:619, 1963.

96. Miler, I. Changes in susceptibility to bacterial endotoxin and infection during the early postnatal period in rats, *Folia Microbiol. (Praha)* 7:223, 1962.

97. Moore, D. M., Cheuk, S. F., Morton, J. D., Berlin, R. D., and Wood, W. B., Jr. Studies on the pathogenesis of fever. XVIII. Activation of leukocytes for pyrogen production, *J. Exp. Med.* 131:179, 1970.

98. Moore, D. M., Murphy, P. A., Chesney, P. J., and Wood, W. B., Jr. Synthesis of endogenous pyrogen by rabbit leukocytes, *J. Exp. Med.* 137:1263, 1973.

99. Movat, H. Z., Fernando, N. V. P.,

Uriuhara, T., and Weiser, W. J. Allergic inflammation. III. The fine structure of collagen fibrils at sites of antigen-antibody interaction in Arthus-type lesions, *J. Exp. Med.* 118:557, 1963.

100. Movat, H. Z., Uriuhara, T., MacMorine, D. L., and Burke, J. S. A permeability factor released from leukocytes after phagocytosis of immune complexes and its possible role in the Arthus reaction, *Life Sci.* 3:1025, 1964.

101. Mulholland, J. H., and Cluff, L. E. The effect of endotoxin upon susceptibility to infection: the role of the granulocyte, *in* M. Landy and W. Braun (eds.), Bacterial Endotoxins, p. 211, Rutgers University Press, New Brunswick, N. J., 1964.

102. Murphy, P. A. An assay method for leukocyte pyrogen, *J. Exp. Med.* 126:745, 1967.

103. Niemetz, J., and Fani, K. Thrombogenic activity of leukocytes, *Blood* 42:47, 1973.

104. Nordlund, J. J., Root, R. K., and Wolff, S. M. Studies on the origin of human leukocytic pyrogen, *J. Exp. Med.* 131:727, 1970.

105. Orange, R. P., and Austen, K. F. Slow reacting substance of anaphylaxis, *in* F. J. Dixon, Jr. and H. G. Kunkel (eds.), Advances in Immunology, vol. 10, p. 105, Academic Press, New York, 1969.

106. Orange, R. P., Valentine, M., and Austen, K. F. Release of slow-reacting substance of anaphylaxis in the rat: polymorphonuclear leukocyte, *Science* 157:318, 1967.

107. Orange, R. P., Valentine, M., and Austen, K. F. Antigen-induced release of slow reacting substance of anaphylaxis (SRS-A^rat^ in rats prepared with homologous antibody, *J. Exp. Med.* 127:767, 1968.

108. Osler, A. G., Lichtenstein, L. M., and Levy, D. A. *In vitro* studies of human reaginic allergy, *in* F. J. Dixon, Jr. and H. G. Kunkel (eds.), Advances in Immunology, vol. 8, p. 183, Academic Press, New York, 1968.

109. Persellin, R. H. Lysosome stabilization by leukocyte granule membrane antiserum, *J. Immunol.* 103:39, 1969.

110. Phelps, P., and McCarty, D. J. Crystal-induced inflammation in

canine joints. II. Importance of polymorphonuclear leukocytes, *J. Exp. Med.* 124:115, 1966.

111. Phelps. P., and McCarty, D. J. Suppressive effects of indomethacin on crystal-induced inflammation in canine joints and on neutrophilic motility *in vitro, J. Pharm. Exp. Therap.* 158:546, 1967.

112. Pruzansky, J. J., and Patterson, R. Subcellular distribution of histamine in human leukocytes, *Proc. Soc. Exp. Biol. Med.* 124:56, 1967.

113. Rafter, G. W., Cheuk, S. F., Krause, D. W., and Wood, W. B., Jr. Studies on the pathogenesis of fever. XIV. Further observations on the chemistry of leukocytic pyrogen, *J. Exp. Med.* 123:433, 1966.

114. Rafter, G. W., Collins, R. D., and Wood, W. B., Jr. Studies on the pathogenesis of fever. VII. Preliminary chemical characterization of leukocytic pyrogen, *J. Exp. Med.* 111:831, 1960.

115. Rajan, K. T. Lysosomes and gout, *Nature* 210:959, 1966.

116. Ranadive, N. S., and Cochrane, C. G. Fractionation and purification of cationic proteins of polymorphonuclear leukocytes, *Fed. Proc.* 26:574, 1967.

117. Ranadive, N. S., and Cochrane, C. G. Isolation and characterization of permeability factors from rabbit neutrophils, *J. Exp. Med.* 128:605, 1968.

118. Riddle, M. J., and Barnhart, M. I. The eosinophil as a source for profibrinolysin in acute inflammation, *Blood* 25:776, 1965.

119. Robertson, P. B., Ryel, R. B., Taylor, R. E., Shyu, K. W., and Fullmer, H. M. Collagenase: localization in polymorphonuclear leukocyte granules in the rabbit, *Science* 177:64, 1972.

120. Root, R. K., Nordlund, J. J., and Wolff, S. M. Factors affecting the quantitative production and assay of the human leukocytic pyrogen, *J. Lab. Clin. Med.* 75:679, 1970.

121. Root, R. K., and Wolff, S. M. Pathogenetic mechanisms in experimental immune fever, *J. Exp. Med.* 128:309, 1968.

122. Rous, P. The relative reaction within living mammalian tissues. II. On the mobilization of acid material within cells, and on the reaction as influenced by the cell state, *J. Exp. Med.* 41:399, 1925.

123. Sarcione, E. J., Bohne, M., and Krauss, S. Evidence for humoral stimulation of serum glycoprotein synthesis by the liver, *Fed. Proc.* 24:230, 1965 (abstract).

124. Scherer, J., and Janoff, A. Mediators of inflammation in leukocyte lysosomes. VII. Observations on mast cell-rupturing agents in different species, *Lab. Invest.* 18:196, 1968.

125. Schramm, G., Westphal, O., and Luderitz, O. Über bakterielle Reizstoffe. III. Mitt: Physikalischchemisches Verhalten eines hochgereinigten Coli-Pyrogens, *Z. Naturforsch.* 7B:594, 1952.

126. Seegal, B. C., Andres, G. A., Hsu, K. C., and Zabriskie, J. B. Studies on the pathogenesis of acute and progressive glomerulonephritis in man by immunofluorescein and immunoferritin techniques, *Fed. Proc.* 24:100, 1965.

127. Seegers, W., and Janoff, A. Mediators of inflammation in leukocyte lysosomes. VI. Partial purification and characterization of a mast cell-rupturing component, *J. Exp. Med.* 124:833, 1966.

128. Smith, R. T., and Thomas, L. Influence of age upon response to meningococcal endotoxin in rabbits, *Proc. Soc. Exp. Biol. Med.* 86:806, 1954.

129. Snell, E. S., and Atkins, E. Interactions of gram-negative bacterial endotoxin with rabbit blood *in vitro, Am. J. Physiol.* 212:1103, 1967.

130. Thomas, L. The role of lysosomes in tissue injury, in B. W. Zweifach, L. Grant, and R. T. McCluskey (eds.), The Inflammatory Process, p. 449, Academic Press, New York, 1965.

131. Thomas, L., and Good, R. A. Studies on the generalized Shwartzman reaction. I. General observations concerning the phenomenon, *J. Exp. Med.* 96:605, 1952.

132. Uriuhara, T., MacMorine, D. R. L., and Franklin, A. E. The pathogenicity of PMN-leukocyte lysosomes in allergic inflammation and tissue injury, *Fed. Proc.* 24:368, 1965 (abstract).

133. Uriuhara, T., and Movat, H. Z. The role of PMN-leukocyte lysosomes in tissue injury, inflammation and hypersensitivity. I. The vascular changes and the role of PMN-leukocytes in the reversed passive Arthus reaction, *Exp. Mol. Pathol.* 5:539, 1966.

134. Ward, P. A., and Cochrane, C. G. Bound complement and immunologic injury of blood vessels, *J. Exp. Med.* 121:215, 1965.

135. Ward, P. A., Cochrane, C. G., and Müller-Eberhard, H. J. The role of serum complement in chemotaxis of leukocytes *in vitro, J. Exp. Med.* 122:327, 1965.

136. Ward, P. A., and Hill, J. H. C'5 chemotactic fragments produced by an enzyme in lysosomal granules of neutrophils, *J. Immunol.* 104:535, 1970.

137. Ward, P. A., and Newman, L. J. A neutrophil chemotactic factor from C'5, *J. Immunol.* 102:93, 1969.

138. Weissmann, G. Lysosomes and joint disease, *Arthritis Rheum.* 9:834, 1966.

139. Weissmann, G. The role of lysosomes in inflammation and disease, *Ann. Rev. Med.* 18:97, 1967.

140. Weissmann, G. Lysosomal mechanisms of tissue injury in arthritis, *N. Engl. J. Med.* 286:141, 1972.

141. Weissmann, G., Becher, B., and Thomas, L. Studies on lysosomes V., *J. Cell Biol.* 22:115, 1964.

142. Weissmann, G., Becher, B., Wiedermann, G., and Bernheimer, A. W. Acute and chronic arthritis produced by intra-articular injections of streptolysin S in rabbits, *Am. J. Pathol.* 46:129, 1965.

143. Weissmann, G., Pras, M., and Rosenberg, L. Arthritis induced by filipin in rabbits, *Arthritis Rheum.* 10:325, 1967.

144. Weissmann, G., and Spilberg, I. Breakdown of cartilage protein-polysaccharide by lysosomes, *Arthritis Rheum.* 11:162, 1968.

145. Weissmann, G., Spilberg, I., and Krakauer, K. Arthritis induced in rabbits by lysates of granulocyte lysosomes, *Arthritis Rheum.* 12:103, 1969.

146. Weissmann, G., Uhr, J. W., and Thomas, L. Acute hypervitaminosis A in guinea pigs. I. Effects on acid hydrolases, *Proc. Soc. Exp. Biol. Med.* 112:284, 1963.

147. Weissmann, G., Zurier, R. B., Spieler, P. J., and Goldstein, I. M. Mechanisms of lysosomal enzyme

release from leukocytes exposed to immune complexes and other particles, *J. Exp. Med.* 134:149s, 1971.

148. Wepsic, H. T., and Hollingsworth, J. W. Effect of drugs on different types of synovial inflammation in the rabbit, *Yale J. Biol. Med.* 41:273, 1968.

149. Wolff, S. M., Kimball, H. R., Perry, S., Root, R. K., and Kappas, A. The biological properties of etiocholanolone, *Ann. Intern. Med.* 67:1268, 1967.

150. Wolff, S. M., Rubenstein, M., Mulholland, J. H., and Alling, D. W. Comparison of hematologic and fe-

brile response to endotoxin in man, *Blood* 26:190, 1965.

151. Wright, D. G., and Malawista, S. E. The mobilization and extracellular release of granular enzymes from human leukocytes during phagocytosis, *J. Cell Biol.* 53:788, 1972.

152. Zieve, P. D., Haghshenass, M., Blanks, M., and Krevans, J. R. Vacuolization of the neutrophil. An aid in the diagnosis of septicemia, *Arch. Intern. Med.* 118:356, 1966.

153. Ziff, M., Gribetz, H. J., and Lospalluto, J. Effect of leukocyte and synovial membrane extracts on cartilage mucoprotein, *J. Clin. Invest.*

39:405, 1960.

154. Zucker-Franklin, D. Electron microscope study of the degranulation of polymorphonuclear leukocytes following treatment with streptolysin, *Am. J. Pathol.* 47:419, 1965.

155. Zucker-Franklin, D., and Hirsch, J. G. Electron microscope studies on the degranulation of rabbit peritoneal leukocytes during phagocytosis. *J. Exp. Med.* 120:569, 1964.

156. Zvaifler, N. Further speculation on the pathogenesis of joint inflammation in rheumatoid arthritis, *Arthritis Rheum.* 13:895, 1970.

Chapter 6 The Eosinophil

The eosinophil was probably first described by T. W. Jones in 1846 when he included a description of a "coarse granular cell" in his report to the Royal Society (95). In 1879 Ehrlich noted the affinity of the coarse granules for acid dyes and christened the cell *eosinophil*. The cell was so attractive to morphologists that in 1914 Schwartz was able to write a monograph about it that contained 2,758 references (163).

Despite the well-documented association of this cell with allergic diseases, its specific functions in the body's economy remain largely unknown. The major roles postulated for the eosinophil are sequestering immune complexes and limiting inflammatory reactions.

The eosinophil clearly has many features in common with the neutrophil in morphogenesis, structure, and metabolism. It also has several distinctive features including surface antigenicity, certain unique enzymes (159), and the longevity of the morphologically mature cell. The factors governing stem cell differentiation along the eosinophilic pathway are largely unknown.

Morphogenesis and Fine Structure

When viewed by electron microscopy, the nuclear morphology of the eosinophil generally appears similar to that of the neutrophil. The known features of the eosinophil that distinguish it from the neutrophil are prominent and distinctive granulation, the presence of only two or three nuclear lobes in the mature cell, a more highly developed Golgi apparatus, and more numerous mitochondria.

In Romanovsky-stained preparations of bone marrow,

the earliest identifiable cell of the eosinophilic series is an eosinophilic promyelocyte that contains 10 or 12 small eosinophilic granules in addition to the more common azurophilic granules (Figs. 6.1 and 6.2) (see Chapter 1). Such cells are very rarely encountered in the examination of the normal bone marrow but are seen, with moderate frequency, in a variety of eosinophilic states.

As maturation proceeds, eosinophilic granules become more prominent and numerous; by the myelocyte stage of development, azurophilic granules are no longer seen. The eosinophilic myelocyte is the least mature cell of the series found with any frequency in normal bone marrow (Fig. 6.3). The eosinophilic metamyelocyte and band forms are slightly smaller than the antecedent myelocyte and generally contain fewer eosinophilic granules (Fig. 6.4). The mature eosinophil usually has a bilobed nucleus and prominent cytoplasmic, eosinophilic granules (Figs. 6.5 and 6.6).

Young Cells

The following characteristics that gauge the maturity of the neutrophilic series serve to stage eosinophils: the degree of condensation of the nuclear chromatin, the state of development of the nucleoli and cytoplasmic granular reticulum, and the granule population of the cytoplasm (208) (see Chapter 1).

The young eosinophil has many of the characteristics of immature granulocytes: a high nuclear-to-cytoplasmic ratio, a large nucleus with diffuse chromatin pattern, and well-developed nucleoli. The cytoplasm has a complex

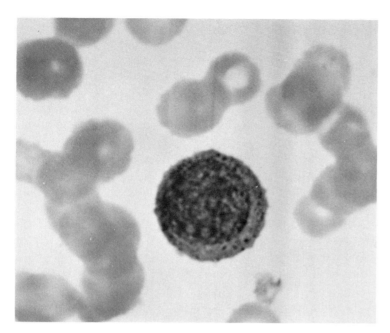

Figure 6.1 Eosinophilic promyelocyte; Wright stain.

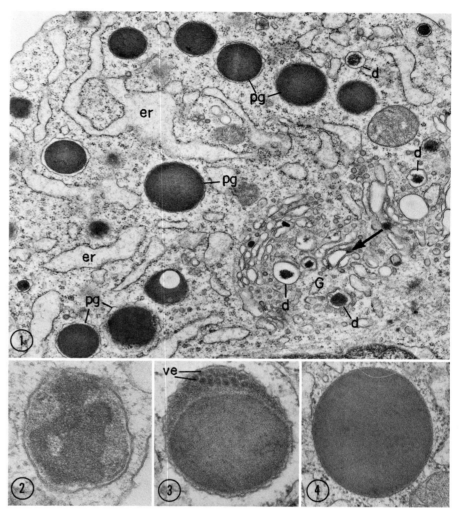

granular endoplasmic reticulum and large mitochondria. Cells of this level of maturity are very rare, whereas cells slightly more advanced in maturation and demonstrating early condensation of nuclear chromatin (Fig. 6.3) are encountered somewhat more frequently.

The most immature eosinophils are recognized by the presence in the cytoplasm of a few homogeneously dense, spherical granules measuring 0.6 to 1.0 micron in diameter (Fig. 6.2). These granules lack the granular crystalloids characteristic of the mature eosinophil. However, a few angular, crystalloid-containing granules soon appear among the spherical granule population of the immature cells. This second granule population consists in irregular, sharp-edged polyhedrons that contain randomly oriented arrays of crystalloids (Fig. 6.3). Such crystalloids are comprised of parallel-stemmed lamellae with no identifiable periodic substructure.

The size of the first populations of homogeneous round granules (0.6 micron) distinguishes them from the homogeneous and smaller primary granules (0.4 micron) of neutrophils and basophils. The homogeneous spherical eosinophil granules are also characterized by relative resistance to crenation and to extraction caused by fixatives. Such artifacts occur readily in neutrophils and basophils.

The homogeneous dense granules of the eosinophil con-

Figure 6.2 Fields from eosinophilic progranulocytes in rabbit bone marrow, illustrating the steps involved in formation of the large (600 to 1,200 millimicrons) primary eosinophil granules.

There are numerous dilated cisternae of the rough ER (*er*), and a prominent Golgi region (*G*) with condensing secretory material. Granule formation appears to occur by condensation of dense material within Golgi cisternae (*arrow*), with subsequent budding of dense-cored vacuoles (*d*) from the inner Golgi cisternae. Several vacuoles then merge into a form with a dense center and lighter periphery containing small vesicles (*ve*) (square 3). The mature or fully condensed granule (*pg*) is spherical with a homogeneous dense content (squares 1 and 4).

The formation of these large primary granules by the eosinophilic progranulocyte resembles the process by which azurophil granules are formed in the PMN progranulocyte. However, the eosinophilic progranulocyte differs from its PMN counterpart in that its ER cisternae (*er*) are shorter and more dilated, its granules are larger and more regularly spherical, and immature granules frequently contain small (~300 Å) vesicles not seen in PMN azurophil granules. Square 1, magnification × 16,000; square 2, × 65,500; square 3, × 52,000; square 4, × 34,500. (From D. F. Bainton and M. G. Farquhar, *J. Cell Biol.* 45:54, 1970. Reprinted by permission of authors and publisher.)

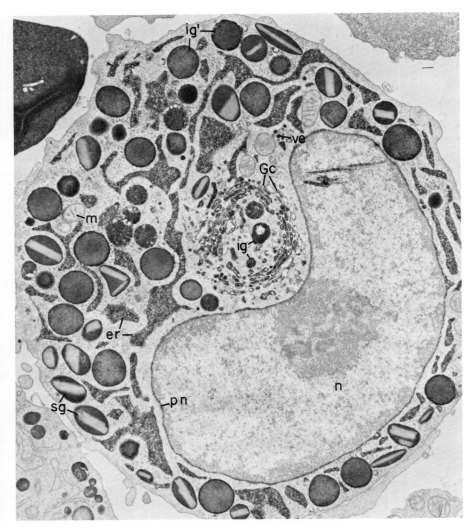

Figure 6.3 Rat eosinophil myelocyte from a preparation incubated for peroxidase. Reaction product appears as a dark, flocculent precipitate that fills the entire rough endoplasmic reticulum (*er*) including the perinuclear cisterna (*pn*), clusters of smooth vesicles (*ve*) at the periphery of the Golgi complex, all the cisternae of the Golgi complex (*Gc*) (shown at a higher magnification in Fig. 6.8), all the immature granules located both in the Golgi region (*ig*) and in the peripheral cytoplasm (*ig'*), and mature granules (*sg*). In mature granules, reaction product is not present in the area occupied by the crystalline bar, which stands out sharply against the dark background provided by the remainder of the reactive granule. Since the section was only lightly stained with lead, ribosomes do not show up and the density of the granules is caused almost entirely by reaction product. Note that no reaction product is seen in the cytoplasmic matrix, the nucleus (*n*), or the mitochondria (*m*). Specimen fixed for three hours at 4° C in glutaraldehyde and incubated one hour at 25° C in Graham and Karnovsky's medium (pH 7.6). Magnification × 12,500. (From D. F. Bainton and M. G. Farquhar, *J. Cell Biol.* 45:54, 1970. Reprinted by permission of authors and publisher.)

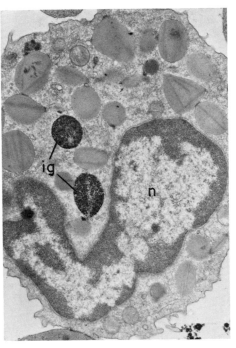

Figure 6.4 Band form of a rabbit eosinophil reacted for acid phosphatase. The only elements that contain reaction product are two immature granules (*ig*). The remainder of the granules, most of which appear fully condensed or mature, are not reactive. Magnification × 10,500. (From D. F. Bainton and M. G. Farquhar, *J. Cell Biol.* 45:54, 1970. Reprinted by permission of authors and publisher.)

tain peroxidase, PAS-reactive material, and acid phosphatase activity. The crystalloid-containing granules have peroxidase activity and also contain zinc and basic proteins (12, 19, 86, 96, 144, 191, 192), the presence of which is required for the aminopeptidase and acid phosphatase activities found in the eosinophil.

Intermediate Cells

Like the intermediate neutrophil, the intermediate eosinophil is characterized by moderately condensed nuclear chromatin and small or absent nucleoli. The cisternae of the granular endoplasmic reticulum of the eosinophil tend to be more dilated than those of the neutrophil, and the mitochondria of the eosinophil are generally larger. Both the homogeneous and crystalline forms of eosinophilic granules are seen in the cytoplasm of the intermediate cell (Fig. 6.3). Granule forms intermediate between these two types have also been identified (88, 140, 205). Because the numbers of each type of granule remain relatively constant during the intermediate stage of development, the following has been suggested: (a) homogeneous granules are continually produced and transformed into

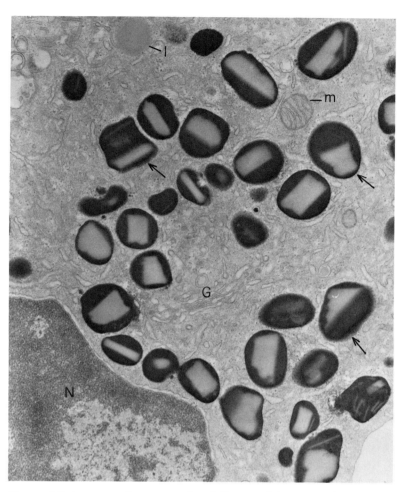

Figure 6.5 A mature human eosinophil reacted for peroxidase. *N* = nucleus, *l* = lipid, *m* = mitochondrion, *G* = Golgi complex. Arrows point to numerous peroxidase-positive granules. Note that the crystalline core of the granules does not contain reaction product. (Photograph courtesy of Dr. Dorothy Bainton.)

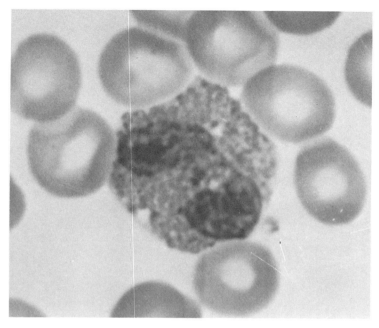

Figure 6.6 A mature human eosinophil from the peripheral blood; Wright stain.

crystalline granules, and (*b*) both types of granules are distributed to the daughter cells with each cell division (cf. 56, 88, 199). The possibility also exists, however, that each type of granule population arises independently.

The evidence for production of granules from the Golgi apparatus in eosinophils is similar to that for neutrophils. Peroxidase activity can be demonstrated in the Golgi, in the cisternae of the granular endoplasmic reticulum, and in both homogeneous and crystalline granules (11, 205) (Figs. 6.7 to 6.9).

Acid phosphatase is probably made in the protein-synthesizing apparatus of the granular reticulum and also packaged in the Golgi. In the early and intermediate eosinophil, Golgi saccules are often distended and have flocculent material of moderate density (Fig. 6.7). Such material is also seen in small vacuoles in the Golgi region and

elsewhere in the cytoplasm. The sequential labeling of Golgi, and then of granules, with tritiated lysine supports the notion of granulogenesis within the Golgi complex (65).

Mature Eosinophils

As in other mature cells of the granulocytic series, the nuclear chromatin of the mature eosinophil is quite condensed and marginated (Fig. 6.5). Nucleoli are absent. Nuclear lobation is less pronounced in the eosinophil than in the neutrophil, and mature eosinophils are generally bilobed. The cytoplasmic reticulum is greatly diminished relative to the highly developed state in the intermediate-staged cell. Mitochondria are fairly abundant and large in the mature eosinophilic leukocyte, unlike the mature neutrophil, suggesting a greater dependence on aerobic metabolism. The granule population of the mature cell is generally restricted to the crystalloid-containing granules (Fig. 6.5).

An autosomal recessive defect of eosinophil morphogenesis has been described. It consists in absence of peroxidase, reduced phospholipids, diminished specific granulation, and hypersegmentation of the nucleus (145, 146). It is not associated with clinical abnormalities.

Species Differences and Eosinophilic Fine Structures

The basic features of eosinophil maturation outlined above are observed in a variety of mammalian species.

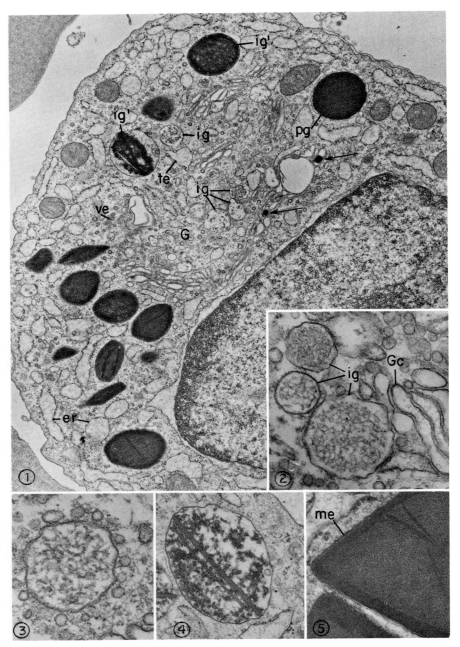

Figure 6.7 Fields from eosinophilic myelocytes in rabbit bone marrow, depicting stages in the formation of specific granules. There is abundant dilated rough endoplasmic reticulum (*er*) and a large Golgi region (*G*) containing many early or immature specific granules (*ig*). At the periphery of the Golgi complex are a number of transitional elements of the ER (*te*) and clusters of small vesicles (*ve*).

Granule formation begins with the appearance of dense (*arrows*) or stringy material within Golgi cisternae. Here numerous immature granules (*ig*) with a flocculent content are present in the Golgi region (squares 1 and 2). As granule formation proceeds, several of these immature granules coalesce into

Progressive condensation and margination of nuclear chromatin, loss of nucleoli, increase and then subsequent diminution in the complexity of the Golgi and granular reticulum, and the production of characteristic granules are hallmarks of eosinophilic maturation in the guinea pig, mouse, cat, rat, and horse, as well as in man. Differences in the morphogenesis of the eosinophilic series among species generally relate either to the evolution of the granule population or to the structure of the granules.

Two forms of eosinophil granules (angular, crystalloid-containing; and spherical, homogeneous, and dense) have been described in the guinea pig (13, 63, 88, 140), mouse (199), rat (13, 18, 140, 205), rhesus monkey (199), and man (21, 31, 60, 64, 106). Differences in the geometry of the crystalloids have been noted between species (21, 63, 134, 136, 140). Periodic structure in the crystalloids has been demonstrated in man (25, 134, 195) and in the rat (18, 134), guinea pig (134), mouse (166), and cat (14, 63). The periodicity varies with the species. The mink has unusual granules with dense, spherical inclusions lacking periodicity. (54, 122), and many of the granules of the gorilla apparently lack crystalloids (91).

Eosinophil Kinetics

The peripheral blood contains only a small fraction of the total eosinophil pool. Hudson's review suggests that for each circulating cell there is a bone marrow reserve of 300 mature and immature cells and between 100 and 300 eosinophils in the tissue (89).

The eosinophil spends three to six days in the bone marrow before release into the circulation. In dogs, its circulating half-life is about 30 minutes compared to a $T_{1/2}$ of four to six hours for the neutrophil (32). The eosinophil probably survives longer in the tissues than does the neutrophil. It survives eight to twelve days in tissue culture, compared to the two- to four-day survival of the neutrophil (137). Once the eosinophil leaves the circulation and enters the tissues, it probably does not return to the blood stream in normal subjects. However, in two pa-

larger forms (square 3 and *ig'*, square 1), condensation occurs, and crystals appear (square 4). Square 5 shows that the forming crystals frequently are found adjacent to the granule membrane (*me*) and parallel to it. Here the membrane follows the contour of the crystal. Square 1 includes a primary granule (*pg*), which appears denser and more regularly round than the condensing specific granules and lacks crystals. Square 1, magnification × 8,500; square 2, × 48,500; square 3, × 56,000; square 4, × 32,500; square 5, × 41,000. (From D. F. Bainton and M. G. Farquhar, *J. Cell Biol.* 45:54, 1970. Reprinted by permission of authors and publisher.)

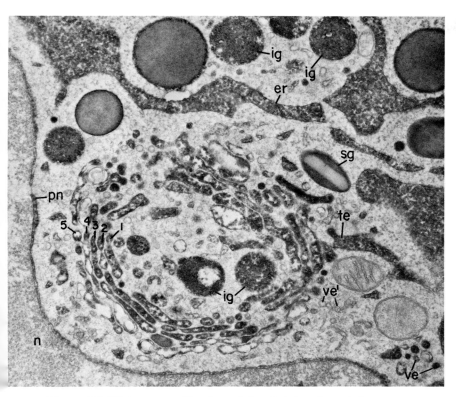

Figure 6.8 Higher magnification of the Golgi region of the eosinophilic myelocyte shown in Fig. 6.3. The localization of peroxidase reaction product in Golgi cisternae and in transitional elements at the periphery of the Golgi complex (*te*) can be seen to better advantage. Note that all five cisternae in the Golgi stack (1–5) are reactive. Reaction product can also be seen in the rough endoplasmic reticulum (*er*), perinuclear cisterna (*pn*), specific granules (*sg*), and immature granules (*ig*), but not in the nucleus (*n*). Many of the small vesicles (*ve*) in the Golgi region contain reaction product, but others (*ve'*) do not. Magnification × 36,000. (From D. F. Bainton and M. G. Farquhar, *J. Cell Biol.* 45:54, 1970. Reprinted by permission of authors and publisher.)

tients with marked eosinophilia, labeled cells began to recirculate within 24 hours of disappearance from the circulation (82).

The bone marrow responds readily to an eosinophilotactic stimulus and is able to begin replenishment of its reserves within two days. Eosinophil production in man normally is confined to the bone marrow. In some animals eosinophilopoiesis occurs in many organs of the reticuloendothelial system. The number of circulating eosinophils roughly indicates the eosinophilopoietic activity. Felarca and Lowell (66) found the total peripheral blood eosinophil count to be less than 250 per cubic millimeter (mean = 100) in a normal population. The level was higher (mean = 202) in patients with allergy.

Diurnal variation of the eosinophil count occurs, with the highest levels at midnight and the lowest levels at noon (188).

Hypoxia may release eosinophils from the marrow (90). Adrenal 11,17-oxycorticosteroids produce eosinopenia in the peripheral blood (84, 149). Administration of epinephrine can also produce eosinopenia, an effect potentiated by glucocorticoids (186). Pretreatment of normal subjects with propranolol blocks the effect of epinephrine on the circulating eosinophil number, suggesting that its action is mediated via beta-adrenergic receptors (100).

Eosinophil Composition and Metabolism

Composition

Clearly, the unusual cytological feature of the eosinophil is the granule system. Archer and Hirsch have shown that half the total protein of the eosinophil is in this cytoplasmic organelle (3). Consequently, considerable attention has been devoted to the study of the composition of the granule population, first by cytochemical techniques and more recently by cell fractionation and biochemical techniques. The major identifiable granule constituents include basic protein or proteins, an oxygenase (peroxidase), and acid phosphatase. Eosinophils of the horse and rat lack lysozyme (3).

The affinity of the eosinophil for "acid" dyes has been attributed to the granule content of an arginine-rich basic protein (70, 165, 193). The function of this protein, or these proteins, is largely unknown. Eosinophil granules apparently lack the bactericidal activity attributed to the cationic protein found in the neutrophil granules of some species (206) (Chapter 4). Recently a low-molecular-weight homogeneous protein accounting for about half of the total granule proteins has been extracted from guinea pig eosinophils (74). This protein lacks peroxidase activity and its functions are unknown.

A high content of zinc extractable from eosinophil granules is thought to be associated with a basic protein or peptide (19, 37, 144, 201).

Eosinophil granules are extremely rich in peroxidase activity (3, 60, 120, 121, 155, 204, 205). The function of this abundant peroxidase activity, long noted in cytochemical studies (76, 189), again is unknown. Neutrophil myeloperoxidase has a microbicidal function (99, 107, 108); it is not known whether eosinophil peroxidase has any bactericidal activity (40, 41).

The eosinophil peroxidase is antigenically distinct and differs in its heme spectrum from the peroxidase enzyme of the neutrophil (159). In the genetic disorder of deficient

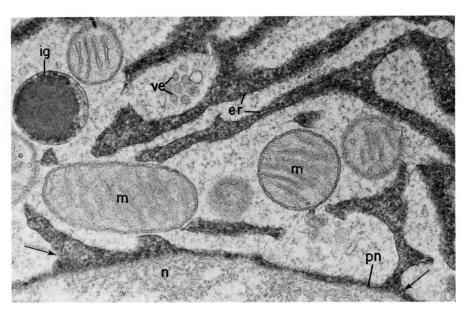

Figure 6.9 The rough endoplasmic reticulum (*er*), including the perinuclear cisterna (*pn*) with which it is continuous (*arrows*), is filled with dense peroxidase reaction product. An immature granule (*ig*) is also reactive. No peroxidase is seen in the cytoplasmic matrix, in the nucleus (*n*), in mitochondria (*m*), or in a cluster of smooth vesicles (*ve*). The ribosomes do not show up in this section, which was lightly stained with lead. Magnification × 44,000. (From D. F. Bainton and M. G. Farquhar, *J. Cell Biol.* 45:54, 1970. Reprinted by permission of authors and publisher.)

myeloperoxidase, eosinophil peroxidase persists although neutrophil and monocyte myeloperoxidase is absent. A familial absence of eosinophil peroxidase also has been described (145). These observations support the notion of divergent granulogenesis in the eosinophilic and neutrophilic cell lines.

High catalase activity in eosinophils has been described, although the methods of study employed have not been wholly satisfactory (1, 92).

Acid phosphatase has been identified histochemically in the granules of both mature and immature eosinophils (72, 147, 148, 164, 182). In the mature cells of most species studied, including man, the general pattern has been one of strong acid phosphatase activity in the homogeneous dense granules and relatively low or absent activity in the crystalloid-containing granules (60, 200, 205). Extraction of eosinophil granule populations reveals a lower acid phosphatase activity than is found in the neutrophil granules (3, 51). In the eosinophil, acid phosphatase activity is associated mainly with a light granule subfraction rather than with the main granule fraction

(120, 121); in other words, probably with the spherical homogeneous granules.

Most histochemical studies have failed to demonstrate alkaline phosphatase activity in eosinophil granules of the rabbit (200). Low levels of activity have been described in the eosinophils of the horse and rat (3, 133, 205), although the data for these species are not unequivocal and may reflect contamination by neutrophil granules (3).

The following granule-associated enzymes have been found in eosinophil-rich fractions of horse and human blood and in guinea pig peritoneal exudate: beta-glucuronidase, cathepsin, aryl sulfatase, ribonuclease, and deoxyribonuclease (3, 120, 121, 185, 193). Lysozyme has not been found in the eosinophil.

Histamine has been described in the eosinophil, but minor contamination with other varieties of leukocytes may have occurred in these studies (77, 78). Plasminogen (profibrinolysin) has also been reported to exist in eosinophils (15, 151). Among the various types of human leukocytes, eosinophils are a rich source of kinin-destroying enzyme activity (kininase) (130).

Metabolism

Relatively little is known about the metabolism of either the developing eosinophil or the mature cell (37, 39, 85). The reason for this paucity of information is the difficulty in obtaining sufficient numbers of pure populations of normal eosinophils for biochemical studies.

The relatively large and abundant mitochondria of the intermediate and mature cell suggest a well-developed aerobic metabolism; however, well-organized studies are difficult to find. In a limited number of analyses of the leukocyte enzymes involved in carbohydrate metabolism, eosinophils were reported to have lower activities than neutrophils of hexokinase (73) and aconitase (184). The rate of glucose utilization is similar in neutrophils and eosinophils (62). Like neutrophils, eosinophils appear to be dependent primarily upon anaerobic mechanisms of energy production for phagocytosis. Inhibitors of glycolytic enzymes, but not of respiration, are effective in suppressing phagocytosis by eosinophils. The stimulation of hexose monophosphate shunt activity provoked by phagocytosis occurs in eosinophils as well as in neutrophils (41).

Glucose utilization by the eosinophil is apportioned roughly as follows: 90 percent is converted to lactic acid, 3 to 6 percent is oxidized to CO_2, and 3 to 4 percent is utilized for glycogen, lipids, and amino acids. Most of the glucose is metabolized by the Embden-Meyerhof pathway and only about 2 percent traverses the pentose shunt. There is little utilization of acetate for lipid synthesis (181).

Functions

Chemotaxis: Interaction with Antigen and Antibody

Eosinophils demonstrate amoeboid motion in culture and move toward certain chemotactic stimuli. Their in vitro chemotactic activity is considerably different from that of neutrophils. In vivo, eosinophils are generally found only in small numbers at sites of acute inflammation, whereas they are often abundant in areas of chronic inflammation —the opposite relation exists for neutrophils.

In vitro, several substances can orient the migration of eosinophils, including histamine (5, 6, 67) and some antigen-antibody complexes (6, 115), and aggregated IgG and IgM in the presence of heat-labile serum factors (105). Ward (194) and Lachmann and his colleagues (104) found that the trimolecular complex of C'5,6,7 had chemotactic activity for eosinophils. Other substances presumed to be involved as chemical mediators of inflammation, such as 5-hydroxytryptamine and bradykinin, are without demonstrable eosinophilotactic activity (7, 8, 98). Kay and his associates (98) have recently isolated an "eosinophil chemotactic factor" (ECF-A) from sensitized guinea pig lung following antigen challenge. This factor has an estimated molecular weight of 500 to 1,000 and is distinct from histamine, from slow-reacting substance of anaphylaxis (SRS-A), and from the trimolecular complex of complement C'5,6,7. In 1953, using lung tissue from an anaphylactically shocked guinea pig, Samter and his colleagues demonstrated passive transfer of a substance chemotactic for eosinophils (161).

In vivo, eosinophils accumulate at the site of histamine injection. When mast cells degranulate and release histamine (67, 152), eosinophils accumulate at the site of release, a phenomenon that is prevented by the prior administration of a histamine antagonist (7).

One of the interesting characteristics of eosinophils is their ability to be attracted by antigen-antibody aggregates and, occasionally, to phagocytize such aggregates (3, 6, 115, 158). Most antigens alone exert relatively little chemotactic attraction for eosinophils and are not taken up by the cells to any great extent (150). Similarly, antibody alone has relatively little effect on these cells.

When injected intraperitoneally in guinea pigs, complexes of precipitating antibody and antigen at equivalence or slight antigen excess stimulate the accumulation of large numbers of eosinophils in the peritoneal cavity (139). Nonprecipitating antigen-antibody complexes are much less effective as chemotactic stimuli (6). In one study, low doses of antigen administered to guinea pigs did not result in any accumulation of eosinophils in the local lymph nodes. However, when the antigen and 7S antibody were introduced into separate epidermal blebs, eosinophils accumulated in the area between the blebs—presumably the site of antigen-antibody interaction (117). These studies were interpreted as indicating that local and systemic eosinophilia may occur in response to antigen-antibody interaction.

Litt demonstrated phagocytosis of immune complexes in a graphic experiment (115, 116). He labeled antibody to bovine serum albumin with green fluorescent dye and labeled bovine serum albumin with red fluorescent dye. He injected the complexes intraperitoneally, and one hour later the eosinophils in the peritoneal fluid fluoresced with the complementary color, yellow.

Under some circumstances antigen alone will cause an eosinophil accumulation, perhaps by inducing local antibody production. For example, Litt (114) showed that a first injection of bovine serum albumin into guinea pigs was followed by eosinophilia in the draining lymph node. The use of other antigens has produced similar results (49, 153, 154, 190). Repeated exposure to the same antigen results in marked eosinophilia at the site of antigen deposition (22, 23, 174, 187) and in the draining regional lymph nodes (49, 114). Eventually, increased numbers of eosinophils appear in the bone marrow and in the blood (30, 87).

When antigen is injected parenterally into a sensitized animal, eosinophils begin to accumulate within 24 hours. They continue to accumulate for a week or more and may persist for months in areas around the granulomatous reactions induced by certain antigens (10, 180). The same phenomenon may occur in sensitized human subjects (57, 69, 81).

It is possible that only certain types of antibody response are capable of inducing eosinophilotaxis. Litt (117) and Kay (97) found that eosinophilia in the guinea pig correlated with γ_1 antibody (that producing passive cutaneous anaphylaxis) rather than with precipitating γ_2 antibody. In a study of patients with penicillin allergy, eosinophilia correlated with reaginic antibody (possibly IgE) rather than with hemagglutinating antibody (IgG, IgM) (207). Similarly, the eosinophilia of helminth infections appears to correlate with the formation of reaginic antibody (156). *As a general rule, eosinophilia is more common in atopic disease associated with increased levels of IgE than with immune diseases mediated by nonreaginic antibody.*

The mechanism whereby antigen-antibody complexes induce eosinophil accumulation is largely unknown. Whether such complexes act by local release of histamine is uncertain. The following three mechanisms have been suggested as leading to the accumulation of eosinophils in tissue: (*a*) chemotactic factors released by the interaction of antigen with anitbody (5, 6, 113, 139, 158, 161); (*b*) chemotactic factors released by delayed hypersensitivity reactions in which mononuclear cells play a role (171, 173); and (*c*) chemotactic factors released by fibrin formation or other large protein aggregates (15, 43, 151, 183).

The chemotactic influence of antigen-antibody aggregates on eosinophils has already been discussed. Aggregates of high-molecular-weight protein may also attract eosinophils. For example, eosinophilia occurs within two to twenty-four hours following injection of high-molecular-weight proteins or polysaccharide (45–48, 50). Eosinophil response to these substances occurs under circumstances in which the participation of antigen and antibody is unlikely. This response is not blocked by reticuloendothelial blockade, X-irradiation, or immunosuppressive drugs. Similar experiments using fibrin as the provocative material have been reported (15, 151). Possibly, any large protein aggregate is chemotactically active for eosinophils, since small polystyrene particles, when coated with protein, will attract these cells (101). The polystyrene particles are active themselves when their size varies between 0.9 and 0.8 micron. Thus it appears that those physical traits that characterize antigen-antibody complexes and various other proteins in microparticulate form are necessary for the generation of a chemotactic influence for eosinophils. The mechanism is unknown, although it has been suggested that the aggregates induce the release of histamine and other chemotactic substances from the leukocytes and tissue cells with which they come into contact.

Eosinophils may interact with other leukocytes. For example, Speirs and Osada (173), using phase contrast photocinemicrography, demonstrated that eosinophils may be attracted toward, and actually penetrate, mononuclear cells. In their experiments disintegrating macrophages were frequently surrounded by eosinophils exhibiting oscillatory and circular movement. Subsequently, large vacuoles appeared in the macrophages prior to their disruption. Eosinophils entered the dying macrophages and were then phagocytized, along with the debris, by other viable macrophages.

Eosinophils thus seem to be attracted to damaged and, perhaps, to intact macrophages in vitro. In vivo, eosinophils may form rosettes around macrophages containing antigen (175). Some evidence suggests that antigen-primed macrophages may produce chemotactic material upon second exposure to antigen (174). Recently evidence has been presented that the eosinophil response to antigen may depend upon the presence of certain lymphoid cells (16, 124).

Phagocytosis

Phagocytosis by eosinophils was probably first observed in 1895 by Mesnil (131). Mammalian eosinophilic leukocytes are capable of ingesting a variety of particles, including antigen-antibody precipitate (2, 3, 138, 158), polystyrene particles (41, 101), ferritin (28), mast cell granules (197), particulate matter in endotoxin preparations (41, 42) (see Fig. 5.1), and bacteria including *Escherichia coli* and *Staphylococcus aureus* (41). Phagocytosis of immune complexes in allergic patients may produce large cytoplasmic vacuoles and degranulation of eosinophils (52). Intraleukocytic inclusions of immunoglobulin may be found in patients with eosinophilia (125).

In general, one can say that phagocytosis in eosinophils resembles that in neutrophils (41, 85, 93). However, the process in eosinophils is less efficient and has a smaller capacity. For example, when a mixture of eosinophils and neutrophils is incubated with *S. aureus* at a ratio of several bacteria to one leukocyte, the neutrophils quickly become engorged with bacteria, whereas the eosinophils ingest only a few organisms (Fig. 6.10).

Phagocytosis by eosinophils appears to involve the same sequence of events as already described for the granulocytes:

(*a*) The energy for particle ingestion is derived from anaerobic metabolism rather than from aerobic metabolism.

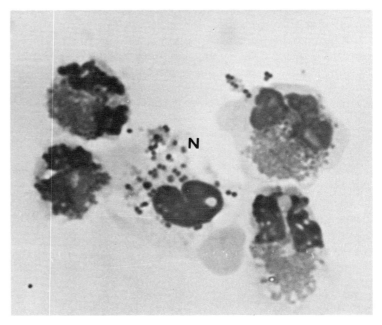

Figure 6.10 Neutrophils and eosinophils from human peripheral blood incubated with *Staphylococcus aureus*. Only the neutrophil (*N*) shows phagocytized microorganisms.

Sodium fluoride and iodoacetate, but not potassium cyanide or dinitrophenol, inhibit particle ingestion (41). The former are glycolytic poisons, the latter interfere with oxidative energy production. Lactic acid production increases with phagocytosis.

(b) Shortly after particle ingestion and vacuole formation, the granules of the eosinophil fuse with the phagocytic vacuole and rupture (4).

(c) Granule enzymes are released into the vacuole. With extensive particle ingestion, these enzymes are also lost from the cell into the surrounding medium (41).

(d) With particle ingestion the hexose monophosphate shunt is stimulated. This stimulation is of roughly the same order of magnitude as that accompanying neutrophil phagocytosis (41).

(e) The incorporation of tritiated uridine into eosinophil RNA is stimulated by phagocytosis in eosinophils as well as neutrophils (41).

(f) Particle ingestion by human eosinophils occurs in a broad pH range—between 5.5 and 8 (41).

(g) Phagocytosis is somewhat more efficient when the eosinophils adhere to a surface than when they are in free suspension. Wood, Smith, and Watson observed that surface phagocytosis by neutrophils may also be a more efficient process than phagocytosis in free suspension. They suggested that surface phagocytosis may require only low levels of opsonizing antibody, whereas phagocytosis by freely suspended cells may require the high levels of antibody that occur late in an infectious process (202).

In addition to the difference in efficiency, there are other minor differences in the phagocytic process of eosinophils and neutrophils. In eosinophils, particle ingestion is more sensitive to inhibition of protein synthesis and to colchicine. Furthermore, intact granules are often extruded from the eosinophilic cell during the phagocytic process.

Relatively little information is available regarding the killing of ingested bacteria by eosinophils. This lack of knowledge stems from the difficulties encountered in obtaining pure populations of eosinophils and also from the greater phagocytic activity of even a small number of contaminating neutrophils. Recent studies indicate that the microbicidal activity of eosinophils against the common pyogenic organisms is considerably less than the activity of neutrophils. Eosinophils phagocytize bacteria but do not kill them well (40).

Eosinophils and Inflammation

Experimental evidence indicates that eosinophils are capable of antagonizing the effects of histamine in the tissues (102, 192). An aqueous extract of eosinophils reduces the edema that follows an intradermal injection of histamine (29). It will also reduce the bronchospasm in guinea pigs that histamine induces (9). Thus some components of eosinophils inhibit both the enhanced capillary permeability and the smooth muscle constriction induced by histamine. Histamine has been shown to be chemically altered by eosinophils in vitro (27). The mechanism of inactivation may involve amine oxidation via the abundant eosinophil peroxidase.

Eosinophil extracts have also been reported to antagonize the edema-producing properties of other presumed chemical mediators of inflammation, including bradykinin (9, 61, 109). Neutrophils of animals and man have been demonstrated to contain bradykinin-inactivating enzyme (kininases) (79, 129); and recently similar enzymes have been described in eosinophils as well (128–130). Kininase activity is maximal at pH 6 to 7 and does not require molecular oxygen for its action. Therefore this activity is distinct from peroxidase activity.

Whether the ability of eosinophils and eosinophil extracts to antagonize chemical mediators of inflammation in the test tube is relevant to their function in the intact animal is not known. One is tempted to speculate, however, that the cells are attracted to certain sites of inflammation in order to exert an "antiphlogistic" effect. For example, in inflammatory sites originating from the interaction of antigen and antibody, mast cells degranulate and release histamine in a multistep response (111). Once histamine is released, eosinophils are attracted to the site and there may counteract the effects of the various soluble mediators—histamine, 5-hydroxytryptamine, and the kinins—thus limiting and circumscribing the inflammatory process.

The eosinophilic response to an inflammatory stimulus, such as an antigen-antibody interaction, may be divided into three temporal phases. First, there is a transient phase of eosinophil accumulation in the tissues, usually occurring within 24 hours of the stimulus (45, 81, 112, 153, 174). Second is a more prolonged phase in which eosinophils continue to accumulate at the site of stimulus for several days or even a week. This phase is generally accompanied by an increase in the numbers of eosinophils in the blood and an increase in the production of eosinophils in the bone marrow (170, 172, 178). The degree of eosinophilia does not necessarily parallel the extent of local eosinophil accumulation at the inflammatory site. This phase of the eosinophil response is affected by the method of antigen priming and the level of circulating antibodies at the time of antigen administration (172, 175, 176, 187). It is also influenced by manipulations such as actinomycin and adrenal steroid hormone administration and by X-irradiation (71, 179). Finally, eosinophils continue to be attracted to the chronic granulomatous inflammatory reaction over a period of weeks or months. This phase may be observed in an experimental model in which particulate antigen is injected (180). Eosinophilia at the site of antigen injection may persist for eight months or more. In addition to eosinophils, plasma cells may be seen at the site of granulomatous reaction. A similar model has been described in which antigenic tetanus toxoid induces a chronic eosinophilic reaction (10). Presumably such models are the experimental counterpart of the chronic eosinophilia that occurs in response to complex antigens such as helminths (135, 196), allografts (127), and certain chemical agents (35, 75, 103), including polysaccharides (46).

The accumulation of eosinophils at an inflammatory site may be inhibited by high doses of adrenal cortico-sterroid (179, 198). This effect is apparently not a result of either the eosinophilolytic effect (169) or the sequestration of eosinophils in the spleen (168). What evidence is available suggests that the chemotactic attraction of eosinophils from the bone marrow is inhibited by high doses of corticosteroids. The mechanism of this phenomenon is obscure.

In a model system of the rat infested by *Trichinella*, the development of eosinophilia is dependent upon a product of thymus-dependent lymphocytes (16). Passive transfer of thoracic duct lymphocytes in inoculated animals produces eosinophilia, whereas thymus cells are ineffective. Cohen and Ward (44) recently have reached similar conclusions regarding lymphocytic requirements in mediating eosinophilotaxis.

The fate of eosinophils in an inflammatory site is of some interest. Apparently very few of the infiltrating cells ever return to the blood stream. Eosinophils accumulate in the draining lymph nodes, where they are engulfed by macrophages. Also, about the second day of an inflammatory lesion which has attracted eosinophils, the cells may be found phagocytized by the local macrophages. Large needle-like crystals (Charcot-Leyden crystals) are found in inflammatory tissues and secretions in association with intact and disintegrating eosinophils (58, 110, 160).

Eosinophilia

Some of the conditions associated with eosinophilia are listed in Table 6.1.

From the foregoing discussion, one may deduce that eosinophilia is apt to be observed in pathological states where there is an interaction between antigen and certain classes of antibody. Examples of such conditions include

Table 6.1 Conditions associated with eosinophilia.

Drug reactions
Iodide sensitivity
Penicillin sensitivity
Parasitosis
Trichinosis
Visceral larva migrans
Tropical eosinophilia
Infections
Leprosy
Brucellosis
Tuberculosis
Fungal infections
Scarlet fever
Malignancies
Carcinoma of the lung
Carcinoma of the ovaries
Carcinoma of the stomach
Hodgkin's disease
Collagen disease
Periarteritis nodosa
Rheumatoid arthritis
"Cutaneous"
Pemphigus
Dermatitis herpetiformis
Loeffler's syndrome
Farmer's lung
Asthma, hay fever
Chronic eosinophilic pneumonia
Leukemia
Chronic myelocytic
Eosinophilic
Eosinophilic endocarditis (Loeffler's endocarditis)
Unknown cause
Idiopathic
Sarcoidosis
Familial

drug reactions, parasitic diseases, certain infectious disorders, collagen diseases, and dermatologic diseases (17, 59, 94). Toxocara catis, the etiologic agent in the "cat sandbox syndrome" (17), may occasionally produce eosinophilia of a magnitude suggesting a hematologic malignancy. It may also be responsible for eosinophilic cystitis occuring with blood eosinophilia (142).

Other disorders where eosinophilia may be associated with immunologic reactions include:

(a) Loeffler's syndrome, which consists in fleeting ("fluchtig") pulmonary infiltrates, blood eosinophilia, and eosinophils in the sputum (118, 141). In some patients, the clinical manifestations are a result of parasites migrating through the lungs as a process of their life cycle (143).

(b) Farmer's lung.

(c) Asthma and hay fever (123). An extreme variant of these disorders may be chronic eosinophilic pneumonia, which is characterized by blood eosinophilia, dyspnea, high fever, and a chronic life-threatening illness (33, 34).

(d) "Tropical eosinophilia," which may represent a reaction to a filarial parasite (55).

(e) Eosinophilia related to cigarette smoke (162).

Blood eosinophilia and pulmonary manifestations are both involved in many of these disorders. An excellent review of diseases resulting from immunologic reactions in the lung has recently been presented (123). Of the four types of allergic reactions responsible for hypersensitivity diseases of lungs (53), two are consistently associated with eosinophilia: IgE dependent reactions and immune complex disease. Pulmonary diseases caused by tissue-specific cytotoxic antibody and by cell-mediated immune reactions are less frequently associated with eosinophilia.

The mechanisms giving rise to the eosinophilia occasionally observed in the malignant diseases periarteritis nodosa and sarcoidosis are unknown, but again may involve complexes of antigen and antibodies.

The question of whether eosinophilic leukemia exists as a primary hematologic neoplasm is of some interest. Until 1960 approximately thirty cases of so-called eosinophilic leukemia had been reported in the world's literature. This "leukemia" had certain rather peculiar features (36). Anemia as well as thrombocytopenia was somewhat rare. In addition, an extremely high incidence of myocardial involvement was reported, and most patients died of either myocardial failure or peripheral embolization. Most of these descriptions of "eosinophilic leukemia" were probably examples of the syndrome *eosinophilic endocarditis*. However, eosinophilic leukemia most likely does exist as a separate disease entity; it is, however, extremely rare and considerably less common than eosinophilic carditis. The statement that eosinophilic leukemia does exist is based on the occurrence of the Philadelphia chromosome in a patient with blood eosinophilia, organomegaly, and diffuse organ infiltration with eosinophils (80). This patient subsequently died in a blast crisis. The entire clinical and pathological picture was compatible with that of chronic granulocytic leukemia. More recent reports of eosinophilic leukemia have been presented (20, 203).

Eosinophilic endocarditis, or "fibroplastic parietal endocarditis with blood eosinophils," was first described by Loeffler in 1936 in the *Swiss Journal of Medicine* (119).

The major clinical features of the original case were significant: peripheral blood eosinophilia, cardiac failure, and peripheral emboli. At autopsy the patient was found to have fibrosis involving the walls of the heart rather than the valves. Both the ventricular walls and the septum were fibrous, and mural thrombi were present. Since the original report of this entity, approximately forty cases have been described. Eosinophilic endocarditis is the usual name applied to the syndrome. The clinical characteristics of these forty cases are summarized in Table 6.2.

A number of more recent descriptions of this interesting disease exist (26, 38, 68, 155, 165); however, its etiology remains obscure (38, 203).

Many cases of eosinophilia cannot be etiologically defined. These are designated as "idiopathic." Idiopathic eosinophilia is generally a benign condition with a good prognosis. A five or more year study following 38 patients with this condition found 32 still living at the end of the study (83). Two patients died of chronic myelocytic leukemia, one of carcinoma of the stomach, and three of apparently unrelated disorders.

Yam (203) recently drew attention to the syndrome of pseudoeosinophilia in which neutrophils may resemble eosinophils. A review of eosinophilias of unknown etiology has appeared in the past few years (209).

Table 6.2 Clinical features of eosinophilic carditis in approximately forty patients.

Age range
  7 to 65 years (usually 30 to 50)
Male/female ratio
  3 to 1
Population
  Negroid and Caucasian
Onset
  Acute or gradual
Duration
  3 months to 6 years (19 of 40 patients died within 12 months)
Manifestations
  Afebrile
  Eosinophilia
  Electrocardiogram
    Nonspecific ST and T changes (16 of 40 patients)
    Left ventricular hypertrophy (3 of 40 patients)
    Possible embolic phenomenon
    Murmur of mitral insufficiency (20 of 40 patients)
    Possible central nervous system signs
Reaction to therapy
  Poor response

Summary

In the light microscope eosinophils are recognized by their distinctive color when stained by Romanovsky dyes. In the electron microscope they are identified by their distinctive granules. Eosinophils share a common progenitor with neutrophils, and the basic features of cellular development and morphogenesis are the same in the two cell lines.

Eosinophils are longer lived than neutrophils and spend the greater part of their life span in the tissues. Eosinophils are phagocytic, but their most striking attribute is interaction with immune complexes. The deposition of such complexes in tissues probably underlies most of the clinically apparent eosinophilias. Eosinophils phagocytize these immune aggregates and may limit the inflammatory reactions incited by them.

Chapter 6 References

1. Archer, G. T. Release of peroxidase from eosinophil granules *in vitro*, *Nature* 194:973, 1962.
2. Archer, G. T., and Bosworth, N. Phagocytosis by eosinophils following antigen-antibody reactions *in vitro*, *Austr. J. Exp. Biol.* 39:157, 1961.
3. Archer, G. T., and Hirsch, J. G. Isolation of granules from eosinophil leukocytes and study of their enzyme content, *J. Exp. Med.* 118:277, 1963.
4. Archer, G. T., and Hirsch, J. G. Motion picture studies on degranulation of horse eosinophils during phagocytosis, *J. Exp. Med.* 118:287, 1963.
5. Archer, R. K. The Eosinophil Leukocytes, F. A. Davis Co., Philadelphia, 1963.
6. Archer, R. K. On the functions of eosinophils in the antigen-antibody reaction, *Br. J. Haematol.* 11:123, 1965.
7. Archer, R. K. Regulatory mechanisms in eosinophil leukocyte production, release, and distribution, *in* A. S. Gordon (ed.), Regulation of Hematopoiesis, p. 917, Appleton-Century-Crofts, New York, 1970.
8. Archer, R. K., and Broome, J. Bradykinin and eosinophils, *Nature* 198:893, 1963.
9. Archer, R. K., Feldberg, W., and Kovacs, B. A. Antihistamine activity in extracts of horse eosinophils, *Br. J. Pharmacol. Chemother.* 18:101, 1962.
10. Athanassiades, T. J., and Speirs, R. S. Formation of antigen-induced granulomas containing plasma cells: a light and electron microscopic study, *J. Reticuloendothel. Soc.* 5:485, 1968.
11. Bainton, D. F., and Farquhar, M. G. Segregation and packaging of granule enzymes in eosinophils, *J. Cell Biol.* 35:6A, 1967 (abstract).
12. Bainton, D. F., and Farquhar, M. G. Differences in enzyme content of azurophil and specific granules of polymorphonuclear leukocytes. I. Histochemical staining of bone marrow smears, *J. Cell Biol.* 39:286, 1968.
13. Bainton, D. F., and Farquhar, M. G. Segregation and packaging of granule enzymes in eosinphilic leukocytes, *J. Cell Biol.* 45:54, 1970.
14. Bargmann, W., and Knoop, A. Über das Granulum des Eosinophilen, *Z. Zellforsch.* 48:130, 1958.
15. Barnhart, M. I., and Riddle, J. M. Cellular localization of profibrinolysin (plasminogen), *Blood* 21:306, 1963.
16. Basten, A., and Beeson, P. B. Mechanism of eosinophilia. II. Role of the lymphocyte, *J. Exp. Med.* 31:1288, 1970.
17. Beaver, P. C., Snyder, C. H., Carrera, G. M., Dent, J. H., and Lafferty, J. W. Chronic eosinophilia due to visceral larva migrans, *Pediatrics* 9:7, 1952.
18. Behnke, O. Demonstration of endogenous peroxidase activity in the electron microscope, *J. Histochem. Cytochem.* 17:62, 1969.
19. Behrens, M., and Marti, H. R. Gewinnung der "eosinophilen Substanz" aus isolierten eosinophilen Granulozyten des Pferdeblutes, *Biochim. Biophys. Acta* 65:551, 1962.
20. Benvenisti, D. S., and Ultmann, J. E. Eosinophilic leukemia. Report of 5 cases and review of literature, *Ann. Intern. Med.* 71:731, 1969.
21. Bessis, M. Structures cellulaires découvertes par le microscope électronique dans les leucocytes, *Rev. Hematol.* 11:295, 1956.
22. Biggart, J. H. Some observations on the eosinophile cell, *J. Pathol. Bacteriol.* 35:799, 1932.
23. Bosworth, N., and Archer, G. T. The eosinophil content of the peritoneal cavity of the rat, *Aust. J. Exp. Biol.* 39:165, 1961.
24. Bresnick, E., and Karjala, R. J. End-product inhibition of thymidine kinase activity in normal and leukemic human leukocytes, *Cancer Res.* 24:841, 1964.
25. Breton-Gorius, J. Structures périodiques dans les granulations éosinophiles et neutrophiles des leucocytes polynucléaires du sang de l'homme, *Nouv. Rev. Fr. Hematol.* 6:195, 1966.
26. Brink, A. J., and Weber, H. W. Fibroplastic parietal endocarditis with eosinophilia, *Am. J. Med.* 34:52, 1963.
27. Broome, J., and Archer, R. K. Effect of equine eosinophils on histamine *in vitro*, *Nature* 193:446, 1962.
28. Bro-Rasmussen, F., and Egeberg, J. The ultrastructure of eosinophilic granulocytes in the peritoneal cavity of rats following injection of ferritin, *Scand. J. Haematol.* 3:257, 1966.
29. Bruce, R. A., and Archer, R. K. Inhibition of histamine oedema in skin by eosinophils, *Lancet* ii:1119, 1962.
30. Campbell, D. H. Experimental eosinophilia with keratin from ascaris suum and other sources, *J. Infect. Dis.* 71:270, 1942.
31. Capone, R. J., Weinreb, E. L., and Chapman, G. B. Electron microscope studies on normal human myeloid elements, *Blood* 23:300, 1964.
32. Carper, H. A., and Hoffman, P. L. The intravascular survival of transfused canine Pelger-Huët neutrophils and eosinophils, *Blood* 27:739, 1966.
33. Carrington, C. B., Addington, W. W., Goff, A. M., Madoff, I. M., Marks, A., Schwaber, J. R., and Gaensler, E. A. Chronic eosinophilic pneumonia, *N. Engl. J. Med.* 280:787, 1969.
34. Chafee, F. H., Ross, J. R., and Gunn, E. M. Eosinophilia in fatal asthma: studies of bone marrow and myocardium, *Ann. Intern. Med.* 17:45, 1942.
35. Chapman, J. S. Eosinophil-stimulating properties of certain chemical substances, *Am. J. Clin. Pathol.* 40:357, 1963.
36. Chen, H. P., and Smith, H. S. Eosinophilic leukemia, *Ann. Intern. Med.* 52:1342, 1960.
37. Cline, M. J. Metabolism of the circulating leukocyte, *Physiol. Rev.* 45:674, 1965.
38. Cline, M. J. Eosinophilia and eosinophilic endocarditis, *Calif. Med.* 111:388, 1969.
39. Cline, M. J. Leukocyte metabolism, *in* A. S. Gordon (ed.), Regulation of Hematopoiesis, p. 1045, Appleton-Century-Crofts, New York, 1970.
40. Cline, M. J. Microbicidal activity of human eosinophils, *J. Reticuloendothel. Soc.* 12:332, 1972.
41. Cline, M. J., Hanifin, J. M., and Lehrer, R. I. Phagocytosis by

human eosinophils, *Blood* 32:922, 1968.

42. Cline, M. J., Melmon, K. L., Davis, W. C., and Williams, H. E. Mechanism of endotoxin interaction with human leucocytes, *Br. J. Haematol.* 15:539, 1968.

43. Cohen, N. S., LoBue, J., and Gordon, A. S. Mechanisms of leukocyte production and release. 8. Eosinophil and neutrophil kinetics in rats, *Scand. J. Haematol.* 4:339, 1967.

44. Cohen, S., and Ward, P. A. *In vitro* and *in vivo* activity of a lymphocyte and immune complex dependent chemotactic factor for eosinophils, *J. Exp. Med.* 133:133, 1971.

45. Cohen, S. G., Kostage, S. T., and Rizzo, A. P. Experimental eosinophilia. IX. Effects of immunosuppressive agents on eosinophil cell responses, *J. Allergy* 39:129, 1967.

46. Cohen, S. G., and Sapp, T. M. Experimental eosinophilia. IV. Eosinotactic influences of polysaccharides, *Exp. Mol. Pathol.* 2:74, 1963.

47. Cohen, S. G., and Sapp, T. M. Polysaccharide effects simulating hypersensitivity response in the rabbit, *Am. J. Physiol.* 207:389, 1964.

48. Cohen, S. G., and Sapp, T. M. Experimental eosinophilia. VIII. Cellular responses to altered globulins within cutaneous tissue, *J. Allergy* 36:415, 1965.

49. Cohen, S. G., Sapp, T. M., and Gallia, A. R. Experimental eosinophilia. V. Specificity of regional lymph node responses to antigen-antibody systems, *Proc. Soc. Exp. Biol. Med.* 113:29, 1963.

50. Cohen, S. G., Sapp, T. M., Rizzo, A. P., and Kostage, S. T. Experimental eosinophilia. VII. Lymph node responses to altered gamma globulins, *J. Allergy* 35:346, 1964.

51. Cohn, Z. A., and Hirsch, J. G. The isolation and properties of the specific cytoplasmic granules of rabbit polymorphonuclear leucocytes, *J. Exp. Med.* 112:983, 1960.

52. Connell, J. T. Morphological changes in eosinophils in allergic disease, *J. Allergy* 41:1, 1968.

53. Coombs, R. R. A., and Gell, P. G. H. Classification of allergic reactions responsible for clinical hypersensitivity and disease, *in* Clinical Aspects of Immunology, 2nd ed., p. 575, Blackwell Scientific Publications, Oxford, 1968.

54. Davis, W. C., Greene, W. B., and Spicer, S. S. Ultrastructure of bone marrow granulocytes in normal and Aleutian mink, *Fed. Proc.* 28:265, 1969 (abstract).

55. Donohugh, D. L. Tropical eosinophilia: an etiologic inquiry, *N. Engl. J. Med.* 269:1357, 1963.

56. Dunn, W. B., Hardin, J. H., and Spicer, S. S. Ultrastructural localization of myeloperoxidase in human neutrophil and rabbit heterophil and eosinophil leukocytes, *Blood* 32:935, 1968.

57. Eidinger, D., Raff, M., and Rose, B. Tissue eosinophilia in hypersensitivity reactions as revealed by the human skin window, *Nature* 196:683, 1962.

58. El-Hashimi, W. Charcot-Leyden crystals, *Am. J. Pathol.* 65:311, 1971.

59. Elsom, K. A., and Ingelfinger, F. J. Eosinophilia and pneumonitis in chronic brucellosis, *Ann. Intern. Med.* 16:995, 1942.

60. Enomoto, T., and Kitani, T. Electron microscopic studies on peroxidase and acid phosphatase reaction in human leukocytes (in normal and leukemic cells and on the phagocytosis), *Acta Haematol. Jap.* 29:554, 1966.

61. Erdös, E. G. Hypotensive peptides: bradykinin, kallidin and elecdoisin, *Adv. Pharmacol.* 4:1, 1966.

62. Esmann, V. Carbohydrate Metabolism and Respiration in Leukocytes from Normal and Diabetic Subjects, Universitetsforlaget, Aarhus, 1962.

63. Fawcett, D. W. An Atlas of Fine Structure: The Cell, Its Organelles and Inclusions, p. 200, W. B. Saunders Co., Philadelphia, 1966.

64. Fedorko, M. Effect of chloroquine on morphology of cytoplasmic granules in maturing human leukocytes—an ultrastructural study, *J. Clin. Invest.* 46:1932, 1967.

65. Fedorko, M. Formation of cytoplasmic granules in human eosinophilic myelocytes: an electron microscopic autoradiographic study, *Blood* 31:188, 1968.

66. Felarca, A. B., and Lowell, F. C. The total eosinophil count in a nonatopic population, *J. Allergy* 40:16, 1967.

67. Fernex, M. The Mast Cell System: Its Relationship to Athero-Sclerosis, Fibrosis and Eosinophils, S. Karger, Basel, 1968.

68. Flannery, E. P., Dillon, D. E., Freeman, M. V. R., Levy, J. D., Dambrosio, U., and Bedynek, J. L. Eosinophilic leukemia with fibrosing endocarditis and short Y chromosome, *Ann. Intern. Med.* 77:223, 1972.

69. Fowler, J. W., and Lowell, F. C. The accumulation of eosinophils as an allergic response to allergen applied to the denuded skin surface, *J. Allergy* 37:19, 1966.

70. Gedigk, P., and Gross, R. *in* H. Braunsteiner and D. Zucker-Franklin (eds.), The Physiology and Pathology of Leukocytes, p. 5, Grune & Stratton, New York, 1962.

71. Geller, B. D., and Speirs, R. S. The effect of actinomycin-D on the haemopoietic and immune response to tetanus toxoid, *Immunology* 15:707, 1968.

72. Ghidoni, J. J., and Goldberg, A. F. Light and electron microscopic localization of acid phosphatase activity in human eosinophils, *Am. J. Clin. Pathol.* 45:402, 1966.

73. Ghiotto, G., Perona, G., DeSandre, G., and Cortesi, S. Hexokinase and TPN-dependent dehydrogenases of leucocytes in leukaemia and other haematological disorders, *Br. J. Haematol.* 9:345, 1963.

74. Gleich, G. J., Loegering, D. A., and Maldonado, J. E. Identification of a major basic protein in guinea pig eosinophil granules, *J. Exp. Med.* 137:1459, 1973.

75. Goswami, P. K. Eosinophil leucocyte reaction to tricycloquinazoline-treated cells and to this chemical, *Nature* 202:1227, 1964.

76. Graham, G. S. Benzidine as a peroxidase reagent for blood smears and tissues, *J. Med. Res.* 39:15, 1918.

77. Graham, H. T., Lowry, O. H., Wheelwright, F., Lenz, M. A., and Parish, H. H., Jr. Distribution of histamine among leukocytes and platelets, *Blood* 10:467, 1955.

78. Graham, H. T., Wheelwright, F.,

Parish, H. H., Jr., Marks, A. R., and Lowry, O. H. Distribution of histamine among blood elements, *Fed. Proc.* 11:350, 1952.

79. Greenbaum, L. M., and Kim, K. S. The kinin-forming and kininase activities of rabbit polymorphonuclear leucocytes, *Br. J. Pharmacol. Chemother.* 29:238, 1967.

80. Gruenwald, H., Kiossoglou, K. A., Mitus, W. J., and Dameshek, W. Philadelphia chromosome in eosinophilic leukemia, *Am. J. Med.* 39:1003, 1965.

81. Halle, C. I., and Lowell, F. C. Diminution of the eosinophilotactic response, a specific effect of injections of allergenic extracts, *J. Allergy* 39:33, 1967.

82. Herion, J. C., Glasser, R. M., Walker, R. I., and Palmer, J. G. Eosinophil kinetics in two patients with eosinophilia, *Blood* 36:361, 1970.

83. Hildebrand, F. L., Christensen, N. A., and Hanlon, D. G. Eosinophilia of unknown cause, *Arch. Intern. Med.* 113:129, 1964.

84. Hills, A. G., Forsham, P. H., and Finch, C. A. Changes in circulating leukocytes induced by the administration of pituitary adrenocorticotrophic hormone (ACTH) in man, *Blood* 3:755, 1948.

85. Hirsch, J. G. Neutrophil and eosinophil leucocytes, *in* B. W. Zweifach, L. Grant, and R. T. McCluskey (eds.), The Inflammatory Process, p. 245, Academic Press, New York, 1965.

86. Horn, R. G., and Spicer, S. S. Sulfated mucopolysaccharide and basic protein in certain granules of rabbit leukocytes, *Lab. Invest.* 13:1, 1964.

87. Hudson, G. Changes in the marrow reserve of eosinophils following reexposure to foreign protein, *Br. J. Haematol.* 9:446, 1964.

88. Hudson, G. Eosinophil granules and cell maturity: electron microscopic observations on guinea-pig marrow, *Acta Haematol.* 36:350, 1966.

89. Hudson, G. Quantitative study of the eosinophil granulocytes, *Semin. Hematol.* 5:166, 1968.

90. Hudson, G., Chin, K. N., and Moffatt, D. J. Changes in eosinophil granulocyte kinetics in severe hypoxia, *Acta Haematol.* 48:58, 1972.

91. Huser, H-J., and Webb, C. M. Variation of the fine structure in granulocytes of great apes, *Experientia* 23:669, 1967.

92. Ichimaru, M. Studies on glycocytes catabolized specially in leukemic cells, *J. Kyushu Hematol. Soc.* 9:722, 1959.

93. Ishikawa, T., Dalton, A. C., and Abresman, C. E. Phagocytosis of candida albicans by eosinophilic leukocytes, *J. Allergy Clin. Immunol.* 49:311, 1972.

94. Jacobs, H. S., Sidd, J. J., Greenberg, B. H., and Lindley, J. F. Extreme eosinophilia with iodide hypersensitivity: report of a case with observations on the cellular composition of inflammatory exudates, *N. Engl. J. Med.* 271:1138, 1964.

95. Jones, T. W. The blood corpuscle considered in its different phases of development in the animal series, Memoir I. Vertebrata Phil. *Trans. R. Soc. Lond.* 136:63, 1846.

96. Kaplow, L. S. Simplified myeloperoxidase stain using benzidine dihydrochloride, *Blood* 26:215, 1965.

97. Kay, A. B. Studies on eosinophil leukocyte migration. II. Factors specifically chemotactic for eosinophils and neutrophils generated from guinea-pig serum by antigen-antibody complexes, *Clin. Exp. Immunol.* 7:723, 1970.

98. Kay, A. B., Stechschulte, D. J., and Austen, K. F. An eosinophil leukocyte chemotactic factor of anaphylaxis, *J. Exp. Med.* 133:602, 1971.

99. Klebanoff, S. J. Iodination of bacteria. A bactericidal mechanism, *J. Exp. Med.* 126:1063, 1967.

100. Koch-Weser, J. Beta adrenergic blockade and circulating eosinophils, *Arch. Intern. Med.* 121:255, 1968.

101. Kostage, S. T., Rizzo, A. P., and Cohen, S. G. Experimental eosinophilia. IX. Cell responses to particles of delineated size, *Proc. Soc. Exp. Biol. Med.* 125:413, 1967.

102. Kovács, A. Antihistaminic effect of eosinophil leukocytes, *Experientia* 6:349, 1950.

103. Kovács, A., and Szijj, I. Experimentell durch Hexadimethrinbromid ausgeloste Eosinophilie bei Ratten, *Folia Haematol.* 86:324, 1966.

104. Lachmann, P. J., Kay, A. B., and

Thompson, R. A. The chemotactic activity for neutrophil and eosinophil leucocytes of the trimolecular complex of the fifth, sixth and seventh components of human complement (C567) prepared in free solution by the "reactive lysis" procedure, *Immunology* 19:895, 1970.

105. Laster, C. E., and Gleich, G. J. Chemotaxis of eosinophils and neutrophils by aggregated immunoglobulins, *J. Allergy Clin. Immunol.* 48:297, 1971.

106. Lazarus, S. S., Vethamnay, V. G., Schneck, L., and Volk, B. W. Fine structure and histochemistry of peripheral blood cells in Niemann-Pick disease, *Lab. Invest.* 17:155, 1967.

107. Lehrer, R. I., and Cline, M. J. Leukocyte myeloperoxidase deficiency and disseminated candidiasis: the role of myeloperoxidase in resistance to candida infection, *J. Clin. Invest.* 48:1478, 1969.

108. Lehrer, R. I., Hanifin, J. M., and Cline, M. J. Defective bactericidal activity in myeloperoxidase-deficient human neutrophils, *Nature* 223:78, 1969.

109. Lewis, G. P. Pharmacological actions of bradykinin and its role in physiological and pathological reactions, *Ann. N.Y. Acad. Sci.* 104:236, 1963.

110. Leyden, E. Zur Kenntis des Bronchial-asthma, *Virchows Arch.* 54:324, 1872.

111. Lichtenstein, L. M., and Osler, A. G. Studies on the mechanisms of hypersensitivity phenomena. IX. Histamine release from human leukocytes by ragweed pollen antigen, *J. Exp. Med.* 120:507, 1964.

112. Litt, M. Studies in experimental eosinophilia. I. Repeated quantitation of peritoneal eosinophilia in guinea pigs by a method of peritoneal lavage, *Blood* 16:1318, 1960.

113. Litt, M. Studies in experimental eosinophilia. III. The induction of peritoneal eosinophilia by the passive transfer of serum antibody, *J. Immunol.* 87:522, 1961.

114. Litt, M. Studies in experimental eosinophilia. V. Eosinophils in lymph nodes of guinea pigs following primary antigenic stimulation, *Am. J. Pathol.* 42:529, 1963.

115. Litt, M. Eosinophils and antigen-antibody reactions, *Ann. N.Y. Acad. Sci.* 116:964, 1964.

116. Litt, M. Studies in experimental eosinophilia. VI. Uptake of immune complexes by eosinophils, *J. Cell Biol.* 23:355, 1964.

117. Litt, M. Studies in experimental eosinophilia. VIII. Int. Cong. Series 162:5:38, Proc. Sixth Cong. Int. Assoc. Allergology, Excerpta Medica, Amsterdam, 1968.

118. Loeffler, W. Zur Differential-diagnose der Lungen Infiltrierungen: über flüchtige Succedan-infiltrate (mit Eosinophilie), *Beitr. Klin. Erforsch. Tuberk.* 79:368, 1932.

119. Loeffler, W. Endocarditis parietalis fibroplastica mit Blut Eosinophile, *Schweiz. Med. Wochenschr.* 66:817, 1936.

120. Lutzner, M. A. Enzymatic specialization of organelles of blood cells, mast cells and platelets, *Fed. Proc.* 23:441, 1964 (abstract).

121. Lutzner, M. A., and Benditt, E. P. Isolation and biochemistry of the granules of the eosinophilic leukocyte of the guinea pig, *J. Cell Biol.* 19:47A, 1963 (abstract).

122. Lutzner, M. A., Tierney, J. H., and Benditt, E. P. Giant granules and widespread cytoplasmic inclusions in a genetic syndrome of Aleutian mink. An electron microscopic study, *Lab. Invest.* 14:2063, 1966.

123. McCombs, R. P. Diseases due to immunologic reactions in the lungs, *N. Engl. J. Med.* 286:1186, 1972.

124. McGarry, M. P., Speirs, R. S., Jenkins, V. K., and Trentin, J. J. Lymphoid cell dependence of eosinophil response to antigen, *J. Exp. Med.* 134:801, 1971.

125. MacSween, J. M., and Langley, G. R. Intraleucocytic immunoglobulin in eosinophilia in man, *Immunology* 21:61, 1971.

126. Mager, M., McNary, W. F., Jr., and Lionetti, F. The histochemical detection of zinc, *J. Histochem. Cytochem.* 1:493, 1953.

127. Marshall, D. C., Friedman, E. A., Goldstein, D. P., Henry, L., and Merrill, J. P. The rejection of skin homografts in the normal human subject. Part I. Clinical observations, *J. Clin. Invest.* 41:411, 1962.

128. Melmon, K. L., and Cline, M. J. Kinins (editorial), *Am. J. Med.* 43:153, 1967.

129. Melmon, K. L., and Cline, M. J. Interaction of plasma kinins and granulocytes, *Nature* 213:90, 1967.

130. Melmon, K. L., and Cline, M. J. The interaction of leukocytes and the kinin system, *Biochem. Pharmacol.* p. 271, 1968 (suppl.).

131. Mesnil, A. Sur le mode de résistance des vertébrés inférieurs aux invasions microbiennes artificielles; contribution à l'étude de l'immunité, *Ann. Inst. Pasteur* 9:301, 1895.

132. Mickenberg, I. D., Root, R. K., and Wolff, S. M. Bactericidal and metabolic properties of human eosinophils, *Blood* 39:67, 1972.

133. Miller, F. *in* R. Uyeda (ed.), Electron Microscopy, vol. 2, p. 71, Maruzen Co., Tokyo, 1966.

134. Miller, F., DeHarven, E., and Palade, G. E. The structure of eosinophil leukocyte granules in rodents and in man, *J. Cell Biol.* 31:349, 1966.

135. Opie, E. L. An experimental study of the relation of cells with eosinophile granulation to infection with an animal parasite (trichina spiralis), *Am. J. Med. Sci.* 127:477, 1904.

136. Osako, R. An electron microscopic observation on the specific granules of eosinophil leukocytes of vertebrates, *Acta Haematol. Jap.* 22:134, 1959.

137. Osgood, E. E. Culture of human marrow: length of life of the neutrophils, eosinophils and basophils of normal blood as determined by comparative cultures of blood and sternal marrow from healthy persons, *J.A.M.A.* 109:933, 1937.

138. Parish, W. E. Investigations in eosinophilia. The influence of histamine antigen-antibody complexes containing γ1 or γ2 globulins, foreign bodies (phagocytosis) and disrupted mast cells, *Br. J. Dermatol.* 82:42, 1970.

139. Parish, W. E., and Coombs, R. R. A. Peripheral blood eosinophilia in guinea-pigs following implantation of anaphylactic guinea-pig and human lung, *Br. J. Haematol.* 14:425, 1968.

140. Pease, D. C. An electron microscopic study of red bone marrow, *Blood* 11:501, 1956.

141. Pepys, J. Hypersensitivity diseases of the lungs due to fungi and organic dusts, Monographs in Allergy, vol. 4, S. Karger, Basel, 1969.

142. Perlmutter, A. D., Edlow, J. B., and Kevy, S. V. Toxocara antibodies in eosinophilic cystitis, *J. Pediatr.* 73:340, 1968.

143. Phills, A., Harrold, A. J., Whiteman, G. V., and Perlmutter, L. Pulmonary infiltrates, asthma and eosinophilia due to *Ascaris Suum* infestation in man, *N. Engl. J. Med.* 286:965, 1972.

144. Pihl, E., Gustafson, G. T., Josefsson, B., and Paul, K. G. Heavy metals in the granules of eosinophilic granulocytes, *Scand. J. Haematol.* 4:371, 1967.

145. Presentey, B. Cytochemical characterization of eosinophils with respect to a newly discovered anomaly, *Am. J. Clin. Pathol.* 51:451, 1969.

146. Presentey, B. Morphologic observations and genetic follow-up of a familial anomaly of eosinophils, *Am. J. Clin. Pathol.* 51:458, 1969.

147. Rabinovitch, M., and Andreucci, D. A histochemical study of "acid" and "alkaline" phosphatase distribution in normal human bone marrow smears, *Blood* 4:580, 1949.

148. Rabinovitch, M., Junqueira, L. C. U., and Mendes, F. T. Cytochemical demonstration of "acid" phosphatase in bone marrow smears, *Science* 107:322, 1948.

149. Recant, L., Hume, D. M., Forsham, P. H., and Thorn, G. W. Studies on the effect of epinephrine on the pituitary-adrenocortical system, *J. Clin. Endocrinol.* 10:187, 1950.

150. Rhodes, J. M., and Lind, I. Antigen uptake *in vivo* by peritoneal macrophages from normal mice and those undergoing primary or secondary responses, *Immunology* 14:511, 1968.

151. Riddle, J. M., and Barnhart, M. I. The eosinophil as a source for profibrinolysin in acute inflammation, *Blood* 25:776, 1965.

152. Riley, J. F. Functional significance of histamine and heparin in tissue

mast cells, *Ann. N.Y. Acad. Sci.* 103:151, 1963.

153. Roberts, A. N. Cellular localization and quantitation of tritiated antigen in mouse lymph nodes during early primary immune response, *Am. J. Pathol.* 49:889, 1966.

154. Roberts, A. N. Rapid uptake of tritiated antigen by mouse eosinophils, *Nature* 210:266, 1966.

155. Roberts, W. C., Liegler, D. G., and Carbone, P. P. Endomyocardial disease and eosinophilia, *Am. J. Med.* 46:28, 1969.

156. Rosenberg, E. B., Polmar, S. H., and Whalen, G. E. Increased circulating IgE in trichinosis, *Ann. Intern. Med.* 75:575, 1971.

157. Rytömaa, T. Organ distribution and histochemical properties of eosinophil granulocytes in rat. I. Histochemical properties. A. Peroxidase activity. Present investigations, *Acta Pathol. Microbiol. Scand.,* vol. 50, 140:79, 1960 (suppl.).

158. Sabesin, S. S. A function of the eosinophil: phagocytosis of antigen-antibody complexes, *Proc. Soc. Exp. Biol. Med.* 112:667, 1963.

159. Salmon, S. E., Cline, M. J., Schultz, J., and Lehrer, R. I. Myeloperoxidase deficiency. Immunologic study of a genetic leukocyte defect, *N. Engl. J. Med.* 282:250, 1970.

160. Samter, M. Charcot-Leyden crystals, *J. Allergy* 18:221, 1947.

161. Samter, M., Kofoed, M. A., and Pieper, W. A factor in lungs of anaphylactically shocked guinea pigs which can induce eosinophilia in normal animals, *Blood* 8:1078, 1953.

162. Schoen, I., and Pizer, M. Eosinophilia apparently related to cigarette smoking, *N. Engl. J. Med.* 27:1344, 1964.

163. Schwartz, E. Die Lehre von der allgemeine und ortlichen "Eosinophilie," *Ergeb. Allg. Pathol.* 17:137, 1914.

164. Seeman, P. M., and Palade, G. E. Acid phosphatase localization in rabbit eosinophils, *J. Cell Biol.* 34:745, 1967.

165. Seligman, A. M., Wasserkrug, H. L., Deb, C., and Hanker, J. S. Osmium-containing compounds with multiple basic or acidic groups as stains for ultra-structure, *J. Histochem. Cytochem.* 16:87, 1968.

166. Sheldon, H., and Zetterquist, H. Internal ultrastructure in granules of white blood cells of the mouse, *Bull. Johns Hopkins Hosp.* 96:135, 1955.

167. Shepherd, A. J. N., Walsh, C. H., Archer, R. K., and Wetherley-Mein, G. Eosinophilia, splenomegaly and cardiac disease, *Br. J. Haematol.* 20:233, 1971.

168. Solomon, D. H., and Humphreys, S. R. Splenic arteriovenous differences in blood cells during the hematologic reaction to adrenal cortical stimulation, *Blood* 6:824, 1951.

169. Speirs, R. S. Physiological approaches to an understanding of the function of eosinophils and basophils, *Ann. N.Y. Acad. Sci.* 59:706, 1955.

170. Speirs, R. S. Advances in the knowledge of the eosinophil in relation to antibody formation, *Ann. N.Y. Acad. Sci.* 73:283, 1958.

171. Speirs, R. S. Function of leukocytes in inflammation and immunity, *in* A. S. Gordon (ed.), Regulation of Hematopoiesis, p. 995, Appleton-Century-Crofts, New York, 1970.

172. Speirs, R. S., and Dreisbach, M. E. Quantitative studies of the cellular responses to antigen injections in normal mice. Technic for determining cells in the peritoneal fluid, *Blood* 11:44, 1956.

173. Speirs, R. S., and Osada, Y. Chemotactic activity and phagocytosis of eosinophils, *Proc. Soc. Exp. Biol. Med.* 109:929, 1962.

174. Speirs, R. S., and Speirs, E. E. Cellular localization of radioactive antigen in immunized and non-immunized mice, *J. Immunol.* 90:561, 1963.

175. Speirs, R. S., and Speirs, E. E. Cellular reactions to reinjection of antigen, *J. Immunol.* 92:540, 1964.

176. Speirs, R. S., and Turner, M. X. The eosinophil response to toxoids and its inhibition by antitoxin, *Blood* 34:320, 1969.

177. Speirs, R. S., and Wenck, U. Eosinophil response to toxoids in actively and passively immunized mice, *Proc. Soc. Exp. Biol. Med.* 90:571, 1955.

178. Speirs, R. S., and Wenck, U. Effect of cortisone on the cellular

response during allergic inflammation, *Acta Haematol.* 17:271, 1957.

179. Speirs, R. S., Wenck, U., and Dreisbach, M. E. Quantitative studies of the cellular responses to antigen injections in adrenalectomized mice, *Blood* 11:56, 1956.

180. Steele, A. S. V., and Rack, J. H. Cellular reaction to polystyrene-protein conjugates, *J. Pathol. Bacteriol.* 89:703, 1965.

181. Stjernholm, R. L., Thomas, P., and Esmann, V. Carbohydrate metabolism in leukocytes. X. Metabolism of the human eosinophil, *J. Reticuloendothel. Soc.* 6:300, 1969.

182. Suzuki, A. Histochemical demonstration of acid phosphatase activity in various blood cells, *Tohoku J. Exp. Med.* 89:27, 1966.

183. Sweet, L. C., Rebuck, J. W., and Noonan, S. M. The role of fibrin in allergen-induced eosinophilotaxis, *J. Allergy* 39:118, 1967 (abstract).

184. Tanaka, K. R., and Valentine, W. N. Aconitase activity of human leukocytes, *Acta Haematol.* 26:12, 1961.

185. Tanaka, K. R., Valentine, W. N., and Fredericks, R. E. Human leucocyte arylsulphatase activity, *Br. J. Haematol.* 8:86, 1962.

186. Thevathason, O. I., and Gordon, A. S. Adrenocortical-medullary interactions on the blood eosinophils, *Acta Haematol.* 19:162, 1958.

187. Turner, M. X., Speirs, R. S., and McLaughlin, J. A. Effect of primary injection site upon cellular and antitoxin responses to subsequent challenging injection, *Proc. Soc. Exp. Biol. Med.* 129:738, 1968.

188. Uhrbrand, H. The number of circulating eosinophils, *Acta Med. Scand.* 160:99, 1958.

189. Undritz, E. Sandoz Atlas of Haematology, Sandoz, Basel, 1952.

190. Vaughn, J. Experimental eosinophilia: local tissue reaction to Ascaris extracts, *J. Allergy* 32:501, 1961.

191. Vercauteren, R. A cytochemical approach to the problem of the significance of blood and tissue eosinophilia, *Enzymologia* 14:340, 1951.

192. Vercauteren, R. The properties of the isolated granules from blood eosinophiles, *Enzymologia* 16:1, 1953.

193. von Brezezinski, D. K. Unter-

suchungen zur Topochemie der eosinophilen leukozyten Granula, *Acta Histochem. (Jena)* 20:343, 1965.

194. Ward, P. A. Chemotaxis of human eosinophils, *Am. J. Pathol.* 54:121, 1969.

195. Watanabe, I., Donahue, S., and Hoggatt, N. Method for electron microscopic studies of circulating human leukocytes and observations on their fine structure, *J. Ultrastruc. Res.* 20:366, 1967.

196. Wells, P. D. Mast cell, eosinophil and histamine levels in nippostrongylus brasiliensis infected rats, *Exp. Parasitol.* 12:82, 1962.

197. Welsh, R. A., and Geer, J. C. Phagocytosis of mast cell granule by the eosinophilic leukocyte in the rat, *Am. J. Pathol.* 35:103, 1959.

198. Wenck, U., and Speirs, R. S. The effect of cortisone on blood leucocytes and peritoneal fluid cells of mice, *Acta Haematol.* 17:193, 1957.

199. Wetzel, B. K. The fine structure and cytochemistry of developing granulocytes, with special reference to the rabbit, *in* A. S. Gordon (ed.), Regulation of Hematopoiesis, p. 769, Appleton-Century-Crofts, New York, 1970.

200. Wetzel, B. K., Spicer, S. S., and Horn, R. G. Fine structural localization of acid and alkaline phosphatases in cells of rabbit blood and bone marrow, *J. Histochem. Cytochem.* 15:311, 1967.

201. Wolff, H. P. Untersuchungen zur Pathophysiologie des Zinkstoffwechsels, *Klin. Wochenschr.* 34:409, 1956.

202. Wood, W. B., Jr., Smith, M. R., and Watson, B. Studies on the mechanism of recovery in pneumococcal pneumonia. IV. The mechanism of phagocytosis in the absence of antibody, *J. Exp. Med.* 84:387, 1946.

203. Yam, L. T. Pseudoeosinophilia, eosinophilic endocarditis and eosinophilic leukemia, *Am. J. Med.* 53:193, 1972.

204. Yamada, E. Electron microscopy of the peroxidase in the granular leucocytes of rat bone marrow, *Arch. Histol. Jap.* 27:131, 1966.

205. Yamada, E., and Yamauchi, R. Some observations on the cytochemistry and morphogenesis of the granulocytes in the rat bone marrow as revealed by electron microscopy, *Acta Haematol. Jap.* 29:530, 1966.

206. Zeya, H. I., and Spitznagel, J. K. Cationic protein-bearing granules of polymorphonuclear leukocytes: separation from enzyme-rich granules, *Science* 163:1069, 1969.

207. Zolov, D. M., and Levine, B. B. Correlation of blood eosinophilia with antibody classes, *Int. Arch. Allergy* 35:179, 1969.

208. Zucker-Franklin, D. Electron microscopic studies of human granulocytes: structural variations related to function, *Semin. Hematol.* 5:109, 1968.

209. Zucker-Franklin, D. Eosinophilia of unknown etiology; a diagnostic dilemma, *Hosp. Pract.* 6:119, 1971.

Chapter 7   The Basophil

The blood basophil was originally described by Ehrlich in 1879 (48) and was also recognized at the turn of the century by Jolly (75, 76), and Maximow (99, 100). Originally called mast leukocytes or blood mast cells, these cells are now generally designated *basophils*. Tissue mast cells, which share many characteristics with basophils, rarely enter the blood and are almost never encountered in the blood smear of man (53).

Structure

Appearance by Light Microscopy

In Romanovsky-stained preparations of human peripheral blood, basophils are distinguished by their large purple or blue-black granules. These granules appear to fill the cytoplasm and partially cover the nucleus (Fig. 7.1), thus obscuring nuclear configuration. The granule content is, at least in part, water soluble. Consequently, the granules may appear to be partially dissolved in the process of fixation and staining, and the cells may then appear to have a vacuolated and slightly acidophilic cytoplasm. The basophil is about 10 microns in diameter (14).

Fine Structure and Morphogenesis

The precursors of the blood basophil have generally been presumed to reside in the bone marrow. This supposition is based on the occurrence of mitotically active immature cellular forms of the basophilic series in the marrow (75, 76, 101). Additionally, proliferation of basophilic precursor cells is observed in the bone marrow in experi-

mental basophilia and in some myeloproliferative disorders (32, 91, 92). Most authors have assumed that the mature basophil derives from an identifiable promyelocyte (43, 101, 109, 128), although other authors have claimed that the cell derives from a separate cell line with a so-called basophiloblast stem cell (154). Differentiation along a basophilic pathway from a still-undifferentiated pluripotent granulocytic precursor probably occurs at the promyelocyte stage of development (Fig. 1.2) (116).

The morphogenesis of the early cells of the basophilic series is basically similar to that of the neutrophilic series. Progressive cellular maturation is denoted by increasing condensation of the nuclear chromatin, loss of highly developed nucleolar structure, and a progressively less complex development of the granular reticulum and Golgi apparatus.

Differentiation into the basophilic series is first identified when the characteristic cytoplasmic granules appear in young and intermediate cells (Fig. 7.2). These granules are soluble in aqueous fixatives (64) and the resulting nonuniform preservation, when viewed in the electron microscope, leads to a varied appearance of the granules in cells of all ages. These morphologically heterogeneous granules are considered representative of a single population that reacts variably to fixation procedures (162). Glutaraldehyde and formaldehyde fixatives generally preserve some granule material that is extremely electron dense, whereas the material appears to be totally extracted by osmium tetroxide alone. The preserved basophil granules vary in size from 0.15 to 0.5 micron in diameter and have

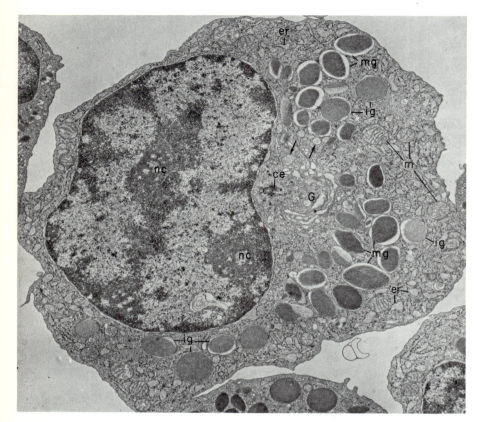

Figure 7.4 Early basophilic myelocyte. This cell is actively forming specific granules. Note the large eccentric nucleus with several nucleoli (*nc*), abundant rough-surfaced endoplasmic reticulum (*er*) with a content of moderate density, and the prominent Golgi complex (*G*) with its associated centriole (*ce*). Several small, immature, or forming granules (*arrows*) are seen in the Golgi region, and a number of larger immature (*ig*) and mature (*mg*) granules are seen in the peripheral cytoplasm. Mitochondria (*m*) are also visible. Magnification × 8,000. (From R. W. Terry, D. F. Bainton, and M. G. Farquhar, *Lab Invest.* 21:65, 1969. Reprinted by permission of authors and publisher.)

Kaung (84) has suggested that the PAS-positive material is restricted to the basophil cytoplasm.

Generally, basophils are described as lacking a sudanophilic (lipid) reaction (1, 63, 132), although contrary reports exist (142). Various oxidative enzymes have been reported in basophil cytoplasm, including the following dehydrogenases: lactic, glucose-6-phosphate, isocitric, beta-hydroxybutyric, and glutamic dehydrogenases. In addition, NADPH and NADH diaphorases are demonstrable (1, 12). The basophils of man, the rabbit, and the guinea pig give a weak histochemical reaction for histamine (1).

The abundant acid hydrolases, alkaline phosphatase, and peroxidase of the neutrophil granules by and large have not been found in the basophil granules (1, 11, 54, 81, 152, 164, 170); a recent report suggests, however, that some peroxidase is present (2). The lack of acid hydrolases also clearly distinguishes the basophil from the tissue mast cell whose granules possess these enzymes (see below). On the basis of these histochemical observations, one can conclude that basophils and tissue mast cells are similar but not identical. To summarize, the following are the major components of basophils derived from histochemical analysis:

Acid mucopolysaccharides: heparin, ? hyaluronic acid
Succinic dehydrogenase
Malic dehydrogenase
Lactic dehydrogenase
Glucose-6-phosphate dehydrogenase
Isocitric dehydrogenase
Beta-hydroxybutyric dehydrogenase
Glutamic dehydrogenase
NADH and NADPH diaphorases
Histamine

Production and Distribution

The paucity of information about the production, distribution, and life-span of the basophil results from technical difficulties in handling and labeling the few cells available in the blood and bone marrow of normal subjects. Based on conclusions drawn largely from morphologic observations, basophils are produced in the bone marrow, released into the circulation where they enjoy a transient residence, and subsequently immigrate into the tissues. Their fate in the tissues is largely unknown. They may be lost from the mucosal surfaces or destroyed at sites of inflammation. The scant information available on basophil kinetics was, for the most part, compiled subsequent to the description of a simple direct method for counting these cells (106).

the peculiar tinctorial quality known as *metachromasia* (1), to be discussed later in this chapter. Heparin is one of the important acid mucopolysaccharide constituents (4). Hyaluronic acid may account for metachromasia, since treatment with testicular hyaluronidase produces a diminution of this staining quality (10). Cytochemical techniques demonstrate that granules also show evidence of an RNA constituent (1, 120). The reason for such a peculiar localization of RNA is unknown. Basophil granules and cytoplasm give a positive periodic acid Schiff reaction of moderate strength; the reaction is wholly or partially diastase labile, indicating the presence of glycogen, glycoproteins, or acid mucopolysaccharides (10, 141, 169).

Figure 7.5 Portion of a basophilic myelocyte with an active Golgi region, containing a number of early-forming granules (*arrows*). During granule development several of these granules apparently aggregate to form larger immature forms of increasing size (ig_1, ig_2, and ig_3), which undergo progressive condensation in the peripheral cytoplasm. The granule contents eventually become organized into the banded patterns characteristic of mature specific granules (*mg*). Portions of centrioles (*ce*), from which microtubules (*mt*) are seen to radiate, are present in the center of the Golgi region. The nucleus (*n*) is visible at the bottom. Magnification × 15,000. (From R. W. Terry, D. F. Bainton, and M. G. Farquhar, *Lab. Invest.* 21:65, 1969. Reprinted by permission of authors and publisher.)

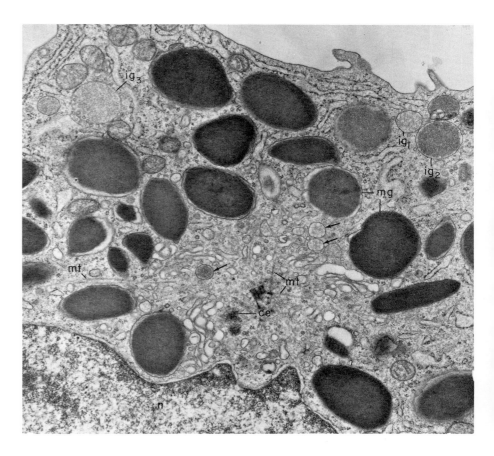

The numbers of circulating basophils are believed to vary with age, being high in the newborn period, reaching the lower adult levels early in childhood, and falling lower with advanced age (7, 73, 103, 104). Mast cell counts appear to follow a similar pattern in the tissues of laboratory animals (13).

The level of circulating basophils is influenced by the hormonal environment and may be altered by endocrine manipulation (23). A single dose of ACTH is reported to cause a fall in the numbers of basophils circulating in man and the rabbit (20, 24, 85). This effect is produced within four hours and is sustained for up to eight hours. It is dependent upon an intact adrenal (148) and can be reproduced by the administration of cortisone or hydrocortisone (40, 41). Prolonged administration of glucocorticoids results in sustained basopenia, which subsides slowly after hormone withdrawal (20). The blood basophils from patients with chronic myelocytic leukemia do not show this normal fall in response to corticoids (85). The mechanism of the basopenia induced by adrenal steroids is not known.

Blood basophils and tissue mast cells are reported to be decreased in thyrotoxicosis (104) and increased in hypothyroidism (30, 66, 104). Basophil numbers return to normal with restoration of the euthyroid state.

Gonadal hormones also influence the blood basophil

Figure 7.6 Mature basophil from the bone marrow. The mature cell differs from the myelocyte of Fig. 7.4 in its smaller size and in that it possesses a bilobed nucleus (*n*) without nucleoli; sparse, rough-surfaced endoplasmic reticulum; an inactive Golgi region (*G*); and a greater number of granules, most of which are mature. Note the presence of a centriole (*ce*) in the Golgi region. Glycogen normally is found in mature cells, but is not visible in this preparation, which was stained in block with uranyl acetate. Magnification × 14,000. (From R. W. Terry, D. F. Bainton, and M. G. Farquhar, *Lab. Invest.* 21:65, 1969. Reprinted by permission of authors and publisher.)

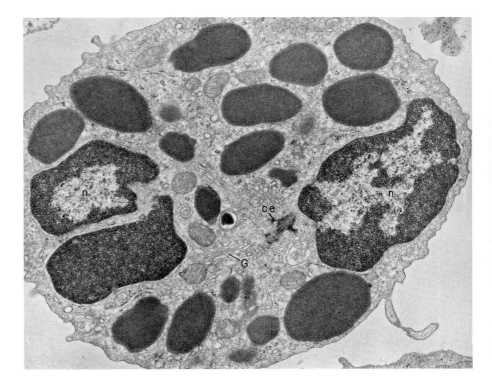

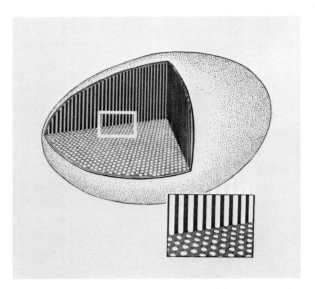

Figure 7.7 Diagrammatic representation of the proposed organization of a mature granule from a basophilic leukocyte of the guinea pig. The views obtained in sections could be explained if the granule contents consisted in a hexagonal lattice or hexagonal arrangement of microfilaments oriented as shown. In sections normal to the hexagon the honeycomb pattern is seen, whereas in the other planes depicted parallel bands are seen. The rectangular lattice pattern, not diagrammed above but illustrated in square 6 of Fig. 7.3, is believed to occur when the hexagonal lattice is cut in grazing section. The inset here depicts an enlarged view of the proposed relation between the hexagons and the parallel bands. (From R. W. Terry, D. F. Bainton, and M. G. Farquhar, *Lab. Invest.* 21:65, 1969. Reprinted by permission of authors and publisher.)

concentration in some mammalian species. Estrogens appear to increase the number, and turnover, of these cells in the circulation, whereas progesterone reduces their number (149, 150). During pregnancy, the blood basophil concentration is reported to be decreased in women and in rabbits (3, 22). A variation in the basophil count with the menstrual cycle has also been claimed (21).

Basophils in the tissues accumulate at sites of inflammation. In normal subjects the relative numbers of basophils to neutrophils at sites of inflammation are roughly proportional to their ratio in the blood; that is, basophils constitute only a few percent of the total inflammatory exudate leukocytes (119, 123, 126). In a variety of diseases, however, basophils are profuse in inflammatory exudates (see below).

Composition and Metabolism

Blood basophils are rich in heparin (16, 97, 129) and histamine (37-39, 129) and thus resemble tissue mast cells. Considerable evidence points to the basophil as the prin-

cipal carrier of blood histamine (39, 54, 58, 158). The histamine is probably synthesized within the basophil rather than acquired from external sources, since the basophil is a rich source of histidine decarboxylase activity (61). The amine is located within the granule fraction of the cell (121). The reactions of basophil-associated histamine are considered in the next section of this chapter.

As noted earlier, basophils lack significant levels of acid or alkaline phosphatase activity, peroxidase activity, and neutral lipid (142, 155). They do have small stores of glycogen. Because of the difficulties encountered in isolating sufficient numbers of these cells for study, relatively little is known about their metabolic activity (33, 34, 142). We know that basophils degranulate under a variety of circumstances, but the detailed cellular mechanisms involved are obscure. Because of their abundant mitochondria, we presume that the mature basophil uses oxidative pathways of energy production to a greater extent than does the neutrophil (33). However, basophils are reported to have less aconitase activity (a tricarboxylic acid enzyme) per cell than the neutrophil (148). Clearly, the metabolism of the mammalian basophil is an area for future exploration.

Functions

The functions of basophils are not known with certainty. Their role in the body's economy has long been accepted as related to their content of pharmacologically active substances such as histamine and heparin. Blood basophils may release the granules containing these pharmacologically active compounds in response to a variety of stimuli. The mast cell, which contains similar agents, degranulates in response to the same stimuli (86, 105, 133, 134). Stimuli producing degranulation include specific antigen added to basophils from sensitized subjects in vivo or in vitro (83, 135, 136), exposure to cold (79), and alimentary hyperlipemia (137). Blood leukocyte histamine is also released by trauma to cells and by proteolytic enzymes (39). Basophils are capable of particle ingestion, but are less avidly phagocytic than neutrophils. During phagocytosis basophil granules appear to "burst throughout the whole of the cell cytoplasm" rather than to lyse around phagocytic vacuoles as is the case with neutrophils (129).

The release of leukocyte histamine by immune complexes may be mediated by the cyclic 3', 5'-adenosine monophosphate (cyclic AMP) system (95). This supposition is based on indirect evidence. Clearly, human granulocytes contain cyclic AMP generating and degrading systems (25), but thus far they have not been delineated in the basophil. Release of histamine by antigen may be related to the binding of IgE to the surface of the basophil (68).

Leukocytes from allergic individuals release histamine upon incubation with the sensitizing antigen (96). When antigen-unresponsive leukocytes from certain nonallergic subjects are incubated in the serum of an allergic donor and subsequently challenged with antigen, histamine is released (93). These observations indicate an interaction of humoral and cellular factors in the antigen-induced release of histamine. Recently, Ishizaka and his colleagues have provided extensive evidence that the humoral factor is immunoglobulin E (67). Antiserum to IgE mimics the effect of added antigen in inducing histamine release (69-71, 94). The basophil appears to be the cell responsible for histamine release. The percentage of recognizable basophils decreases in the blood of allergic individuals incubated with antigen (122) as a result of degranulation (62). Radioactive IgE appears to bind preferentially to human basophils (70). The distribution of bound IgE is influenced by temperature (145) and by cations (15).

After injecting rabbits with antigen to induce serum sickness, immune complexes appear in the circulation. Additionally, the homocytotropic IgE antibody that is formed binds to basophils. Leukocyte suspensions containing these basophils, when combined with antigen, release soluble factors that cause platelets to clump and to release vasoactive amines (36). It is the interaction of IgE and basophils that is critical in the initiation process (18). Basophils may thus be involved in certain types of tissue injuries induced by immune complexes.

In vitro, basophils from sensitized subjects degranulate in response to antigens (80, 134, 138). Chan and Yoffey (32) and Winqvist (166) reported that the numbers of basophils in the blood and bone marrow increase with repeated antigenic challenge. Eventually, however, the numbers of basophils equal or fall below preimmunization levels. In the rabbit and guinea pig, basophils, as well as eosinophils, accumulate at the sites of antigen deposition (8, 9, 56, 113, 114).

The release of histamine by basophils and mast cells may be modulated by agents that influence the cellular levels of cyclic AMP. Agents or maneuvers that increase cellular cyclic AMP tend to retard allergic histamine release (25, 26, 112).

Some types of delayed hypersensitivity reactions in experimental animals are characterized by extensive infiltration of basophilic leukocytes (44), although such infiltration is unusual in the classic models of delayed hypersensitivity (42, 153). The basophilic reaction is influenced by the mode of antigen administration (44, 45, 125) and is best accomplished without the use of complete Freund's adjuvant. Basophilic infiltration may occur in allergic contact dermatitis reactions of man (45, 46). After a patch test

with an allergen, initial perivascular accumulation of lymphocytes is followed by an influx of basophils and, subsequently, of eosinophils. Increased vascular permeability occurs during the course of the reaction. The role of homocytotropic antibody (IgE), which is bound to the basophil in the pathogenesis of this reaction, is not yet clearly defined (68).

Beyond these few observations, relatively little is known about basophil function. Because basophils share certain prominent constituents with tissue mast cells, in particular histamine and heparin, one is tempted to speculate that the two cell types share a common role in inflammatory responses to certain physical factors, such as cold, and to antigens. In this speculation, the mast cells constitute the fixed tissue component of the response and the blood basophils constitute the mobile component. Because of their greater abundance, accessibility, and susceptibility to tissue culture techniques, mast cells have been studied more extensively than basophils. Their responses to a variety of conditions have been well documented. In areas where information is available, the basophil and tissue mast cells usually behave in a similar manner. However, these similarities should not lead to the conclusion that the cells possess identical physiologic responses. We cannot know this as a fact until more information is available on the basophil.

Similarities to Tissue Mast Cells
Von Recklinghausen in 1863 (159) was probably the first person to document the presence of mast cells in the connective tissues of man. Mast cells subsequently have been identified in a variety of species ranging from sponges to primates (127). The introduction of analine dye staining techniques permitted both the observation of prominent granules in mast cells (47, 48) and their identification in the connective tissues of most vertebrate, and many invertebrate, species (102). The mast cell granules stain purple with basic analine dyes, changing the shade of the dye. Ehrlich called this phenomenon *metachromasia*, and the granules are often referred to as *metachromatic granules*. Like the granules of the basophil, mast cell granules contain histamine and heparin and also are rich in zinc (5, 87), which is released by mast cell degranulation. Compound 48/80, the histamine-releasing agent, breaks the histamine-heparin-zinc complex (87). The histamine and heparin content of the mast cell is probably found only in the granules. Lagunoff and his associates (90) analyzed isolated granules from the mast cells of the rat and found that the dry weight is comprised of 30 percent heparin, 1.3 percent phospholipids, 33 percent basic proteins, and 9.6 percent histamine. The granules also

contain a chymotrypsin-like protein. Radioactive sulfate, which is incorporated into the structure of the heparin molecule, labels mast cells rapidly (77, 98).

In addition to heparin and histamine, the mast cells of rats and mice contain serotonin (5-hydroxytryptamine) (17, 161). Human mast cells may contain 5-hydroxytryptophan in addition to heparin and histamine (144). In sheep and cattle, mast cell granules contain dopamine (50, 157). Enzymes that have been demonstrated in mast cells by histochemical techniques include alkaline phosphatase (111), histidine decarboxylase (131), phosphatidase, acid phosphatase, peroxidase, and beta-glucuronidase (130). Proteases with trypsin- and alpha-chymotrypsin-like activity have also been identified in mast cells (82, 89), as well as leucyl aminopeptidase (28). Mast cells may possess fibrinolytic activity (49, 157).

These observations indicate that although basophils and mast cells share the property of metachromasia and are both rich in histamine and heparin, they differ in several respects. Basophils lack the hydrolytic enzymes and peroxidase that are a conspicuous part of the mast cells' armamentarium. Furthermore, no evidence points to a common origin for these two cell species (102). Nevertheless, the fixed tissue mast cell and the circulating basophil respond to a variety of stimuli with a similar release of the inflammatory mediator, histamine. The degranulation of basophils in response to cold and specific antigens has already been cited. Degranulation of the mast cells by the synthetic amine 48/80 or by antigen appears to be an energy-requiring process, which is blocked by anaerobiasis or metabolic inhibitors (156). Phospholipase-A provokes a similar energy-dependent degranulation response in mast cells.

The mast cells degranulate under a variety of other circumstances, of which the best studied is the anaphylactic reaction. The observation that mast cells disrupt in anaphylactic reactions was probably first made by Jacques and Waters (74), who studied anaphylactic shock in dogs. A subsequent, more detailed study by Stuart (143), which embraced several mammalian species, characterized this response by demonstrating rupture and disappearance of cells, and extracellular dispersion of granules. Mast cells can be passively sensitized by antibody in vitro and then degranulated with subsequent addition of antigen (107, 108). A good correlation appears to exist between mast cell rupture and histamine release in anaphylaxis. A partial explanation of the interaction of mast cells with antigen and antibody was provided by the recent observation that mast cells possess receptors for certain classes of immunoglobulins (151). We have recently observed the retention of surface receptors for immunoglobulin in a mast

cell tumor growing in tissue culture (Fig. 7.8) (35). This retention occurred despite a loss of other differentiated mast cell functions. The role of the mast cell in anaphylaxis was reviewed by Mota in 1963 (108), and its biosynthetic pathways were reviewed by Green and Day in the same year (59).

Colchicine, vinblastine, and griseofulvin inhibit release of histamine from peritoneal mast cells, whereas deuterium oxide potentiates its release. These agents alter the degree of organization of certain cytoplasmic structural elements such as microtubules. It has been suggested that these elements are involved in mast cell degranulation (57). Mast cells may play a role in the pulmonary response to hypoxia (60).

Basophils in Disease

Basophils are difficult to enumerate because of their rarity in normal blood. In 1953 Moore and James described a direct method for counting the number of basophils in a cubic millimeter of blood (106). They used a selective staining technique. Various modifications of this technique have been described since (65, 88, 139, 149).

In certain nonneoplastic diseases, basophils are believed to be unusually prominent in inflammatory exudates following nonspecific stimuli. For example, basophils are reported to accumulate in skin window preparations (sterile glass cover slips placed over a superficial skin abrasion) in diseases such as ulcerative colitis, regional ileitis, and interstitial cystitis (78, 123, 124) and in certain

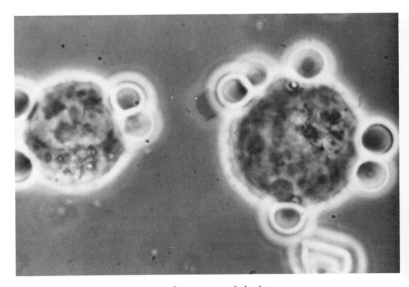

Figure 7.8 Demonstration of immunoglobulin receptors on a mouse mast cell. Sheep erythrocytes were coated with IgG antibody. The sensitized erythrocytes form rosettes around the central mast cell. Phase microscopy.

skin diseases, including Bechet's syndrome, eczema, contact dermatitis, and photosensitivity (8, 9, 55).

In ulcerative colitis, blood basophilia is not prominent despite increased migration of these cells into skin window preparations. In interstitial cystitis, increased numbers of basophils and tissue mast cells are found in the mucosa of the bladder (123).

Increased numbers of circulating basophils have been described in a number of disease states, including hypersensitivity and myxedema. Myeloproliferative disorders, including polycythemia vera and chronic myelocytic leukemia, have also been reported to show this increase of circulating basophils (31, 78, 134, 139). High levels of basophils are observed in the tissues of patients with certain myeloproliferative diseases, especially chronic myelocytic leukemia. In certain cases of chronic myelocytic leukemia the basophilia may reach such striking proportions that they suggest a diagnosis of basophilic leukemia (110, 140). Interestingly, tissue inflammatory exudates in such patients may contain neutrophils, but only rarely basophils (123).

Low levels of basophils in the circulation have been described in association with a variety of states: acute hypersensitivity reactions, such as anaphylactic shock; and severe stress such as myocardial infarction, glucocorticoid administration, and hyperthyroidism (139).

Chapter 7 References

1. Ackerman, G. A. Cytochemical properties of the blood basophilic granulocyte, *Ann. N.Y. Acad. Sci.* 103:376, 1963.
2. Ackerman, G. A., and Clark, M. A. Ultrastructural localization of peroxidase activity in human basophil leukocytes, *Acta Haematol.* 45:280, 1971.
3. Albritton, E. C. Standard Values in Blood, W. B. Saunders Co., Philadelphia, 1953.
4. Amann, R., and Martin, H. Blutmastzellen und Heparin, *Acta Haematol.* 25:209, 1961.
5. Amann, R., and Werle, E. Über Komplexe von Heparin mit Histamin und anderen Di- und Polyaminen, *Klin. Wochenschr.* 34:207, 1956.
6. Anderson, D. R. Ultrastructure of normal and leukemic leukocytes in human peripheral blood, *J. Ultrastruct. Res.* 9:1, 1966 (suppl.).
7. Angeli, G., Tedeschi, G., and Cavazzuti, F. Studio sul comportamento dei basofili ematici in soggetti di età avanzata, *Acta Gerontol.* 5:28, 1955.
8. Aspegren, N., Fregert, S., and Rorsman, H. Basophil leukocytes in allergic eczematous contact dermatitis, *Int. Arch. Allergy* 23:150, 1963.
9. Aspegren, N., Fregert, S., and Rorsman, H. Basophil leukocytes at sites of intracutaneous tuberculin test reactions, *Int. Arch. Allergy* 24:35, 1964.
10. Astaldi, G., Rondanelli, E. G., and Bernardelli, E. Recherches cytochimiques sur la moelle osseuse et le sang d'une leucémie à basocytes, *Rev. Hematol.* 8:105, 1953.
11. Austin, J. H., and Bischel, M. A histochemical method for sulfatase activity in hemic cells and organ imprints, *Blood* 17:216, 1961.
12. Balogh, K., Jr., and Cohen, R. B. Histochemical demonstration of diaphorases and dehydrogenases in normal human leukocytes and platelets, *Blood* 17:491, 1961.
13. Bates, E. O. A quantitative study and interpretation of the occurrence of basophile (mast) cells in the subcutaneous tissue of the albino rat, *Anat. Rec.* 61:231, 1935.
14. Bauer, J. D. *In* S. Frankel, S. Reitman, and A. C. Sonnenwirth (eds.), Gradwohl's Clinical Laboratory Methods and Diagnosis, vol. 1, p. 549, C. V. Mosby Co., St. Louis, 1970.
15. Becker, K. E., Ishizaka, T., Metzger, H., Ishizaka, K., and Grimley, P. M. Surface IgE on human basophils during histamine release, *J. Exp. Med.* 138:394, 1973.
16. Behrens, M., and Taubert, M. Der Nachweis von Heparin in den basophilen Leukocyten, *Klin. Wochenschr.* 30:76, 1952.
17. Benditt, E. P., Wong, R. L., Arase, M., and Roeper, E. 5-Hydroxytryptamine in mast cells, *Proc. Soc. Exp. Biol. Med.* 90:303, 1955.
18. Benveniste, J., Henson, P. M., and Cochrane, C. G. Leukocyte-dependent histamine release from rabbit platelets. The role of IgE, basophils and a platelet-activating factor, *J. Exp. Med.* 136:1356, 1972.
19. Bessis, M., and Thiery, J-P. Electron microscopy of human white blood cells and their stem cells, *Int. Rev. Cytol.* 12:199, 1961.
20. Boseila, A-W. A. Influence of corticotrophin on the circulating basophils in the rabbit, *Acta Endocrinol.* 29:355, 1958.
21. Boseila, A-W. A. The normal count of basophil leucocytes in human blood, *Acta Med. Scand.* 163:525, 1959.
22. Boseila, A-W. A. Normal count and physiological variability of rabbit blood basophils, *Experientia* 15:149, 1959.
23. Boseila, A-W. A. Hormonal influence on blood and tissue basophilic granulocytes, *Ann. N.Y. Acad. Sci.* 103:394, 1963.
24. Boseila, A-W. A., and Uhrbrand, H. Basophil-eosinophil relationship in human blood. Studies on the effect of corticotrophin, *Acta Endocrinol.* 28:49, 1958.
25. Bourne, H. R., Lehrer, R. I., Cline, M. J., and Melmon, K. L. Cyclic 3', 5'-adenosine monophosphate in the human leukocyte: synthesis, degradation, and effects on neutrophil candidacidal activity, *J. Clin. Invest.* 50:920, 1971.
26. Bourne, H. R., Lichtenstein, L. M., and Melmon, K. L. Pharmacologic control of allergic histamine release *in vitro*: evidence for an inhibitory role of 3',5'-adenosine monophosphate in human leukocytes, *J. Immunol.* 108:695, 1972.
27. Bourne, H. R., Melmon, K. L., and Lichtenstein, L. M. Histamine augments leukocyte adenosine 3',5'-monophosphate and blocks antigenic histamine release, *Science* 173:743, 1971.
28. Braun-Falco, O., and Salfeld, K. Leucine aminopeptidase activity in mast cells, *Nature* 183:51, 1959.
29. Braunsteiner, H. Mast cells and basophilic leukocytes, *in* H. Braunsteiner and D. Zucker-Franklin (eds.), The Physiology and Pathology of Leukocytes, p. 46, Grune & Stratton, New York, 1962.
30. Braunsteiner, H., Höfer, R., Thumb, N., and Vetter, H. Untersuchungen über die basophilen Leukocyten bei Schilddrüsenkrankheiten, *Klin. Wochenschr.* 37:250, 1959.
31. Braunsteiner, H., and Thumb, N. Quantitative Veränderungen der Blutbasophilen und ihre klinische Bedeutung, *Acta Haematol.* 20:339, 1958.
32. Chan, B. S. T., and Yoffey, J. M. The basophil cells of guinea-pig bone marrow and their response to horse serum, *Immunology* 3:237, 1960.
33. Cline, M. J. Metabolism of the circulating leukocyte, *Physiol. Rev.* 45:674, 1965.
34. Cline, M. J. Leukocyte metabolism, *in* A. S. Gordon (ed.), Regulation of Hematopoiesis, p. 1045, Appleton-Century-Crofts, New York, 1970.
35. Cline, M. J., and Warner, N. L. Immunoglobulin receptors on a mouse mast cell tumor, *J. Immunol.* 108:339, 1972.
36. Cochrane, C. G. Mechanisms involved in the deposition of immune complexes in tissues, *J. Exp. Med.* 134:75s, 1971.
37. Code, C. F. The source in blood of the histamine-like constituent, *J. Physiol.* (*Lond.*) 90:349, 1937.
38. Code, C. F. The histamine-like activity of white blood cells, *J. Physiol.* (*Lond.*) 90:485, 1937.
39. Code, C. F. The histamine content of white blood cells, *in* J. L. Tullis (ed.), Blood Cells and Plasma Proteins, p. 292, Academic Press, New York, 1953.
40. Code, C. F., and Mitchell, R. G. Histamine, eosinophils and baso-

phils in the blood, *J. Physiol.* 136:449, 1957.

41. Code, C. F., Mitchell, R. G., and Kennedy, J. C. The effect of cortisone on the number of circulating basophils and eosinophils: is there a relationship between these cells? *Proc. Mayo Clin.* 29:200, 1954.

42. Dale, H. H., and Laidlaw, P. P. Histamine shock, *J. Physiol.* 52:355, 1919.

43. Downey, H. Heteroplastic development of eosinophil leucocytes and of hematogenous mast cells in bone marrow of guinea-pig, *Anat. Rec.* 8:135, 1914.

44. Dvorak, H. F., Dvorak, A. M., Simpson, B. A., Richerson, H. B., Leskowitz, S., and Karnovsky, M. J. Cutaneous basophil hypersensitivity. II. A light and electron microscopic description, *J. Exp. Med.* 132:558, 1970.

45. Dvorak, H. F., and Mihm, M. C., Jr. Basophilic leukocytes in allergic contact dermatitis, *J. Exp. Med.* 135:235, 1972.

46. Dvorak, H. F., Simpson, B. A., Bast, R. C., Jr., and Leskowitz, S. Cutaneous basophil hypersensitivity. III. Participation of the basophil in hypersensitivity to antigen-antibody complexes, delayed hypersensitivity and contact allergy, passive transfer, *J. Immunol.* 107:138, 1971.

47. Ehrlich, P. Beiträge zur Kenntnis der Anilinfärbungen, *Arch. Mikr. Anat.* 13:263, 1877.

48. Ehrlich, P. Beiträge zur Kenntnis der granulierten Bindegewebzellen und der eosinophilen Leukocyten, *Arch. Anat. Physiol.* 3:166, 1879.

49. Ende, N., and Auditore, J. Fibrinolytic activity of human tissues and dog mast cell tumors, *Am. J. Clin. Pathol.* 36:16, 1961.

50. Falck, B., Nystedt, T., Rosengren, E., and Stenflo, J. Dopamine and mast cells in ruminants, *Acta Pharmacol. Toxicol.* 21:51, 1964.

51. Fawcett, D. W. An Atlas of Fine Structure: The Cell, Its Organelles and Inclusions, W. B. Saunders Co., Philadelphia, 1966.

52. Fedorko, M. E., and Hirsch, J. G. Crystalloid structure in granules of guinea pig basophils and human mast cells, *J. Cell Biol.* 26:973, 1965.

53. Fernex, M. The Mast Cell System, Its Relationship to Atherosclerosis, Fibrosis and Eosinophils, S. Karger, Basel, 1968.

54. Fredericks, R. E., and Moloney, W. C. The basophilic granulocyte, *Blood* 14:571, 1959.

55. Fregert, S., and Rorsman, H. Basophil leukocytes in intracutaneous test reactions to metals, *J. Invest. Dermatol.* 41:361, 1963.

56. Fulton, J. E., Jr., and Derbes, V. J. Basophil leukocyte infiltration in the positive tuberculin skin test in man, *J. Invest. Dermatol.* 43:125, 1964.

57. Gillespie, E., Levine, R. J., and Malawista, S. E. Histamine release from rat peritoneal mast cells: inhibition by colchicine and potentiation by deuterium oxide, *J. Pharmacol. Exp. Ther.* 164:158, 1968.

58. Graham, H. T., Lowry, O. H., Wheelwright, F., Lenz, M. A., and Parish, H. H., Jr. Distribution of histamine among leukocytes and platelets, *Blood* 10:467, 1955.

59. Green, J. P., and Day, M. Biosynthetic pathways in mastocytoma cells in culture and *in vivo*, *Ann. N.Y. Acad. Sci.* 103:334, 1963.

60. Haas, F., and Bergofsky, E. H. Role of the mast cell in the pulmonary pressor response to hypoxia, *J. Clin. Invest.* 51:3154, 1972.

61. Hartman, W. J., Clark, W. G., and Cyr, S. D. Histidine decarboxylase activity of basophils from chronic myelogenous leukemic patients. Origin of blood histamine, *Proc. Soc. Exp. Biol. Med.* 107:123, 1961.

62. Hastie, R. The antigen-induced degranulation of basophil leukocytes from atopic subjects, studied by phase-contrast microscopy, *Clin. Exp. Immunol.* 8:45, 1971.

63. Hayhoe, F. G. J. The cytochemical demonstration of lipids in blood and bone-marrow cells, *J. Pathol. Bacteriol.* 65:413, 1953.

64. Horn, R. G., and Spicer, S. S. Sulfated mucopolysaccharide and basic protein in certain granules of rabbit leukocytes, *Lab. Invest.* 13:1, 1964.

65. Inagaki, S. Studies on the fixing, staining and counting methods for basophil leukocytes, *Acta Haematol. Jap.* 18:635, 1955.

66. Inagaki, S. The relationship between the level of circulating basophil leucocytes and thyroid function, *Acta Endocrinol.* 26:477, 1957.

67. Ishizaka, K. Human reaginic antibodies, *Ann. Rev. Med.* 21:187, 1970.

68. Ishizaka, K., and Ishizaka, T. The significance of immunoglobulin E in reaginic hypersensitivity, *Ann. Allergy* 28:189, 1970.

69. Ishizaka, K., Ishizaka, T., and Lee, E. H. Biologic function of the Fc fragments of E myeloma protein, *Immunochemistry* 7:687, 1970.

70. Ishizaka, K., Tomioka, H., and Ishizaka, T. Mechanisms of passive sensitization. I. Presence of IgE and IgG molecules on human leukocytes, *J. Immunol.* 105:1459, 1970.

71. Ishizaka, T., Ishizaka, K., Gunnar, S., Johansson, O., and Bennich, H. Histamine release from human leukocytes by anti-γE antibodies, *J. Immunol.* 102:884, 1969.

72. Ito, T. Electron microscopic observation on myeloid leukemic cells, with special reference to the findings resembling to virus infection, *Acta Haematol. Jap.* 21:631, 1958.

73. James, G. W. III, Wright, D. U., Wilkerson, V., and Shellenberg, R. Observations on the absolute basophil count in health and disease, *Clin. Res. Proc.* 3:31, 1955.

74. Jaques, L. B., and Waters, E. T. The identity and origin of the anticoagulant of anaphylactic shock in the dog, *J. Physiol.* 99:454, 1941.

75. Jolly, M. Recherches sur la division indirecte des cellules lymphatiques granuleuses de la moelle des os, *Arch. Anat. Microbiol.* 3:168, 1900.

76. Jolly, M. J. Clasmatocytes et mastzellen, *C. R. Soc. Biol.* (Paris) 52:609, 1900.

77. Jorpes, J. E., and Gardell, S. On heparin monosulfuric acid, *J. Biol. Chem.* 176:267, 1948.

78. Juhlin, L. Basophil leukocytes in ulcerative colitis, *Acta Med. Scand.* 173:351, 1963.

79. Juhlin, L., and Shelley, W. B. Role of mast cell and basophil in cold urticaria with associated systemic reactions, *J.A.M.A.* 177:371, 1961.

80. Juhlin, L., and Westphal, O. Degranulation of basophil leukocytes in a case of milk allergy, *Acta Derm. Venereol.* 42:273, 1962.

81. Kaplow, L. S. Simplified myeloperoxidase stain using benzidine di-

hydrochloride, *Blood* 26:215, 1965.

82. Katayama, Y., and Eude, M. Atee- and tame-esterases of human mast cell, *Fed. Proc.* 23:392, 1964.

83. Katz, H. I., Gill, K. A., Baxter, D. L., and Moschella, S. L. Indirect basophil degranulation test in penicillin allergy, *J.A.M.A.* 188:351, 1964.

84. Kaung, D. T. Periodic acid-Schiff reaction in human basophilic leucocytes, *Acta Haematol.* 42:269, 1969.

85. Kelemen, E., and Bikich, G. Insufficiency of acute response of basophil and eosinophil leukocytes and of blood histamine after the administration of ACTH and cortisone in untreated myelocytic leukaemia, *Acta Haematol.* 15:202, 1956.

86. Keller, R. Tissue mast cells in immune reaction, *Monogr. Allergy* 2:144, 1966.

87. Kerp, L. Bedeutung von Zink für die Histaminspeicherung in Mastzellen, *Int. Arch. Allergy* 22:112, 1963.

88. Kovacs, G. S. A simple direct method for absolute basophil and eosinophil counts from the same blood sample, *Folia Haematol.* 5:166, 1961.

89. Lagunoff, D., and Benditt, E. P. Histochemical examinations of chymotrypsin-like esterases, *Nature* 192:1198, 1961.

90. Lagunoff, D., Phillips, M. T., Iseri, O. A., and Benditt, E. P. Isolation and preliminary characterization of rat mast cell granules, *Lab. Invest.* 13:1331, 1964.

91. Leder, L. D. Über die selektive fermentcytochemische Darstellung von neutrophilen myelosicher Zellen und Gewebsmastzellen im Paraffinschnitt, *Klin. Wochenschr.* 42:553, 1964.

92. Leder, L. D. Der Blutmonocyt, Springer-Verlag, Berlin, 1967.

93. Levy, D. A., and Osler, A. G. Studies on the mechanisms of hypersensitivity phenomena. XIV. Passive sensitization *in vitro* of human leukocytes to rag weed pollen antigen, *J. Immunol.* 97:203, 1966.

94. Lichtenstein, L. M., Levy, D. A., and Ishizaka, K. *In vitro* reversed anaphylaxis: characteristics of anti-IgE mediated histamine release, *Immunology* 19:831, 1970.

95. Lichtenstein, L. M., and Margolis, S. Histamine release *in vitro*: inhibition by catecholamines and methylxanthines, *Science* 161:902, 1968.

96. Lichtenstein, L. M., and Osler, A. G. Studies on the mechanisms of hypersensitivity phenomena. IX. Histamine release from human leukocytes by rag weed pollen antigen, *J. Exp. Med.* 120:507, 1964.

97. Martin, H., and Roka, L. Zur Frage des Heparingehaltes der Blutmastzellen des Menschen, *Acta Haematol.* 10:26, 1953.

98. Marx, W., and Spolter, L. Zur Kenntnis der Heparinbiosynthese, *Helv. Physiol. Pharmacol. Acta* 19:C85, 1962.

99. Maximow, A. Ueber entzündliche Bindegewebsneubildung bei der weissen Ratte und die dabei auftretenden Veränderungen der Mastzellen und Fettzellen, *Beitr. Pathol. Anat.* 35:93, 1904.

100. Maximow, A. Untersuchungen über Blut und Bindegewebe. III. Die embryonale Histogenese des Knochenmarks der Saugetiere, *Arch. Mikr. Anat.* 76:1, 1910.

101. Maximow, A. Untersuchungen über Blut und Bindegewebe. VI. Ueber Blutmastzellen, *Arch. Mikr. Anat.* 83:247, 1913.

102. Michels, N. A. The mast cells, *in* H. Downey (ed.), Downey Handbook of Haematology, vol. 1, p. 232, Paul B. Hoeber, New York, 1938.

103. Mitchell, R. G. Circulating-basophilic leucocyte counts in the newborn, *Arch. Dis. Child.* 30:130, 1955.

104. Mitchell, R. G. Basophilic leucocytes in children in health and disease, *Arch. Dis. Child.* 33:193, 1958.

105. Mongar, J. L., and Schild, H. O. Cellular mechanisms in anaphylaxis, *Physiol. Rev.* 42:226, 1962.

106. Moore, J. E. III, and James, G. W. III. A simple direct method for absolute basophil leucocyte count, *Proc. Soc. Exp. Biol. Med.* 82:601, 1953.

107. Mota, I. Effect of antigen and octylamine on mast cells and histamine content of sensitized guinea-pig tissues, *J. Physiol.* 147:425, 1959.

108. Mota, I. Mast cells and anaphylaxis, *Ann. N.Y. Acad. Sci.* 103:264, 1963.

109. Naegeli, O. Lehrbuch der Blutkrankheiten und Blutdiagnostik, Springer-Verlag, Berlin, 1931.

110. Nan, R. C., and Hoagland, H. C. A myeloproliferative disorder manifested by persistent basophilia, granulocytic leukemia and erythroleukemic phases, *Cancer* 28:662, 1971.

111. Noback, C. R., and Montagna, W. Some histochemical aspects of the mast cell with special reference to alkaline phosphatase and cytochrome oxidase, *Anat. Rec.* 96:279, 1946.

112. Orange, R. P., Austen, W. G., and Austen, K. F. Immunological release of histamine and slow-reacting substance of anaphylaxis from human lung. I. Modulation by agents influencing cellular levels of cyclic 3',5'-adenosine monophosphate, *J. Exp. Med.* 134:136s, 1971.

113. Osada, Y., and Ogawa, S. Experimental basophilia and eosinophilia in rabbit produced by immunization with egg albumin, *Bull. Inst. Publ. Health (Tokyo)* 10:205, 1961.

114. Osada, Y., and Ogawa, S. Basophilia and eosinophilia in blood and peritoneal cavity produced by intraperitoneal challenging injection in the immunized guinea pig, *Bull. Inst. Publ. Health (Tokyo)* 13:1, 1964.

115. Osako, R. An electron microscopic observation on the specific granules of eosinophil leukocytes of vertebrates, *Acta Haematol. Jap.* 22:134, 1959.

116. Parwaresch, M. R., Leder, L. D., and Dannenberg, K. E. G. On the origin of human basophilic granulocytes, *Acta Haematol.* 45:273, 1971.

117. Pease, D. C. Marrow cells seen with the electron microscope after ultrathin sectioning, *Rev. Hematol.* 10:300, 1955.

118. Pease, D. C. An electron microscopic study of red bone marrow, *Blood* 11:501, 1956.

119. Perillie, P. E., and Finch, S. C. The local exudative cellular response in leukemia, *J. Clin. Invest.* 39:1353, 1960.

120. Perry, S., and Reynolds, J. Methyl-green-pyronin as a differential nu-

cleic acid stain for peripheral blood smears, *Blood* 11:1132, 1956.

121. Pruzansky, J. J., and Patterson, R. Stability of human leukocyte granules which contain histamine, *J. Immunol.* 100:1165, 1968.

122. Pruzansky, J. J., and Patterson, R. Decrease in basophils after incubation with specific antigens of leukocytes from allergic donors, *Int. Arch. Allergy Appl. Immunol.* 38:522, 1970.

123. Rebuck, J. W., and Crowley, J. H. A method of studying leukocytic functions *in vivo*, *Ann. N.Y. Acad. Sci.* 59:757, 1955.

124. Rebuck, J. W., Hodson, J. M., Priest, R. J., and Barth, C. L. Basophilic granulocytes in inflammatory tissues of man, *Ann. N.Y. Acad. Sci.* 103:409, 1963.

125. Richerson, H. B. Cutaneous basophil (Jones-Mote) hypersensitivity after "tolerogenic" doses of intravenous ovalbumin in the guinea pig, *J. Exp. Med.* 134:630, 1971.

126. Riis, P. The Cytology of Inflammatory Exudate, Munksgaard, Copenhagen, 1959.

127. Riley, J. F. The Mast Cells, E. and S. Livingstone Co., Edinburgh, 1959.

128. Ringoen, A. R. The mast leucocytes in the adult guinea pig under experimental conditions, *Am. J. Anat.* 31:319, 1923.

129. Sampson, D., and Archer, G. T. Release of histamine from human basophils, *Blood* 29:722, 1967.

130. Schauer, A. Die Mastzelle. Veröffentlichung aus der morphologischen Pathologie, no. 68. Gustav Fischer Verlag, Stuttgart, 1964.

131. Schayer, R. W. Histidine decarboxylase in mast cells, *Ann. N.Y. Acad. Sci.* 103:164, 1963.

132. Sheehan, H. L., and Storey, G. W. An improved method of staining leucocyte granules with sudan black B, *J. Pathol. Bacteriol.* 59:336, 1947.

133. Shelley, W. B. Adventures with the basophil, *J. Invest. Dermatol.* 39:277, 1962.

134. Shelley, W. B. Methods of observing the basophil leucocyte degranulation response, *Ann. N.Y. Acad. Sci.* 103:427, 1963.

135. Shelley, W.B., and Caro, W. A. Detection of anaphylactic sensitivity by the basophil degranulation response, *J.A.M.A.* 182:172, 1962.

136. Shelley, W. B., and Comaish, J. S. New test for penicillin allergy fluorometric assay of histamine release, *J.A.M.A.* 192:36, 1965.

137. Shelley, W. B., and Juhlin, L. Degranulation of the basophil in man induced by alimentary lipemia, *Am. J. Med. Sci.* 242:211, 1961.

138. Shelley, W. B., and Juhlin, L. A new test for detecting anaphylactic sensitivity: the basophil reaction, *Nature* 191:1056, 1961.

139. Shelley, W. B., and Parnes, H. M. The absolute basophil count, *J.A.M.A.* 192:368, 1965.

140. Shohet, S. B., and Blum, S. F. Coincident basophilic myelogenous leukemia and pulmonary tuberculosis, *Cancer* 22:173, 1968.

141. Smith, C. Glycogen in basophilic leucocytes in human blood smears, *Proc. Soc. Exp. Biol. Med.* 72:209, 1949.

142. Storti, E., and Perugini, S. Cytochemical researches on the lipids of the hematic cells with particular attention to those of acute leukosis, *Acta Haematol.* 5:321, 1951.

143. Stuart, E. G. Mast cell responses to anaphylaxis, *Anat. Rec.* 112:394, 1952.

144. Sturm, A., Jr., and Stüttgen, G. Nachweis von 5-hydroxytryptophan in menschlichen Mastzellen, *Klin. Wochenschr.* 40:199, 1962.

145. Sullivan, A. L., Grimley, P. M., and Metzger, H. Electron microscopic localization of immunoglobulin E on the surface membrane of human basophils, *J. Exp. Med.* 134:1403, 1971.

146. Tanaka, K. R., and Valentine, W. N. Aconitase activity of human leukocytes, *Acta Haematol.* 26:12, 1961.

147. Terry, R. W., Bainton, D. F., and Farquhar, M. G. Formation and structure of specific granules in basophilic leukocytes of the guinea pig, *Lab. Invest.* 21:65, 1969.

148. Thonnard-Neumann, E. The influence of hormones on the basophilic leukocytes. A review, *Acta Haematol.* 25:261, 1961.

149. Thonnard-Neumann, E. Studies of basophils: variations with age and sex, *Acta Haematol.* 30:221, 1963.

150. Thonnard-Neumann, E. Studies of basophils: basophilic leukocytes and gonadal activity in the rabbit, *Acta Haematol.* 32:358, 1964.

151. Tigelaar, R. E., Vaz, N. M., and Ovary, Z. Immunoglobulin receptors on mouse mast cells, *J. Immunol.* 106:661, 1971.

152. Tokué, K. The blood mast cell and its oxidase and peroxidase reaction, *J. Exp. Med.* 12:459, 1929.

153. Turk, J. L. Delayed Hypersensitivity, John Wiley and Sons, New York, 1967.

154. Undritz, E. Sandoz Atlas of Hematology, Sandoz, Basel, 1952.

155. Undritz, E. Die Alius-Grignaschi-Anomalie: der erblichkonstitutionelle Peroxydasedefekt der Neutrophilen und Monozyten, *Blut* 14:129, 1966.

156. Uvnäs, B. Mechanism of histamine release in mast cells, *Ann. N.Y. Acad. Sci.* 103:278, 1963.

157. Uvnäs, B. Release processes in mast cells and their activation by injury, *Ann. N.Y. Acad. Sci.* 116:880, 1964.

158. Valentine, W. N., Lawrence, J. S., Pearce, M. L., and Beck, W. S. The relationship of the basophil to blood histamine in man, *Blood* 10:154, 1955.

159. von Recklinghausen, F. Ueber Eiter- und Bindegewebskörperchen, *Virchows Arch. (Pathol. Anat.)* 28:157, 1863.

160. Watanabe, I., Donahue, S., and Hoggatt, N. Method for electron microscopic studies of circulating human leukocytes and observations on their fine structure, *J. Ultrastruct. Res.* 20:366, 1967.

161. West, G. B., and Parratt, J. R. Hydroxytryptamine and the skin, *Arch. Dermatol.* 76:336, 1957.

162. Wetzel, B. K. The fine structure and cytochemistry of developing granulocytes, with special reference to the rabbit, *in* A. S. Gordon (ed.), Regulation of Hematopoiesis, p. 769, Appleton-Century-Crofts, New York, 1970.

163. Wetzel, B. K., Horn, R. G., and Spicer, S. S. Fine structural studies on the development of heterophil, eosinophil, and basophil granulocytes in rabbits, *Lab. Invest.* 16:349, 1967.

164. Wetzel, B. K., Spicer, S. S., and Horn, R. G. Fine structural localization of acid and alkaline phos-

phatases in cells of rabbit blood and bone marrow, *J. Histochem. Cytochem.* 15:311, 1967.

165. Winqvist, G. Experimental production of basophil granulocytes in the guinea pig, *Exp. Cell Res.* 19:7, 1960.

166. Winqvist, G. The ultrastructure of the granules of the basophil granulocyte, *Z. Zellforsch.* 52:475, 1960.

167. Winqvist, G. Electron microscopy of the basophilic granulocyte, *Ann.* *N.Y. Acad. Sci.* 103:352, 1963.

168. Winqvist, G. The formation of specific granules in myelocytes, Proc. 9th Congr. Eur. Soc. Haematol., Lisbon, Part II/IC, p. 129, 1963.

169. Wislocki, G. B., Rheingold, J. J., and Dempsey, E. W. The occurrence of the periodic acid-Schiff reaction in various normal cells of blood and connective tissue, *Blood* 4:562, 1949.

170. Yamada, E., and Yamauchi, R. Some observations on the cyto-

chemistry and morphogenesis of the granulocytes in the rat bone marrow as revealed by electron microscopy, *Acta Haematol. Jap.* 29:530, 1966.

171. Zucker-Franklin, D. Electron microscopic study of human basophils, *Blood* 29:878, 1967.

172. Zucker-Franklin, D. Electron microscopic studies of human granulocytes: structural variations related to function, *Semin. Hematol.* 5:109, 1968.

B The Abnormal Granulocyte

Chapter 8 Abnormalities of Neutrophil Function

The mature cells of the neutrophilic granulocyte series must perform three integrated functions in their role as a defensive unit against microbial invaders: directed movement toward the invading particle, phagocytosis, and killing of the microorganism. The first two functions require extracellular "humoral" factors, including immunoglobulin opsonin and complement components found in the blood plasma (see Chapter 4). The killing function at present is known to require only the leukocyte, not external factors.

A breakdown in any one of the three integrated functions clearly would result in impaired host defenses and enhanced susceptibility to infection. Such a breakdown might arise from either an extrinsic humoral abnormality or an intrinsic leukocyte defect. There is an obvious analogy between extrinsic and intrinsic leukocyte defects and extracorpuscular and intracorpuscular red cell abnormalities.

Extrinsic Defects: Abnormalities in the Environment of the Neutrophil

The movement of neutrophils toward a bacterium or other particle is dependent upon release of chemotactically active substances from that particle. At least four chemotactically active factors have been identified: (a) the activated trimolecular complex of the fifth (C5), sixth (C6), and seventh (C7) components of complement (174); (b) a heat-labile, dialyzable substance formed by the action of plasmin on C3 (171), with a molecular weight of about 6,000; (c) cleavage products formed by the action of tissue protease on C3 (69); and (d) products released into the culture medium by a variety of bacterial species (177).

The chemotactic response of rabbit neutrophils appears to require cellular esterase (173). In addition, directed movement by the neutrophil requires an appropriate osmotic environment (28), an intact energy metabolism, and probably an intact and functional microtubular cellular skeleton (109, 111) (see Chapter 4). Once the particle is encountered by the phagocytic leukocyte, its subsequent ingestion often requires that the particle's surface be coated with opsonins, which may include immunoglobulin, complement components, noncomplement thermolabile substances, and basic peptides (71, 128, 146, 169). The coating probably provides for intimate contact between the leukocyte and the particle. In the case of immunoglobulin and complement opsonins, this may occur by means of receptors on the cell surface that specifically recognize these substances (Fig. 8.1). Once the intimate contact is established, and provided the neutrophil has an intact glycolytic energy metabolism, the particle may then be engulfed.

Glycolysis, and not respiration, clearly provides the energy necessary for the phagocytic activity of neutrophils (34, 81), as well as eosinophils (37) and monocytes (38). Particle ingestion by these cells proceeds in the absence of oxygen and in the presence of inhibitors of oxidative phosphorylation. The carbohydrate source for glycolytic energy is either exogenous glucose or other simple sugars, or the endogenous glycogen stores of the neutrophil (33, 81).

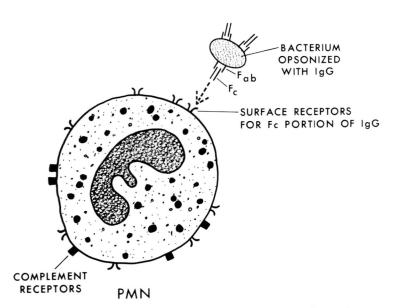

Figure 8.1 Schematic representation of receptors on the surface of a neutrophil (PMN) that interact with complement components and with the Fc portion of IgG molecules.

An additional requirement for phagocytosis is a hospitable osmotic and cationic environment.

The foregoing indicates that the functional defects of neutrophilic leukocytes arising from extrinsic causes will be manifest as abnormalities of migration (chemotaxis), or of phagocytosis. Causes of such defects may include abnormalities of the immunoglobulin or complement system, drugs or toxins interacting with the leukocyte surface, energy metabolism, or locomotive mechanism (Table 8.1).

Opsonin Deficiencies

The opsonizing activity of specific antibodies arising from previous infection or vaccination is critical in promoting leukocyte phagocytosis. The Fab portion of the IgG antibody molecule is necessary for its interaction with antigenic sites on the surface of the bacterium. For opsonic activity, an intact Fc portion of the molecule is necessary as well (144) (see Chapters 4 and 16). The Fc portion of the molecule interacts with receptors on the surface of the phagocytic leukocyte (102). This phenomenon is illustrated in Fig. 8.1.

A variety of disorders is associated with impaired immunoglobulin and specific antibody synthesis and consequently with abnormal opsonic activity in serum. These disorders include acquired abnormalities as well as congenital and usually genetic deficiencies of the immunoglobulin-producing system (see Chapter 18). An example of the congenital anomalies is the Bruton type of

agammaglobulinemia (27, 152, 158). The acquired abnormalities of immunoglobulin production are often associated with malignant disorders of the lymphoreticular system, such as chronic lymphocytic leukemia and multiple myeloma (42, 56) (see Chapters 19 and 20).

Repeated infection suffered by patients with agammaglobulinemia, and by some patients with chronic lymphocytic leukemia, may result primarily from deficiency of heat-stable immunoglobulin opsonins and the consequent failure of the leukocyte defense mechanism. The neutrophils themselves appear normal in their ability to kill. When measured in normal serum, neutrophil function in hypogammaglobulinemia is normal (119). Only when suspended in the patient's serum do the neutrophils show impaired phagocytosis. In some patients with these disorders, the propensity to infection may be partially corrected by replacement therapy with gammaglobulin.

The sera of patients with sickle cell anemia have reduced amounts of heat-labile opsonins for type 25 pneumococci (188). Such patients may fail to utilize fully the alternate pathway of complement activation (76). This abnormality, combined with the functional asplenia of sickle cell anemia patients (140), may underlie the enhanced susceptibility of these patients to pneumococcal sepsis and meningitis.

Low-birth-weight infants may have low serum opsonic activity. Leukocyte function is normal when cells of such infants are tested in adult serum (58), but abnormal when tested in their own serum. Patients with osteomyelitis

Table 8.1 Extrinsic defects in neutrophil function arising from an abnormal environment.

Opsonin deficiencies
    Congenital and acquired agammaglobulinemia
    Multiple myeloma
    Chronic lymphocytic leukemia
    (?) Sickle cell disease
    Immunologic suppression
    Low-birth-weight infants
Abnormalities of the complement system
    C'3 deficiency
    C'5 deficiency
Drugs and toxins
    Adrenocorticosteroids
    Ethanol
    Cytotoxic drugs
    S. aureus protein A
    Staphylococcal alpha toxin
Hyperosmolarity
    In the renal medulla
    Diabetic ketoacidosis

and established infection also may have low levels of heat-stable IgG opsonic activity (183).

Abnormalities of the Complement System

The studies of Wright and Douglas in 1904 pointed out that phagocytosis of certain microbial organisms is promoted by heat-labile serum factors (189). Hirsch and Strauss (71) observed that certain heat-labile opsonins were distinct from immunoglobulin antibodies and from the heat-labile complement sequence necessary for immune hemolysis. More recent investigations implicate the third and fifth components of complement in the phagocytosis of pneumococci (159, 162). As seen in Fig. 8.1, these complement components may interact with binding sites for complement on the surface of the phagocytic leukocytes (93).

Complement components are also necessary for chemotaxis. For example, a trimolecular complex of C5, C6, and C7 is generated by the addition of antigen-antibody precipitate to serum (174). This complex is chemotactic for neutrophils. Other chemotactic factors of low molecular weight are generated by the cleavage of C'3 by plasma (171) and C5 by trypsin (176).

Complement deficiencies in man may be manifest by abnormal leukocyte chemotactic response and impaired phagocytosis, with a consequent enhanced susceptibility to infection. Alper and his co-workers (4) recently described a young adult with Klinefelter's syndrome and a lifelong history of recurrent bacterial infections. The C3 (beta-1-C globulin) in his serum was reduced in amount and was inactive. The serum failed both to support normal levels of phagocytosis of pneumococci and to generate chemotactic factors normally. Normal serum, but not C3, corrected these deficiencies. The conclusion was that the patient probably lacked a serum factor, as yet uncharacterized, required for normal function and stability of C3.

Miller and co-workers (123, 124) described an infant with a history of eczemoid dermatitis and recurrent systemic infection. The sera of the patient, her mother, and various relatives were deficient in opsonization and in chemotactic activities. The deficiencies were corrected by normal serum or purified C5. Although this patient's susceptibility to infection has been ascribed to a deficiency of C5, some relatives with a similar deficiency gave no history of repeated infections.

Ward and Schlegel (177) described a four-year-old child with recurrent respiratory and cutaneous infections who had a serum factor that inhibited neutrophil chemotactic response.

In diseases with frequently encountered low levels of serum complement activity (for example, systemic lupus erythematosus) it is not known whether abnormal levels of serum-opsonizing and chemotactic activity are also demonstrable. This should be a fruitful field of inquiry. For example, patients with cirrhosis of the liver may have reduced levels of serum complement components and a circulating inhibitor of leukocyte chemotaxis (46).

Drugs, Toxins, and Abnormal Osmolarity

The methods of assessing leukocyte migration, inflammation, and chemotactic response in vivo are still exceedingly crude. A number of studies have utilized either migration into a skin window, made by placing a sterile glass cover slip over a superficially abraded area of skin (147) or migration into a superficial blister. Using these relatively unsophisticated techniques, investigators have reported that adrenocorticosteroids (23, 142), ethanol (25), and diabetic ketoacidosis (25, 141) interfere with neutrophil response. Hydrocortisone and cortisone are reported to block chemotactic response to trimolecular complement components (170) and also to inhibit bactericidal activity and postphagocytic oxidative activity in neutrophils (114).

Antimetabolites used in cancer chemotherapy are also said to inhibit local inflammatory responses in man (66). Alcohol inhibits leukocyte mobilization, but not phagocytic or killing activity (25). The laboratory tool cytochalasin B reversibly inhibits phagocytosis and associated metabolic changes (112) and alters certain membrane transport systems (194). Concanavalin A is another such inhibitory agent (20). Levorphanol (a morphine-like drug) may inhibit phagocytosis and some of the associated metabolic phenomena (190). If the effect of these agents or diseases is functionally significant, they then provide pathogenic bacteria with an advantage for initiating and spreading a nidus of inflammation.

Production of substances that interfere with chemotaxis or phagocytosis may be another mechanism by which certain microorganisms protect themselves and become virulent. For example, in the absence of specific opsonins, the large polysaccharide coat of pneumococci or *Cryptococcus neoformans* inhibits phagocytosis of the organism (160). Protein A of *Staphylococcus aureus* can interfere with the Fc component of the IgG immunoglobulin molecule and thereby inhibit its opsonic activity (48). Staphylococcal alpha toxin apparently causes neutrophil degranulation (108), and other staphylococcal toxins as well as streptococcal M protein may be injurious to granulocytes (15, 60).

High osmolarity impairs neutrophil phagocytosis. This may account for the impaired phagocytic activity observed in diabetic ketoacidosis (25, 141), and it almost certainly accounts for the abnormal leukocyte accumulation and phagocytosis within the renal medulla that occurs in certain disease states such as diabetes mellitus (29, 91). It may also explain why pyelonephritis is so frequently refractory to all therapy (32). Patients with chronic renal failure who are maintained on chronic hemodialysis exhibit normal neutrophil phagocytic and bactericidal activity (64).

Intrinsic Neutrophil Defects

As is outlined in detail in Chapter 4, the known microbicidal mechanisms used by mammalian neutrophils include (a) aerobic hydrogen peroxide generation and superoxide (126, 139); (b) interaction of hydrogen peroxide and the enzyme myeloperoxidase; and (c) in some species, a series of antimicrobial cationic proteins (70, 161, 165, 191–193). The known intrinsic neutrophil defects are shown in Table 8.2.

Defects of Hydrogen Peroxide Generation

Chronic Granulomatous Disease of Childhood First described in 1957 by Landing and Shirkey (92) and by Berendes, Bridges, and Good (19), chronic granulomatous disease (CGD) is a rare familial disorder whose major manifestations are susceptibility to severe infection and infiltration of the tissues by lipid pigmented histiocytes (50, 87, 122). The infections are often caused by microorganisms of limited virulence (26, 30). The original cases were all male children, and the inheritance pattern X-linked (186). Later, however, a variant disease that involved females and had a different pattern of hereditary transmission was also described (6, 11, 143).

Onset of disease usually occurs during infancy and almost always within the first two years of life, although one teen-age case has been reported (113, 115). Infectious complications include pneumonia, meningitis, suppurative adenitis, conjunctivitis, rhinitis, sinusitis, skin infections, and septicemia (30, 78). The range of organisms in-

Table 8.2 Intrinsic neutrophil defects.

Defective hydrogen peroxide generation
   Chronic granulomatous disease
   Complete glucose-6-phosphate dehydrogenase deficiency
   (?) Pyruvate kinase deficiency
Other enzyme deficiencies
   Myeloperoxidase deficiency
Unknown mechanisms
   Acute leukemia
   Overwhelming infection

volved in these infections is great; in addition to the common *Staphylococci* and coliforms, infections with *Actinomycetes* and *Candida* have also been described. The mortality rate is high, even in the era of antibiotics, and 18 of 28 patients described by Johnston and McMurry (78) were dead before the age of seven years.

In 1967 Holmes, Quie, and their collaborators provided a basis for understanding the pathogenesis of this disease (73, 145). They demonstrated that leukocytes from infected patients phagocytized bacteria normally, but failed to kill the ingested organisms (Fig. 8.2). They also demonstrated that these leukocytes have a remarkable metabolic defect: they fail to develop the respiratory burst and increment in glucose-1-^{14}C oxidation and in hydrogen peroxide generation that normally accompany particle ingestion (10, 12, 73) (Fig. 8.3). More recently a defect in the generation of superoxide radicals has been added to the list of abnormalities of oxidative metabolism (43). This metabolic failure occurs despite normal postphagocytic degranulation (55, 82). In the typical X-linked form of this disease, the clinically asymptomatic mothers have an intermediate defect in neutrophil function (186) and two populations of peripheral leukocytes—one normal and one defective (88, 185).

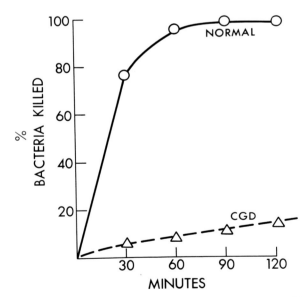

Figure 8.2 Effect of incubating *Staphylococcus aureus* 502A with peripheral blood leukocytes from normal subjects and from a patient with chronic granulomatous disease (CGD). The percentage of bacteria phagocytized and killed with time is shown. By 60 minutes, more than 90 percent of the added bacteria had been killed by normal leukocytes. Leukocytes from the patient with CGD were deficient in their ability to kill the ingested microorganisms.

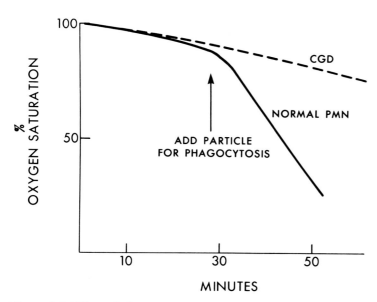

Figure 8.3 Effect of phagocytosis on oxygen consumption by normal neutrophils (PMNs) and by neutrophils from a patient with chronic granulomatous disease (CGD). Oxygen saturation in a suspension of leukocytes is measured. After addition of a particle for phagocytosis, the oxygen saturation of the solution containing normal neutrophils fell abruptly as these cells utilized oxygen. No such increased oxygen utilization was apparent with phagocytosis by the CGD cells.

Evidence indicates that defective hydrogen peroxide generation and reduced bacterial killing are linked in chronic granulomatous disease. Provision of an exogenous source of hydrogen peroxide corrects the bactericidal abnormality of the neutrophil (77). Furthermore, hydrogen-peroxide–producing bacteria, such as *Streptococci*, *Pneumococci*, and *Lactobacilli*, are killed almost normally by CGD leukokytes (80, 88, 113). These observations provide the strongest lines of evidence that the principle neutrophil killing mechanism involves hydrogen peroxide generation and perhaps superoxide. In addition to the bactericidal impairment, CGD neutrophils have decreased virucidal (107) and fungicidal activity (83, 95, 97).

To establish the diagnosis of chronic granulomatous disease requires two types of data: evidence for a leukocyte killing defect, and evidence for an abnormal neutrophil oxidative response to particle phagocytosis.

Evidence for a bactericidal defect generally has been obtained by demonstrating an abnormal fall in viable colony count following phagocytosis (71, 106) (Fig. 8.2). More recently, simpler tests such as dye exclusion by viable *Candida* (95, 97) (Fig. 8.4) or inhibition of tritiated thymidine incorporation by replicating bacteria (35) have also

been used. Defects in monocyte killing capacity have been described as well in chronic granulomatous disease (45, 95, 150).

The most direct way of demonstrating an abnormality of oxidative metabolism in chronic granulomatous disease cells is to measure oxygen consumption before and after particle ingestion (Fig. 8.3) with either an oxygen electrode or a Warburg apparatus. The extent of conversion of glucose-1-C^{14} to $C^{14}O_2$ and of formate -C^{14} to $C^{14}O_2$ may also be used. The iodination of phagocytized bacteria may be used also as a measure of the ability of phagocytic neutrophils to produce H_2O_2 (88). These are relatively complex tests. Consequently, many investigators have used a simple dye test. Nitroblue tetrazolium is reduced to an insoluble blue product that accumulates in normal leukocytes after phagocytosis. Although CGD leukocytes ingest normally, they fail to reduce nitroblue tetrazolium (NBT) and little blue color is formed (Fig. 8.5). Microscopy allows for qualitative expression of the results (120, 127, 136), and spectrophotometry produces quantitative results when NBT is extracted chemically (11).

The mechanism of the abnormality, or abnormalities, of postphagocytic oxygen metabolism in chronic granulo-

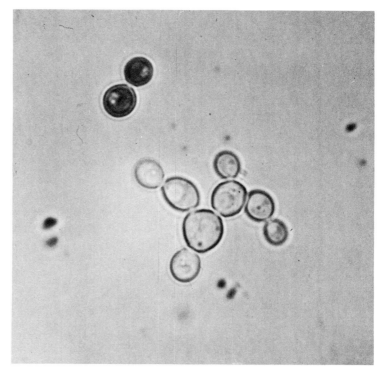

Figure 8.4 Viable fungi (*Candida albicans*) distinguished from dead fungi by their ability to exclude the dye methylene blue. This simple test of viability can be used to measure the capacity of leukocytes to kill this microorganism.

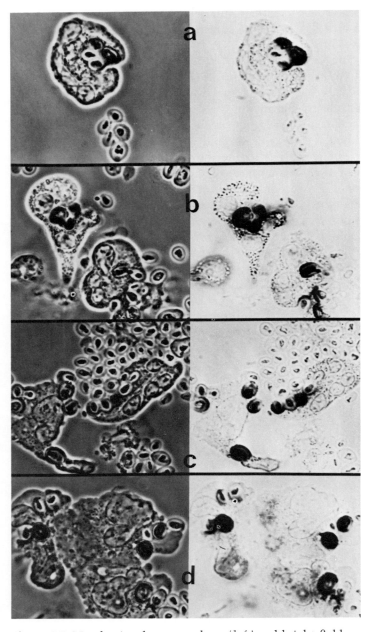

Figure 8.5 Nearly simultaneous phase (*left*) and bright field (*right*) photomicrographs of a normal neutrophil (*a*), eosinophil and neutrophil (*b*), neutrophil and monocyte (*c*), and neutrophil and two monocytes (*d*) 20 minutes after incubation with zymosan and nitroblue tetrazolium (NBT) on a glass slide under a cover slip. Dye reduction is observed only on and around phagocytized zymosan; extracellular zymosan is not stained. (From D. G. Nathan, R. L. Baehner, and D. K. Weaver, *J. Clin. Invest.* 48:1895, 1969. Reprinted by permission of authors and publisher.)

matous disease is not known for certain. It has been suggested (9) and denied (73) that leukocytes of this disease have abnormally low levels of NADH oxidase. Baehner and Karnovsky (9) postulated that a very early postphagocytic step involves activation of NADH oxidase, and they suggested that the increase in hexose monophosphate shunt activity is a secondary phenomenon. Strauss and his co-workers (166) proposed that the initial postphagocytic events center around the activation of glutathione reductase with hexose monophosphate shunt stimulation as a primary event. Whether or not this is the case, it appears that one could restore oxygen consumption, hexose monophosphate shunt activity, and hydrogen peroxide generation to near-normal levels in CGD leukocytes by providing them with an electron acceptor such as phenazine or methylene blue (73). The most recent, and I believe the best, evidence favors an abnormality of NADPH oxidase as the defect in the typical form of chronic granulomatous disease (72). The pathways of glucose oxygen utilization and hydrogen peroxide generation were illustrated in Fig. 4.11.

Chronic granulomatous disease is probably a disease syndrome resulting from the common manifestation of abnormal leukocyte oxidative metabolism, which in turn may result from any of several enzymic defects within the cell. This theory is suggested by the increasing heterogeneity of the patient population described as having defects. For example, leukocyte defects resembling those of chronic granulomatous disease have been reported in association with other abnormalities, including impaired leukotaxis (177) and selective immunoglobulin deficiency (52). Male patients whose mothers have no detectable leukocyte defects may have a non-X-linked disease (89, 115). Similarly, intraleukocytic defects in females must reflect a mode of inheritance other than X-linked (6, 7, 143). "Job's syndrome" may be a clinical variant of chronic granulomatous disease manifested by recurrent cold staphylococcal abscesses that occur from birth in red-haired, fair-skinned girls (14, 44). In one female patient with a variant syndrome, leukocyte glutathione peroxidase deficiency was observed (74). In some patients there may be an anomalous, unstable leukocyte glucose-6-phosphate dehydrogenase (17), although this observation is open to question (148). Further investigation should enable us to classify these varying clinical syndromes (57, 87, 149) more precisely in terms of their specific subcellular defects.

Other Defects in Hydrogen Peroxide Generation Recently some preliminary reports describing neutrophil killing defects in association with other abnormalities of

Table 8.3 Comparison of normal, CGD, and G6PD-deficient neutrophils during phagocytosis.

Type of neutrophil	Change in nitroblue tetrazolium (NBT)	Glucose-1-^{14}C → ^{14}CO$_2$ with phagocytosis	H$_2$O$_2$ production	Correction of oxidative abnormalities by methylene blue
Normal	Yes	↑	↑	—
CGD	No	No	No	Yes
G6PD	No	No	No	No

oxygen metabolism have appeared. In one of the variants of the red blood cell glucose-6-phosphate dehydrogenase deficiency that affects Caucasians, the levels of this enzyme activity are also low in leukocytes. In such affected individuals, enzyme activity in the white cells is generally reduced to about 20 percent of normal—an insufficient decrease for production of any significant abnormality of carbohydrate metabolism. Occasionally, however, enzyme activity is undetectable in leukocytes. A female patient with such an abnormality suffered from hemolytic anemia and recurrent infections. A six-year-old boy with a similar abnormality but compensated hemolysis also had impaired defenses (8). Their neutrophils did not kill several species of bacteria normally. Because they lacked the first enzyme of the pathway, no detectable hexose monophosphate shunt activity occurred in either resting or phagocytic leukocytes; methylene blue did not stimulate the oxidative pathway. These observations suggest than an intact, direct glucose oxidative pathway is necessary for bacterial killing. A comparison of metabolic alterations in G6PD-deficient and chronic granulomatous disease neutrophils is given in Table 8.3.

Deficient Myeloperoxidase

How are the postphagocytic oxygen bursts, hexose monophosphate shunt activity, and hydrogen peroxide generation of the normal neutrophil linked to bacterial killing? One suggestion is that the neutrophil granule enzyme myeloperoxidase, in the presence of hydrogen peroxide, oxidizes intracellular halide and produces a substance lethal for ingested bacteria (84, 85). This may be accomplished by iodination of the microbial cell wall, (84), by the production of aldehydes from the decarboxylation of amino acids (167), or perhaps by other mechanisms. The iodination reaction may not be the critical factor in bacterial killing. For example, blocking of the iodination reaction with 0.01 M ascorbic acid does not block the killing of bacteria. Notwithstanding the uncertainty of the iodination mechanism, *the available evidence favors a critical*

role for hydrogen peroxide and myeloperoxidase in the neutrophil microbicidal system (118).

Myeloperoxidase constitutes between 3 and 5 percent of the dry weight of the neutrophil and a lesser fraction in the monocyte (33). It catalyzes the reaction AH$_2$ + H$_2$O$_2$ → A + 2H$_2$O, where AH$_2$ is any of a variety of electron donors. The characteristics of the enzyme have been summarized in Chapter 3.

The thesis that myeloperoxidase is critical to the neutrophil's killing of ingested microorganisms was closely examined in a patient with a hereditary deficiency of this enzyme (86, 98, 101). The patient had been in generally good health until the age of forty-nine, when he developed systemic infection with *Candida albicans*. His neutrophils could phagocytize the yeasts normally but failed to kill them (Fig. 8.6). Ultimately the inability to kill was traced to a specific lack of the neutrophil and monocyte enzyme myeloperoxidase (98, 155). This deficiency was simple to demonstrate histochemically (Fig. 8.7) as well as biochemically (Fig. 8.8). Neutrophils from the patient had a slower than normal rate of killing *Staphylococcus aureus* and *Serratia marcescens*, but ultimately killed almost all ingested bacteria (Fig. 8.9). The patient's sister had no detectable leukocyte myeloperoxidase (not shown in figure); his four sons had between 25 and 50 percent of the normal level (Fig. 8.8). None of these subjects has suffered from recurrent infection.

Thus far, five patients with hereditary myeloperoxidase deficiency have been reported, including two pairs of sib-

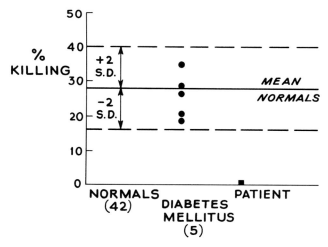

Figure 8.6 The killing of phagocytized *Candida* by polymorphonuclear leukocytes from 42 normal subjects, from 5 patients with diabetes mellitus, and from a patient with genetic deficiency of neutrophil peroxidase. The killing assay was that of Fig. 8.4 and reference 97.

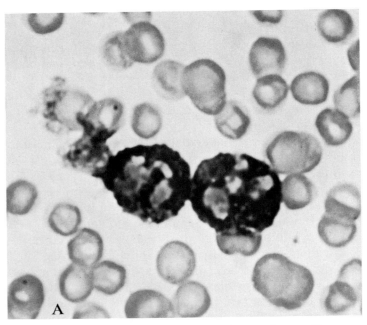

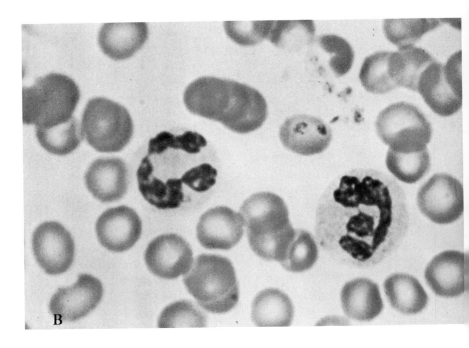

Figure 8.7 Human neutrophils stained for myeloperoxidase. The neutrophils in Fig. 8.7A are normal; those in Fig. 8.7B are from a patient with a genetic absence of myeloperoxidase.

lings (63, 98, 168). Except for the patient with *C. albicans* infection, the defect has been an incidental finding and none of the subjects has a history of recurrent infection.

In addition to the hereditary form of myeloperoxidase deficiency, a presumably acquired form of the disorder in association with other hematologic abnormalities has been reported. In this acquired form, normal and myelo-

peroxidase-deficient granulocytes coexist in the bone marrow and circulate in the blood (5, 68, 100).

From these observations it appears that myeloperoxidase plays a critical role in the killing of certain fungi, but is of secondary importance in the killing of most bacteria (94). The lack of serious recurrent bacterial infection in myeloperoxidase-deficient subjects supports this thesis.

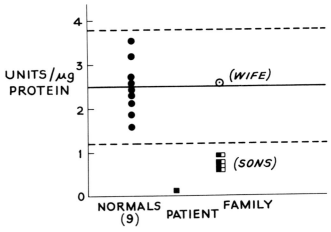

Figure 8.8 Level of myeloperoxidase activity of white cell homogenates from nine normal subjects, a patient with a genetic deficiency of myeloperoxidase, his wife, and his four sons.

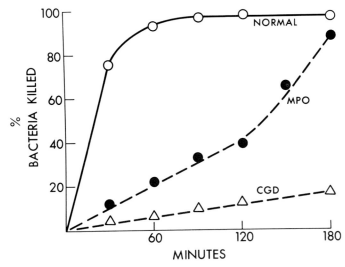

Figure 8.9 The killing of *Staphylococcus aureus* 502A by normal leukocytes, leukocytes from a patient with genetic absence of myeloperoxidase (MPO), and from a patient with chronic granulomatous disease (CGD). The relatively greater defect in killing ability of CGD neutrophils is shown.

Table 8.4 Comparison of two intrinsic neutrophil defects.

Feature	Chronic granulomatous disease	Myeloperoxidase deficiency
Age of onset of symptoms	Infancy or early childhood	Never or adult life
Manifestations	Recurrent severe bacterial and fungal infections	None or susceptibility to opportunistic fungi
Cellular defect	H_2O_2 generation	Absent myeloperoxidase
Inheritance	X-linked, sporadic male and female	Autosomal recessive
Diagnosis	Nitroblue tetrazolium test; impaired phagocytic oxygen burst; microbial killing	Peroxidase stain

The contrast between the clinical course of myeloperoxidase deficiency and chronic granulomatous disease is striking. The differences in neutrophil-associated defects between these two disorders are summarized in Table 8.4.

Other Defects of Unknown Mechanism

A wide variety of patients have impaired antimicrobial defenses and suffer from repeated infections. Such patients often have organisms that are nonvirulent for normal man. These infections are spoken of as *opportunistic infections*. They occur when host defenses are obviously impaired—for example, with agranulocytosis from hematologic disease or cancer chemotherapy; with immunologic suppression in a renal transplant recipient; and with the previously described hereditary abnormalities of the immunoglobulin or complement system. In addition, a number of disorders exist in which a leukocyte defect is certain or probable, but in which the mechanism of that defect is not known.

Chediak-Higashi Syndrome The Chediak-Higashi syndrome (CHS) is a rare familial disorder characterized by partial oculocutaneous albinism, photophobia, nystagmus, abnormal granulations in neutrophils and other cells, and enhanced susceptibility to both bacterial and viral infection (16, 31, 47, 59, 67, 156, 164, 178). Affected children surviving the repeated infections often develop lymphoid malignancy (54, 134, 135). Granulocytopenia is frequent in advanced disease states (22). The pattern of inheritance is autosomal recessive.

The circulating neutrophilic granulocytes and mono-cytes of affected patients contain giant granules (see figures in Chapter 9). Similar giant lysosomal structures are found in a variety of somatic cells (51–53, 90, 103, 180, 182, 187). Long-term "lymphoblastoid" cell lines have been established in patients with CHS (20). These show the characteristic granule abnormality (22). Rarely, virus-like particles have been observed in the leukocytes (181).

Inclusions similar to those of CHS patients have been found in the cells of the Aleutian mink (CHS mink) (105), a strain of partial albino Hereford cattle (CHS cattle) (132), and a strain of beige mice (CHS mice) (104, 129). Like the human patients, the cattle and mink suffer from repeated severe infections; the beige mice do not (18, 132, 133). CHS mink are more susceptible to infections from a variety of microbial species: *S. aureus* (65), *Pasteurella multocida*, cornebacterium species (131), and Aleutian disease virus (61). Postmortem examination of CHS cattle often reveals disseminated bacterial abscesses (131).

Interestingly, no significant variation from normal has been observed in the amount of bactericidal cationic proteins or the activities of acid phosphatase, cathepsin, or glucuronidase in leukocytes from CHS cattle and mink (131, 132). The white cells from patients with this disorder may have moderate increases in alkaline phosphatase, PAS-reactive material, and sphingolipid turnover (79, 154). The giant granules of the neutrophils of CHS patients and mink are more stable than are normal granules during phagocytosis (131, 151). One may be tempted to equate the clinically apparent increased susceptibility to infection with the obvious morphologic abnormalities of the neutrophilic leukocytes. However, most studies have failed to demonstrate obvious impairment of CHS leukocyte bactericidal activity (132, 184), and immunologic parameters are generally within normal limits (134). The precise aberration in host defense mechanism has not been defined. Some evidence suggests ineffective granulopoiesis in this syndrome (79).

Acute Leukemia Recently developed techniques for evaluating the microbicidal function of individual leukocytes in a mixed population (35, 95, 97) were illustrated in Fig. 4.14. Use of these techniques has led to the observation that the morphologically mature neutrophils of some patients with acute myelocytic leukemia have impaired ability to kill certain species of fungi and bacteria (35, 99, 157) (see Fig. 4.15). This impairment does not seem to be the result of chemotherapy exclusively and may be an intrinsic feature of the disease state. The mechanism of the deficiency is not known, although evidence suggests that it is associated with low levels of lysosomal enzyme activity (99). The defect is particularly striking in some mononuclear phagocytes of patients with acute myelo-monocytic leukemia. These cells possibly phagocytize bacteria normally, but fail to kill them. The intracellular bacteria may be sequestered and protected from the bactericidal action of administered antibiotics. This observation could, in part, explain the resistance of bacterial infection to antibiotics in such patients. Children with acute lymphoblastic leukemia undergoing craniospinal irradiation may also have defective phagocytic leukocytes (13).

Newborn Infants Neonates and, particularly, premature infants may have an increased susceptibility to infection. Reports of leukocyte phagocytic and microbicidal abnormalities in this age group are conflicting (39, 41, 49, 121, 137). Spontaneous nitroblue tetrazolium reduction by leukocytes from both premature and full-term neonates is high (40, 137, 138).

Severe Burns Leukocytes from patients with serious thermal burns may be defective in microbicidal capacity (2, 3) and deficient in certain granular enzymes (1).

Severe Infection Leukocytes from some patients with severe infection may have a diminished microbicidal capacity (2, 36, 163). The reasons for this defect are not clear. It has been suggested that as a result of increased demands for marrow granulocyte production, granule and granule enzyme formation may be impaired (62).

In bacterial infection there may be an increased spontaneous reduction of NBT (75, 116, 136). Chemotaxis may be impaired in severe infection, perhaps as a result of prior ingestion of antigen-antibody complexes (125).

Drugs and Toxins A variety of drugs may deleteriously influence neutrophil microbicidal activity in vitro and perhaps in vivo (36, 87). These include salicylates (130), corticosteroids (114, 120), colchicine (110, 111), methimazole (88), polyene antifungal antibiotics (179), pharmacologic agents that increase neutrophil cyclic adenosine monophosphate (24, 117) and certain sulfonamides (96). Of these the sulfonamide effects have been best studied; the drugs appear to interfere with the MPO-H_2O_2 system.

Summary

The neutrophilic leukocyte is highly specialized to carry out its primary function—the localization and killing of microorganisms. To perform this role, it must coordinate directed locomotion, phagocytosis, and mobilization of intracellular microbicidal systems. These systems are interlocking and complex. For locomotion and phagocytosis the leukocyte depends upon glycolytic energy and hospitable environment. For killing it utilizes both oxygen-dependent and oxygen-independent systems. Abnormalities in these systems may be induced by drugs, acquired in hematologic diseases, or inherited. At present, the best-understood abnormalities are those of the extracellular opsonin systems and of the intracellular oxygen-dependent microbicidal mechanism. With the rapid rate of research in this field, one may anticipate better understanding soon of other leukocyte defense systems.

Chapter 8 References

1. Alexander, J. W. Serum and leukocyte lysosomal enzymes, *Arch. Surg.* 95:482, 1967.
2. Alexander, J. W., Hegg, M., and Altemeier, W. A. Neutrophil function in selected surgical disorders, *Ann. Surg.* 168:447, 1968.
3. Alexander, J. W., and Wixson, D. Neutrophil dysfunction and sepsis in burn injury, *Surg. Gynecol. Obstet.* 130:431, 1970.
4. Alper, C. A., Abramson, N., Johnston, R. B., Jr., Jandl, J. H., and Rosen, F. S. Increased susceptibility to infection associated with abnormalities of complement-mediated functions and of the third component (C3), *N. Engl. J. Med.* 282:349, 1970.
5. Arakawa, T., Wada, Y., Hayashi, T., Kakizaki, R., Chida, N., Chiba, R., and Konno, T. Uracil-uric refractory anemia with peroxidase negative neutrophils, *Tohoku J. Exp. Med.* 87:52, 1965.
6. Azimi, P. H., Bodenbender, J. C., Hintz, R. L., and Kontras, S. B. Chronic granulomatous disease in three female siblings, *J.A.M.A.* 206:2865, 1968.
7. Azimi, P. H., Bodenbender, J. C., Hintz, R. L., and Kontras, S. B. Chronic granulomatous disease in three sisters *Lancet* 1:208, 1968.
8. Baehner, R. L., Johnston, R. B., Jr., and Nathan, D. G. Comparative study of the metabolic and bactericidal characteristics of severely glucose-6-phosphate dehydrogenase-deficient polymorphonuclear leukocytes and leukocytes from children with chronic granulomatous disease, *J. Reticuloendothel. Soc.* 12:150, 1972.
9. Baehner, R. L., and Karnovsky, M. L. Deficiency of reduced nicotinamide-adenine dinucleotide oxidase in chronic granulomatous disease, *Science* 162:1277, 1968.
10. Baehner, R. L., and Nathan, D. G. Leukocyte oxidase: defective activity in chronic granulomatous disease, *Science* 155:835, 1967.
11. Baehner, R. L., and Nathan, D. G. Quantitative nitroblue tetrazolium test in chronic granulomatous disease, *N. Engl. J. Med.* 278:971, 1968.
12. Baehner, R. L., Nathan, D. G., and

Karnovsky, M. L. Correction of metabolic deficiencies in the leukocytes of patients with chronic granulomatous disease, *J. Clin. Invest.* 49:865, 1970.
13. Baehner, R. L., Neiburger, R. G., Johnson, D. E., and Murrmann, S. M. Transient bactericidal defect of peripheral blood phagocytes from children with acute lymphoblastic leukemia receiving craniospinal irradiation, *N. Engl. J. Med.* 289:1209, 1973.
14. Bannatyne, R. M., Skowron, P. N., and Weber, J. L. Job's syndrome — a variant of chronic granulomatous disease, *J. Pediatr.* 75:236, 1969.
15. Beachy, E. H., and Stollerman, G. H. Toxic effects of streptococcal M protein on platelets and polymorphonuclear leukocytes in human blood, *J. Exp. Med.* 134:351, 1971.
16. Béguez-César, A. Neutropenia cronica maligna familiar con granulaciones atipicas de los leucocitos, *Bol. Soc. Cuba Pediatr.* 15:900, 1943.
17. Bellanti, J. A., Cantz, B. E., and Schlegel, R. J. Accelerated decay of glucose-6-phosphate dehydrogenase activity in chronic granulomatous disease, *Pediatr. Res.* 4:405, 1970.
18. Bennett, J. M., Blume, R. S., and Wolff, S. M. Characterization and significance of abnormal leukocyte granules in the beige mouse: a possible homologue for Chediak-Higashi Aleutian trait, *J. Lab. Clin. Med.* 73:235, 1969.
19. Berendes, H., Bridges, R. A., and Good, R. A. A fatal granulomatous disease of childhood. The clinical study of a new syndrome, *Minn. Med.* 40:309, 1957.
20. Berlin, R. D. Effect of concanavalin A on phagocytosis, *Nature (New Biol.)* 235:44, 1972.
21. Blume, R. S. The Chediak-Higashi syndrome: continuous suspension cultures derived from peripheral blood, *Blood* 33:821, 1969.
22. Blume, R. S., Bennett, J. M., Yankee, R. A., and Wolff, S. M. Defective granulocyte regulation in the Chediak-Higashi syndrome, *N. Engl. J. Med.* 279:1009, 1968.
23. Boggs, D. R., Athens, J. W., Cartwright, G. E., and Wintrobe, M. M. The effect of adrenal glucocorticosteroids upon the cellular composition of inflammatory ex-

udates, *Am. J. Pathol.* 44:763, 1964.
24. Bourne, H. R., Lehrer, R. I., Cline, M. J., and Melmon, K. L. Cyclic 3', 5'-adenosine monophosphate in the human leukocyte: synthesis, degradation, and effects on neutrophil candidacidal activity, *J. Clin. Invest.* 50:920, 1971.
25. Brayton, R. G., Stokes, P. E., Schwartz, M. S., and Louria, D. B. Effect of alcohol and various diseases on leukocyte mobilization, phagocytosis and intracellular bacterial killing, *N. Engl. J. Med.* 282:123, 1970.
26. Bridges, R. A., Berendes, H., and Good, R. A. A fatal granulomatous disease of childhood: the clinical, pathological, and laboratory features of a new syndrome, *Am. J. Dis. Child.* 97:387, 1959.
27. Bruton, O. C. Agammaglobulinemia, *Pediatrics* 9:722,1952.
28. Bryant, R. E., DesPrez, R. M., VanWay, M. H., and Rogers, D. E. Studies on human leukocyte motility. I. Effects of alterations in pH, electrolyte concentration, and phagocytosis on leukocyte migration, adhesiveness, and aggregation, *J. Exp. Med.* 124:483, 1966.
29. Bryant, R. E., Sutcliffe, M. C., and McGee, Z. A. Effect of osmolalities comparable to those of the renal medulla on function of human polymorphonuclear leukocytes, *J. Infect. Dis.* 126:1, 1972.
30. Carson, M. J., Chadwick, D. L., Brubaker, C. A., Cleland, R. S., and Landing, B. H. Thirteen boys with progressive septic granulomatosis, *Pediatrics* 35:405, 1965.
31. Chediak, M. Nouvelle anomalie leucocytaire de caractère constitutionnel et familial, *Rev. Hematol.* 7:362, 1952.
32. Chernew, I., and Braude, A. I. Depression of phagocytosis by solutes in concentrations found in the kidney and urine, *J. Clin. Invest.* 41:1945, 1962.
33. Cline, M. J. Metabolism of the circulating leukocyte, *Physiol. Rev.* 45:674, 1965.
34. Cline, M. J. Leukocyte metabolism, *in* A.S. Gordon (ed.), Regulation of Hematopoiesis, vol. 2, p. 1045, Appleton-Century-Crofts, New York, 1970.
35. Cline, M. J. A new white cell test

that measures individual phagocyte function in a mixed population. I. A neutrophil defect in acute myelocytic leukemia, *J. Lab. Clin. Med.* 81:311, 1973.

36. Cline, M. J. Influence of drugs and disease on phagocyte function, *in* W. Braun (ed.), "Nonspecific" Factors Influencing Host Resistance, p. 73, Paul Ehrlich Society, S. Karger, Basel, 1973.

37. Cline, M. J., and Lehrer, R. I. Phagocytosis by human moncytes, *Blood* 32:423, 1968.

38. Cline, M. J., Hanifin, J. M., and Lehrer, R. I. Phagocytosis by human eosinphils, *Blood,* 32:922, 1968.

39. Cocchi, P., and Marianelli, L. Phagocytosis and intracellular killing of pseudomonas aeruginosa in premature infants, *Helv. Paediatr. Acta* 22:110, 1967.

40. Cocchi, P., Mori, S., and Becattini, A. N.B.T. tests in premature infants, *Lancet* 2:1426, 1969.

41. Coen, R., Grush, O., and Kauder, E. Studies of bactericidal activity and metabolism of the leukocyte in full-term neonates, *J. Pediatr.* 75:400, 1969.

42. Cone, L., and Uhr, J. W. Immunological deficiency disorders associated with chronic lymphocytic leukemia and multiple myeloma, *J. Clin. Invest.* 43:2241, 1964.

43. Curnutte, J. T., Whitten, D. M., and Babior, B. M. Defective leukocyte superoxide production in chronic granulomatous disease, *N. Engl. J. Med.* 290:593, 1974.

44. Davis, S. D., Schaller, J., and Wedgwood, R. J. Job's syndrome: recurrent, "cold," staphylococcal abscesses, *Lancet* 1:1013, 1966.

45. Davis, W. C., Huber, H., Douglas, S. D., and Fudenberg, H. H. A defect in circulating mononuclear phagocytes in chronic granulomatous disease of childhood, *J. Immunol.* 101:1093, 1968.

46. DeMeo, A. N., and Andersen, B. R. Defective chemotaxis associated with a serum inhibitor in cirrhotic patients, *N. Engl. J. Med.* 286:735, 1972.

47. Dent, P. B., Fish, L. A., White, J. G., and Good, R. A. Chediak-Higashi syndrome: observations on the nature of the associated malig-

nancy, *Lab. Invest.* 15:1634, 1966.

48. Dossett, J. H., Kronvall, G., Williams, R. C., Jr., and Quie, P. G. Protein A: an antiphagocytic factor of staphylococcus aureus, *J. Clin. Invest.* 48:21a, 1969.

49. Dossett, J. H., Williams, R. C., Jr., and Quie, P. G. Studies on interaction of bacteria serum factors and polymorphonuclear leukocytes in mothers and newborns, *Pediatrics* 44:49, 1969.

50. Douglas, S. D. Analytic review: disorders of phagocytic function, *Blood* 35:851, 1970.

51. Douglas, S. D., Blume, R. S., and Wolff, S. M. Fine structural studies of leukocytes from patients and heterozygotes with Chediak-Higashi syndrome, *Blood* 33:527, 1969.

52. Douglas, S. D., Davis, W. C., and Fudenberg, H. H. Granulocytopathies: pleomorphism of neutrophil dysfunction, *Am. J. Med.* 46:901, 1969.

53. Efrati, P., and Danon, D. Electronmicroscopical study of bone marrow cells in a case of Chediak-Higashi-Steinbrinck syndrome, *Br. J. Haematol.* 15:173, 1968.

54. Efrati, P., and Jonas, W. Chediak's anomaly of leukocytes in malignant lymphoma associated with leukemic manifestations—case report with necropsy, *Blood* 13:1063, 1958.

55. Elsbach, P., Zucker-Franklin, D., and Sansaricq, C. Increased lecithin synthesis during phagocytosis by normal leukocytes and by leukocytes of a patient with chronic granulomatous disease, *N. Engl. J. Med.* 280:1319, 1969.

56. Fahey, J. L., Scoggins, R., Utz, J. P., and Szwed, C. F. Infection, antibody response and gamma globulin components in multiple myeloma and macroglobulinemia, *Am. J. Med.* 35:698, 1963.

57. Ford, D. K., Price, G. E., Culling, C. F. A., and Vassar, P. S. Familial lipochrome pigmentation of histiocytes with hyperglobulinemia, pulmonary infiltration, splenomegaly, arthritis and susceptibility to infection, *Am. J. Med.* 33:478, 1962.

58. Forman, M. L., and Stiehm, E. R.

Impaired opsonic activity but normal phagocytosis in low birth-weight infants, *N. Engl. J. Med.* 281:926, 1969.

59. Gilloon, J. R., Pease, G. L., and Mills, S. D. Chediak-Higashi anomaly of the leukocytes—report of a case, *Proc. Mayo Clin.* 35:635, 1960.

60. Gilson, V. M., and Donahue, J. A. Leukocytotoxic activity of toxin from the 80/81 strain of Staphylococcus aureus, *J. Bacteriol.* 95:2409, 1968.

61. Gorham, J. R., et al. Some observations on the natural occurrence of Aleutian disease, *in* Natl. Inst. Neurol. Dis. Blind Monogr. No. 2, Slow, latent and temperate virus infections, p. 279, U.S. Government Printing Office, Washington, D.C., 1965.

62. Graham, G. S. The neutrophilic granules of the circulating blood in health and in disease—a preliminary report, *N.Y. State J. Med.* 20:46, 1920.

63. Grignaschi, V. J., Sperperato, A. M., Etcheverry, M. J., and Macario, A. J. L. Un neuvo cuadro citoquimico: negatividad espontanea de las reaciones de peroxidasas, oxidasas y lipido en la progenie neutrofila y en los monocitos de dos hermanos, *Rev. Asoc. Med. Argent.* 77:218, 1963.

64. Guckian, J. C., Karrh, L. R., Copeland, J. L., et al. Phagocytosis by polymorphonuclear leukocytes in patients with renal failure on chronic hemodialysis, *Texas Rep. Biol. Med.* 29:193, 1971.

65. Helgebostad, A. The Aleutian disease, *Fur Trade J. Can.* 40:10, 1963.

66. Hersh, E. M., Wong, V. G., and Freireich, E. J. Inhibition of the local inflammatory response in man by antimetabolites, *Blood* 27:38, 1966.

67. Higashi, O. Congenital gigantism of peroxidase granules—first case ever reported of qualitative abnormality of peroxidase, *Tohoku J. Exp. Med.* 59:315, 1954.

68. Higashi, O., Katsuyama, N., and Satodate, R. A case with hematological abnormality characterized by the absence of peroxidase activity in blood polymorphonuclear

leukocytes, *Tohoku J. Exp. Med.* 87:77, 1965.

69. Hill, J. H., and Ward, P. A. C3 leukotactic factors produced by a tissue protease, *J. Exp. Med.* 130:505, 1969.

70. Hirsch, J. G. Further studies on preparation and properties of phagocytin, *J. Exp. Med.* 111:323, 1960.

71. Hirsch, J. G., and Strauss, B. Studies on heat-labile opsonin in rabbit serum, *J. Immunol.* 92:145, 1964.

72. Hohn, D. C., and Lehrer, R. I. Identification of the defect in X-linked chronic granulomatous disease, *Clin. Res.* 22:394A, 1974.

73. Holmes, B., Page, A. R., and Good, R. A. Studies of the metabolic activity of leukocytes from patients with a genetic abnormality of phagocytic function, *J. Clin. Invest.* 46:1422, 1967.

74. Holmes, B., Park, B. H., Malawista, S. E., Quie, P. G., Nelson, D. L., and Good, R. A. Chronic granulomatous disease in females: a deficiency of leukocyte glutathione peroxidase, *N. Engl. J. Med.* 283:217, 1970.

75. Humbert, J. R., Jr., Kurtz, M. L., and Hathaway, W. E. Increased reduction of nitroblue tetrazolium by neutrophils of newborn infants, *Pediatrics* 45:125, 1970.

76. Johnson, R. B., Jr., Newman, S. L., and Struth, A. G. An abnormality of the alternate pathway of complement activation in sickle-cell disease, *N. Engl. J. Med.* 288:803, 1973.

77. Johnston, R. B., Jr., and Baehner, R. L. Improvement of leukocyte bactericidal activity in chronic granulomatous disease, *Blood* 35:350, 1970.

78. Johnston, R. B., Jr., and McMurry, J. S. Chronic familial granulomatosis: report of five cases and review of the literature, *Am. J. Dis. Child.* 114:370, 1967.

79. Kanfer, J. N. Alteration of sphingolipid metabolism in leukocytes from patients with the Chediak-Higashi syndrome, *N. Engl. J. Med.* 279:410, 1968.

80. Kaplan, E. L., Laxdal, T., and Quie, P. G. Studies of polymorphonuclear leukocytes from patients with chronic granulomatous disease of

childhood: bactericidal capacity for streptococci, *Pediatrics* 41:591, 1968.

81. Karnovsky, M. L. Metabolic basis of phagocytosis, *Physiol. Rev.* 42:143, 1962.

82. Kauder, E., Kahle, L. L., Moreno, H., and Partin, J. C. Leukocyte degranulation and vacuole formation in patients with chronic granulomatous disease of childhood, *J. Clin. Invest.* 47:1753, 1968.

83. Kim, M-H., Rodey, G. E., Good, R. A., Chilgren, R. A., and Quie, P. G. Defective candidacidal capacity of polymorphonuclear leukocytes in chronic granulomatous disease of childhood, *J. Pediatr.* 75:300, 1969.

84. Klebanoff, S. J. Iodination of bacteria. A bactericidal mechanism, *J. Exp. Med.* 126:1063, 1967.

85. Klebanoff, S. J. Myeloperoxidase-halide-hydrogen peroxide antibacterial system, *J. Bacteriol.* 95:2131, 1968.

86. Klebanoff, S. J. Myeloperoxidase: Contribution to the microbicidal activity of intact leukocytes, *Science* 169:1095, 1970.

87. Klebanoff, S. J. Intraleukocytic microbicidal defects, *Ann. Rev. Med.* 22:39, 1971.

88. Klebanoff, S. J., and White, L. R. Iodination defect in the leukocytes of a patient with chronic granulomatous disease of childhood, *N. Engl. J. Med.* 280:460, 1969.

89. Kontras, S. B., and Bass, J. C. Chronic granulomatous disease, *Lancet* 2:646, 1969.

90. Kritzler, R. A., Terner, J. Y., Lindenbaum, J., Magidson, J., Williams, R., and Preisig, R. Chediak-Higashi syndrome: cytologic and serum lipid observations in a case and family, *Am. J. Med.* 36:583, 1964.

91. Lancaster, M. G., and Allison, F., Jr. Studies on the pathogenesis of acute inflammation. VII. The influence of osmolality upon the phagocytic and clumping activity by human leukocytes, *Am. J. Pathol.* 49:1185, 1966.

92. Landing, B. H., and Shirkey, H. S. A syndrome of recurrent infection and infiltration of viscera by pigmented lipid histiocytes, *Pediatrics* 20:431, 1957.

93. Lay, W. H., and Nussenzweig, V.

Receptors for complement on leukocytes, *J. Exp. Med.* 128:991, 1968.

94. Lehrer, R. I. Antifungal effects of peroxidase systems, *J. Bacteriol.* 99:361, 1969.

95. Lehrer, R. I. Measurement of candidacidal activity of specific leukocyte types in mixed cell populations — I. Normal, myeloperoxidase-deficient, and chronic granulomatous disease neutrophils, *Infect. Immun.* 2:42, 1970.

96. Lehrer, R. I. Inhibition by sulfonamides of the candidacidal activity of human neutrophils, *J. Clin. Invest.* 50:2498, 1971.

97. Lehrer, R. I., and Cline, M. J. Interaction of Candida albicans with human leukocytes and serum, *J. Bacteriol.* 98:996, 1969.

98. Lehrer, R. I., and Cline, M. J. Leukocyte myeloperoxidase deficiency and disseminated candidiasis: the role of myeloperoxidase in resistance to Candida infection, *J. Clin. Invest.* 48:1478, 1969.

99. Lehrer, R. I., and Cline, M. J. Leukocyte candidacidal activity and resistance to systemic candidiasis in patients with cancer, *Cancer* 27:1211, 1971.

100. Lehrer, R. I., Goldberg, L. S., Apple, M. A., and Rosenthal, N. P. Refractory megaloblastic anemia with myeloperoxidase deficient neutrophils, *Ann. Intern. Med.* 76:447, 1972.

101. Lehrer, R. I., Hanifin, J., and Cline, M. J. Defective bactericidal activity in myeloperoxidase-deficient human neutrophils, *Nature* 223:78, 1969.

102. LoBuglio, A. F., Cotran, R. S., and Jandl, J. H. Red cells coated with immunoglobulin G: binding and sphering by mononuclear cells in man, *Science* 158:1582, 1967.

103. Lockman, L. A., Kennedy, W. R., and White, J. G. The Chediak-Higashi syndrome: electrophysiological and electron microscopic observations on the peripheral neuropathy, *J. Pediatr.* 70:942, 1967.

104. Lutzner, M. A., Lowrie, C. T., and Jordan, H. W. Giant granules in leukocytes of the beige mouse, *J. Hered.* 58:299, 1967.

105. Lutzner, M. A., Tierney, J. H., and

Benditt, E. P. Giant granules and widespread cytoplasmic inclusions in a genetic syndrome of Aleutian mink: an electron microscopic study, *Lab. Invest.* 14:2063, 1966.

106. Maaløe, O. On the Relation between Alexin and Opsonin, Munksgaard, Copenhagen, 1946.

107. MacFarlane, P. S., Speirs, A. L., and Sommerville, R. G. Fatal granulomatous disease of children and benign lymphocytic infiltration of the skin (congenital dysphagocytosis), *Lancet* 1:408, 1967.

108. Maheswaran, S. K., Frommes, S. P., and Lindorfer, R. K. Ultrastructural changes in neutrophils treated with staphylococcal alpha toxin, *Can. J. Microbiol.* 15:128, 1969.

109. Malawista, S. E. The action of colchicine in acute gout, *Arthritis Rheum.* 8:752, 1965.

110. Malawista, S. E., and Bensch, K. G. Human polymorphonuclear leukocytes: demonstration of microtubules and effect of colchicine, *Science* 156:521, 1967.

111. Malawista, S. E., and Bodel, P. The dissociation by colchicine of phagocytosis from increased oxygen consumption in human leukocytes, *J. Clin. Invest.* 46:786, 1967.

112. Malawista, S. E., Gee, J. B. L., and Bensch, K. G. Cytochalasin B reversibly inhibits phagocytosis: functional, metabolic and ultrastructural effects in human blood and rabbit alveolar macrophages, *Yale J. Biol. Med.* 44:286, 1971.

113. Mandell, G. L., and Hook, E. W. Leukocyte function in chronic granulomatous disease of childhood: studies on a seventeen-year-old boy, *Am. J. Med.* 47:473, 1969.

114. Mandell, G. L., Rubin, W., and Hook, E. W. The effect of an NADH oxidase inhibitor (hydrocortisone) on polymorphonuclear leukocyte bactericidal activity, *J. Clin. Invest.* 49:1381, 1970.

115. Mattison, R. A., Gooch, W. M., III, Kurt, W. L., Guelzow, B. A., and South, M. A. Chronic granulomatous disease of childhood in a 17-year-old boy, *J. Pediatr.* 76:890, 1970.

116. Matula, G., and Paterson, P. Y. Spontaneous *in vitro* nitro blue tetrazolium reduction: a discriminatory test for bacterial infection in adults, *J. Clin. Invest.* 49:62a, 1970.

117. May, C. D., Levine, B. B., and Weissmann, G. Effects of compounds which inhibit antigenic release of histamine and phagocytic release of lysosomal enzyme on glucose utilization by leukocytes in humans, *Proc. Soc. Exp. Biol. Med.* 133:758, 1970.

118. McRipley, R. J., and Sbarra, A. J. Role of the phagocyte in host-parasite interactions—XII. Hydrogen peroxidase–myeloperoxidase bactericidal system in the phagocyte, *J. Bacteriol.* 94:1425, 1967.

119. Mickenberg, I. D., Root, R. K., and Wolff, S. M. Leukocytic function in hypogammaglobulinemia, *J. Clin. Invest.* 49:1528, 1970.

120. Miller, D. R., and Kaplan, H. G. Decreased nitroblue tetrazolium dye reduction in the phagocytes of patients receiving prednisone, *Pediatrics* 45:861, 1970.

121. Miller, M. E. Phagocytosis in the newborn infant: humoral and cellular factors, *J. Pediatr.* 74:255, 1969.

122. Miller, M. E. Enhanced susceptibility to infection, *Med. Clin. North Am.* 54:713, 1970.

123. Miller, M. E., and Nilsson, U. R. A familial deficiency of the phagocytosis-enhancing activity of serum related to a dysfunction of the fifth component of complement (C5), *N. Engl. J. Med.* 282:354, 1970.

124. Miller, M. E., Seals, J., Kaye, R., and Levitsky, L. C. A familial, plasma-associated defect of phagocytosis. A new cause of recurrent bacterial infections, *Lancet* 2:60, 1968.

125. Mowat, A. G., and Baum, J. Polymorphonuclear leucocyte chemotaxis in patients with bacterial infections, *Br. Med. J.* 3:617, 1971.

126. Mukherjee, A. K., Paul, B., Strauss, R., and Sbarra, A. J. The role of the phagocyte in host-parasite interactions. XV. Effects of H_2O_2 and x-irradiation on the bactericidal activities of phagocyte fractions, *J. Reticuloendothel. Soc.* 5:529, 1968.

127. Nathan, D. G., Baehner, R. L., and Weaver, D. K. Failure of nitroblue tetrazolium reduction in the phagocyte vacuoles of leukocytes in chronic granulomatous disease, *J. Clin. Invest.* 48:1895, 1969.

128. Nickerson, D. S., Kazmierowski, J. A., Dossett, J. H., Williams, R. C.,

and Quie, P. G. Studies of immune and normal opsonins during experimental staphylococcal infection in rabbits, *J. Immunol.* 102:1235, 1969.

129. Oliver, C., and Essner, E. Distribution of anomalous lysosomes in the beige mouse: a homologue of Chediak-Higashi syndrome, *J. Histochem. Cytochem.* 21:218, 1973.

130. Pachman, L. M. The effect of salicylate on the function and metabolism of peripheral blood leukocytes, *Fed. Proc.* 29:492, 1970.

131. Padgett, G. A. Neutrophilic function in animals with the Chediak-Higashi syndrome, *Blood* 29:906, 1967.

132. Padgett, G. A., Reiquam, C. W., Gorham, J. R., Henson, J. B., and O'Mary, C. C. Comparative studies on the Chediak-Higashi syndrome, *Am. J. Pathol.* 51:553, 1967.

133. Padgett, G. A., Reiquam, C. W., Henson, J. B., and Gorham, J. R. Comparative studies of susceptibility to infection in the Chediak-Higashi syndrome, *J. Pathol. Bacteriol.* 95:509, 1968.

134. Page, A. R., Berendes, H., Warner, J., and Good, R. A. The Chediak-Higashi syndrome, *Blood* 20:330, 1962.

135. Page, A. R., Hansen, A. E., and Good, R. A. Occurrence of leukemia and lymphoma in patients with agammaglobulinemia, *Blood* 21:197, 1963.

136. Park, B. H., Fikrig, S. M., and Smithwick, E. M. Infection and nitroblue-tetrazolium reduction by neutrophils, *Lancet* 2:532, 1968.

137. Park, B. H., Holmes, B., and Good, R. A. Metabolic activities in leukocytes of newborn infants, *J. Pediatr.* 76:237, 1970.

138. Park, B. H., Holmes, B. M., Rodey, G. E., and Good, R. A. Nitroblue-tetrazolium test in children with fatal granulomatous disease and newborn infants, *Lancet* 1:157, 1969.

139. Paul, B., Strauss, R., and Sbarra, A. J. The role of the phagocyte in host-parasite interactions, *J. Reticuloendothel. Soc.* 5:538, 1968.

140. Pearson, H. A., Spencer, R. P., and Cornelius, E. A. Functional asplenia in sickle-cell anemia, *N. Engl. J. Med.* 281:923, 1969.

141. Perillie, P. E., Nolan, J. P., and

Finch, S. C. Studies of the resistance to infection in diabetes mellitus: local exudative cellular response, *J. Lab. Clin. Med.* 59:1008, 1962.

142. Peters, W. P., Holland, J. F., Hansjoeg, S., Rhomberg, W., and Banerjee, T. Corticosteroid administration and localized leukocyte mobilization in man, *N. Engl. J. Med.* 286:342, 1972.

143. Quie, P. G., Kaplan, E. L., Page, A. R., Gruskay, F. L., and Malawista, S. E. Defective polymorphonuclear-leukocyte function and chronic granulomatous disease in two female children, *N. Engl. J. Med.* 278:976, 1968.

144. Quie, P. G., Messner, R. P., and Williams, R. C., Jr. Phagocytosis in subacute bacterial endocarditis: localization of the primary opsonic site to Fc fragment, *J. Exp. Med.* 128:553, 1968.

145. Quie, P. G., White, J. G., Holmes, B., and Good, R. A. *In vitro* bactericidal capacity of human polymorphonuclear leukocytes: diminished activity in chronic granulomatous disease of childhood, *J. Clin. Invest.* 46:668, 1967.

146. Rabinovitch, M. Phagocytosis: the engulfment stage, *Semin. Hematol.* 5:134, 1968.

147. Rebuck, J. W., and Crowley, J. H. A method of studying leukocytic functions *in vivo, Ann. N.Y. Acad. Sci.* 59:757, 1955.

148. Rodey, G. E., Jacob, H. S., Holmes, B., McArthur, J. R., and Good, R. A. Leucocyte G.-6-P.D. levels and bactericidal activity, *Lancet* 1:355, 1970.

149. Rodey, G. E., Park, B. H., Ford, D. K., Gray, B. H., and Good, R. A. Defective bactericidal activity of peripheral blood leukocytes in lipochrome histiocytosis, *Am. J. Med.* 49:322, 1970.

150. Rodey, G. E., Park, B. H., Windhorst, D. B., and Good, R. A. Defective bactericidal activity of monocytes in fatal granulomatous disease, *Blood* 33:813, 1969.

151. Root, R. K., Blume, R. S., and Wolff, S. M. Abnormal leukocyte function in the Chediak-Higashi syndrome, *Clin. Res.* 16:335, 1968.

152. Rosen, F. S., and Janeway, C. A. The gammaglobulins. III. The antibody deficiency syndromes, *N. Engl. J. Med.* 275:709, 769; 1966.

153. Ruddle, F., Ricciuti, F., McMorris, F. A., Tischfield, J., Creagan, R., Darlington, G., and Chen, T. Somatic cell genetic assignment of peptidase C and the Rh linkage group to chromosome A-1 in man, *Science* 176:1429, 1972.

154. Sadan, N., Yaffe, D., Rozenszaun, L., Adar, H., Soroker, B., and Efrati, P. Cytochemical and genetic studies in four cases of Chediak-Higashi-Steinbrinck syndrome, *Acta Haematol.* 34:20, 1965.

155. Salmon, S. E., Cline, M. J., Schultz, J., and Lehrer, R. I. Myeloperoxidase deficiency: immunologic study of a genetic leukocyte defect, *N. Engl. J. Med.* 282:250, 1970.

156. Saraiva, L. G., Azevedo, M., Correa, J. M., Carvalho, G., and Prospero, J. D. Anomalous panleukocytic granulation, *Blood* 14:1112, 1959.

157. Sbarra, A. J., Shirley, W., Selvaraj, R. J., McRipley, R. J., and Rosenbaum, E. The role of the phagocyte in host-parasite interactions. III. The phagocytic capabilities of leukocytes from myeloproliferative and other neoplastic disorders, *Cancer Res.* 25:1199, 1965.

158. Seligmann, M., Fudenberg, H. H., and Good, R. A. Editorial. A proposed classification of primary immunologic deficiencies, *Am. J. Med.* 45: 817, 1968.

159. Shin, H. S., Smith, M. R., and Wood, W. B., Jr. Heat-labile opsonins to pneumococcus—II. Involvement of C3 and C5, *J. Exp. Med.* 130:1229, 1969.

160. Sia, R. H. P. Studies on pneumococcus growth inhibition. VI. The specific effect of pneumococcus soluble substance on the growth of pneumococci in normal serum-leucocyte mixtures, *J. Exp. Med.* 43:633, 1926.

161. Skarnes, R. C., and Watson, D. W. Characterization of leukin: an antibacterial factor from leucocytes active against gram-positive pathogens, *J. Exp. Med.* 104:829, 1956.

162. Smith, M. R., and Wood, W. B., Jr. Heat-labile opsonins to pneumococcus. I. Participation of complement, *J. Exp. Med.* 130:1209, 1969.

163. Solberg, C. O., and Hellum, K. B. Neutrophil granulocyte function in bacterial infections, *Lancet* 2:727, 1972.

164. Spencer, W. H., and Hogan, M. J. Ocular manifestations of Chediak-Higashi syndrome; report of a case with histopathologic examination of ocular tissues, *Am. J. Ophthalmol.* 50:1197, 1960.

165. Spitznagel, J. K., and Zeya, H. I. Basic proteins and leukocyte lysosomes as biochemical determinants of resistance to infection, *Trans. Assoc. Am. Physicians* 77:126, 1964.

166. Strauss, R. R., Paul, B. B., Jacobs, A. A., and Sbarra, A. J. The role of the phagocyte in host-parasite interactions. XIX. Leukocytic glutathione reductase and its involvement in phagocytosis, *Arch. Biochem. Biophys.* 135:265, 1969.

167. Paul, B. B., Jacobs, A. A., Strauss, R. R., and Sbarra, A. J. The role of the phagocyte in host-parasite interactions. XX. Restoration of x-irradiation phagocytic damage by endotoxin or polyadenylic-polyuridylic acids, *J. Reticuloendothel. Soc.* 7:743, 1970.

168. Undritz, E. Die Alius-Grignaschi-Anomalie: der erblichkonstitutionelle Peroxydasedefekt der Neutrophilen und Monozyten, *Blut* 14:129, 1966.

169. Ward, H. K., and Enders, J. F. An analysis of the opsonic and tropic action of normal and immune sera based on experiments with the pneumococcus, *J. Exp. Med.* 57:527, 1933.

170. Ward, P. A. The chemosuppression of chemotaxis, *J. Exp. Med.* 124:209, 1966.

171. Ward, P. A. A plasmin-split fragment of C'3 as a new chemotactic factor, *J. Exp. Med.* 126:189, 1967.

172. Ward, P. A. Chemotaxis of mononuclear cells, *J. Exp. Med.* 128:1201, 1968.

173. Ward, P. A., and Becker, E. L. Mechanisms of the inhibition of chemotaxis by phosphonate esters, *J. Exp. Med.* 125:1001, 1967.

174. Ward, P. A., Cochrane, C. G., and Muller-Eberhard, H. J. Further studies on the chemotactic factor of complement and its formation *in vivo, Immunology* 11:141, 1966.

175. Ward, P. A., Lepow, I. H., and Newman, L. J. Bacterial factors chemotactic for polymorphonuclear

leukocytes, *Am. J. Pathol.* 52:725, 1968.

176. Ward, P. A., and Newman, L. J. A neutrophil chemotactic factor from human C'5, *J. Immunol.* 102:93, 1969.

177. Ward, P. A., and Schlegel, R. J. Impaired leucotactic responsiveness in a child with recurrent infections, *Lancet* 2:344, 1969.

178. Weary, P. E., and Bender, A. S. Chediak-Higashi syndrome with severe cutaneous involvement, *Arch. Intern. Med.* 119:381, 1967.

179. Weissmann, G. The effects of steroids and drugs on lysosomes, *in* J. T. Dingle and H. B. Fell (eds.), Lysosomes in Biology and Pathology, p. 276, North-Holland Publishing Co., Amsterdam, 1969.

180. White, J. G. The Chediak-Higashi syndrome: a possible lysosomal disease, *Blood* 28:143, 1966.

181. White, J. G. Virus-like particles in the peripheral blood cells of two patients with Chediak-Higashi syndrome, *Cancer* 19:877, 1966.

182. White, J. G. The Chediak-Higashi syndrome: cytoplasmic sequestration in circulating leukocytes, *Blood* 29:435, 1967.

183. Williams, R. C., Jr., Dossett, J. H., and Quie, P. G. Comparative studies of immunoglobulin opsonins in osteomyelitis and other established infections, *Immunology* 17:249, 1969.

184. Windhorst D. B. Studies on a hereditary defect involving lysosomal structure, *Fed. Proc.* 25:358, 1966.

185. Windhorst, D. B., Holmes, B., and Good, R. A. A newly defined x-linked trait in man with demonstration of the Lyon effect on carrier females, *Lancet* 1:737, 1967.

186. Windhorst, D. B., Page, A. R., Holmes, B., Quie, P. G., and Good, R. A. The pattern of genetic transmission of the leukocyte defect in fatal granulomatous disease of childhood, *J. Clin. Invest.* 47:1026, 1968.

187. Windhorst, D. B., Zelickson, A. S., and Good, R. A. Chediak-Higashi syndrome: hereditary gigantism of cytoplasmic organelles, *Science* 151:81, 1966.

188. Winkelstein, J. A., and Drachman, R. H. Deficiency of pneumococcal serum opsonizing activity in sickle-cell disease, *N. Engl. J. Med.* 279:459, 1968.

189. Wright, A. E., and Douglas, S. R. An experimental investigation on the role of the blood fluids in connection with phagocytosis, *Proc. R. Soc.* 72:357, 1904.

190. Wurster, N., Elsbach, P., Simon, E. J., Pettis, P., and Lebow, S. The effects of the morphine analogue levorphanol on leukocytes, *J. Clin. Invest.* 50:1091, 1971.

191. Zeya, H. I., and Spitznagel, J. K. Antimicrobial specificity of leukocyte lysosomal cationic proteins, *Science* 154:1049, 1966.

192. Zeya, H. I., and Spitznagel, J. K. Arginine-rich proteins of polymorphonuclear leukocyte lysosomes: antimicrobial specificity and biochemical heterogeneity, *J. Exp. Med.* 127:927, 1968.

193. Zeya, H. I., and Spitznagel, J. K. Cationic protein-bearing granules of polymorphonuclear leukocytes: separation from enzyme-rich granules, *Science* 163:1069, 1969.

194. Zigmond, S. H., and Hirsch, J. G. Cytochalasin B: inhibition of D-2-deoxyglucose transport into leukocytes and fibroblasts, *Science* 176:1432, 1972.

Chapter 9   Abnormalities of Neutrophil Production, Destruction, and Morphogenesis

In considering abnormalities in the number of circulating neutrophils, it is both convenient and logical to consider three factors: (*a*) the rate of granulocyte production, (*b*) the rate of granulocyte destruction or utilization, and (*c*) the distribution of granulocytes among the various compartments within the vascular space. Low numbers of circulating neutrophils (neutropenia) can result from any of the following: diminished production, excessive utilization, shifts of cells out of the circulating pool, or some combination of these events. Similarly, an increased number of circulating granulocytes (granulocytosis) results from either excessive cellular production or from shifts of cells into the circulating pool (Fig. 9.1).

The laboratory techniques used in evaluating the rate of granulopoiesis, granulocyte loss, and compartmental distribution were summarized in Chapter 2. These techniques include bone marrow cellularity, peripheral leukocyte count, cell labeling studies with radio-labeled diiso-propyl-fluorophosphate and ^{51}chromium, and lysozyme concentration in serum and urine.

In addition to the quantity of neutrophils, one must be concerned with their quality. In Chapter 8 we considered abnormalities of granulocyte phagocytic and microbicidal function. These abnormalities are subtle in the sense that they are not readily apparent from a simple examination of a stained smear of peripheral blood. They require sophisticated tests of leukocyte function. In this chapter we shall also consider *peculiar leukocytes*—cells whose morphologic abnormalities usually are readily apparent on stained smears of blood. These abnormalities, resulting from disordered morphogenesis of granulocytes within the bone marrow, may be either congenital or acquired.

Neutropenias

Definitions and Clinical Features

Neutropenia means a reduction below the normal range in the numbers of circulating neutrophils. The term *granulocytopenia* is often used synonymously, although strictly speaking, granulocytopenia means reduced numbers of all granulocytes, including neutrophils, eosinophils, and basophils. The term *agranulocytosis* is often used to designate a very severe degree of neutropenia.

The absolute number of circulating neutrophils is calculated as a product of the total leukocyte count and the percentage of neutrophils in the differential leukocyte count. The normal range varies with age and race (35, 48).

We shall be using a kinetic classification of the neutropenias and shall sequentially consider disorders of leukocyte production, disorders of excessive neutrophil destruction, combinations of these abnormalities, and finally, the relatively rare neutropenias resulting from abnormalities of distribution (Table 9.1).

The clinical manifestations of neutropenia vary with the magnitude of the reduction in granulocyte numbers and granulocyte reserve. Symptoms are rarely manifest when the neutrophil count exceeds 1,000/mm³. The risk of infection is moderately increased when the count is from 500 to 1,000 neutrophils per cubic millimeter. Below 500 cells the risk is greatly increased.

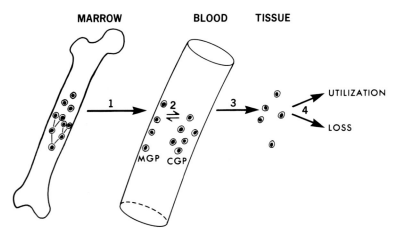

Figure 9.1 Schematic approach to the evaluation of granulocytosis and granulocytopenia. Granulocytosis may result from increased granulocyte proliferation or mobilization from the bone marrow reserves (*1*), from shifts of cells from the marginal granulocyte pool (MGP) to the circulating granulocyte pool (CGP) (*2*), or, theoretically, from decreased mobilization from the blood (*3*).

Granulocytopenia may result from inadequate proliferation of granulocyte precursors in the marrow or diminished mobilization from bone marrow stores (*1*), from shifts of cells from the circulating to the marginal granulocyte pool (*2*), or from excessive loss or utilization of granulocytes in the tissues (*3* and *4*).

Frequent sites of infection are the lungs, oro- and nasopharynx, sinuses, and genitourinary tract. Such infections occurring in granulocytopenic patients are often refractory to antibiotic therapy. As might be anticipated, decreased neutrophil mobilization into areas of inflammation occurs in severe neutropenic states (77). In part, mononuclear phagocytes may compensate for a decrease in numbers of granulocytes. Recent evidence suggests that intact monocyte function may be critically important in children with chronic neutropenia (15).

Comprehensive summaries of the leukocyte counts of the healthy adult, child, and fetus respectively may be found in the reviews of Zacharski and his colleagues (378), Wintrobe (369), and Playfair and his associates (270). The neutrophil number in normal Caucasians may be higher than that in normal blacks (35).

Underproduction Neutropenias

Table 9.2 classifies neutropenias that arise from inadequate granulopoiesis in the bone marrow. Neutropenias arising from insufficient granulopoiesis are characterized by reduced granulocyte turnover rates (GTR). In this condition, granulocyte survival in the circulation may be normal or reduced. The marginal and circulating granulocyte pools and the marrow storage pools are all reduced in size. Neutrophil mobilization in response to endotoxin or inflammation is impaired (21). The myeloid elements of

Table 9.1 Kinetic classification of the neutropenic disorders.

| | Blood granulocytes | | | | |
Disorder	CGP[a]	MGP[b]	$T_{1/2}$ in circulation	Marrow reserve	Granulocyte turnover rate
Underproduction neutropenia	↓	↓	Normal or ↓	↓	↓
Excessive granulocyte destruction or utilization	↓	↓	↓	↑ or normal	↑ or normal; rarely ↓
Shift neutropenia	↓	↑	Normal	Normal	Normal

[a] Circulating granulocyte pool.   ↓Reduced.
[b] Marginal granulocyte pool.   ↑Increased.

Table 9.2 Causes of neutropenias related to underproduction by the bone marrow.

Bone marrow injury
  Cytotoxic drugs (such as nitrogen mustard)
  Irradiation
  Drugs interfering with precursor cell metabolism (for example, phenazines or chloramphenicol)
  Immune injury
Bone marrow replacement
Nutrition
  Vitamin B_{12}
  Folic acid
Abnormalities probably involving the control of granulopoiesis
  Familial cyclic neutropenia
  Gray-collie syndrome
Congenital abnormalities of myelogenesis of unknown etiology
  Fanconi's anemia
  Familial benign neutropenia (Gänsslen)
  Infantile genetic agranulocytosis (Kostmann)
Acquired abnormalities of granulogenesis of unknown etiology
  Paroxysmal nocturnal hemoglobinuria
  Collagen disease
  Cirrhosis

the bone marrow are reduced, and the differential count may shift toward more immature forms.

Causes of bone marrow injury and neutropenia include cytotoxic drugs, irradiation, replacement by tumor cells, and nutritional deficiencies. Abnormalities of granulopoietic control mechanisms also may result in diminished granulocyte production.

Bone Marrow Injury   Injury to the hematopoietic cells of the bone marrow may result from a variety of agents. Some of these are easy to identify; others are still not known.

Cytotoxic drugs and irradiation.   Replicating cells are generally the primary target of drugs used in cancer chemotherapy and immunosuppression (131). The principal toxicity of these drugs arises from their interruption of the replicative sequence of normal hematopoietic precursors, with resultant neutropenia, thrombocytopenia, and anemia. The commonly used classes of agents that produce these effects are alkylating drugs, antimetabolites such as 6-mercaptopurine and methotrexate, vinca alkaloids, nitrosoureas, antibiotics such as actinomycin D, and procarbazine (46, 59). Neutropenia is frequently observed in patients with malignant disease who undergo chemotherapy with cytotoxic agents, and it is one of the chief parameters used as a guide in drug dosage schedules. Hypoplasia of the bone marrow generally reflects marrow injury (Fig. 9.2) and underproduction of neutrophils.

Irradiation of bone marrow has an effect similar to that produced by cytotoxic drugs. The targets for ionizing irradiation are the replicating hematopoietic cells and the vascular endothelium of the bone marrow (68, 106, 151).

Neutropenia arising from the use of cytotoxic drugs or ionizing irradiation can occur in all individuals, provided the dosage is sufficiently high and administration is sufficiently prolonged.

Noncytotoxic drugs.   Neutropenia from bone marrow suppression occurs frequently with the use of a variety of drugs that are not ordinarily considered cytotoxic. Obviously, these "noncytotoxic" drugs do produce cellular injury in susceptible individuals. The variability of myeloid response to these drugs is generally much greater than the highly predictable response to alkylating agents or to other known cytotoxic drugs. Agents reported to be associated with myelosuppression are listed in Table 9.3. Identifying drugs that produce granulocytopenia is difficult because of inadequate reporting and the simultaneous use of multiple drugs, and also because the contribution of underlying disease may be difficult to define. These problems have been summarized in a number of reports (51, 146, 165, 266, 368).

Drugs and classes of drugs most frequently associated with neutropenia and other evidence of myelosuppression include phenothiazines, chloramphenicol, thiouracil derivatives, methimazole, sulfonamides, phenylbutazone, and anticonvulsants. The mechanism of myelosuppression by these drugs is not known (268). Some clearly cause myelosuppression based on interference with cell metabolism; others are thought to invoke immunologic reactions. Unfortunately, definitive proof that immunologic drug reactions result in underproduction of neutrophils has been difficult to obtain.

Most of the drugs cited in Table 9.3 have potent metabolic effects that might, in susceptible individuals, lead to impaired cell replication and viability. Susceptibility might result from genetic or acquired lack of drug detoxification systems, lack of alternate metabolic pathways around a drug-induced block, unusual drug binding, or kinetics of distribution and excretion. Perhaps other as yet undefined mechanisms are also involved (234, 268).

Some authors have classified drug-induced neutropenias as "antimetabolite type" or as "idiosyncratic type" (107). However, such a classification does not seem useful until more information is available on the mechanism of myelosuppression caused by noncytotoxic drugs. The term "idiosyncratic" is not meaningful. It would be logical to divide the drugs in Table 9.3 into those causing myelosuppression by interference with cell metabolism (57) and those operating by immunologic mechanisms. However, the techniques available for defining the latter are still too imprecise to attempt such a classification with security.

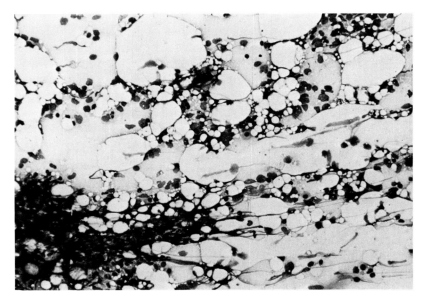

Figure 9.2 Hypoplasia of the bone marrow reflecting drug-induced bone marrow injury.

Table 9.3 Drugs other than cytotoxic agents associated with myelosuppression and neutropenia.

Drugs	References
Antimicrobial agents	
Chloramphenicol	140, 302, 311, 376, 377
Sulfonamides	11, 211, 328
Ampicillin	133, 139
Streptomycin	252
Ristocetin	246
Gentamicin	38
Lincomycin	250
Griseofulvin	100
Cephalothin	93
Dapsone	199, 349
Nitrofurantoin	201
Amphotericin	204
Phenothiazines	
Mepazine, promazine, etc.	109, 160, 181, 217, 267
Dibenzazepine compounds	
Imipramine, etc.	65, 177
Antihistamines	
Pyribenzamine, etc.	45, 145
Anticonvulsants	
Tridione	226, 319
Antithyroid drugs	
Methimazole, thiouracil derivatives	10, 213, 365
Anti-inflammatory	
Indomethacin	52, 229
Phenylbutazone	111, 210, 220
Gold salts	176, 198
Diuretics	
Thiazide	148
Ethacrynic acid	8, 355
Mercurial diuretics	184
Acetazolamide (Diamox)	260
Hypoglycemic agents (sulfonamide derivatives)	
Tolbutamide	7
Chlorpropamide	321
Miscellaneous	
Penicillamine	63
Phenindione	334
Cinchopen	327
Hydroxychloroquine	54, 271, 274
Quinidine	16
Procaine amide	191, 332, 356
Allopurinol	94
Propranolol	244

The mechanism of a few drugs in producing myelosuppression is known with reasonable detail. Agranulocytosis produced by phenothiazines appears related to dose of drug. Onset of agranulocytosis is rare before the tenth day of drug therapy and is unlikely to develop if it has not occurred by the ninetieth day. In susceptible individuals the drug inhibits DNA synthesis, with resultant bone marrow hypoplasia (267, 269). The current estimate of incidence of agranulocytosis resulting from the use of phenothiazine drugs is about 1 in 1,200 (181, 267). Certain phenothiazine derivatives may be implicated as a cause of agranulocytosis more frequently than any other group of drugs in common use.

Chloramphenicol may also inhibit protein and nucleic acid synthesis in hematopoietic cells (358, 377). In some individuals leukemia has developed following bone marrow suppression induced by chloramphenicol and phenylbutazone (111).

In contrast to the rather slow development of granulocytopenia after the initiation of therapy with phenothiazines, chloramphenicol, and phenylbutazone, a rapid fall is sometimes observed with aminopyrine administration. This drug may cause a rapid destruction of leukocytes in the peripheral blood, with associated fever, chills, and circulatory collapse. The syndrome resembles that produced by rapid leukocyte destruction from leukoagglutinins (33) and may have an immunologic reaction as its basis.

The list of drugs associated with the development of neutropenia is continually increasing, so that Table 9.3 is necessarily incomplete. When a suspicious drug history is obtained, the physician should consult the current Registry on Blood Dyscrasias published by the Council on Drugs of the American Medical Association.

In addition to drugs, a number of chemicals may produce agranulocytosis on the basis of bone marrow injury. Often the agranulocytosis is associated with the suppression of other hematopoietic elements. Characteristically, the bone marrow is hypocellular and contains few residual hematopoietic elements. Some of these compounds, such as benzol, have been associated with the subsequent development of leukemia. A partial list of chemical toxins appears in Table 9.4.

Few detailed studies of leukocyte kinetics are available on myelosuppression induced by noncytotoxic drugs. Bishop and his co-workers (21) studied a patient with butazolidine-induced neutropenia. In this patient total body granulocyte pool was about 20 percent of the mean normal value, and the circulating granulocyte pool and marrow reserve both were about one-third of normal. The clearance of neutrophils from the circulation was normal, but the granulocyte turnover rate (the measure of granulo-

Table 9.4 Chemical compounds that have been associated with agranulocytosis.

Compound	References
Benzol, benzene	295, 306, 322, 350
Arsenic	192, 364
Nitrous oxide	256
Thioglycolic acid	64
DDT	292, 375
Dinitrophenol	127
Thiocyanate	113
Bismuth	307
Carbon tetrachloride and other organic solvents	301, 329
Thorotrast	249

cyte production) was only one-tenth of normal. In view of the severe depression of granulocyte turnover rate, it is interesting that the marrow cellularity estimated by biopsy was normal. This observation points up the inadequacy of the routine clinical method of evaluating bone marrow granulocyte production on a morphologic basis.

Bone Marrow Replacement Neutropenia resulting from diminished production is seen in a number of malignant disorders where the bone marrow is infiltrated with tumor cells (71, 265). This phenomenon has been called *myelophthisis.* Bone marrow replacement resulting in neutropenia is more often seen in hematologic malignancies such as acute leukemia, lymphoma, and multiple myeloma, than in nonhematologic neoplasms. Among the "solid tumors," bone marrow infiltration and replacement probably occur most frequently in carcinoma of the lung and breast (Fig. 9.3) and in neuroblastoma. Neutropenia may be seen also in myelofibrosis with myeloid metaplasia (Fig. 9.4), a condition where the normal hematopoietic elements of the bone marrow are replaced by fibrous tissue.

In their investigation of leukocyte kinetics in neutropenic states, Bishop and his colleagues (21) studied two patients with acute myelocytic leukemia and one with multiple myeloma. The mature neutrophils of these patients had normal disappearance time from the blood, but their granulocyte turnover rates varied from 10 to 30 percent of normal.

Nutritional Deficiencies The generalized nutritional deficiencies that occur with starvation or anorexia nervosa may produce myelosuppression and neutropenia (259, 310). The bone marrow is usually hypocellular. Low levels

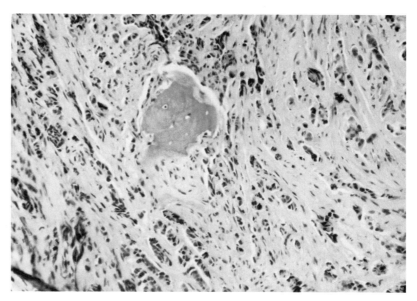

Figure 9.3 A bone marrow cavity replaced by carcinoma of the breast and fibrous tissue. A bone spicule is seen in the center of the figure.

of circulating neutrophils may also accompany the megaloblastic anemias of vitamin B_{12} and folic acid deficiency (99, 108, 262) and the hypochromic anemia of severe iron deficiency. Although the circulating granulocytes and the granulocyte reserve are reduced in severe megaloblastic anemia, serious infections are rare (330). Correction of the

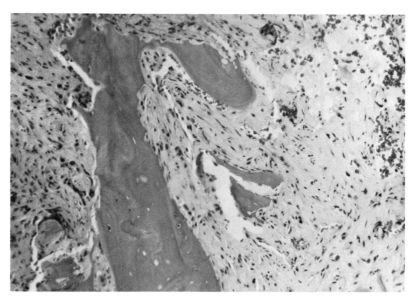

Figure 9.4 A bone marrow biopsy from a patient with myelofibrosis showing increased fibrous tissue surrounding a bony spicule.

nutritional status rectifies the leukopenia in these disorders. In starvation, the recovery of neutrophils may be quite slow (three months or more) after refeeding (310), whereas correction of the neutropenia occurring in severe vitamin B$_{12}$ and folic acid deficiency is usually rapid. Deficiencies of vitamin B$_{12}$ and folate presumably interfere with nucleic acid synthesis of myeloid precursors in the bone marrow and lead to inadequate granulopoiesis. Ineffective granulopoiesis (that is, intrameduallary destruction of young granulocytes) may also be characteristic of these disorders (107). Abnormal nuclear lobulation with hypersegmented neutrophils is common in abnormal DNA synthesis and may result from either nutritional deficiency or antimetabolite drugs such as cytosine arabinoside or 6-mercaptopurine (Fig. 9.5).

In 1964 Schwachman and his colleagues described a syndrome in five children characterized by pancreatic insufficiency and anemia, thrombocytopenia, and granulocytopenia of variable severity (299). The finding of bone marrow hypoplasia suggested that the pancytopenia was a result of decreased cell production. Since then a number of investigators have contributed observations on this interesting syndrome (27, 43, 60, 195, 233, 240, 273). Its characteristics are (*a*) hereditary transmission not sex-linked; (*b*) onset early in life; (*c*) steatorrhea; (*d*) failure to thrive; (*e*) frequent infection; (*f*) occasional associated anomalies such as epiphyseal dysplasia; and (*g*) neutropenia in the range of 200 to 400/mm^3.

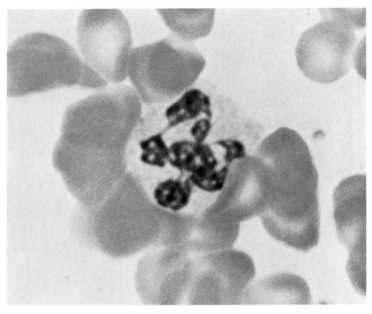

Figure 9.5 A neutrophil showing excessive nuclear lobulation (hypersegmented neutrophil).

Whether the neutropenia results from nutritional deficiencies secondary to steatorrhea or is related to some other abnormality has not been determined with certainty. Other hypoplastic neutropenias with accompanying constitutional disorders are known. In some instances there may be a factor in the serum that is cytotoxic for neutrophils (233). Bone marrow hyperplasia, rather than hypoplasia, has been noted in some patients. For the present, until more information is available, this disease may be classified as an underproduction neutropenia.

Abnormal Control Mechanisms

Cyclic neutropenia. The term periodic diseases was introduced by Reimann (281) as a designation for a number of diseases sharing the feature of regularly recurrent manifestations. Based on relatively little evidence, these periodic diseases have been suggested as reflecting underlying intrinsic body rhythms. One of these disorders is cyclic neutropenia, a disease entity characterized by periodic oscillation of the neutrophil count (6, 116, 141, 235, 238, 254, 280). The oscillations are based on cyclic changes in bone marrow production and release of neutrophils. The periodicity is generally between 19 and 21 days, but may be as short as 14 days or as long as 30 days. Usually the disorder is familial; occasionally it is associated with either an underlying hematologic neoplasm (243, 293) or with other diseases (238). In some cases hematopoietic cell lines other than the neutrophil are involved in the cyclic process, suggesting that control mechanisms at the stem cell level may be disordered.

Cyclic neutropenia probably was first described by Leale in 1910 (196); by 1963 at least 42 cases had been recognized (281). Morley and his co-workers in 1967 added another 20 patients (238). Clinical manifestations nearly always appear before age ten years. The disease generally runs a benign course, although death from infection occurred in 4 out of 42 cases. Reimann noted that splenectomy or adrenocorticosteroids produced improvement in some cases, but never effected a cure. Subsequently, Brodsky and his co-workers (34) described one patient in whom hematologic improvement followed treatment with testosterone.

Symptoms attributable to neutropenia include fever, oral ulcerations, and skin infections. Periodontal disease is prominent in some families (316, 353). Symptoms are rarely seen when the neutrophil count is in excess of 500/mm^3 (238).

Monocytosis has been described in about half the reported cases of cyclic neutropenia. It may occur at the time of minimum neutrophil count (238). Eosinophilia may also occur (95, 238, 254, 348).

In 1966 Morley observed a 14- to 23-day cycle of neutrophil levels in some normal males (237). He suggested that granulopoiesis is probably controlled by a negative feedback circuit containing an inherent time delay. Such a system is subject to oscillation and theoretically could account for cycling in normal subjects and exaggerated cycling in patients with cyclic neutropenia. The model developed by King-Smith and Morley (179, 180) (see Fig. 2.6) contains two feedback loops from the blood neutrophil concentration: one controlling bone marrow production of neutrophils, the other controlling rate of release from the storage compartments in the marrow. Morley and Stohlman (239) tested this model by producing mild bone marrow depression in dogs with cyclophosphamide and, subsequently, induced cyclic neutropenia. A similar negative feedback system has been postulated as accounting for the spontaneous cyclic leukocytosis sometimes observed in chronic myelocytic leukemia (351).

If this model is correct, it would suggest that cyclic neutropenia may not be a single disease entity; rather, it may be a family of diseases of diverse etiology sharing the common feature of an exaggeration of the normal tendency of neutrophil numbers to oscillate. In theory, a partial failure at any point in the feedback loop from neutrophil to stem cell could result in cyclic neutropenia, provided the slope of neutrophil production remained fairly steep. This possibility is suggested by the occasional nonfamilial occurrence (238, 280), and by the heterogeneity of manifestations from family to family in the familial form of the disorder.

Presently, the mechanisms of humoral regulation of granulopoiesis are largely unknown. On the basis of in vitro studies of granulocytic clonal growth, it has been suggested that there may be positive control of granulopoiesis by cells or substances contained in the peripheral blood (284). The blood monocyte may be the principal source of stimulatory activity for colony growth (126). As we come to understand the normal controls of granulopoiesis, we may better understand the mechanisms involved in cyclic neutropenia.

The gray-collie syndrome. The gray-collie syndrome is a lethal disease of collie dogs characterized by hair-coat abnormalities, malabsorption (366), and cyclic neutropenia (205). Correlated with episodes of neutropenia are infectious complications including septicemia, arthritis, enteritis, and respiratory infections. Death usually occurs in puppyhood or early adult life. Surviving animals

may develop amyloidosis. Neutropenic cycles may average 10 or 11 days and are followed by rebound granulocytosis and monocytosis. Neutrophils are normal by light and electron microscopy (55).

This disorder in gray collies has many features in common with human familial neutropenia. In both disorders cyclic phenomena may involve hematopoietic cells in addition to the neutrophil series. Periodicity may be an expression of mild bone marrow failure in the canine, as well as the human, disease (75). Dale and his colleagues (74, 76) have suggested that this syndrome is caused by a defect of hematopoietic regulation at the stem cell level and have presented ultrastructural evidence of defective granulogenesis (303).

Congenital Abnormalities of Myelogenesis of Unknown Etiology A large number of congenital disorders of neutrophil production share the features of being rare, exotic, and of unknown etiology. Table 9.5 provides a tabulation of the better documented of these disorders.

Hereditary neutropenia (Kostmann). In 1956 Kostmann described congenital neutropenia in several Swedish families with a history of consanguinity (183). The pattern of inheritance was autosomal recessive. The clinical course was dramatic; many of the patients died in early childhood of overwhelming sepsis. The bone marrow aspirates in this disorder are cellular and are characterized by a "maturation arrest" with absence of mature

Table 9.5 Congenital disorders of myelogenesis of unknown etiology.

Disease	Inheritance	References
Hereditary neutropenia (Kostmann's syndrome)	Autosomal recessive	1, 123, 183, 194, 218, 228, 373
Familial benign neutropenia (Gänsslen)	Autosomal dominant	29, 72, 85, 86, 118
Familial severe neutropenia (Hitzig)	Autosomal dominant	157
Reticular dysgenesis (alymphocytic neutropenia)	Uncertain	84, 110, 124
Neutropenia, abnormal cellular immunity, and cartilage-hair hypoplasia	Familial	207
Agammaglobulinemia and dysgammaglobulinemia	Variable or uncertain; see Chapter 18	3, 129, 161, 203, 335
Familial neutropenia related to deficiency of a plasma factor	Uncertain	22
Chronic hypoplastic neutropenia	Uncertain	4, 311
Neutropenia associated with various constitutional defects	Uncertain	40, 120, 352

myeloid forms. In addition to peculiar nuclear lobation, cytoplasmic vacuolization of myeloid cells and monocytes frequently occurs. In one case marrow granulocytic precursor activity was decreased and compensatory defense systems, including monocytes and serum immunoglobulins, were thought to be activated (373).

Familial benign neutropenia (Gänsslen). In 1941 Gänsslen described a familial neutropenia with an autosomal dominant mode of inheritance and a benign course (118). In this, and in subsequently described cases, the bone marrow cellularity was normal with a decrease in granulocytic cells beyond the myelocyte stage. Because of the benign clinical course, granulocytopenia may not be recognized until late in life. About one-half of the patients have had monocytosis, and some have had slight eosinophilia. Overlap of this syndrome with Fanconi's anemia has been suggested (17, 122). The relation between familial benign neutropenia and the neutropenic disorder observed in Yemenite Jews (86) is uncertain. In the latter disease the number of granulocyte progenitors in the marrow appears to be normal (230).

Familial severe neutropenia. In 1959 Hitzig described severe chronic familial neutropenia associated with hypergammaglobulinemia (157). Inheritance was autosomal dominant. In these and subsequently described patients (200, 288), characteristics of the syndrome included severe infections (particularly oral infections), monocytosis, maturation arrest of the bone marrow, and severe peripheral neutropenia. The relation between this disorder and familial benign neutropenia is uncertain.

Reticular dysgenesis (alymphocytic neutropenia). In 1959 DeVaal and Seynhaeve (84), and later Gitlin and his colleagues (110, 124), described a disorder associated with thymic alymphoplasia that was characterized by a complete absence of leukocytes. In addition to abnormalities of lymphoid tissues, myeloid precursor cells either are absent from the bone marrow or, more rarely, show a maturation arrest. The clinical disease is a spectrum varying from rapidly lethal aleukocytosis to a somewhat milder, but still fatal, variant called thymic alymphoplasia (115, 124). Both bacterial and viral infections are frequent, the latter probably arising from impaired immunity. This disorder probably results from a congenital decrease of hematopoietic stem cells.

Neutropenia, abnormal cellular immunity, and cartilage-hair hypoplasia. Cartilage-hair hypoplasia is a syndrome of short-limbed dwarfism and abnormally fine hair described in a study of Old Order Amish by McKusick and his colleagues (214). An unusual susceptibility to severe Varicella infection was noted. In detailed studies of two infection-prone children (207), neutropenia with failure of myelocytic maturation and persistent lymphopenia with abnormal cellular immunity were documented. The immunologic defect is probably the major factor contributing to a susceptibility to viral infection in affected children.

Agammaglobulinemia and dysgammaglobulinemia. Some patients with immunologic deficiency disease (see Chapter 18) have an associated abnormality of granulocyte production. In 1956 Good and Zak (129) described a group of eight patients with agammaglobulinemia, six of whom had "aregenerative neutropenia" that was transient in three, persistent in two, and cyclic in one. Subsequently, other investigators have described additional immunologic abnormalities in association with neutropenia (161, 203, 335). In one patient injection of gamma globulin was associated with improvement in the neutropenia (3).

Bone marrow aspirates in affected patients usually have been cellular, often with a maturation arrest. Whether neutropenia in these patients results from decreased production alone or decreased production in association with increased utilization is not always certain. Both mechanisms probably contribute to the neutropenia in at least some patients (161).

As might be anticipated, abnormalities in two antibacterial defense systems give rise to severe infections in these patients. In a family described by Lonsdale and his colleagues (203), three siblings died of infection before age three years.

Familial neutropenia possibly caused by deficiency of a plasma factor. In 1962 Bjure and his colleagues described two brothers with chronic neutropenia with onset at infancy (22). The bone marrow showed a decrease in granulocytes beyond the myelocyte stage. Cultivation of marrow in normal plasma in vitro resulted in myeloid proliferation, whereas cultivation in autologous plasma resulted in little cellular proliferation. Infusion of normal plasma in one brother led to transient increase in blood neutrophils. The inference from these observations is that the children lacked a serum factor necessary for normal myelopoiesis.

Chronic hypoplastic neutropenia. Adams and Witts (4), and Spaet and Dameshek (318), described patients with chronic neutropenia with decreased myeloid precursors in the bone marrow. The onset of disease generally occurrred early in adult life, but in one case it developed in childhood. The neutropenia generally was of moderate severity. In some patients there was a compensatory monocytosis. Splenectomy was of no benefit. There is no evidence for a hereditary factor, and the etiology of this syndrome is unknown.

Neutropenia associated with constitutional defects. Hypoplastic neutropenia has been described in association with a variety of constitutional defects (40, 120, 352). The genesis of the neutropenia is unknown in these disorders, and there is no reason to suppose that the multiple syndromes share a common pathogenesis.

Acquired Abnormalities of Granulocyte Production of Unknown Etiology

Paroxysmal nocturnal hemoglobinuria. Paroxysmal nocturnal hemoglobinuria (PNH) is a disorder of unknown etiology that may affect all hematopoietic lines. Its most prominent manifestation is generally hemolytic anemia (286). Leukopenia, and particularly granulocytopenia, occurs sometime in the course of the disease in more than half of the patients with PNH and may be associated with severe infection. Granulocytopenia usually occurs with a hypoplastic bone marrow and is assumed to result from underproduction of leukocytes.

The defect of this disorder may well be in a primitive hematopoietic progenitor cell, since certain red cell enzymes are abnormal, platelets are defective, and neutrophil alkaline phosphatase is often reduced (57, 333). It has been suggested that this disorder involves a defect of the granulocyte membrane, since PNH neutrophils are abnormally sensitive to antibody and complement (12).

PNH has followed drug-induced bone marrow hypoplasia (275). The drug-induced disease has the same characteristics as the more usual disorder with no known inciting agent. One suspects that all forms of this disease follow some type of injury to primitive hematopoietic cells of the bone marrow.

Disseminated lupus erythematosus. Neutropenia is frequently one of the clinical manifestations of systemic lupus (147). Little information is available on the mechanism of this leukopenia. Bishop and his colleagues (21) studied one patient with lupus and neutropenia: they found a granulocyte production rate less than 10 percent of normal and a normal half-life of granulocytes in the circulation. Interestingly, the bone marrow cellularity was considered to be normal, and the myeloid/erythroid ratio in the marrow was greatly increased. Unfortunately, little clinical information is available on this patient. Some patients with disseminated lupus erythematosus and neutropenia may have accelerated granulocyte destruction. One of the patients with suspected lupus studied by the same investigators did have splenomegaly and a markedly shortened blood granulocyte half-life.

Cirrhosis. Hepatic cirrhosis from diverse causes is occasionally associated with neutropenia. Based on analysis of the clinical data, the mechanism causing the neutropenia generally has been assumed to be accelerated cell destruction resulting from splenomegaly and "hypersplenism" secondary to portal vein hypertension. This is almost certainly the situation in some cirrhotic patients with neutropenia. However, Bishop and his colleagues (21) studied one patient in whom plasma clearance of granulocytes was delayed rather than accelerated and in whom the granulocyte production rate was about 25 percent of normal. This observation suggests that underproduction of neutrophils may be the pathogenetic mechanism underlying neutropenia in some cirrhotic patients.

In 1968 Rubin and his colleagues (289) described a syndrome of hepatitis and aplastic anemia characterized by bone marrow failure, neutropenia, and associated with icteric hepatitis and possibly anicteric hepatitis. Injury of the marrow by virus was suggested as a possible etiology.

Idiopathic neutropenia (agranulocytosis). Some of the patients with underproduction neutropenia do not fit any of the categories we have considered thus far. These cases occur sporadically rather than in families. The clinical manifestations and infectious complications vary with the severity of the neutropenia. The disease syndrome may merge into that of idiopathic aplastic anemia, where all the hematopoietic elements of the bone marrow are affected (154, 301). As might be anticipated, leukokinetic studies in at least some of these patients show diminished rates of granulocyte production (21). Some patients have diminished granulocyte survival as well.

Excessive Granulocyte Destruction

Thus far we have considered disorders in which underproduction of neutrophils in the bone marrow is the principal cause of lower-than-normal numbers of circulating neutrophils. Now we shall consider disorders in which neutropenia results primarily from excessive destruction of cells in the circulation or in the tissues.

Neutropenia develops if the peripheral depletion rate exceeds the bone marrow production rate. Excessive granulocyte utilization may result from splenic sequestration and destruction of cells, immunologic injury, mechanical trauma, or loss of cells in areas of inflammation.

The Concept of Hypersplenism Few concepts in clinical medicine are so vague as *hypersplenism* (167). A good working definition, however, is the reduction of one or more of the cellular elements of the peripheral blood that is associated with splenomegaly and that is corrected by removal of the spleen. One variant of this syndrome is *splenic neutropenia* (370), in which granulocytopenia and severe infections are associated with splenomegaly and are corrected by splenectomy.

The reduction of circulating neutrophils or other cellular elements in hypersplenism is generally thought to occur by their sequestration in an enlarged spleen (9, 88, 169). For example, when splenic artery and splenic vein blood is sampled in patients with hypersplenism, the leukocyte count is lower on the venous side (374).

Understanding the mechanism of cellular sequestration in the spleen requires a knowledge of the complex vascular anatomy of this organ (360, 361). The red pulp contains vascular spaces lined with phagocytic reticuloendothelial cells. Sequestration and stasis within these spaces, followed by phagocytosis, are the presumed mechanisms of blood cell removal in hypersplenism. As the blood percolates through the vascular channels of the spleen, the cells must pass through a unique fenestrated basement membrane, which separates the splenic cords from the lumen of the sinuses (362).

Splenic enlargement and hypersplenism may result from several causes: (a) increased pressure in the portal vein from thrombosis or cirrhosis of the liver (21, 23); (b) chronic infection or parasitic diseases such as tuberculosis and malaria (49); (c) malignant proliferative diseases such as leukemia and lymphoma; (d) myelofibrosis with myeloid metaplasia (21); (e) metabolic storage diseases such as Gaucher's (222); and (f) chronic hemolytic anemia such as hereditary spherocytosis (167). Splenic neutropenia can also occur in rare disorders such as Weber-Christian disease (21). In some instances the cause of the splenomegaly may be obscure and the disorder may be referred to as primary splenic neutropenia (89, 371).

The development of splenomegaly in certain hemolytic anemias may be an example of "work hypertrophy." In hemolysis the workload of the spleen increases as large numbers of damaged or defective erythrocytes are removed. The organ increases in size to compensate. The result is an enlarged spleen, which efficiently traps even normal, undamaged erythrocytes. A cycle of progressive cell destruction ensues (168, 170). The spleen seems to lose its discriminatory ability as it enlarges, removing leukocytes and platelets as well as erythrocytes. Similarly, as the phagocytic reticuloendothelial cells of the spleen proliferate in response to other indigestible materials, the organ may indiscriminately remove circulating cellular elements. Examples of this phenomenon may be seen in Gaucher's disease and in the experimental model of methyl cellulose injection (255). These are examples of "work hyperplasia," rather than "work hypertrophy," since there is an increase in spleen cell number rather than in the size of the individual cells.

Studies of DFP^{32}-labeled leukocytes in patients with hypersplenic granulocytopenia indicate the presence of large splenic granulocyte pools (277, 291), whereas normal subjects have no significant splenic storage pools of granulocytes. Patients with cirrhosis and splenomegaly often have a shortened granulocyte survival and normal, decreased, or increased rates of granulocyte production (21).

Immunologic Neutropenia Immunologic injury of neutrophils can result either from antibody, which interacts directly with some component of the cell surface, or with some extracellular antigen as, for example, a drug.

Drug-associated immunologic injury. The classic example that is usally cited for drug-induced immunologic injury of neutrophils is aminopyrine, a drug no longer in common use (79, 142, 215, 336, 380). Moeschlein and Wagner (232) suggested that this drug acts as a hapten, which links to the leukocyte surface. Antibody to the drug may be present in the circulation without deleterious effect until the drug is administered. When aminopyrine is given, the interaction of antibody with the leukocyte-bound drug results in cell agglutination and sequestration in the pulmonary capillary bed, and probably in other vascular filtration beds such as the spleen. The resultant neutropenia provokes a bone marrow response which may or may not compensate for the excessive destruction. "Marrow exhaustion," which was observed in some of the early cases, probably represented depletion of a critical nutrient such as folic acid.

Although the exact mechanism of immunologic injury to leukocytes is unknown, these are some of the suggested mechanisms: (a) the antibody interacts directly with the drug, which is bound to the cell surface; (b) the antibody interacts with antigen in the fluid phase of the blood and the immune complex adsorbs to the cell surface; (c) the antibody coats the cell surface and then reacts with administered antigen. The second of these suggested mechanisms is the most likely.

Since the description of aminopyrine agranulocytosis, a number of drugs have been linked to immunologic injury of granulocytes (146, 232). These include mercurial diuretics (184), phenylbutazone (363), chlorpromazine (158), and alpha-methyl dopa (56). Evidence that all of these drugs produce neutropenia by immune mechanisms is not especially convincing.

Other immunologic neutropenias. The neutropenic condition thought to arise from maternal-fetal incompatibility is called *neonatal isoimmunization neutropenia* (30, 143, 171, 193, 287). This subject has recently been reviewed by Nymand and his associates (248). The presumed mechanism of neutropenia is transplacental passage of antibody from the mother to fetal leukocytes. The condition is most commonly seen in women with repeated opportunities of exposure to antigen derived from the father as a result of multiple pregnancies. The situation is analogous to erythroblastosis fetalis, in which maternal antibody is directed against antigens present on fetal erythrocytes. Neutropenia in the neonate may be severe and may persist for six to twelve weeks. However, maternal leukoagglutinins having no deleterious effect on the newborn may also exist (2, 143, 258).

A condition related to neonatal isoimmunization neutropenia is one in which transient neonatal neutropenia is observed in infants born of granulocytopenic mothers (305, 320). Maternal systemic lupus erythematosus may be the most common disorder in which this phenomenon occurs.

In postnatal life, leukoagglutinins have been observed in a variety of disorders (80, 231, 341, 354). These include systemic lupus erythematosus, rheumatoid arthritis, and Felty's syndrome. The leukoagglutinins are most commonly observed in the patient transfused many times (257). In such patients transfusion of blood containing leukocytes may result in severe febrile reactions.

It is not certain that the presence of leukoagglutinins in the adult indicates that the patient's own neutrophils are being rapidly destroyed. In some instances, however, leukoagglutinins clearly are correlated with shortened granulocyte survival (138).

Felty's Syndrome and Systemic Lupus Erythematosus
Leukopenia is frequent in systemic lupus erythematosus (SLE) (96, 147) and is part of the complex of rheumatoid arthritis and splenomegaly that defines Felty's syndrome (61, 83, 104). Felty's syndrome occurs in about 1 percent of patients with rheumatoid arthritis (61). Other features of this syndrome may include weight loss, malaise, anemia, thrombocytopenia, lymphadenopathy, leg ulcers, and frequent infections (236).

In both systemic lupus and Felty's syndrome, more than one mechanism may be operative in reducing granulocyte survival. Two that are possible are circulating leukoagglutinins (102) and splenomegaly with hypersplenism (24, 39, 47). In both Felty's syndrome and SLE, granulocyte survival in the circulation may be reduced. In patients with Felty's syndrome there may be a low ratio of the circulating granulocyte pool to the total body granulocyte pool, indicating sequestration of granulocytes in the spleen. In some patients with lupus, and perhaps some with Felty's syndrome, diminished granulocyte production contributes to the development of neutropenia (21).

A number of reports on the results of splenectomy in Felty's syndrome are available. In 1968 Sandusky, Rudolf, and Leavell (294) reviewed 104 cases reported in the English language literature. Forty-six cases subsequently were added in other series (24, 236, 251, 290). Immediately following splenectomy, the neutrophil count rises to normal levels in about 80 percent of patients (236). However, some of these patients subsequently relapse, with the result that a long-term beneficial effect is achieved in only 60 to 70 percent. Retrospective studies generally have shown a decreased incidence of infection following splenectomy (137).

Perfusion and Surface-induced Neutrophil Injury   Severe neutropenia has been noted during the first hour of hemodialysis with several types of hemodialyzers (134, 174). The neutrophil count usually returns to normal or supernormal levels within $1\frac{1}{2}$ to 3 hours. This return is the result of reentry of cells from the marginated granulocyte pools and entry of new cells from bone marrow stores (37). The mechanism of granulocyte sequestration during the neutropenic phase is unclear; disappearance of almost all neutrophils from the circulation occurs when no more than 5 or 10 percent of the total blood volume could have traversed the dialysis coil. Toren and his colleagues (339) suggested that a soluble substance was released into the blood, leading to granulocyte sequestration in the lung.

In addition to the experience with the hemodialyzer, other clinical (130, 206) and experimental (117) studies indicate that leukocytes may be susceptible to perfusion-induced injury. For example, use of pump oxygenators of the type used in heart-lung bypass procedures may lead to transient drops in leukocyte count. Similar drops may be seen with bubble, film, and membrane oxygenators (32, 117, 188, 189). Both rheological (flow) factors and foreign surface effects traumatize nucleated blood cells. Granulocytes may also adhere to a plastic surface (150).

In addition to a decrease in the numbers of granulocytes induced by perfusion, morphologic abnormalities, including vacuolization, ragged cytoplasm, and distortion of nuclear lobulation, may be seen. The damaged cells have decreased phagocytic activity.

Miscellaneous Disorders with Increased Granulocyte Destruction   In 1964 Krill and his colleagues described a nine-year-old girl with chronic idiopathic granulocytopenia characterized by active marrow myelopoiesis, impaired granulocyte release, and a shortened granulocyte survival time (185). The mature neutrophils were morphologically abnormal. In the same year Zuelzer described a ten-year-old girl with granulocytopenia, evidence for intramedullary death of leukocytes, and decreased viability of granulocytes (382). Morphologic and functional abnormalities of the mature cells were prominent. He called

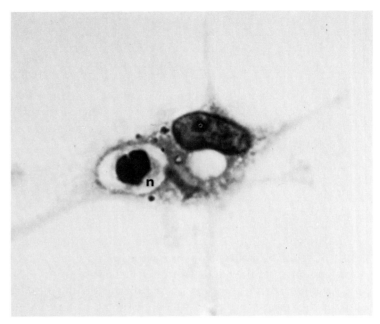

Figure 9.6 A macrophage containing a phagocytized neutrophil (*n*) undergoing degeneration (from a patient with histiocytic medullary reticulosis).

the disorder *myelokathexis.* The pathogenetic mechanisms of these two disorders are unknown.

In histiocytic medullary reticulosis, a rare malignant disorder (see Chapter 27), phagocytosis of leukocytes by malignant reticuloendothelial cells may occur (Fig. 9.6). Erythrophagocytosis, often considered the hallmark of this disease, is generally more prominent than leukophagocytosis. It has been suggested, but not proven, that leukophagocytosis may contribute to the neutropenia sometimes observed in this interesting disorder (242).

Neutropenia from a Combination of Increased Destruction and Diminished Production

Many of the neutropenic disorders that we have considered thus far as arising *primarily* from either diminished production or enhanced utilization may in fact involve both mechanisms to some degree. For example, Felty's syndrome is primarily a disorder of granulocyte utilization, but decreased granulocyte production may contribute to the neutropenia in some patients. The same phenomenon probably exists in neutropenias associated with vitamin B_{12} and folic acid deficiency (99, 219).

The severe neutropenias associated with overwhelming bacterial and mycobacterial infection may be another example of multiple causal factors. Bone marrow hypoplasia and "toxic" changes in the neutrophil may be seen with such infections (107, 178, 241, 297). The occurrence of

granulocytopenia during the course of severe infection generally has grave prognostic implications. A similar pattern of marrow hypoplasia in the alcoholic patient with severe sepsis may be seen, and it is suspected that in this circumstance both diminished production and increased utilization contribute to the neutropenia (31, 212).

Finally, the rare familial disorder known as Chediak-Higashi syndrome may show the abnormalities of both production and destruction (25). This disorder is described in more detail below.

Abnormal Distribution of Neutrophils

Neutropenia apparently can result from a shift of cells from the circulating pool into the marginal pool. This disorder has been called *shift neutropenia.* Bishop and his colleagues (21) observed that in subjects with minimal to moderate neutropenia (greater than 1,000 neutrophils per cubic millimeter), the neutropenia may reflect a shift of cells into the marginal sites. In these subjects the neutrophil level tends to fluctuate from neutropenic to normal levels and, in some cases, can be increased by epinephrine injection. The diseases that these patients suffered included Weber-Christian disease, cirrhosis, Felty's syndrome, idiopathic hemolytic anemia, macroglobulinemia, and multiple myeloma. In malaria, granulocytes may be released prematurely from the marrow, with a subsequent shift of circulating cells into the marginal pool (78).

Neutrophilia

Definitions

Neutrophilia is defined as an increase above normal in the number of circulating neutrophils. In the adult this generally means more than 8,000 cells of the neutrophilic series per cubic millimeter. The term *granulocytosis* is often used interchangeably, although strictly speaking it refers to an increase in all types of granulocytes—neutrophils, eosinophils, and basophils. *Leukocytosis* refers to an absolute increase in the concentration of leukocytes in the peripheral blood without reference to cell type or level of maturity. A *leukemoid reaction* is a leukocytosis resembling leukemia but arising from another cause such as infection (187). In the adult, 10,000 leukocytes per cubic millimeter may be taken as the upper limit of normal.

Mechanisms of Neutrophilia

There are several possible mechanisms that might cause an increase in the number of neutrophils in the circulation: (*a*) a sustained increase in cell production by the bone marrow; (*b*) a transient increase in neutrophil release from stores in the bone marrow; (c) a reduced rate of egress of cells from the circulation; and (d) a shift of cells from the marginal to the circulating granulocyte pool (50, 69, 70).

Acute granulocytic reactions generally involve release of cells from marrow storage pools and a shift of cells from the marginal to the circulating pool (263). These reactions generally occur within a few hours following the application of a stimulus such as administration of endotoxin or a pyrogenic steroid, or a febrile transfusion reaction. The mechanisms of leukocyte release under these circumstances are uncertain, although a number of leukocytosis-inducing blood "factors" have been proposed as the possible control mechanism (19, 28, 132, 175, 223, 285, 324). Blood flow factors also may be important in a shift of cells into the circulation.

Chronic granulocytosis usually reflects increased production of cells within the bone marrow proliferative compartment. This mechanism probably accounts for the granulocytosis associated with lithium carbonate therapy for manic depressive psychosis (338). With some stimuli such as glucocorticoids, reduced egress of cells from the circulation and shifts of cells from the marginal pool may contribute to neutrophilia (20). Chronic infection may also involve these multiple mechanisms of producing granulocytosis and immature neutrophils in the circulation ("shift to the left"). Chronic granulocytosis may persist for weeks or months. Very high concentrations of neutrophils do not in themselves seem to have much influence on the flow properties of the blood (325).

The neutrophilia associated with polycythemia vera, infection, or myelofibrosis is usually associated with increases in total blood granulocyte pool, in circulating granulocyte pool, and granulocytic turnover rate, and often delayed egress of cells from the circulation (14).

A number of hypothetical humoral factors that stimulate granulopoiesis have been described (69, 70, 114, 132, 175, 202, 245, 285, 312, 323, 331, 342). Despite this plethora of humoral regulators, none has emerged as being clearly an important control mechanism.

Neutrophilia and the Differential Diagnosis of Leukemoid Reaction

In this section we shall consider neutrophilic disorders arising from an identifiable physical or chemical stimulus or associated with inflammatory disease. Neutrophilia occurring in such circumstances has been designated *reactive neutrophilia*. A list of conditions in which reactive neutrophilia has been described is given in Table 9.6. The myeloproliferative disorders in which neutrophilia occurs and in which neither an identifiable physical or chemical

Table 9.6 Causes of neutrophilia.

Causes	References
Infectious and parasitic diseases, including bacterial, fungal, viral, mycobacterial, and rickettsial diseases	36, 58, 97, 156, 159, 162, 187, 314, 326, 343, 372
Inflammatory diseases of uncertain etiology: rheumatoid arthritis, colitis, thyroiditis, vasculitis, acute gout	155, 156, 159, 313
Malignant disease: Hodgkin's disease, renal cell carcinoma, infiltration of the marrow	42, 44, 53, 92, 103, 156, 224, 304, 367, 379
Drugs and chemicals: corticosteroids, epinephrine, etiocholanolone, ethylene glycol, venoms, histamine, mercury poisoning, lithium carbonate	20, 66, 92, 105, 114, 125, 155, 225, 338, 367
Physical stimuli: exercise, burns, cold, trauma, electric shock, labor, pregnancy, anoxia, ozone	13, 26, 67, 119, 190, 282
Emotional stress, probably mediated via hormonal stimuli	227
Metabolic disorders: diabetic ketoacidosis, thyroid storm, eclampsia	340, 367
Hematologic disorders: acute hemolytic anemia, myeloproliferative disorders, hemorrhage, postsplenectomy, transfusion reactions, therapy of megaloblastic anemia	73, 159, 187, 208, 276, 283, 300
Miscellaneous: hepatic necrosis, familial urticaria, certain congenital disorders, exfoliative dermatitis, chronic idiopathic leukocytosis, hereditary and familial leukocytosis	62, 98, 276, 317, 337, 357, 369

agent nor an inflammatory disease can be identified are considered in the next section of this chapter and in Chapters 10 and 11.

When the magnitude of the reactive neutrophilia or granulocytosis is such as to suggest leukemia, the term *leukemoid reaction* is used. Leukemoid reactions usually involve granulocytic elements—rarely lymphocytic. These reactions must be considered in the differential diagnosis of leukemia (see Chapter 11). Among the causes of neutrophilia presented in Table 9.6, only a few are sometimes confused with granulocytic leukemia. These include: (a) "solid" tumors, particularly those involving the bone marrow, such as carcinoma of the breast, bronchus, and kidney; (b) chronic intracellular infections, such as tuberculosis; and (c) some drug reactions. Figure 9.7 is a peripheral blood smear of a patient with a severe penicillin reaction.

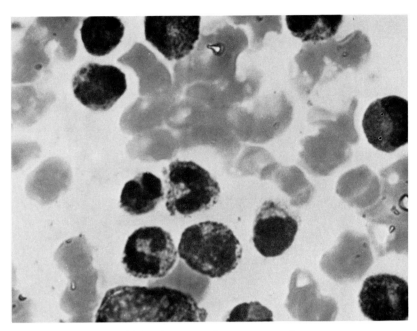

Figure 9.7 Peripheral blood smear of a patient with a severe penicillin reaction; Wright stain.

Shift Neutrophilia

The term *shift neutrophilia* indicates an increased number of neutrophils per cubic millimeter of blood without a concomitant increase in the total blood granulocyte pool. The phenomenon results from a shift of cells from the marginal to the circulating pool. Stimuli such as exercise, epinephrine, and etiocholanolone may cause such a shift. It is quite likely that the persistent leukocytosis that follows splenectomy also reflects a shift in the distribution of cells (208).

The Peculiar Neutrophil: Abnormal Morphogenesis

Inherited Abnormalities of Leukocyte Morphology

A number of inherited disorders with associated morphologically abnormal neutrophils exist. In some, neutrophil function is deranged; in others, it is apparently normal.

Hereditary Hypersegmentation and Hereditary Macropolycytes In 1954 and later Undritz described a hypersegmentation of the neutrophils inherited as an autosomal dominant without other associated clinical abnormalities (344, 345, 347). A similar condition involving eosinophils exists. In these conditions the mean nuclear index exceeds four lobes per cell, whereas the normal is slightly less than three.

In 1960 Davidson and his colleagues described an inherited anomaly of giant neutrophils. No other clinical

abnormalities are associated, and the neutrophils are probably normal in function. These cells, which have twice the normal neutrophil volume, are also hypersegmented (82).

The existence of an inherited disorder of anomalous nuclear appendages has been described (81, 82) and may occasionally be encountered in routine blood smears (see Fig. 9.8).

Pelger-Huët Anomaly This anomaly of neutrophil morphogenesis is characterized by failure of normal development of the nuclear lobes (261). It is transmitted as a simple autosomal dominant characteristic and is fairly common in the general population—about 1 in 6,000 people (163, 164). The heterozygotes have mature neutrophils with bilobed nuclei (Fig. 9.9). Homozygotes have mature neutrophils with round nuclei containing clumped chromatin (18).

In 1969 Schneiderman and his colleagues (296) described a family with two unusual autosomal dominant conditions: muscular dystrophy and Pelger-Huët anomaly. Family studies suggested that these abnormalities were linked on the same chromosome. Interestingly, the appearance of the Pelger phenomenon usually antedated that of the muscular dystrophy. Subjects carrying the gene for muscular dystrophy, which was destined to be manifest in later life, were marked at birth by the Pelger-Huët anomaly.

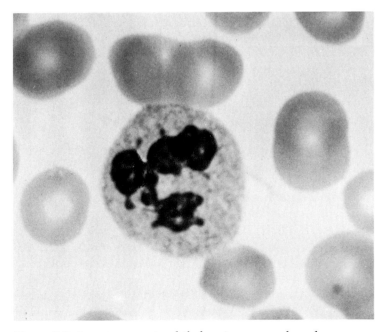

Figure 9.8 A mature neutrophil showing unusual nuclear appendages.

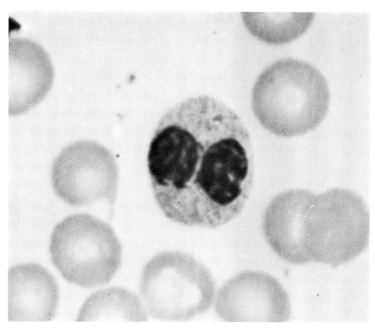

Figure 9.9 A mature neutrophil with a bilobed nucleus (from a patient with heterozygous Pelger-Huët anomaly).

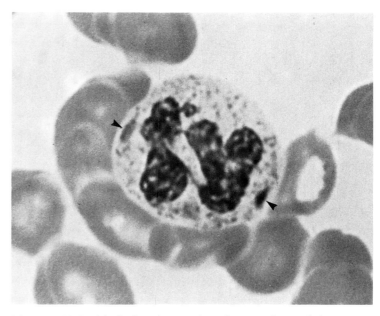

Figure 9.10 Döhle bodies (*arrows*) in the periphery of the cytoplasm of a mature neutrophil.

The morphologically abnormal neutrophils of this anomaly have no apparent functional impairment (346). A similar neutrophil anomaly described in rabbits may be associated with other congenital anomalies (144). As will be described below, morphologically abnormal leukocytes resembling those of the Pelger-Huët anomaly may be seen in several diseases.

May-Hegglin Anomaly May (221) and subsequently Hegglin (149) described a clinical entity characterized by large, bizarre platelets; leukopenia; and neutrophils containing one or two large intracytoplasmic inclusions known as Döhle bodies (Fig. 9.10). Similar inclusions of dense fibrils 50 Å in diameter may be seen in a variety of acquired disorders (172). They may consist of RNA and ribosomes (197, 359).

A number of studies (253, 264, 359) have confirmed the familial nature of this condition and suggested a dominant mode of inheritance. In some families with the disorder chromosomal abnormalities occur (41), but this is not a universal finding (121). About one-third of reported cases have thrombocytopenia. Many of these are asymptomatic (264, 298, 359), but others have a hemorrhagic diathesis (253). Abnormalities of platelet function have also been demonstrated (197).

Alder-Reilly Anomaly The Alder-Reilly anomaly of neutrophils is part of a constellation of clinical manifesta-

tions arising from disordered polysaccharide metabolism 5, 278, 279). Giant "granules" are seen in neutrophils in association with other anomalies such as gargoylism (112). Similar granules may be observed in monocytes and lymphocytes.

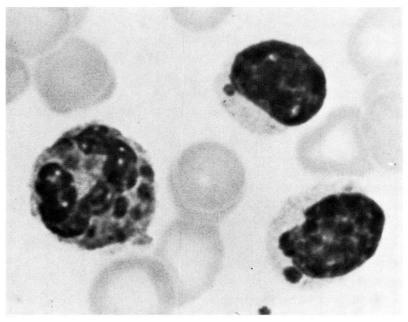

Figure 9.11 Enlarged granules (lysosomes) in a neutrophil and lymphocytes from a patient with Chediak-Higashi syndrome.

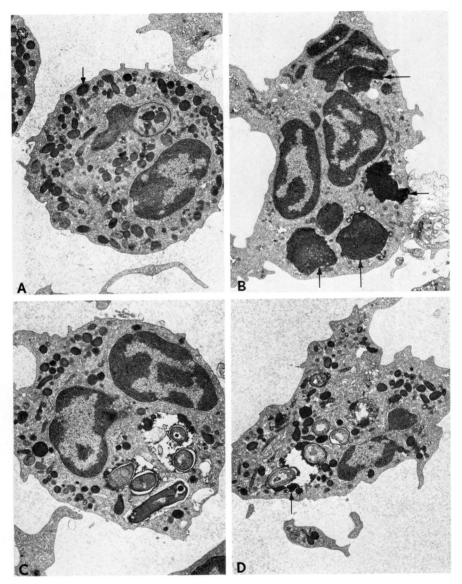

Figure 9.12 Electron micrographs of granulocytes histochemically stained for peroxidase activity. *A* shows a normal granulocyte and *B* a Chediak-Higashi syndrome granulocyte without ingested particles. Arrows point to peroxidase-positive lysosomes. *C* and *D* show representative sections of normal granulocytes 15 minutes after mixing with *Staphylococcus aureus*. Note the dark staining peroxidase activity in phagosomes surrounding bacteria and evidence of active degranulation (*arrow* in *D*). (From R. K. Root, A. S. Rosenthal, and D. J. Balestra, *J. Clin. Invest.* 51:649, 1972. Reprinted by permission of authors and publisher.)

Chediak-Higashi Syndrome In this disorder giant granules are seen in the neutrophils and other leukocytes (Figs. 9.11 to 9.13), and giant lysosomes occur in other cells throughout the body. Leukopenia and increased susceptibility to infection are common (25, 186). There may be increased destruction of granulocytes within the marrow. Patients surviving repeated infections often die of hematologic malignancy. Because the neutrophils of this anomaly are believed to be defective in function, as well as morphologically abnormal, they have been described in more detail in Chapter 8.

Acquired Abnormalities of Granulocyte Morphogenesis

Hypersegmentation and Macropolycytes Hypersegmentation of the mature neutrophils (see Fig. 9.5) and larger than normal granulocytes at all levels of maturation occur in patients with deficiency of vitamin B_{12} or folic acid. Such enlargement is not restricted to granulocytes, but is observed in other dividing cells throughout the body. Similar changes may be induced by antimetabolite drugs, which interfere with DNA synthesis. Examples of such drugs in common use are 6-mercaptopurine, cytosine arabinoside, and methotrexate. Chronic infection may also produce marcrocytes (272).

Pseudo-Pelger-Huët Anomaly Morphologic changes resembling the Pelger-Huët anomaly have been described in the neutrophils of several myeloproliferative diseases (91, 308). Single reports have associated this anomaly with severe myxedema (309), influenza (101), and sulfisoxazole therapy (173).

Döhle Bodies Döhle bodies are large, pale blue, intracytoplasmic inclusions of granulocytes (see Fig. 9.10). Usually located in the inner rim of the cytoplasm, they occur following chemotherapy and in a variety of disorders, including infection, trauma, burns, and malignant diseases (90, 166).

"Toxic" Granulation and Vacuolization Coarse "toxic" granules in the cytoplasm of neutrophils sometimes occur in association with vacuolization and may be seen in a variety of conditions (Figs. 9.14 to 9.16). They most commonly accompany infections, serious burns, and acute inflammatory diseases (209, 272). Vacuolization may be a laboratory hint of the presence of septicemia (381).

The pathogenesis of toxic granules and their significance have been discussed in Chapter 1. The mechanism of vacuole production is uncertain. In some cases the vacuoles may represent phagocytic vacuoles in which the

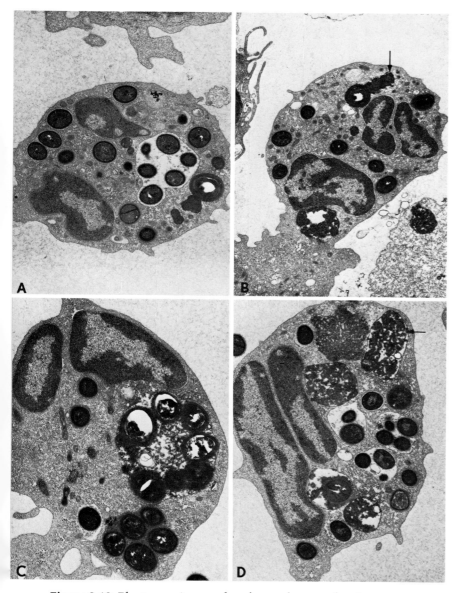

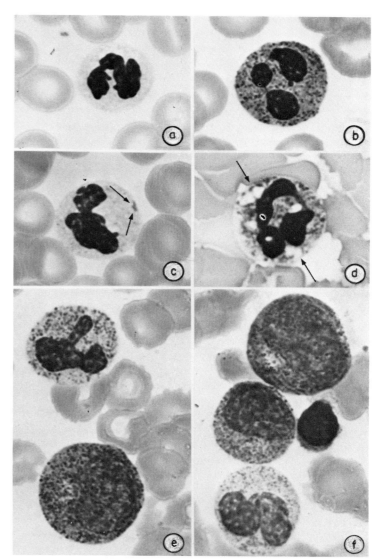

Figure 9.13 Electron micrographs of granulocytes that have phagocytized *Staphylococcus aureus* and are histochemically stained for peroxidase. *A* and *B* depict sections of Chediak-Higashi syndrome granulocytes taken 15 minutes after mixing with staphylococci. Note the lack of peroxidase activity around most phagosomes, with the exception of those into which giant lysosomes (*arrows*) appear to be discharging their contents. In *C* a normal granulocyte is shown 60 minutes after mixing with staphylococci and demonstrates phagosomal fusion with peroxidase activity in the phagosomes and a lack of peroxidase-positive granules in the cytoplasm. *D* shows a Chediak-Higashi syndrome granulocyte after the same time interval and displays the persistence of structurally intact peroxidase-positive giant lysosomes (*arrows*). Peroxidase activity can be seen in some, but not all, phagosomes. (From R. K. Root, A. S. Rosenthal, and D. J. Balestra, *J. Clin. Invest.* 51:649, 1972. Reprinted by permission of authors and publisher.)

Figure 9.14 Section *a:* Normal blood neutrophil, Wright-stained for 4 minutes. Magnification × 1,860.

Section *b:* Normal blood neutrophil, Wright-stained for 60 minutes. Granules are deeply stained and appear similar to those visible in toxic cells. Magnification × 2,000.

Section *c:* Döhle body (*arrows*) within cytoplasm of a blood neutrophil, Wright-stained for 4 minutes. Magnification × 2,000.

Section *d:* Cytoplasmic vacuolization (*arrows*) in toxic blood neutrophil, Wright-stained for 4 minutes. Magnification × 2,000.

Section *e:* Toxic granulation in mature neutrophil and metamyelocyte from blood smear of a bacteremic patient, Wright-stained for 4 minutes. Magnification × 2,000.

Section *f:* Bone marrow smear from patient with toxic neutrophils in peripheral blood. Azurophilic granules of neutrophil precursors resemble toxic granules in mature neutrophil. Wright-stained for 4 minutes. Magnification × 2,000. (From C. E. McCall, I. Katayama, R. S. Cotran, and M. Finland, *J. Exp. Med.* 129:267, 1969. Reprinted by permission of authors and publisher.)

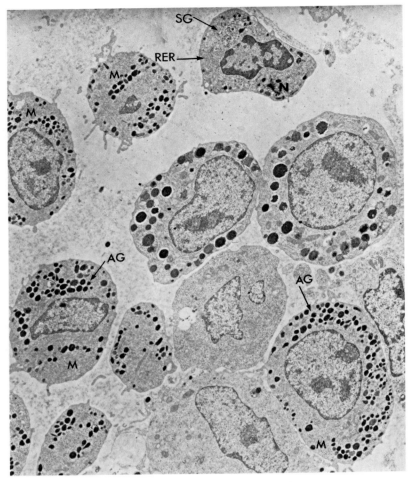

Figure 9.15 Electron micrograph of bone marrow from a patient with bacteremia. Cells labeled *M* are immature neutrophil precursors. Note numerous large, dense granules (*AG*). Cell labeled *N* is a more mature neutrophil showing a group of specific granules (*SG*) and an aggregate of rough endoplasmic reticulum (*RER*). Magnification × 4,500. (From C. E. McCall, I. Katayama, R. S. Cotran, and M. Finland, *J. Exp. Med.* 129:267, 1969. Reprinted by permission of authors and publisher.)

organism has been digested. Vacuolated neutrophils are common in exudative joint fluids, especially in rheumatoid arthritis (216).

Other Acquired Abnormalities   The lobe count of the polymorphonuclear leukocyte is reduced in congenital hypothroidism and with therapy returns to normal levels (182). In addition to the acquired neutrophil anomalies that are obvious on Romanovsky-stained smears (315), there are other abnormalities that may be detected only by special histochemical techniques (333) or by osmotically stressing the cells (247).

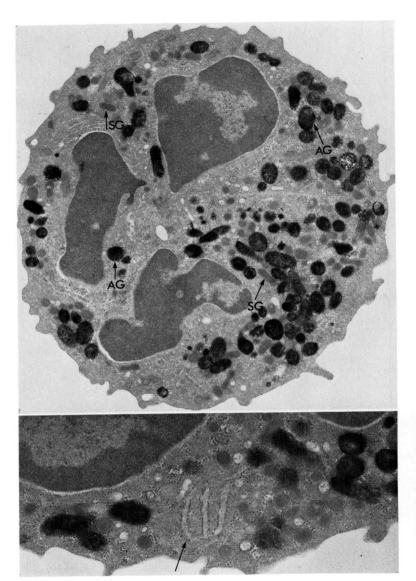

Figure 9.16 *Top:* Electron micrograph of toxic neutrophil reacted for peroxidase. Large dense azurophilic granules (*AG*) are peroxidase-positive and most specific granules (*SG*) are peroxidase-negative. Lead stain. Magnification × 21,000. *Bottom:* Toxic neutrophil reacted for peroxidase. The arrays of rough endoplasmic reticulum (*arrow*) are peroxidase-negative. Lead stain. Magnification × 25,000. (From C. E. McCall, L. Katayama, R. S. Cotran, and M. Finland, *J. Exp. Med.* 129:267, 1969. Reprinted by permission of authors and publisher.)

Summary and Perspectives in Therapy

To better understand diseases with too many or too few neutrophils, a knowledge of the normal production and distribution of these cells in needed. The neutropenias and neutrophilias may be classified on the basis of abnormalities of cell production, abnormalities of cell survival, or abnormalities of distribution within the various compartments of the body. Once such a classification is made, the cause of the abnormality should be determined. In this chapter several congenital and acquired diseases of neutrophil production and kinetics have been catalogued, and various abnormalities of neutrophil morphogenesis have been discussed. Familiarity with the fundamentals of the morphologic development of granulocytes (set forth in Chapter 1) facilitates a better understanding of these diseases.

Some of the disorders of neutrophil morphogenesis have associated clinical manifestations. All the neutropenic syndromes are characterized by enhanced susceptibility to infection when the granulocyte count is sufficiently reduced. The therapy for such neutropenic diseases is generally two-pronged: specific therapy directed at the underlying cause of the disease, and supportive therapy directed at the infectious complications. The latter approach generally encompasses appropriate antibiotic treatment. Only recently has another modality of therapy been introduced—replacement therapy. In principle, one should be able to apply the same techniques to granulocyte replacement as have been applied to red cell transfusion. The major hurdles to be crossed in leukocyte transfusion are procurement technology and histocompatibility factors. Procurement techniques recently have improved to the point where reasonable numbers of granulocytes may be transfused into neutropenic recipients (87, 135, 136, 153). In addition, the histocompatibility factors necessary for successful transfusion are becoming clarified (128).

Another type of approach to the problem of a functionally abnormal or quantitatively reduced hematopoietic stem cell pool is bone marrow transplantation. This technique has been applied successfully to the treatment of bone marrow failure. The current status of bone marrow transplantation will be discussed briefly in Chapter 21.

Chapter 9 References

1. Aarskog, D. Infantile congenital aneutrocytosis, *Arch. Dis. Child.* 36:511, 1961.

2. Abildgaard, H., and Jensen, K. G. The influence of maternal leucocyte antibodies on infants, *Scand. J. Haematol.* 1:47, 1964.

3. Ackerman, B. D. Dysgammaglobulinemia: report of a case with a family history of a congenital gamma globulin disorder, *Pediatrics* 34:211, 1964.

4. Adams, E. B., and Witts, L. J. Chronic agranulocytosis, *Q. J. Med.* 18:173, 1949.

5. Alder, A. Über Konstitutionell bedingte Granulationsveränderungen der Leukocyten, *Dtsch. Arch. Klin. Med.* 183:372, 1939.

6. Alestig, K. Cyclic agranulocytosis treated with steroids, *Acta Med. Scand.* 169:253, 1961.

7. A.M.A. Council on Drugs. Registry on adverse reactions, tabulation of reports, panel on hematology, Chicago, 1964.

8. A.M.A. Council on Drugs. Evaluation of a new oral diuretic agent. Ethacrynic acid and ethacrynate sodium (edecrin and edecrin sodium), *J.A.M.A.* 208:2327, 1969.

9. Amorosi, E. L. Hypersplenism, *Semin. Hematol.* 2:249, 1965.

10. Amrhein, J. A., Kenny, F. M., and Ross, D. Granulocytopenia, lupus-like syndrome and other complications of propylthiouracil therapy, *J. Pediatr.* 76:54, 1970.

11. Arrowsmith, W. R., Binkley, B., and Moore, C. V. Fatal agranulocytosis following the intraperitoneal implantation of sulfanilamide crystals, *Ann. Intern. Med.* 21:323, 1944.

12. Aster, R. H., and Enright, S. E. A platelet and granulocyte membrane defect in paroxysmal nocturnal hemoglobinuria: usefulness for the detection of platelet antibodies, *J. Clin. Invest.* 48:1199, 1969.

13. Athens, J. W. Tagging white blood cells, *J.A.M.A.* 198:43, 1966.

14. Athens, J. W., Haab, O. P., Raab, S. O., Boggs, D. R., Ashenbrucker, H. E., Cartwright, G. E., and Wintrobe, M. M. Leukokinetic studies. XI. Blood granulocyte kinetics in polycythemia vera, infection and myelofibrosis, *J. Clin. Invest.* 44:778, 1965.

15. Baehner, R. L., and Johnston, R. B., Jr.: Monocyte function in children with neutropenia and chronic infections, *Blood* 40:31, 1972.

16. Barzel, U. S. Quinidine-sulfate-induced hypoplastic anemia and agranulocytosis, *J.A.M.A.* 201:325, 1967.

17. Baumann, Th. Konstitutionelle Panmyelophthise mit multiplen Abartungen (Fanconi-Syndrom), *Ann. Paediatr.* 177:65, 1951.

18. Begemann, N. H., and Campagne, A. van L. Homozygous form of Pelger-Huët's nuclear anomaly in man, *Acta Haematol.* 7:295, 1952.

19. Bierman, H. R. Characteristics of leukopoietin G in animals and man, *Ann. N.Y. Acad. Sci.* 113:753, 1964.

20. Bishop, C. R., Athens, J. W., Boggs, D. R., Warner, H. R., Cartwright, G. E., and Wintrobe, M. M. Leukokinetic studies. XIII. A non-steady-state kinetic evaluation of the mechanism of cortisone-induced granulocytosis, *J. Clin. Invest.* 47:249, 1968.

21. Bishop, C. R., Rothstein, G., Ashenbrucker, H. E., and Athens, J. W. Leukokinetic studies. XIV. Blood neutrophil kinetics in chronic steady-state neutropenia, *J. Clin. Invest.* 50:1678, 1971.

22. Bjure, J., Nilsson, L. R., and Plum, C. M. Familial neutropenia possibly caused by deficiency of a plasma factor, *Acta Paediatr.* 51:497, 1962.

23. Blackman, A., Grace, N., Chandler, H., Iber, F., and Greenberg, M. Hypersplenism in cirrhosis: measurements of portal pressure, spleen size and circulating blood cell disappearance rates, *Clin. Res.* 17:298, 1969.

24. Blendis, L. M., Ansell, I. D., Jones, K. L., Hamilton, E., and Williams, R. Liver in Felty's syndrome, *Br. Med. J.* 1:131, 1970.

25. Blume, R. S., Bennett, J. M., Yankee, R. A., and Wolff, S. M. Defective granulocyte regulation in the Chediak-Higashi syndrome, *N. Engl. J. Med.* 279:1009, 1968.

26. Bobb, G. A., and Fairchild, E. J. Neutrophil-to-lymphocyte ratio as indicator of ozone exposure, *Toxicol. Appl. Pharmacol.* 11:558, 1967.

27. Bodian, M., Sheldon, W., and Lightwood, R. Congenital hypoplasia of the exocrine pancreas, *Acta Paediatr.* 53:282, 1964.

28. Boggs, D. R., Marsh, J. C., Chervenick, P. A., Cartwright, G. E., and Wintrobe, M. M. Neutrophil releasing activity in plasma of normal human subjects injected with endotoxin, *Proc. Soc. Exp. Biol. Med.* 127:689, 1968.

29. Bousser, J., and Neyde, R. La neutropénie familiale, *Sangre* 18:521, 1947.

30. Braun, E. H., Buckwold, A. E., Emson, H. E., and Russell, A. V. Familial neonatal neutropenia with maternal leucocyte antibodies, *Blood* 16:1745, 1960.

31. Brayton, R. G., Stokes, P. E., Schwartz, M. S., and Louria, D. B. Effect of alcohol and various diseases on leukocyte mobilization, phagocytosis and intracellular bacterial killing, *N. Engl. J. Med.* 282:123, 1970.

32. Brinsfield, D. E., Hopf, M. A., Geering, R. B., and Galletti, P. M. Hematological changes in long-term perfusion, *J. Appl. Physiol.* 17:531, 1962.

33. Brittingham, T. E., and Chaplin, H., Jr. Febrile transfusion reactions caused by sensitivity to donor leukocytes and platelets, *J.A.M.A.* 165:819, 1957.

34. Brodsky, I., Reimann, H. A., and Dennis, L. H. Treatment of cyclic neutropenia with testosterone, *Am. J. Med.* 38:802, 1965.

35. Broun, G. O., Jr., Herbig, F. K., and Hamilton, J. R. Leukopenia in Negroes, *N. Engl. J. Med.* 275:1410, 1966.

36. Brown, H. W. Basic Clinical Parasitology, 3rd ed., Appleton-Century-Crofts, New York, 1969.

37. Brubaker, L. H., and Nolph, K. D. Mechanisms of recovery from neutropenia induced by hemodialysis, *Blood* 38:623, 1971.

38. Brun, J., Perrin-Fayolie, M., and Sedallian, A. La Gentamycine en pneumologie. Etude clinique et bacteriologique, *Lyon Med.* 218:1263, 1967.

39. Brunner, C. M., and Davis, J. S. IV. Characteristics of antinuclear factors in Felty's syndrome, *Arthritis Rheum.* 13:33, 1970.

40. Bryan, H. G., and Nixon, R. K. Dyskeratosis congenita and familial

pancytopenia, *J.A.M.A.* 192:203, 1965.

41. Buchanan, J. G., Pearce, L., and Wetherley-Mein, G. The May-Hegglin anomaly. A family report and chromosome study, *Br. J. Haematol.* 10:508, 1964.

42. Burnham, C. F. Hodgkin's disease. With special reference to its treatment by irradiation, *J.A.M.A.* 87:1445, 1926.

43. Burke, V., Colebatch, J. H., Anderson, C. M., and Simons, M. J. Association of pancreatic insufficiency and chronic neutropenia in childhood, *Arch. Dis. Child.* 42:147, 1967.

44. Burkett, L. L., Cox, M. L., and Fields, M. L. Leukoerythroblastosis in the adult, *Am. J. Clin. Pathol.* 44:494, 1965.

45. Cahan, A. M., Meilman, E., and Jacobson, B. M. Agranulocytosis following pyrabenzamine, *N. Engl. J. Med.* 241:865, 1949.

46. Calabresi, P., and Welch, A. D. Cytotoxic drugs, hormones, and radioactive isotopes, *in* L. S. Goodman and A. Gilman (eds.), The Pharmacological Basis of Therapeutics, p. 1345, Macmillan, New York, 1965.

47. Calabresi, P., Edwards, E. A., and Schilling, R. F. Fluorescent antiglobulin studies in leukopenic and related disorders, *J. Clin. Invest.* 38:2091, 1959.

48. Cartwright, G. E. Diagnostic Laboratory Hematology, 3rd, ed., Grune & Stratton, New York, 1963.

49. Cartwright, G. E., Athens, J. W., Haab, O. P., Raab, S. O., Boggs, D. R., and Wintrobe, M. M. Blood granulocyte kinetics in conditions associated with granulocytosis, *Ann. N.Y. Acad. Sci.* 113:963, 1964.

50. Cartwright, G. E., Chung, H-L., and Chang, A. Studies on the pancytopenia of kala-azar, *Blood* 3:249, 1948.

51. Casey, T. P. Drug-induced blood dyscrasias, *N.Z. Med. J.* 67:599, 1968.

52. Chapman, R. A. Suspected adverse reactions to indomethacin, *Can. Med. Assoc. J.* 95:1156, 1966.

53. Chen, H. P., and Walz, D. V. Leukemoid reaction in the bone marrow, associated with malignant neoplasms, *Am. J. Clin. Pathol.* 29:345, 1958.

54. Chernof, D., and Taylor, K. S. Hydroxychloroquine-induced agranulocytosis, *Arch. Dermatol.* 97:163, 1968.

55. Cheville, N. F. Amyloidosis associated with cyclic neutropenia in the dog, *Blood* 31:111, 1968.

56. Clark, K. G. A. Haemolysis and agranulocytosis complicating treatment with methyldopa, *Br. Med. J.* 4:94, 1967.

57. Cline, M. J. Metabolism of the circulating leukocyte, *Physiol. Rev.* 45:674, 1965.

58. Cline, M. J. Hematologic manifestations of tuberculosis, *Calif. Med.* 106:215, 1967.

59. Cline, M. J. Cancer Chemotherapy, W. B. Saunders Co., Philadelphia, 1971.

60. Colebatch, J. H., Anderson, C. M., Simons, M. J., and Burke, V. Neutropenia and pancreatic disorder, *Lancet* 2:496, 1965.

61. Collier, R. L., and Brush, B. E. Hematologic disorder in Felty's syndrome. Prolonged benefits of splenectomy, *Am. J. Surg.* 112:869, 1966.

62. Colman, R. W., and Shein, H. M. Leukemoid reaction, hyperuricemia, and severe hyperpyrexia complicating a fatal case of acute fatty liver of the alcoholic, *Ann. Intern. Med.* 57:110, 1962.

63. Corcos, J. M., Soler-Bechara, J., Mayer, K., Freyberg, R. H., Goldstein, R., and Jaffe, I. Neutrophilic agranulocytosis during administration of penicillamine (2 cases), *J.A.M.A.* 189:265, 1964.

64. Cotter, L. H. Thioglycolic acid poisoning in connection with the "cold wave" process, *J.A.M.A.* 131:592, 1946.

65. Crammer, J. L., and Elkes, A. Agranulocytosis after desipramine, *Lancet* 1:105, 1967.

66. Cream, J. J. Prednisolone-induced granulocytosis, *Br. J. Haematol.* 15:259, 1968.

67. Cress, C. H., Clare, F. B., and Gellhorn, E. The effect of anoxic and anemic anoxia on the leucocyte count, *Am. J. Physiol.* 140:299, 1943.

68. Cronkite, E. P., Bond, V. P., and Conard, R. A. The hematology of ionizing radiation, *in* C. F. Behrens, E. R. King, and J. W. J. Carpenter (eds.), Atomic Medicine, p. 189,

Williams & Wilkins Co., Baltimore, 1969.

69. Cronkite, E. P., and Fliedner, T. M. Medical progress: granulopoiesis, *N. Engl. J. Med.* 270:1347, 1964.

70. Cronkite, E. P., and Fliedner, T. M. Medical progress: granulopoiesis (concl.), *N. Engl. J. Med.* 270:1403, 1964.

71. Custer, R. P. Leukopenia: a guide toward pathogenesis, *Postgrad. Med.* 38:536, 1965.

72. Cutting, H. O., and Lang, J. E. Familial benign chronic neutropenia, *Ann. Intern. Med.* 61:876, 1964.

73. Dacie, J. V. The Haemolytic Anaemias: Congenital and Acquired, Pt. II. The Auto-immune Haemolytic Anaemias, 2nd ed., p. 360, Grune & Stratton, New York, 1962.

74. Dale, D. C., Alling, D. W., and Wolff, S. M. Cyclic hematopoiesis: the mechanism of cyclic neutropenia in grey collie dogs, *J. Clin. Invest.* 51:2197, 1972.

75. Dale, D. C., Kimball, H. R., and Wolff, S. M. Studies of cyclic neutropenia in grey collie dogs, *Clin. Res.* 18:402, 1970.

76. Dale, D. C., Ward, S. B., Kimball, H. R., and Wolff, S. M. Studies of neutrophil production and turnover in grey collie dogs with cyclic neutropenia, *J. Clin. Invest.* 51:2190, 1972.

77. Dale, D. C., and Wolff, S. M. Skin window studies of the acute inflammatory responses of neutropenic patients, *Blood* 38:138, 1971.

78. Dale, D. C., and Wolff, S. M. Studies of the neutropenia of acute malaria, *Blood* 41:197, 1973.

79. Dameshek, W., and Colmes, A. The effect of drugs in the production of agranulocytosis with particular reference to amidopyrine hypersensitivity, *J. Clin. Invest.* 15:85, 1936.

80. Dausset, J. Auto-antileukocyte ribosomal fraction in leukoneutropenias, *Ann. N.Y. Acad. Sci.* 124:550, 1965.

81. Davidson, W. M. Inherited variations in leukocytes, *Semin. Hematol.* 5:255, 1968.

82. Davidson, W. M., Milner, R. D. G., and Lawlor, S. D. Giant neutrophil leukocytes: an inherited anomaly, *Br. J. Haematol.* 6:339, 1960.

83. de Gruchy, G. C., and Langley,

G. R. Felty's syndrome, *Aust. Ann. Med.* 10:292, 1961.

84. deVaal, O. M., and Seynhaeve, V. Reticular dysgenesia, *Lancet* 2:1123, 1959.

85. De Vries, A., Peketh, L., and Joshua, H. Leukaemia and agranulocytosis in a member of a family with hereditary leukopenia, *Acta Med. Orient* 17:26, 1958.

86. Djaldetti, M., Joshua, H., and Kalderon, M. Familial leukopenia-neutropenia in Yemenite Jews. Observations on eleven families, *Bull. Res. Counc. Israel J. Exp. Med.* 9E:24, 1961.

87. Djerassi, I., Kim, J. S., et al. Filtration leukophoresis for separation and concentration of transfusable amounts of normal human granulocytes, *J. Med. (Basel)* 1:358, 1970.

88. Doan, C. A. Hypersplenism, *Bull. N.Y. Acad. Med.* 25:625, 1949.

89. Doan, C. A., Bruce, M. D., and Wiseman, K. Hypersplenic cytopenic syndromes: a 25 year experience with special reference to splenectomy, *in* A. R. Jones, Proc. VIth Int. Cong. Int. Soc. Hematol., p. 429, Grune & Stratton, New York, 1956.

90. Döhle, H. Leukocyteneinschluse bei Scharlach, *Zentralbl. Bakteriol.* 61:63, 1911.

91. Dorr, A. D., and Moloney, W. C. Acquired pseudo-Pelger anomaly of granulocytic leukocytes, *N. Engl. J. Med.* 261:742, 1959.

92. Downey, H., Major, S. G., and Noble, J. F. Leukemoid blood pictures of the myeloid type, *Folia Haematol.* 41:493, 1930.

93. Cephalothin (Keflin): medical letter, *Drug Ther. Bull.* 7:6, 1965.

94. Allopurinol for gout, *Drug Ther. Bull.* 4:41, 1966.

95. Duane, G. W. Periodic neutropenia, *Arch. Intern. Med.* 102:462, 1958.

96. Dubois, E. L. The clinical picture of systemic lupus erythematosus, *in* E. L. Dubois (ed.), Lupus Erythematosus, p. 136, McGraw-Hill, New York, 1966.

97. Dubos, R. J., and Hirsch, J. G. (eds.), Bacterial and Mycotic Infections of Man, 4th ed., J. B. Lippincott, Philadelphia, 1965.

98. Editorial. An odd leukaemia-like disease, *Br. Med. J.* 2:376, 1966.

99. Editorial. Megaloblastic leukopenia, *N. Engl. J. Med.* 277:50, 1967.

100. Elgart, M. L. Griseofulvin. A review of the literature and summary of present usage, *Med. Ann. D.C.* 36:331, 1967.

101. Elliott, P. W., and Blackford, F. Nuclear alterations of the cells in peripheral blood associated with the virus of Influenza A-1 Asian infection and inoculation, *J. Indiana State Med. Assoc.* 51:1651, 1958.

102. Faber, V., and Preben, E. Leucocyte-specific anti-nuclear factors in patients with Felty's syndrome, rheumatoid arthritis, systemic lupus erythematosus and other disease, *Acta Med. Scand.* 179:257, 1966.

103. Fahey, R. J. Unusual leukocyte responses in primary carcinoma of the lung, *Cancer* 4:930, 1951.

104. Felty, A. R. Chronic arthritis in the adult, associated with splenomegaly and leucopenia, *Bull. Johns Hopkins Hosp.* 35:16, 1924.

105. Filkins, J. P., and DiLuzio, N. R. Heparin protection in endotoxin shock, *Am. J. Physiol.* 214:1074, 1968.

106. Finch, S. C. Recognition of radiation-induced late bone marrow changes, *Ann. N.Y. Acad. Sci.* 145:748, 1967.

107. Finch, S. C. Granulocytopenia, *in* W. J. Williams, E. Beutler, A. J. Erslev, and R. W. Rundles (eds.), Hematology, p. 628, McGraw-Hill, New York, 1972.

108. Fink, M. E., and Finch, S. C. Serum muramidase and granulocyte turnover, *Proc. Soc. Exp. Biol. Med.* 127:365, 1968.

109. Fiore, J. M., and Noonan, F. M. Agranulocytosis due to mepazine (phenothiazine), *N. Engl. J. Med.* 260:375, 1959.

110. Fireman, P., Johnson, H. A., and Gitlin, D. Presence of plasma cells and γ_1M-globulin synthesis in a patient with thymic alymphoplasia, *Pediatrics* 37:485, 1966.

111. Fraumeni, J. F., Jr. Bone marrow depression induced by chloramphenicol or phenylbutazone. Leukemia and other sequelae, *J.A.M.A.* 201:828, 1967.

112. Fricker-Alder, H. Die aldersche Granulationsanomalie. Nachuntersuchungen des erstbeschriebene Falles und Überblick über den heutigen Stand der Kenntnisse, *Schweiz. Med. Wochenschr.* 88:989, 1958.

113. Frohman, L. A., and Klocke, F. J. Recurrent thiocyanate intoxication with pancytopenia, hypothroidism and psychosis, *N. Engl. J. Med.* 268:701, 1963.

114. Fukuta, H., and Hattori, K. Studies on leukocytosis due to the injection of chlorophyllin derivatives. I. Experimental studies on leukocyte neuroregulatory mechanism, *Kyushu J. Med. Sci.* 12:21, 1961.

115. Fulginiti, V. A., Kempe, C. H., Hathaway, W. E., Pearlman, D. S., Sieber, O. F., Eller, J. J., Joyner, J. J., Sr., and Robinson, A. Progressive vaccinia in immunologically deficient individuals, *in* D. Bergsma (ed.), Immunologic Deficiency Diseases in Man (Birth Defects Original Article Series), vol. 4, no. 1, p. 129, National Foundation, New York, 1968.

116. Fullerton, H. W., and Duguid, H. L. D. A case of cyclical agranulocytosis with marked improvement following splenectomy, *Blood* 4:269, 1949.

117. Galletti, P. M. Laboratory experience with 24 hour partial heart-lung bypass, *J. Surg. Res.* 5:97, 1965.

118. Gänsslen, M. Konstitutionelle familiäre Leukopenie (Neutropenie), *Klin. Wochenschr.* 20:922, 1941.

119. Garrey, W. E., and Bryan, W. R. Variations in white blood cell counts, *Physiol. Rev.* 15:597, 1935.

120. Gasser, C. Die Pathogenese der essentiellen chronischen Granulocytopenie in Kindesalter auf Grund der Knochenmarksbefunde, *Helv. Paediatr. Acta* 7:426, 1952.

121. Gausis, N., Fortune, D. W., and Whiteside, M. G. The May-Hegglin anomaly. A case report and chromosome studies, *Br. J. Haematol.* 16:619, 1969.

122. Genz, H. Klinische Beobachtungen und Untersuchungen bei einem Fall von Fanconi-anämie, *Arch. Kinderheilkd.* 145:237, 1952.

123. Gilman, P. A., Jackson, D. P., and Guild, H. G. Congenital agranulocytosis: prolonged survival and terminal acute leukemia, *Blood* 34:827, 1969.

124. Gitlin, D., Vawter, G., and Craig, J. M. Thymic alymphoplasia and con-

genital aleukocytosis, *Pediatrics* 33:184, 1964.

125. Godwin, H. A., Zimmerman, T. S., Kimball, H. R., Wolff, S. M., and Perry, S. The effect of etiocholanolone on the entry of granulocytes into the peripheral blood, *Blood* 31:461, 1968.

126. Golde, D. W., and Cline, M. J. Identification of the colony-stimulating cell in human peripheral blood, *J. Clin. Invest.* 51:2981, 1972.

127. Goldman, A., and Haber, M. Acute complete granulopenia with death due to dinitrophenol poisoning, *J.A.M.A.* 107:2115, 1936.

128. Goldstein, I. M., Eyre, H. J., Terasaki, P. I., et al. Leukocyte transfusions: role of leukocyte alloantibodies in determining transfusion response, *Transfusion* 11:19, 1971.

129. Good, R. A., and Zak, S. J. Disturbances in gamma globulin synthesis as "experiments of nature," *Pediatrics* 18:109, 1956.

130. Goodman, J. S., Schaffner, W., Collins, H. A., Battersby, E. J., and Koenig, M. G. Infection after cardiovascular surgery. Clinical study including examination of antimicrobial prophylaxis, *N. Engl. J. Med.* 278:117, 1968.

131. Goodman, L. S., and Gilman, A. (eds.), The Pharmacological Basis of Therapeutics, 3rd ed., Macmillan, New York, 1965.

132. Gordon, A. S., Handler, E. S., Siegel, C. D., Dornfest, B. S., and LoBue, J. Plasma factors influencing leukocyte release in rats, *Ann. N.Y. Acad. Sci.* 113:766, 1964.

133. Graf, M., and Tarlov, A. Agranulocytosis with monohistiocytosis associated with ampicillin therapy, *Ann. Intern. Med.* 69:91, 1968.

134. Gral, T., Schroth, P., DePalma, J. R., and Gordon, A. Leukocyte dynamics with three types of hemodialyzers, *Trans. Am. Soc. Artif. Intern. Organs* 15:45, 1969.

135. Graw, R. G., Jr., Herzig, G. P., Eisel, R. J., and Perry, S. Leukocyte and platelet collection from normal donors with the continuous flow blood cell separator, *Transfusion* 11:94, 1971.

136. Graw, R. G., Jr., Herzig, G. P., Perry, S., and Henderson, E. S. Normal granulocyte transfusion

therapy, *N. Engl. J. Med.* 287:367, 1972.

137. Green, R. A., and Fromke, V. L. Splenectomy in Felty's syndrome, *Ann. Intern. Med.* 64:1265, 1966.

138. Greenberg, M. S., Zanger, B., and Wong, H. Studies in granulocytopenic subjects, *Blood* 30:891, 1967.

139. Grossman, E. R. Ampicillin reaction, *Am. J. Dis. Child.* 112:609, 1966.

140. Gussoff, B. D., and Lee, S. L. Chloramphenicol-induced hematopoietic depression: a controlled comparison with tetracycline, *Am. J. Med. Sci.* 251:8, 1966.

141. Hahneman, B. M., and Alt, H. L. Cyclic neutropenia in a father and daughter, *J.A.M.A.* 168:270, 1958.

142. Halpern, B. N., Holtzer, A., Liacopoulos, P., and Meyer, J. Allergy to pyrazolone derivatives (amonipyrine) with evidence of a reaginic type antibody, *J. Allergy* 29:1, 1958.

143. Halvorsen, K. Neonatal leucopenia due to fetomaternal leucocyte incompatibility, *Acta Paediatr. Scand.* 54:86, 1965.

144. Harin, H. Beiträge zur Morphologie und Genetik der Pelger-Anomalie bei Mensch und Kaninchen, *Z. Menschl. Vererb.* 30:501, 1952.

145. Harter, J. G. Current drug therapy: antihistaminics: tailoring dosage to suit patients, *Clin. Pharmacol. Ther.* 6:553, 1965.

146. Hartl, W. Drug allergic agranulocytosis (Schultz's disease), *Semin. Hematol.* 2:313, 1965.

147. Harvey, A. M., Shulman, L. E., Tumulty, P. A., Conley, C. L., and Schoenrich, E. H. Systemic lupus erythematosus: review of the literature and clinical analysis of 138 cases, *Medicine* 33:291, 1954.

148. Havard, C. W. H. A reappraisal of the thiazide diuretics, *Curr. Med. Drugs* 7:14, 1966.

149. Hegglin, R. Gleichzeitige konstitutionelle Veränderungen an Neutrophilen und Thrombozyten, *Helv. Med. Acta* 12:439, 1945.

150. Hegyeli-Johnsson, R. I., et al. *in* R. Hegyeli (ed.), Proc. Artificial Heart Program Conf., p. 203, U.S. Govt. Printing Office, Washington, D.C., 1969.

151. Hellman, S., and Grate, H. E. X-ray and alkylating agents alter differen-

tiation of surviving hematopoietic cells, *Blood* 38:174, 1971.

152. Hellman, S., Grate, H. E., and Chaffey, J. T. Effects of radiation on the capacity of the stem cell compartment to differentiate into granulocytic and erythrocytic progeny, *Blood* 34:141, 1969.

153. Herzig, G. P., Root, R. K., and Graw, R. G., Jr. Granulocyte collection by continuous-flow filtration leukapheresis, *Blood* 39:554, 1972.

154. Heyn, R. M., Ertel, I. J., and Tubergen, D. G. Course of acquired aplastic anemia in children treated with supportive care, *J.A.M.A.* 208:1372, 1969.

155. Hill, J. M., and Duncan, C. N. Leukemoid reactions, *Am. J. Med. Sci.* 201:847, 1941.

156. Hilts, S. V., and Shaw, C. C. Leukemoid blood reactions, *N. Engl. J. Med.* 249:434, 1953.

157. Hitzig, W. H. Familiäre Neutropenie mit dominanten Erbgang und Hypergammaglobulinämie, *Helv. Med. Acta* 26:779, 1959.

158. Hoffman, G. C., Hewlett, J. S., and Garzón, F. L. A drug-specific leucoagglutinin in a fatal case of agranulocytosis due to chlorpromazine, *J. Clin. Pathol.* 16:232, 1963.

159. Holland, P., and Mauer, A. M. Myeloid leukemoid reactions in children, *Am. J. Dis. Child.* 105:568, 1963.

160. Hollister, L. E., Caffey, E. M., Jr., and Klett, C. J. Abnormal symptoms, signs and laboratory tests during treatment with phenothiazine derivatives, *Clin. Pharmacol. Ther.* 1:284, 1960.

161. Hong, R., Schubert, W. K., Perrin, E. V., and West, C. D. Antibody deficiency syndrome associated with beta-2 macroglobulinemia, *J. Pediatr.* 61:831, 1962.

162. Horsfall, F. L., and Tamm, I. (eds.), Viral and Rickettsial Infections of Man, 4th ed., J. B. Lippincott, Philadelphia, 1965.

163. Huët, G. J. Familial abnormality of leukocytes, *Ned. Tijdschr. Geneeskd.* 75:5956, 1931.

164. Huët, G. J. Über eine bisher unbekannte familiäre Anomalie der Leukocyten, *Klin. Wochenschr.* 11:1264, 1932.

165. Huguley, C. M., Jr. Hematological reactions, *J.A.M.A.* 196:408, 1966.

166. Itoga, T., and Laszlo, J. Döhle bodies and other granulocytic alterations during chemotherapy and cyclophosphamide, *Blood* 20:668, 1962.

167. Jacob, H. S. Hypersplenism, *in* W. J. Williams, E. Beutler, A. J. Ersle, and R. W. Rundles (eds.), Hematology, p. 511, McGraw-Hill, New York, 1972.

168. Jacob, H. S., MacDonald, R. A., and Jandl, J. H. Regulation of spleen growth and sequestering function, *J. Clin. Invest.* 42:1476, 1963.

169. Jandl, J. H., and Aster, R. H. Increased splenic pooling and the pathogenesis of hypersplenism, *Am. J. Med. Sci.* 253:383, 1967.

170. Jandl, J. H., Files, N. M., Barnett, S. B., and MacDonald, R. A. Proliferative response of the spleen and liver to hemolysis, *J. Exp. Med.* 122:299, 1965.

171. Jensen, K. G. Transplacental passage of leucocyte agglutinin occurring on account of pregnancy, *Dan. Med. Bull.* 7:55, 1960.

172. Jordan S. W., and Larsen, W. E. Ultrastructural studies of the May-Hegglin anomaly, *Blood* 25:921, 1965.

173. Kaplan, J. M., and Barrett, O'N., Jr. Reversible pseudo-Pelger anomaly related to sulfisoxazole therapy, *N. Engl. J. Med.* 277:421, 1967.

174. Kaplow, L. S., and Goffinet, J. A. Profound neutropenia during the early phase of hemodialysis, *J.A.M.A.* 203:1135, 1968.

175. Katz, R., Gordon, A. S., and Lapin, D. M. Mechanisms of leukocyte production and release. VI. Studies on the purification of the leukocytosis-inducing factor (LIF), *J. Reticuloendothel. Soc.* 3:103, 1966.

176. Kiczak, J., and Wichert, K. A cured case of agranulocytosis caused by gold therapy, *Pol. Arch. Med. Wewn.* 33:85, 1963.

177. Klerman, G. L., and Cole, J. O. Clinical pharmacology of imipramine and related antidepressant compounds, *Pharmacol. Rev.* 17:101, 1965.

178. Kilbridge, T. M., Gonnella, J. S., and Bolan, J. T. Pancytopenia and death. Disseminated anonymous mycobacterial infection. *Arch. Intern. Med.* 120:38, 1967.

179. King-Smith, E. A., and Morley, A. A. A computer model for the mammalian (human) leucocyte system, Proc. 20th Ann. Conf. on Engineering in Med. and Biol., vol. 9, sect. 19, abst. 9, N.Y. Inst. of Electrical and Electronics Engineers, Boston, 1967.

180. King-Smith E. A., and Morley, A. A. Computer simulation of granulopoiesis: normal and impaired granulopoiesis, *Blood* 36:254, 1970.

181. Kinross-Wright, J. The current status of phenothiazines, *J.A.M.A.* 200:461, 1967.

182. Kiossoglou, K. A., Bilalis, P., Nicolaidis, A., et al. Polymorphonuclear lobe counts in congenital hypothyroidism, *J. Pediatr.* 82:162, 1973.

183. Kostmann, R. Infantile genetic agranulocytosis (agranulocytosis infantilis hereditaria), *Acta Paediatr.* 105:1, 1956 (suppl.).

184. Koszewski, B. J., and Hubbard, T. F. Immunologic agranulocytosis due to mercurial diuretics, *Am. J. Med.* 20:958, 1956.

185. Krill, C. E., Jr., Smith, H. D., and Mauer, A. M. Chronic idiopathic granulocytopenia, *N. Engl. J. Med.* 270:973, 1964.

186. Kritzler, R. A., Terner, J. Y., Lindenbaum, J. L., Magidson, J., Williams, R., Preisig, R., and Phillips, G. B. Chediak-Higashi syndrome. Cytologic and serum lipid observations in a case and family, *Am. J. Med.* 36:583, 1964.

187. Krumbhaar, E. B. Leukemoid blood pictures in various clinical conditions, *Am. J. Med. Sci.* 172:519, 1926.

188. Kusserow, B., Larrow, R., and Nichols, J. Metabolic and morphological alterations in leukocytes following prolonged blood pumping, *Trans. Am. Soc. Artif. Intern. Organs* 15:40, 1969.

189. Kusserow, B., Larrow, R., and Nichols, J. Perfusion- and surface-induced injury in leukocytes, *Fed. Proc.* 30:1516, 1971.

190. Kuvin, S. F., and Brecher, G. Differential neutrophil counts in pregnancy, *N. Engl. J. Med.* 266:877, 1962.

191. Kwan, V. W. Procaine amide-induced leukopenia, *J. Am. Geriatr. Soc.* 17:404, 1969.

192. Kyle, R. A., and Pease, G. L. Hematologic aspects of arsenic intoxication, *N. Engl. J. Med.* 273:18, 1965.

193. Lalezari, P., Nussbaum, M., Gelman, S., and Spaet, T. H. Neonatal neutropenia due to maternal isoimmunization, *Blood* 15:236, 1960.

194. Lang, J. E., and Cutting, H. O. Infantile genetic agranulocytosis, *Pediatrics* 35:596, 1965.

195. Launiala, K., Furuhjelm, U., Hjelt, L., and Visakorpi, J. K. A syndrome with pancreatic achylia and granulocytopenia, *Acta Paediatr. Scand.* 177:28, 1967 (suppl.).

196. Leale, M. Recurrent furunculosis in an infant showing an unusual blood picture, *J.A.M.A.* 54:1854, 1910.

197. Lechner, K., Breddin, K., Moser, K., Stockinger, L., and Wenzel, E. May-Hegglinsche Anomalie, *Acta Haematol.* 42:303, 1969.

198. Lee, J. C., Dushkin, M., Eyring, E. J., Engleman, E. P., and Hopper, J., Jr. Renal lesions associated with gold therapy: light and electron microscopic studies, *Arthritis Rheum.* 8:1, 1965.

199. Levine, P. H., and Weintraub, L. R. Pseudoleukemia during recovery from Dapsone-induced agranulocytosis, *Ann. Intern. Med.* 68:1060, 1968.

200. Levine, S. Chronic familial neutropenia with marked periodontal lesions: report of a case, *Oral Surg.* 12:310, 1959.

201. Levy, S. B., Meyers, B., and Mellin, H. Reversible granulocytopenia in a patient with polycythemia vera taking nitrofurantoin, *J. Mt. Sinai Hosp.* 36:26, 1969.

202. Linman, J. W. Factors controlling hemopoiesis: thrombopoietic and leukopoietic effects of "anemic" plasma, *J. Lab. Clin. Med.* 59:262, 1962.

203. Lonsdale, D., Deodhar, S. D., and Mercer, R. D. Familial granulocytopenia and associated immunoglobulin abnormality, Report of three cases in young brothers, *J. Pediatr.* 71:790, 1967.

204. Louria, D. B. The treatment of endocarditis, *Am. Heart J.* 66:429, 1963.

205. Lund, J. E., Padgett, G. A., and Ott, R. L. Cyclic neutropenia in grey collie dogs, *Blood* 29:452, 1967.

206. Lundström, M., Olsson, P., Unger,

P., and Ekestrom, S. Effect of extracorporeal circulation on hematopoiesis and phagocytosis, *J. Cardiovasc. Surg.* 4:664, 1963.

207. Lux, S. E., Johnston, R. B., Jr., August, C. S., Say, B., Penchaszadeh, V. B., Rosen, F. S., and McKusick, V. A. Chronic neutropenia and abnormal cellular immunity in cartilage-hair hypoplasia, *N. Engl. J. Med.* 282:231, 1970.

208. McBride, J. A., Dacie, J. V., and Shapley, R. The effect of splenectomy on the leucocyte count, *Br. J. Haematol.* 14:225, 1968.

209. McCall, C. E., Katayama, I., Cotran, R. S., and Finland, M. Lysosomal and ultrastructural changes in human "toxic" neutrophils during bacterial infection, *J. Exp. Med.* 129:267, 1969.

210. McCarthy, D. D., and Chalmers, M. B. Hematologic complications of phenylbutazone therapy: review of the literature and report of 2 cases, *Can. Med. Assoc. J.* 90:1061, 1964.

211. McCluskey, H. B. Corticotropin (ACTH) in treatment of agranulocytosis following sulfisoxazole therapy, *J.A.M.A.* 152:232, 1953.

212. McFarland, W., and Libre, E. P. Abnormal leukocyte response in alcoholism, *Ann. Intern. Med.* 59:865, 1963.

213. McGavack, T. H., and Chevalley, J. Untoward hematologic responses to the antithyroid compounds, *Am. J. Med.* 17:36, 1954.

214. McKusick, V. A., Eldridge, R., Hostetler, J., Ruangluit, U., and Egeland, J. A. Dwarfism in the Amish. II. Cartilage-hair hypoplasia, *Bull. Johns Hopkins Hosp.* 116:285, 1965.

215. Madison, F. W., and Squier, T. L. The etiology of primary granulocytopenia (agranulocytic angina), *J.A.M.A.* 102:755, 1934.

216. Malinin, T. I., Pekin, T. J., Jr., Baur, H., and Zvaifler, N. J. Vacuoles in synovial fluid leukocytes, *Am. J. Clin. Pathol.* 45:728, 1966.

217. Mandel, A., and Gross, M. Agranulocytosis and phenothiazines, *Dis. Nerv. Syst.* 29:32, 1968.

218. Matsaniotis, N., Kiossoglou, K. A., Karpouzas, J., and Anastasea-Vlachou, K. Chromosomes in Kostmann's disease, *Lancet* 2:104, 1966.

219. Mauer, A. M., and Krill, C. E. A study of the mechanisms for granulocytopenia, *Ann. N.Y. Acad. Sci.* 113:1003, 1964.

220. Mauer, E. F. The toxic effects of phenylbutazone (Butazolidin). Review of the literature and report of the twenty-third death following its use, *N. Engl. J. Med.* 253:404, 1955.

221. May, R. Leukocyteneinschlüsse, *Dtsch. Arch. Klin. Med.* 96:1, 1909.

222. Matoth, Y., and Fried, K. Chronic Gaucher's disease. Clinical observations on 34 patients, *Isr. J. Med. Sci.* 1:521, 1965.

223. Menkin, V. Factors concerned in the mobilization of leukocytes in inflammation, *Ann. N.Y. Acad. Sci.* 59:956, 1955.

224. Meyer, L. M., and Rotter, S. D. Leukemoid reaction (hyperleukocytosis) in malignancy, *Am. J. Clin. Pathol.* 12:218, 1942.

225. Michaelson, A. K. Severe leukemoid reaction after promazine-induced agranulocytosis (1 case), *J. Fla. Med. Assoc.* 45:1418, 1959.

226. Michelstein, I., and Weiser, N. J. Fatal agranulocytosis due to trimethadione (Tridione), *Arch. Neurol. Psychiat.* 62:358, 1949.

227. Milhorat, A. T., Small, S. M., and Diethelm, O. Leukocytosis during various emotional states, *Arch. Neurol. Psychiat.* 47:779, 1942.

228. Miller, D. R., Freed, B. A., and Lapey, J. D. Congenital neutropenia: report of a fatal case in a Negro infant with leukocyte function studies, *Am. J. Dis. Child.* 115:337, 1968.

229. Millington, D. Leucopenia and indomethacin, *Br. Med. J.* 1:49, 1966.

230. Mintz, U., and Sachs, L. Normal granulocyte colony-forming cells in the bone marrow of Yemenite Jews with genetic neutropenia, *Blood* 41:745, 1973.

231. Moeschlin, S. Immunological granulocytopenia and agranulocytosis: clinical aspects, *Acta Med. Scand.* 312:518, 1956 (suppl.).

232. Moeschlin, S., and Wagner, K. Agranulocytosis due to the occurrence of leukocyte-agglutinins (Pyramidon and cold agglutinins), *Acta Haematol.* 8:29, 1952.

233. Möller, E., Olin, P., and Zetterström, R. Neutropenia and insufficiency of the exocrine pancreas, *Acta Paediatr. Scand.* 177:29, 1967 (suppl.).

234. Moltusky, A. G. Drug reactions, enzymes and biochemical genetics, *J.A.M.A.* 165:835, 1957.

235. Monto, R. W., Shafer, H. C., Brennan, M. J., and Rebuck, J. W. Periodic neutropenia treated by adrenocorticotrophic hormone and splenectomy, *N. Engl. J. Med.* 246:893, 1952.

236. Moore, R. A., Brunner, C. M., Sandusky, W. R., et al. Felty's syndrome: long-term follow-up after splenectomy, *Ann. Intern. Med.* 75:381, 1971.

237. Morley, A. A. A neutrophil cycle in healthy individuals, *Lancet* 2:1220, 1966.

238. Morley, A. A., Carew, J. P., and Baikie, A. G. Familial cyclical neutropenia, *Br. J. Haematol.* 13:719, 1967.

239. Morley, A. A., and Stohlman, F., Jr. Cyclophosphamide-induced cyclical neutropenia, *N. Engl. J. Med.* 282:643, 1970.

240. Mozziconacci, P., Boisse, J., Attal, C., Pham-Huu-Trung, Guy-Grand, D., and Griscelli, C. Hypoplasie du pancréas exocrine avec troubles hématologiques. Absence du cellules A dans les îlots de Langerhans, *Arch. Fr. Pediatr.* 24:741, 1967.

241. Mulholland, J. H., and Cluff, L. E. The effect of endotoxin upon susceptibility to infection: the role of the granulocyte, *in* M. Landy and W. Braun (eds.), Bacterial Endotoxins, p. 211, Rutgers University Press, New Brunswick, N.J., 1964.

242. Natelson, E. A., Lynch, E. C., Hettig, R. A., and Alfrey, C. P., Jr. Histiocytic medullary reticulosis. The role of phagocytosis in pancytopenia, *Arch. Intern. Med.* 122:223, 1968.

243. Natelson, R. P. Cyclic neutropenia with giant follicular lymphoblastoma and lymphosarcoma. Report of a case with splenectomy, *Blood* 8:923, 1953.

244. Nawabi, I. U., and Ritz, N. D. Agranulocytosis due to propranolol, *J.A.M.A.* 223:1376, 1973.

245. Nettleship, A. Leucocytosis associated with acute inflammation, *Am. J. Clin. Pathol.* 8:398, 1938.

246. Newton, R. M., and Ward, V. G. Leukopenia associated with ris-

tocetin (Spontin) administration, *J.A.M.A.* 166:1956, 1958.

247. Nir, E., Efrati, P., and Danon, D. The osmotic fragility of human leucocytes in normal and in some pathological conditions, *Br. J. Haematol.* 18:237, 1970.

248. Nymand, G., Heron, I., Jensen, K. G., and Lundsgaard, A. Occurrence of cytotoxic antibodies during pregnancy, *Vox Sang.* 21:21, 1971.

249. Oberling, J. M., et al. Thorotrastose post-angiographique et agranulocytose chronique, *Nouv. Rev. Fr. Hematol.* 13:291, 1973.

250. O'Connell, C. J., and Plaut, M. E. Intravenous lincomycin in high doses, *Curr. Ther. Res.* 11:478, 1969.

251. O'Neill, J. A., Scott, H. W., Jr., Billings, F. T., and Foster, J. H. The role of splenectomy in Felty's syndrome, *Ann. Surg.* 167:81, 1968.

252. Oppenheim, M., and de Meyer, G. Granulo- und Thrombo-cytopenie infolge Streptomycin-behandlung, *Schweiz. Med. Wochenschr.* 79:1187, 1949.

253. Oski, F. A., Naiman, J. L., Allen, D. M., and Diamond, L. K. Leukocytic inclusions—Döhle bodies—associated with platelet abnormality (the May-Hegglin anomaly): report of a family and review of the literature, *Blood* 20:657, 1962.

254. Page, A. R., and Good, R. A. Studies on cyclic neutropenia: a clinical and experimental investigation, *Am. J. Dis. Child.* 94:623, 1957.

255. Palmer, J. G., Eichwald, E. J., Cartwright, G. E., and Wintrobe, M. M. The experimental production of splenomegaly, anemia and leucopenia in albino rats, *Blood* 8:72, 1953.

256. Parbrook, G. D. Leucopenic effects of prolonged nitrous oxide treatment, *Br. J. Anaesth.* 39:119, 1967.

257. Payne, R. Leukocyte agglutinins in human sera. Correlation between blood transfusions and their development, *Arch. Intern. Med.* 99:587, 1957.

258. Payne, R. Neonatal neutropenia and leukoagglutinins, *Pediatrics* 33:194, 1964.

259. Pearson, H. A. Marrow hypoplasia in anorexia nervosa, *J. Pediatr.* 71:211, 1967.

260. Pearson, J. R., Binder, C. I., and Neber, J. Agranulocytosis following Diamox therapy, *J.A.M.A.* 157:339, 1955.

261. Pelger, K. Demonstratie van een paar zeldzaam voorkomende typen van bloedlichaampjes en bespreking der patienten, *Discuss. Med. Tijdschr. Geneesk.* 72:1178, 1928.

262. Perillie, P. E., Kaplan, S. S., and Finch, S. C. Significance of changes in serum muramidase activity in megaloblastic anemia, *N. Engl. J. Med.* 277:10, 1967.

263. Perry, S., Weinstein, I. M., Craddock, C. G., Jr., and Lawrence, J. S. Rates of appearance and dissappearance of white blood cells in normal and in various disease states, *J. Lab. Clin. Med.* 51:101, 1958.

264. Petz, A., Smith, I., and Nelson, N. The May-Hegglin anomaly: a study of three cases, *Clin. Res.* 8:215, 1960.

265. Pisciotta, A. V. Clinical and pathologic effects of space-occupying lesions of the bone marrow, *Am. J. Clin. Pathol.* 20:915, 1950.

266. Pisciotta, A. V. Drug-induced bone marrow damage, *in* S. E. Bjorkman (ed.), Aplastic Anemia, Series Haematologica, vol. 5, p. 64, Munksgaard, Copenhagen, 1965.

267. Pisciotta, A. V. Agranulocytosis induced by certain phenothiazine derivatives, *J.A.M.A.* 208:1862, 1969.

268. Pisciotta, A. V. Drug-induced leukopenia and aplastic anemia, *Clin. Pharmacol. Ther.* 12:13, 1971.

269. Pisciotta, A. V. Studies on agranulocytosis. IX. A biochemical defect in chlorpromazine-sensitive marrow cells, *J. Lab. Clin. Med.* 78:435, 1971.

270. Playfair, J. H. L., Wolfendale, M. R., and Kay, H. E. M. The leucocytes of peripheral blood in the human foetus, *Br. J. Haematol.* 9:336, 1963.

271. Polano, M. K., Cats, A., and van Olden, G. A. J. Agranulocytosis following treatment with hydroxychloroquine sulphate, *Lancet* 1:1275, 1965.

272. Ponder, E., and Ponder, R. The cytology of the polymorphonuclear leucocyte in toxic conditions, *J. Lab. Clin. Med.* 28:316, 1942.

273. Pringle, E. M., Young, W. F., and

Haworth, E. M. Syndrome of pancreatic insufficiency, blood dyscrasia and metaphyseal dysplasia, *Proc. R. Soc. Med.* 61:776, 1968.

274. Propp, R. P., and Stillman, J. S. Agranulocytosis and hydroxychloroquine, *N. Engl. J. Med.* 277:492, 1967.

275. Quagliana, J. M., Cartwright, G. E., and Wintrobe, M. M. Paroxysmal nocturnal hemoglobinuria following drug-induced aplastic anemia, *Ann. Intern. Med.* 61:1045, 1964.

276. Randall, D. L., Reiquam, C. W., Githens, J. H., and Robinson, A. Familial myeloproliferative disease. A new syndrome closely simulating myelogenous leukemia in childhood, *Am. J. Dis. Child.* 110:479, 1965.

277. Reed, I. L., Barry, P., Wong, H., and Greenberg, M. S. Granulocyte turnover in patients with cirrhosis, *Clin. Res.* 14:325, 1966.

278. Reilly, W. A. The granules in the leukocytes in gargoylism, *Am. J. Dis. Child.* 62:489, 1941.

279. Reilly, W. A., and Lindsay, S. Gargoylism (lipochondrodystrophy): a review of clinical observations in eighteen cases, *Am. J. Dis. Child.* 75:595, 1948.

280. Reimann, H. A. Periodic disease: a probable syndrome including periodic fever, benign paroxysmal peritonitis, cyclic neutropenia and intermittent arthralgia, *J.A.M.A.* 136:239, 1948.

281. Reimann, H. A. Periodic Diseases, F. A. Davis Co., Philadelphia, 1963.

282. Rey, J. J., and Wolf, P. L. Extreme leucocytosis in accidental electric shock, *Lancet* 1:18, 1968.

283. Ritchie, G. M. Extensive myeloid response during folic acid therapy in megaloblastic anaemia of pregnancy, *J. Clin. Pathol.* 5:329, 1952.

284. Robinson, W. A., and Otsuka, A. Production of granulocyte colony stimulating activity by human WBC and subcellular localization, *in* D. W. van Bekkum and K. A. Dicke (eds.), In Vitro Culture of Hemopoietic Cells, p. 266, Radiobiological Institute TNO, Rijswijk, 1972.

285. Robinson, W. A., and Pike, B. L. Leukopoietic activity in human urine, *N. Engl. J. Med.* 282:1291, 1970.

286. Rosse, W. F. Erythrocyte disorders—paroxysmal nocturnal hemoglobinuria, *in* W. J. Williams, E. Beutler, A. J. Erslev, and R. W. Rundles (eds.), Hematology, p. 460, McGraw-Hill, New York, 1972.

287. Rossi, J. P., and Brandt, I. K. Transient granulocytopenia of the newborn associated with sepsis due to *Shigella alkalescens* and maternal leukocyte agglutinins, *J. Pediatr.* 56:639, 1960.

288. Rossman, P. L., and Hummer, G. J. Chronic neutropenia in siblings: the effect of steroids, *Ann. Intern. Med.* 52:242, 1960.

289. Rubin, E., Gottleib, C., and Vogel, P. Syndrome of hepatitis and aplastic anemia, *Am. J. Med.* 45:88, 1968.

290. Ruderman, M., Miller, L. M., and Pinals, R. S. Clinical and serologic observations on 27 patients with Felty's syndrome, *Arthritis Rheum.* 11:377, 1968.

291. Sacchetti, G., et al. Quantitation and distribution of neutrophilic granulocytes after splenectomy, X Int. Cong. Int. Soc. Haematol., Stockholm, 1964 (abstract).

292. Sanchez-Medal, L., Castanedo, J. P., and Garcia-Rojas, F. Insecticides and aplastic anemia, *N. Engl. J. Med.* 269:1365, 1963.

293. Sandella, J. F. Cyclic acute agranulocytosis: report of a case with improvement after splenectomy, *Ann. Intern. Med.* 35:1365, 1951.

294. Sandusky, W. R., Rudolf, L. E., and Leavell, B. S. Splenectomy for control of neutropenia in Felty's syndrome, *Ann. Surg.* 167:744, 1968.

295. Savilahti, M. Mehr als 100 Vergiftungsfälle durch Benzol in einer Schuhfabrik, *Arch. Gewerbepathol. Gewerbehyg.* 15:147, 1956.

296. Schneiderman, L. J., Sampson, N. L., Schoene, W. C., and Haydon, G. B. Genetic studies of a family with two unusual autosomal dominant conditions: muscular dystrophy and Pelger-Huët anomaly, *Am. J. Med.* 46:380, 1969.

297. Schofield, T. P. C., Talbot, J. M., Bryceson, A. D. M., and Parry, E. H. O. Leucopenia and fever in the "Jarisch-Herxheimer" reaction of louse-borne relapsing fever, *Lancet* 1:58, 1968.

298. Scholer, H., Imhof, H., and Schnös, M. Beobachtungen an einem weiterem Träger der May-Hegglinschen Anomalie der Leukocyten und Blutplättchen, *Schweiz. Med. Wochenschr.* 90:1269, 1960.

299. Schwachman, H., Diamond, L. K., Oski, F. A., and Khaw, K-T. The syndrome of pancreatic insufficiency and bone marrow dysfunction, *J. Pediatr.* 65:645, 1964.

300. Sclare, G., and Cragg, J. A leukaemoid blood picture in megaloblastic anaemia of the puerperium, *J. Clin. Pathol.* 11:45, 1958.

301. Scott, J. L., Cartwright, G. E., and Wintrobe, M. M. Acquired aplastic anemia: an analysis of thirty-nine cases and review of the pertinent literature, *Medicine* 38:119, 1959.

302. Scott, J. L., Finegold, S. M., Belkin, G. A., and Lawrence, J. S. A controlled double-blind study of the hematologic toxicity of chloramphenicol, *N. Engl. J. Med.* 272:1137, 1965.

303. Scott, R. E., Dale, D. C., et al. Cyclic neutropenia in grey collie dogs, *Lab. Invest.* 28:514, 1973.

304. Scott, W. P., and Vaughn, J. Chemotherapy incidental to a leukemoid reaction, *N.C. Med. J.* 29:380, 1968.

305. Seip, M. Systemic lupus erythematosus in pregnancy with haemolytic anaemia, leucopenia and thrombocytopenia in the mother and her newborn infant, *Arch. Dis. Child.* 35:364, 1960.

306. Selling, L. Benzol as a leucotoxin. Studies on the degeneration and regeneration of the blood and haematopoietic organs, *Johns Hopkins Hosp. Rep.* 17:83, 1916.

307. Sézary, A., and Boucher, G. Agranulocytose bismuthique, *Bull. Mem. Soc. Med. Hosp. Paris* 47:1795, 1931.

308. Shanbrom, E., Collins, Z., and Miller, S. "Acquired" Pelger-Huët cells in blood dyscrasias, *Am. J. Med. Sci.* 240:732, 1960.

309. Shanbrom, E., and Tanaka, K. R. Acquired Pelger-Huët granulocytes in severe myxedema, *Acta Haematol.* 27:289, 1962.

310. Shapiro, Y. L. Changes in differential leukocyte count in prolonged total alimentary starvation, *Fed. Proc.* 23, Transl. 447, 1964 (suppl.).

311. Sheba, C. Risks of chloramphenicol? *Lancet* 1:1007, 1967.

312. Shen, S. C., and Hoshino, T. Study of humoral factors regulating the production of leukocytes. I. Demonstration of a "Neutropoietic" in the plasma after administration of triamcinolone to rats, *Blood* 17:434, 1961.

313. Short, C. L., Bauer, W., and Reynolds, W. E. Rheumatoid Arthritis: A Definition of the Disease and a Clinical Description Based on a Numerical Study of 293 Patients and Controls, p. 352, Harvard University Press, Cambridge, Mass., 1957.

314. Skårberg, K. O., Lagerlöf, B., and Reizenstein, P. Leukaemia, leukaemoid reaction and tuberculosis, *Acta Med. Scand.* 182:427, 1967.

315. Smith, H. Unidentified inclusions in haemopoietic cells, congenital atresia of the bile ducts and livedo reticularis in an infant: ? a new syndrome, *Br. J. Haematol.* 13:695, 1967.

316. Smith, J. F. Cyclic neutropenia, *Oral Surg.* 18:312, 1964.

317. Smith, L. G., and Herring, W. B. Hereditary leukemoid reaction, *Clin. Res.* 19:432, 1971.

318. Spaet, T. H., and Dameshek, W. Chronic hypoplastic neutropenia, *Am. J. Med.* 13:35, 1952.

319. Sparberg, M. Diagnostically confusing complications of diphenylhydantoin therapy: a review, *Ann. Intern. Med.* 59:914, 1963.

320. Stefanini, M., Mele, R. H., and Skinner, D. Transitory congenital neutropenia: a new syndrome. Report of two cases, *Am. J. Med.* 25:749, 1958.

321. Stein, J. H., Hamilton, H. E., and Sheets, R. F. Agranulocytosis caused by chlorpropamide, *Arch. Intern. Med.* 113:186, 1964.

322. Steinberg, B. Bone marrow regeneration in experimental benzene intoxication, *Blood* 4:550, 1949.

323. Steinberg, B. Mechanism of hematopoiesis: hematopoietic effects of serum albumin, *Arch. Pathol.* 67:489, 1959.

324. Steinberg, B., and Martin, R. A. Plasma factor increasing circulating leukocytes, *Am. J. Physiol.* 161:14, 1950.

325. Steinberg, M. H., and Charm, S. E.

Effect of high concentrations of leukocytes on whole blood viscosity, *Blood* 38:299, 1971.

326. Stephens, D. J. The occurrence of myelocytes in the peripheral blood in lobar pneumonia, *Am. J. Med. Sci.* 188:332, 1934.

327. Sternlieb, P., and Eisman, S. H. Toxic hepatitis and agranulocytosis due to cinchophen, *Ann. Intern. Med.* 47:826, 1957.

328. Stevens, A. R., Jr. Agranulocytosis induced by sulfaguanidine, *Arch. Intern. Med.* 123:428, 1969.

329. Straus, B. Aplastic anemia following exposure to carbon tetrachloride, *J.A.M.A.* 155:737, 1954.

330. Strausz, I., Barcsak, J., Kékes, E., and Szebeni, A. Prednisolone-induced acute changes in circulating neutrophil granulocytes. III. In cases of pernicious anemia, *Haematologica* 2:109, 1968.

331. Strausz, I., Kékes, E., and Szebeni, A. Mechanism of prednisolone-induced leucocytosis in man, *Acta Haematol.* 33:40, 1965.

332. Talmers, F. N., and Telmos, A. J. A case report: procaine amide hydrochloride (Pronestyl) induced agranulocytosis, *Mich. Med.* 64:655, 1965.

333. Tanaka, K. R., Valentine, W. N., Fredricks, R. E. Diseases or clinical conditions associated with low leucocyte alkaline phosphatase, *N. Engl. J. Med.* 262:912, 1960.

334. Tashjian, A. H., Jr., and Leddy, J. P. Agranulocytosis associated with phenindione: a case report with review of the literature, *Arch. Intern. Med.* 105:121, 1960.

335. Thiele, H. G., and Frenzel, H. G. Immunoglobulin-Mangel-syndrom und Agranulocytose bei Thymom, *Schweiz. Med. Wochenschr.* 97:1606, 1967.

336. Thierfelder, S., Magis, C., Saint-Paul, M., and Dausset, J. Die Pyramidon-agranulozytose: eine immunhamatologische Studie, *Dtsch. Med. Wochenschr.* 89:506, 1964.

337. Tindall, J. P., Beeker, S. K., and Rosse, W. F. Familial cold urticaria. A generalized reaction involving leukocytosis, *Arch. Intern. Med.* 124:129, 1969.

338. Tisman, G., Herbert, V., and Rosenblatt, S. Evidence that lithium induces human granulocyte proliferation: elevated serum vitamin B$_{12}$ binding capacity in vivo and granulocyte colony proliferation in vitro, *Br. J. Haematol.* 24:767, 1973.

339. Toren, M., Goffinet, J. A., and Kaplow, L. S. Pulmonary bed sequestration of neutrophils during hemodialysis, *Blood* 36:337, 1970.

340. Tullis, J. L. Effects of experimental hypertonia on circulating leukocytes, *J. Clin. Invest.* 26:1098, 1947.

341. Tullis, J. L. Prevalence, nature and identification of leukocyte antibodies, *N. Engl. J. Med.* 258:569, 1958.

342. Turner, D. L., Miller, F. R., and Flint, J. S. The concentration of myelokentric and lymphokentric acids from serum and plasma of leukemic patients, *J. Natl. Cancer Inst.* 14:439, 1953.

343. Twomey, J. J., and Leavell, B. S. Leukemoid reactions to tuberculosis, *Arch. Intern. Med.* 116:21, 1965.

344. Undritz, E. Les malformations héréditaires des éléments figurés du sang, *Le Sang* 25:296, 1954.

345. Undritz, E. Eine neue Sippe mit erblichkonstitutioneller Hochsegmentierung der Neutrophilenkerne, *Schweiz. Med. Wochenschr.* 88:1000, 1958.

346. Undritz, E., and de Sepibus, C. Das Resultat der Nachuntersuchung der vor 25 Jahren im Wallis gefundenen ersten schweizer Sippe mit Pelger-Huëtscher kernanomalieder Blutkörperchen und derzeitiger Stand der Erforschung der Anomalie, *Schweiz. Med. Wochenschr.* 87:1258, 1957.

347. Undritz, E., and Schäli, H. Eine neue Sippe mit erblichkonstitutioneller Hochsegmentierung der Neutrophilenkerne und das Knochenmarkbild beim homozygoten Träger dieser Anomalie, *Schweiz. Med. Wochenschr.* 94:1365, 1964.

348. Vahlquist, B. Cyclic agranulocytosis: report of a case with a short survey of the disease, *Acta Med. Scand.* 170:531, 1946 (suppl.).

349. Viani, H., and Holland, P. D. J. The control of Dapsone Heinz-body anaemia with adrenal corticosteroids, *Br. J. Dermatol.* 76:63, 1964.

350. Vigliani, E. C., and Saita, G. Benzene and leukemia, *N. Engl. J. Med.* 271:872, 1964.

351. Vodopick, H., Rupp, E. M., Edwards, C. L, Goswitz, F. A., and Beauchamp, J. J. Spontaneous cyclic leukocytosis and thrombocytosis in chronic granulocytic leukemia, *N. Engl. J. Med.* 286:284, 1972.

352. Vrtilek, M. R. Das Bild der chronischen Granulocytopenie im Kindesalter, *Helv. Paediatr. Acta* 7:207, 1952.

353. Wade, A. B., and Stafford, J. L. Cyclical neutropenia, *Oral Surg.* 16:1443, 1963.

354. Walford, R. L. Leukocyte Antigens and Antibodies, Grune & Stratton, New York, 1960.

355. Walker, J. G. Fatal agranulocytosis complicating treatment with ethacrynic acid. Report of a case, *Ann. Intern. Med.* 64:1303, 1966.

356. Wang, R. I. H., and Schuller, G. Agranulocytosis following procainamide administration, *Am. Heart J.* 78:282, 1969.

357. Ward, H. N., and Reinhard, E. H. Chronic idiopathic leukocytosis, *Ann. Intern. Med.* 75:193, 1971.

358. Ward, H. P. The effect of chloramphenicol on RNA and heme synthesis in bone marrow cultures, *J. Lab. Clin. Med.* 68:400, 1966.

359. Wassmuth, D. R., DeGroote, J. W., Hamilton, H. E., and Sheets, R. F. An anomaly of granulocytes and platelets: a newly established hereditary entity, *J. Lab. Clin. Med.* 58:969, 1961.

360. Weiss, L. The structure of fine splenic arterial vessels in relation to hemoconcentration and red cell destruction, *Am. J. Anat.* 111:131, 1962.

361. Weiss, L. The spleen, in R. Greep (ed.), Histology, McGraw-Hill, New York, 1965.

362. Weiss, L. The structure of the normal spleen, *Semin. Hematol.* 2:205, 1965.

363. Weissmann, G., and Xefteris, E. D. Phenylbutazone leukopenia, *Arch. Intern. Med.* 103:957, 1959.

364. Wheelihan, R. Y. Granulocytic aplasia of the bone marrow following the use of arsenic, *Am. J. Dis. Child.* 35:1032, 1928.

365. Willcox, P. H. Antithyroid treatment: a personal series, *Postgrad. Med. J.* 43:146, 1967.

366. Windhorst, D. B., Lund, J. E., Decker, J., and Swatez, I. Intestinal

malabsorption in the gray collie syndrome. *Fed. Proc.* 26:260, 1967.

367. Wintrobe, M. M. Diagnostic significance of changes in leukocytes, *Bull. N.Y. Acad. Med.* 15:223, 1939.

368. Wintrobe, M. M. The problems of drug toxicity in man: a view from the hematopoietic system, *Ann. N.Y. Acad. Sci.* 123:316, 1965.

369. Wintrobe, M. M. Clinical Hematology, 6th, ed., p. 282, Lea & Febiger, Philadelphia, 1967.

370. Wiseman, B. K., and Doan, C. A. A newly recognized granulopenic syndrome caused by excessive leukolysis and successfully treated by splenectomy, *J. Clin. Invest.* 18:473, 1939.

371. Wiseman, B. K., and Doan, C. A. Primary splenic neutropenia; a newly recognized syndrome, closely related to congenital hemolytic icterus and essential thrombocytopenic purpura, *Ann. Intern. Med.* 16:1097, 1942.

372. Withers, K. L. Leukaemoid reactions in disseminated nonreactive tuberculosis: a review of the literature with a report of a case, *Med. J. Aust.* 2:142, 1964.

373. Wriedt, K., Kauder, E., and Mauer, A. M. Failure of myeloid differentiation as a cause of congenital neutropenia, *J. Pediatr.* 68:839, 1966.

374. Wright, C. S., Doan, C. A., Bouroncle, B. A., Zollinger, R. M. Direct splenic arterial and venous blood studies in the hypersplenic syndromes before and after epinephrine, *Blood* 6:195, 1951.

375. Wright, C. S., Doan, C. A., and Haynie, H. C. Agranulocytosis occurring after exposure to a D.D.T. pyrenthrum aerosol bomb, *Am. J. Med.* 1:562, 1946.

376. Yunis, A. A., and Bloomberg, G. R. Chloramphenicol toxicity: clinical features and pathogenesis, *in* C. V. Moore and E. B. Brown (eds.), Progress in Hematology, vol. 4, p. 138, Grune & Stratton, New York, 1964.

377. Yunis, A. A., and Harrington, W. J. Patterns of inhibition by chloramphenicol of nucleic acid synthesis in human bone marrow and leukemic cells, *J. Lab. Clin. Med.* 56:831, 1960.

378. Zacharski, L. R., Lila, R. E., and Linman, J. W. Leukocyte counts in healthy adults, *Am. J. Clin. Pathol.* 56:148, 1971.

379. Zarafonetis, C. J. D., and Joseph, R. R. Bronchogenic carcinoma with adrenal metastases and leukemoid reaction: probable noncontribution of leukocytosis to elevated serum alkaline phosphatase, *Am J. Med. Sci.* 242:750, 1961.

380. Zernechel, C. F. Aminopyrine and agranulocytosis. Review and report of six cases, *N.C. Med. J.* 28:91, 1967.

381. Zieve, P. D., Haghshenass, M., Blanks, M., and Krevans, J. R. Vacuolization of the neutrophil, *Arch. Intern. Med.* 118:356, 1966.

382. Zuelzer, W. W. "Myelokathexis"—a new form of chronic granulocytopenia, *N. Engl. J. Med.* 270:699, 1964.

Chapter 10 Chronic Myelocytic Leukemia and Chronic Myeloproliferative Disorders

The collective term *chronic myeloproliferative disorders* encompasses a group of diseases including chronic myelocytic leukemia, polycythemia vera, myelofibrosis with myeloid metaplasia, and essential thrombocythemia. Use of this term does not imply that the disorders share a common etiology or pathogenesis. It does imply, however, that the disorders are all characterized by a chronic excessive proliferation of one or more bone marrow elements: granulocytes, erythrocytes, megakaryocytes, or stromal cells. This proliferation occurs within the bone marrow and/or certain extramedullary sites, especially the spleen and liver (56, 57, 204). The clinical abnormalities that result from the proliferation of a given hematopoietic cell line are similar in several of the myeloproliferative disorders. These common clinical abnormalities, coupled with a propensity for splenomegaly and hyperuricemia, seem to justify grouping these disorders. However, some authors question the validity of the concept of overlapping myeloproliferative disorders (87) and instead consider each disease entity separately.

Proliferation of bone marrow cell lines may be described on the one hand as *reactive* and on the other as *idiopathic* or *agnogenic*. Reactive proliferations are usually in response to known causes and may involve a single cell line or several lines. They are generally acute and self-limited. An example of a reactive proliferation is the bone marrow response to hemorrhage or hemolysis, which predominantly involves the erythrocytic series but may also involve the megakaryocyte and granulocyte lines. Another example is the bone marrow response to acute pyogenic infection; in this situation the marrow response is predominantly granulocytic.

In contrast, the idiopathic or agnogenic proliferation of hematopoietic cell lines has no known cause and is generally sustained rather than acute. Furthermore, these proliferations are not self-limited; that is, they result in an excessive production of cells so that normal levels are exceeded in tissues and in the circulation. In general, a return to the original normal hematologic status does not occur in chronic myeloproliferative syndromes; the process usually is inexorably progressive and often shows a tendency to accelerate with time.

The chronic myeloproliferative disorders customarily are classified as shown in Table 10.1 (56–58). However, clinical diseases transitional between two or more of these disorders are often seen. This is not surprising, considering that in each disorder several cell lines may be affected by the proliferative process and also that the clinical symptomatology reflects the result of such proliferation. In Table 10.1 the predominant proliferating cell line for each disorder is indicated.

Clinical diseases transitional between the *chronic* myeloproliferative disorders and the *acute* myeloproliferative disorders (acute myelocytic leukemia, acute monocytic leukemia, and Di Guglielmo's syndrome, Chapter 11) also are occasionally observed by hematologists. Furthermore, clinical disease may in the course of time undergo transition from a typical chronic myeloproliferative process to an acute process. For example, a transition from chronic myelocytic leukemia to acute leukemia or

Table 10.1 Classification of chronic myeloproliferative disorders.

Disease	Predominant proliferating cell line
Chronic myelocytic leukemia	Granulocyte
Chronic eosinophilic leukemia	Eosinophil
Chronic basophilic leukemia	Basophil
Polycythemia rubra vera	Erythrocyte
Essential thrombocytosis	Megakaryocyte
Agnogenic myeloid metaplasia	Variable extramedullary hematopoiesis

from polycythemia vera to acute leukemia is not uncommon.

In most modern classifications, chronic myeloproliferative disorders are distinguished from lymphoproliferative disorders such as acute and chronic lymphocytic leukemia, the various lymphomas, and infectious mononucleosis. Little overlap occurs between the hematologic features of the chronic myeloproliferative and lymphoproliferative disorders. Rarely, however, mixed proliferation of lymphoid and other cell lines is seen (37).

The interrelationship of the disorders that constitute the acute and chronic myeloproliferative syndromes and lymphoproliferative syndromes may be better understood with reference to the interrelation of the various hematopoietic cell lines (Fig. 10.1; see also Fig. I.1). Clearly, a pluripotent hematopoietic stem cell exists that is capable of repleting lymphoid and myeloid tissues in ir-

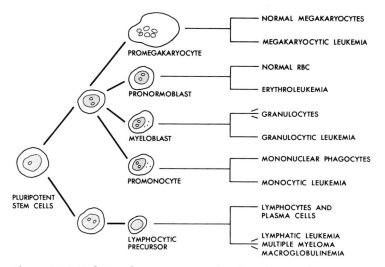

Figure 10.1 Relation between normal and malignant hematopoietic cell lines and a common pluripotent stem cell. In each cell series, normal cellular differentiation has a neoplastic counterpart.

radiated animals. Evidence summarized in Chapter 2 suggests that the commitment to differentiation along a given pathway is made relatively early in cell differentiation. The branch point for differentiation into either granulocytic or monocytic lines is beyond the branch point for determining lymphoid vs nonlymphoid differentiation.

Chronic Myelocytic Leukemia

Some of the synonyms for the term chronic myelocytic leukemia are chronic myelogenous leukemia, chronic granulocytic leukemia, and chronic neutrophilic leukemia.

Incidence

A knowledge of the incidence of chronic myelocytic leukemia and other leukemias comes from sources such as hospital series (170), analyses of death certificates (102, 131, 176), and the use of special schemes such as tumor registries (46, 65). There are, however, limitations to these methods of collecting data (65, 184, 193), and the true incidence of the disease is not known. Chronic, as well as acute, leukemia is worldwide in distribution, although considerable differences are recognized in different geographic areas (221). The available data on incidence of chronic myelocytic leukemia will be considered in this chapter, and the data for all types of leukemia will be reviewed in Chapter 11. The data available on a specific morphologic type of leukemia are not so reliable as the data covering leukemias in general (96, 125, 193).

In 1917 Ward (210) assembled what was probably the earliest comprehensive series of patients of leukemia. His source was 729 reported cases of leukemia. By his analysis, 34 percent had chronic myelocytic leukemia, 11.5 percent had chronic lymphocytic leukemia, and the remainder had acute leukemia. Considerably lower estimates of the relative frequency of chronic myelocytic leukemia have been reported from more recent analyses of death certificates (96), although a figure of 37 percent was found in one modern hospital series (170). Probably the best compilation of data on the relative incidence of chronic myelocytic leukemia among the leukemias can be found in Wintrobe's textbook of hematology (218); there the figure given in 26.6 percent.

The peak age incidence for chronic myelocytic leukemia in series published before 1937 was thirty years (138, 169). This is a considerably younger age than more modern series would suggest (96, 125, 217). In most studies published in the last twenty years the median age incidence of chronic myelocytic leukemia has been in the mid-forties. A tendency for leukemia to occur at progressively greater ages has been the recent experience of all countries for which statistics are available, with the notable exception of Japan (53, 58, 186).

Although chronic myelocytic leukemia is generally a disease of adults, it occurs also in childhood and has been reported as early as the first few weeks of life (164). It may account for about 5 percent of childhood leukemias (8). Occasional familial occurrence of this disease has been recorded (211).

In most early series of chronic myelocytic leukemia cases there is a predominance of males, with observed ratios of males to females varying between about 1.2 to 1 and 1.4 to 1 (124, 138, 169, 218). In more recent series the ratio is nearer unity (96, 177).

Clinical Features

Probably the earliest recorded case of chronic myelocytic leukemia is that reported by Neumann in 1870 (149). The clinical features of chronic myelocytic leukemia may be classified as typical or atypical. In large series of patients there is a correlation between the presence of typical features and of the characteristic chromosomal abnormality (see 194 and the section later in this chapter on the Philadelphia chromosome). Features of the typical case of chronic myelocytic leukemia will be considered first, followed by a discussion of some of the atypical variants.

Onset   The onset of chronic myelocytic leukemia is generally insidious, rarely acute. The patient's first complaints often are related to symptomatology associated with anemia or splenomegaly. He may complain of dyspnea, palpitation, pedal edema, abdominal fullness, or left upper quadrant pain or discomfort. More rarely he may note left shoulder pain and abdominal pain from splenic infarcts early in the disease. At the clinical onset of disease, symptoms are more often systemic than localized in a specific organ. The complaints are of loss of energy, malaise, loss of appetite, and sometimes of night sweats. Infrequently, the patient is almost or wholly asymptomatic, and an elevated granulocyte count is observed on incidental examination (218, 219). Very rarely, symptoms are referable to a single organ such as the skin or gastrointestinal tract.

Although a variable degree of splenomegaly usually is demonstrable, a physical examination at the clinical onset of disease may show few other abnormalities (104).

Progression   With the passage of time and progression of the disease, symptoms referable to hematologic cell abnormalities and to local organ infiltration become increasingly prominent, provided the disease is not controlled by therapy. In uncontrolled disease progressive anemia with associated weakness and shortness of breath may become severe. Abnormalities in platelet numbers and function resulting from the disease process itself, or chemotherapy, become more frequent and result in hemorrhagic manifestations.

Infections as a consequence of granulocyte abnormality are rare in early- or intermediate-stage disease, although granulocytopenia may result from either overly vigorous therapy or transition of the disease to a more acute form.

In untreated disease progressive splenic enlargement and splenic infarctions become prominent. Splenomegaly may be appreciated by the patient as a fullness, especially after meals, or as a "dragging" sensation in the left upper quadrant. Splenic infarction is noted as left shoulder pain or localized abdominal pain consequent to perisplenitis and peritoneal involvement. A friction rub can generally be heard in such circumstances. More serious complications of splenic infarction are intra-abdominal hemorrhage and splenic rupture. With progressive disease the spleen may be moderately or massively enlarged and appear to fill the entire abdomen and extend into the pelvis. At this stage of disease the spleen is usually hard and nontender unless infarcted. The liver also shows moderate or marked enlargement.

In uncontrolled progressive disease, localized organ involvement may be prominent. Direct skin infiltration by leukemic cells producing an erythematous maculopapular rash is not uncommon in advanced disease (71, 84, 93) and may be a poor prognostic sign. Bone lesions, including periosteal infiltration and lytic lesions, are rare in chronic myelocytic leukemia, but when present they may be a prominent feature of the clinical disease (173). Hypercalcemia may occur (6). The appearance of osseous lesions often is associated with rapid clinical deterioration and either progressive pancytopenia or so-called "blast crisis" (39). Osteosclerosis also has been described in a patient with chronic myelocytic leukemia (117).

Lymphadenopathy may occur during the terminal acute transition of the disease (68), but otherwise is not prominent. Priapism, probably the consequence of local obstruction to blood flow, is a relatively rare occurrence (94), as is a prominent gastrointestinal involvement (220) or ascites with Banti's syndrome (40). Prominent pulmonary involvement, although rare, has been described (95, 116). At any time during the course of the disease, clinically symptomatic hyperuricemia with joint or renal manifestations may occur. Occasionally myelofibrosis develops (27, 117, 188).

Two points should be made about the progressive phase

of chronic myelocytic leukemia. First, in the uncontrolled disease a rough parallelism occurs between the granulocyte level, the size of the spleen, and clinical symptomatology. This phenomenon stands in contrast to the situation in chronic lymphocytic leukemia where there is often no such parallelism between symptomatology and the white blood count. Second, the signs and symptoms of progressive disease are only rarely seen in most modern medical centers, where the disease is kept under control with chemotherapy until terminal transition occurs. Many of the descriptions of progressive disease are located in the older medical literature. Those patients whose granulocyte count can be maintained near normal levels tend to experience minimal symptoms from their disease. Therefore, the modern physician generally observes and tries to maintain a *modified* natural history of disease which is considerably different from the natural history of uncontrolled disease.

Terminal Events   The most common preterminal event observed in the course of the modified natural history of chronic myelocytic leukemia is transition to "blast crisis," a term designating a disease syndrome essentially indistinguishable from acute myelocytic leukemia. When such transition occurs, the manifestations are those resulting from the loss of normal blood elements (anemia, granulocytopenia, thrombocytopenia) with consequent increased susceptibility to infection and hemorrhage as well as localized infiltrations of skin and viscera. Even meningeal leukemia has been observed at this stage (122). Symptomatology is considered in detail in the description of acute myelocytic leukemia (see Chapter 11). Death at this stage is usually from hemorrhage or infection.

Very rarely, chronic myelocytic leukemia may present as blast crisis (25). Although blast crisis may superficially resemble uncontrolled acute myelocytic leukemia, there appear to be fundamental differences between these disease processes: (*a*) the in vitro proliferative characteristics of acute leukemic and chronic myelocytic leukemic cells differ (92); (*b*) the control of erythropoiesis appears to be autonomous in blast crisis (182, 183); and (*c*) generally, blast crisis is less responsive to chemotherapeutic control (33).

Hematologic Features

Onset   The hematocrit, the red cell, and the reticulocyte count are usually near normal levels in the early stages of chronic myelocytic leukemia. Typically the platelet count is elevated and may be 1,000,000/mm³ or more. The granulocyte count is also elevated. In the symptomatic patient it is usually greater than 50,000 and may be in excess of

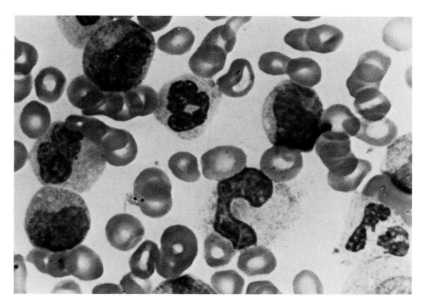

Figure 10.2 Peripheral blood smear from a patient with chronic myelocytic leukemia in relapse.

500,000/mm³. In the asymptomatic patient it is often less than 50,000. The increased numbers of leukocytes and platelets produce a striking increase in the size of the buffy coat seen when blood is centrifuged in hematrocrit tubes.

The blood smear shows predominance of granulocytes at all stages of maturation, but particularly at or beyond the myelocyte stage (Fig. 10.2). Mature neutrophils are abundant. When the granulocyte count is high, moderate numbers of myeloblasts and promyelocytes may be seen in the peripheral blood, although they usually constitute less than 5 percent of the total circulating granulocytes. Even in very early disease, when the granulocyte count is high, leukocyte alkaline phosphatase activity is low or absent (see below).

Basophils are almost always present in greater than normal numbers and may be increased relative to other granulocytes (Fig. 10.3). In some variants of chronic myelocytic leukemia they are the predominant cell (148, 178).

Bizarre and abnormally large platelets may appear in the peripheral blood, as well as neutrophils with abnormal granulation (59) (see Fig. 10.4). At the time of diagnosis the bone marrow usually is densely packed with granulocytes at all stages of maturation up to the mature neutrophil. The myeloid/erythroid ratio is greatly increased. Megakaryocytes appear to be more abundant than normal (Fig. 10.5). Lipid-laden histiocytes resembling Gaucher cells have been described in the bone marrow of patients with chronic myelocytic leukemia (1, 179) and may be

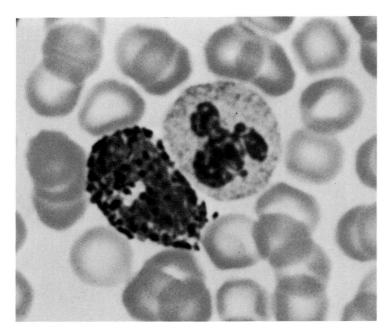

Figure 10.3 A polymorphonuclear leukocyte and a basophil in the peripheral blood of a patient with chronic granulocytic leukemia.

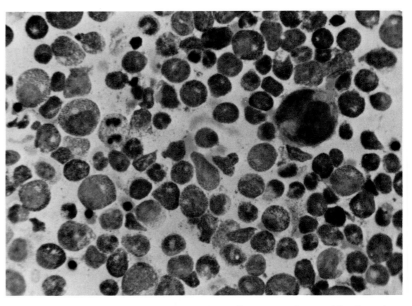

Figure 10.5 Bone marrow aspirate from a patient with chronic myelocytic leukemia in relapse. Note the densely packed marrow and the young megakaryocytes. Giemsa stain.

seen in Fig. 10.6. Glucocerebroside, a constituent of red and white cell membranes, is the lipid that accumulates in both disorders (111, 179). The lipid accumulation in leukemic patients appears to result from an increased turnover of hematopoietic cells rather than from a defect in the enzyme glucocerebrosidase (111).

Progression When the disease is kept under control by therapy, the hematologic abnormalities may revert to normal. When the disease is uncontrolled, however, the hematologic abnormalities become progressively more severe. A normochromic normocytic anemia develops in most patients, which is attributable to short erythrocyte survival and inadequate marrow erythropoietic response to anemia. In some patients the enlarged spleen is a site of excessive erythrocyte destruction (50). Fetal hemoglobin concentration may be increased (135). Antibody-induced hemolysis is rare. The platelet count tends to remain elevated until the terminal stages of disease.

Terminal Events At the time of transition to an acute form of leukemia, progressively increasing numbers of myeloblasts and other immature forms appear in the bone marrow and circulation (Fig. 10.7). The typical hematologic features of acute myelocytic leukemia then supervene. The anemia becomes more severe and the platelet count falls as megakaryocytes disappear from the bone marrow. The terminal blood picture as a rule is indistin-

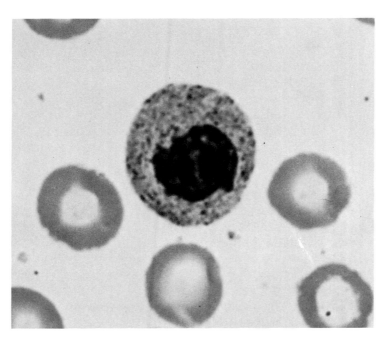

Figure 10.4 A myelocyte in the peripheral blood of a patient with chronic myelocytic leukemia, showing abnormal nuclear configuration and abnormal cytoplasmic granulation. Contrast this figure with the normal early metamyelocyte seen in Fig. 1.6.

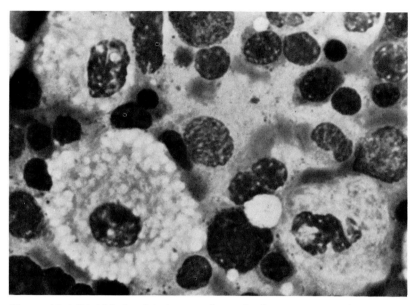

Figure 10.6 Lipid-laden histiocytes from the bone marrow of a patient with chronic myelocytic leukemia. The appearance of these cells closely resembles those of patients with Gaucher's disease.

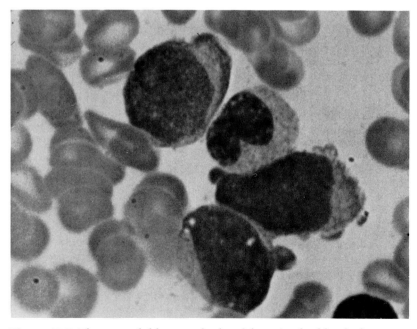

Figure 10.7 Three myeloblasts and a band form in the blood of a patient with chronic myelocytic leukemia undergoing blast transformation.

guishable from acute myelocytic leukemia. This late phase, often termed the blast crisis, probably results from acute transformation of a single clone of hematopoietic cells (146). Rarely, the transition is erythroblastic rather than myeloblastic (182).

Differential Diagnosis

When the patient with chronic myelocytic leukemia first consults a physician because of nonspecific symptoms of malaise and weakness, or symptoms referable to splenomegaly, the diagnostic possibilities are legion. However, once the physician performs a blood count and observes granulocytosis and often thrombocytosis, the diagnostic possibilities are much more circumscribed. When the triad of extreme granulocytosis with many mature neutrophils, splenomegaly, and thrombocytosis is documented, the differential diagnoses include chronic myelocytic leukemia, other chronic myeloproliferative disorders, and diseases with "reactive" granulocytosis or so-called "leukemoid reactions."

On the basis of clinical manifestations and peripheral blood hematology, myelofibrosis with myeloid metaplasia is the chronic myeloproliferative disorder most commonly confused with chronic myelocytic leukemia. This disorder is easily distinguished from chronic myelocytic leukemia simply by examining a needle biopsy specimen of the bone marrow; in myeloid metaplasia the marrow space is fibrotic, in chronic myelocytic leukemia it is densely infiltrated with granulocyte precursors. Furthermore, the characteristic abnormalities of erythrocyte morphology seen in myeloid metaplasia are relatively rare in chronic myelocytic leukemia. In addition, the Philadelphia chromosome is present in chronic myelocytic leukemia and absent in myeloid metaplasia.

The leukemoid reactions may be divided into those associated with malignant disease, those associated with microbial infection, and those occurring in other inflammatory and hematologic diseases.

Malignant conditions in which high levels of circulating granulocytes are sometimes observed include disseminated carcinoma of the lung (72) and carcinoma of the breast with bone marrow involvement, as well as other cancers (30, 101, 165, 174, 203). Generally such tumors produce neutrophilic leukemoid reactions only when they have spread to the bone marrow.

The relation between tuberculosis and various myeloproliferative disorders is of some interest (48, 178). For instance, the association between tuberculosis and myelosclerosis seems to be greater than can be accounted for by chance alone. Leukemoid reactions can occur in tuberculosis; however, it is unlikely that mycobacterial disease ever causes chronic myelocytic leukemia (55, 74, 88, 132, 154, 197).

Leukemoid blood pictures may also be associated with acute infections such as pneumonia and meningococcal meningitis (103, 105, 121). Inflammatory diseases that may occasionally resemble chronic myelocytic leukemia in their hematologic manifestations include some of the collagen vascular diseases and acute hemolytic disease (121). A patient with fulminant cirrhosis with minimal jaundice, whose disease resembled chronic myelocytic leukemia, has been described (52). Other reported causes of neutrophilic leukemoid reactions include eclampsia (218) and mercury poisoning (67). Drug reactions and acute hemolytic reactions can also simulate leukemia.

It should be stressed that those diseases producing a leukemoid picture are only very rarely serious diagnostic considerations for the patient with chronic myelocytic leukemia. Obvious clinical and hematologic features of the leukemoid reactions distinguish them from chronic myelocytic leukemia. These features include the usual absence of prominent basophilia and the absence of the very prominent increase in megakaryocytes in the bone marrow. Furthermore, only rarely do the diseases cited have associated levels of granulocytes in the range encountered in chronic myelocytic leukemia; moderate neutrophilia is more common. The definitive distinction between chronic myelocytic leukemia and leukemoid reactions from other causes rests on the presence of the Philadelphia chromosome anomaly and the neutrophil alkaline phosphatase reaction. The neutrophil alkaline phosphatase activity almost always is low in the mature neutrophils of active chronic myelocytic leukemia and usually is high in reactive leukocytoses (126). The Philadelphia chromosome anomaly appears to be unique to chronic myelocytic leukemia. Disorders sometimes associated with leukemoid reactions are summarized below:

Infections
  Tuberculosis
  Pneumococcal pneumonia
  Meningococcal meningitis
Malignant diseases
  Carcinoma of the lung, breast, kidney
  Hodgkin's disease
Inflammatory diseases
  Collagen-vascular diseases
Miscellaneous causes
  Fulminant cirrhosis
  Eclampsia
  Acute hemolysis
  Drug reactions

Prognosis

Remissions in chronic leukemia by X-irradiation or chemotherapy have been obtained for nearly three-quarters of a century (127, 160). Consequently, it is not possible to obtain a contemporary series of untreated patients to demonstrate the natural history of chronic myelocytic leukemia. In the 1920s, Minot and his colleagues concluded that the duration of disease they were observing was not significantly modified by the therapy then available (138). A similar conclusion was reached in several later studies (58, 192). A study published in 1939 (219) gave a figure of 3.3 years for median survival from onset of symptoms. In 1954 Tivey (192) drew together a large series with 1,090 cases of chronic myelocytic leukemia seen between 1929 and 1951. He found that survival curves showed a skewed deviation, so that they could not be expressed in terms of mean and standard deviations; analysis of median survival was, however, satisfactory. Median survival from clinical onset of disease to death was 2.7 years, with a range of 2.6 to 2.8 in this study. However, this analysis probably underestimated duration of disease, since patients still living at the time of the analysis were not included in the calculation of survival time. One other point made by this study was that survival times in chronic myelocytic and chronic lymphocytic leukemia were quite similar (cf. 123).

The studies of Feinlieb and MacMahon (73) reported a median total survival of 19.4 months in a series of chronic leukemias (both chronic myelocytic and chronic lymphocytic) collected between 1943 and 1952. These data suggest that shortened survival is not uncommon in chronic myelocytic leukemia. On the other hand, a substantial number of patients with chronic myelocytic leukemia live five to ten years or longer (138, 163, 219). In Tivey's series (192) 22 percent of patients with either form of chronic leukemia lived longer than five years after diagnosis. Spontaneous remission is exceedingly rare but not unknown in chronic myelocytic leukemia (138). Existence of severe thrombocytopenia during the course of illness is regarded as a poor prognostic sign.

Now that the disease can be well controlled by therapy, death from anemia or splenic rupture is a relatively rare occurrence, although death from drug-induced marrow aplasia as a result of too vigorous therapy is not so rare. *At present, the usual preterminal occurrence is the appearance of cellular immaturity with a development of blastic crisis and resistance to therapy* (100, 110, 145, 215). Once blastic crisis supervenes, 75 percent of patients are dead within six months. Average survival time in the patients developing blast crisis is twenty-four months from initial diagnosis of chronic leukemia (110).

The Philadelphia Chromosome and Atypical Variants of Chronic Myelocytic Leukemia

An abnormal marker chromosome in chronic myelocytic leukemia was originally described by Nowell and Hungerford in 1960 (150, 151) and quickly confirmed by others (76, 112). It was called the Philadelphia — or Ph[1] — chromosome. The Ph[1] chromosome is derived from a chromosome of pair 22 through loss of a variable portion of the long arm (36). With the exception of its occurrence in a few cases of acute leukemia (113, 134, 194), the Ph[1] chromosome abnormality is restricted to patients with chronic myelocytic leukemia. It appears to be the only consistent chromosomal anomaly found in any malignant disease. In 85 to 90 percent of patients with chronic myelocytic leukemia the Ph[1] chromosome is found in most, if not all, nucleated marrow hematopoietic cells, even when the disease is in remission (213). The abnormality is observed in erythroid and megakaryocytic precursors, as well as in granulocyte precursors (45). Evidence suggests that these multiple cell lines are affected (see Fig. 10.1) because of a loss of genetic material in a common stem cell precursor (4, 195). The disease probably results from malignant transformation in a single pluripotent precursor cell (75). The lymphoid cells of patients with chronic myelocytic leukemia do not share the Ph[1] abnormality, and fibroblasts from subcutaneous tissue and bone marrow also are negative (5, 133). Spleen granulocyte precursors, on the other hand, have the abnormality (181).

In 10 to 15 percent of patients with chronic myelocytic leukemia the Ph[1] chromosome is not detectable. Such patients may have no chromosomal abnormality of the hematopoietic cells. The correlation between cytogenetic abnormality and clinical disease is best summarized in a recent study of 179 patients (213). The median survival of patients with the Ph[1] chromosome abnormality was 31 to 40 months. Median survival of patients who were either Ph[1]-negative or Ph[1]-negative with other chromosomal anomalies was 12 to 15 months. This difference in survival and prognosis has been recognized in several studies, as has the general refractiveness of Ph[1]-negative disease to therapy (164, 171, 194).

Chronic myelocytic leukemia in the pediatric age range is often Ph[1] chromosome-negative (99, 164, 213) and lacks the characteristic leukocyte alkaline phosphatase abnormality (167). The prognosis of the juvenile type of chronic myelocytic leukemia is poor, and response to therapy is often marginal (8, 99, 164).

Ph[1]-negative disease may have many atypical features distinguishing it from the classical disease picture. For example, patients have been seen with Ph[1]-negative chronic

Table 10.2 Characteristics of Ph[1]-positive and Ph[1]-negative chronic myelocytic leukemia.

Characteristic	Ph[1]-positive	Ph[1]-negative
Median age	52	65
Male/female ratio	Equal	Male > female
Initial WBC count	Variable	<150,000
Initial platelet count	Normal, high	Normal, low
Presentation	Variable	More ill
Marrow M/E ratio	>20–30:1	<20–30:1
Median survival	3–4 years	<2 years

myelocytic leukemia characterized by densely packed bone marrow and tissue infiltration, but little peripheral blood leukocytosis. The differences between Ph[1]-positive and Ph[1]-negative disease are summarized in Table 10.2.

Chromosomal abnormalities in chronic myelocytic leukemia other than the Ph[1] abnormality are most often found in chromosome groups 6 to 12 (115, 152, 155, 213). Occasional patients may have cell lines with double Ph[1] chromosomes (79, 114, 213).

The appearance, late in the disease, of chromosomal abnormalities other than the Ph[1] chromosome generally signals the preterminal stage and the occurrence of primitive cells in the circulation (120, 157, 213). In contrast, aneuploidy and other chromosomal abnormalities early in the disease do not appear to alter prognosis or survival (213). It has been suggested that the development of high frequencies of hyperdiploid Ph[1]-positive cells is involved in the hematologic and clinical progression of chronic myelocytic leukemia (156, 157).

The Ph[1] chromosome abnormality repeatedly has been reported in one member of a pair of monozygotic twins (9, 66, 91, 107). Therefore it is presumably a postzygous abnormality. Weiner described a family with a high incidence of leukemia: the Ph[1] chromosome was found in blood cell metaphases of family members who did not have clinical evidence of chronic myelocytic leukemia (211) and has recently been observed in bone marrow cells of a patient before the appearance of overt clinical disease (32).

The Malignant Granulocyte

Production, Distribution, and Function

When peripheral blood leukocytes from patients with chronic myelocytic leukemia are labeled with ^{32}P-diisopropylfluorophosphate (Chapter 2) and returned to the patient, they disappear from the circulation at an abnormally slow rate (3, 81). Their mode of disappearance varies considerably, depending in part on the hematologic status of the patient at the time of study (83). Patients in remission have normal or near-normal leukocyte kinetics; patients in relapse have abnormal kinetics. Cell fractionation studies by Galbraith indicate that the intravascular life-span of the mature neutrophils is greatly prolonged when the disease is in relapse (81–83). This kinetic abnormality reflects mainly a cellular defect in the malignant granulocyte, but also an "environmental" abnormality in leukemic patients. Other investigators have felt that the prolonged blood clearance time of granulocytes in chronic myelocytic leukemia in relapse reflects mainly cellular immaturity (3).

Additional kinetic studies suggest that malignant granulocytes reenter the bone marrow parenchyma, whereas normal neutrophils do not (42, 82, 147). This property of malignant granulocytes may reflect their tendency to be sequestered in extravascular compartments from which they recirculate (69, 82). Sequestration in and recirculation from the spleen may explain why splenic irradiation often produces a remission in chronic myelocytic leukemia.

Since the intravascular residence time of leukemic granulocytes is greatly prolonged, the levels of circulating cells are higher than might be anticipated from the increased granulocyte turnover rate. For example, the total body granulocyte pool is greatly expanded in chronic myelocytic leukemia in relapse (10 to 150 times normal). The blood granulocyte disappearance time is 4 to 12 times normal. Consequently (see Chapter 2), the granulocyte turnover rate, a measure of granulocyte production, is only 3 to 6 times the normal rate (3).

Granulopoiesis clearly occurs in the spleen and liver of patients with active chronic myelocytic leukemia, as well as in their bone marrow (29, 43, 141, 180). When blast crisis supervenes in chronic myelocytic leukemia, the kinetic pattern of leukocyte behavior resembles that found in acute leukemia in relapse (90).

Several authors recently have commented on the occasional occurrence of cyclic leukocytosis in chronic myelocytic leukemia (144, 175, 206) and it is plotted in Fig. 10.8. The striking cyclic changes in granulopoiesis occasionally may be accompanied by cyclic changes in thrombopoiesis (206). An examination of the mechanisms of cyclic granulopoiesis was presented in Chapter 9.

Leukocyte mobilization into sites of inflammation may be impaired in patients with chronic myelocytic leukemia (7). In general, only mature neutrophils and band forms are mobilized (21, 108, 158).

The morphologically mature neutrophils of patients with chronic myelocytic leukemia appear to be normal in

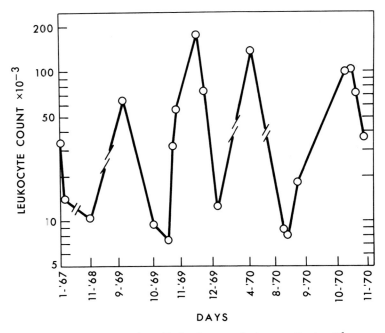

Figure 10.8 Pattern of cyclic leukocytosis in a patient with chronic myelocytic leukemia. (Modified from R. K. Shadduck, A. Winkelstein, and N. G. Nunna, *Cancer* 29:399, 1972.)

their ability to phagocytize and kill microorganisms (109). The normal phagocyte function probably accounts for the rarity of bacterial infections during the early and progressive phase of the disease (214). Leukocytes from chronic myelocytic leukemia have been used successfully as replacement therapy for patients with neutropenia from bone marrow failure (78, 172).

Metabolism

Carbohydrate and Amino Acid Metabolism The rates of glucose utilization and lactate production are lower in the granulocytes of patients with chronic myelocytic leukemia than in normal leukocytes (11–15, 134). In an attempt to define the mechanism of the abnormally low glycolytic rate of certain leukemic leukocytes, individual enzymes of the Embden-Meyerhoff pathway have been analyzed. In white cells isolated from patients with chronic myelocytic leukemia, activities of five of these enzymes have been reported as abnormally low, whereas the levels of five other enzymes were either normal or increased (13–15, 85, 205). Despite differences in the levels of activity of some of the glycolytic enzymes found in normal and leukemic white cells, the enzymes appear to be identical when Michaelis constant and pH activity curves are used as criteria (10, 11, 63, 64).

Increased levels of glutamic acid dehydrogenase activity

(208, 209) and low levels of glyoxalase (130) are reported to occur in white cells isolated from patients with chronic myelocytic leukemia.

Another abnormality in carbohydrate metabolism of chronic myelocytic leukemia granulocytes is a lower-than-normal concentration of cellular glycogen, although their ability to synthesize glycogen in vitro is unimpaired (202). Abnormally low periodic acid Schiff reactivity corresponds to the low glycogen (79). In contrast, neutrophil glycogen concentration is increased in granulocytosis associated with infection and polycythemia vera (200, 201, 207).

In addition to these reported abnormalities of carbohydrate metabolism, abnormalities in enzyme control of amino acid metabolism in chronic myelocytic leukemia have been described. For example, levels of leukocyte glutamic-oxalacetic transaminase activity have been reported for normal granulocytes, mononuclear cells, and white cells of acute leukemia and "reactive" leukocytosis (22). Waisman (208) found normal levels of this enzyme in white cells from patients with chronic myelocytic leukemia, but other investigators have found increased levels in this condition.

A higher degree of arginase activity has been reported in some (23), but not all (187), studies of white cells of patients with chronic myelocytic leukemia (cf. 24, 166).

A striking feature of the amino acid metabolism of leukocytes from patients with chronic myelocytic leukemia is the very high levels of histamine that may be present in the blood (51, 185, 189, 198, 199, 222). Almost certainly this arises from the enzymatic decarboxylation of histidine by large numbers of circulating basophils (see Chapters 3 and 7). Lesser elevations of blood histamine are found in polycythemia vera (200). It is interesting that remarkably few symptoms can actually be correlated with the increased levels of histamine observed in the chronic myeloproliferative disorders (185).

DNA, Lipid, Protein, and Mineral Metabolism   Most of the important abnormalities that have been described in cellular purine, pyrimidine, lipid metabolism, nucleic acid, and protein metabolism in chronic myelocytic leukemia can be explained on the basis of cellular immaturity alone (see Chapter 3). A few cannot. For example, the molecular configuration of mitochondrial DNA from chronic granulocytic leukemia leukocytes exists in an abnormal circular dimer form (44). Another interesting observation of unknown significance is the occurrence of low levels of zinc in leukocytes from patients with chronic myelocytic leukemia and myeloid metaplasia (60–62, 77, 86).

Vitamin Metabolism   Formate-activating enzyme and dihydrofolate reductase activities are increased in leukocytes of patients with chronic myelocytic leukemia, but not chronic lymphocytic leukemia (16, 139, 216). These enzymes appear to have the same physical properties in leukemic cells as in normal white cells (16–19). Whether these abnormalities of enzyme are a function of malignancy or of cellular immaturity is still unknown.

The most dramatic of the documented abnormalities of vitamin metabolism in chronic myelocytic leukemia is that concerned with vitamin B_{12}. Human leukocytes carry significant amounts of vitamin B_{12}. In patients with chronic myelocytic leukemia in relapse, and in some individuals with polycythemia vera and nonmalignant leukocytosis, the serum–vitamin-B_{12} binding capacity is markedly increased above normal (35, 38, 98, 136, 161). In 1955 Mollin and Ross (142) reported that the breakdown products of granulocytes from patients with chronic myelocytic leukemia were capable of binding vitamin B_{12} in vitro (cf. 190).

There are two well-defined vitamin B_{12} binding proteins in serum: transcobalamin I and II (97, 106). The increased serum binding capacity in chronic myelocytic leukemia results mainly from an increase in transcobalamin I (162). A third vitamin B_{12} protein originating in granulocytes may exist (34). Recent evidence suggests that cells as primitive as promyelocytes may also produce transcobalamin I (162).

Mature normal neutrophils have a high Co^{60}-vitamin B_{12} binding capacity. Immature granulocytes and eosinophils have only a limited binding capacity (137). The disintegration products of mature neutrophils thus may be important in the increased vitamin B_{12} binding capacity of serum in patients with chronic myelocytic leukemia and polycythemia vera (137, 142).

Granule Enzymes   During the chronic phase of the disease, chronic myelocytic leukemia cells are rich in granules and granular enzymes. The elevated levels of serum lysozyme occasionally observed in this disorder may reflect granulocyte turnover (38). Irradiation-induced cell destruction may result in massive lysozymuria (191).

In subjects with nonmalignant granulocytosis, the activity of alkaline phosphatase in the mature neutrophil tends to be higher than normal (47). In contrast, alkaline phosphatase activity usually is low or absent in the neutrophils of patients with chronic myelocytic leukemia in relapse (47, 118). Despite intensive study, the relation between the abnormal enzyme activity and the occurrence of the Ph[1] chromosome still is not clear (47, 118, 167). Other disorders in which low leukocyte alkaline

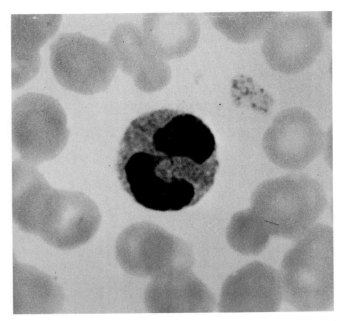

Figure 10.9 A mature neutrophil with a bilobed nucleus from the peripheral blood of a patient with chronic myelocytic leukemia. The cell closely resembles those seen in the Pelger-Huët anomaly.

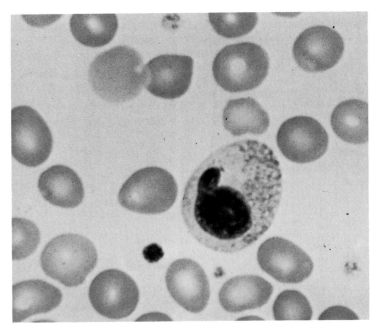

Figure 10.10 An eosinophil showing abnormal nuclear configuration in the peripheral blood of a patient with chronic myelocytic leukemia.

phosphatase have been described (47, 118, 140) are listed below:

Chronic myelocytic leukemia
Agnogenic myeloid metaplasia (occasional)
Di Guglielmo syndrome (occasional)
Paroxysmal nocturnal hemoglobinuria
Idiopathic thrombocytopenic purpura
Aplastic anemia (occasional)
Sarcoidosis (occasional)

Granulocytes in Other Myeloproliferative Disorders

Increased numbers of granulocytes are seen in a variety of chronic myeloproliferative disorders including polycythemia rubra vera and myeloid metaplasia. Abnormal granulocyte forms are frequently encountered in the circulation of patients with these disorders. For example, bilobed mature neutrophils (Fig. 10.9) and mature granulocytes with diminished granulation or other abnormalities of nuclear configuration (Fig. 10.10) are often demonstrable.

At the turn of the century, Türk noted that leukocytosis frequently accompanies polycythemia vera (196). Many of the patients described by Osler in 1908 (153) had leukocyte counts in excess of 10,000/mm³. In another early series about two-thirds of the patients with polycythemia vera had moderate elevation of the granulocyte count (128). This observation is so common it is rarely mentioned by modern authors. Occasionally the leuko-

cyte count may exceed 50,000/mm³ and the blood picture may resemble chronic myelocytic leukemia (168). The leukocyte alkaline phosphatase may be normal in polycythemia; however, when the granulocyte count is elevated, enzyme activity generally is increased (2).

The neutrophils of patients with polycythemia vera often have an increased concentration of glycogen and an elevated rate of glycogenolysis (84, 129, 207). Resting glucose-1-C oxidation and oxygen consumption are increased in polycythemia leukocytes. The metabolic changes accompanying phagocytosis also may be greater (28, 54).

The leukocyte count may be increased in 40 to 50 percent of patients with myelofibrosis and decreased in another 10 to 20 percent (26, 89, 159, 218). Myelocytes, promyelocytes, and, occasionally, myeloblasts may be found in the circulation. The leukocyte alkaline phosphatase is usually high or normal, rarely low (20, 47). Increased numbers of stem cells may circulate in the blood of patients with myelofibrosis (41).

Principles of Management of Chronic Myelocytic Leukemia

Objectives of Therapy

The available modalities of treatment of chronic myelocytic leukemia probably do not significantly prolong life.

However, treatment unquestionably makes the patient more comfortable and improves his capacity to function; the objective of treatment is to maintain the patient symptom-free for as long a period as possible without risking complications arising from therapy.

Because of the parallelism between symptom status and the degree of peripheral blood granulocytosis, the level of the white blood count is used as a guide to treatment. Simply stated, *therapy is directed toward maintaining the white blood count at or near the normal level.*

Modes of Therapy

Two types of treatment have proved effective in chronic myelocytic leukemia: chemotherapy and splenic irradiation. The level of the white blood count is effectively reduced by a number of drugs, including alkylators, 6-mercaptopurine, hydroxyurea, colcemide, trimethyl-colchicinic acid, dibromomannitol, and daunomycin (49); only the first three have had widespread clinical use. The most widely used drug is busulfan (Myleran^R). In the occasional case unresponsive to busulfan, hydroxyurea and 6-mercaptopurine are the alternative drugs of choice.

Busulfan is given orally until the white blood count reaches approximately 20,000/mm³. At that time the dose is reduced by one-half, and the drug is discontinued when the white blood count reaches 10,000 to 12,000/mm³. Busulfan therapy is not resumed until the white count rises above approximately 15,000/mm³. The lowest dose that will keep the white blood count at about 10,000/mm³ is used for maintenance therapy (49,100). A careful watch is kept on the platelet count during treatment, since it may sometimes fall abruptly. Induction of a normal hematologic status may take three to six weeks, and occasionally longer.

Hematopoietic suppression is the principal toxicity from drug therapy. Other toxic side effects of busulfan therapy include pulmonary fibrosis, skin pigmentation, and a syndrome resembling Addison's disease (49).

Occasionally, patients have a disease that is refractory to treatment with busulfan (100). Such patients can be treated with 6-mercaptopurine. This drug is somewhat more difficult to use: control is not so smooth, and unpredictable thrombocytopenia may occur.

An often neglected observation is that splenic irradia-

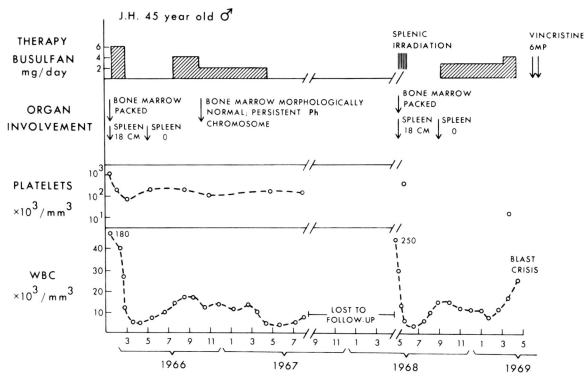

Figure 10.11 The monthly sequence of therapy and response in a patient with chronic myelocytic leukemia. The patient was treated initially with busulfan and subsequently with splenic irradiation followed by busulfan. This treatment became ineffective, and blast transformation occurred. (Modified from M. J. Cline, Cancer Chemotherapy, p. 141, W. B. Saunders Co., Philadelphia, 1971.)

tion is approximately as effective as busulfan in the treatment of chronic myelocytic leukemia (143). Small doses of 200 to 600 rads in seven to ten days can produce a striking decrease in the size of the spleen, a concomitant fall in the peripheral white blood count, and a return of the bone marrow to a morphologically normal status (119). Such a remission may last for many months, or occasionally, years. When subsequent relapses occur, the patient can again be given a course of radiation therapy, although it is usually less effective than the initial course. Splenectomy also has a place when thrombocytopenia complicates the course of chronic granulocytic leukemia (31). A few clinics still use radioactive phosphorus in the treatment of chronic myelocytic leukemia. This form of therapy cannot be recommended as superior to drug treatment.

Remissions induced by either drugs or irradiation are associated with the return of the leukocyte alkaline phosphatase to normal, although the Philadelphia chromosome persists in the marrow.

Unless the patient dies of complications of his disease or of therapy, the clinical picture of blast crisis eventually supervenes. The precise treatment of blast crisis is still uncertain, although in general it is treated in the same way as acute myelocytic leukemia (see Chapter 11). Busulfan and splenic irradiation are of no value during this phase of the disease.

The management of a patient with chronic myelocytic leukemia is illustrated in Fig. 10.11. Zubrod (223), who recently reviewed new developments in the treatment of chronic myelocytic leukemia, states, "The slower pace of the chronic leukemias has led to this curious situation: even though these diseases are 100 percent fatal, physicians have chosen to treat symptoms rather than use the available drugs (plus X-irradiation) in an attempt to eradicate the leukemic cells." He has thus succinctly summarized the existing situation with regard to treatment of chronic myelocytic leukemia. It is to be hoped that a more vigorous approach will be used in future treatment of this uniformly fatal disease.

Chapter 10 References

1. Albrecht, M. "Gaucher-Zellen" bei chronisch myeloischer Leukämie, *Blut* 13:169, 1966.
2. Anstey, L., Kemp, N. H., Stafford, J. L., and Tanner, R. K. Leucocyte alkaline-phosphatase activity in polycythemia rubra vera, *Br. J. Haematol.* 9:91, 1963.
3. Athens, J. W., Raab, S. O., Haab, O. P., Boggs, D. R., Ashenbrucker, H., Cartwright, G. E., and Wintrobe, M. M. Leukokinetic studies. X. Blood granulocyte kinetics in chronic myelocytic leukemia, *J. Clin. Invest.* 44:765, 1965.
4. Baikie, A. G. The Philadelphia chromosome, *Lancet* i:556, 1964.
5. Baikie, A. G., Court-Brown, W. M., Buckton, K. E., Harnden, D. G., Jacobs, P. A., and Tough, I. M. A possible specific chromosome abnormality in human chronic myeloid leukaemia, *Nature* 188:1165, 1960.
6. Ballard, H. S., and Marcus, A. J. Hypercalcemia in chronic myelogenous leukemia, *N. Engl. J. Med.* 282:663, 1970.
7. Banerjee, T. K., Senn, H., and Holland, J. F. Comparative studies on localized leukocyte mobilization in patients with chronic myelocytic leukemia, *Cancer*, 29:637, 1972.
8. Barrett, O'N., Jr., Conrad, M., and Crosby, W. H. Chronic granulocytic leukemia in childhood, *Am. J. Med. Sci.* 240:587, 1960.
9. Bauke, J. Chronic myelocytic leukemia. Chromosome studies of a patient and his non-leukemic identical twin, *Cancer* 24:643, 1969.
10. Beck, W. S. Leukocyte glycolysis: an investigation of the factors controlling the rate behavior in multienzyme systems, *Ann. N.Y. Acad. Sci.* 75:4, 1958.
11. Beck, W. S. The control of leukocyte glycolysis, *J. Biol. Chem.* 232:251, 1958.
12. Beck, W. S. Occurrence and control of the phosphogluconate oxidation pathway in normal and leukemic leukocytes, *J. Biol. Chem.* 232:271, 1958.
13. Beck, W. S., and Valentine, W. N. The aerobic carbohydrate metabolism of leukocytes in health and leukemia. I. Glycolysis and respiration, *Cancer Res.* 12:818, 1952.
14. Beck, W. S., and Valentine, W. N. The aerobic carbohydrate metabolism of leukocytes in health and leukemia. II. The effect of various substrates and coenzymes on glycolysis and respiration, *Cancer Res.* 12:823, 1952.
15. Beck, W. S., and Valentine, W. N. The carbohydrate metabolism of leukocytes: a review, *Cancer Res.* 13:309, 1953.
16. Bertino, J. R., Donohue, D. M., Simmons, B., Gabrio, B. W., Silber, R., and Huennekens, F. M. The "induction" of dihydrofolic reductase in leucocytes and erythrocytes of patients treated with amethopterin, *J. Clin. Invest.* 42:466, 1963.
17. Bertino, J. R., Gabrio, B. W., and Huennekens, F. M. Dihydrofolic reductase in human leukemic leukocytes, *Biochem. Biophys. Res. Commun.* 3:461, 1960.
18. Bertino, J. R., Gabrio, B. W., and Huennekens, F. M. Increased activity of leukocyte dihydrofolic reductase in amethopterin-treated patients, *Clin. Res.* 9:103, 1961.
19. Bertino, J. R., Silber, R., Freeman, M., Alenty, A., Albrecht, M., Gabrio, B. W., and Huennekens, F. M. Studies on normal and leukemic leukocytes. IV. Tetrahydrofolate-dependent enzyme systems and dihydrofolate reductase, *J. Clin. Invest.* 42:1899, 1963.
20. Better, O., Brandstaetter, S., Padeh, B., and Bianu, G. Myeloid metaplasia: clinical, laboratory and cytogenetic observations, *Isr. Med. J.* 23:162, 1964.
21. Boggs, D. R. The cellular composition of inflammatory exudates in human leukemias, *Blood* 15:466, 1960.
22. Borel, C., Frie, J., Horvath, G., Montri, S., and Vannotti, A. Etude comparée du métabolisme du polynucléaire et de la cellule mononucléé chez l'homme, *Helv. Med. Acta* 26:785, 1959.
23. Borghetti, A., and Scarpioni, L. Sull' attività arginasica nei leucociti, *Rass. Fisiopat. Clin.* 27:941, 1955.
24. Borghetti, A., and Scarpioni, L. Attività arginasica dei leucociti umani, *Enzymologia* 17:338, 1956.
25. Bornstein, R. S., Nesbit, M., and Kennedy, B. J. Chronic myelogenous leukemia presenting in blastic crisis, *Cancer* 30:939, 1972.
26. Bouroncle, B. A., and Doan, C. A. Myelofibrosis. Clinical, hematologic and pathologic study of 110 patients, *Am. J. Med. Sci.* 243:697, 1962.
27. Bowen, P., and Lee, C. S. N. Ph[1] chromosome in the diagnosis of chronic myeloid leukemia: report of a case with features simulating myelofibrosis, *Bull. Johns Hopkins Hosp.* 113:1, 1963.
28. Brandt, L. Studies on the phagocytic activity of neutrophilic leukocytes, *Scand. J. Haematol.* 2:1, 1967 (suppl.).
29. Brandt, L., and Schnell, C. R. Granulopoiesis in bone marrow and spleen in chronic myeloid leukemia, *Scand. J. Haematol.* 6:65, 1969.
30. Burham, C. F. Hodgkin's disease with especial reference to its treatment by irradiation, *J.A.M.A.* 87:1445, 1926.
31. Canellos, G. P. Splenectomy for thrombocytopenia in chronic granulocytic leukemia, *Cancer* 29:660, 1972.
32. Canellos, G. P., and Whang-Peng, J. Philadelphia-chromosome-positive preleukaemic state, *Lancet* ii:1227, 1972.
33. Canellos, G. P., Whang-Peng, J., Schnipper, L., and Brown, C. H. Prolonged cytogenetic and hematologic remission of blastic transformation in chronic granulocytic leukemia, *Cancer* 30:288, 1972.
34. Carmel, R. Vitamin B_{12}-binding protein abnormality in subjects without myeloproliferative disease. II. The presence of a third vitamin B_{12}-binding protein in serum, *Br. J. Haematol.* 22:53, 1972.
35. Carmel, R., and Coltman, C. A., Jr. Non-leukemic elevation of serum vitamin B_{12} and B_{12}-binding capacity levels resembling that in chronic myelogenous leukemia, *J. Lab. Clin. Med.* 78:289, 1971.
36. Caspersson, T., Gahrton, G., Lindsten, J., and Zech, L. Identification of the Philadelphia chromosome as a number 22 by quinacrine mustard fluorescence analysis, *Exp. Cell Res.* 63:238, 1970.
37. Castleman, B., and McNeely, B. U. Case records of the Massachusetts General Hospital. Case 2-1969, *N. Engl. J. Med.* 280:97, 1969.
38. Catovsky, D., Galton, A. G.,

Griffin, C., Hoffbrand, A. V., and Szur, L. Serum lysozyme and vitamin B$_{12}$ binding capacity in myeloproliferative disorders, *Br. J. Haematol.* 21:661, 1971.

39. Chabner, B. A., Haskell, C. M., and Canellos, G. P. Destructive bone lesions in chronic granulocytic leukemia, *Medicine* 48:401, 1969.

40. Cheney, G. Chronic myelogenous leukemia with ascites resembling Banti's syndrome; with a report of two cases, *Acta Med. Scand.* 81:14, 1934.

41. Chervenick, P. A. Increase in circulating stem cells in patients with myelofibrosis, *Blood* 41:67, 1973.

42. Chikkappa, G., and Galbraith, P. R. Studies on the exchange of leukocytes between blood and bone marrow in chronic myelogenous leukemia, *Can. Med. Assoc. J.* 97:64, 1967.

43. Clarkson, B., Ota, K., O'Connor, A., and Karnovsky, D. A. Production of granulocytes by the spleen in chronic granulocytic leukemia, *J. Clin. Invest.* 42:924, 1963.

44. Clayton, D. A., and Vinograd, J. Complex mitochondrial DNA in leukemic and normal human myeloid cells, *Proc. Natl. Acad. Sci. U.S.A.* 62:1077, 1969.

45. Clein, G. P., and Flemans, R. J. Involvement of the erythroid series in blastic crises of chronic myeloid leukemia, *Br. J. Haematol.* 12:754, 1966.

46. Clemmesen, J., Busk, Th., and Nielsen, A. The topographical distribution of leukemia and Hodgkin's disease in Denmark 1942–46, *Acta Radiol.* 37:223, 1952.

47. Cline, M. J. The metabolism of the circulating leukocyte, *Physiol. Rev.* 45:674, 1965.

48. Cline, M. J. Medical staff conference. Hematologic manifestations of tuberculosis, *Calif. Med.* 106:215, 1967.

49. Cline, M. J. Cancer Chemotherapy, p. 137, W. B. Saunders Co., Philadelphia, 1971.

50. Cline, M. J., and Berlin, N. I. Patterns of anemia in chronic myelocytic leukemia, *Cancer* 16:624, 1963.

51. Code, C. F. The histamine-like activity of white blood cells, *J. Physiol. (Lond.)* 90:485, 1937.

52. Colman, R. W., and Shein, H. M. Leukemoid reaction, hyperuricemia, and severe hyperpyrexia complicating a fatal case of acute fatty liver of the alcoholic, *Ann. Intern. Med.* 57:110, 1962.

53. Cooke, J. V. The occurrence of leukemia, *Blood* 9:340, 1954.

54. Cooper, M. R., DeChatelet, L. R., McCall, C. E., and Spurr, C. L. The activated phagocyte of polycythemia vera, *Blood* 40:366, 1972.

55. Corr, W. P., Jr., Kyle, R. A., and Bowie, E. J. W. Hematologic changes in tuberculosis, *Am. J. Med. Sci.* 248:709, 1964.

56. Dameshek, W. Editorial: some speculations on the myeloproliferative syndromes, *Blood,* 6:372, 1951.

57. Dameshek, W. The Myeloproliferative Disorders, in Proc. 3rd National Cancer Congress, p. 383, J. B. Lippincott, Philadelphia, 1956.

58. Dameshek, W., and Gunz, F. Leukemia, 2nd ed., p. 356, Grune & Stratton, New York, 1964.

59. Darte, J. M., Dacie, J. V., and McSorley, J. G. A. Pelger-like leucocytes in chronic myeloid leukaemia, *Acta Haematol.* 12:117, 1954.

60. Dennes, E., Tupper, R., and Wormall, A. Zinc content of erythrocytes and leucocytes of blood of normal and leukaemic subjects, *Nature* 187:302, 1960.

61. Dennes, E., Tupper, R., and Wormall, A. The zinc content of erythrocytes and leucocytes of blood from normal and leukaemic subjects, *Biochem. J.* 78:578, 1961.

62. Dennes, E., Tupper, R., and Wormall, A. Studies on zinc in blood. Transport of zinc and incorporation of zinc in leucocytes, *Biochem. J.* 82:466, 1962.

63. Dioguardi, N., Agostoni, A., and Fiorelli, G. Characterization of lactic dehydrogenase in cells of myeloid leukemia, *Enzymol. Biol. Clin.* 2:116, 1963.

64. Dioguardi, N., Agostoni, A., Fiorelli, G., and Lomanto, B. Characterization of lactic dehydrogenase of normal human granulocytes, *J. Lab. Clin. Med.* 61:713, 1963.

65. Dorn, H. F., and Cutler, S. J. Morbidity from cancer in the United States, Publ. Health Monogr. 25, U.S. Govt. Printing Office, Washington, D.C., 1955.

66. Dougan, L., Scott, I. D., and Woodliff, H. J. A pair of twins, one of whom has chronic granulocytic leukemia, *J. Med. Genet.* 3:217, 1966.

67. Downey, H., Major, S. G., and Noble, J. F. Leukemoid blood pictures of the myeloid type, *Folia Haematol.* 41:493, 1930.

68. Duvall, C. P., Carbone, P. P., Bell, W. R., Whang, J., Tjio, J. H., and Perry, S. Chronic myelocytic leukemia with two Philadelphia chromosomes and prominent peripheral lymphadenopathy, *Blood* 29:652, 1967.

69. Duvall, C. P., and Perry, S. The use of 51-chromium in the study of leukocyte kinetics in chronic myelocytic leukemia, *J. Lab. Clin. Med.* 71:614, 1968.

70. Engel, E., and McKee, L. C. Double Ph[1] chromosomes in leukaemia, *Lancet* ii:337, 1966.

71. Epstein, E., and MacEachern, K. Dermatologic manifestations of the lymphoblastoma-leukemia group, *Arch. Intern. Med.* 60:867, 1937.

72. Fahey, R. J. Unusual leukocyte responses in primary carcinoma of the lung, *Cancer* 4:930, 1951.

73. Feinlieb, M., and MacMahon, B. Variation in the duration of survival of patients with the chronic leukemias, *Blood* 15:332, 1960.

74. Feldman, W. H., and Stasney, J. Leukemoid response of tuberculous rabbits to administration of tuberculin, *Am. J. Med. Sci.* 193:28, 1934.

75. Fialkow, P. J., Gartler, S. M., and Yoshida, A. Clonal origin of chronic myelocytic leukemia in man, *Proc. Natl. Acad. Sci. U.S.A.* 58:1468, 1967.

76. Fitzgerald, P. H., Adams, A., and Gunz, F. W. Chronic granulocytic leukemia and the Philadelphia chromosome, *Blood* 21:183, 1963.

77. Fredericks, R. E., Tanaka, K. R., and Valentine, W. N. Variations of human blood cell zinc in disease, *J. Clin. Invest.* 43:304, 1964.

78. Freireich, E. J., Levin, R. H., Whang, J., Carbone, P. P., Bronson, W., and Morse, E. E. The function and fate of transfused leukocytes from donors with chronic myelocytic leukemia in leukopenic recipients, *Ann. N.Y. Acad. Sci.* 113:1081, 1964.

79. Gahrton, G., Brandt, L., Franzén, S., and Nordén, Å. Cytochemical variants of neutrophil leukocyte populations in chronic myelocytic leukaemia, *Scand. J. Haematol.* 6:365, 1969.

80. Gahrton, G., and Zettergerg, A. Glycogen synthesis in normal leukemic and polycythemic leukocytes, *Acta Med. Scand.* 180:497, 1966.

81. Galbraith, P. R. Studies on the longevity, sequestration and release of the leukocytes in chronic myelogenous leukemia, *Can. Med. Assoc. J.* 95:511, 1966.

82. Galbraith, P. R. Granulocyte kinetic studies in chronic myelogenous leukemia, *Natl. Cancer Inst. Monogr.* 30:121, 1969.

83. Galbraith, P. R., and Abu-Zahra, H. T. Granulopoiesis in chronic granulocytic leukaemia, *Br. J. Haematol.* 22:135, 1972.

84. Gates, O. Cutaneous tumors in leukemia and lymphoma, *Arch. Dermatol. Syph.* 37:1015, 1938.

85. Ghiotto, G., Perona, G., Desandre, G., and Cortesi, S. Hexokinase and TPN-dependent dehydrogenases of leukocytes in leukaemia and other haematological disorders, *Br. J. Haematol.* 9:345, 1963.

86. Gibson, J. G. II, Valee, B. L., Fluharty, R. G., and Nelson, J. E. Studies of the zinc content of the leucocytes in myelogenous leukemia, *Un. Int. Clin. contra Cancr. Acta* 6:1102, 1950.

87. Glasser, R. M., and Walker, R. I. Transitions among the myeloproliferative disorders, *Ann. Intern. Med.* 71:285, 1969.

88. Glasser, R. M., Walker, R. I., and Herion, J. C. The significance of hematologic abnormalities in patients with tuberculosis, *Arch. Intern. Med.* 125:691, 1970.

89. Glew, R. H., Haese, W. H., and McIntyre, P. A. Myeloid metaplasia with myelofibrosis. The clinical spectrum of extramedullary hematopoiesis and tumor formation, *Johns Hopkins Med. J.* 132:253, 1973.

90. Godwin, H. A., Zimmerman, T. S., and Perry, S. Peripheral leukocyte kinetic studies of acute leukemia in relapse and remission and chronic myelocytic leukemia in blastic crises, *Blood* 31:686, 1968.

91. Goh, K-O., Swisher, S. N., and Herman, E. C., Jr. Chronic myelocytic leukemia and identical twins. Additional evidence of the Philadelphia chromosome as a post zygotic abnormality, *Arch. Intern. Med.* 120:214, 1967.

92. Golde, D. W., and Cline, M. J. Human preleukemia. Identification of a maturation defect in vitro, *N. Engl. J. Med.* 288:1083, 1973.

93. Goldhamer, S. M., and Barney, B. F. Myelogenous leukemia with cutaneous involvement, *J.A.M.A.* 107:1041, 1936.

94. Graw, R. G., Jr., Skeel, R. T., and Carbone, P. P. Priapism in a child with chronic granulocytic leukemia, *J. Pediatr.* 74:788, 1969.

95. Green, R. A., and Nichols, N. J. Pulmonary involvement in leukemia, *Ann. Rev. Resp. Dis.* 80:833, 1959.

96. Gunz, F. W., and Hough, R. F. Acute leukemia over the age of fifty: a study of its incidence and natural history, *Blood* 11:882, 1956.

97. Hall, C. A. Vitamin B_{12}-binding proteins of man, *Ann. Intern. Med.* 75:297, 1971.

98. Hall, C. A., and Finkler, A. E. Vitamin B_{12}-binding protein in polycythemia vera plasma, *J. Lab. Clin. Med.* 73:60, 1969.

99. Hardisty, R. M., Speed, D. E., and Till, M. Granulocytic leukaemia in childhood, *Br. J. Haematol.* 10:551, 1964.

100. Haut, A., Abbott, W. S., Wintrobe, M. M., and Cartwright, G. E. Busulfan in the treatment of chronic myelocytic leukemia. The effect of long term intermittent therapy, *Blood* 17:1, 1961.

101. Hensler, L. Hohe Leukocytose durch Karzinom, *Schweiz. Med. Wochenschr.* 83:1032, 1953.

102. Hewitt, D. Some features of leukaemia mortality, *Br. J. Prev. Soc. Med.* 9:81, 1955.

103. Hilts, S. V., and Shaw, C. C. Leukemoid blood reactions, *N. Engl. J. Med.* 249:434, 1953.

104. Hoffman, W. J., and Craver, L. F. Chronic myelogenous leukemia; value of irradiation and its effect on the duration of life, *J.A.M.A.* 97:836, 1931.

105. Holland, P., and Mauer, A. M. Myeloid leukemoid reactions in chil-

dren, *Am. J. Dis. Child.* 105:568, 1963.

106. Hom, B., Olesen, H., and Lous, P. Fractionation of vitamin B_{12} binders in human serum, *J. Lab. Clin. Med.* 68:958, 1966.

107. Jacobs, E. M., Luce, J. K., and Cailleau, R. Chromosome abnormalities in human cancer. Report of a patient with chronic myelocytic leukemia and his nonleukemic monozygotic twin, *Cancer* 19:869, 1966.

108. Jaffé, R. H. Morphology of inflammatory defense reactions in leukemia, *Arch. Pathol.* 14:177, 1932.

109. Kalinske, R. W., and Hoeprich, P. D. Engulfment and bactericidal capabilities of peripheral blood leukocytes in chronic leukemias, *Cancer* 23:1094, 1969.

110. Karanas, A., and Silver, R. T. Characteristics of the terminal phase of chronic granulocytic leukemia, *Blood* 32:445, 1968.

111. Kattlove, H. E., Williams, J. C., Gaynor, E., Spivack, M., Bradley, R. M., and Brady, R. O. Gaucher cells in chronic myelocytic leukemia: an acquired abnormality, *Blood* 33:379, 1969.

112. Kinlough, M. A., and Robson, H. N. Study of chromosomes in human leukaemia by a direct method, *Br. Med. J.* 2:1052, 1961.

113. Kiossoglou, K. A., Mitus, W. J., and Dameshek, W. Chromosomal aberrations in acute leukemia, *Blood* 26:610, 1965.

114. Kiossoglou, K. A., Mitus, W. J., and Dameshek, W. Two Ph[1] chromosomes in acute granulocytic leukemia. A study of two cases, *Lancet* ii:665, 1965.

115. Kiossoglou, K. A., Mitus, W. J., and Dameshek, W. Cytogenetic studies in the chronic myeloproliferative syndrome, *Blood* 28:241, 1966.

116. Klatte, E. C., Yardley, J., Smith, E. B., Rohn, R., and Campbell, J. A. The pulmonary manifestations and complications of leukemia, *Am. J. Roentgenol.* 89:598, 1963.

117. Krauss, S. Chronic myelocytic leukemia with features simulating myelofibrosis with myeloid metaplasia, *Cancer* 19:1321, 1966.

118. Krauss, S. The Philadelphia chromosome and leukocyte alkaline phosphatase in chronic myelocytic

leukemia and related disorders, *Ann. N.Y. Acad. Sci.* 155:983, 1968.

119. Krebs, C., and Bichel, J. Results of roentgen treatment in chronic myelogenous leukemia, *Acta Radiol.* 28:697, 1947.

120. Krompotic, E., Lewis, J. P., and Donnelly, W. J. Chromosome aberrations in two patients with chronic granulocytic leukemia undergoing acute transformation, *Am. J. Clin. Pathol.* 49:161, 1968.

121. Krumbhaar, E. B. Leukemoid blood pictures in various clinical conditions, *Am. J. Med. Sci.* 172:519, 1926.

122. Kwaan, H. C., Pierre, R. V., and Long, D. L. Meningeal involvement as first manifestation of acute myeloblastic transformation in chronic granulocytic leukemia, *Blood* 33:348, 1969.

123. Lawrence, J. H. The treatment of chronic leukemia, *Med. Clin. North Am.* 38:525, 1954.

124. Lawrence, J. H., Dobson, R. L., Low-Beer, B. V. A., and Brown, B. R. Chronic myelogenous leukemia, *J.A.M.A.* 136:672, 1948.

125. Lea, A. J., and Abbatt, J. D. The changing pattern of Leukaemia, *Lancet* i:389, 1957.

126. Leonard, B. J., Israëls, M. C. G., and Wilkinson, J. F. Alkaline phosphatase in the white cells in leukaemia and leukaemoid reactions, *Lancet* i:289, 1958.

127. Lissauer, Dr. Zwei Falle von Leucaemie, *Berlin Klin. Wochenschr.* 2:403, 1865.

128. Lucas, W. S. Erythremia, or polycythemia with chronic cyanosis and splenomegaly, *Arch. Intern. Med.* 10:597, 1912.

129. Luganova, I. S., and Seits, I. F. Glycogen content and metabolism in normal and leukemic human leukocytes, *Fed. Proc.* 22 (transl.), 447, 1964 (suppl.).

130. McKinney, G. R., and Rundles, R. W. Lactate formation and glyoxalase activity in normal and leukemic leukocytes *in vitro, Cancer Res.* 16:67, 1956.

131. MacMahon, B., and Koller, E. K. Ethnic differences in the incidence of leukemia, *in* A. R. Jones, Proc. VIth Int. Cong. Int. Soc. Hematol., p. 60, Grune & Stratton, New York, 1956.

132. McNutt, D. R., and Fudenberg, H.

H. Disseminated scotochromogen infection and unusual myeloproliferative disorder, *Ann. Intern. Med.* 75:737, 1971.

133. Maniatis, A. K., Amsel, S., Mitus, W. J., and Coleman, N. Chromosome pattern of bone marrow fibroblasts in patients with chronic granulocytic leukemia, *Nature* 222:1278, 1969.

134. Mastrangelo, R., Zuelzer, W., and Thompson, R. I. The significance of the Ph¹ chromosome in acute myeloblastic leukemia: serial cytogenetic studies in a critical case, *Pediatrics* 40:834, 1967.

135. Maurer, H. S., Vida, L. N., and Honig, G. R. Similarities of the erythrocytes in juvenile chronic myelogenous leukemia to fetal erythrocytes, *Blood* 39:778, 1972.

136. Meyer, L. M., Bertcher, R. W., and Cronkite, E. P. Serum Co⁶⁰ vitamin B₁₂ binding capacity in some hematologic disorders, *Proc. Soc. Exp. Biol. Med.* 96:360, 1957.

137. Meyer, L. M., Cronkite, E. P., Miller, I. F., Mulzoc, C. W., and Jones, I. Co⁶⁰ vitamin B₁₂ binding capacity of human leukocytes, *Blood* 19:339, 1962.

138. Minot, G. R., Buckman, T. E., and Isaacs, R. Chronic myelogenous leukemia: age incidence, duration, and benefit derived from irradiation, *J.A.M.A.* 82:1489, 1924.

139. Misra, D. K. A direct assay for dihydrofolate reductase in human leukocytes, *Blood,* 23:572, 1964.

140. Mitus, W. J., and Kiossoglou, K. A. Leukocyte alkaline phosphatase in myeloproliferative syndrome, *Ann. N.Y. Acad. Sci.* 155:976, 1968.

141. Moeschlin, S. Myelocytic leucoses (chronic myeloid leukemia) *in* Spleen Puncture (A. Piney, transl.), p. 130, Grune & Stratton, New York, 1951.

142. Mollin, D. L., and Ross, G. I. M. Serum vitamin B₁₂ concentrations in leukaemia and in some other haematological conditions, *Br. J. Haematol.* 1:155, 1955.

143. Monfardini, S., et al. Survival in chronic myelogenous leukemia: influence of treatment and extent of disease at diagnosis, *Cancer* 31:492, 1973.

144. Morley, A. A., Baikie, A. G., and Galton, D. A. G. Cyclic leucocytosis as evidence for retention of

normal homeostatic control in chronic granulocytic leukaemia, *Lancet* ii:1320, 1967.

145. Morrow, G. W., Jr., Pease, G. L., Stroebel, C. F., and Bennett, W. A. Terminal phase of chronic myelogenous leukemia, *Cancer* 18:369, 1965.

146. Motonura, S., Ogi, K., and Horie, M. Monoclonal origin of acute transformation of chronic myelogenous leukemia, *Acta Haematol.* 49:300, 1973.

147. Moxley, J. H. III, Perry, S., Weiss, G. H., and Zelen, M. Return of leucocytes to the bone marrow in chronic myelocytic leukaemia, *Nature* 208:1281, 1965.

148. Nau, R. C., and Hoagland, H. C. A myeloproliferative disorder manifested by persistent basophilia, granulocytic leukemia and erythroleukemic phases, *Cancer* 28:662, 1971.

149. Neumann, E. Ein Fall von Leukamie mit Erkrankung des Knochenmarkes, *Arch. Heilkd.* 11:1, 1870.

150. Nowell, P. C., and Hungerford, D. A. Chromosome studies on normal and leukemic human leukocytes, *J. Natl. Cancer Inst.* 25:85, 1960.

151. Nowell, P. C., and Hungerford, D. A. A minute chromosome in human chronic granulocytic leukemia, *Science* 132:1497, 1960.

152. Nowell, P. C., and Hungerford, D. A. Chromosome studies in human leukemia. IV. Myeloproliferative syndrome and other atypical myeloid disorders, *J. Natl. Cancer Inst.* 29:911, 1962.

153. Osler, W. A clinical lecture on erythraemia (polycythaemia with cyanosis, maladie De Vaquez), *Lancet* i:143, 1908.

154. Oswald, N. C. Acute tuberculosis and granulocytic disorders, *Br. Med. J.* 2:1489, 1963.

155. Pedersen, B. Two cases of chronic myeloid leukaemia with presumably identical 47-chromosome cell-lines in the blood, *Acta Pathol. Microbiol. Scand.* 61:497, 1964.

156. Pederson, B. Influence of hyperdiploidy on Ph¹ prevalence response to therapy in chronic myelogenous leukaemia, *Br. J. Haematol.* 14:507, 1968.

157. Pedersen, B. Relation between karyotype and cytology in chronic

myelogenous leukaemia, *Scand. J. Haematol.* 8:494, 1971.

158. Perillie, P. E., and Finch, S. C. The local exudative cellular response in leukemia, *J. Clin. Invest.* 39:1353, 1960.

159. Pitcock, J. A., Reinhard, E. H., Justus, B. W., and Mendelsohn, R. S. A clinical and pathological study of seventy cases of myelofibrosis, *Ann. Intern. Med.* 57:73, 1962.

160. Pusey, W. A. Report of cases treated with roentgen rays, *J.A.M.A.* 38:911, 1902.

161. Raccuglia, G., and Sacks, M. S. Vitamin B_{12} binding capacity of normal and leukemic sera, *J. Lab. Clin. Med.* 50:69, 1957.

162. Rachmilewitz, B., Rachmilewitz, M., Moshkowitz, B., and Gross, J. Serum transcobalamin in myeloid leukemia, *J. Lab. Clin. Med.* 78:275, 1971.

163. Rák, K., Csapó, G., Macher, A., and Török, G. Chronic granulocytic leukaemia with unusual long duration, *Folia Haematol.* 9:131, 1964.

164. Reisman, L. E., and Trujillo, J. M. Chronic granulocytic leukemia of childhood. Clinical and cytogenetic studies, *J. Pediatr.* 62:710, 1963.

165. Retief, F. P. Leuco-erythroblastosis in the adult, *Lancet* i:639, 1964.

166. Reynolds, J., Follette, J. H., and Valentine, W. N. The arginase activity of erythrocytes and leukocytes with particular reference to pernicious anemia and thalassemia major, *J. Lab. Clin. Med.* 50:78, 1957.

167. Rosen, R. B., and Nishiyama, H. Leukocyte alkaline phosphatase in chronic granulocytic leukemia of childhood, *Ann. N.Y. Acad. Sci.* 155:992, 1968.

168. Rosenthal, N., and Bassen, F. A. Course of polycythemia, *Arch. Intern. Med.* 62:903, 1938.

169. Rosenthal, N., and Harris, W. Leukemia: its diagnosis and treatment, *J.A.M.A.* 104:702, 1935.

170. Rubnitz, A. S. Leukemia cases at the University of Nebraska hospital. Statistical analysis and review of all records of leukemic cases treated at the university hospital from January 1933 to January 1951, *Nebr. Med. J.* 37:95, 1952.

171. Sandberg, A. A., Ishihara, T., Crosswhite, L. H., and Hauschka, T. S. Comparison of chromosome constitution in chronic myelocytic leu-kemia and other myeloproliferative disorders, *Blood* 20:393, 1962.

172. Schwarzenberg, L., Mathé, G., De Grouchy, J., De Nava, C., De Vries, J., Amiel, J. L., Cattan, A., Schneider, M., and Schlumberger, J. R. White blood cell transfusions, *Isr. J. Med. Sci.* 1:925, 1965.

173. Scott, R. B. The surgical aspects of the lymphomata, *Ann. R. Coll. Surg. Engl.* 22:178, 1958.

174. Sears, W. G. The blood in Hodgkin's disease with special reference to eosinophilia, *Guy's Hosp. Rep.* 82:40, 1932.

175. Shadduck, R. K., Winkelstein, A., and Nunna, N. G. Cyclic leukemic cell production in CML, *Cancer* 29:399, 1972.

176. Shimkin, M. B. Hodgkin's disease mortality in the United States, 1921–1951; race, sex, and age distribution. Comparison with leukemia, *Blood* 10:1214, 1955.

177. Shimkin, M. B., Mettier, S. R., and Bierman, H. R. Myelocytic leukemia: an analysis of incidence, distribution and fatality 1910–1948, *Ann. Intern. Med.* 35:194, 1951. Lymphocytic leukemia: an analysis of frequency distribution and mortality at the University of California hospital 1913–1947, *Ann. Intern. Med.* 39:1254, 1953.

178. Shohet, S. B., and Blum, S. F. Coincident basophilic chronic myelogenous leukemia and pulmonary tuberculosis, *Cancer* 22:173, 1968.

179. Smith, W. C., Kaneshiro, M. M., Goldstein, B. D., Parker, J. W., and Lukes, R. J. Gaucher cells in chronic granulocytic leukemia, *Lancet* ii:780, 1968.

180. Söderström, N. Fine-needle Aspiration Biopsy Used as a Direct Adjunct in Clinical Diagnostic Work, Almquist and Wiksell, Stockholm, and Grune & Stratton, New York, 1966.

181. Spiers, A. S. D., and Baikie, A. G. Chronic granulocytic leukaemia: demonstration of the Philadelphia chromosome in cultures of spleen cells, *Nature* 208:497, 1965.

182. Srodes, C. H., Hyde, E. H., and Boggs, D. R. Autonomous erythropoiesis during erythroblastic crisis of chronic myelocytic leukemia, *J. Clin. Invest.* 52:512, 1973.

183. Srodes, C. H., Hyde, E. F., Pan, S. F., Chervenick, P. A., and Boggs, D. R. Cytogenetic studies during remission of blastic crisis in a patient with chronic myelocytic leukaemia, Scand. J. Haematol. 10:130, 1973.

184. Steiner, P. E. An evaluation of the cancer problem, *Cancer Res.* 12:455, 1952.

185. Suzuki, S., Ishida, F., Kono, T., and Muranaka, M. Histamine contents of blood plasma and cells in patients with myelogenous leukemia, *Cancer* 28:384, 1971.

186. Takeda, K. International union against cancer. Geographical pathology of leukaemia in Japan, *Un. Int. Clin. contra Cancr. Acta* 16:1629, 1960.

187. Tanaka, K. R., and Valentine, W. N. The arginase activity of human leukocytes, *J. Lab. Clin. Med.* 56:754, 1960.

188. Tanzer, J., Najean, Y., Jacquillat, C., Ripault, J., and Chome, J. Fibrose médullaire et érythroblastose splénique dans la leucémie myéloïde chronique, *Nouv. Rev. Fr. Hematol.* 7:801, 1967.

189. Thiersch, J. B. Histamine and histaminase in chronic myeloid leukaemia of man. I. Histamine in the blood of chronic myeloid leukaemia, *Aust. J. Exp. Biol. Med. Sci.* 25:73, 1947.

190. Thomas, J. W., and Anderson, B. B. Vitamin B_{12} content of normal and leukaemic leucocytes, *Br. J. Haematol.* 2:41, 1956.

191. Tischendorf, F. W., Ledderose, G., Müller, D., Roywall, D., and Williams, W. Chronische Myelosen mit massiver Lysozymurie unter Milzbestrahlung, *Klin. Wochenschr.* 50:250, 1972.

192. Tivey, H. The prognosis for survival in chronic granulocytic and lymphocytic leukemia, *Am. J. Roentgenol.* 72:68, 1954.

193. Tivey, H. The natural history of untreated acute leukemia, *Ann. N.Y. Acad. Sci.* 60:322, 1954.

194. Tjio, J. H., Carbone, P. P., Whang, J., and Frei, E. III. The Philadelphia chromosome and chronic myelogenous leukemia, *J. Natl. Cancer Inst.* 36:567, 1966.

195. Tough, I. M., Jacobs, P. A., Court-Brown, W. M., Baikie, A. G., and Williamson, E. R. D. Cytogenetic studies on bone marrow in chronic

myeloid leukaemia, *Lancet* i:844, 1963.

196. Türk, W. Beiträge zur Kenntnis des Symptomenbildes: Polycythämie mit Milztumor und Zyanose, *Wien. Klin. Wochenschr.* 17:153, 1904.

197. Twomey, J. J., and Leavell, B. S. Leukemoid reactions to tuberculosis, *Arch. Intern. Med.* 116:21, 1965.

198. Valentine, W. N. The biochemistry and enzymatic activities of leukocytes in health and disease, *in* L. M. Tocantins (ed.), Progress in Hematology, vol. 1, p. 293, Grune & Stratton, New York, 1956.

199. Valentine, W. N. The metabolism of the leukemic leukocyte, *Am. J. Med.* 28:699, 1960.

200. Valentine, W. N., Beck, W. S., Follette, J. H., Mills, H., and Lawrence, J. S. Biochemical studies in chronic myelocytic leukemia, polycythemia vera and other idiopathic myeloproliferative disorders, *Blood* 7:959, 1952.

201. Valentine, W. N., Follette, J. H., and Lawrence, J. S. The glycogen content of human leukocytes in health and various disease states, *J. Clin. Invest.* 32:251, 1953.

202. VanderWende, C., Miller, W. L., and Glass, S. A. Glycogen metabolism of normal and leukemic leukocytes, *Life Sci.* 3:223, 1964.

203. Vaughan, J. M. Leuco-erythroblastic anaemia, *J. Pathol. Bacteriol.* 42:541, 1936.

204. Vaughan, J. M., and Harrison, C. W. Leuco-erythroblastic anaemia and myelosclerosis, *J. Pathol. Bacteriol.* 48:339, 1939.

205. Vetter, Von K. Über das Verhalten von Fermenten in normalen und pathologischen menschlichen Leukozyten, *Acta Haematol.* 26:344, 1961.

206. Vodopick, H., Rupp, E. M., Edwards, C. L., Goswitz, F. A., and Beauchamp, J. J. Spontaneous cyclic leukocytosis and thrombocytosis in chronic granulocytic leukemia, *N. Engl. J. Med.* 286:284, 1972.

207. Wagner, R. Studies on the physiology of the white blood cell: the glycogen content of leukocytes in leukemia and polycythemia, *Blood* 2:235, 1947.

208. Waisman, H. A. Some aspects of amino acid metabolism in leukemia, *in* J. W. Rebuck, F. H. Bethell, and R. W. Monto (eds.), The Leukemias: Etiology, Pathophysiology and Treatment, p. 339, Academic Press, New York, 1957.

209. Waisman, H. A., Monder, C., and Williams, J. N., Jr. Glutamic acid dehydrogenase and transaminase of leucemic and nonleucemic leucocytes, *Fed. Proc.* 14:299, 1955.

210. Ward, G. The infective theory of acute leukaemia, *Br. J. Child. Dis.* 14:10, 1917.

211. Weiner, L. A family with high incidence of leukemia and unique Ph[1] chromosome findings, *Blood* 26:871, 1965.

212. Weiner, L. B., and Osserman, K. E. Studies in myasthenia gravis: demonstration of presence of immunofluorescence in serums correlated with clinical findings, *Ann. N.Y. Acad. Sci.* 135:644, 1966.

213. Whang-Peng, J., Canellos, G. P., Carbone, P. P., and Tjio, J. H. Clinical implications of cytogenetic variants in chronic myelocytic leukemia (CML), *Blood* 32:755, 1968.

214. Whang-Peng, J., Perry, S., and Knutsen, T. Maturation and phagocytosis by chronic myelogenous leukemia cells *in vitro*. A prelimi-

nary report, *J. Natl. Cancer Inst.* 38:969, 1967.

215. Wildhack, R. Beitrag zu den Terminalstadien der chronischen Myelose, *Folia Haematol.* 5:349, 1961.

216. Wilmanns, W. Bestimmung, Eigenschaften und Bedeutung der Dihydrofolsäure-Reductase in den weissen Blutzellen bei Leukämien, *Klin. Wochenschr.* 40:533, 1962.

217. Windeyer, B. W., and Stewart, J. W. The leukaemias, *in* S. Cade (ed.), Malignant Disease and its Treatment by Radium, 2nd ed., vol. 4, p. 347, John Wright and Sons, Bristol, England, 1952.

218. Wintrobe, M. M. Clinical Hematology, 6th ed., p. 982, Lea & Febiger, Philadelphia, 1967.

219. Wintrobe, M. M., and Hasenbush, L. L. Chronic leukemia. The early phase of chronic leukemia, the results of treatment and the effects of complicating infections; a study of eighty-six adults, *Arch. Intern. Med.* 64:701, 1939.

220. Wintrobe, M. M., and Mitchell, D. M. Atypical manifestations of leukaemia, *Q. J. Med.* 9:67, 1940.

221. World Health Organization: Cas et décès dus a des maladies infectieuses déclarés dans divers pays, *Epidemiol. and Vital Statistics Rep.* 8:34, 1955.

222. Youman, J. D., Taddeini, L., and Cooper, T. Histamine excess symptoms in basophilic chronic granulocytic leukemia, *Arch. Intern. Med.* 131:560, 1973.

223. Zubrod, C. G. New developments in the chemotherapy of the leukemias and lymphomas, *in* E. Jaffe (ed.), Plenary Session Papers, XIIth Congr. Int. Soc. Hematol., p. 32, The Society, New York, 1968.

Chapter 11   Acute Myelocytic Leukemia

Acute leukemia probably was first described by Friedreich in 1857 (72); however, it was not until Naegeli described the myeloblast in 1900 (158) that a distinction was made between acute leukemia of lymphocytic origin and acute leukemia of myelogenous (granulocytic) origin. In 1913 Reschad and Schilling-Torgau (174) described a case of what may have been monocytic leukemia. In the 1940s and 1950s Di Guglielmo (51, 52) drew attention to an acute hemoproliferative disorder that appeared to involve predominantly the erythroid series.

From what we know of the common origin of several hematopoietic cell lines, it is not surprising that an overlap between acute myeloproliferative disorders is frequently observed. The pluripotent stem cell precursor that gives rise to the hematopoietic cells has been discussed in Chapter 2 and illustrated in Figs. I.1 and 10.1. The branch point between lymphoid cells and other hematopoietic cell lines occurs early, whereas the branch point between granulocytic and monocytic differentiation occurs later. Consequently, combined proliferation of granulocytic and mononuclear elements is common in acute myelocytic leukemia; this variant is often designated myelomonocytic leukemia. Abnormalities of red cell and megakaryocyte proliferation and differentiation also are common in acute myelocytic leukemia (26). The phenomenon of the combined proliferation of several cell lines in the acute myeloproliferative disorders is illustrated by the frequent termination of acute erythroleukemia in a clinical syndrome indistinguishable from acute myelocytic leukemia. On the other hand, abnormalities of

lymphocyte proliferation in patients with acute myelocytic leukemia are relatively uncommon.

The proliferating cells of some patients are so undifferentiated that classification into lymphocytic or granulocytic categories cannot be made with certainty. Such leukemias are described by a variety of names, including undifferentiated acute leukemia and acute stem cell leukemia.

For the purposes of this chapter, the term *acute myelocytic leukemia* or AML (synonyms: acute myelogenous leukemia, acute myeloblastic leukemia, and acute granulocytic leukemia) will be used to describe that acute hemoproliferative disorder in which the predominant proliferating cells are myeloblasts, promyelocytes, and other young cells of the granulocytic series. However, one should be aware that immature monocytes and abnormalities of red cell precursors are the rule rather than the exception in acute myelocytic leukemia. Since myelomonocytic leukemia by and large is similar in its clinical manifestations, natural history, and response to therapy, it will be considered as part of the spectrum of acute myelocytic leukemia. Only at the extreme end of the spectrum, when monocytes and histiocytes predominate, does the clinical picture differ somewhat. This entity, monocytic leukemia, is discussed in Chapter 27.

With these considerations in mind, acute myelocytic leukemia may be defined as a neoplastic disorder characterized by (*a*) infiltration of the bone marrow and other organs by immature cells of the granulocytic series, (*b*) reduction of the normal hematopoietic cell precursors in the bone marrow with resultant anemia, granulocytopenia, and thrombocytopenia, and (c) a rapidly fatal course resulting from infection, bleeding, or anemia if the disease is untreated.

Incidence and Etiologic Considerations

Incidence

It is extremely difficult to find a figure for the average annual death rate from acute myelocytic leukemia in the United States. In one study published in 1958, the average annual death rate from all types of leukemias between 1951 and 1955 was 7.7 per 100,000 for males and 5.3 for females (83, 161). Expressed another way, leukemia (all types) accounts for about 4 percent of all malignant neoplasms in males and 3 percent in females (5, 209).

Such studies showed a dramatic increase in the incidence of leukemia from about 1920 to 1950. However, the changing diagnostic criteria and the greater dissemination of medical facilities may account for this increase in reported cases (182). In more recent series, the reported rates of increase in leukemia cases have not been so marked as in those reported between 1920 and 1940 (67, 119, 237).

As a rough approximation, about 25 percent of all cases of leukemia are in the acute myelocytic or monocytic categories. In an analysis of more than 10,000 cases of leukemia examined over a 22-year period, 46 percent were acute; of these, equal numbers fell into either the acute myelocytic or acute lymphocytic category (43). In another

series of 565 patients, acute myelocytic and monocytic leukemia together constituted 25 percent of all cases of leukemia (17).

Wintrobe's compilation of data (234) from five large series totaling 3,051 patients gives a roughly similar incidence: acute myelocytic leukemia, 16.9 percent; acute monocytic leukemia, 7.8 percent. The myelocytic variety has been slightly more frequent in males in these series.

The sharp peak for leukemia incidence for ages three to four years occurring in white American children appears to be specific for acute lymphocytic leukemia (21). A less pronounced peak for acute myelocytic leukemia occurs at adolescence (131). Acute myelocytic leukemia is observed in all ages from infancy through the ninth decade. After the first five years of life, the curve of incidence increases slowly throughout life, reaches a shallow peak between ages sixty and seventy-five, and declines thereafter. A similar pattern is seen in the curve of acute monocytic leukemia (43). Data for incidence of leukemia by age are summarized in Table 11.1.

Etiologic Considerations

Radiation, Chemicals, and Viruses   Although the etiology of acute myelocytic leukemia still is unknown, certain factors have been associated with an unusually high incidence. For example, high-dose irradiation is positively associated with a high incidence of acute and chronic myelocytic leukemia (65). Studies of patients with ankylosing spondylitis treated with X ray (22) and patients with polycythemia vera treated with X ray or radioactive phosphorus (154) have a high risk of developing acute myelocytic leukemia. Analyses of the survivors of the atomic bombings of Hiroshima and Nagasaki strongly support the concept of the correlation between irradiation and leukemogenesis (12). Studies in animals concerned with radiation leukemogenesis are also available (224).

Evidence regarding the effect of preconceptual parental irradiation on the subsequent development of chromosomal aberrations and leukemia in the offspring is controversial (4, 91, 113, 140, 147, 194, 201, 215). Some studies suggest that diagnostic irradiation during pregnancy may double the risk of the offspring developing childhood leukemia; other studies fail to confirm such a relationship.

There is a characteristic correlation between radiation dosage and the subsequent incidence of leukemia (147). However, exceptions to this rule have been noted. An excessive incidence of leukemia was noted in women receiving relatively low doses of pelvic irradiation for menorrhagia (55), whereas other women receiving high doses for cervical cancer did not demonstrate such an increase

Table 11.1 Distribution of morphologic classes of leukemia by age: 1965 to 1969.

Morphologic classification	All ages	Under 15	15–34	35–54	55–64	65 and over
Number of cases	4,019	804	407	639	627	1,542
Percent classified as—						
Acute:	61	95	80	57	50	43
Lymphocytic	17	57	24	8	4	4
Myelocytic	25	10	34	30	30	25
Monocytic	9	3	11	13	12	9
Acute NOS[a]	10	25	11	6	4	4
Chronic:	39	5	20	43	50	57
Lymphocytic	23	2	3	21	30	38
Myelocytic	15	2	16	21	19	17
Leukemia NOS[a]	1	1	1	1	1	2

SOURCE: L. M. Axtell, S. J. Cutler, and M. H. Myers, End Results in Cancer, rept. 4, DHEW publ. (NIH) 73-272, 1972.

[a] Not otherwise specified.

(114). This apparent paradox may be resolved by an ongoing study of a large number of women who received ovarian irradiation for benign gynecologic disease (65).

Reasonably good evidence demonstrates that exposure to benzene and related compounds may predispose to acute leukemia and aplastic anemia (48, 218). There are rare reports of marrow aplasia and subsequent development of leukemia associated with phenylbutazone treatment (117) and chloramphenicol (20, 38, 64). For example, in a survey of 124 patients with chloramphenicol-associated bone marrow aplasia, four developed leukemia (65). Chromosomal abnormalities also have been linked with chloramphenicol (20, 180). All these chemical agents with leukemogenic potential share with X ray the propensity for depressing the normal bone marrow and inducing chromosomal anomalies.

In vitro studies (152) and numerous animal experiments have indicated the possibility of a viral etiology for some or all cases of human leukemia. Prime examples are the murine leukemias caused by oncogenic RNA viruses (95). The proponents of a viral etiology for human leukemia received strong support when the association between Epstein-Barr virus and Burkitt's lymphoma and infectious mononucleosis was uncovered (61, 81, 82, 108). However, as outlined in Chapter 21, this association by no means proves that the herpes-like virus is leukemogenic (80).

Further support for the concept of a viral etiology of human leukemia has resulted from numerous studies of oncogenic RNA viruses (75, 89, 136, 198, 217), and from the finding of reverse transcriptase activity and RNA sequences in leukemic cells that are homologous with sequences in the mouse leukemia agent (104). The reverse transcriptase enzyme activity thus far has been restricted to oncogenic RNA viruses and a few "slow" viruses that cause neurologic disease. The presence of this enzyme is presumptive evidence for the presence of an oncogenic RNA virus in human leukemia. However, definitive evidence for a viral etiology in human acute leukemia is extremely difficult to obtain. No clear etiologic association with Epstein-Barr virus (a DNA virus) has been obtained thus far, and infection with Epstein-Barr virus occurring first in the course of acute leukemia has been documented (47). Whether the oncogenic RNA viruses have a role in the etiology of human leukemia at present remains unknown. Their possible role in the etiology of human leukemia is reviewed more completely in Chapter 21.

Genetic Factors   Several congenital disorders have a higher-than-normal incidence of acute leukemia, both lymphocytic and myelocytic. For example, the frequency of leukemia in Down's syndrome has been estimated to be some twenty-fold greater than normal (145, 151, 206, 222). This estimate is probably higher than the true incidence, since other disorders of granulopoiesis may occur in this syndrome and be mistaken for acute leukemia. However, the risk of leukemia in mongoloid children is probably greater than in the normal population. Variants of Down's syndrome with mongolism, erythroleukemia, and a characteristic chromosomal anomaly have recently been described (118). The characteristic chromosomal aberration of G-trisomy in Down's syndrome is thought to result from meiotic nondisjunction prior to conception. This association raises the question of whether the extra chromosome plays a role in leukemogenesis. Strictly speaking, Down's syndrome is a noninheritable disorder resulting from a meiotic accident.

Additional conditions in which aneuploidy occurs with possible increases in the incidence of leukemia include Klinefelter's syndrome (67, 193, 242) and other disorders (24). Aneuploidy was found in three of twenty-five children with leukemia and no somatic anomalies (19). In other studies, a high incidence of both chronic and acute myelocytic leukemia was found in individuals with prezygotic chromosomal anomalies (170).

There are diseases inherited in an autosomal recessive pattern with increased chromosomal breakage and rearrangement, as well as increased incidence of leukemia (149). For example, in one series of patients with Bloom's syndrome (dwarfism, impaired intellectual development, unusual facies, and photosensitive facial rash), three of twenty-three developed acute leukemia (192).

Aplastic anemia associated with multiple congenital anomalies (Fanconi's syndrome) may also involve an increased susceptibility to leukemia (14, 49, 85), and acute leukemia has been well documented in ataxia telangiectasia (98, 103).

It has often been speculated that the increased incidence of leukemia in patients with chromosomal abnormalites occurs because cells with such abnormalities are more readily transformed by oncogenic viruses (1, 152). The cellular chromosomes of patients with Fanconi's anemia are also more susceptible to radiation damage than are normal cells (110).

An association between leukemia and certain genetic diseases of the skeletal system has been suggested but not proven. For example, there are scattered case reports of childhood leukemia occurring in association with Kippel-Feil syndrome (207), achondroplasia (66), Marfan's syndrome (173), and a variant of Ellis-van Creveld syndrome (146).

Evidence suggests that genetic factors may be involved

in leukemogenesis, in addition to their role in the afore-mentioned and poorly understood syndromes. For instance, the concordance rate of leukemia among identical twins is 20 percent, whereas it is negligible among fraternal twins (141, 150). Furthermore, leukemia may occur repeatedly in some families (3, 96, 175). Whether this occurrence is based on genetic or environmental factors is not known (124).

Except for these special syndromes of familial leukemia, the importance of genetic factors to the etiology of human leukemia must still be determined (182, 241). Any genes involved in leukemogenesis apparently are part of a complex polygenic system (216, 241).

There are several diseases, usually considered to be acquired, that carry a greater-than-normal risk of leukemia. This association is strong in the case of polycythemia vera (154) and weak in the case of hyperthyroidism (184) and perhaps Hodgkin's disease (61, 126). In these diseases radioiosotopes and chemotherapeutic agents that may cause chromosomal damage are used in therapy. Pernicious anemia is said to carry a small increased risk of leukemia (13). Acute leukemia has also been reported in association with paroxysmal nocturnal hemoglobinuria (111). Other birth and social factors may be associated with leukemogenesis (63).

Hematologic Features

In acute myelocytic leukemia the peripheral leukocyte count is usually elevated, but may be normal or even low. The latter variant is known as *aleukemic leukemia*. Aleukemic leukemia may be the presenting form of the disease in 40 to 60 percent of patients with acute myelocytic leukemia. When the white count is elevated, it may reach very high levels of several hundred thousand per cubic millimeter. Immature cells constitute between 5 and 100 percent of the circulating leukocytes (Fig. 11.1). As a rule, mature neutrophils are reduced in numbers; only rarely are they increased. Eosinophilia or basophilia is infrequently present (17).

Anemia is the rule in acute myelocytic leukemia. It is generally normocytic, occasionally macrocytic. Polychromatophilia and normoblasts in the peripheral blood are common, although the level of reticulocytes is rarely in excess of 3 percent. Reduced numbers of normoblasts are found in the bone marrow, and megaloblasts and abnormal erythroid precursors are sometimes seen. The mechanisms of anemia in this disease are complex. Often red cell survival is shortened with no compensatory increase in marrow erythropoietic activity (159, 166, 214, 226).

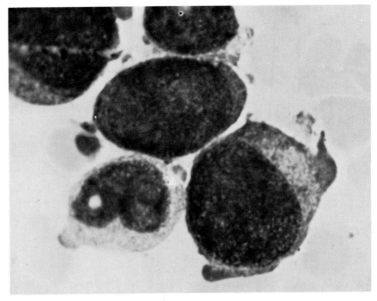

Figure 11.1 Myeloblasts and a band form from the peripheral blood of a patient with acute myeloblastic leukemia; Giemsa stain.

Recent in vivo erythrokinetics with tritiated thymidine in patients with acute myelocytic leukemia suggests a decrease in the size of the stem cell compartment available for erythroid differentiation (34, 76). One report indicates diminished erythropoietin production in myeloblastic leukemia in relapse, with return to normal in remission (239). Leukopoietic activity also may be diminished (176).

Thrombocytopenia occurs in over 90 percent of acute leukemic patients (234). Platelets may be large and bizarre in shape. Bleeding time is prolonged, the tourniquet test is positive, and clot retraction is poor. The frequency of hemorrhagic manifestations increases when the platelet count falls below 50,000/mm³. At a given low platelet count, the incidence of serious bleeding increases as the leukocyte count rises to high levels. Defects in platelet function have been demonstrated (71).

Although fibrinolysins and fibrinolytic purpura occasionally have been demonstrated in patients with acute myelocytic leukemia (25, 135, 167), hemorrhage is only rarely related to abnormalities of coagulation factors, except in acute promyelocytic leukemia. In this variant of the disease, atypical promyelocytes are preponderant in the bone marrow and blood (50). They are visible in Fig. 11.2. A syndrome resembling disseminated intravascular coagulation with hypofibrinogenemia and reduced levels of factors V, VIII, and X may be seen in this disorder (41, 92, 93, 128).

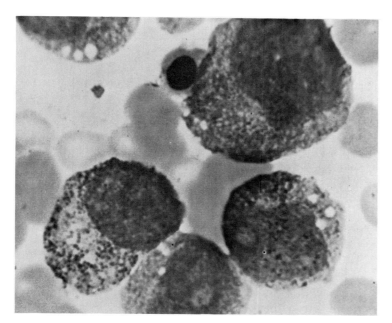

Figure 11.2 Cells from the bone marrow of a patient with acute promyelocytic leukemia. Note the prominent nucleoli and cytoplasmic granulation.

In acute myelocytic leukemia the marrow is crowded with myeloblasts, promyelocytes, and undifferentiated cells. The fat spaces are obliterated, as demonstrated in Fig. 11.3. Little granulocytic differentiation is seen. The megakaryocytes and erythroid cells are reduced in numbers. Megaloblastic changes are often seen in the erythroid series. Few other conditions present this composite morphologic picture of the bone marrow, although drug injury occasionally may produce a similar but not identical picture (134).

Morphology

The majority of immature cells in acute myelocytic leukemia resemble myeloblasts and promyelocytes (see Chapter 1 and Figs. 11.1, 11.2, and 11.4). These malignant cells have the following features: the nucleus/cytoplasm ratio is quite high; the nucleus is round to oval with a fine chromatin structure; the nucleoli are large and distinct, and may be multiple; the cytoplasm is deep blue and, in the case of the myeloblast, has no granules. Cells identified as promyelocytes may have distinctive cytoplasmic, splinter-shaped granules (208).

A characteristic, but not invariant, feature of the immature cells of myelocytic leukemia is the presence of Auer bodies (69); as seen in Fig. 11.5, these are needle or rod-like cytoplasmic inclusions that stain red with Romanovsky stain. They have peroxidase, acid phosphatase

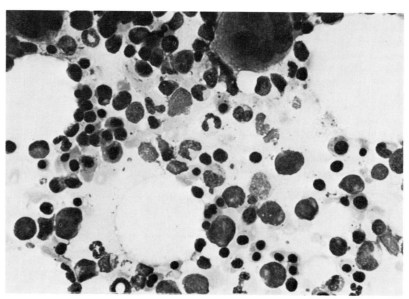

Fig. 11.3A

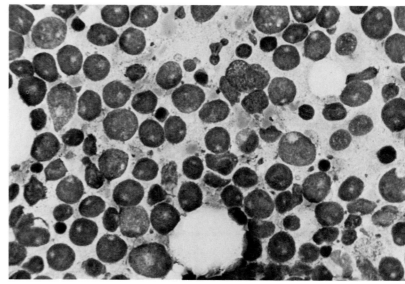

Fig. 11.3B

Figure 11.3 Bone marrow aspirate from a normal subject and from a patient with acute myelocytic leukemia. In Fig. 11.3A, the normal subject, note the relation of cellularity to fat spaces and the heterogeneity of cell types. In Fig. 11.3B there are fewer fat spaces, cellularity is increased, and the cell types are relatively homogeneous.

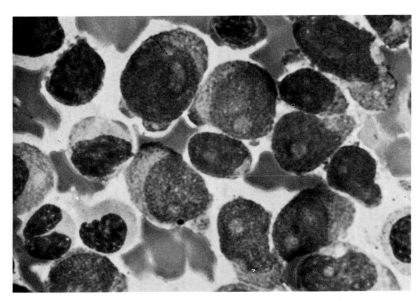

Figure 11.4 A group of myeloblasts in the bone marrow of a patient with acute myelocytic leukemia. Note the prominent nucleoli and the large, round nuclei with fine chromatin structure.

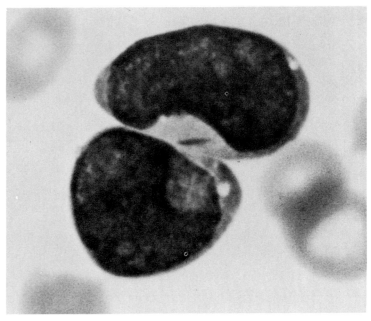

Figure 11.5 Two myeloblasts from the blood of a patient with acute myelocytic leukemia. One contains a prominent cytoplasmic Auer rod.

activity, and probably a high mucopolysaccharide content (see Chapter 1). Auer bodies probably are abnormal developments of the primary granules. Their presence may be diagnostic of myelogenous or monocytic leukemia although, rarely, they have been described in other conditions (129).

Cells resembling Pelger-Huët, with bilobed nuclei (see Chapter 9), may be seen in acute, as well as chronic, myeloproliferative disorders (45, 56, 130). Leukemic myeloblasts with lipid-containing cytoplasmic vacuoles occur occasionally (168).

Cytochemistry

The cytochemistry of acute leukemic cells is quite complex and is influenced by the line of origin of the predominant cell type and the degree of heterogeneity of the cellular population with regard to maturation. Ultimately the biochemical reactions depend upon the structural and enzyme components of the leukocyte. In Chapter 1 we considered the cytochemical reactions of normal and malignant granulocytes in the context of cellular morphogenesis and formation of granules. Here it is appropriate to consider the cytochemical properties of malignant myeloblasts, monoblasts, lymphoblasts, and erythroblasts. Such distinctions are important, both for clinical diagnosis and for understanding some of the biologic properties of these malignant cells.

Some of the major cytochemical reactions of blast cells are summarized in Table 11.2 and discussed below (101, 102, 144). The periodic acid Schiff (PAS) reaction tests for the presence of glycogen or glycoprotein. This reaction may be negative or moderately positive in myeloblasts. When positive, the reaction produced is finely granular. In contrast, the reaction product, when present in lymphoblasts, tends to be coarse with block deposits against a clear cytoplasmic background (101).

Table 11.2 Cytochemical reactions of leukemic cells.

Type of cell	PAS reaction	Sudano-philia	Perox-idase	Nuclear aryl sulfatase	α-naphthyl esterase
Myeloblasts and promyelocytes	0 to +; fine	+ to +++; coarse	+ to ++	0	0 to +
Monoblasts	0 to +++; fine to moderate	+ to ++; fine	+	0	++ to +++
Lymphoblasts	0 to ++; coarse	0	0	++	0
Erythroblasts	++ to ++++; variable	0	0	---	---

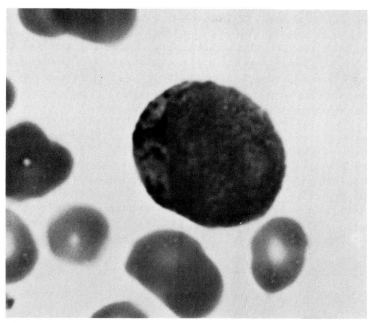

Fig. 11.6A

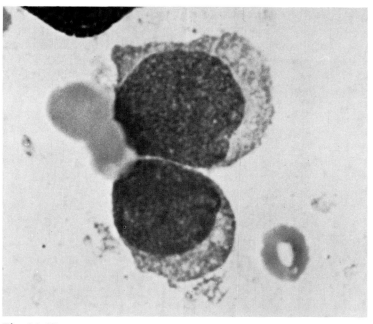

Fig. 11.6B

Figure 11.6 Primitive cells from the blood of patients with acute myelocytic leukemia (Fig. 11.6A) and acute lymphocytic leukemia (Fig. 11.6B), stained for peroxidase and counterstained with Giemsa. In Fig. 11.6A note the dense, cytoplasmic, peroxidase-positive material, which is not present in Fig. 11.6B.

Lymphoblasts rarely show sudanophilia (lipid staining), whereas myeloblasts often have coarse, sudanophilic material. Generally, a high percentage of myeloblasts and promyelocytes are positive with sudan black stain; in occasional cases only a rare cell is positive. Promyelocytes tend to stain more heavily than myelocytes. Similarly, myeloblasts and monoblasts—if sufficiently differentiated to have granules—have peroxidase activity, whereas lymphoblasts lack this enzyme (Fig. 11.6) If the early granulocytes are not sufficiently differentiated to the stage of granule production, they will also lack this enzymatic activity.

Lymphoblasts are said to be unique in demonstrating nuclear aryl sulfatase activity (59, 127).

A variety of esterase activities is demonstrable in hemic cells, the pattern among different cell lines being determined by the substrate employed (181). With alpha-naphthyl acetate, monoblasts and monocytes are strongly positive, whereas early granulocytes and lymphoblasts are weakly positive or negative. With naphthol AS-D, the positive reactions are confined to the granulocytic series.

The addition of acidic dye such as chromotrope 2R to Romanovsky stains may result in nucleolar staining characteristics that help differentiate among the different types of acute leukemic cells (84, 186).

Proliferation

Monti and his colleagues (155), using tritiated thymidine, first observed that myeloblasts in acute leukemia have a lower labeling index (percentage of cells with nuclear labeling) than do precursor cells in normal bone marrow. This observation challenged the long-held concept of rapid and uncontrolled proliferation of a completely autonomous population of leukemic cells. It is now clear that the fraction of the leukemic cell population that is replicating is smaller than the comparable fraction of normal bone marrow precursor cells and that the generation time of acute leukemic cells is equal to, or more prolonged than, that of normal bone marrow cells (28, 31, 32, 34, 77, 94, 120, 143, 196).

Were the leukemic cell population to expand logarithmically, it would follow the pattern shown in Fig. 11.7A. However, it does not. Rather, as shown in Fig 11.7B, the rate of growth diminishes as the total tumor cell mass increases (11, 191, 204). Such a pattern of growth is said to follow Gompertzian growth kinetics. It is also the type of pattern found in regenerating normal tissues (169). It appears, therefore, that leukemic cells are not wholly autonomous and that their proliferation is influenced by external factors.

One may ask what the significance of this phenomenon

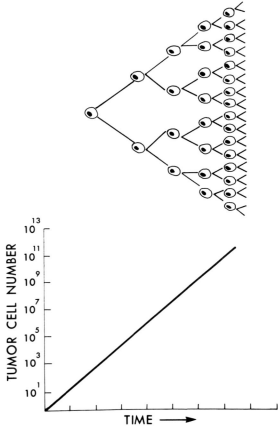

Fig. 11.7A

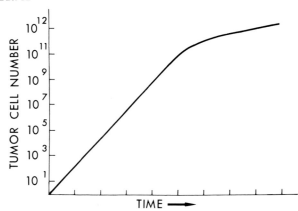

Fig. 11.7B

Figure 11.7 Increase in tumor cell numbers with time. If all leukemic cells proliferated without any restrictions on growth and without any significant cell death, the increase would be exponential, as indicated in Fig. 11.7A. The observed increase, shown in Fig. 11.7B, is not exponential, but tends to level off at the higher numbers of tumor cells.

of Gompertzian growth kinetics is for leukemic patients. It probably means that if the size of a leukemic population is reduced by chemotherapy or irradiation, the residual cell population will expand more rapidly. This appears to be correct: a higher bone marrow labeling index with tritiated thymidine has been found in the leukemic bone marrow immediately following either the induction of a remission (77, 160) or following extracorporeal irradiation (27).

In both acute myelocytic and acute lymphoblastic leukemia, a pulse of tritiated thymidine predominantly labels the large blast cells (Fig. 11.8), suggesting that these constitute the replicating pool of cells (94, 196). It is thought that the proliferating blast cells are not self-maintaining but, after one or two divisions, become smaller and enter a nonproliferating compartment. The smaller blast cells with a lower proliferative rate may later reenter the rapidly proliferating compartment (73). Thus, initial labeling studies of myeloblastic leukemic cells were interpreted as indicating a smaller proliferating cell pool and a larger nonproliferating pool. However, when tritiated thymidine was continuously infused into a patient with myeloblastic leukemia for twenty days, 99 percent of the leukemic marrow cells were labeled (29, 33). This observation indicates that essentially all the blast cells may enter the proliferating pool, a phenomenon illustrated in Fig. 11.9. The proliferating cells probably do not cross the placental barrier (139).

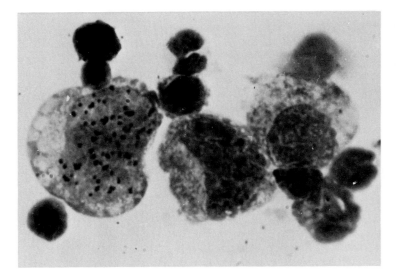

Figure 11.8 Two large blast cells from the bone marrow of a patient with acute myelocytic leukemia labeled with tritiated thymidine. The slide containing the cells was coated with photographic emulsion, exposed for ten days, developed, and stained with Giemsa.

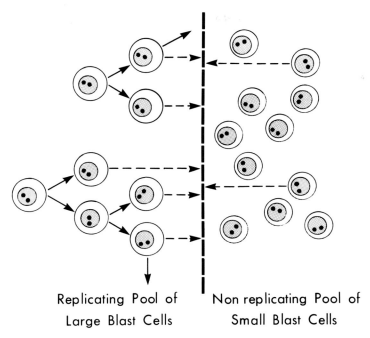

Replicating Pool of   Non replicating Pool of
Large Blast Cells   Small Blast Cells

Figure 11.9 Schematic representation of a replicating pool of large leukemic blast cells and a nonreplicating pool of smaller blast cells. After a few divisions, the large cells enter the pool of smaller cells. Over a period of time the small cells gradually reenter the proliferating pool.

The principal abnormality of the leukemic myeloblast appears to be the failure to mature normally to a differentiated end cell incapable of further division. The consequence of this abnormality is that essentially all the leukemic cells retain the ability to divide. Accumulation of neoplastic cells in the bone marrow, blood, and tissues results.

Some leukemic myeloblasts are capable of maturation in vitro (87) and presumably in vivo as well. Inferential evidence suggests that the later stages of granulopoiesis may be impaired, along with the early steps in differentiation. For example, the time required for myelocytes to mature and for their progeny to traverse the marrow granulocyte reserve and the blood stream is usually prolonged in acute myelocytic leukemia (74). Additionally, the "mature" neutrophils produced by patients with acute leukemia may be functionally defective, presumably as a result of aberrant maturation (35).

Cytogenetics

The outstanding features of the chromosomal changes in acute leukemia are the large numbers of different chromosomes that may be abnormal, and the protean nature of the changes (187–189). In a recent series, 41 percent of 95 adult patients with acute leukemia had abnormal karyo-

types in their leukemic cells (100). Similar figures have been found in other series (213). No specific chromosomal abnormalities can be said to characterize acute myelocytic leukemia (6, 190); however, in any given patient the chromosomal changes generally remain constant. This situation contrasts with that of the patients with chronic myelocytic leukemia, most of whom have the same specific cytogenetic abnormality in the leukocytes until blast crisis occurs. When blast transformation occurs, various aneuploid cytogenetic abnormalities are found in association with the characteristic Ph[1] chromosome (189, 211).

Hart and her colleagues (100) made several observations in cytogenetic studies of a large series of adults with acute leukemia: (a) the frequency of chromosomal abnormalities correlated roughly with increasing leukocytosis; (b) hypoploidy and chromosomal deletions from groups D and E were associated with an adverse prognosis and poorer response to therapy. Conversely, patients with an extra D or E chromosome had a better prognosis; (c) as time of observation was prolonged and as leukemic cell infiltration of blood and bone marrow increased, the frequency of chromosomal aberrations also increased; (d) marrow leukemic cell aneuploidy tended to disappear with remission and recur with relapse; and (e) deletion of G-group chromosomes occurred more frequently than could be expected by chance alone. This last observation is of interest in that abnormalities of G-group chromosomes are associated also with chronic myelocytic leukemia and Down's syndrome, a condition with a predisposition to acute leukemia (148).

Unusually high frequencies of group D and E chromosomal abnormalities have been observed in patients with acute myelocytic leukemia (121, 227). Children with acute erythroleukemia may have a high frequency of C-group chromosomal abnormalities (58).

Chromosomal abnormalities in myeloblastic leukemia cannot be consistently related to the use of chemotherapeutic agents. Of the anticancer drugs, BCNU (a nitrosourea derivative) has been shown to produce random persistent cytogenetic abnormality (99).

The occurrence of a chromosomal abnormality in a variety of "preleukemic" disorders may favor the development of leukemia (164). Such disorders include polycythemia vera and idiopathic pancytopenia.

The presence of a chromosomal abnormality in the bone marrow of patients with acute myelocytic leukemia may adversely affect prognosis (185).

The relation between a detectable chromosomal abnormality and the genesis of acute leukemia is unknown. As Sandberg and his colleagues have stated, "To equate cloning or selection of a fairly stable and definable karyotypic profile by an established human cancer with direct participation of the chromosomal aberrations in cancer development appears to be unwise and unfounded at the present state of our knowledge regarding carcinogenesis" (188). In addition to the cytogenetic abnormalities, recent evidence suggests that leukemic lymphoblasts and myeloblasts may have distinctive antigens on their surface (132, 177).

Clinical Features and Natural History

Clinical Features

As in the other acute leukemias (see Chapters 21 and 27), the major clinical manifestations of myeloblastic leukemia are related to infiltration of the bone marrow and displacement of the normal hematopoietic cells. Anemia, thrombocytopenia with bleeding, and granulocytopenia with enhanced susceptibility to infection account for the major clinical features of this disease.

Bleeding may be manifest as petechial hemorrhages of skin and mucous membranes, as hemorrhage from the nasopharynx or gastrointestinal tract, or as oozing from venapuncture sites. A hemorrhagic diathesis may be especially prominent in acute promyelocytic leukemia as a result of depletion of clotting factors (7, 10, 172), but this problem may occur in other types of acute myelocytic leukemia as well (93). Initiation of the clotting process with subsequent depletion of clotting factors may result from release of a leukocyte procoagulant (123).

Infections are protean in nature, including bacterial, viral (for example, cytomegalovirus), and other pathogens (such as *Pneumocystis carinii*), and fungi (23). Infections result from granulocytopenia, malfunctioning granulocytes (35) and immunologic abnormalities secondary to drug therapy.

Organ infiltration by leukemic cells produces the characteristic hepatosplenomegaly. Splenic infarcts with a friction rub and perisplenitis may occur. Splenic enlargement may, rarely, be a result of infection rather than leukemic infiltration (16). Some degree of lymphadenopathy usually is present, although lymph node involvement in myeloblastic leukemia is not so prominent as in the lymphocytic leukemias.

Sternal tenderness is the rule when the disease is in relapse (39); spontaneous bone pain infrequently may dominate the clinical situation. Bone involvement may take the form of lytic or sclerotic lesions, tumors, arthritis, or osteomyelitis (40, 157, 233, 236). Occasionally hypercalcemia is associated with bone reabsorption. Hypocalcemia has been described also in acute leukemia, most commonly the childhood variety (116).

The skin may be directly infiltrated by leukemic cells, as well as being involved by hemorrhage and infection. The resultant lesions may assume a variety of forms, including papules, nodules, and exfoliative lesions (15, 236).

The gastrointestinal tract may be involved by hemorrhage, infection with bacteria or fungi, or by direct leukemia infiltration. Perforation of the bowel, although not common, has been observed at one time or another by most students of this disease. Perirectal abscess is a frequent, and occasionally fatal, complication of myeloblastic leukemia.

Microscopy frequently shows evidence of cellular infiltration in the heart. However, clinically significant infiltration with disturbances of conduction or heart failure are distinctly uncommon. These cardiac manifestations may be observed secondary to therapy with drugs such as daunomycin. Even though the lungs may be infiltrated by leukemic cells in a patchy or diffuse manner, bleeding and infection are more common as causes of clinical or roentgenographic pulmonary manifestation.

Urogenital involvement may be manifested by hematuria, pyelonephritis, perinephric abscess, prostate infiltration, and priapism. The last may be caused by stasis in, or thrombosis of, the spaces of the corpora cavernosa (115, 125, 138, 199, 220). Although microscopic cellular infiltration of the kidneys is common, direct impairment of renal function by this mechanism is rare. A more common, and frequently preventable, renal complication is uric acid nephropathy. Hyperuricemia results from the rapid turnover in nucleic acids associated with leukemic cell proliferation. Uric acid is poorly soluble in an acid urine. Under conditions of extreme hyperuricemia, crystals of uric acid may precipitate in the renal tubules, resulting in renal damage and anuria. This complication is relatively easy to prevent by a program of high fluid intake, urine alkalinization, and allopurinol (36). It is difficult to treat, however, once azotemia is established.

The variants of acute myelocytic leukemia in which monoblasts are predominant may have extreme degrees of lysozymuria and evidence of proximal renal tubule dysfunction (165, 171, 202, 230) (see Chapter 27). Another metabolic complication of acute leukemia is severe lactic acidosis (221).

Lesions of the nervous system, in acute myelocytic leukemia, may take the form of tumors, disseminated infiltration, thrombosis, hemorrhage, or infection. Any part of the nervous system may be involved, including the brain, spinal cord, meninges, and cranial and peripheral nerves (156, 162, 163, 197, 232).

Hemorrhagic complications in the central nervous system are quite common. Meningeal leukemia is rare in acute myelocytic leukemia when compared to its frequency in lymphoblastic leukemia. However, with longer durations of survival, we are now seeing this complication in myelocytic leukemia with increasing frequency. Generally, the diagnosis of meningeal involvement is easily made from the cytology of the spinal fluid (203).

Natural History

Acute myelocytic leukemia is almost invariably acute in onset. The patient may notice fatigue, exertional dyspnea, palpitations, fever, or bleeding tendency developing over the course of several weeks. Less commonly, the initial manifestations are related to infiltration by leukemic cells of parenchymal organs. Occasionally the clinical course is so abrupt that only a few hours intervene between the first hemorrhagic manifestations and fatal hemorrhagic complications.

An alternative pattern of clinical onset of disease is the following. Leukemia may become manifest by a long prodromal period in which a variety of hematopoietic disturbances occur, including refractory anemia, variable leukopenia, and sometimes thrombocytopenia. The marrow may be hypercellular with "left shift" or, less commonly, hypocellular. When leukemia is clearly diagnosable at this stage, the condition is generally designated *smoldering leukemia*. When the hematopoietic disturbance is present but the morphologic alterations are insufficient to allow a definitive diagnosis of acute leukemia, the condition is generally designated *preleukemia* (183). Inevitably, both the preleukemic and smoldering leukemic variants evolve into typical acute leukemia.

During the preleukemic phase it may be very difficult to predict whether the hematopoietic disorder will evolve to leukemia or to another condition such as refractory anemia. Chromosomal abnormalities may be present during the preleukemic phase. It is probable that abnormalities of hematopoietic cell differentiation exist during this phase and may be used to establish a diagnosis before overt leukemia becomes manifest (88).

Once preleukemia makes the transition to acute leukemia, the course of disease is quite typical—untreated disease advances rapidly and progressively until death occurs. Similarly, smoldering leukemia may pursue a low-grade subacute course until transition to typical acute leukemia occurs.

Median survival in myeloblastic leukemia was two months or less in the period before effective therapy was developed (210). Only rarely has this unmodified natural history been seen in the United States since 1953. Today the natural history is modified by drug treatment.

The untreated disease customarily is acute at onset, progressing rapidly and inexorably with a continuously

Table 11.3 Survival in acute myelocytic leukemia.

Years	Principal therapy[a]	Median survival (mos.)	References
	Childhood AML		
1937–53	Support only	<2	210
1944–60	P, Mtx, 6-MP	4	17
1955–59	P, Mtx, 6-MP	4–7	105, 240
1963–68	Ara-C, MeGAG, V + DN	13	105, 106
	Adult AML		
1937–53	Supportive care	<2	210
1953–65	P, 6-MP, V, Mtx	4–5	44, 105, 142
1963–66	P, 6-MP, V, Mtx, MeGAG, Ara-C	6	105, 106
1966–72	P, 6-MP, V, Mtx, DN, 6-TG, Ara-C	>10	79, 106, 133, 231

[a] P = prednisone; Mtx = methotrexate; 6-MP = 6-mercaptopurine; Ara-C = cytosine arabinoside; MeGAG = methylglyoxal-bis-guanylhydrazone; V = vincristine; DN = daunorubicin; 6-TG = 6-thioguanine.

rising white count, increasing organomegaly, and fatal outcome. Death is usually from bleeding, infection, or, more rarely, from complications of anemia or perforation of a viscus (109). Once in a great while spontaneous remissions or remissions following infection or administration of blood products have been reported (205). Trials with viral infection or administration of fresh blood products have conferred no consistent benefit (225, 228).

Today the physician sees a modified natural history. He may even see very long-term survivors (122). Generally, high white blood counts are reduced by drug treatment, and normal or low counts are the rule even in advanced disease. The availability of platelet transfusions at many institutions has greatly reduced the incidence of hemorrhage (53, 97, 200). Effective drugs against the common bacterial pathogens and *Staphylococcus* have reduced these as prominent causes of mortality (109). Infection with gram-negative bacteria, opportunistic fungal pathogens, viruses, and protozoa has risen to the fore as the cause of death.

In Table 11.3 are recorded the changing statistics over time of survival with acute myelocytic leukemia and the changing pattern of drug management.

Principles of Therapy

Strategy of the Attack

The object of therapy in acute myelocytic leukemia is to prolong life and improve the quality of life. The available data strongly suggest that these goals are correlated with induction of a hematologic remission—that is, the return of blood and bone marrow to normal status and disappear-

Table 11.4 Drugs useful in the treatment of AML.

Agent	Class of compounds	References
6-mercaptopurine	Antimetabolite	70, 137
6-thioguanine	Antimetabolite	78
Methotrexate	Antimetabolite	54, 70
Cytosine arabinoside	Antimetabolite	105
Vincristine	Plant alkaloid	37
Daunorubicin	Antibiotic	8

ance of any evidence of compromised organ function (60, 112). The strategy of current therapy is to combine two or more drugs, each of which is effective alone, in an intensive regimen to induce rapid control of disease (30, 106). Once remission is induced, its duration is prolonged by cyclic readministration of combinations of effective drugs. Examples of drugs that have proven to have some efficacy in the control of myeloblastic leukemia are listed in Table 11.4. Various other agents have been used with limited success (36, 137).

The principles of management of acute leukemia are discussed in more detail in Chapter 21 and embrace specific chemotherapy, supportive measures, innovative immunotherapy, and bone marrow transplantation. With the use of drug combinations and intensive reinduction schedules, both the frequency of remission induction and the median duration of survival of patients with acute myelocytic leukemia have increased (5), as we have seen in Table 11.3. Specific regimens of drug administration may be found in recent texts (36, 137) and in the following references: 9, 18, 30, 42, 106, and 229.

Summary

Acute myelocytic leukemia is an acute myeloproliferative disorder characterized by accumulation of immature cells of the granulocytic series. Concomitant abnormalities of erythropoiesis and thrombopoiesis are common. The generation time of leukemic cells is not abnormally short, nor is the fraction of proliferating cells unusually high. The defect in the malignant cells appears to be a failure of maturation to normal nonproliferating end cells. This defect results in excessive accumulation of the leukemic cells in the bone marrow, blood, and tissues. Essentially all of the neoplastic cells are capable of entering the proliferative compartment. Abnormalities of morphogenesis of leukemic myeloid cells result in abnormal morphology (for instance, Auer rods) as well as abnormal function. Their accumulation in the bone marrow results in diminished numbers of normal granulocytes and megakaryocytes. The consequent complications of infection and bleeding are the hallmarks of untreated acute leukemia.

The etiology of acute myelocytic leukemia is presently unknown; however, the evidence points increasingly to a principal pathogenetic role for RNA tumor viruses. The relation between such agents and the frequently observed abnormalities of chromosome structure are still obscure. Although patterns of chromosomal abnormalities are observed, no single aberration is characteristic of acute myelocytic leukemia.

The typical pattern of untreated acute leukemia is one of inexorable progression. Modern therapy utilizes several chemotherapeutic agents in combination, with the objective of inducing and maintaining hematologic remission.

Chapter 11 References

1. Aaronson, S. A., and Todaro, G. J. SV40 T antigen induction and transformation in human fibroblast cell strains, *Virology* 36:254, 1968.
2. Ackerman, G. A. Microscopic and histochemical studies on the Auer bodies in leukemic cells, *Blood* 5:847, 1950.
3. Anderson, R. C. Familial leukemia (a report of leukemia in five siblings, with a brief review of the genetic aspects of this disease), *Am. J. Dis. Child.* 81:313, 1951.
4. Awa, A. A., Bloom, A. D., Yoshida, M. C., Neriishi, S., and Archer, P. G. Cytogenetic study of the offspring of atom bomb survivors, *Nature* 218:367, 1968.
5. Axtell, L. M., Cutler, S. J., and Myers, M. H. End Results in Cancer, rept. 4, DHEW publ. (NIH) 73–272, 1972.
6. Baikie, A. G., Jacobs, P. A., McBride, V. A., and Tough, I. M. Cytogenetic studies in acute leukemia, *Br. Med. J.* 1:1564, 1961.
7. Baker, W. G., Bang, N. U., Nachman, R. L., Raafat, F., and Horowitz, H. I. Hypofibrinogenic hemorrhage in acute myelogenous leukemia treated with heparin, *Ann. Intern. Med.* 61:116, 1964.
8. Bernard, J., Boiron, M., and Jacquillat, C. Rubidomycin in 400 patients with leukemia and other malignancies, p. 5, XII Congress Int. Soc. Hematol., 1968.
9. Bernard, J., Jacquillat, C., and Weil, M. Treatment of the acute leukemias, *Semin. Hematol.* 9:181, 1972.
10. Bernard, J., Lasneret, J., Chrome, J., Levy, J. P., and Boiron, M. A cytological and histological study of acute promyelocytic leukemia, *J. Clin. Pathol.* 16:319, 1963.
11. Bierman, H. R. Hypothesis: the leukemias—proliferative or accumulative?, *Blood* 30:238, 1967.
12. Bizzozero, O. J., Jr., Johnson, K. G., and Ciocco, A. Radiation-related leukemia in Hiroshima and Nagasaki, 1946-1964. I. Distribution, incidence and appearance time, *N. Engl. J. Med.* 274:1095, 1966.
13. Blackburn, E. K., Callender, S. T., Dacie, J. V., Doll, R., Girdwood, R. H., Mollin, D. L., Saracci, R., Stafford, J. L., Thompson, R. B., Varadi, S., and Wetherley-Mein, G. Possible association between pernicious anaemia and leukaemia: a prospective study of 1,625 patients with a note on the very high incidence of stomach cancer, *Int. J. Cancer* 3:163, 1968.
14. Bloom, G. E., Warner, S., Gerald, P. S., and Diamond, L. K. Chromosome abnormalities in constitutional aplastic anemia, *N. Engl. J. Med.* 274:8, 1966.
15. Bluefarb, S. M. Leukemia Cutis, Charles C Thomas, Springfield, Ill., 1960.
16. Bodey, G. P., DeJongh, D., Isassi, A., and Freireich, E. J. Hypersplenism due to disseminated candidiasis in a patient with acute leukemia, *Cancer* 24:417, 1969.
17. Boggs, D. R., Wintrobe, M. M., and Cartwright, G. E. The acute leukemias, *Medicine* 41:163, 1962.
18. Boiron, M., Weil. M., Jacquillat, C., et al. Daunorubicin in the treatment of acute myelocytic leukaemia, *Lancet* i:330, 1969.
19. Borges, W. H., Nicklas, J. W., and Hamm, C. W. Prezygotic determinants in acute leukemia, *J. Pediatr.* 70:180, 1967.
20. Brauer, M. J., and Dameshek, W. Hypoplastic anemia and myeloblastic leukemia following chloramphenicol therapy. Report of three cases, *N. Engl. J. Med.* 277:1003, 1967.
21. Brown, W. M. C., and Doll, R. Leukaemia in childhood and young adult life. Trends in mortality in relation to aetiology, *Br. Med. J.* 2:981, 1961.
22. Brown, W. M. C., and Doll, R. Mortality from cancer and other causes after radiotherapy for ankylosing spondylitis, *Br. Med. J.* 2:1327, 1965.
23. Burke, P. S., and Coltman, C. A., Jr. Multiple pulmonary aspergillomas in acute leukemia, *Cancer* 28:1289, 1971.
24. Castoldi, G. L., Grusovin, G. D., Scapoli, G. L., and Spanedda, R. Association of multiple haematological disorders (acute myeloblastic leukaemia, paraproteinaemia and thalassaemia) in a 46, XX/46, XXqi female, *Acta Haematol.* 46:294, 1971.
25. Cattan, A., Schwarzenberg. L., Amiel, J. L., et al. Syndrome de fibrinogénopénie au cours de leucémies aiguës. Rôle déterminant des cellules leucémiques. Étude *in vitro* de leur pouvoir fibrinolytique, *Rev. Fr. Etude Clin. Biol.* 11:155, 1966.
26. Chan, B. W. B., Flemans, R. J., and Zbinden, G. Acute leukemia with megakaryocytic predominance, *Cancer* 28:1343, 1971.
27. Chan, B. W. B., Hayhoe, F. G. J., and Bullimore, J. A. Effect of extracorporeal irradiation of the blood on bone marrow activity in acute leukaemia, *Nature* 221:972, 1969.
28. Clarkson, B. A review of recent studies of cellular proliferation, *Natl. Cancer Inst. Monogr.* 30:81, 1969.
29. Clarkson, B., cited by S. Perry and R. C. Gallo, in A. S. Gordon (eds.), Regulation of Hematopoiesis, p. 1226, Appleton-Century-Crofts, New York, 1970.
30. Clarkson, B. D. Acute myelocytic leukemia in adults, *Cancer* 30:1572, 1972.
31. Clarkson, B., and Fried, J. Changing concepts of treatment in acute leukemia, *Med. Clin. North Am.* 55:561, 1971.
32. Clarkson, B., Fried, J., Strife, A., Sakai, Y., Ota, K., and Ohkita, T. Studies of cellular proliferation in human leukemia. III. Behavior of leukemic cells in three adults with acute leukemia given continuous infusions of ^{3}H-thymidine for 8 or 10 days, *Cancer* 25:1237, 1970.
33. Clarkson, B., Ohkita, T., Ota, K., et al. Studies of cellular proliferation in acute leukemia, *J. Clin. Invest.* 44:1035, 1965.
34. Clarkson, B., Ohkita, T., Ota, K., et al. Studies of cellular proliferation in human leukemia. I. Estimation of growth rates of leukemic and normal hematopoietic cells in two adults with acute leukemia given simple injections of tritiated thymidine, *J. Clin. Invest.* 46:506, 1967.
35. Cline, M. J. A new white cell test that measures individual phagocyte function in a mixed population. I. A neutrophil defect in acute myelocytic leukemia, *J. Lab. Clin. Med.* 81:311, 1973.
36. Cline, M. J., and Haskell, C. M. Cancer Chemotherapy, 2nd ed., W. B. Saunders Co., Philadelphia, 1975.
37. Cline, M. J., and Rosenbaum, E. Prediction of *in vivo* cytotoxicity of

chemotherapeutic agents by their *in vitro* effect on leukocytes from patients with acute leukemia, *Cancer Res.* 28:2516, 1968.

38. Cohen, T., and Creger, W. P. Acute myeloid leukemia following seven years of aplastic anemia induced by chloramphenicol, *Am. J. Med.* 43:762, 1967.

39. Craver, L. F. Tenderness of sternum in leukemia, *Am. J. Med. Sci.* 174:799, 1927.

40. Craver, L. F., and Copeland, M. M. Changes of the bones in the leukemias, *Arch. Surg.* 30:639, 1935.

41. Croizat, P., and Favre-Gilly, J. Les aspects du syndrome hémorragique des leucémies, à propos de 12 cas de thrombocytopénie et d'un cas de fibrinopénie, *Le Sang* 20:417, 1949.

42. Crowther, D., Bateman, C. J., Vartan, C. P., et al. Combination chemotherapy using L-asparaginase, daunorubicin and cytosine arabinoside in adults with acute myelogenous leukaemia, *Br. Med. J.* 4:513, 1970 (suppl.).

43. Cutler, S. J., Axtell, L., and Heise, H. Ten thousand cases of leukemia: 1940-62, *J. Natl. Cancer Inst.* 39:993, 1967.

44. Dameshek, W., Necheles, T. F., and Finkel, H. E. Survival in myeloblastic leukemia of adults, *N. Engl. J. Med.* 275:700, 1966.

45. Darte, J. M., Dacie, J. V., and McSorley, J. G. A. Pelger-like leukocytes in chronic myeloid leukaemia, *Acta Haematol.* 12:117, 1954.

46. Dawson, D. M., Rosenthal, D. S., and Moloney, W. C. Neurological complications of acute leukemia in adults: changing rate, *Ann. Intern. Med.* 79:541, 1973.

47. Deardorff, W. L., Gerber, P., and Vogler, W. R. Infectious mononucleosis in acute leukemia with rising Epstein-Barr virus antibody titers, *Ann. Intern. Med.* 72:235, 1970.

48. DeGowin, R. L. Benzene exposure and aplastic anemia followed by leukemia 15 years later, *J.A.M.A.* 185:748, 1963.

49. de Grouchy, J. Generic diseases, chromosome rearrangements and malignancy, *Ann. Intern. Med.* 65:603, 1966.

50. Didisheim, P., Trombold, J. S., Vandervoort, L. E., and Mibashan, R. S. Acute promyelocytic leukemia with fibrinogen and factor V deficiencies, *Blood* 23:717, 1964.

51. Di Guglielmo, G. Les maladies érythrémiques, *Rev. Hematol.* 1:355, 1946.

52. Di Guglielmo, G., and Ferrara, A. Contributo alla diagnostica delle malattie eritremiche ed eritroleucemiche, *Hematologica* 41:605, 1956.

53. Djerassi, I., and Farber, S. Control and prevention of hemorrhage: platelet transfusion, *Cancer Res.* 25:1499, 1965.

54. Djerassi, I., Farber, S., Abir, E., and Neikirk, W. Continuous infusion of methotrexate in children with acute leukemia, *Cancer* 20:233, 1967.

55. Doll, R., and Smith, P. G. The longterm effects of X-irradiation in patients treated for metropathia haemorrhagica, *Br. J. Radiol.* 41:362, 1968.

56. Dorr, A. E., and Moloney, W. C. Acquired pseudo-Pelger anomaly of granulocytic leukocytes, *N. Engl. J. Med.* 261:742, 1959.

57. Dougan, L., and Woodliff, H. J. Acute leukaemia associated with phenylbutazone treatment. A review of the literature and report of a further case, *Med. J. Aust.* 1:217, 1965.

58. Dyment, P. G., Melnyk, J., and Brubaker, C. A. A cytogenetic study of acute erythroleukemia in children, *Blood* 32:997, 1968.

59. Ekert, H., and Denett, X. An evaluation of nuclear arylsulphatase activity as an aid to the cytological diagnosis of acute leukaemia, *Aust. Ann. Med.* 15:152, 1966.

60. Ellison, R. R., Holland, J. F., Weil, M., Jacquillat, C., Boiron, M., Bernard, J., Sawitsky, A., Rosner, F., Gussoff, B., Silver, R. T., Karanas, A., Cuttner, J., Spurr, C. L., Hayes, D. M., Blom, J., Leone, L. A., Haurani, F., Kyle, R., Hutchison, J. L., Forcier, R. J., and Moon, J. H. Arabinosyl cytosine: a useful agent in the treatment of acute leukemia in adults, *Blood* 32:507, 1968.

61. Evans, A. S., Niederman, J. C., and McCollum, R. W. Seroepidemiologic studies of infectious mononucleosis with EB virus, *N. Engl. J. Med.* 279:1121, 1968.

62. Ezdinli, E. Z., Sokal, J. E., Aungst, C. W., Untae, K., and Sandberg, A. A. Myeloid leukemia in Hodgkin's disease: chromosomal abnormalities, *Ann. Intern. Med.* 71:1097, 1969.

63. Fasal, E., Jackson, E. W., and Klauber, M. R. Birth characteristics and leukemia in childhood, *J. Natl. Cancer Inst.* 47:501, 1971.

64. Fraumeni, J. F., Jr. Bone marrow depression induced by chloramphenicol or phenylbutazone. Leukemia and other sequelae, *J.A.M.A.* 201:828, 1967.

65. Fraumeni, J. F., Jr. Clinical epidemiology of leukemia, *Semin. Hematol.* 6:250, 1969.

66. Fraumeni, J. F., Jr., and Manning, M. D. Achondroplasia and leukaemia, *Br. Med. J.* 3:680, 1967.

67. Fraumeni, J. F., Jr., and Miller, R. W. Epidemiology of human leukemia: recent observations, *J. Natl. Cancer Inst.* 38:593, 1967.

68. Fraumeni, J. F., Jr., and Miller, R. W. Leukemia mortality: downturn rates in the United States, *Science* 155:1126, 1967.

69. Freeman, J. A. Origin of Auer bodies, *Blood* 27:499, 1966.

70. Frei, E. III, Freireich, E. J., Gehan, E., Pinkel, D., Holland, J. F., Selawry, O., Haurani, F., Spurr, C. L., Hayes, D. M., James, G. W., Rothberg, H., Sodee, D. B., Rundles, R. W., Schroeder, L. R., Hoogstraten, B., Wolman, I. J., Traggis, D. G., Cooper, T., Gendel, B-R., Ebaugh, F., and Taylor, R. Studies of sequential and combination antimetabolite therapy in acute leukemia: 6-mercaptopurine and methotrexate, from the acute leukemia group B, *Blood* 18:431, 1961.

71. Friedman, I. A., Schwartz, S. D., and Leithold, S. L. Platelet function defects with bleeding. Early manifestation of acute leukemia, *Arch. Intern. Med.* 113:177, 1964.

72. Friedreich, N. Ein neuer Fall von Leukämie, *Virchows Arch. Pathol. Anat.* 12:37, 1857.

73. Gabutti, V., Pileri, A., Tarocco R. P., et al. Proliferative potential of out-of-cycle leukaemic cells, *Nature* 224:375, 1969.

74. Galbraith, P. R., and Advincula, E. G. Observations on the myelocyte to tissue transit time (MTT) in acute leukaemia and other prolifer-

ative disorders, *Br. J. Haematol.* 22:453, 1972.

75. Gallo, R. C., Smith, R. G., Whang-Peng, J., et al. RNA tumor viruses, DNA polymerases and oncogenesis: some selective effects of rifampicin derivatives, *Medicine* 51:159, 1972.
76. Gavosto, F., Gabutti, V., Masera, P., et al. The problem of anaemia in the acute leukemias. Kinetic studies, *Eur. J. Cancer* 6:33, 1970.
77. Gavosto, F., Pileri, A., and Pegoraro, L. Proliferation kinetics of acute leukemia cells in relation to the chemotherapy, *Acta Genet. Med. Gemellol. (Roma)* 17:30, 1968.
78. Gee, T. S., Yu, K-P., Augustin, B. T., Krakoff, I. H., and Clarkson, B. D. Combination therapy of adult acute leukemia with thioguanine (TG) and 1-B-D-arabinofuranosylcytosine (CA), *Proc. Am. Assoc. Cancer Res.* 9:23, 1968.
79. Gee, T. S., Yu, K-P., and Clarkson, B. D. Treatment of adult acute leukemia with arabinosylcytosine and thioguanine, *Cancer* 23:1019, 1969.
80. Gerber, P. Activation of Epstein-Barr virus by 5-bromodeoxyuridine in "virus-free" human cells, *Proc. Natl. Acad. Sci. U.S.A.* 69:83, 1972.
81. Gerber, P., et al. Infectious mononucleosis: complement-fixing antibodies to herpes-like virus associated with Burkitt lymphoma, *Science* 161:173, 1968.
82. Gerber, P., and Hoyer, B. H. Induction of cellular DNA synthesis in human leucocytes by Epstein-Barr virus, *Nature* 231:46, 1971.
83. Gilliam, A. G., and Walter, W. A. Trends of mortality from leukemia in the United States 1921-1955, *Public Health Rept.* 73:773, 1958.
84. Gillis, E. M., and Baikie, A. G. Method for the demonstration of nucleoli in lymphocytes and other blood and bone marrow cells, *J. Clin. Pathol.* 17:573, 1964.
85. Gmyrek, D., Witkowski, R., Syllm-Rapoport, I., and Jacobasch, G. Chromosomal aberrations and abnormalities of red-cell metabolism in a case of Fanconi's anaemia before and after development of leukaemia, *Ger. Med. Mon.* 13:105, 1968.
86. Goldberg, A. F. Acid phosphatase activity in Auer bodies, *Blood* 24:305, 1964.

87. Golde, D. W., and Cline, M. J. Growth of human bone marrow in liquid culture, *Blood* 41:45, 1973.
88. Golde, D. W., and Cline, M. J. Human preleukemia: identification of a maturation defect in vitro, *N. Engl. J. Med.* 288:1083, 1973.
89. Goodman, N. C., and Spiegelman, S. Distinguishing reverse transcriptase of an RNA tumor virus from other known DNA polymerases, *Proc. Natl. Acad. Sci. U.S.A.* 68:2203, 1971.
90. Gottfried, E. L. Lipid patterns of leukocytes in health and disease, *Semin. Hematol.* 9:241, 1972.
91. Graham, S., Levin, M. L., Lilienfeld, A. M., Schuman, L. M., Gibson, R., Dowd, J. E., and Hempelmann, L. Preconception, intrauterine, and postnatal irradiation as related to leukemia, *Natl. Cancer Inst. Monogr.* 19:347, 1966.
92. Gralnick, H. R., and Abrell, E. Studies of the procoagulant and fibrinolytic activity of promyelocytes in acute promyelocytic leukaemia, *Br. J. Haematol.* 24:89, 1973.
93. Gralnick, H. R., Marchesi, S., and Givelber, H. Intravascular coagulation in acute leukemia: clinical and subclinical abnormalities, *Blood* 40:709, 1972.
94. Greenberg, M. L., Chanana, A. D., Cronkite, E. P., et al. The generation time of human leukemic myeloblasts, *Lab. Invest.* 26:245, 1972.
95. Gross, L. Oncogenic Viruses, 2nd ed., Pergamon Press, New York, 1970.
96. Gunz, F. W., Fitzgerald, P. H., Crossen, P. E., MacKenzie, I. S., Powles, C. P., and Jensen, G. R. Multiple cases of leukemia in a sibship, *Blood* 27:482, 1966.
97. Han, T., Stutzman, L., Cohen, E., and Kim, U. Effect of platelet transfusion on hemorrhage in patients with acute leukemia. An autopsy study, *Cancer* 19:1937, 1966.
98. Harley, R. D., Baird, H. W., and Craven, E. M. Ataxia-telangiectasia. Report of seven cases, *Arch. Ophthalmol.* 77:582, 1967.
99. Harrod, E. K., and Cortner, J. A. Prolonged survival of lymphocytes with chromosomal defects in children treated with 1, 3-bis (2-

chloroethyl)-1-nitrosourea, *J. Natl. Cancer Inst.* 40:269, 1968.
100. Hart, J. S., Trujillo, J. M., Freireich, E. J., George, S. L., and Frei, E. III. Cytogenetic studies and their clinical correlates in adults with acute leukemia, *Ann. Intern. Med.* 75:353, 1971.
101. Hayhoe, F. G. J. Cytochemical aspects of leukemia and lymphoma, *Semin. Hematol.* 6:261, 1969.
102. Hayhoe, F. G. J., Quaglino, D., and Doll, R. The Cytology and Cytochemistry of Acute Leukaemias, M. R. C. spec. rep. ser. 304, H. M. S. O., London, 1964.
103. Hecht, F., Koler, R. D., Rigas, D. A., Dahnke, G. S., Case, M. P., Tisdale, V., and Miller, R. W. Leukaemia and lymphocytes in ataxia-telangiectasia, *Lancet* ii:1193, 1966.
104. Hehlmann, R., Kufe, D., and Spiegelman, S. RNA in human leukemic cells related to the RNA of a mouse leukemia virus, *Proc. Natl. Acad. Sci. U.S.A.* 69:435, 1972.
105. Henderson, E. S. Treatment of acute leukemia, *Ann. Intern. Med.* 69:628, 1968.
106. Henderson, E. S. Treatment of acute leukemia, *Semin. Hematol.* 6:271, 1969.
107. Henderson, E. S., Serpick, A., Leventhal, B., and Henry, P. Cytosine arabinoside infusions in adult and childhood acute myelocytic leukemia, *Proc. Am. Assoc. Cancer Res.* 9:29, 1968.
108. Henle, G., Henle, W., and Diehl, V. Relation of Burkitt's tumor-associated herpes-type virus to infectious mononucleosis, *Proc. Natl. Acad. Sci. U.S.A.* 59:94, 1968.
109. Hersh, E. M., Bodey, G. P., Nies, B. A., et al. Causes of death in acute leukemia. A ten-year study of 414 patients from 1954–1963. *J.A.M.A.* 193:105, 1965.
110. Higurashi, M., and Conen, P. E. In vitro chromosomal radiosensitivity in Fanconi's anemia, *Blood* 38:336, 1971.
111. Holden, D., and Lichtman, H. Paroxysmal nocturnal hemoglobinuria with acute leukemia, *Blood* 33:283, 1969.
112. Holland, J. F. Progress in the treatment of acute leukemia, in Perspectives in Leukemia, p. 217, Grune & Stratton, New York, 1968.

113. Hoshino, T., Kato, H., Finch, S. C., and Hrubec, Z. Leukemia in offspring of atomic bomb survivors, *Blood* 30:719, 1967.

114. Hutchison, G. B. Leukemia in patients with cancer of the cervix uteri treated with radiation. A report covering the first 5 years of an international study, *J. Natl. Cancer Inst.* 40:951, 1968.

115. Jaffe, N., and Kim, B. S. Priapism in acute granulocytic leukemia, *Am. J. Dis. Child.* 118:619, 1969.

116. Jaffe, N., Paed, D., Kim, B. S., and Vawter, G. F. Hypocalcemia—a complication of childhood leukemia, *Cancer* 29:392, 1972.

117. Jensen, M. K., and Roll, K. Phenylbutazone and leukaemia, *Acta Med. Scand.* 178:505, 1965.

118. Juberg, R. C., and Jones, B. The Christchurch chromosome (Gp⁻), *N. Engl. J. Med.* 282:292, 1970.

119. Keogh, E. V., and McCall, C. Mortality from leukaemia in Victoria, 1946 to 1955: a report from the central cancer registry, *Melbourne, Med. J. Aust.* 2:632, 1958.

120. Killmann, S-A. Acute leukemia: the kinetics of leukemic blast cells in man. An analytical review, *Ser. Haematol.* 1:38, 1968.

121. Kiossoglou, K. A., Mitus, W. J., and Dameshek, W. Chromosomal aberrations in acute leukemia, *Blood* 26:610, 1965.

122. Klaassen, D. J., Choi, O. S., and Barrett, K. E.: Acute leukemia long-term survival, *Cancer* 29:622, 1972.

123. Kociba, G. J., and Griesemer, R. A. Disseminated intravascular coagulation induced with leukocyte procoagulant, *Am. J. Pathol.* 69:407, 1972.

124. Kolmeier, K. H., and Bayrd, E. D. Familial leukemia: report of instance and review of the literature, *Mayo Clin. Proc.* 38:523, 1963.

125. Kulka, H. Leukämischer Priapismus der Klitoris unter dem Bilde eines Carcinoms, *Arch. Gynaekol.* 149:450, 1932.

126. Lacher, M. J., and Sussman, L. N. Leukemia and Hodgkin's disease, *Ann. Intern. Med.* 59:369, 1963.

127. Lawrinson, W., and Gross, S. Nuclear arylsulfatase activity in primitive hemic cells, *Lab. Invest.* 13:1612, 1964.

128. Laws, W. C., Bohannon, R. A., Robinson, A. J., and Aggeler, P. M. Acute promyelocytic leukemia with hypofibrinogenemia, *Calif. Med.* 109:219, 1968.

129. Leavell, B. S., and Twomey, J. Possible leukemoid reaction in disseminated tuberculosis: report of a case with Auer rods, *Trans. Am. Clin. Climatol. Assoc.* 75:166, 1963.

130. Leder, L-D. A case of acute leukemia with pseudo-Pelger cells containing Auer bodies, *Acta Haematol.* 42:58, 1969.

131. Lee, J. A. H. Acute myeloid leukaemia in adolescents, *Br. Med. J.* 1:988, 1961.

132. Leventhal, B. G., Halterman, R. H., Rosenberg, E. B., and Herberman, R. B. Immune reactivity of leukemia patients to autologous blast cells, *Cancer Res.* 32:1820, 1972.

133. Levi, J. A., Vincent, P. C., and Gunz, F. W. Combination chemotherapy of adult acute nonlymphoblastic leukemia, *Ann. Intern. Med.* 76:397, 1972.

134. Levine, P. H., and Weintraub, L. R. Pseudoleukemia during recovery from Dapsone-induced agranulocytosis, *Ann. Intern. Med.* 68:1060, 1968.

135. Lewis, J. H., Burchenal, J. H., Ellison, R. R., Ferguson, J. H., Palmer, J. H., Murphy, M. L., and Zucker, M. B. Studies of hemostatic mechanisms in leukemia and thrombocytopenia, *Am. J. Clin. Pathol.* 28:433, 1957.

136. Livingston, D. M., et al. Affinity chromatography of RNA-dependent DNA polymerase from RNA tumor viruses on a solid phase immunoadsorbent, *Proc. Natl. Acad. Sci. U.S.A.* 69:393, 1972.

137. Livingstone, R. B., and Carter, S. K. Single Agents in Cancer Chemotherapy, p. 173, IFI/Plenum, New York, 1970.

138. Locke, E. A., and Minot, G. R. Hematuria as a symptom of systemic disease, *J.A.M.A.* 83:1311, 1924.

139. Loewenstein, D., Hughes, W. L., Hofer, K. G., et al. Impenetrability of the mouse placenta to maternal leukaemia cells, *Nature* 231:389, 1971.

140. MacMahon, B. Prenatal x-ray exposure and childhood cancer, *J. Natl. Cancer Inst.* 28:1173, 1962.

141. MacMahon, B., and Levy, M. A. Prenatal origin of childhood leukemia. Evidence from twins, *N. Engl. J. Med.* 270:1082, 1964.

142. Mangalik, A., Boggs, D. R., Wintrobe, M. M., and Cartwright, G. E. The influence of chemotherapy on survival in acute leukemia. III. A comparison of patients treated during 1958-1964 with those treated in two sequentially preceding periods, *Blood* 27:490, 1966.

143. Mauer, A. M., Saunders, E. F., and Lampkin, B. C. The nature and causes of variability of proliferative activity in marrow cell population in human acute leukemia, *in* The Proliferation and Spread of Neoplastic Cells, p. 358, Williams & Wilkins Co., Baltimore, 1968.

144. Melnick, P. J. Histochemical enzymology of leukaemic cells, *in* G. D. Amromin (ed.), Pathology of Leukaemia, p. 125, Harper & Row, New York, 1968.

145. Merrit, D. H., and Harris, J. S. Mongolism and acute leukemia. A report of four cases, *Am. J. Dis. Child.* 92:41, 1956.

146. Miller, D. R., Newstead, G. J., and Young, L. W. Perinatal leukemia with a possible variant of the Ellis-van Creveld syndrome, *J. Pediatr.* 74:300, 1969.

147. Miller, R. W. Radiation, chromosomes and viruses in the etiology of leukemia. Evidence from epidemiologic research, *N. Engl. J. Med.* 271:30, 1964.

148. Miller, R. W. Relation between cancer and congenital defects in man, *N. Engl. J. Med.* 275:87, 1966.

149. Miller, R. W. Persons with exceptionally high risk of leukemia, *Cancer Res.* 27:2420, 1967.

150. Miller, R. W. Deaths from childhood cancer in sibs, *N. Engl. J. Med.* 279:122, 1968.

151. Miller, R. W., and Fraumeni, J. F., Jr. Down's syndrome and neonatal leukemia, *Lancet* ii:404, 1968.

152. Miller, R. W., and Todaro, G. J. Viral transformation of cells from persons at high risk of cancer, *Lancet* i:81, 1969.

153. Miras, C. J., Mantzos, J. D., and Levis, G. M. The isolation and partial characterization of glycolipids of normal human leucocytes, *Biochem. J.* 98:782, 1966.

154. Modan, B., and Lilienfeld, A. M. Polycythemia vera and leukemia—the role of radiation treatment. A study of 1222 patients, *Medicine (Baltimore)* 44:305, 1965.

155. Monti, A., Maloney, M. A., Weber, C. L., and Patt, H. H. Comparison of cell renewal in normal and leukemic states, *Blood* 18:793, 1961.

156. Moore, E. W., Thomas, L. B., Shaw, R. K., and Freireich, E. J. The central nervous system in acute leukemia: a post-mortem study of 17 consecutive cases with particular reference to hemorrhages, leukemic infiltrations and the syndrome of meningeal leukemia, *Arch. Intern. Med.* 105:451, 1960.

157. Moseley, J. E. Patterns of bone change in the leukemias and myelosclerosis, *J. Mt. Sinai Hosp.* 28:1, 1961.

158. Naegeli, O. Ueber rothes Knochenmark und Myeloblasten, *Dtsch. Med. Wochenschr.* 26:287, 1900.

159. Nathan, D. G., and Berlin, N. I. Studies of the rate of production and life span of erythrocytes in acute leukemia, *Blood* 14:935, 1959.

160. Necheles, T. F., Maniatis, A., and Allen, D. M. Studies on cellular proliferation in childhood acute leukemia, *Proc. Am. Assoc. Cancer Res.* 9:54, 1968.

161. Neumann, G. Die Sterblichkeit an Leukämie und Aleukämie in der Bundesrepublik Deutschland von 1948–1956, *Dtsch. Med. Wochenschr.* 84:191, 1959.

162. Nies, B. A., Malmgren, R. A., Chu, E. W., Del Vecchio, P. R., Thomas, L. B., and Freireich, E. J. Cerebrospinal fluid cytology in patients with acute leukemia, *Cancer* 18:1385, 1965.

163. Nies, B. A., Thomas, L. B., and Freireich, E. J. Meningeal leukemia: a follow-up study, *Cancer* 18:546, 1965.

164. Nowell, P. C. Marrow chromosome studies in "pre leukemia," *Cancer* 28:513, 1971.

165. Osserman, E. F., and Lawlor, D. P. Serum and urinary lysozyme (muramidase) in monocytic and myelomonocytic leukemia, *J. Exp. Med.* 124:921, 1966.

166. Pengelly, C. D. R., and Wilkinson, J. F. The frequency and mechanism of haemolysis in the leukaemias, reticuloses and myeloproliferative diseases, *Br. J. Haematol.* 8:343, 1962.

167. Perugini, S., Gobbi, F., Ascari, E., et al. Fibrinolytic purpura in acute myelogenous leukemia, *Haematol. Latina* 4:15, 1961.

168. Polliack, A., and Timberg, R. Electron microscopy of leukaemic myeloblasts with numerous lipid-containing vacuoles, *Scand. J. Haematol.* 9:437, 1972.

169. Post, J., and Hoffman, J. Cell renewal patterns, *N. Engl. J. Med.* 279:248, 1968.

170. Prigozhina, E. L., Stavrovskaya, A. A., Zakharov, A. F., Lelikova, G. P., and Streljukhina, N. V. Congenital anomalies of the karyotype in human acute leukaemia, *Vopr. Onkol.* 14:58, 1968.

171. Pruzanski, W., and Platts, M. E. Serum and urinary proteins, lysozyme (muramidase) and renal dysfunction in mono- and myelomonocytic leukemia, *J. Clin. Invest.* 49:1694, 1970.

172. Quigley, H. Peripheral leukocyte thromboplastin in promyelocytic leukemia, *Fed. Proc.* 26:648, 1967.

173. Reisman, L. E., Mitani, M., and Zuelzer, W. W. Chromosome studies in leukemia. I. Evidence for the origin of leukemic stem lines from aneuploid mutants, *N. Engl. J. Med.* 270:591, 1964.

174. Reschad, H., and Schilling-Torgau, V. Ueber eine neue Leukämie durch echte Uebergangsformen (Splenozyten-leukämie) und ihre Bedeutung für die Selbstständigkeit dieser Zellen, *Munch. Med. Wochenschr.* 60:1981, 1913.

175. Rigby, P. G., Pratt, P. T., Rosenlof, R. C., and Lemon, H. M. Genetic relationships in familial leukemia and lymphoma, *Arch. Intern. Med.* 121:67, 1968.

176. Robinson, W. A., and Pike, B. L. Leukopoietic activity in human urine. The granulocytic leukemias, *N. Engl. J. Med.* 282:1291, 1970.

177. Rosenberg, E. B. Lymphocyte cytotoxicity reactions to leukemia-associated antigens in identical twins, *Int. J. Cancer* 9:648, 1972.

178. Rosenthal, D. S., and Moloney, W. C. The treatment of acute granulocytic leukemia in adults, *N. Engl. J. Med.* 286:1176, 1972.

179. Rosner, F., Glidewell, O., Ellison, R. R., et al. Failure of hydroxyurea (NSC-32065) and prednisone (NSC-10023) in the treatment of acute myelocytic leukemia, *Cancer Chemother. Rep.* 55:199, 1971.

180. Rowley, J. D., Blaisdell, R. K., and Jacobson, L. O. Chromosome studies in preleukemia. I. Aneuploidy of group C chromosomes in three patients, *Blood* 27:782, 1966.

181. Rozenszajn, L., Leibovich, M., Shoham, D., and Epstein, J. The esterase activity in megaloblasts, leukaemic and normal haemopoietic cells, *Br. J. Haematol.* 14:605, 1968.

182. Rucknagel, D. L. Epidemiologic and genetic features of leukaemia in the United States, *N. Z. Med. J.* 65:869, 1966 (suppl.).

183. Saarni, M. I., and Linman, J. W. Preleukemia. The hematologic syndrome preceding acute leukemia, *Am. J. Med.* 55:38, 1973.

184. Saenger, E. L., Thoma, G. E., and Tompkins, E. A. Incidence of leukemia following treatment of hyperthyroidism. Preliminary report of the cooperative thyrotoxicosis therapy follow-up study, *J.A.M.A.* 205:855, 1968.

185. Sakurai, M., and Sandberg, A. A. Prognosis of acute myeloblastic leukemia: chromosomal correlation, *Blood* 41:93, 1973.

186. Salsbury, A. J. Nucleolar staining in the differentiation of acute leukaemias, *Br. J. Haematol.* 13:768, 1967.

187. Sandberg, A. A. The chromosomes and causation of human cancer and leukemia, *Cancer Res.* 26:2064, 1966.

188. Sandberg, A. A., Bross, I. D. J., Takagi, N., and Schmidt, M. L. Chromosomes and causation of human cancer and leukemia. IV. Vectorial analysis, *Cancer* 21:77, 1968.

189. Sandberg, A. A., and Hossfeld, D. K. Chromosomal abnormalities in human neoplasia, *Ann. Rev. Med.* 21:379, 1970.

190. Sandberg, A. A., Takagi, N., Sofuni, T., and Crosswhite, L. H. Chromosomes and causation of human cancer and leukemia. V. Karyotypic aspects of acute leukemia, *Cancer* 22:1268, 1968.

191. Saunders, E. F., Lampkin, B. C., and Mauer, A. M. Variation of proliferative activity in leukemic cell populations of patients with acute leukemia, *J. Clin. Invest.* 46:1356, 1967.

192. Sawitsky, A., Bloom, D., and German, J. Chromosomal breakage and acute leukemia in congenital telangietatic erythema and stunted growth, *Ann. Intern. Med.* 65:487, 1966.

193. Schade, H., Schoeller, L., and Schultze, K. W. D-Trisomie (Pätau-Syndrom) mit kongenitaler myeloischer Leukämie, *Med. Welt* 50:2690, 1962.

194. Schull, W. J., and Neel, J. V. Maternal radiation and mongolism, *Lancet* i:537, 1962.

195. Schull, W. J., and Neel, J. V. *In* The Effects of Inbreeding in Japanese Children, Harper & Row, New York, 1965.

196. Schumacher, H. R., McFeely, A. E., Davis, K. D., and Maugel, T. K. The acute leukemic cell. IV. DNA synthesis in peripheral blood and bone marrow, *Am. J. Clin. Pathol.* 56:508, 1971.

197. Schwab, R. S., and Weiss, S. Neurologic aspect of leukemia, *Am. J. Med. Sci.* 189:766, 1935.

198. Scolnick, E. M., Parks, W. P., Todaro, G. J., et al. Immunological characterization of primate C-type virus reverse transcriptases, *Nature (New Biol.)* 235:35, 1972.

199. Shapiro, J. H., Ramsay, C. G., Jacobson, H. G., Botstein, C. C., and Allen, L. B. Renal involvement in lymphomas and leukemias in adults, *Am. J. Roentgenol.* 88:928, 1962.

200. Shively, J. A., et al. Transfusion of platelet concentrates prepared from acidified platelet-rich plasma, *Transfusion* 6:302, 1966.

201. Sigler, A. T., Lilienfeld, A. M., Cohen, B. H., and Westlake, J. E. Radiation exposure in parents of children with mongolism (Down's syndrome), *Bull. Johns Hopkins Hosp.* 117:374, 1965.

202. Skarin, A. T., Matsuo, Y., and Moloney, W. C. Muramidase in myeloproliferative disorders terminating in acute leukemia, *Cancer* 29:1336, 1972.

203. Skeel, R. T., Yankee, R. A., and Hendersen, E. S. Meningeal leukemia, *J.A.M.A.* 205:863, 1968.

204. Skipper, H. E. Kinetic considerations associated with therapy of solid tumors, *in* The Proliferation and Spread of Neoplastic Cells, p. 213, Williams & Wilkins Co., Baltimore, 1968.

205. Southam, C. M., Craver, L. F., Dargeon, H. W., and Burchenal, J. H. A study of the natural history of acute leukemia with special reference to the duration of the disease and the occurrence of remissions, *Cancer* 4:39, 1951.

206. Stewart, A., Webb, J., and Hewitt, D. A survey of childhood malignancies, *Br. Med. J.* 1:1495, 1958.

207. Stransky, E. Perinatal leukaemia. A review, *Acta Paediatr. Acad. Sci. Hung.* 8:121, 1967.

208. Tan, H. K. Ultrastructural studies in acute promyelocytic leukemia, *Blood* 39:628, 1972.

209. Third National Cancer Survey, 1969 Incidence, Preliminary Report, DHEW Publ. (NIH) 72, 1971.

210. Tivey, H. The natural history of untreated acute leukemia, *Ann. N.Y. Acad. Sci.* 60:322, 1954.

211. Tjio, J. H., Carbone, P. P., Whang, J., et al. The Philadelphia chromosome and chronic myelogenous leukemia, *J. Natl. Cancer Inst.* 36:567, 1966.

212. Tough, I. M., Court Brown, W. M., Baikie, A. G., Buckton K. E., Harnden, D. G., Jacobs, P. A., and Williams, J. A. Chronic myeloid leukaemia: cytogenetic studies before and after splenic irradiation, *Lancet* ii:115, 1962.

213. Trujillo, J. M., et al. Cytogenetic contributions to the study of human leukemias, *in* Leukemia-Lymphoma, p. 105, Yearbook Publishers, Chicago, 1970.

214. Tudhope, G. R. The survival of red cells and the causation of anaemia in leukaemia, *Scott. Med. J.* 4:342, 1959.

215. Uchida, I. A., Holunga, R., and Lawler, C. Maternal radiation and chromosomal aberrations, *Lancet* ii:1045, 1968.

216. Veale, A. M. O. Polygenic inheritance, *N. Z. Med. J.* 67:344, 1968.

217. Verma, I. M., Meuth, N. L., Bromfeld, E., et al. Covalently linked RNA-DNA molecule as initial product of RNA tumour virus DNA polymerase, *Nature (New Biol.)* 233:131, 1971.

218. Vigliani, E. C., and Saita, G. Benzene and leukemia, *N. Engl. J. Med.* 271:872, 1964.

219. Vogler, W. R. 1, 3-bis (2-chloroethyl)-1-nitrosourea (BCNU) and cytosine arabinoside (CA) combination in acute leukemia, *Proc. Am. Assoc. Cancer Res.* 9:74, 1968.

220. Voigt, K-G., and Helbig, W. Pathologie der Nieren bei Leukämien, *Folia Haematol.* 81:121, 1964.

221. Wainer, R. A., Wiernik, P. H., and Thompson, W. L. Metabolic and therapeutic studies of a patient with acute leukemia and severe lactic acidosis of prolonged duration, *Am. J. Med.* 55:255, 1973.

222. Wald, N., Borges, W. H., Li, C. C., Turner, J. H., and Harnois, M. C. Leukaemia associated with mongolism, *Lancet* i:1228, 1961.

223. Walters, T. R., Aur, R. J. A., Hernandez, K., Vietti, T., and Pinkel, D. 6-azauridine in combination chemotherapy of childhood acute myelocytic leukemia, *Cancer* 29:1057, 1972.

224. Warren, S., and Gates, O. The induction of leukemia and life shortening in mice by continuous low-level external gamma radiation, *Radiation Res.* 47:480, 1971.

225. Wetherley-Mein, G., and Cottom, D. G. Fresh blood transfusion in leukaemia, *Br. J. Haematol.* 2:25, 1956.

226. Wetherley-Mein, G., Epstein, I. S., Foster, W. D., and Grimes, A. J. Mechanisms of anaemia in leukaemia, *Br. J. Haematol.* 4:281, 1958.

227. Whang-Peng, J., Henderson, E. S., Knutsen, T., Freireich, E. J., and Gart, J. J. Cytogenetic studies in acute myelocytic leukemia with special emphasis on the occurrence of Ph¹ chromosome, *Blood* 36:448, 1970.

228. Wheelock, E. F., and Dingle, J. H. Observations on the repeated administration of viruses to a patient with acute leukemia. A preliminary report, *N. Engl. J. Med.* 271:645, 1964.

229. Whitecar, J. P., Jr., Bodey, G. P., Freireich, E. J., et al. Cyclophosphamide, vincristine, cytosine

arabinoside and prednisone (COAP) combination chemotherapy for acute leukemia in adults, *Cancer Chemother. Rep.* 56:543, 1972.

230. Wiernik, P. H., and Serpick, A. A. Clinical significance of serum and urinary muramidase activity in leukemia and other hematologic malignancies, *Am. J. Med.* 46:330, 1969.

231. Wiernik, P. H., and Serpick, A. A. A randomized clinical trial of daunorubicin and a combination of prednisone, vincristine, 6-mercaptopurine and methotrexate in adult acute nonlymphocytic leukemia, *Cancer Res.* 32:2023, 1972.

232. Wilhyde, D. E., Jane, J. A., and Mullan, S. Spinal epidural leukemia, *Am. J. Med.* 34:281, 1963.

233. Windholz, F., and Foster, S. E. Bone sclerosis in leukemia and in non-leukemic myelosis, *Am. J. Roentgenol.* 61:61, 1949.

234. Wintrobe, M. M. Clinical Hematology, 6th ed., p. 985, Lea & Febiger, Philadelphia, 1967.

235. Wintrobe, M. M. Clinical Hematology, 6th ed., p. 1017, Lea & Febiger, Philadelphia, 1967.

236. Wintrobe, M. M., and Mitchell, D. M. Atypical manifestations of leukaemia, *Q. J. Med.* 9:67, 1940.

237. Wood, E. E. A survey of leukaemia in Cornwall, 1948–1959, *Br. Med. J.* 1:1760, 1960.

238. Working Party on the Evaluation of Different Methods of Therapy in Leukemia. Treatment of acute leukemia in adults: comparison of steroid therapy at high and low dosage in conjunction with 6-mercaptopurine, *Br. Med. J.* 1:7, 1963.

239. Zaizov, R., and Matoth, Y. The pathogenesis of anemia in acute leukemia, *Isr. J. Med. Sci.* 7:1025, 1971.

240. Zuelzer, W. W. Implications of long-term survival in acute stem cell leukemia of childhood treated with composite cyclic therapy, *Blood* 24:477, 1964.

241. Zuelzer, W. W., and Cox, D. E. Genetic aspects of leukemia, *Semin. Hematol.* 6:228, 1969.

242. Zuelzer, W. W., Thompson, R. I., and Mastrangelo, R. Evidence for a genetic factor related to leukemogenesis and congenital anomalies: chromosomal aberrations in pedigree of an infant with partial D trisomy and leukemia, *J. Pediatr.* 72:367, 1968.

PART II Lymphocytes and Plasma Cells

A The Normal Lymphocyte and Plasma Cell

Chapter 12 Morphogenesis of the Lymphoid System

Much of hematology has been based on the concept that cells may be recognized and classified by morphologic criteria. An extension of this basic concept is that in considering the relationship between cells of a series, transitional forms are characterized by morphologic features that are intermediate between those of cells at either end of the series. In the past few years this concept has been contested, particularly in relation to recognizing and classifying cells of the lymphoid series. It is now apparent that morphologically similar cells may have different functions, life cycles, and metabolism. Furthermore, the concept that morphologically intermediate cells are transitional in maturation and function may be invalid for cells of the lymphocytic series.

Evidence accrued in recent investigations demonstrates clearly that the cells morphologically identified as small lymphocytes constitute several populations that are heterogeneous in function and life cycle. The same may be true for cells designated as large lymphocytes, and for a variety of intermediate forms.

This chapter will be concerned with the morphologic features of lymphocytes as they have been traditionally identified by hematologists and, more recently, by immunologists. In addition, the morphogenesis of the lymphoid system as a whole and the interrelationships of its parts will be described. Chapters 13 to 15 will attempt to identify the functionally heterogeneous subpopulations of morphologically homogeneous lymphocytes. The interrelationships among the cells of the lymphoid cell series are extremely complex and even today there are large gaps in our knowledge. Any organizational framework for these cells must still be considered provisional.

A simplified scheme of the relation of cells of the lymphoid series to other hematopoietic cells is given in Fig. 12.1. The lymphoid cell line traces its origin to *pluripotent stem cells.* These are hematopoietic cells that are self-replicating and capable of giving rise to *unipotent committed stem cells* (180). The latter are destined for development along one or another hematopoietic pathways: erythroid, granulocytic, megakaryocytic, or lymphoid. The commitment to one of these pathways is probably determined by the microenvironment of the organ in which the stem cell develops (cf. 112). For example, stem cells developing in the bone marrow may give rise to granulocytic or erythroid progeny, whereas others developing in thymus or lymphoid tissues may give rise to lymphoid cells. Neither the pluripotent nor the committed hematopoietic stem cell has been identified morphologically with certainty.

The small lymphocyte represents one pathway of development of committed stem cells. The small lymphocyte (Fig. 12.2) ordinarily does not replicate. It is arrested in the G_1 phase of the cell cycle or is in G_0. Under an appropriate stimulus, such as specific antigen, it transforms to a large, metabolically more active cell (Figs. 12.3 and 12.4). This activated cell has been called by a variety of names including "activated lymphocyte" and "large pyroninophil cell." The latter term derives from the staining of the abundant cytoplasmic RNA by methyl green pyronine. The activated lymphocyte is a dividing cell. Under some

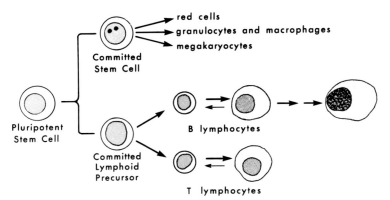

Figure 12.1 Relation of lymphoid cells to other hematopoietic cell lines. Lymphoid cell, red cell, granulocyte, macrophage, and megakaryocyte precursors arise from a common pluripotent stem cell. Once commitment to a lymphoid precursor is made, local microenvironment factors—and perhaps humoral factors—influence the development along a B-lymphocyte or a T-lymphocyte pathway. B lymphocytes are the precursors of immunoglobulin-producing plasma cells. Small T lymphocytes may undergo reversible transformation to larger, more active lymphoid cells.

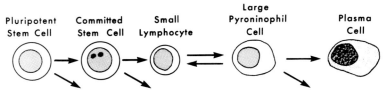

Figure 12.3 Schematic representation of the B-lymphocyte pathway of development. A committed lymphoid stem cell arises from a pluripotent stem cell capable of giving rise to multiple hematopoietic cell lines. The committed stem cell is capable of cell replication, as well as differentiation to a small lymphocyte. Under appropriate activating circumstances, the small lymphocyte may undergo reversible transformation to a large, pyroninophilic cell. The pyroninophil may divide and ultimately give rise to mature plasma cells.

circumstances (see Fig. 12.5) it can give rise to a plasma cell (19). The mature plasma cell is an end cell committed to immunoglobulin synthesis and no longer capable of replication.

In an alternative pathway of development, some small lymphocytes (T cells in Fig. 12.1) give rise to activated lymphocytes that are incapable of differentiating to plasma cells. The potential pathway of differentiation of the small lymphocyte again appears to be influenced by the organ microenvironment in which it develops (112). The bone marrow, the thymus gland, and in birds the bursa of Fabricius, contain microenvironments critical in influencing lymphoid cell differentiation.

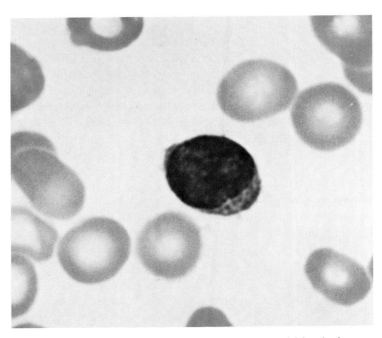

Figure 12.2 A small lymphocyte in the peripheral blood of a normal subject; Wright stain.

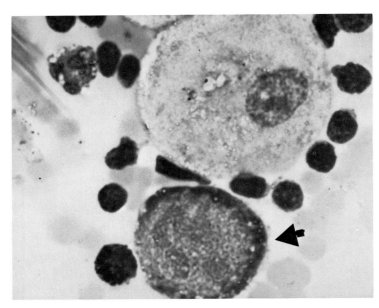

Figure 12.4 A lymphocyte activated by antigen (*arrow*). Other unstimulated small lymphocytes are seen surrounding a large, pale macrophage. Giemsa stain.

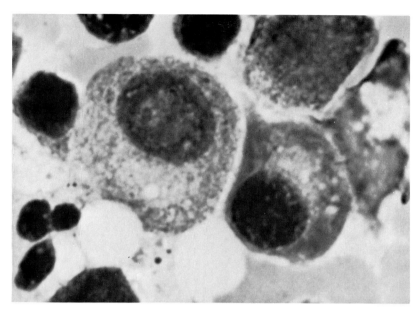

Figure 12.5 Two plasma cells in the bone marrow of a normal subject. Note the eccentric nuclei and the perinuclear clear zone, which represents the Golgi apparatus.

The relation between the development of lymphocytes and other hematopoietic cells in embryonic development is illustrated in Fig. 12.6. Ultimately the origin of the lymphocytes, like that of the other blood cells, can be traced back to the embryonic yolk sac (28, 112, 166).

Cellular Elements of the Lymphoid System

Lymphocytes are the central cells in immunity. They range in size from approximately 5 to greater than 15 μ. It

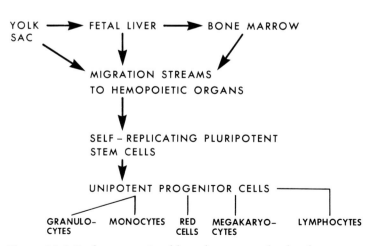

Figure 12.6 Embryogenesis of lymphocytes and other hematopoietic cell lines. The ultimate source of all hematopoietic cells is the fetal yolk sac.

is a common, if somewhat arbitrary, practice to group them as small (5 to 8 μ), medium (8 to 12 μ), and large (12 to 15 μ).

Small Lymphocytes

The population of small lymphocytes comprises a number of subpopulations of differing potential and functional capabilities. Viewed by light microscopy, the Romanovsky-stained small lymphocyte of the blood (see Fig. 12.2) has a deeply stained round or oval nucleus consisting of densely aggregated chromatin (heterochromatin). The nuclear membrane is distinct, and occasionally one or two nucleolar remnants may be seen. The nucleus is eccentrically located in blue cytoplasm, which is scanty compared to the nucleus; often only a thin rim is seen. It is usually clear, but may contain a few small reddish granules.

Electron micrographic studies of small lymphocytes (81, 183) (Fig. 12.7) reveal that the cytoplasm contains small or moderate numbers of mitochondria, and occasional vesicles. No well-defined endoplasmic reticulum or Golgi bodies are apparent, and only isolated ribosomes are seen (16). The nucleus often has a slight invagination, with a small nucleolus usually present. When stained with Janus green, the mitochondria appear as short thick rods that often lie either opposite or over the nuclear indentation, or else encircle the nucleus. Certain ultrastructural features may distinguish thymus-derived and thymus-independent lymphoid cells (108).

Preparations of living lymphocytes reveal that the cells are motile, but move more slowly than granulocytes. They usually have a single cytoplasmic protrusion. This structure produces a "hand-mirror" appearance with the nucleus at the larger end (Fig. 12.8); the direction of movement is away from the handle (101-103). No specific tropism in lymphocyte movement has been established (70), except for a tendency to move toward any mitosing cell that is entering telophase (80). Locomotion is amoeboid in character (95, 152). Cinephotomicrographic studies of lymphocytes indicate that the cytoplasmic tail is used to contact debris, other cells, or other surfaces in the lymphocyte environment. The tail process is called a uropod; from it extend threadlike projections called microspikes (Figs. 12.8 and 12.9). The uropod also contains microtubules, mitochondria, rough endoplasmic reticulum, and pinocytic vacuoles. It is through the uropod and its microspikes that the lymphocyte explores its environment. This tail region may be most active in pinocytosis, resembling the tail region of amoebae in this respect (179).

The surface of the lymphocyte viewed by the scanning electron microscope is covered with microvilli. The char-

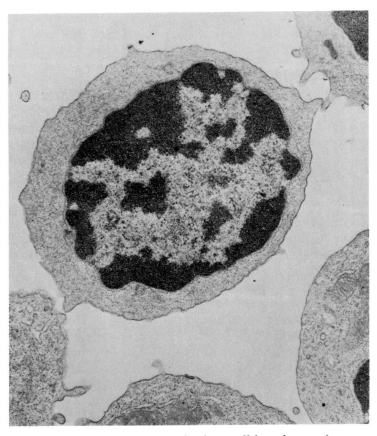

Figure 12.7 Electron micrograph of a small lymphocyte from mouse spleen. Magnification × 12,000. (From L-T. Chin, A. Eden, V. Nussenzweig, and L. Weiss, *Cell. Immunol.* 4:279, 1972. Reprinted by permission of authors and publisher.)

acter and distribution of these microvilli are said to be different in the functionally distinct subpopulations of lymphocytes (B cells and T cells) (96).

Medium and Large Lymphocytes

Lymphocytes in this category vary in size between 8 and 15 μ in Wright-stained smears of peripheral blood. The nuclear pattern resembles that of the typical small lymphocyte, but the chromatin pattern tends to be less dense and the small nuceoli may be more prominent (Fig. 12.10). The cytoplasm is more abundant than that of the small lymphocyte and may contain a few reddish granules. In preparations of living cells viewed by phase microscopy, the nucleus is round, oval, or reniform.

Lymphoblasts

Lymphoblasts are almost never observed in the peripheral blood of normal individuals, and only rarely in the bone marrow. However, preparations from lymph nodes and spleen often contain primitive lymphoid cells resembling

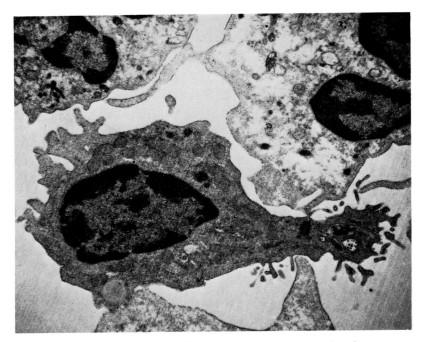

Figure 12.8 The motile lymphocyte in vitro has the characteristic hand-mirror appearance. The narrow region remote from the nucleus of the cell is known as the uropod and contains numerous microspikes. (From W. McFarland, *Science* 163:818, 1969. Reprinted by permission of author and publisher.)

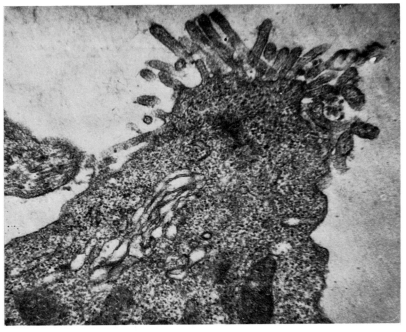

Figure 12.9 High-power magnification of the uropod region of a motile lymphocyte, showing luxuriant microspikes. (From W. McFarland, *Science* 163:818, 1969. Reprinted by permission of author and publisher.)

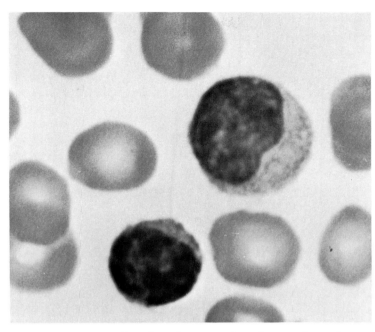

Figure 12.10 A small and medium-size lymphocyte from the peripheral blood of a normal subject; Wright stain.

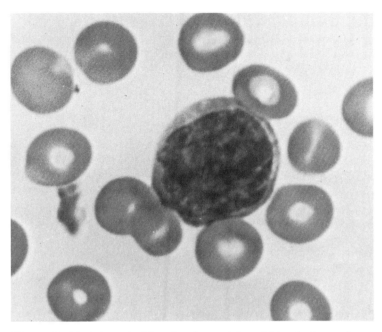

Figure 12.11 A lymphoblast in the peripheral blood of a patient with acute lymphocytic leukemia; Wright stain.

those seen in the circulation of patients with acute lymphoblastic leukemia (Fig. 12.11). The lymphoblast is 12 to 20 μ in diameter and is characterized by the following: (a) a large nucleus with a finer chromatin structure than that of the mature cell, (b) a well-defined nuclear membrane, and (c) one or two prominent nucleoli. The clear blue cytoplasm rarely contains inclusions. However, short, thick, rodlike mitochondria are prominent in supravitally stained preparations. Living cells are motile and may demonstrate the hand-mirror appearance characteristic of the mature cell. The fine structure seen in the electron microscope has few distinctive features (Fig. 12.12).

Plasma Cells

The mature plasma cell (see Fig. 12.5), seen in Wright-stained preparations, is a medium to large spherical or oval cell (8 to 20 μ in diameter) with a relatively small, round or oval eccentric nucleus. The nuclear chromatin is condensed in large masses, often arranged in a wheel-spoke fashion. The cytoplasm is characteristically sky blue and often has a perinuclear clear zone. The cytoplasm frequently contains inclusions and sometimes is vacuolated. When acidophilic hyaline inclusions are numerous, the cells are sometimes referred to as *Russell body cells* (Fig. 12.13).

In supravitally stained preparations the nucleus is eccentrically located and mitochondria are numerous. When viewed by electron microscopy, a striking feature of the

cytoplasm of mature plasma cells is the great development in lamellar form of the rough endoplasmic reticulum. The Golgi apparatus also is highly developed and is responsible for the cytoplasmic perinuclear clear area. Moderate numbers of mitochondria are seen in the cytoplasm. The nucleus shows a well-delineated nucleolus. These features are seen in Figs. 12.14 to 12.16. The life cycle of plasma cells from young to mature forms is shown schematically in Fig. 12.17.

Intermediate and Transitional Forms

It is presently thought (22) that both plasma cells and small lymphocytes are derived from large, pyroninophilic cells called blast cells (see Figs. 12.1, 12.3, and 12.4). Whether a single blast cell has the potential of developing into either a lymphocyte or a plasma cell or is restricted in its potential differentiation to a single cell type has not been determined. The steps from the large pyroninophilic cell to the small lymphocyte are not unidirectional. The process can, under certain circumstances, go in the reverse direction and small lymphocytes can give rise to the larger pyroninophils (19, 149) (see Fig. 12.3).

For example, in 1962 J. L. Gowans (55) used the purest available preparations of lymphocytes obtained from the thoracic duct drainage of two strains of inbred rats. He labeled the cells isotopically and injected a single parental lymphocyte line into F$_1$ hybrid animals to provoke a fatal graft-versus-host reaction. Four hours after injection, col-

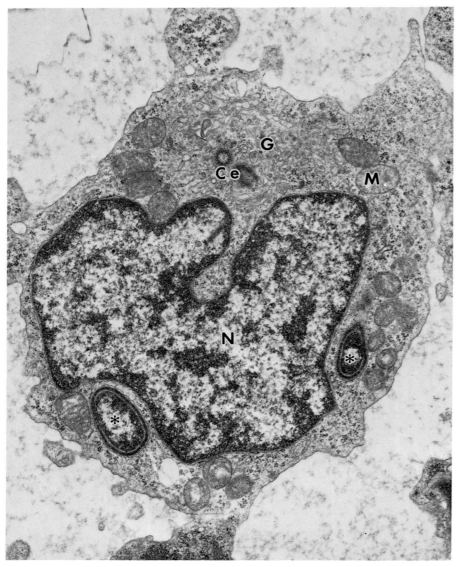

Figure 12.12 A lymphoblast from the peripheral blood of a leukemic child. Note the condensation of the chromatin of the nucleus (*N*) and two isolated nuclear blebs with lamellar chromatin (*). In the Golgi area (*G*) are two centrioles (*Ce*). The rest of the cytoplasm has scattered polyribosomes, small vesicles, and large round mitochondria (*M*). (From Y. Tanaka and J. R. Goodman, Electron Microscopy of Human Blood Cells, Harper & Row, New York, 1972. Reprinted by permission of authors and publisher.)

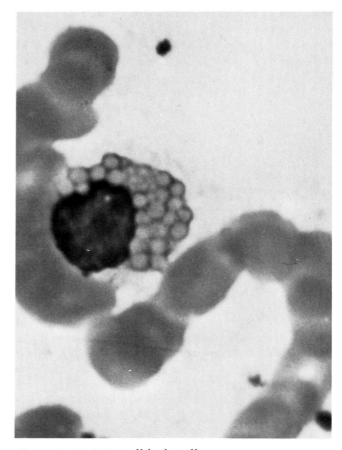

Figure 12.13 A Russell body cell.

lections of labeled small lymphocytes were seen in the primary follicles of lymph nodes and the white pulp of the spleen. By 24 hours the same areas contained heavily labeled, large, pyroninophilic cells with prominent nucleoli. Since a nuclear ^{3}H-thymidine label generally is not transferable from cell to cell, these observations suggest a conversion of small lymphocytes into intermediate and blast cells.

An in vitro model (Fig. 12.18) of the conversion of small lymphocytes to blast cells is the blastogenic stimulation of small lymphocytes induced by nonspecific mitogens such as phytohemagglutinin (31, 107, 131) and specific antigens such as tuberculin (146). Antilymphocyte serum (27, 60) and mixed leukocyte cultures, where lymphocytes from genetically unrelated individuals are co-cultivated, also convert small lymphocytes to large blast cells (13).

Electron micrographs of the large cells in the thoracic duct of man, the rabbit, and the rat show some cells with numerous vesicles, mitochondria, and a well-developed Golgi apparatus, but little endoplasmic reticulum; that is, cells that appear to be intermediate between lymphocytes and plasma cells (Fig. 12.19A). Other cells show definite development of the endoplasmic reticulum (Fig. 12.19B) and are more closely related to plasma cells (106, 183).

The same spectrum of cells progressing from those with little endoplasmic reticulum (lymphocyte-like) to those with highly developed endoplasmic reticulum and Golgi apparatus (plasma-cell–like) are observed in lymphocytes stimulated to blastogenic transformation by some mitogens. Similarly, cells circulating in the lymph fluid early in the immune response (64–67, 79, 93) and cells producing antibody at the center of hemolytic plaques (69, 73) show only minimal development of endoplasmic reticulum; in other words, they more closely resemble intermediate lymphocytes than plasma cells. However, a variety of intermediate forms differentiating toward typical mature plasma cells can be observed as well.

Cells intermediate between large lymphoid cells and smaller plasma cells have been called *transitional cells.* These cells are capable of antibody synthesis. Cells at different stages of the maturation cycle of plasma cells from transitional cells are shown in Fig. 12.17.

In addition to the relatively clear evidence for differentiation along the lymphocyte–plasma-cell axis, occasional claims have been made that lymphocytes can transform into fibroblasts and macrophages. However, these claims have not stood the test of time and more extensive investigation (58, 128).

The erythrocytes, granulocytes, and platelet precursors of patients with chronic myelocytic leukemia carry the Philadelphia chromosome; dividing lymphocytes lack this marker. This observation suggests that lymphocytes branch off from a common progenitor stem cell sooner than the cells of other blood lines (see Chapters 1, 2, and 10 and Fig. 12.1).

Simply stated, *existing evidence favors the hypothesis that some circulating lymphocytes are capable of differentiating within the hematopoietic cell series, but they are not capable of differentiating to cells outside this series.*

Development of Lymphoid Tissue

Central and Peripheral Lymphoid Tissues

Available evidence indicates that two major types of peripheral lymphoid tissue may be found in higher vertebrates, each dependent upon a different primordial organ for development. One tissue consisting primarily of small lymphocytes is involved in antigen recognition and cellular immune reactions, including delayed hypersensitivity reactions (see Chapters 15–17). This peripheral lymphoid tissue is derived in part from the thymus and is also

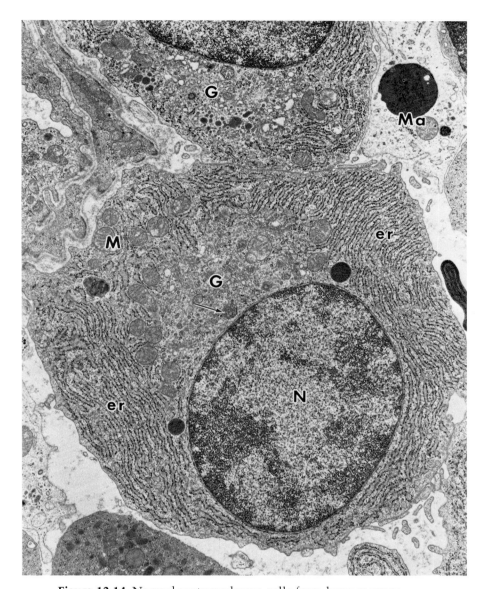

Figure 12.14 Normal mature plasma cells from bone marrow. The large cell with an eccentrically located nucleus (*N*) has extensive areas of endoplasmic reticulum (*er*), a large Golgi zone (*G*), several mitochondria (*M*), and multivesicular structure (*arrow*). Variable-sized vesicles contain material of differing density in the Golgi area, some of which may correspond to the azurophilic granules seen by light microscopy. This is evident in the top cell. The nucleus has some chromatin concentrated around its periphery, a characteristic of the maturing cell. Electron-dense particles and part of a macrophage (*Ma*) are in the right upper corner, as well as a blood vessel (*left upper corner*). (From Y. Tanaka and J. R. Goodman, Electron Microscopy of Human Blood Cells, Harper & Row, New York, 1972. Reprinted by permission of authors and publisher.)

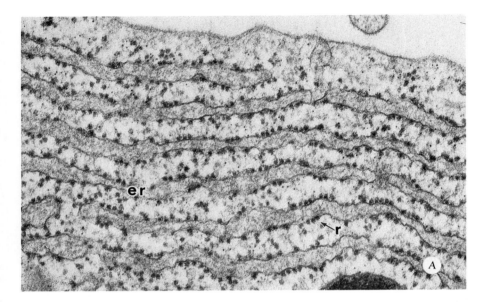

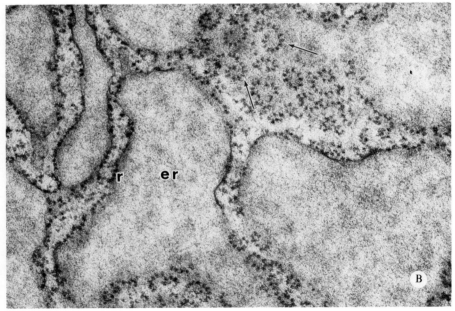

Figure 12.15 Mature plasma cells. Figure 12.15A shows lamellar arrangement of endoplasmic reticulum (*er*). The ribosomes (*r*) are only on the outside of the membrane pair, and a small amount of protein material is present in cisternae. Particles dispersed in cytoplasm are ferritin granules. Magnification × 52,000. Figure 12.15B shows distended endoplasmic reticulum (*er*) that contains amorphous material, presumably globulin produced by this structure. The orderly lamellar structure seen is disrupted as the cisternae enlarge. The plane of section cut some endoplasmic membranes perpendicular to their surface; they appear as sharp lines with dots of ribosomal (*r*) RNA on one surface, while the angle of cut in other areas is tangential. Membranes cut at an angle of less than 30° usually are not visualized by electron microscopy. These latter locations show

dependent upon the thymus for its full development. Consequently, it has been referred to as *thymus-dependent lymphoid tissue.* The lymphocytes of this system have been designated *T cells* (Fig. 12.1).

The second major type of peripheral lymphoid tissue consists mainly of plasma cells, and large pyroninophilic lymphocytes and small lymphocytes. This lymphoid tissue is the chief source of immunoglobulin and has been termed the *immunoglobulin-producing system.* The precise embryonic source of the immunoglobulin-producing system in most higher vertebrates is not definitively known. Its source is known with a reasonable degree of certainty only in the chicken, in which species the bursa of Fabricius (a hind-gut organ) contains the primordial immunoglobulin-producing cells.

The immunoglobulin-producing systems of higher mammals appear to be associated with lymphoid cells derived from the bone marrow; such bone-marrow–derived lymphocytes are designated *B lymphocytes* (Fig. 12.1).

The Thymus

The microenvironment of the thymus in some manner conditions lymphocytes along a certain pathway of potential development. The T lymphocytes play only a minor direct role in the synthesis of immunoglobulin antibody. They are critically important, however, in interacting with B lymphocytes in the immunoglobulin response to some antigens. T lymphocytes are also the principal mediators of cellular immune responses. The mechanisms by which the thymus exerts this influence are discussed in subsequent sections.

Anatomic Considerations Detailed consideration of the architecture of the thymus is beyond the scope of this book. The interested reader may wish to consult the excellent reviews available on the subject, particularly those of Metcalf (39, 110), Clark (26), and Weiss (173).

Based on electron micrographic studies, Clark interprets the thymus as an epithelial organ honeycombed by nests of proliferating lymphocytes in the cortex. The medulla is irregularly infiltrated with lymphocytes and other cells associated with the blood vascular supply. Thus the cortical area is comprised of "packets" of closely packed, multiplying lymphocytes and occasional macrophages completely enclosed in a capsule of epithelial cells (Figs. 12.20

the rosette arrangement (*arrows*) of ribosomal RNA particles on the membrane surface. (From Y. Tanaka and J. R. Goodman, Electron Microscopy of Human Blood Cells, Harper & Row, New York, 1972. Reprinted by permission of authors and publisher.)

and 12.21). The cortical area has a minimal amount of supporting collagenous and elastic tissue. Metcalf also identifies the presence of periodic-acid-Schiff–positive phagocytic cells (macrophages) in the perivascular wall. He regards the reticuloendothelial cells of the cortex and medulla as representing a single tissue and suggests that the distribution of lymphocytes is determined by hormonal and vascular factors.

With aging, the mammalian thymus steadily decreases in both relative and absolute size. This decrease involves primarily the cortex, rather than the medulla (68, 110). In man, both cortex and medulla are progressively replaced by fatty tissue.

Embryology In reptiles, thymic primordia arise from gill pouches I, II, and III, and in some, IV (46). In the majority of placental mammals, the thymus arises from the third pouch. Most of the definitive studies of thymic embryology have been made in the mouse (8–11). In this species the early morphologic evidence of embryonic thymic development is a proliferation of gut epithelial cells in the area of the third and fourth pharyngeal pouches—the same area of primitive thymic development as in the lamprey eel. It was originally proposed that in the mouse, the gut epithelial cells become lymphocytes, provided mesenchymal cells are available (8–11, 14). This conclusion is probably erroneous, and other workers have preferred the view (Figs. 12.21 and 12.22) that mesenchymal cells from outside the thymus infiltrate the primordial epithelial tissue and there proliferate into lymphocytes (61, 62, 106, 137). In the mouse, stem cells enter the thymic rudiment from the blood stream between the tenth and eleventh day of gestation (137).

It appears, therefore, that there exists a complex interaction between the thymic epithelial primordium and primitive mesenchymal cells and that the thymus is necessary for the differentiation of certain classes of lymphocytes. Once formed, the thymic lymphoid cells differentiate into smaller cells recognizable as lymphocytes (14).

A critically important observation is the following: during the embryonic period of thymic development, peripheral lymphoid tissues (such as lymph nodes and spleen) develop stroma and structural organization, but are not yet populated with lymphoid cells (3, 17, 53). *Thus, mammalian lymphocytes first make their appearance in the thymus.*

Effect of Thymectomy Several mammalian species are born with the lymphoid system at that stage of development in which the thymus is present, but the peripheral lymphoid tissues are not yet populated. Thymectomy of

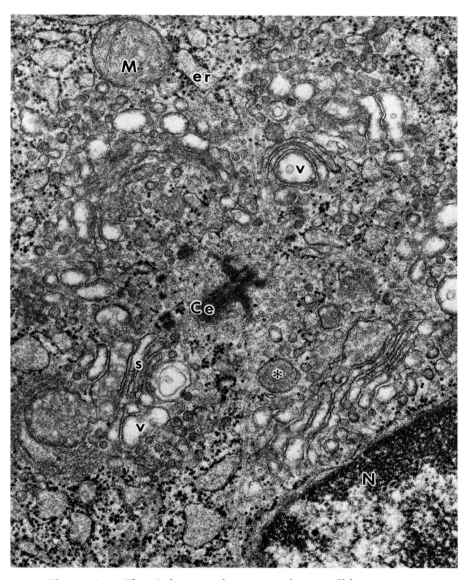

Figure 12.16 This Golgi area of a mature plasma cell has a tangentially cut centriole (*Ce*). There are many small and larger vesicles (*v*), which contain amorphous material (*asterisk*). A portion of the flattened sacs (*s*) or vesicles typical of Golgi structures are also seen. A mitochondrion (*M*) is located near outer edge of the Golgi zone. Some Golgi vesicles near rough-surfaced endoplasmic reticulum (*er*) appear to be connected to membranes with scattered ribosomal particles. A portion of the nucleus (*N*) is seen in the lower right corner. (From Y. Tanaka and J. R. Goodman, Electron Microscopy of Human Blood Cells, Harper & Row, New York, 1972. Reprinted by permission of authors and publisher.)

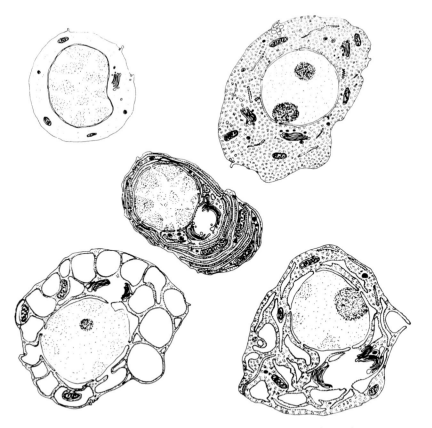

Figure 12.17 In this schematic, several stages in the life cycle of plasma cells are shown. At the upper left is a cell, lymphocytic in form, which may be a plasma cell precursor. The upper right-hand cell is a blast form. It has polyribosomes, segments of rough endoplasmic reticulum, nucleoli, nuclear pores, and other cellular elements indicative of protein synthesis. Antibody may be present in the perinuclear space and in the lumen of the rough endoplasmic reticulum. The lower cells, right and left, are clearly plasmacytic, of intermediate or transitional character. They have dilated perinuclear spaces and dilated endoplasmic reticulum that both contain antibody. Indeed, the continuity of the outer nuclear membrane and the endoplasmic reticulum is shown. The cell in the center is the classic small plasma cell, displaying polarized nucleus and cytoplasm, distribution of heterochromatin in chunks along the inner nuclear membrane, prominent cytocentrum including Golgi and centrioles, and deeply basophilic or pyroninophilic (= RNA) cytoplasm. This cell is a near-terminal form, past the peak of antibody production. The intermediate cells produce most of the antibody. (From L. Weiss, The Cells and Tissues of the Immune System. Structure, Functions, Interactions, page 158, Prentice-Hall, Inc., Englewood Cliffs, New Jersey, 1972. Reprinted by permission of author and publisher.)

the newborn of these species, including the mouse, rat, and hamster, interferes with subsequent maturation of the peripheral lymphoid tissues. Such neonatally thymectomized animals fail to develop normal homograft immunity and do not achieve normal levels of circulating antibodies to administered antigens (51, 86, 116, 156).

Some species, such as the dog, are born with well-developed peripheral lymphoid tissue, and neonatal thymectomy has relatively little effect on the immune response (88). Chickens and rabbits are intermediate with respect to the development of a thymus-dependent peripheral lymphoid tissue at birth (4, 5, 7, 59, 85, 171). In these species neonatal thymectomy has some adverse effect on the attainment of full immunologic competence, but does not comepletely abolish it. In order to define thymus-dependent peripheral tissues in the rabbit and the chicken it is necessary to irradiate the newborns to destroy the peripheral tissues already developed at the time of birth (33).

In neonatally thymectomized, irradiated rabbits, the thymus-dependent peripheral lymphoid areas fail to develop. These areas include cuffs of small lymphocytes around the germinal centers of lymph nodes (paracortical areas) and the lymphoid follicles of the spleen, as well as peripheral blood lymphocytes (148). The regions are therefore identified as *thymus dependent*. Similar treatment of newborn chicks results in lymphopenia in the circulating

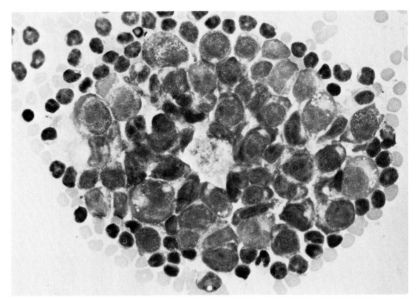

Figure 12.18 A cluster of transformed lymphocytes activated by phytohemagglutinin. Smaller untransformed lymphocytes are seen at the periphery of the cluster. Large transformed cells occupy the center surrounding a pale-staining macrophage.

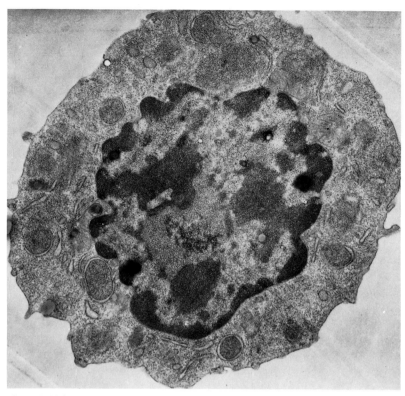

Fig. 12.19A

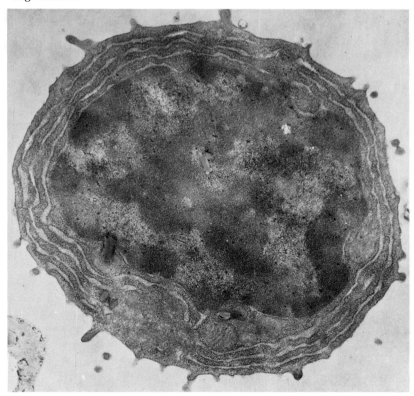

Fig. 12.19B

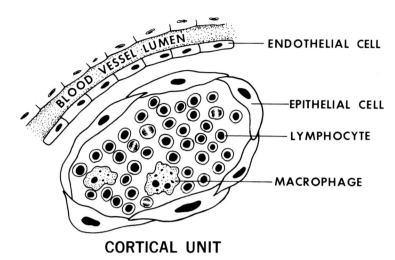

Figure 12.20 A thymic packet. The cortical unit is comprised of lymphoid cells and macrophages surrounded by epithelial cells.

blood and some depletion of the splenic white pulp (33, 84).

In animals deprived of the thymus and thymus-dependent peripheral lymphoid tissues the immunoglobulin-producing system is largely intact and serum immunoglobulin concentrations are generally normal, or elevated (12, 82). Similarly, in the human disorder known as DiGeorge's syndrome (see Chapter 18), in which the thymus is absent because of defective embryogenesis, serum immunoglobulin levels are normal (41, 78, 98, 163). Despite this apparent intactness of immunoglobulin synthesis, thymus-deprived animals and patients have moderate impairment of specific antibody synthesis. For example, they do not produce normal amounts of antibody against a variety of antigens, including tetanus toxoid, sheep erythrocytes, bacteriophage, and bovine serum al-

Figure 12.19 Two types of antibody-producing cells. The one in Fig. 12.19A is large and most commonly found in efferent lymph and thoracic duct. Note the central location of the nucleus, with irregular outline and condensed chromatin. The short and widened channels of endoplasmic reticulum are sectioned at various angles. Figure 12.19B shows a small, antibody-producing cell from the blood. The large central nucleus also shows an irregular outline and condensed chromatin. The relatively small cytoplasm contains few mitochondria and a large, well-developed Golgi body, and is organized into parallel lamellae of widened endoplasmic reticulum. Magnifications: Fig. 12.19A, × 18,000; Fig. 12.19B, × 18,300. (From K. Hummeler, T. N. Harris, N. Tomassini, M. Hechtel, and M. B. Farber, *J. Exp. Med.* 124:255, 1966. Reprinted by permission of authors and publisher.)

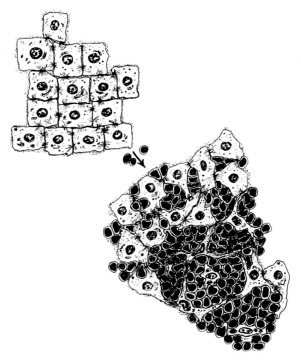

Figure 12.21 Thymic epithelium plus lymphocytes equals thymic epithelial reticular cells. (From L. Weiss, The Cells and Tissues of the Immune System. Structure, Functions, Interactions, page 82, Prentice-Hall, Inc., Englewood Cliffs, New Jersey, 1972. Reprinted by permission of author and publisher.)

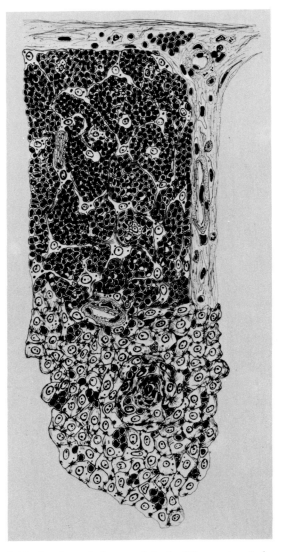

Figure 12.22 Portion of thymus lobule. The cortex is heavily infiltrated with lymphocytes. As a result, the epithelial cells become stellate and remain attached to one another by desmosomes (Fig. 12.21). The medulla is closer to a pure epithelium, although it too is commonly infiltrated by lymphocytes. A large thymic corpuscle, consisting of concentrically arranged epithelial cells, is figured. The capsule and trabecula are rich in connective tissue fibers (mainly collagen) and contain blood vessels and variable numbers of plasma cells, granulocytes, and lymphocytes. (From L. Weiss, The Cells and Tissues of the Immune System. Structure, Functions, Interactions, page 81, Prentice-Hall, Inc., Englewood Cliffs, New Jersey, 1972. Reprinted by permission of author and publisher.)

bumin (4, 74, 141, 145, 164), whereas they do produce normal or nearly normal antibody titers against hemocyanin and whole bacterial antigens (15, 145, 148). Thymus-deprived animals and patients have, in addition to a partial defect in humoral antibody production, seriously impaired cellular immune responses. This latter defect predisposes them to recurrent serious infections; patients with the DiGeorge syndrome usually die in infancy.

Studies on experimental thymic ablation and the naturally occurring thymic aplasia support the concept that the thymus is required for the full development of the immune system. *The thymus-dependent lymphoid tissue has the major role in cellular immune responses*, such as the delayed hypersensitivity reaction and graft rejection. However, *the thymus-dependent system clearly must interact with the immunoglobulin-producing system for the production of specific antibody*. Possible mechanisms of this interaction are explored further in Chapter 15.

The major clinical and laboratory aspects of neonatal thymectomy or congenital absence of the thymus are the following:

Decreased numbers of recirculating lymphocytes

Patchy decrease in lymphocytes in paracortical areas of lymph nodes and periarteriolar sheaths of spleen

Impaired cellular immune responses, including delayed rejection of allogeneic grafts

Impaired humoral immune response to certain antigens (foreign red cells and proteins)

High mortality in the first few months (mice) or years (man) of life

Increased susceptibility to infectious agents with stunting of growth (stunting not observed in thymectomized "germ-free" animals)

Increased susceptibility to certain chemical and viral carcinogens

Certain features of the syndrome of neonatal thymectomy are probably the result of impaired immunlogic defenses, plus secondary bacterial, or possibly viral, infections. Neonatal thymectomy in germ-free mice, for instance, is not followed by lethal runt diesease. When asepsis breaks down, runt disease appears in four to eight weeks (105, 177).

Neonatally thymectomized mice may be restored to normal by grafting of a syngeneic or, under appropriate circumstances, an allogeneic thymus. Injections of approximately 10^7 syngeneic spleen or lymph node cells will also reconstitute such animals (118), as well large numbers of thymocytes (75). Bone marrow cells, even in very large numbers, usually are ineffective (36).

Cellular and Humoral Effects of the Thymus On the basis of the observations cited above, one may logically ask how the thymus influences the development of certain peripheral lymphoid tissues. At least two mechanisms exist.

First, the thymus appears to influence the development of certain lymphoid tissues by the elaboration of a humoral substance (37, 94, 117, 136).

Second, thymic lymphocytes leave the thymus to populate the thymus-dependent areas of peripheral lymph nodes and the spleen (9, 21, 71, 154).

Humoral mechanism. The hypothesis that the thymus produces a humoral substance necessary for proper development of the lymphoid system evolved from Metcalf's observations (109) that extract of mouse and human thymus, as well as plasma from patients with chronic lymphocytic leukemia and plasma from preleukemic mice, produced a temporary lymphocytosis when injected into baby mice. More evidence pointing to the existence of a thymic humoral factor was provided primarily by experiments in which thymic tissue encased in cell-im-

permeable Millipore chambers permitted development of peripheral lymphoid tissue in neonatally thymectomized rodents (94, 136). It has been shown that administration of bone marrow together with Millipore-enclosed thymus tissue or with thymic extract can restore the immune system of thymectomized, lethally irradiated adult mice (120, 157). Since lymphocytes do not long sustain viability in such chambers, the putative humoral substance is probably produced by the thymic epithelial cells.

Despite evidence obtained during the past nine years, which indicates that a thymic humoral substance does exist, there has been relatively little accomplished toward purifying and characterizing the putative hormone. Recently, however, this field of investigation has been gaining in momentum (50, 91, 157, 176), and it has recently been shown that T-cell differentiation can be induced by nonthymic agents such as cyclic AMP and poly A:U (155).

Colonization. Early studies of thymic development and neonatal thymectomy by Auerbach (8, 9) and Miller (118) were interpreted as indicating that the thymus was involved in the provision of cells differentiated for immune function and that such cells colonized the peripheral lymphoid organs. Direct evidence for this colonization has been very difficult to obtain. In 1964 Nossal (129) labeled the cells of the superficial thymus of the guinea pig with tritiated thymidine and three to four days later observed heavily labeled, small lymphocytes in the spleen and lymph nodes. Other investigators obtained similar results when they compared the distribution of labeled lymphocytes after intrathymic injection of tritiated thymidine with the distribution of labeled lymphocytes after intraperitoneal injection (97). In a more direct experiment, Weissman and others used microneedles to inject tritiated thymidine into the thymus and, at the same time, administered an intravenous infusion of unlabeled thymidine (87, 174). This technique produced a highly selective labeling of thymocytes and confirmed the colonization concept.

Suspensions of radioactively labeled thymocytes, when injected intravenously into syngeneic mice, lodge in lymph nodes and the spleen in the same manner as lymphocytes from the thoracic duct or lymph nodes (43, 44, 47, 121, 130); however, labeled thymocytes more frequently "home" in thymus-dependent areas than do other labeled lymphocytes (144).

Abundant evidence shows that thymus grafts implanted seven to ten days after neonatal thymectomy or irradiation liberate the cells that colonize lymph nodes and spleen. Such cells can be recognized by markers such as distinctive chromosomal patterns (38, 119, 130). The lymphocytes of the peripheral lymphoid tissue containing the marker of the thymus donor will proliferate appropriately under the stimulus of an antigen.

The cells of the thymic cortex have a very high mitotic activity, only slightly less than the epithelial cells of the small intestine. After labeling thymocytes by either a single pulse of tritiated thymidine or repeated injections over several days, the labeled cells disappear from the gland over a period of two to three days (20, 121). Part of the disappearance of labeled cells can be attributed to the migration of cells from the glands; the rest appears to be caused by intrathymic destruction of cells (22, 110, 111, 121). Neither the precise mechanism of the rapid cell proliferation and in situ destruction nor its "purpose" is known. Burnet has suggested that the phenomenon is related to the thymus "as a source of new immune patterns" and that the intrathymic death of cells is a mechanism whereby a "massive turnover of cells in the thymus is achieved with only minor contribution of metabolites from the circulating blood" (22).

Some evidence indicates that the thymus, in addition to serving as a source of immunocytes for colonizing peripheral lymphoid tissues, may serve as a site for differentiation of immunocytes. For example, although syngeneic bone marrow cells injected into a thymectomized, lethally irradiated mouse will save the animal's life, they will not reconstitute its immunologic capacity. When the same mouse cells are injected into a similarly irradiated, but not thymectomized, animal, they will restore immunologic capacity as well (120). The thymus of the irradiated, but not thymectomized, animal before bone marrow infusion contains no thymocytes, but does show preservation of the epithelial elements of the gland. By three weeks after marrow infusion the thymus has recovered almost completely and thymocytes are present (115). It appears, therefore, that the immunologic reconstitution of an irradiated mouse by bone marrow cells is dependent upon the thymus.

Do bone marrow stem cells normally populate the thymus? Osmond and Everett (135) demonstrated that the small lymphocytes of the bone marrow were constantly being produced in, and subsequently leaving, the marrow cavity. A single injection of tritiated thymidine will label 40 percent of the bone marrow lymphocytes within 72 hours. Chromosomally labeled bone marrow cells injected intravenously in mice may first be identified in the host thymus and later in the lymph nodes and spleen (100). Perhaps the best evidence for traffic of bone marrow cells through the thymus comes from the parabiotic studies of Harris and his colleagues (72). In a pair of animals united for five weeks, the thymus glands contained 12 to 13 per-

cent of mitoses resulting from the partner's cells. The cells came through the circulation, probably from the bone marrow, since firm evidence shows that cells from the spleen, lymph nodes, and thoracic duct do not establish themselves in the thymus (56).

Burnet (22) summarized a number of observations relative to the cellular traffic through the thymus:

a) Cells of bone marrow origin readily establish themselves and multiply in the thymus; b) neither thymocytes, thoracic duct lymphocytes, nor lymph node cells can lodge and multiply in the thymus; c) thymocytes do not recirculate in the rat in the way that thoracic lymphocytes do; d) thymocytes injected in adequate doses can i) reconstitute immune capacity in a thymectomized mouse, ii) give rise to a graft-versus-host reaction, and iii) give an immunologic response against injected heterologous cells; and e) that none of these faculties is shown by normal syngeneic bone marrow.

These last characteristics of the thymocytes will be considered in the next section.

Thymoctytes: Immunologic Activity and Serologic Reactions When cell suspensions are prepared from murine thymus glands, probably well over 90 percent are cortical thymocytes, plus a scattering of small lymphocytes from the medulla, macrophages, and plasma cells. Thymus cells from an immunized rabbit do not transfer antibody-producing capacity to an irradiated recipient animal. Similar results are obtained in mice, in which species thymocytes are only 2 to 10 percent as effective as the same number of spleen cells in transferring antitoxin production (159). Similarly, peripheral lymphocytes, but not thymocytes, produce antibody when implanted with antigen in Millipore chambers (76).

In contrast to this evidence against antibody production by thymocytes, thymocytes can restore immune capacity in neonatally thymectomized mice (75, 182) and can mount a graft-versus-host reaction in certain species (29, 165).

Thymocytes possess antigens not found in other lymphoid cells, but regularly found in certain mouse leukemia cell lines (150). In 1964 Reif and Allen (151) produced cytotoxic sera by immunizing C_3H mice with AKR thymocytes and AKR mice with C_3H thymocytes. They identified two antigens. The first, designated theta-AKR, was found in thymocytes of mouse strains AKR and RF and in four of six AKR leukemia lines. The second antigen, designated theta-C_3HeB/Fe, was found in the thymocytes of all other mouse strains tested.

At about the same time Old and his colleagues (132, 133) characterized an antigen (TL) present in the thymocytes of strains A and C_{58} mice and in many leukemic lines. Normal thymocytes of AKR, C_3H and $C_{57}BL$ lacked the TL antigen, but several leukemia lines arising in these strains were TL-positive.

From these data it appears that in the mouse a small number of antigens are unique to thymocytes and thymus-derived lymphocytes and are not found in other normal lymphocytes. The same antigens may be found in certain leukemic lines. Peripheral lymphoid cells may also have the antigen, but in considerably lesser amounts than the thymocytes (151).

Interestingly, brain tissue is quite rich in thymic antigen (151). Antisera against thymocytes have been produced by immunizing rabbits against mouse or rat thymic homogenates (127, 153). Such antisera may produce lymphopenia and a decrease in the number of germinal centers in the spleen.

Recent evidence suggests that there may be multiple populations of thymus-derived lymphocytes (18, 92). For example, Cantor and Asofsky have demonstrated that in the mouse two distinct populations of T cells cooperate in graft-versus-host reaction (24, 25).

Bursa of Fabricius

Up to now we have been concerned with the contributions of the thymus gland to the full development of immune capacities. Clearly the thymus is concerned with the full expression of both humoral and cellular immune responses; however, the effects of early thymectomy or congenital absence of the thymus are seen most strikingly in deficits of cellular immune responses and of certain thymus-dependent areas of peripheral lymphoid tissues. Many attempts have been made to define and locate a primordial central lymphoid tissue responsible for full development of the peripheral immunoglobulin-producing system in higher vertebrates.

Thus far, studies using the chicken as the experimental animal have been the most rewarding. This species possesses the bursa of Fabricius, a hind-gut organ, which develops as an epithelial sac budding from the dorsal region of the cloaca. Beginning about the fourteenth day of incubation, lymphocytes appear in the wall of the bursa. They continue to develop there until about the fourth month of postnatal age, when the bursa undergoes involution (1, 2, 48, 49, 122). The bursal lymphocytes may originate from the gut epithelial cells lining the bursa, but more likely they originate from cells migrating in from the blood. In any event, a multilobular lymphoid organ develops, which reaches a maximum size of 1.5 to 2 gm and which atrophies at sexual maturity. Premature atrophy or interference with development can be achieved

with androgenic hormones such as testosterone (113, 170).

From studies of bursa-ablated animals one can define, in the chicken at least, the bursa-dependent lymphoid tissues as: (*a*) large, pyrininophilic lymphoid cells in discrete splenic lymphoid follicles, and (*b*) plasma cells scattered throughout the white pulp of the spleen (33–35, 148; see also refs. 43, 89, 90, 114, 143, 160, 178, 181).

Removal of the bursa from a newly hatched chick impedes, but does not wholly prevent, the development of the bursal-dependent peripheral lymphoid tissues (124, 142). Complete eradication of bursal-dependent tissues requires X-irradiation, in addition to bursectomy. Chickens completely deprived of bursa-dependent tissues show severe depression of 7S and 19S serum immunoglobulins and are incapable of producing antibody even in response to intense antigen stimulus (33, 172). Chickens bursectomized, but not irradiated, show partial reduction of serum immunoglobulins (99, 134, 171).

Animals which are bursectomized and irradiated still show evidence of preserved cellular immunity despite a severe restriction of immunoglobulin synthesis (33). Thus, bursectomized chickens with intact thymus glands can reject homografts and their cells can initiate graft-versus-host reactions in appropriate recipients. Hormonal bursectomy producing minimal damage to the thymus gland also inhibits antibody production, but leaves homograft rejection virtually intact (6, 125, 126, 162, 171).

These observations are consistent with the hypothesis that the bursal system is critical to the development of immunoglobulin-producing lymphoid tissues (33, 83) in a manner analogous to the thymus and the cellular immune systems. The bursa is thought to "seed" immunocompetent cells to peripheral sites, where they become antibody-producing cells (23, 123, 167); however, bursal lymphocytes may themselves form antibody to certain antigens (168).

The search for the equivalent of a bursal system in higher mammals has yielded many suggestions, including the human tonsils, the intestinal Peyer's patches, and the concentrated lymphoid tissues around the appendix (32, 147, 161). To date, however, there is no definite evidence for the existence of a precisely equivalent system in higher mammals. Studies described in detail in Chapter 15 indicate that in higher mammals the bone-marrow–derived (B) lymphocyte is primarily responsible for development of the immunoglobulin-producing system.

Phylogenetic Development of the Lymphoid System

Phylogenetic studies have been a major means of identifying the cellular components of the immune system and the interaction of these components. The hagfish is one of the most primitive of vertebrate life forms. This species was originally thought to lack all identifiable lymphoid tissue, including a thymus, and any identifiable immunologic responses (52, 138–140). More recent studies suggest that a primitive immune system is, in fact, present in the hagfish.

In the lamprey, a somewhat more highly developed vertebrate, a rudimentary lymphoid system is present. Foci of lymphoid cells in the epithelium of the pharyngeal gutter from the second to the fifth pharyngeal pouches probably represent a primitive thymus. Lymphocytes of various sizes occur in the peripheral blood, and clusters of lymphoid cells are seen in the spleen of the lamprey. Functionally, this species has some measure of gamma globulin and can form small amounts of antibody against selected antigens. The lamprey also possesses the capacity to develop delayed hypersensitivity reactions and reject skin homografts (45, 138).

Further along the phylogenetic scale is the guitar fish, a primitive elasmobranch. It has a thymus comparable in development to that of higher mammals. Sharks have a well-defined plasma-cell system (45). A well-developed immunoglobulin-producing system comparable to that of higher primates probably first appeared in the primitive polyodon fishes (45). Reptiles have a highly developed immune system (30). Several good reviews of the phylogeny of the immune response have been published in recent years (30, 40, 42, 63, 77, 158).

Summary

The cellular elements of the lymphoid system include small, medium, and large lymphocytes, lymphoblasts, plasma cells, and cells transitional between lymphocytes and plasma cells. Routine morphology and ultrastructure may be insufficient to define functionally distinct subpopulations of small and intermediate lymphocytes.

The interrelationships among these various cell types is complex. Plasma cells normally are end cells. Small lymphocytes usually are nonreplicating, but may be activated to divide by appropriate immunologic stimulus. Their subsequent differentiation to plasma cells or to other lymphoid cells is determined by the subpopulation of origin of the small lymphocyte.

Two major types of lymphoid tissues have been identified in higher vertebrates: (a) the thymus-dependent system, which has the major role in cellular immune reactions, and (b) the immunoglobulin-producing system. In chickens, the bursa of Fabricius provides the microenvironment for development of the immunoglobulin-producing system.

Chapter 12 References

1. Ackerman, G. A. Electron microscopy of the bursa of Fabricius of the embryonic chick with particular reference to the lympho-epithelial nodules, *J. Cell. Biol.* 13:127, 1962.

2. Ackerman, G. A., and Knouff, R. A. Lymphocytopoiesis in the bursa of Fabricius, *Am. J. Anat.* 104:163, 1959.

3. Archer, O. K., Kelly, W. D., Papermaster, B. W., and Good, R. A. Further morphological and immunological studies on the role of the thymus in immunobiology, *Fed. Proc.* 22:599, 1963.

4. Archer, O. K., and Pierce, J. C. Role of thymus in development of the immune response, *Fed. Proc.* 20:26, 1961.

5. Archer, O. K., Pierce, J. C., Papermaster, B. W., and Good, R. A. Reduced antibody response in thymectomized rabbits, *Nature* 195:191, 1962.

6. Aspinall, R. L., and Meyer, R. K. Effect of steroidal and surgical bursectomy and surgical thymectomy on the skin homograft reaction in chickens, *in* R. A. Good and A. E. Gabrielsen (eds.), The Thymus in Immunobiology, p. 376, Hoeber-Harper, New York, 1964.

7. Aspinall, R. L., Meyer, R. K., Graetzer, M. A., and Wolfe, H. R. Effect of thymectomy and bursectomy on the survival of skin homografts in chickens, *J. Immunol.* 90:872, 1963.

8. Auerbach, R. Morphogenetic interactions in the development of the mouse thymus gland, *Dev. Biol.* 2:271, 1960.

9. Auerbach, R. Experimental analysis of the origin of cell types in the development of the mouse thymus, *Dev. Biol.* 3:336, 1961.

10. Auerbach, R. Developmental studies of mouse thymus and spleen, *Natl. Cancer Inst. Monogr.* 11:23, 1963.

11. Auerbach, R. Experimental analysis of mouse thymus and spleen morphogenesis, *in* R. A. Good and A. E. Gabrielsen (eds.), The Thymus in Immunobiology, p. 95, Hoeber-Harper, New York, 1964.

12. Azar, H. A. Discussion following

thymectomy in rabbit and mouse: consideration of time of lymphoid peripheralization, *in* R. A. Good and A. E. Gabrielsen (eds.), The Thymus in Immunobiology, p. 414, Hoeber-Harper, New York, 1964.

13. Bach, F., and Hirschhorn, K. Lymphocyte interaction: a potential histocompatibility test in vitro, *Science* 143:813, 1964.

14. Ball, W. D. A quantitative assessment of mouse thymus differentiation, *Exp. Cell Res.* 31:82, 1963.

15. Barnett, J. A., Souda, L. L., and Sanford, J. P. Persistence of immunologic competence against bacterial antigen in thymectomized rats, *J. Lab. Clin. Med.* 62:856, 1963.

16. Bernhard, W., and Granboulan, N. *In* G. E. W. Wolstenholme and M. O'Connor (eds.), Ciba Foundation Symposium on the Cellular Aspects of Immunity, p. 92, Churchill, London, 1960.

17. Block, M. IV. The blood forming tissues and blood of the new born opossum (Didelphys virginiana), *Ergeb. Anat. Entwicklungsgesch.* 37:237, 1964.

18. Boldt, D., Skinner, A. M., and Kornfeld, S. Studies of two subpopulations of human lymphocytes differing in responsiveness to concanavalin A, *J. Clin. Invest.* 51:3225, 1972.

19. Bosman, C., and Feldman, J. D. Cytology of immunologic memory, *J. Exp. Med.* 293:281, 1968.

20. Bryant, B. J., and Kelly, L. S. Autoradiographic studies of leukocyte formation, *Proc. Soc. Exp. Biol. Med.* 99:681, 1958.

21. Burnet, F. M. Role of the thymus and related organs in immunity, *Br. Med. J.* 2:807, 1962.

22. Burnet, F. M. Cellular Immunology, p. 339, Cambridge University Press, Cambridge, England, 1969.

23. Cain, W. A., Cooper, M. D., Van Alten, P. J., and Good, R. A. Development and function of the immunoglobulin-producing system. II. Role of the bursa in the development of humoral immunological competence, *J. Immunol.* 102:671, 1969.

24. Cantor, H., and Asofsky, R. Synergy among lymphoid cells mediating the graft-versus-host response. II. Synergy in graft-versus-

host reactions produced by Balb-c lymphoid cells of differing anatomic origin, *J. Exp. Med.* 131:235, 1970.

25. Cantor, H., Asofsky, R., and Talal, N. Synergy among lymphoid cells mediating the graft-versus-host response. I. Synergy in graft-versus-host reactions produced by cells from NZB-Bl mice, *J. Exp. Med.* 131:223, 1970.

26. Clark, S. L., Jr. The thymus in mice of strain 129/J studied with the electron microscope, *Am. J. Anat.* 112:1, 1963.

27. Cline, M. J., and Fudenberg, H. H. Defective RNA synthesis in lymphocytes from patients with primary agammaglobulinemia, *Science* 150:311, 1965.

28. Cline, M. J., and Moore, M. A. S. Embryonic origin of the mouse macrophage, *Blood* 39:842, 1972.

29. Cohen, M. W., Thorbecke, G. J., Hochwald, G. M., and Jacobson, E. G. Induction of graft-versus-host reaction in newborn mice by injection of newborn or adult homologous thymus cells, *Proc. Soc. Exp. Biol. Med.* 114:242, 1963.

30. Cohen, N. Reptiles as models for the study of immunity and its phylogenesis, *J. Am. Vet. Med. Assoc.* 159:1662, 1971.

31. Cooper, E. H., Barkhan, P., and Hale, A. J. Mitogenic activity of phytohemagglutinin, *Lancet* ii:210, 1961.

32. Cooper, M. D., Gabrielsen, A. E., Peterson, R. D. A., and Good, R. A. Ontogenetic development of the germinal centers and their function-relationship to the bursa of Fabricius, *in* H. Cottier, N. Odartchenko, R. Schindler, and C. C. Congdon (eds.), Germinal Centers in Immune Responses, p. 28, Springer-Verlag, New York, 1967.

33. Cooper, M. D., Peterson, R. D. A., and Good, R. A. Delineation of the thymic and bursal lymphoid systems in the chicken, *Nature* 205:143, 1965.

34. Cottier, H., Keiser, G., Odartchenko, N., Hess, M., and Stoner, R. D. De novo formation and rapid growth of germinal centers during secondary antibody responses to tetanus toxoid in mice, *in* H. Cottier, N. Odartchenko, R. Schindler,

and C. C. Congdon (eds.), Germinal Centers in Immune Responses, p. 270, Springer-Verlag, New York, 1967.

35. Cottier, H., Odartchenko, N., Schindler, R., and Congdon, C. C. (eds.), Germinal Centers in Immune Responses, Springer-Verlag, New York, 1967.

36. Cross, A. M., Leuchars, E., and Miller, J. F. A. P. Studies on the recovery of the immune response in irradiated mice thymectomized in adult life, *J. Exp. Med.* 119:837, 1964.

37. Dalmasso, A. P., Martinez, C., Sjodin, K., and Good, R. A. Studies on the role of the thymus in immunobiologic reconstitution of immunologic capacity in mice thymectomized at birth, *J. Exp. Med.* 118:1089, 1963.

38. Davies, A. J. S., Leuchars, E., Wallis, V., and Koller, P. The mitotic response of thymus-derived cells to antigenic stimulus, *Transplantation* 4:438, 1966.

39. Defendi, V., and Metcalf, D. (eds.) The Thymus, *Wistar Inst. Symp. Monogr.* 2, Philadelphia, 1964.

40. Diener, E. Evolutionary aspects of immunity and lymphoid organs in vertebrates, *Transplant. Proc.* 2:309, 1970.

41. DiGeorge, A. M. Congenital absence of the thymus and its immunological consequences, concurrence with congenital hypoparathyroidism, *in* R. A. Good and D. Bergsma (eds.), Immunologic Deficiency Diseases in Man, p. 116, National Foundation Press, New York, 1968.

42. Evans, E. E. Antibody response in amphibia and reptilia, *Fed. Proc.* 22:1132, 1963.

43. Everett, N. B., and Tyler (Caffrey), R. W. Radioautographic studies of reticular and lymphoid cells in germinal centers of lymph nodes, *in* H. Cottier, N. Odartchenko, R. Schindler, and C. C. Congdon (eds.), Germinal Centers in Immune Responses, p. 145, Springer-Verlag, New York, 1967.

44. Fichtelius, K-E. On the fate of the lymphocyte, *Acta Anat. Suppl.* 19:1, 1953.

45. Finstad, J., Papermaster, B. W., and Good, R. A. Evolution of the im-

mune response. II. Morphologic studies on the origin of the thymus and organized lymphoid tissue, *Lab. Invest.* 13:490, 1964.

46. Fraser, E. A., and Hill, J. P. The development of the thymus, epithelial bodies and thyroid in the marsupialia. I. Trichosurus vulpecula, *Proc. R. Soc. Lond. (Biol.)* 88:100, 1915.

47. Gesner, B. M., and Gowans, J. L. The fate of lethally irradiated mice given isologous and heterologous thoracic duct lymphocytes, *Br. J. Exp. Pathol.* 43:431, 1962.

48. Glick, B. Normal growth of the bursa of Fabricius in chickens, *Poult. Sci.* 35:843, 1956.

49. Glick, B., Chang, T. S., and Jaap, R. G. The bursa of Fabricius and antibody production, *Poult. Sci.* 35:224, 1956.

50. Goldstein, A. L., Guha, A., Zatz, M. M., Hardy, M. A., and White, A. Purification and biological activity of thymosin, a hormone of the thymus gland, *Proc. Natl. Acad. Sci. U.S.A.* 69:1800, 1972.

51. Good, R. A., Dalmasso, A. P., Martinez, C., Archer, O. K., Pierce, J. C., and Papermaster, B. W. The role of the thymus in development of immunologic capacity in rabbits and mice, *J. Exp. Med.* 116:773, 1962.

52. Good, R. A., and Papermaster, B. W. Phylogeny of the immune response. I. The agnathan, polystotrema stouti, *Fed. Proc.* 20:26, 1961.

53. Good, R. A., and Papermaster, B. W. Ontogeny and phylogeny of adaptive immunity, *Adv. Immunol.* 4:1, 1964.

54. Gowans, J. L. The recirculation of lymphocytes from blood to lymph in the rat, *J. Physiol. Lond.* 146:54, 1959.

55. Gowans, J. L. The fate of parental strain small lymphocytes in F_1 hybrid rats, *Ann. N.Y. Acad. Sci.* 99:432, 1962.

56. Gowans, J. L., Gesner, B. M., and McGregor, D. D. The immunological activity of lymphocytes, *in* G. E. W. Wolstenholme and M. O'Connor (eds.), Biological Activity of the Leucocyte, Ciba Foundation Study Group No. 10, p. 32, Little, Brown and Co., New York, 1961.

57. Gowans, J. L., and Knight, E. J. The route of recirculation of lymphocytes in the rat, *Proc. R. Soc. Lond.* 159:257, 1964.

58. Gowans, J. L., and McGregor, D. D. The immunological activities of lymphocytes, *Prog. Allergy* 9:1, 1965.

59. Graetzer, M. A., Wolfe, H. R., Aspinall, R. L., and Meyer, R. K. Effect of thymectomy and bursectomy on precipitin and natural hemagglutinin production in the chicken, *J. Immunol.* 90:878, 1963.

60. Gräsbeck, R., Nordman, C., and de la Chapelle, A. Mitogenic action of antileucocyte immune serum on peripheral leucocytes in vitro, *Lancet* ii:385, 1963.

61. Grégoire, C. Recherches sur la symbiose lymphoepithéliale au niveau du thymus du mammifère, *Arch. Biol. Paris* 46:717, 1935.

62. Grégoire, C. The cultivation in living organisms of the thymus epithelium of the guinea-pig and rat, *Q. J. Microbiol. Sci.* 99:511, 1958.

63. Grey, H. M. Phylogeny of immunoglobulins, *Adv. Immunol.* 10:51, 1969.

64. Hall, J. G., and Morris, B. Effect of X-irradiation of the popliteal lymph-node on its output of lymphocytes and immunological responsiveness, *Lancet* i:1077, 1964.

65. Hall, J. G., and Morris, B. The origin of the cells in the efferent lymph from a single lymph node, *J. Exp. Med.* 121:901, 1965.

66. Hall, J. G., Morris, B., Moreno, G. D., and Bessis, M. C. The ultrastructure and function of the cells in lymph following antigenic stimulation, *J. Exp. Med.* 125:91, 1967.

67. Hallander, H., and Danielsson, D. In vitro production of antibodies by thoracic duct lymphocytes, *Acta Pathol. Microbiol. Scand.* 56:75, 1962.

68. Hammar, J. A. Die normal-morphologische Thymusforschung im letzten Vierteljahre, Barth, Leipzig, 1936.

69. Hannoun, C., and Bussard, A. E. Antibody production by cells in tissue culture. I. Morphological evolution of lymph node and spleen cells in culture, *J. Exp. Med.* 123:1035, 1966.

70. Harris, H. Role of chemotaxis in

inflammation, *Physiol. Rev.* 34:529, 1954.

71. Harris, J. E., and Ford, C. E. Cellular traffic of the thymus: experiments with chromosome markers. Evidence that the thymus plays an instructional part, *Nature* 201:884, 1964.

72. Harris, J. E., Ford, C. E., Barnes, D. W. H., and Evans, E. P. Evidence from parabiosis for an afferent stream of cells, *Nature* 201:886, 1964.

73. Harris, T. N., Hummeler, K., and Harris, S. Electron microscopic observations on antibody-producing lymph node cells, *J. Exp. Med.* 123:161, 1966.

74. Hess, M. W., Cottier, H., and Stoner, R. D. Primary and secondary antitoxin responses in thymectomized mice, *J. Immunol.* 91:425, 1963.

75. Hilgard, H. R., Yunis, E., and Martinez, C. Treatment of wasting in thymectomized mice with splenic or thymic cells, *Fed. Proc.* 23:287, 1964.

76. Holub, M., Říha, I., and Kamarýtová, V. Immunological competence of different stages of the lymphoid cell, *in* J. Šterzl (ed.), Molecular and Cellular Basis of Antibody Formation, Czechoslovak Acad. Sci., p. 447, Academic Press, New York, 1965.

77. Horton, J. D. Ontogeny of the immune system in amphibians, *Am. Zool.* 11:219, 1971.

78. Huber, J., Cholnoky, P., and Zoethout, H. E. Congenital aplasia of parathyroid glands and thymus, *Arch. Dis. Child.* 42:190, 1967.

79. Hulliger, L., and Sorkin, E. Formation of specific antibody by circulating cells, *Immunology* 9:391, 1965.

80. Humble, J. G., Jayne, W. H. W., and Pulvertaft, H. J. V. Biological interaction between lymphocytes and other cells, *Br. J. Haematol.* 2:283, 1956.

81. Hummeler, K., Harris, T. N., Tomassini, N., Hechtel, M., and Farber, M. B. Electron microscopic observations on antibody-producing cells in lymph and blood, *J. Exp. Med.* 124:255, 1966.

82. Humphrey, J. H., Parrott, D. M. V., and East, J. Studies on globulin and antibody production in mice thymectomized at birth, *Immunology* 7:419, 1964.

83. Jaffe, W. P., and Fechheimer, N. S. Cytology, cell transport and the bursa of Fabricius, *Nature* 212:92, 1966.

84. Janković, B. D., and Isaković, R. Role of the thymus and the bursa of Fabricius in immune reactions in chickens. I. Changes in lymphoid tissues of chickens surgically thymectomized at hatching, *Int. Arch. Allergy* 24:278, 1964.

85. Janković, B. D., and Išvaneski, M. Experimental allergic encephalomyelitis in thymectomized, bursectomized and normal chickens, *Int. Arch. Allergy* 23:188, 1963.

86. Janković, B. D., Waksman, B. H., and Arnason, B. G. Role of the thymus in immune reactions in rats. I. The immunologic response to bovine serum albumin (antibody formation Arthus reactivity and delayed hypersensitivity) in rats thymectomized or splenectomized at various times after birth, *J. Exp. Med.* 116:159, 1962.

87. Joel, D. D., Hess, M. W., and Cottier, H. Magnitude and pattern of thymic lymphocyte migration in neonatal mice, *J. Exp. Med.* 135:907, 1972.

88. Kelly, W. D. The thymus and lymphoid morphogenesis in the dog, *Fed. Proc.* 22:600, 1963.

89. Keuning, F. J., and Bos, W. H. Regeneration patterns of lymphoid follicles in the rabbit spleen after sublethal X-irradiation, *in* H. Cottier, N. Odartchenko, R. Schindler, and C. C. Congdon (eds.), Germinal Centers in Immune Responses, p. 250, Springer-Verlag, New York, 1967.

90. Koburg, E. Cell production and cell migration in the tonsil, *in* H. Cottier, N. Odartchenko, R. Schindler, and C. C. Congdon (eds.), Germinal Centers in Immune Responses, p. 176, Springer-Verlag, New York, 1967.

91. Komuro, K., and Boyse, E. A. In vitro demonstration of thymic hormone in the mouse by conversion of precursor cells into lymphocytes, *Lancet* i:740, 1973.

92. Konda, S., Nakao, Y., and Smith, R. T. Immunologic properties of mouse thymus cells. Identification of T cell functions within a minor, low-density subpopulation, *J. Exp. Med.* 136:1461, 1972.

93. Landy, M., Sanderson, R. P., Bernstein, M. T., and Jackson, A. L. Antibody production by leucocytes in peripheral blood, *Nature* 204:1320, 1964.

94. Levey, R. H., Trainin, N., and Law, L. W. Evidence for function of thymic tissue in diffusion chambers implanted in neonatally thymectomized mice. Preliminary report, *J. Natl. Cancer Inst.* 31:199, 1963.

95. Lewis, W. H. Locomotion of lymphocytes, *Bull. Johns Hopkins Hosp.* 49:29, 1931.

96. Lin, P. S., Cooper, A. G., and Wortis, H. H. Scanning electron microscopy of human T-cell and B-cell rosettes, *N. Engl. J. Med.* 289:548, 1973.

97. Linna, J., and Stillström, J. Migration of cells from the thymus to the spleen in young guinea pigs, *Acta Pathol. Microbiol. Scand.* 68:465, 1966.

98. Lischner, H. W., Punnett, H. H., and DiGeorge, A. M. Lymphocytes in congenital absence of the thymus, *Nature* 214:580, 1967.

99. Long, P. L., and Pierce, A. E. Role of cellular factors in the mediation of immunity to avian coccidiosis (Eimeria tenella), *Nature* 200:426, 1963.

100. Loutit, J. F. Immunological and trophic functions of lymphocytes, *Lancet* ii:1106, 1962.

101. McFarland, W. Microspikes on the lymphocyte uropod, *Science* 163:818, 1969.

102. McFarland, W., and Heilman, D. H. Lymphocyte foot appendage: its role in lymphocyte function and in immunological reactions, *Nature* 205:887, 1965.

103. McFarland, W., Heilman, D. H., and Moorhead, J. F. Functional anatomy of the lymphocyte in immunological reactions in vitro, *J. Exp. Med.* 124:851, 1966.

104. McGregor, D. D., and Gowans, J. L. The antibody response of rats depleted of lymphocytes by chronic drainage from the thoracic duct, *J. Exp. Med.* 117:303, 1963.

105. McIntire, K. R., Sell, S., and Miller,

J. F. A. P. Pathogenesis of the post-neonatal thymectomy wasting syndrome, *Nature* 204:151, 1964.

106. Marchesi, V. T., and Gowans, J. L. The migration of lymphocytes through the endothelium of venules in lymph nodes: an electron microscope study, *Proc. R. Soc. Lond.* 159:283, 1964.

107. Marshall, W. H., and Roberts, K. B. The growth and mitosis of human small lymphocytes after incubation with a phytohaemagglutinin, *Q. J. Exp. Physiol.* 48:146, 1963.

108. Matter, A., Lisowska-Bernstein, B., Ryser, J. E., et al. Mouse thymus-independent and thymus-derived lymphoid cells. II. Ultrastructural studies, *J. Exp. Med.* 136:1008, 1972.

109. Metcalf, D. The thymic origin of the plasma lymphocytosis stimulating factor, *Br. J. Cancer* 10:442, 1956.

110. Metcalf, D. The thymus: its role in immune responses, leukemia development and carcinogenesis, Recent Results in Cancer Research No. 5, Springer-Verlag, Berlin, 1966.

111. Metcalf, D., and Brumby, M. The role of the thymus in the ontogeny of the immune system, *J. Cell. Physiol.* 67 (suppl. 1):149, 1966.

112. Metcalf, D., and Moore, M. A. S. Haemopoietic Cells, p. 312, North-Holland Publishing Co., Amsterdam, 1971.

113. Meyer, R. K., Rao, M. A., and Aspinall, R. L. Inhibition of the development of the bursa of Fabricius in the embryos of the common fowl by 19-nortestosterone, *Endocrinology* 64:890, 1959.

114. Micklem, H. S., and Brown, J. A. H. Germinal centers, allograft sensitivity and iso-antibody formation in skin allografted mice, *in* H. Cottier, N. Odartchenko, R. Schindler, and C. C. Congdon (eds.), Germinal Centers in the Immune Response, p. 277, Springer-Verlag, New York, 1967.

115. Micklem, H. S., Ford, C. E., Evans, E. P., and Gray, J. Interrelationships of myeloid and lymphoid cells: studies with chromosome-marked cells transfused into lethally irradiated mice, *Proc. R. Soc. Lond.* 165:78, 1966.

116. Miller, J. F. A. P. Immunological

function of the thymus, *Lancet* ii:748, 1961.

117. Miller, J. F. A. P. Role of the thymus in transplantation immunity, *Ann. N.Y. Acad. Sci.* 99:340, 1962.

118. Miller, J. F. A. P. Effect of neonatal thymectomy on the immunological responsiveness of the mouse, *Proc. R. Soc. Lond.* 156:415, 1962.

119. Miller, J. F. A. P. Immunity and the thymus, *Lancet* i:43, 1963.

120. Miller, J. F. A. P., Doak, S. M. A., and Cross, A. M. Role of the thymus in recovery of the immune mechanism in the irradiated adult mouse (28170), *Proc. Soc. Exp. Biol. Med.* 112:785, 1963.

121. Mims, C. A. Experiments on the origin and fate of lymphocytes, *Br. J. Exp. Pathol.* 43:639, 1962.

122. Moore, M. A. S., and Owen, J. J. T. Experimental studies on the development of the bursa of Fabricius, *Dev. Biol.* 14:40, 1966.

123. Motika, E. J., and Van Alten, P. J. Alterations in the kinetics of hemagglutinin formation following embryonic bursectomy, *J. Immunol.* 107:512, 1971.

124. Mueller, A. P., Wolfe, H. R., and Cote, W. P. Antibody studies in hormonally and surgically bursectomized chickens, *in* R. A. Good and A. E. Gabrielsen (eds.), The Thymus in Immunobiology, p. 359, Hoeber-Harper, New York, 1964.

125. Mueller, A. P., Wolfe, H. R., and Meyer, R. K. Precipitin production in chickens. XXI. Antibody production in bursectomized chickens and in chickens injected with 19-nortestosterone on the fifth day of incubation, *J. Immunol.* 85:172, 1960.

126. Mueller, A. P., Wolfe, H. R., Meyer, R. K., and Aspinall, R. L. Further studies on the role of the bursa of Fabricius in antibody production, *J. Immunol.* 88:354, 1962.

127. Nagaya, H., and Sieker, H. O. Allograft survival: effect of antiserums to thymus glands and lymphocytes, *Science* 150:1181, 1961.

128. Nettesheim, P., and Makinodan, T. Differentiation of lymphocytes undergoing an immune response in diffusion chambers, *J. Immunol.* 94:868, 1965.

129. Nossal, G. J. V. Studies on the rate of seeding of lymphocytes from the

intact guinea pig thymus, *Ann. N.Y. Acad. Sci.* 120:171, 1964.

130. Nossal, G. J. V., and Gorrie, J. Studies on the emigration of thymic cells in young guinea pigs, *in* R. A. Good and A. E. Gabrielsen (eds.), The Thymus in Immunobiology, p. 288, Hoeber-Harper, New York, 1964.

131. Nowell, P. C. Phytohemagglutinin: an initiator of mitosis in cultures of normal human leukocytes, *Cancer Res.* 20:462, 1960.

132. Old, L. J., Boyse, E. A., and Stockert, E. Antigenic properties of experimental leukemias. I. Serological studies in vitro with spontaneous and radiation-induced leukemias, *J. Natl. Cancer Inst.* 31:977, 1963.

133. Old, L. J., Boyse, E. A., and Stockert, E. Mouse leukaemias. Typing of mouse leukaemias by serological methods, *Nature* 201:777, 1964.

134. Ortega, L. G., and Der, B. K. Studies of agammaglobulinemia induced by ablation of the bursa of Fabricius, *Fed. Proc.* 23:546, 1964.

135. Osmond, D. G., and Everett, N. B. Radioautographic studies of bone marrow lymphocytes in vivo and in diffusion chamber cultures, *Blood* 23:1, 1964.

136. Osoba, D., and Miller, J. F. A. P. Evidence for a humoral thymus factor responsible for the maturation of immunological faculty, *Nature* 199:653, 1963.

137. Owen, J. J. T., and Ritter, M. A. Tissue interaction in the development of thymus lymphocytes, *J. Exp. Med.* 129:431, 1969.

138. Papermaster, B. W., Condie, R. M., Finstad, J., and Good, R. A. Evolution of the immune response. I. The phylogenetic development of adaptive immunologic responsiveness in vertebrates, *J. Exp. Med.* 119:105, 1964.

139. Papermaster, B. W., Condie, R. M., Finstad, J. K., Good, R. A., and Gabrielsen, A. E. Phylogenetic development of adaptive immunity, *Fed. Proc.* 22:1152, 1963.

140. Papermaster, B. W., Condie, R. M., and Good, R. A. Immune response in the California hagfish, *Nature* 196:355, 1962.

141. Papermaster, B. W., Dalmasso, A.

P., Martinez, C., and Good, R. A. Suppression of antibody forming capacity with thymectomy in the mouse, *Proc. Soc. Exp. Biol. Med.* 111:41, 1962.

142. Papermaster, B. W., Friedman, D. I., and Good, R. A. Relationship of the bursa of Fabricius to immunologic responsiveness and homograft immunity in the chicken (27423), *Proc. Soc. Exp. Biol. Med.* 110:62, 1962.

143. Parrott, D. M. V. The integrity of the germinal center: an investigation of the differential localization of labeled cells in lymphoid organs, *in* H. Cottier, N. Odartchenko, R. Schindler, and C. C. Congdon (eds.), Germinal Centers in Immune Responses, p. 168, Springer-Verlag, New York, 1967.

144. Parrott, D. M. V., de Sousa, M. A. B., and East, J. Thymus-dependent areas in the lymphoid organs of neonatally thymectomized mice, *J. Exp. Med.* 123:191, 1966.

145. Parrott, D. M. V., and East, J. Studies on a fatal wasting syndrome of mice thymectomized at birth, *in* R. A. Good and A. E. Gabrielsen (eds.), The Thymus in Immunobiology, p. 523, Hoeber-Harper, New York, 1964.

146. Pearmain, G., Lycette, R. R., and Fitzgerald, P. H. Tuberculin-induced mitosis in peripheral blood leucocytes, *Lancet* i:637, 1963.

147. Perey, D. Y. E., Cooper, M. D., and Good, R. A. Lymphoepithelial tissues of the intestine and differentiation of antibody production, *Science* 161:265, 1968.

148. Peterson, R. D. A., Cooper, M. D., and Good, R. A. The pathogenesis of immunologic deficiency diseases, *Am. J. Med.* 38:579, 1965.

149. Polgar, P. R., and Kibrick, S. Origin of small lymphocytes following blastogenesis induced by short-term PHA-stimulation, *Nature* 225:857, 1970.

150. Raff, M. C. Theta isoantigen as a marker of thymus-derived lymphocytes in mice, *Nature* 224:378, 1969.

151. Reif, A. E., and Allen, J. M. V. The AKR thymic antigen and its distribution in leukemias and nervous tissues, *J. Exp. Med.* 120:413, 1964.

152. Rich, A. R., Lewis, M. R., and Win-trobe, M. M. The activity of the lymphocyte in the body's reaction to foreign protein, as established by the identification of the acute splenic tumor cell, *Bull. Johns Hopkins Hosp.* 65:311, 1939.

153. Russe, H. P., and Crowle, A. J. A comparison of thymectomized and antithymocyte serum-treated mice in their development of hypersensitivity to protein antigens, *J. Immunol.* 94:74, 1965.

154. Sainte-Marie, G., and Leblond, C. P. Cytologic features and cellular migration in the cortex and medulla of thymus in the young adult rat, *Blood* 23:275, 1964.

155. Scheid, M. P., Hoffmann, M. K., Komuro, K., et al. Differentiation of T cells induced by preparations from thymus and by nonthymic agents, *J. Exp. Med.* 138:1027, 1973.

156. Sherman, J. D., Adner, M. M., and Dameshek, W. Effect of thymectomy on the golden hamster (Mesocricetus auratus). II. Studies of the immune response in thymectomized and splenectomized non-wasted animals, *Blood* 23:375, 1964.

157. Small, M., and Trainin, N. Contribution of a thymic humoral factor to the development of an immunologically competent population from cells of mouse bone marrow, *J. Exp. Med.* 134:786, 1971.

158. Smith, R. T., Miescher, P. A., and Good, R. A. Phylogeny of Immunity, University of Florida Press, Gainesville, 1966.

159. Stoner, R. D., and Bond, V. P. Antibody formation by transplanted bone marrow, spleen, lymph nodes and thymus cells in irradiated recipients, *J. Immunol.* 91:185, 1963.

160. Süssdorf, D. H. Repopulation of the spleen of X-irradiated rabbits by tritium-labeled lymphoid cells of the shielded appendix, *J. Infect. Dis.* 107:108, 1960.

161. Sutherland, D. E. R., Archer, O. K., and Good, R. A. Role of the appendix in development of immunologic capacity, *Proc. Soc. Exp. Biol. Med.* 115:673, 1964.

162. Szenberg, A., and Warner, N. L. Immunological function of thymus and bursa of Fabricius, *Nature* 194:146, 1962.

163. Taitz, L. S., Zarate-Salvador, C., and Schwartz, E. Congenital absence of the parathyroid and thymus glands in an infant (III and IV pharyngeal pouch syndrome), *Pediatrics* 38:412, 1966.

164. Taylor, R. B. Immunological competence of thymus cells after transfer to thymectomized recipients, *Nature* 199:873, 1963.

165. Thorbecke, G. J., and Cohen, M. W. Immunological competence and responsiveness of the thymus, *in* V. Defendi and D. Metcalf (eds.), The Thymus, p. 33, *Wistar Inst. Symp. Monogr.* 2, Philadelphia, 1964.

166. Tyan, M. L., and Herzenberg, L. A. Studies on the ontogeny of the mouse immune system, *J. Immunol.* 101:446, 1968.

167. Van Alten, P. J., Cain, W. A., Good, R. A., and Cooper, M. D. Gamma globulin production and antibody synthesis in chickens bursectomized as embryos, *Nature* 217:358, 1968.

168. Van Alten, P. J., and Meuwissen, H. J. Production of specific antibody by lymphocytes of the bursa of Fabricius, *Science* 176:45, 1972.

169. Van Furth, R. The formation of immunoglobulins by human tissues in vitro, doctoral thesis, Leiden, 1964.

170. Warner, N. L., and Burnet, F. M. The influence of testosterone treatment on the development of the bursa of Fabricius in the chick embryo, *Aust. J. Biol. Sci.* 14:580, 1961.

171. Warner, N. L., Szenberg, A., and Burnet, F. M. The immunological role of different lymphoid organs in the chicken. I. Dissociation of immunological responsiveness, *Aust. J. Exp. Biol. Med. Sci.* 40:373, 1962.

172. Warner, N. L., Uhr, J. W., Thorbecke, G. J., and Ovary, Z. Immunoglobulins, antibodies and the bursa of Fabricius: induction of agammaglobulinemia and the loss of all antibody-forming capacity by hormonal bursectomy, *J. Immunol.* 103:1317, 1969.

173. Weiss, L. The Cells and Tissues of the Immune System. Structure, Functions, Interactions, Prentice-Hall, Englewood Cliffs, N.J., 1972.

174. Weissman, I. L. Thymus cell migration, *J. Exp. Med.* 126:291, 1967.

175. Wesslén, T. Studies on the rôle of lymphocytes in antibody production, *Acta Derm. Venereol. (Stockh.)* 32:265, 1952.

176. White, A., and Goldstein, A. L. Is the thymus an endocrine gland? Old problem, new data, *Perspect. Biol. Med.* 11:475, 1968.

177. Wilson, R., Sjodin, K., and Bealmear, M. The absence of wasting in thymectomized germfree (axenic) mice (29545), *Proc. Soc. Exp. Biol. Med.* 117:237, 1964.

178. Wissler, R. W., Robson, M. J., Fitch, F., Nelson, W., and Jacobson, L. O. The effects of spleen shielding and subsequent splenectomy upon antibody formation in rats receiving total-body X-irradiation, *J. Immunol.* 70:379, 1953.

179. Wolpert, L., and O'Neill, C. H. Dynamics of the membrane of amoeba proteus studied with labelled specific antibody, *Nature* 196:1261, 1962.

180. Wu, A. M., Till, J. E., Siminovitch, L., and McCulloch, E. A. Cytological evidence for a relationship between normal hematopoietic colony-forming cells and cells of the lymphoid system, *J. Exp. Med.* 127:455, 1968.

181. Yoffrey, J. M., Hanks, G. A., and Kelly, L. Some problems of lymphocyte production, *Ann. N.Y. Acad. Sci.* 73:47, 1958.

182. Yunis, E. J., Hilgard, H. R., Martinez, C., and Good, R. A. Studies on immunologic reconstitution of thymectomized mice, *J. Exp. Med.* 121:607, 1965.

183. Zucker-Franklin, D. The ultrastructure of cells in human thoracic duct lymph, *J. Ultrastruct. Res.* 9:325, 1963.

Chapter 13   Production and Distribution of Lymphocytes

Lymphocytes comprise a family of cells differing in size, morphologic characteristics, origin, life cycle, and migration patterns. As discussed in Chapters 2 and 12 and illustrated in Fig. I.1, lymphoid cells and myeloid hematopoietic cells probably share a common progenitor stem cell (35, 82, 127). Classification of lymphocyte subpopulations based solely on morphologic grounds has not been possible. As Yoffey and Courtice have suggested (129), lymphocytes must be identified not by positive cytologic features, but by the absence of features present in other white cells—for example, specific granulation and nuclear lobation. Despite these limitations, modern techniques of studying cell kinetics and migration have permitted a preliminary analysis of the heterogeneous family of lymphoid cells (44).

Cronkite and Chanana (18) listed the following as major technical advances in the study of the kinetic behavior of lymphocytes: (a) the use of radioisotopes in the study of biological systems and to demonstrate the existence of long- and short-lived lymphocytes (47, 94); (b) the introduction of mitotic arresting agents (22); and (c) the application of tritiated thymidine in the study of lymphocyte proliferation (116).

The Small Lymphocyte: A Heterogeneous Population

Small lymphocytes may be divided into two major populations: short-lived and long-lived (9, 66). Most available evidence supports the premise that the long-lived population is homogeneous in migration pattern and life cycle.

The short-lived small lymphocyte is probably heterogeneous in these respects (32).

The Long-lived Small Lymphocyte

Pool Size and Distribution   The following are the major characteristics of long-lived lymphocytes:

Constitute the major cell of the recirculating lymphocyte pool
Apparently identical to thymus-derived (T) lymphocytes
Constitute the antigen-reactive cell population
Life-span of months to years, depending on the species
Distribution in paracortical areas of lymph nodes and white pulp of spleen
Presumed functions: precursor of antigen-reactive cells; cellular immunity; immunologic memory

Caffrey and his colleagues (9) were the first to define a "mobilizable lymphocyte pool" among the lymphocyte populations of the rat. This pool was lost by thoracic duct drainage until a low steady-state output was achieved—usually in two to three days. The number of lymphocytes lost by this technique was approximately one-half the total small lymphocytes of the animal (30). Subsequently, a "recirculating lymphocyte pool" was defined as the population of small lymphocytes that migrates from the blood via the postcapillary venules (43) to reach and traverse the lymph node and enter the efferent lymph, thus reentering the circulation.

Both the mobilizable lymphocyte pool and the recirculating lymphocyte pool of the rat contain roughly 1×10^7 cells per gram of body weight. They may not be identical populations of cells (42), although firm evidence shows that the major cellular component of both of these pools is the long-lived small lymphocyte. This evidence is based on repopulation of irradiated lymph nodes (4) and the equilibrium of radioactively labeled small lymphocytes among various organs in growing animals (30).

Long-lived lymphocytes are found in lymph nodes deep in the cortex in paracortical areas, in the medullary sinuses, in the efferent lymphatics, and as a corona around the germinal centers (32). They are also found in the loose white pulp of the spleen (43).

As noted in the previous chapter, neonatal thymectomy in an animal such as the mouse results in depletion in these areas of lymph nodes and spleen. Thus *the thymus-dependent areas are the same as those populated by long-lived lymphocytes* (5, 32, 95, 96, 124). In contrast, the red pulp of the spleen, the bone marrow lymphocytes, and the germinal centers of lymph nodes appear to be relatively unaffected by neonatal thymectomy. Areas depleted by neonatal thymectomy are also depleted by extracorporeal irradiation of the blood (14, 18).

These observations may be taken as inferential evidence that the thymus-dependent lymphocytes and the long-lived lymphocyte population are identical. They do not exclude the possibility that some B cells may also be long-lived.

Thymic Origin of the Long-lived Lymphocyte   The neonatally thymectomized animal has a decreased mobilizable lymphocyte pool (84) and decreased numbers of small lymphocytes in the thoracic duct lymph (99). This reduction is in the long-lived T-cell population, whereas short-lived small lymphocytes and large lymphocytes are present in normal numbers (99). Adult thymectomy has an effect similar to neonatal thymectomy, but less pronounced (78, 83, 110, 128). This suggests that the long-lived thymus-derived lymphocytes may be produced in postnatal life as well as during the fetal and neonatal period. As mentioned in Chapter 12, the thymus-derived lymphocytes of certain species have unique antigenic markers, which distinguish them from B lymphocytes (97).

Antigen Reactivity   The term "antigen-reactive cell" (ARC) probably was first coined by Miller and Mitchell (85) in reference to the lymphoid population, which reacts to antigen by proliferation. One variety of ARC appears to be the same as the long-lived T lymphocyte (21, 84, 86).

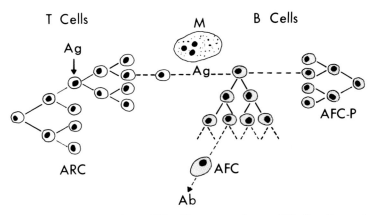

Figure 13.1 Interaction of T cells, macrophages (*M*), B cells, and antigen (*Ag*) in antibody (*Ab*) production. *ARC* = antigen-reactive cell; *AFC* = antibody-forming cell; *AFC-P* = antibody-forming cell precursor.

Although the ARC usually is formally equated with a subpopulation of T cells, it is clear that B cells also may interact with antigen as a result of antibody immunoglobulin present at the cell surface.

The antigen-reactive lymphocyte is the most sensitive to the effects of antilymphocytic sera (31, 71) and comprises the majority of small lymphocytes in the blood and thoracic duct fluid. Recently there has been some progress in separating the long-lived T cell from the short-lived B cell (3).

The immunologic reactions of the long-lived T lymphocytes are considered in detail in Chapter 15. The basic aspects of the role of this cell in the production of antibody in response to antigen are illustrated in Fig. 13.1. Long-lived T cells probably constitute one source of *immunologic memory cells* (45); B-cell subpopulations constitute another source. After exposure to an antigen, B memory cells begin proliferating well before the peak of response of B antibody-forming cells (126). When exposed to an appropriate antigen, an antigen-reactive cell is stimulated to proliferate and produces a clone of cells like itself. The ARC interacts with antigen and, under some circumstances, with macrophages to provide an environment for replication of B cells and their differentiation to lymphoid cells and plasma cells that produce specific antibody immunoglobulin. The long-lived ARC is necessary for reaction to only certain classes of antigen. B cells may respond directly to antigens that have a large number of repeating identical determinants, allowing for multivalent binding to receptors on their surface. Examples of such directly reacting antigens are polymerized flagellin and certain polysaccharides.

Life-span Continuous infusion of tritiated thymidine in rats demonstrated a median life-span of about one month for small lymphocytes; 5 to 8 percent of the cells had a life-span of more than nine months (100). In this study small lymphocytes labeled nonuniformly and appeared to comprise at least two populations differing in labeling intensity and turnover.

Little and his colleagues (66) demonstrated that the small-lymphocyte population of the rat can be divided into lymphocytes with relatively short life-span and those with life-spans greater than one year.

In adult women, small lymphocytes are reported to have a mean life-span of 530 ± 64 days (89).

The Short-lived Small Lymphocyte

As noted earlier, short-lived small lymphocytes comprise a heterogeneous population of cells varying in origin, life-span, distribution, and probably function. The life-span of short-lived lymphocytes in the circulation of the rat varies between a few hours and approximately five days (30). Somewhere between 5 and 15 percent of the normal small lymphocytes in the thoracic duct lymph of the mouse are short lived. Neonatal thymectomy has little effect on this population (99). After the mobilizable lymphocyte pool has been collected by chronic thoracic duct drainage, short-lived lymphocytes continue to appear for several days.

Short-lived lymphocytes may be found in several locations:

Blood   about 15 percent of small-
Thoracic duct lymph   lymphocyte population
Thymus gland
Bone marrow
Germinal centers of lymph nodes
Spleen

In the rat, the lymphocytes with a short life-span in the blood stream accumulate in acutely inflamed tissues (58). Recent evidence suggests that some short-lived lymphocytes interact with macrophages in mediating certain cellular immune reactions (67).

Turnover in the Thymus The turnover of small lymphocytes in the thymus has been studied by repeated injections of tritiated thymidine to label all cells entering DNA synthesis (30, 69). In both the rat and the mouse, approximately 50 percent of cells become labeled by 36 hours, indicating a very high renewal rate for this population. After cessation of tritiated thymidine administra-

tion, labeled cells leave the thymus or are destroyed in situ in a random fashion (that is, logarithmically and without respect to cell age). From these data it could be calculated that in the rat the turnover rate of thymic lymphocytes is sufficient to replace the organ every 2.5 days. This of course is an extraordinarily high cellular turnover rate. Its possible significance has been discussed in Chapter 12.

Various experiments indicate that the great majority of cells formed in the thymus die in situ (78, 79, 90, 99) and that less than 5 percent enter the blood and lymphoid organs (30). Labeling studies indicate that this subpopulation that migrates from the thymus is part of the long-lived lymphocyte pool (64, 96) rather than the very short-lived pool of intrathymic lymphocytes. Thus it is important to distinguish these short-lived thymocytes from the long-lived T lymphocytes, which are conditioned by, and migrate from, the thymus.

Turnover in the Bone Marrow Everett and Caffrey (29) have presented evidence that the half-renewal time of small lymphocytes in the bone marrow is 24 hours—a turnover rate even faster than that of thymocytes. Over 95 percent of the small lymphocytes in the bone marrow apparently are formed from cell proliferation in situ (29, 93). Many of these lymphocytes enter the circulation.

The bone-marrow–derived lymphocytes (B cells) appear to be precursors of the antibody-forming cells, which are thought to be mainly plasma cells (23, 91) (see Fig. 13.1). The B cells do not themselves appear to be completely competent immunologically, in that they do not confer graft-vs-host reactivity (6) or restore immunologic competence to an irradiated recipient animal (1). After migrating from the bone marrow, these cells are found in the germinal centers and medullary cords of lymph nodes, which are the the primary sites of 19S antibody production (74). They are also found in the thoracic duct lymph, where they may be the precursor of the antibody-forming cells found in this site. The B cell is probably the lymphocyte species that is sensitive to the action of corticosteroids (17, 28).

The two critical unanswered questions regarding the short-lived small lymphocyte are first, what is the significance of the high turnover rate of in situ death of the thymic lymphocytes, and second, is the presumed pathway from bone marrow lymphocyte to blast cell to antibody-forming cell correct?

The known characteristics of short-lived small lymphocytes are summarized below:

Constitute a heterogeneous population of cells, including thymocytes and bone-marrow–derived (B) lymphocytes

Found in small numbers in the blood and thoracic duct and in other sites

Life-span: generally less than 5 days; in some murine species less than 24 hours

Functions: many unknown; some probably precursors of antibody-forming cells

Blast Cells

Early morphologic hematologists recognized a large cell distributed in the bone marrow, spleen, and lymphoid tissue (including the thymus). The cell, called the blast cell or hemocytoblast by these early morphologists, was large and had a low nucleus/cytoplasm ratio relative to the small lymphocyte (Fig. 13.2). The blast cell had a high proliferative capacity, as indicated by the frequency of mitoses. Subsequent thymidine labeling studies have confirmed this high proliferative rate and indicate a generation time of 112 hours for blast cells in the lymph nodes, spleen, and thymus of murine species (69, 98).

Labeling studies with tritiated thymidine of blast cells in mesenteric lymph nodes of the rat indicate that as many as 50 percent of these cells may be in DNA synthesis at a given time (98). Subsequent analysis of the distribution of radioactive label has shown that the progeny of the blast cell were also blast cells. Thus there was evi-

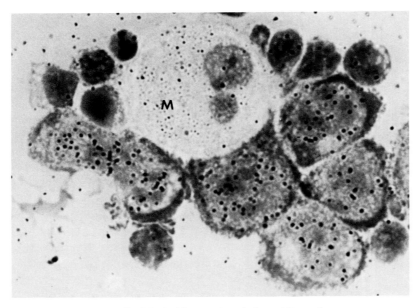

Figure 13.2 Blast cells labeled by tritiated thymidine. A macrophage (*M*) is seen in the center of the cluster.

dence that the majority of blast cells arose from cells of similar morphology rather than via transformation of small lymphocytes. Similarly, large and medium lymphocytes, which have been designated transitional cells because of their intermediate morphologic characteristics, appear to be self-sustaining populations (32, 106).

Everett and Tyler (32) have summarized evidence that long-lived small lymphocytes infrequently transform to blast cells in vivo. Only a small percentage of lymphocytes respond to specific antigenic stimuli by blastogenic transformation in vitro (15, 70, 121). It is apparent, of course, that only a very few small lymphocytes need to undergo transformation for a great number of blast cells to accumulate rapidly. If the initially generated blast cells are self-sustaining and if the generation time is 12 hours, then 2^6 cells would accumulate from a single transformation in 3 days, and 2^{10} cells in 5 days—provided, of course, that there is no cell loss. The generation time may in fact be considerable shorter than this 12-hour period. The life cycle of splenic blast cells from primed donors exposed to antigen in vitro has been demonstrated to have a generation time of only 8 to 9 hours during the transition from latent period to log phase growth. The G_1 phase is about an hour; the mitotic time, about a half-hour (33, 107, 123). Under certain circumstances mitotic time may be as short as 18 minutes (20). Only a few of these blast cells recirculate (120).

Whether or not the blast cell is a precursor of the plasma cell has been the subject of considerable debate since the first definitive expression of this concept by Maximow in 1932 (73). The subject has been considered in some detail in Chapter 12.

Plasma Cells

The plasma cell response to antigenic stimuli is analyzed in Chapters 15 and 16. At this point in the description of the lymphoid cell subpopulations and their kinetic responses, it is important to know the cardinal features of plasma cell proliferation in response to antigen.

An anamnestic antigenic stimulus calls forth extensive mitoses of lymphoid cells within the lymph nodes and spleen. Antibody response is generally detectable within two to three days of the antigenic stimulus and reaches peak values at about the fifth day (52, 113). Electron microscopic analysis of lymph nodes during this period suggests a differentiation of some lymphoid cells to plasma cells. The percentage of plasma cells in the nodes follows a pattern corresponding roughly to that of the antibody response (109). However, there is no synchrony between the wave of mitosis in response to antigen and the development of plasma cells (114, 115). A large number of antibody-producing cells leave the lymph node via the efferent lymphatics during the secondary response. The peak efflux is at about the fourth to fifth post-stimulus day (10, 19, 46).

Little is known about the life-span of the morphologically mature plasma cell. Recently Mattioli and Tomasi (72) have demonstrated a half-life of 4.7 days for mouse intestinal IgA-producing plasma cells. They also observed a maximum life-span of seven to eight weeks for intestinal IgA cells and splenic plasma cells producing IgA, IgG, and IgM.

Migration Pathways

The blood and lymph provide the highways for traffic of lymphocytes within the tissues. Many of the lymphoid cells of the body use the blood and/or lymph to migrate from one hematopoietic organ to another. This traffic is critical for the development and maintenance of the normal immunologic system (2, 34, 38, 40, 46, 81, 85, 117, 118–120, 122). In addition, lymphocytes accumulate in inflammatory exudates where they may express their immunologic reactivity (68, 92, 102). Newly formed small lymphocytes may be preferentially attracted to such inflamed sites (58).

Lymphocytes may be mobilized from lymphoid tissues into the blood stream by certain bacterial vaccines (87). Fetal lymphocytes may pass into the maternal circulation (111).

The major known migration pathways of the lymphocyte are illustrated in Fig. 13.3.

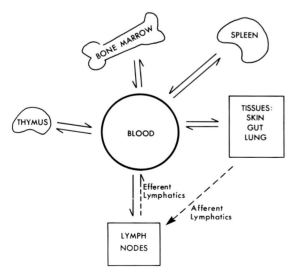

Figure 13.3 Migration pathways of lymphocytes.

General Considerations

The lymphocyte population of the body is highly mobile. A single lymphocyte may traverse the major circulation in the following manner: from the thoracic duct it passes into the blood and enters a lymph node follicle through the cuboidal epithelium of postcapillary venules (Fig. 13.4). The lymphocyte then percolates through channels of the lymph node into the cortex, eventually reaching those lymph sinuses associated with the medullary cords. It enters the efferent lymph vessels at the hilus of the node (Fig. 13.5). Following the course of the efferent lymphatics of the node, the lymphocyte gradually moves to the more central lymph nodes of the chain and thence into the main lymphatic trunk and once again into the blood. A number of alternatives to this major circulation exist. Lymphocytes are constantly being destroyed or lost

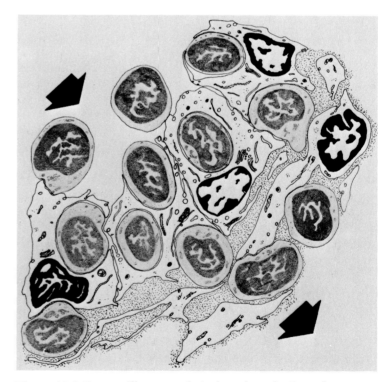

Figure 13.4 Postcapillary venule in lymph node. Lymphocytes pass through the high endothelium, both through the endothelial cytoplasm and between the endothelial cells. Their movement is from the lumen of the venule into the node (*arrows*). The endothelium of these vessels tends to be high where lymphocytic passage is active and low where it is not. (From L. Weiss, The Cells and Tissues of the Immune System. Structure, Functions, Interactions, page 45, Prentice-Hall, Inc., Englewood Cliffs, New Jersey, 1972. Reprinted by permission of author and publisher.)

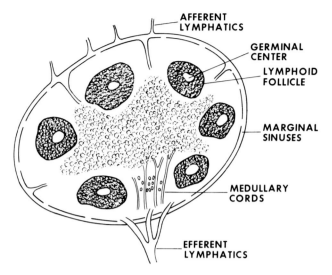

AFFERENT LYMPHATICS

GERMINAL CENTER

LYMPHOID FOLLICLE

MARGINAL SINUSES

MEDULLARY CORDS

EFFERENT LYMPHATICS

Figure 13.5 Schematic representation of the anatomy of a lymph node.

through mucosal surfaces such as those of the gastrointestinal and respiratory tracts. Newly formed lymphocytes are constantly generated within the germinal centers of the lymph nodes and pass rapidly into the circulation.

It is apparent that this circulation will distribute lymphocytes widely throughout the major lymphocyte-bearing areas of the body, including the lymph nodes, spleen, Peyer's patches, tonsils, mucosal surfaces, and thymus. The long-lived T cell is the most abundant cellular component of this recirculating population. The long-lived small lymphocyte population behaves like a single pool of cells with respect to kinetic behavior and recirculation (120). The short-lived lymphocytes in the thoracic duct have only a limited recirculation.

Lymph Node Recycling

The concept of lymphocytes recycling from blood to lymph has a long history (18, 41, 43, 61). Lymph nodes constitute the principal route of recirculation of small lymphocytes from blood to lymph (43). The postcapillary venule (see Fig. 13.4) has been identified as the site of lymphocyte egress from the blood (43, 60, 108), and electron microscopic studies of Marchesi and Gowans (69) suggest passage of lymphocytes through epithelial lining cells.

In contrast to this clear knowledge of the mechanism of lymphocyte passage from the blood, the mechanism of release from lymph nodes into the efferent lymphatics is not known definitively. One suggestion is that there is passive release of cells into the medullary sinuses as a

result of population pressure (112). This phenomenon has been called "desquamation," and the concentration of outflowing lymphocytes has been called a "mud stream" (112). Within the lymph node the lymphocyte population is heterogeneous. It has been estimated that about 60 percent of the cells belong to the readily mobilizable pool (30).

Migration to the Spleen

The concentration of lymphocytes in the splenic vein is higher than that in the artery, suggesting that there is a net input of lymphocytes from the spleen into the blood (24, 26, 27). Ford (37) has shown that the lymphocytes recycle through the spleen with a minimal transit time of two to three hours and at a rate proportional to their blood concentration. The route of migration within the spleen appears to involve trapping of lymphocytes in the periarteriolar sheath of the marginal zone and then entrance into the white pulp (39). Ford (36) has documented an extensive migration pathway involving recycling of cells to the spleen, thoracic duct, lymph, and lymph nodes. Chaperon and his colleagues (11), as well as Tyler and Everett (120), have traced the migration of lymphoid cells and antibody-forming cells between spleen, thymus, and bone marrow; and Cannon and Wissler (10) have identified antibody-forming cells leaving the spleen following an immune response.

Bone Marrow

The bone marrow is a major site of proliferation of small lymphocytes (16, 29, 49, 93). There is some migration of lymphocytes from other sites to the bone marrow (54), although its magnitude is probably not so great as the efflux of cells from the bone marrow (8). Hudson and Yoffey (50) have demonstrated by electron microscopy that lymphocytes migrate between sinusoidal endothelial cells of the marrow. Linna and Liden (65), and more recently Tyler and Everett (120), have shown that under relatively stable conditions there is a migration of labeled bone marrow lymphocytes to the spleen, to other bone marrow sites, to lymph nodes, and to skin areas involved in delayed hypersensitivity reactions. Studies in irradiated animals have demonstrated a relatively slow migration of cells from bone marrow to both the thymus and the lymph nodes (35, 82). Most of the bone marrow lymphocytes of the guinea pig have a short life-span and a rapid turnover rate (104); a small subpopulation has a slower turnover rate (103, 105). In the mouse about 75 percent of cells have a rapid turnover rate and about 8 percent have a very slow turnover rate (101).

Thymic Migration

The very high production rate of lymphoid cells in the thymus must be balanced by cell egress or in situ death in order to maintain a steady-state balance (12, 30, 55, 56, 77). In 1966 Metcalf speculated that over 90 percent of the thymocytes of newborn animals died in situ (76). This very high figure has been challenged by other studies (12, 80). The magnitude of intrathymic death as opposed to migration of thymocytes appears to be a function of the age of the animal. Migration is probably of greater importance during fetal and early postnatal life (80).

Lymphocytes leave the thymus through both the blood vessels and the lymphatics. In young adult mice, thymocytes move from the outer cortical zone into the perivascular lymphatics via the corticomedullary junction (7, 48). They then pass into the efferent lymphatic channels (59). Lymphocytes may also leave the thymus via the veins (62–64, 88, 90, 125). The daily output of cells from the thymus is approximately four times the number in the circulation (18, 25). This observation may explain the fall in blood lymphocyte count following thymectomy (13, 75).

The distribution of cells leaving the thymus to populate thymic-dependent areas of the lymph nodes and spleen has already been commented upon (18, 51). Labeled cells from the thymus occasionally have been found in the thoracic duct, indicating that they enter the recycling pool of small lymphocytes (39). When ³H-thymidine is injected into the thymus glands of neonatal mice, labeled cells subsequently are widely distributed in lymphoid tissues. Joel and his colleagues (53) found that the majority of lymphocytes present within mesenteric lymph nodes (74 percent) and Peyer's patches (61 percent), and a large proportion of those within the popliteal nodes (40 percent) and spleen (26 percent) were of thymic origin. A fraction of these thymus-derived cells in the periphery enter a nonproliferative phase for at least seven days, while others divide.

Summary

The small-lymphocyte population is heterogeneous and comprises at least two major subpopulations: the long-lived small lymphocyte population and the short-lived. The former is relatively homogeneous and is composed primarily of thymus-derived T cells. The short-lived population is more heterogeneous; it is derived in part from bone marrow lymphoid precursors (B cells).

The long-lived T cells are concerned with antigen reactivity and form the memory cell population. They constitute the bulk of cells found in the recirculating lymphocyte pool migrating between blood, lymph fluid, various lymphoid organs, and the tissues. The short-lived lymphocytes may migrate also to various lymphoid organs such as the thymus and lymph nodes. The bone-marrow-derived lymphocyte is the precursor of transitional antibody-forming lymphocytes and plasma cells.

An unexplained phenomenon in the study of lymphocyte kinetics is the very high turnover rate of thymocytes. Many of these thymic lymphocytes die in situ and never leave the thymus gland.

Chapter 13 References

1. Aisenberg, A. C., and Wilkes, B. Immunologic status of thymectomized adult rats, *J. Immunol.* 93:75, 1964.
2. Auerbach, R. Embryogenesis of immune systems, *in* G. E. W. Wolstenholme and R. Porter (eds.), Ciba Foundation Symposium on the Thymus. Experimental and Clinical Studies, p. 39, Little, Brown and Co., Boston, 1966.
3. Basten, A., Sprent, J., and Miller, J. F. A. P. Receptor for antibody-antigen complexes used to separate T cells from B cells, *Nature (New Biol.)* 235:178, 1971.
4. Benninghoff, D. L., Tyler, R. W., and Everett, N. B. Repopulation of irradiated lymph nodes by recirculating lymphocytes, *Radiat. Res.* 37:381, 1969.
5. Bierring, F. Quantitative investigations on the lymphomyeloid system in thymectomized rats, *in* G. E. W. Wolstenholme and M. O'Connor (eds.), Ciba Foundation Symposium on Haemopoiesis, p. 185, Little, Brown and Co., Boston, 1960.
6. Billingham, R. E., Brown, J. B., De-Fendi, V., Silvers, W. K., and Steinmuller, D. Quantitative studies on the induction of tolerance of homologous tissues and on runt disease in the rat, *Ann. N.Y. Acad. Sci.* 87:457, 1960.
7. Borum, K. Pattern of cell production and cell migration in mouse thymus studied by autoradiography, *Scand. J. Haematol.* 5:339, 1968.
8. Brahim, F., and Osmond, D. G. Migration of bone marrow lymphocytes demonstrated by selective bone marrow labeling with thymidine-H³, *Anat. Rec.* 168:139, 1970.
9. Caffrey, R. W., Rieke, W. O., and Everett, N. B. Radioautographic studies of small lymphocytes in the thoracic duct of the rat, *Acta Haematol.* 28:145, 1962.
10. Cannon, D. C., and Wissler, R. W. Spleen cell migration in the immune response of the rat, *Arch. Pathol.* 84:109, 1967.
11. Chaperon, E. A., Selmer, J. C., and Claman, H. N. Migration of antibody-forming cells and antigen-sensitive precursors between spleen, thymus, and bone marrow, *Immunology* 14:553, 1968.
12. Claesson, M. H. Quantitative studies on the normal decay of lymphocytes in the thymolymphatic system, *Scand. J. Haematol.* 6:87, 1969.
13. Clark, W. G. B., Williams, C. B., and Yoffey, J. M. Thoracic duct lymphocytes following thymectomy in the guinea pig, *J. Lab. Clin. Med.* 67:439, 1966.
14. Cottier, H., Cronkite, E. P., Jansen, C. R., Rai, K. R., Singer, S., and Sipe, C. R. Studies on lymphocytes. III. Effects of extracorporeal irradiation of the circulating blood upon the lymphoreticular organs in the calf, *Blood* 24:241, 1964.
15. Coulson, A. S., and Chalmers, D. G. Response of human blood lymphocytes to tuberculin PPD in tissue culture, *Immunology* 12:417, 1967.
16. Craddock, C. G. Bone marrow lymphocytes of the rat as studied by autoradiography, *Acta Haematol.* 33:19, 1965.
17. Craddock, C. G., Winkelstein, A., Matsuyuki, Y., and Lawrence, J. S. The immune response to foreign red blood cells and the participation of short-lived lymphocytes, *J. Exp. Med.* 125:1149, 1967.
18. Cronkite, E. P., and Chanana, A. D. Lymphocytopoiesis, *in* T. J. Greenwalt and G. A. Jamieson (eds.), Formation and Destruction of Blood Cells, p. 284, J. B. Lippincott, Philadelphia, 1970.
19. Cunningham, A. J., Smith, J. B., and Mercer, E. H. Antibody formation by single cells from lymph nodes and efferent lymph of sheep, *J. Exp. Med.* 124:701, 1966.
20. Cunningham, L., Cottier, H., Wagner, H. P., Cronkite, E. P., Jansen, C. R., Rai, K. R., and Safier, S. Studies on lymphocytes. VIII. Short in vivo mitotic time of basophilic lymphoid cells in the thoracic duct of calves after simulated or effective extra-corporeal irradiation of circulating blood, *Exp. Cell Res.* 47:479, 1967.
21. Davis, A. J. S., Carter, R. L., Leuchars, E., Wallis, V., and Koller, P. C. The morphology of immune reactions, in normal, thymec-tomized and reconstituted mice. I. The response to sheep erythrocytes, *Immunology* 16:57, 1969.
22. Dustin, P. J. Remarques sur l'analyse quantitative de la croissance mitotique par la méthode stathmocinetique, *Rev. Belg. Pathol.* 25:402, 1956.
23. Ellis, S. T., Gowans, J. L., and Howard, J. C. Cellular events during the formation of antibody, *Cold Spring Harbor Symp. Quant. Biol.* 32:395, 1967.
24. Ernstrom, U., Gyllensten, L., and Sandberg, G. Regulation of output of lymphocytes from the spleen. 1. A quantitative investigation in normal, sham-operated and thymectomized guinea-pigs, *Acta Pathol. Microbiol. Scand.* 76:43, 1969.
25. Ernstrom, U., and Larsson, B. Export and import of lymphocytes in the thymus during steroid-induced involution and regeneration, *Acta Pathol. Microbiol. Scand.* 70:371, 1967.
26. Ernstrom, U., and Sandberg, G. Migration of splenic lymphocytes, *Acta Pathol. Microbiol. Scand.* 72:379, 1968.
27. Ernstrom, U., and Sandberg, G. Regulation of output of lymphocytes from the spleen. 2. A quantitative investigation in sham-operated and thymectomized guinea-pigs during steroid-induced involution and regeneration, *Acta Pathol. Microbiol. Scand.* 76:52, 1969.
28. Esteban, J. N. The differential effect of hydrocortisone on the short-lived small lymphocyte, *Anat. Rec.* 162:349, 1968.
29. Everett, N. B., and Caffrey, R. W. Radiographic studies of bone marrow small lymphocytes, *in* J. M. Yoffey (ed.), The Lymphocyte in Immunology and Haemopoiesis, p. 108, Edward Arnold, London, 1967.
30. Everett, N. B., Caffrey, R. W., and Reike, W. O. Recirculation of lymphocytes, *Ann. N.Y. Acad. Sci.* 113:887, 1964.
31. Everett, N. B., Schwartz, M. R., Tyler, R. W., and Perkins, W. D. Observations relative to the mechanism of action of antilymphocyte serum, *Fed. Proc.* 29:212, 1970.

32. Everett, N. B., and Tyler, R. W. Quantitative aspects of lymphocyte formation and destruction, *in* T. J. Greenwalt and G. A. Jamieson (eds.), Formation and Destruction of Blood Cells, p. 264, J. B. Lippincott, Philadelphia, 1970.

33. Fliedner, T. M., Keese, M., Cronkite, E. P., and Robertson, J. S. Cell proliferation in germinal centers of the rat spleen, *Ann. N.Y. Acad. Sci.* 113:578, 1964.

34. Ford, C. E. Traffic of lymphoid cells in the body, *in* G. E. W. Wolstenholme and R. Porter (eds.), Ciba Foundation Symposium on the Thymus. Experimental and Clinical Studies, p. 131, Little, Brown and Co., Boston, 1966.

35. Ford, C. E., Micklem, H. S., Evans, E. P., Gray, J. G., and Oyden, D. A. The inflow of bone marrow cells to the thymus: studies with part body irradiated mice injected with chromosome-marked bone marrow and subjected to antigenic stimulation, *Ann. N.Y. Acad. Sci.* 129:283, 1966.

36. Ford, W. L. The immunological and migratory properties of the lymphocytes recirculating through the rat spleen, *Br. J. Exp. Pathol.* 50:257, 1969.

37. Ford, W. L. The kinetics of lymphocyte recirculation within the rat spleen, *Cell Tissue Kinet.* 2:171, 1969.

38. Ford, W. L., and Gowans, J. L. The role of the lymphocyte in antibody formation. II. The influence of lymphocyte migration on the initiation of antibody formation in the isolated, perfused spleen, *Proc. R. Soc.* 168:244, 1967.

39. Goldschneider, I., and McGregor, D. D. Migration of lymphocytes and thymocytes in the rat. II. Circulation of lymphocytes and thymocytes from blood to lymph, *Lab. Invest.* 18:397, 1968.

40. Goodman, J. W., and Hodgson, G. S. Evidence for stem cells in the peripheral blood of mice, *Blood* 19:702, 1962.

41. Gowans, J. L. The recirculation of lymphocytes from blood to lymph in the rat, *J. Physiol. (Lond.)* 146:54, 1959.

42. Gowans, J. L. Life-span, recirculation, and transformation of lymphocytes, *Int. Rev. Exp. Pathol.* 5:1, 1966.

43. Gowans, J. L., and Knight, E. J. The route of re-circulation of lymphocytes in the rat, *Proc. Roy. Soc. (Biol.)* 159:257, 1964.

44. Gowans, J. L., and McGregor, D. D. The immunological activities of lymphocytes, *Prog. Allergy* 9:1, 1965.

45. Gowans, J. L., and Uhr, J. W. The carriage of immunological memory by small lymphocytes in the rat, *J. Exp. Med.* 124:1017, 1966.

46. Hall, J. G., Morris, B., Moreno, G. D., and Bessis, M. C. The ultrastructure and function of the cells in lymph following antigenic stimulation, *J. Exp. Med.* 125:91, 1967.

47. Hersey, P. The separation and [51]chromium labeling of human lymphocytes with in vivo studies of survival and migration, *Blood* 38:360, 1971.

48. Hinrichsen, K. Zellteilungen und Zelländerungen im Thymus der erwachsenen Maus, *Z. Zell Forsch.* 68:427, 1965.

49. Hudson, G., Osmond, D.G., and Roylance, P. J. Cell-populations in the bone marrow of the normal guinea-pig, *Acta Anat.* 53:234, 1963.

50. Hudson, G., and Yoffey, J. M. The passage of lymphocytes through the sinusoidal endothelium of guinea-pig bone marrow, *Proc. Roy. Soc. (Biol.)* 165:486, 1966.

51. Iorio, R. J., Chanana, A. D., Cronkite, E. P., and Joel, D. D. Studies on lymphocytes. XVI. Distribution of bovine thymic lymphocytes in the spleen and lymph nodes, *Cell Tissue Kinet.* 3:161, 1970.

52. Jerne, N. K., Nordin, A. A., and Henry, C. The agar plaque technique for recognizing antibody-producing cells, *in* B. Amos and H. Koprowski (eds.), Cell-Bound Antibodies, p. 109, Wistar Inst. Press, Philadelphia, 1963.

53. Joel, D. D., Hess, M. W., and Cottier, H. Magnitude and pattern of thymic lymphocyte migration in neonatal mice, *J. Exp. Med.* 135:907, 1972.

54. Keiser, G., Cottier, N., Odart-Chenko, B., and Bond, V. P. Autoradiographic study on the origin and fate of small lymphoid cells in

the dog bone marrow: effect of femoral artery clamping during in vivo availability, *Blood* 24:254, 1964.

55. Kindred, J. E. A quantitative study of the hemopoietic organs of young albino rats, *Am. J. Anat.* 67:99, 1940.

56. Kindred, J. E. A quantitative study of the hemopoietic organs of young adult albino rats, *Am. J. Anat.* 71:207, 1942.

57. Koster, F. The mediator of cellular immunity. II. Migration of immunologically committed lymphocytes into inflammatory exudates, *J. Exp. Med.* 133:400, 1971.

58. Koster, F., and McGregor, D. D. Rat thoracic duct lymphocytes: types that participate in inflammation, *Science* 167:1137, 1970.

59. Kotani, M., Seiki, K., Yamashita, A., and Horii, I. Lymphatic drainage of thymocytes to the circulation in the guinea pig, *Blood* 27:511, 1966.

60. Kuczynski, M. H., and Goldmanns, E. Untersuchungen über cellulare Vorgänge im Gefolge des Verdauungsprozesses auf Grund nachgelassener Präparate dargestellt und durch neue Versuche ergänzt, *Virchows Arch. (Pathol. Anat.)* 239:185, 1922.

61. Lance, E. M., and Taub, R. N. Segregation of lymphocyte populations through differential migration, *Nature* 221:841, 1969.

62. Larsson, B. Changes in blood flow through the thymus in steroid-treated guinea-pigs with calculation of thymic export and import of lymphocytes, *Acta Pathol. Microbiol. Scand.* 70:385, 1967.

63. Larsson, B. Export and import of ^{3}H-thymidine-labelled lymphocytes in the thymus of normal and steroid-treated guinea-pigs, *Acta Pathol. Microbiol. Scand.* 70:390, 1967.

64. Linna, T. J. Transport of tritium-labelled DNA from the thymus to other lymphoid organs in rabbits under normal conditions and after administration of endotoxin, *Int. Arch. Allergy Appl. Immunol.* 31:313, 1967.

65. Linna, T. J., and Liden, S. Cell migration from the bone marrow to the spleen in young guinea pigs,

Int. Arch. Allergy Appl. Immunol. 35:35, 1969.

66. Little, J. R., Brecher, G., Bradley, T. R., and Rose, S. Determination of lymphocyte turnover by continuous infusion of H³ thymidine, *Blood* 19:236, 1962.

67. McGregor, D. D., Koster, F. T., and Mackaness, G. B. The short lived small lymphocyte as a mediator of cellular immunity, *Nature* 228:855, 1970.

68. McGregor, D. D., Koster, F. T., and Mackaness, G. B. The mediator of cellular immunity. I. The life-span and circulation dynamics of the immunologically committed lymphocyte, *J. Exp. Med.* 133:389, 1971.

69. Marchesi, V. T., and Gowans, J. L. The migration of lymphocytes through the endothelium of venules in lymph nodes: an electron microscope study, *Proc. R. Soc. Lond. (Biol.)* 159:283, 1964.

70. Marshall, W. M., Valentine, F. T., and Lawrence, H. S. Cellular immunity in vitro. Clonal proliferation of antigen-stimulated lymphocytes, *J. Exp. Med.* 130:327, 1969.

71. Martin, W. J., and Miller, J. F. A. P. Cell to cell interaction in the immune response. IV. Site of action of antilymphocyte globulin, *J. Exp. Med.* 128:855, 1969.

72. Mattioli, C. A., and Tomasi, T. B., Jr. The life span of IgA plasma cells from the mouse intestine, *J. Exp. Med.* 138:452, 1973.

73. Maximow, A. The lymphocytes and plasma cells, *in* E. V. Cowdry (ed.), Special Cytology, vol. 2, p. 601, Hafner Publishing Co., New York, 1932.

74. Mellors, R. C., and Korngold, L. The cellular origin of human immunoglobulins, *J. Exp. Med.* 118:387, 1963.

75. Metcalf, D. The effect of thymectomy on the lymphoid tissues of the mouse, *Br. J. Haematol.* 6:324, 1960.

76. Metcalf, D. The nature and regulation of lymphopoiesis in the normal and neoplastic thymus, *in* G. E. W. Wolstenholme and R. Porter (eds.), Ciba Foundation Symposium on the Thymus, p. 242, Little, Brown and Co., Boston, 1966.

77. Metcalf, D. Lymphocyte kinetics in the thymus, *in* J. M. Yoffey (ed.), The Lymphocyte in Immunology, and Haemopoiesis, p. 333, Edward Arnold, London, 1967.

78. Metcalf, D., and Brumby, M. The role of the thymus in the ontogeny of the immune response, *J. Cell Physiol.* 67, suppl. 1:149, 1966.

79. Metcalf, D., and Wakonig-Vaartaja, R. Stem cell replacement in normal thymus grafts, *Proc. Soc. Exp. Biol. Med.* 115:731, 1964.

80. Michalke, W. D., Hess, M. W., Riedwyl, H., Stoner, R. D., and Cottier, H. Thymic lymphopoiesis and cell loss in newborn mice, *Blood* 33:541, 1969.

81. Micklem, H. S., and Ford, C. E. Proliferation of injected lymph node and thymus cells in lethally irradiated mice, *Transplantation* 26:436, 1960.

82. Micklem, H. S., Ford, C. E., Evans, E. P., and Gray, J. Interrelationships of myeloid and lymphoid cells: studies with chromosome-marked cells transfused into lethally irradiated mice, *Proc. R. Soc. Lond. (Biol.)* 165:78, 1966.

83. Miller, J. F. A. P. Effect of neonatal thymectomy on the immunological responsiveness of the mouse, *Proc. R. Soc. Lond. (Biol.)* 156:415, 1962.

84. Miller, J. F. A. P., and Mitchell, G. F. Influence of the thymus on antigen-reactive cells and their precursors, *in* J. Dausset, J. Hamburger, and G. Mathe (eds.), Advances in Transplantation, p. 79, Scandinavian University Books, Munksgaard, 1967.

85. Miller, J. F. A. P., and Mitchell, G. F. Cell to cell interaction in the immune response. I. Hemolysin-forming cells in neonatally thymectomized mice reconstituted with thymus or thoracic duct lymphocytes, *J. Exp. Med.* 128:801, 1968.

86. Mitchell, G. F., and Miller, J. F. A. P. Cell to cell interaction in the immune response. II. The source of hemolysin-forming cells in irradiated mice given bone marrow and thymus or thoracic duct lymphocytes, *J. Exp. Med.* 128:821, 1968.

87. Morse, S. I., and Bray, K. K. The occurrence and properties of leukocytosis and lymphocytosis-

stimulating material in the supernatant fluids of Bordetella pertussis cultures, *J. Exp. Med.* 129:523, 1969.

88. Murray, R. G., and Woods, P. A. Studies on the fate of lymphocytes, *Anat. Rec.* 150:113, 1964.

89. Norman, A., Sasaki, M. S., Ottoman, R. E., and Fingerhut, A. G. Lymphocyte lifetime in women, *Science* 147:745, 1965.

90. Nossal, G. J. V. Studies on the rate of seeding of lymphocytes from the intact guinea pig thymus, *Ann. N.Y. Acad. Sci.* 120:171, 1964.

91. Nossal, G. J. V., Cunningham, A., Mitchell, G. F., and Miller, J. F. A. P. Cell to cell interaction in the immune response. III. Chromosomal marker analysis of single antibody-forming cells in reconstituted, irradiated or thymectomized mice, *J. Exp. Med.* 128:839, 1968.

92. Oppenheim, J. J., Zbar, B., and Rapp, H. Specific inhibition of tumor cell DNA synthesis in vitro by lymphocytes from peritoneal exudate of immunized syngeneic guinea pigs, *Proc. Natl. Acad. Sci. U.S.A.* 66:1119, 1970.

93. Osmond, D. G., and Everett, N. B. Radioautographic studies of bone marrow lymphocytes in vivo and in diffusion chamber cultures, *Blood* 23:1, 1964.

94. Ottesen, J. On the age of human white cells in peripheral blood, *Acta Physiol. Scand.* 32:75, 1954.

95. Parrott, D. M. V., and de Sousa, M. A. B. The persistence of donor-derived cells in thymus grafts, lymph nodes and spleens of recipient mice, *Immunology* 13:193, 1967.

96. Parrott, D. M. V., de Sousa, M. A. B., and East, J. Thymus-dependent areas in the lymphoid organs of neonatally thymectomized mice, *J. Exp. Med.* 123:191, 1966.

97. Raff, M. C. Theta isoantigen as a marker of thymus-derived lymphocytes in mice, *Nature* 224:378, 1969.

98. Rieke, W. O., Caffrey, R. W., and Everett, N. B. Rates of proliferation and interrelationships of cells in the mesenteric lymph node of the rat, *Blood* 22:674, 1963.

99. Rieke, W. O., and Schwartz, M. R. The proliferative and immunologic

potential of thoracic duct lymphocytes from normal and thymectomized rats, *in* J. M. Yoffey (ed.), The Lymphocyte in Immunology, and Haemopoiesis, p. 224, Edward Arnold, London, 1967.

100. Robinson, S. H., Brecher, G., Laurie, I. S., and Haley, J. E. Leukocyte labeling in rats during and after continuous infusion of tritiated thymidine; implications for lymphocyte longevity and DNA reutilization, *Blood* 26:281, 1965.

101. Röpke, C., and Everett, N. B. Small lymphocyte populations in the mouse bone marrow, *Cell Tissue Kinet.* 6:499, 1973.

102. Rosenstreich, D. L., Blake, J. T., and Rosenthal, A. S. The peritoneal exudate lymphocyte. I., *J. Exp. Med.* 134:1170, 1971.

103. Rosse, C. Two morphologically and kinetically distinct populations of lymphoid cells in the bone marrow, *Nature* 227:73, 1970.

104. Rosse, C. Lymphocyte production and life-span in the bone marrow of the guinea pig, *Blood* 38:372, 1971.

105. Rosse, C. Migration of long-lived lymphocytes to the bone marrow and other lympho-myeloid tissues in normal parabiotic guinea pigs, *Blood* 40:90, 1972.

106. Rosse C., and Yoffey, J. M. The morphology of the transitional lymphocyte in guinea-pig bone marrow, *J. Anat.* 102:113, 1967.

107. Sado, T., and Makinodan, T. The cell cycle of blast cells involved in secondary antibody response, *J. Immunol.* 93:696, 1964.

108. Sainte-Marie, G., Sin, Y. M., and Chan, C. The diapedesis of lymphocytes through post capillary venules of rat lymph nodes, *Rev. Can. Biol.* 26:141, 1967.

109. Schoenberg, M. D., Moore, R. D., Stavitsky, A. B., and Gusdon, J. P. Differentiation of antibody forming cells in lymph nodes during the anamnestic response, *J. Cell. Physiol.* 71:133, 1968.

110. Schooley, J. C., and Kelly, L. S. Influence of the thymus on the output of thoracic-duct lymphocytes, *in* R. A. Good and A. E. Gabrielsen (eds.), The Thymus in Immunobiology, p. 236, Harper & Row, New York, 1964.

111. Schroder, J., and de la Chapelle, A. Fetal lymphocytes in the maternal blood, *Blood* 39:153, 1972.

112. Soderstrom, N., and Stenstrom, A. Outflow paths of cells from the lymph node parenchyma to the efferent lymphatics, *Scand. J. Haematol.* 6:186, 1969.

113. Stavitsky, A. B., and Wolf, B. Mechanisms of antibody globulin synthesis by lymphoid tissue in vitro, *Biochim. Biophys. Acta* 27:4, 1958.

114. Sterzl, J. Immunological tolerance as the result of terminal differentiation of immunologically competent cells, *Nature* 209:416, 1966.

115. Tannenberg, W. J. K. Induction of 19S antibody synthesis without stimulation of cellular proliferation, *Nature* 214:293, 1967.

116. Taylor, J. H., Woods, P. S., and Hughes, W. L. The organization and duplication of chromosomes as revealed by autoradiographic studies using tritium-labeled thymidine, *Proc. Natl. Acad. Sci. U.S.A.* 43:122, 1957.

117. Taylor, R. B. Pluripotential stem cells in mouse embryo liver, *Br. J. Exp. Pathol.* 46:376, 1965.

118. Tyan, M. L., Cole, L. J., and Nowell, P. C. Fetal liver and thymus: roles in the ontogenesis of the mouse immune system, *Transplantation* 4:79, 1966.

119. Tyler, R. W., and Everett, N. B. A radioautographic study of hemopoietic repopulation using irradiated parabiotic rats: relation to the stem cell problem, *Blood* 28:873, 1966.

120. Tyler, R. W., and Everett, N. B. Radioautographic study of cellular migration using parabiotic rats, *Blood* 39:249, 1972.

121. Tyler, R. W., Ginsburg, H., and Everett, N. B. The response of rat thoracic duct lymphocytes cultured on mouse monolayers, *in* W. O. Rieke (ed.), Proc. 3rd Annual Leukocyte Culture Conf., p. 451, Appleton-Century-Crofts, New York, 1969.

122. Umiel, T., Globerson, A., and Auerbach, R. Role of the thymus in the development of immunocompetence of embryonic liver cells in vitro, *Proc. Soc. Exp. Biol. Med.* 129:598, 1968.

123. Vincent, P. C., Borner, G., Chanana, A. D., Cronkite, E. P., Greenberg, M. L., Joel, D. D., Schiffer, L. M., and Stryckmans, P. A. Studies on lymphocytes. XIV. Measurement of DNA synthesis time in bovine thoracic duct lymphocytes by analysis of labeled mitoses and by double labeling, before and after extracorporeal irradiation of the lymph, *Cell Tissue Kinet.* 2:235, 1969.

124. Waksman, B. H., Arnason, B., and Jankovic, B. Role of the thymus in immune reactions in rats. III. Changes in the lymphoid organs of thymectomized rats, *J. Exp. Med.* 116:187, 1962.

125. Weissman, I. L. Thymus cell migration, *J. Exp. Med.* 126:291, 1967.

126. Williamson, A. R., McMichael, A. J., and Zitron, I. N. B memory cells in the propagation of stable clones of antibody-forming cells, *in* E. E. Sercarz, A. R. Williamson, and C. F. Fox (eds.), The Immune System. Genes, Receptors, Signals, p. 387, Academic Press, New York, 1974.

127. Wu, A. M., Till, J. E., Siminovitch, L., and McCulloch, E. A. Cytological evidence for a relationship between normal hematopoietic colony-forming cells and cells of the lymphoid systems, *J. Exp. Med.* 127:455, 1968.

128. Yoffey, J. M. Quantitative Cellular Haematology, Charles C Thomas, Springfield, Ill., 1960.

129. Yoffey, J. M., and Courtice, F. C. Lymphatics, Lymph and Lymphoid Tissue, Edward Arnold, London, 1956.

Chapter 14   Composition and Metabolism
of Lymphocytes and Plasma Cells

Relatively little information is available on most areas relating to the metabolism of normal lymphoid cells. Until quite recently, no reliable techniques had been developed for separating lymphocytes from other leukocytes (146). Normal plasma cells still are unobtainable in quantity. Because of the commitment of lymphoid and plasma cells to the synthesis of immunoglobulin and effector substances, attention has focused on protein and nucleic acid synthesis at the expense of other areas of metabolism.

It has been established in preceding chapters that the population of cells designated *lymphocytes* is actually several subpopulations of cells. Some of these are short-lived, others are long-lived. Some are destined to differentiate and become mature plasma cells committed to immunoglobulin synthesis; others, when appropriately activated, will take part in cellular immune reactions. When not activated, the small lymphocyte has little DNA synthetic or mitotic activity and is said to be in a prolonged G_1 or G_0 state. When exposed to appropriate antigen or nonspecific mitogen, certain lymphocytes enlarge and become metabolically more active. This process is called *transformation* or *blastogenesis*. Clearly the composition and metabolism of the lymphocyte reflect its state of activation.

Respiration: Carbohydrate, Lipid, and Energy Metabolism

Small lymphocytes have only small numbers of mitochondria, scattered ribosomes, and no well-defined endoplasmic reticulum or Golgi bodies (Chapter 12). From these morphologic features one can reasonably extrapolate that the small lymphocytes have a low rate of respiration and protein synthesis. They have only small stores of glycogen relative to the neutrophil (88, 151, 172, 173, 200) and show little staining with lipophilic dyes (17). However, they are capable of glycogen and fatty acid synthesis (73). Like the granulocyte, the lymphocyte probably has the enzymatic machinery for chain elongation of pre-existing fatty acids (16).

Unstimulated lymphocytes have a lower rate of oxygen consumption than do neutrophils, monocytes, or macrophages (88, 102, 184, 201). Similarly, among all these cells, the rate of glycolysis is lowest in the resting lymphocyte (56, 171, 201). Ascorbic acid and dinitrophenol can increase the rate of respiration (136).

In addition to a glycolytic pathway, lymphocytes apparently have an intact hexose monophosphate shunt (116). This pentose pathway probably accounts for only a few percent of total glucose utilization under normal conditions (73). Glucose uptake may be influenced by alpha adrenergic stimulation (66).

About 60 percent of the total carbon dioxide evolved from lymphocytes derives from decarboxylation of pyruvate, about 20 to 25 percent from the tricarboxylic acid cycle, and the rest from the pentose cycle (73).

Leukemic lymphoblasts and normal lymphocytes transformed by phythohemagglutinin have surface receptors for insulin. These may play an important role in cell growth and proliferation (98).

The total lipid of the lymphocyte is only about 11×10^{-12} gm/cell, which is approximately one-half the total lipid found in the neutrophil (63, 64). Phospholipids are the predominant species and lymphocytes are rich in lecithins (16, 63, 82). The normal mature lymphocyte contains about twice the amount of lipid as the cells of both chronic lymphocytic leukemia and lymphoblastic leukemia (63). This difference is attributable to the greater amounts of cholesterol esters in the normal cells.

Protein Synthesis

Little is known about the amino acid or protein metabolism of the small lymphocyte, although considerable information is available on the protein synthetic mechanisms of the immunoglobulin-synthesizing plasma cell.

One interesting feature of the amino acid metabolism of certain neoplastic lymphoid cells is their low synthetic capacity for L-asparagine. For most cells of the body, this is a nonessential amino acid; for neoplastic lymphoid cells, however, L-asparagine is required from the extracellular medium in vitro or from the extracellular fluid in vivo (21, 71, 124). In the treatment of lymphoblastic leukemia, asparaginase is used to reduce blood levels of L-asparagine and thereby deprive the lymphoblasts of this amino acid (see Chapter 21). Normal lymphoid cells and plasma cells may have a requirement also for exogenous L-asparagine, since asparaginase therapy has an immunosuppressive effect.

Lymphocytes produce a number of acid hydrolases that are lysosomal in distribution (19).

Immunoglobulin Synthesis and Assembly

The major focus in the protein metabolism of lymphocytic cells has been on the mechanisms of immunoglobulin synthesis and assembly. As outlined in Chapter 16, immunoglobulin molecules are composed of subunits of heavy and light chains. Protein synthesis in all mammalian cells takes place on polyribosomes, which are groups of individual ribosomes linked together by a messenger RNA molecule (166). The heavy (H) and light (L) chain subunits of the immunoglobulin molecules are synthesized on different-sized classes of polyribosomes in both myeloma cells and immunized lymph nodes (13, 123, 166, 175, 194, 205). The polyribosomes for heavy chains have a sedimentation rate of approximately 270 S; and those for light chains, of approximately 190 S. The details of immunoglobulin synthesis may be found in Chapter 16 and in the following references: 9, 10, 23, 96, 101, 169, 170, 175–177.

In human lymphoid cell lines synchronized in culture, production of immunoglobulins G and M is greatest

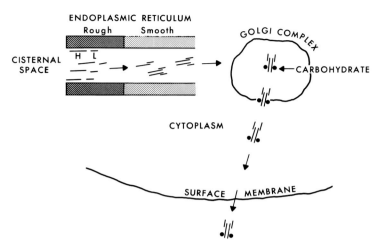

Figure 14.1 A possible model of the secretion of immunoglobulins. Heavy and light chains are synthesized and joined in the endoplasmic reticulum. The carbohydrate moiety is thought to be added in the Golgi complex, which transports the completed immunoglobulin into the cytoplasm; from there it is transported through the surface membrane to the exterior.

during the late G_1 and S phases of the cell cycle. Little synthesis occurs around the time of mitosis, indicating that transcription of the immunoglobulin genes takes place during a limited part of the mitotic cycle (22).

The sequence of events for immunoglobulin synthesis has been elucidated mainly in secretory plasma cells. However, lymphocytic cells lacking a well-developed rough endoplasmic reticulum also are capable of IgG synthesis (4, 43, 106, 177). Some lymphoma lines that synthesize IgM but do not secrete immunoglobulin may have the vast majority of polyribosomes in the free or unbound state (69, 177). Although immunoglobulin may be present at the surface of such cells, it is not secreted into the extracellular fluid.

The precise mechanism of secretion of immunoglobulin to the outside of the cell is not known. A model system based on currently known facts is shown in Fig. 14.1.

Membrane Proteins

In both normal and neoplastic lymphoid cells the proteins of the surface membrane exist in a dynamic state. They are released from the surface and replenished by a process requiring cellular respiration and active protein synthesis (36).

Recently, the reaction of antibodies to cell surface antigens has been reported to result in the formation of "caps" of immune complexes (195, 208). These caps are usually visualized by fluorescence microscopy or electron microscopy as markers localized to one region of the cell surface. They are thought to result from aggregations of surface antigens floating free on the plasma membrane, subject to movement in the plane of the membrane. Cap formation is dependent upon active cell metabolism. Edidin and Weiss (46) have suggested that only cells such as lymphocytes and fibroblasts that have leading ruffled membranes are capable of driving antigen-antibody aggregates to form caps.

There has been some effort to analyze the chemical composition of lymphocyte membranes by quantitative chemical analysis as well as by ultrastructural studies (111). Antisera specific for lymphocytes in the dividing phase have been developed (196).

Nucleic Acid Metabolism

The DNA content of the small lymphocyte, like that of other diploid cells, is approximately 8×10^{-12} gm/cell. The RNA content is approximately 2.5×10^{-12} gm/cell. Therefore the normal RNA/DNA ratio of lymphocytes is about 0.32 (62, 132). This value contrasts with the RNA/DNA ratio of 1.0 or more found in most mammalian cells (107). The morphologic counterpart of this low RNA content is a paucity of ribosomes scattered in a scanty cytoplasm. About one-half of the lymphocyte RNA is found within the nucleus (132).

A unique species of DNA found in human lymphocytes constitutes about 0.5 percent of the total DNA content. It is associated with the cytoplasmic membranes. Like other DNA species, it is synthesized in the nucleus during the S phase, but in contrast to the nuclear DNA it is then transported to the plasma membrane (67). Its function is unknown.

The small lymphocyte of the circulation does not divide and shows little DNA synthetic activity in its "basal" state (117). Although a small amount of incorporation of thymidine into DNA occurs in the basal state, it is not certain whether this represents new DNA synthesis or repair of existing DNA (86). When activated by nonspecific mitogens, the blood lymphocyte begins active synthesis of both RNA and DNA. As originally observed by Baney, Vazquez, and Dixon (5), the development of antibody-producing plasma cells similarly requires intervening DNA synthesis and mitotic division of antigen-stimulated precursor lymphoid cells. One may reasonably postulate, therefore, that some populations of lymphocytes have the potential for full expression of nucleic synthetic capacity.

The major pathways of pyrimidine and purine biosynthesis in leukocytes (27, 30, 31) were briefly reviewed in Chapter 3. A critical feature of nucleic acid metabolism in these cells is the existence of both a de novo pathway

and a salvage pathway for pyrimidine biosynthesis, but an absence of the enzymes for the early steps of purine synthesis. The activities of deoxythymidine phosphorylase, pyrimidine deoxyribosyl transferase, deoxyadenosine deaminase, and purine nucleoside phosphorylase are present at low levels in lymphocytes of normal subjects and patients with chronic lymphocytic leukemia (58). The deoxycytidine pathway has been studied in these cells as well (149). Activities for methylation of DNA purines and pyrimidines are high in lymphoblasts and low in chronic lymphocytic leukemic cells (180).

Lymphocytes probably handle interconversions of the completed purine bases in the same manner as other somatic cells. For example, lymphoid cell lines have been established from patients with the Lesch-Nyhan syndrome. Their lymphoid cells are deficient in the enzyme hypoxanthine-guanine phosphoribosyltransferase (25).

The major features of assembly of purines and pyrimidines into RNA were summarized in Chapter 3 under the discussion of granulocyte metabolism. The same discussion is applicable to lymphoid cells and is depicted schematically in Fig. 14.2 (28, 31, 37, 75, 99, 103, 132, 181, 183). The nucleolus is the site of synthesis of 45 S and 32 S precursor molecules of ribosomal RNA. The mature ribosomal RNA molecules (28 S and 18 S) are later found in the cytoplasm. The conversion of 45 S ribosomal precursor molecules to 32 S and 18 S RNA requires about two and a half to three hours (197), a slow rate compared to other mammalian cells in cultures (65). Much of the 18 S ribosomal RNA made within the nucleus is degraded at this site and never reaches the cell cytoplasm. Survival of

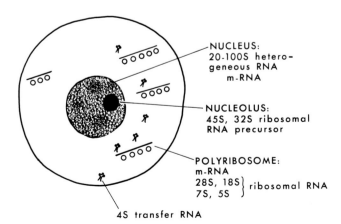

Figure 14.2 Schematic representation of the RNA metabolism of a lymphocyte. The nucleolus is the site of synthesis of ribosomal RNA precursors. The nucleus is the site of synthesis of messenger RNA and heterogeneous RNA.

newly formed 18S RNA is dependent upon the continuous synthesis of a protein or proteins (40).

The other RNA components of the cell, including heterogeneous (Hrn RNA, 20 to 100S) RNA, messenger RNA, and 4S transfer RNA, are made in the nucleus. The heterogeneous nucleus RNA has a short half-life of 90 to 120 minutes. Most is degraded within the nucleus, never reaching the cytoplasm (132). The function of heterogeneous RNA is largely unknown. It may represent RNA copies of repeated sequences of polydeoxyribonucleotides found in abundance in human DNA (20, 115).

Recent studies indicate that heterogeneous nuclear RNA contains the messenger RNA precursor that codes for amino acid sequences of immunoglobulin. Recently a nuclear premessenger RNA coding for immunoglobulin heavy chain has been isolated (188). A presumptive messenger has also been identified (92). Multiple sequences of adenylic acid appear to be associated with this messenger both in the nuclear Hrn RNA and in the cytoplasm (185). This observation was made by injecting RNA from a plasma cell tumor that contained poly-A–rich sequences into *xenopus* eggs and demonstrating that such eggs can synthesize heavy and light immunoglobulin chains.

Stevens and Williamson (186, 187) have recently presented evidence that immunoglobulin can interact with messenger RNA for heavy chain. This interaction provides a mechanism for the laboratory purification of messenger and, more importantly, may be a physiologic means of controlling the translation of messenger RNA.

Production of Hrn RNA constitutes the bulk of RNA synthesis; ribosomal RNA amounts for only about 4 percent of the total production (38, 39). A similar pattern of RNA synthesis has been noted in lymphocytes from patients with chronic lymphocytic leukemia (75).

The rate of RNA synthesis in leukemic lymphoblasts is extremely high, whereas normal unstimulated peripheral blood lymphocytes have a low rate of RNA synthesis and turnover (28, 182, 197). The abnormal lymphocytes of patients with infectious mononucleosis, as well as those of some patients with lymphosarcoma, have very high rates of RNA and DNA synthesis (28, 34, 51, 167).

Abnormal nucleic acid response of peripheral blood lymphocytes to activating agents has been described in agammaglobulinemia (33, 198), Down's syndrome (1), multiple myeloma (164), macroglobulinemia (164), and chronic lymphocytic leukemia (72, 162). Studies of nucleic acid hybridization have shown that chronic lymphocytic leukemia lymphocytes may have a species of RNA absent in normal lymphocytes (131).

Nucleic acid synthesis in human lymphoblasts is very sensitive to interruption of protein synthesis (30). Treat-

ment of lymphoblasts in vitro with cyclohexamide or puromycin rapidly reduces incorporation of uridine into RNA and thymidine into DNA, a pattern similar to that of other mammalian cells in tissue culture (50).

Relatively little progress has been made in purifying the leukocyte enzymes involved in DNA or RNA synthesis and repair; however, Wolff and his colleagues (207) reported the partial characterization of DNA-dependent RNA polymerase activity of nuclei from peripheral blood lymphocytes. Other authors have identified magnesium- and manganese-dependent RNA polymerase activities in these cells (70,91), as well as DNA polymerases (109, 110, 153). More recently, several investigators have studied the RNA-dependent DNA polymerase activity of leukemic blast cells (57, 59, 153, 165) and normal lymphocytes transformed with phytohemagglutinin (18). As discussed in Chapter 21, this enzyme activity sometimes may indicate the presence in such cells of an oncogenic RNA virus. Another recently identified lymphocyte enzyme perhaps characteristic of T cells and many populations of leukemic lymphoblasts is terminal deoxynucleotidyl transferase (114).

Lymphocytes have mechanisms for repairing damage to DNA. Such mechanisms may be inhibited by agents that act as co-carcinogens (60, 86).

Steroid Interaction

In many species the glucorcorticoids of the adrenal exert a lympholytic effect. This effect may be exerted on distinct subpopulations of lymphocytes (203). Although steroids have been known since 1944 to exert an influence on the structure and function of lymphoid tissues (44, 45), the mechanism of their lympholytic action still is largely unknown. Normal and malignant lymphoid tissues can metabolize cortisol to biologically inactive products (14). In vitro, steroids can inhibit RNA and protein synthesis in lymphoid cells, and this inhibition has been suggested as ultimately resulting in the killing of these cells in vivo (119, 204). Interference with RNA synthesis may occur via the inhibition of RNA polymerase (55, 91). Cortisol binds to lymphoid cell nuclei and nuclear histones (192, 206).

Another possible mechanism by which steroids may produce lympholysis is through blocking of glucose transport and/or phosphorylation (129) and, perhaps, the transport of other compounds. This interference may be related to the interaction of steroids with cytoplasmic receptors of lymphoid cells. A number of studies suggest that the toxic effect of glucocorticoids may be mediated by inhibition of transport (6, 89, 120–122, 126, 156, 158, 191).

Glucocorticoids are known to exert their effect on lymphoid target cells whether or not the cells are in a proliferative state as, for example, after phytohemagglutinin stimulation (24). Steroids are said to be "cell-cycle nonspecific" in their effect on lymphoid target cells; they are distinguished in their mode of action from "cell-cycle specific" agents such as methotrexate, whose major cytotoxic effects are exerted during the period when the neoplastic cell is synthesizing DNA.

The metabolic effects of steroids on lymphoid cells may result from either: (a) glucocorticoid actions that can be demonstrated at physiological concentrations and are triggered by the interaction of steroid with glucocorticoid-specific receptors in the cell cytoplasm, or (b) nonspecific effects of steroids that are unrelated to glucocorticoid potency, develop only at high concentrations, and may not be physiologically or pharmacologically significant (128, 130).

Many hormonally active tissues contain cytoplasmic receptors for steroids. For example, estrogen receptors have been identified in uterine and breast tissues (68, 87), and androgen receptors exist in the prostate (2). Similar cortisol receptors have been demonstrated in lymphoid tissues (100, 130) including lymphoblasts (108). After the steroid binds to the receptor in the cytoplasm, the complex then migrates and binds to receptors in the nucleus (161).

An important, relatively recent observation is that the responsiveness of lymphoid tumors to glucocorticoids may be determined by the presence or absence of these specific steroid receptors at the cell surface (12, 94, 159). This observation obviously has important implications for the treatment of lymphoid neoplasms, since glucocorticoids are used extensively for this class of malignancy (32). Baxter and Forsham, as well as Claman, recently have reviewed the tissue effects of glucocorticoids (11, 26).

Lymphocyte Activation

Lymphocytes cultured in vitro rarely synthesize DNA and rarely divide. Addition of phytohemagglutinin (PHA), an extract of the kidney bean (*Phaseolus vulgaris*), stimulates the majority of the cells to enlarge, synthesize DNA, and undergo mitosis within 48 to 72 hours (133). The cells increase their cytoplasmic volume and, also, the number of free ribosomes increases. The Golgi apparatus increases in size and complexity and nucleoli become prominent (84, 193, 209).

These activated cells resemble the large pyroninophilic (RNA-staining) lymph node cells that appear after antigenic stimulation in vivo (134, 137, 199). Similar

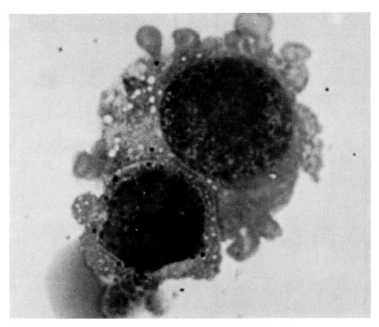

Figure 14.3 Activated lymphocytes cultured with phytohemagglutinin for 72 hours. The smaller cell has incorporated tritiated thymidine, and grains may be observed over the nucleus.

changes, although of smaller magnitude, are observed when specific antigen is added to sensitized lymphocytes in vitro (48, 138). Morphologic changes preceding mitosis are barely detectable by the end of the first 24 hours of culture. In the next 24 to 48 hours, large pyronine-staining blast cells appear (Fig. 14.3) (49, 168).

Activation of lymphocytes by a specific antigen or a nonspecific mitogen is characterized by a multiplicity of metabolic changes: increased RNA, protein, and DNA synthesis; increased pyrimidine nucleotide synthesis; changes in isozyme pattern and phosphorylation of nuclear protein; increased glucose utilization by several pathways; and changes in lysosomal enzymes (190). Among this multitude of biochemical changes, those that are primary and critical to leukocyte activation are difficult to identify. Conversion of the lymphocyte from a resting G_0 cell to a replicating cell clearly requires activation of the DNA synthetic mechanism, although the "switch-on" device is still unidentified. Proposed mechanisms of activation include release of lysosomal enzymes with attack on nuclear chromatin (78), and mediation of activation via the cyclic-AMP system of the lymphocyte (77, 118, 152). The enzyme that degrades cyclic-AMP (phosphodiesterase) is localized in the lymphocyte membrane (42). To date, neither has been solidly established as the mechanism of activation.

Among the earliest metabolic changes induced by phy-

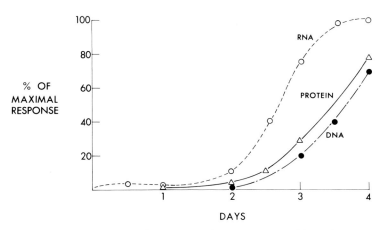

Figure 14.4 Sequence of events in the activation of lymphocytes by mitogen. After addition of phytohemagglutinin to lymphocytes cultured in vitro, the synthesis of RNA increases before any detectable change in the synthetic rates for protein and DNA.

tohemagglutinin is an exponential increase in RNA and RNA precursor synthesis (41, 113, 127, 197), and an increase in acetylation of nuclear chromatin (140) and phosphorylation and dephosphorylation of nuclear proteins (95, 160). The physical characteristics of deoxyribonucleoprotein alter with activation (93). DNA may be excreted from the cell (155). Within 2 to 4 hours after the addition of phytohemagglutinin, DNA-dependent RNA polymerase activity increases (70). Somewhat later, as shown in Fig. 14.4, there is an increase in protein synthesis (83, 127, 174). Whether this increased synthesis includes gamma globulin is not entirely clear in the literature (61).

Polydispersed RNA, which has a short half-life and is not a precursor of ribosomal RNA, comprises most of the RNA synthesized in the system during the first 20 hours after stimulation (37). A new species of low-molecular RNA may also be made in the lymphocyte during blastogenic transformation (80). The heterogeneously sedimenting nuclear RNA has an average base composition similar to that of DNA (43 percent guanine plus cytosine). It has sometimes been designated *giant* nuclear RNA since its sedimentation coefficient may be as large as 100 S (3, 202).

Within 4 hours of the addition of mitogen, dramatic changes occur in carbohydrate metabolism, including increased glucose utilization, pyruvate and lactate production, and glycogen synthesis (73). By 24 hours, considerable glycogen accumulates in the cells (141) and the activities of some enzymes involved in glucose catabolism are increased (8, 78, 142). Overall carbon dioxide production

is increased (73, 81), as is fatty acid synthesis. Changes dependent upon oxygen concentration occur in lactic dehydrogenase isozymes (74, 147, 148). Some of these changes in carbohydrate metabolism depend also on concomitant protein synthesis.

Changes in phospholipid metabolism may occur within minutes or hours following the addition of phytohemagglutinin. These may be caused by the interaction of mitogen with the lymphocyte membrane (52–54, 82, 90, 97, 112) and may be important in inducing changes in membrane functions such as pinocytosis (154), potassium uptake (145), and transport of other molecules (125).

These early changes in cell metabolism caused by mitogen are followed by an increase in DNA synthesis, which reaches significant levels between 60 and 70 hours after addition of phytohemagglutinin (127). The concomitants of this increased DNA synthesis are increases in activity of DNA polymerase (109, 110) and of thymidine and TMP kinases (110, 150). RNA-dependent DNA polymerase activity has been reported to increase also (139). Mitosis then follows. The sequence of changes in RNA protein and DNA synthesis are seen in Fig. 14.4 (127). Concomitant with augmented DNA synthesis, DNA polymerase activity increases 30- to 100-fold (109, 110). Rather surprisingly, acid phosphatase activity increases at about the same time (24 to 48 hours), and acid phosphatase-rich granules appear in the cytoplasm (76, 78, 79). ATP'ase activity also increases (47). If 6-mercaptoethanol is added during the period of DNA synthesis, polyploidy and chromosome aberrations result (85).

Many of the events reported in phytohemagglutinin-stimulated lymphocytes have been documented also when the cells are activated by antigen (15) or certain heavy metals (163). Lymphoid cells from animals immunized 24 hours previously show enhanced synthesis of several species of RNA, including ribosomal (28 S and 18 S) and rapidly labeled, unstable, 6 to 12 S RNA (35, 105). Interestingly, spleen cells from hyperimmune rabbits continue to synthesize antibody in vitro for at least 18 hours after RNA synthesis has been interrupted by actinomycin-D (104). This observation suggests a messenger RNA for antibody synthesis with a relatively long half-life.

The activation of lymphocytes by phytohemagglutinin may be inhibited by oubain (144) and by mycoplasma infection (7).

Plasma Cells

Except for detailed knowledge of the synthesis and assembly of immunoglobulins, relatively little is known about the metabolism of plasma cells.

Histochemical studies reveal the presence of succinic dehydrogenase, cytochrome oxidase, and acid phosphatase; and the absence of alkaline phosphatase and free lipid. Only small amounts of glycogen and phospholipids are present (143). The cells possess the machinery for the tricarboxylic acid cycle and glycolysis as well as for the pentose shunt pathway (189).

Summary

The important features of lymphocyte–plasma-cell metabolism relate to (a) the metabolic changes associated with blast transformation; (b) the synthesis, assembly, and secretion of immunoglobulins; and (c) the interaction of certain classes of lymphocytes with the adrenoglucocorticoids.

Chapter 14 References

1. Agarwal, S. S., Blumberg, B. S., Gerstley, B. J. S., London, W. T., Sutnick, A. I., and Loeb, L. A. DNA polymerase activity as an index of lymphocyte stimulation: studies in Down's syndrome, *J. Clin. Invest.* 49:161, 1970.
2. Anderson, K. M., and Liao, S. Selective retention of dihydrotestosterone by prostatic nuclei, *Nature* 219:277, 1968.
3. Attardi, G., Parnas, H., Hwang, M. I. H., and Attardi, B. Giant-sized rapidly labeled nuclear ribonucleic acid and cytoplasmic messenger ribonucleic acid in immature duck erythrocytes, *J. Mol. Biol.* 20:145, 1966.
4. Avrameas, S., and Leduc, E. H. Detection of simultaneous antibody synthesis in plasma cells and specialized lymphocytes in rabbit lymph nodes, *J. Exp. Med.* 131:1137, 1970.
5. Baney, R. N., Vazquez, J. J., and Dixon, F. J. Cellular proliferation in relation to antibody synthesis, *Proc. Soc. Exp. Biol. Med.* 109:1, 1962.
6. Baran, D. T., Lichtman, M. A., and Peck, W. A. Alpha-aminoisobutyric acid transport in leukemic lymphocytes: in vitro characteristics and inhibition by cortisol and cycloheximide, *J. Clin. Invest.* 51:2181, 1972.
7. Barile, M. F., and Leventhal, B. G. Possible mechanism for mycoplasma inhibition of lymphocyte transformation induced by phytohemagglutinin, *Nature* 219:751, 1968.
8. Barker, B. E., and Farnes, P. Histochemistry of blood cells treated with pokeweed mitogen, *Nature* 214:787, 1967.
9. Baumal, R., Potter, M., and Scharff, M. D. Synthesis, assembly and secretion of gamma globulin in mouse myeloma cells. III. *J. Exp. Med.* 134:1316, 1971.
10. Baumal, R., and Scharff, M. Synthesis, assembly and secretion of IgG$_{2a}$ by the mouse plasma cell tumors MOPC173 and MOPC494, *Fed. Proc.* 29:577, 1970 (abstract).
11. Baxter, J. D., and Forsham, P. H. Tissue effects of glucocorticoids, *Am. J. Med.* 53:573, 1972.
12. Baxter, J. D., Harris, A. W., Tomkins, G. M., and Cohn, M. Glucocorticoid receptors in lymphoma cells in culture: relationship to glucocorticoid killing activity, *Science* 171:189, 1971.
13. Becker, M. J., and Rich, A. Polyribosomes of tissues producing antibodies, *Nature* 212:142, 1966.
14. Berliner, M. L., and Dougherty, T. F. Interconversion of cortisol and cortisone by normal and leukemic murine lymphocytes, *Acta Un. Int. Cancr.* 20:1133, 1964.
15. Black, M. M., and Ansley, H. R. Antigen-induced changes in lymphoid cell histones, *J. Cell Biol.* 26:201, 1965.
16. Blomstrand, R. Fatty acid synthesis in human lymphocytes, *Acta Chem. Scand.* 20:1122, 1966.
17. Bloom, M. L., and Wislocki, G. B. The localization of lipids in human blood and bone marrow cells, *Blood* 5:79, 1950.
18. Bobrow, S. N., Smith, R. G., Reitz, M. S., and Gallo, R. C. Stimulated normal human lymphocytes contain a ribonuclease-sensitive DNA polymerase distinct from viral RNA-directed DNA polymerase, *Proc. Natl. Acad. Sci. U.S.A.* 69:3228, 1972.
19. Bowers, W. E. Lysosomes in rat thoracic duct lymphocytes, *J. Exp. Med.* 136:1394, 1972.
20. Britten, R. J., and Kohne, D. E. Repeated sequences in DNA, *Science* 161:529, 1968.
21. Broome, J. D. Evidence that the L-asparaginase of guinea pig serum is responsible for its antilymphoma effects; I. Properties of the L-asparaginase of guinea pig serum in relation to those of the antilymphoma substance, *J. Exp. Med.* 118:99, 1963.
22. Buell, D. N., and Fahey, J. L. Limited periods of gene expression in immunoglobulin synthesizing cells, *Science* 164:1524, 1969.
23. Buxbaum, J., Solla, S., Scharff, M. D., and Franklin, E. C. Synthesis and assembly of immunoglobulins by malignant human plasmacytes and lymphocytes. II. Heterogeneity of assembly in cells producing IgM proteins, *J. Exp. Med.* 133:1118, 1971.
24. Caron, G. A. Prednisolone inhibition of DNA synthesis by human lymphocytes induced in vitro by phytohemagglutinin, *Int. Arch. Allergy Appl. Immunol.* 32:191, 1967.
25. Choi, K. W., and Bloom, A. D. Biochemically marked lymphocytoid lines: establishment of Lesch-Nyhan cells, *Science* 170:89, 1970.
26. Claman, H. N. Corticosteroids and lymphoid cells, *N. Engl. J. Med.* 287:388, 1972.
27. Cline, M. J. Metabolism of the circulating leukocyte, *Physiol. Rev.* 45:674, 1965.
28. Cline, M. J. Ribonucleic acid biosynthesis in human leukocytes: the fate of rapidly labeled RNA in normal and abnormal leukocytes, *Blood* 28:650, 1966.
29. Cline, M. J. Isolation and characterization of RNA from human leukocytes, *J. Lab. Clin. Med.* 68:33, 1966.
30. Cline, M. J. Leukocyte metabolism, *in* A. S. Gordon (ed.), Regulation of Hematopoiesis, p. 1045, Appleton-Century-Crofts, New York, 1970.
31. Cline, M. J. Metabolism of RNA in normal and leukemic leukocytes, *Acta Haematol.* 45:174, 1971.
32. Cline, M. J. Adrenal steroids in leukemia and lymphoma, *Cancer Chemother. Rep.* 58:521, 1974.
33. Cline, M. J., and Fudenberg, H. H. Defective RNA synthesis in lymphocytes from patients with primary agammaglobulinemia, *Science* 150:311, 1965.
34. Cline, M. J., and MacKenzie, M. R. Synthesis of macroglobulins in vitro, *Nature* 214:496, 1967.
35. Cohen, E. P. Partial characterization by molecular hybridization of RNAs from immunocompetent cells exposed to antigen, *Nature* 221:685, 1969.
36. Cone, R. E., Marchalonis, J. J., and Rolley, R. T. Lymphocyte membrane dynamics, *J. Exp. Med.* 134:1373, 1971.
37. Cooper, H. L. Ribonucleic acid metabolism in lymphocytes stimulated by phytohemagglutinin, *J. Biol. Chem.* 243:34, 1968.
38. Cooper, H. L. Alterations in RNA metabolism in lymphocytes during the shift from resting state to active growth, *in* R. Baserga (ed.), Biochemistry of Cell Division, Charles C Thomas, Springfield, Ill., 1969.

39. Cooper, H. L. Ribosomal ribonucleic acid production and growth regulation in human lymphocytes, *J. Biol. Chem.* 244:1946, 1969.

40. Cooper, H. L., and Gibson, E. M. Control of synthesis and wastage of ribosomal ribonucleic acid in lymphocytes, *J. Biol. Chem.* 246:5059, 1971.

41. Cooper, H. L., and Rubin, A. D. RNA metabolism in lymphocytes stimulated by phytohemagglutinin: initial responses to phytohemagglutinin, *Blood* 25:1014, 1965.

42. Coulson, A. S., and Kennedy, L. A. Lymphocyte membrane enzymes. II. Cyclic 3′, 5′-adenosine monophosphatase located on unstimulated human small lymphocyte nuclear membranes, *Blood* 38:485, 1971.

43. De Petris, S., and Karlsbad, G. Localization of antibodies by electron microscopy in developing antibody-producing cells, *J. Cell Biol.* 26:759, 1965.

44. Dougherty, T., and White, A. Influence of hormones on lymphoid tissue structure and function. Role of pituitary adrenotrophic hormone in regulation of lymphocytes and other cellular elements of the blood, *Endocrinology* 35:1, 1944.

45. Dougherty, T., and White, A. Evaluation of alterations produced in lymphoid tissue by pituitary adrenal cortical secretion, *J. Lab. Clin. Med.* 32:584, 1947.

46. Edidin, M., and Weiss, A. Antigen cap formation in cultured fibroblasts: a reflection of membrane fluidity and of cell motility, *Proc. Natl. Acad. Sci. U.S.A.* 69:2456, 1972.

47. Ellegaard, J., and Dimitrov, N. V. ATP-ase activity of lymphocytes from normal individuals and patients with cancer, *Cancer* 30:881, 1972.

48. Elves, M. W., Roath, S., and Israëls, M. C. G. The response of lymphocytes to antigen challenge in vitro, *Lancet* i:806, 1963.

49. Elves, M. W., and Wilkinson, J. F. The effects of phytohaemagglutinin on normal and leukaemic leucocytes when cultured in vitro, *Exp. Cell Res.* 30:200, 1963.

50. Ennis, H. L. Synthesis of ribonucleic acid in L cells during inhibition of protein synthesis by cycloheximide, *Mol. Pharmacol.* 2:543, 1966.

51. Epstein, L. B., and Brecher, G. DNA and RNA synthesis of circulating atypical lymphocytes in infectious mononucleosis, *Blood* 25:197, 1965.

52. Fisher, D. B., and Mueller, G. C. An early alteration in the phospholipid metabolism of lymphocytes by phytohemagglutinin, *Proc. Natl. Acad. Sci. U.S.A.* 60:1396, 1968.

53. Fisher, D. B., and Mueller, G. C. The stepwise acceleration of phosphatidyl choline synthesis in phytohemagglutinin-treated lymphocytes, *Biochim. Biophys. Acta* 176:316, 1969.

54. Fisher, D. B., and Mueller, G. C. N-acetyl-D-galactosamine inhibits the early phospholipid response by lymphocytes to phytohemagglutinin, *Nature* 221:566, 1969.

55. Fox, K. E., and Gabourel, J. D. Effect of cortisol on the RNA polymerase system of rat thymus, *Mol. Pharmacol.* 3:479, 1967.

56. Frei, J., Borel, C., Horvath, G., Cullity, B., and Vannotti, A. Enzymatic studies in the different types of normal and leukemic human white cells, *Blood* 18:317, 1961.

57. Gallo, R. C. RNA-dependent DNA polymerase in viruses and cells: views on the current state, *Blood* 39:117, 1972.

58. Gallo, R. C., and Perry, S. The enzymatic mechanisms for deoxythymidine synthesis in human leucocytes. IV. Comparisons between normal and leukemic leukocytes, *J. Clin. Invest.* 48:105, 1969.

59. Gallo, R. C., Yang, S. S., and Ting, R. C. RNA dependent DNA polymerase of human acute leukaemic cells, *Nature* 228:927, 1970.

60. Gaudin, D., Gregg, R. S., and Yielding, K. L. DNA repair inhibition: a possible mechanism of action of co-carcinogens, *Biochem. Biophys. Res. Commun.* 45:630, 1971.

61. Girard, J. P. Antibody synthesis in vitro by human peripheral lymphocytes, *Int. Arch. Allergy Appl. Immunol.* 32:294, 1967.

62. Glen, A. C. A. Measurement of DNA and RNA in human peripheral blood lymphocytes, *Clin. Chem.* 13:299, 1967.

63. Gottfried, E. L. Lipids of human leukocytes: relation to cell type, *J. Lipid Res.* 8:321, 1967.

64. Gottfried, E. L. Lipid patterns of leukocytes in health and disease, *Semin. Hematol.* 9:241, 1972.

65. Greenberg, H., and Penman, S. Methylation and processing of ribosomal RNA in HeLa cells, *J. Mol. Biol.* 21:527, 1966.

66. Hadden, J. W., Hadden, E. M., and Good, R. A. Alpha adrenergic stimulation of glucose uptake in human erythrocyte, lymphocyte and lymphoblast, *Exp. Cell Res.* 68:217, 1971.

67. Hall, M. R., Meinke, W., Goldstein, D. A., and Lerner, R. A. Synthesis of cytoplasmic membrane-associated DNA in lymphocyte nucleus, *Nature (New Biol.)* 234:227, 1971.

68. Hamilton, T. H. Control by estrogen of genetic transcription and translation, *Science* 161:649, 1968.

69. Hammond, E. Ultrastructural characteristics of surface IgM reactive malignant lymphoid cells, *Exp. Cell Res.* 59:359, 1970.

70. Handmaker, S. D., and Graef, J. W. The effect of phytohemagglutinin on the DNA-dependent RNA polymerase activity of nuclei isolated from human lymphocytes, *Biochim. Biophys. Acta* 199:95, 1970.

71. Handschumacher, R. E. Mechanisms of control of tumor growth: asparaginase and asparagine analogs, *in* Exploitable Molecular Mechanisms of Neoplasia, 22nd Annual Symposium on Fundamental Cancer Research, M. D. Anderson Hospital, Houston, Tex., 1968.

72. Havemann, K., and Rubin, A. D. The delayed response of chronic lymphocytic leukemia lymphocytes to phytohemagglutinin in vitro, *Proc. Soc. Exp. Biol. Med.* 127:668, 1968.

73. Hedeskov, C. J. Early effects of phytohemagglutinin on glucose metabolism of normal human lymphocytes, *Biochem. J.* 110:373, 1968.

74. Hellung-Larsen, R., and Andersen, P. Kinetics of oxygen-induced changes in lactate dehydrogenase

isoenzymes of human lymphocytes in culture, *Exp. Cell Res.* 54:201, 1969.

75. Henry, P., Reich, P., Karon, M., and Weissman, S. M. Characteristics of RNA synthesized in vitro by lymphocytes of chronic lymphocytic leukemia, *J. Lab. Clin. Med.* 69:47, 1967.
76. Hirschhorn, K., and Hirschhorn, R. Role of lysosomes in the lymphocyte response, *Lancet* i:1046, 1965.
77. Hirschhorn, R., Grossman, J., and Weissmann, G. Effect of cyclic 3'-5'-adenosine monophosphate and theophyline on lymphocyte transformation, *Proc. Soc. Exp. Biol. Med.* 133:1361, 1970.
78. Hirschhorn, R., Hirschhorn, K., and Weissmann, G. Appearance of hydrolase rich granules in human lymphocytes induced by phytohemagglutinin and antigens, *Blood* 30:84, 1967.
79. Hirschhorn, R., Kaplan, J. M., Goldberg, A. F., Hirschhorn, K., and Weissmann, G. Acid phosphatase-rich granules in human lymphocytes induced by phytohemagglutinin, *Science* 147:55, 1965.
80. Howard, E., and Stubblefield, E. Low molecular weight nuclear RNA in phytohemagglutinin treated and untreated human lymphocytes, *Exp. Cell Res.* 70:460, 1972.
81. Hrachovec, J. P. The effect of phytohemagglutinin on glucose-V-C^{14} oxidation by peritoneal and blood white cells of the rat, *J. Cell Physiol.* 67:399, 1966.
82. Huber, H., Strieder, N., Winkler, H., Reiser, G., and Koppelstaetter, K. Studies on the incorporation of ^{14}C-sodium acetate into the phospholipids of phytohemagglutinin-stimulated and unstimulated lymphocytes, *Br. J. Haematol.* 15:203, 1968.
83. Huber, H., Winkler, H., Reiser, G., Huber, C., Gabl, F., and Braunsteiner, H. Eigenschaften und subcelluläre Lokalisation neugebildeter proteine menschlicher Lymphocyten in vitro mit und ohne Phytohämagglutinin Zausatz, *Klin. Wochenschr.* 45:204, 1967.
84. Inman, D. R., and Cooper, E. H. Electron microscopy of human lymphocytes stimulated by phyto-

haemagglutinin, *J. Cell Biol.* 19:441, 1963.
85. Jackson, J. F., and Killander, D. DNA synthesis in phytohemagglutinin-stimulated human leukocyte cultures treated with B-mercaptoethanol, *Exp. Cell Res.* 33:459, 1964.
86. Jacobs, A. J., O'Brien, R. L., Parker, J. W., and Paolilli, P. DNA repair following exposure of human lymphocytes to 4-nitroquinoline-1-oxide, *Int. J. Cancer* 10:118, 1972.
87. Jensen, E. V., and Jacobson, H. I. Basic guides to the mechanisms of estrogen action, *in* G. Pincus (ed.), Recent Progress in Hormone Research, vol. 18, p. 387, Academic Press, New York, 1962.
88. Karnovsky, M. L. Metabolic basis of phagocytic activity, *Physiol. Rev.* 42:143, 1962.
89. Kattwinkel, J., and Munck, A. Activities *in vitro* of glucocorticoids and related steroids on glucose uptake by rat thymus cell suspensions, *Endocrinology* 79:387, 1966.
90. Kay, J. E. Phytohemagglutinin: an early effect on lymphocyte lipid metabolism, *Nature* 219:172, 1968.
91. Kehoe, J. M., Lust, G., and Beisel, W. R. Lymphoid tissue-corticosteroid interaction: an early effect on both Mg^{2+}-Mn^{2+}-activated RNA polymerase activities, *Biochim. Biophys. Acta* 174:761, 1969.
92. Kemper, B., and Rich, A. Identification of presumptive histone messenger RNA in rapidly labelled polysomal RNA of mouse myelomas, *Biochim. Biophys. Acta* 319:364, 1973.
93. Killander, D., and Rigler, R. Activation of deoxyribonucleoprotein in human leucocytes stimulated by phytohemagglutinin, *Exp. Cell Res.* 54:163, 1969.
94. Kirkpatrick, A. F., Milholland, R. J., and Rosen, F. Stereospecific glucocorticoid binding to subcellular fractions of the sensitive and resistant lymphosarcoma P 1798, *Nature (New Biol.)* 232:216, 1971.
95. Kleinsmith, L. J., Allfrey, V. G., and Mirsky, A. E. Phosphorylation of nuclear protein early in the course of gene activation in lymphocytes, *Science* 154:780, 1966.

96. Knopf, P. M., Parkhouse, R. M. E., and Lennox, E. S. Biosynthesis of units of an immunoglobulin heavy chain, *Proc. Natl. Acad. Sci. U.S.A.* 58:2288, 1967.
97. Kornfeld, S., and Kornfeld, R. Solubilization and partial characterization of a phytohemagglutinin receptor site from human erythrocytes, *Proc. Natl. Acad. Sci. U.S.A.* 63:1439, 1969.
98. Krug, U., Krug, F., and Cuatrecasas, P. Emergence of insulin receptors on human lymphocytes during in vitro transformation, *Proc. Natl. Acad. Sci. U.S.A.* 69:2604, 1972.
99. Kuechler, E., and Rich, A. Two rapidly labeled RNA species in the polysomes of antibody-producing lymphoid tissue, *Proc. Natl. Acad. Sci. U.S.A.* 63:520, 1969.
100. Lang, R. F., and Stevens, W. Evidence for intranuclear receptor sites for cortisol in lymphatic tissue, *J. Reticuloendothel. Soc.* 7:294, 1970.
101. Laskov, R., and Scharff, M. D. Synthesis, assembly, and secretion of gamma globulin by mouse myeloma cells, I., *J. Exp. Med.* 131:515, 1970.
102. Laszlo, J. Energy metabolism of human leukemic lymphocytes and granulocytes, *Blood* 30:151, 1967.
103. Lazda, V. A. The metabolism of messenger RNA synthesized after primary immunization, *J. Immunol.* 101:359, 1968.
104. Lazda, V. A., and Starr, J. L. The stability of messenger ribonucleic acid in antibody synthesis, *J. Immunol.* 95:254, 1965.
105. Lazda, V. A., Starr, J. L., and Rachmeler, M. The synthesis of ribonucleic acid during early antibody induction, *J. Immunol.* 101:349, 1968.
106. Leduc, E. H., Avrameas, S., and Bouteille, M. Ultrastructural localization of antibody in differentiating plasma cells, *J. Exp. Med.* 127:109, 1968.
107. Leslie, I. The nucleic acid content of tissues and cells, *in* E. Chargaff and J. N. Davidson (eds.), The Nucleic Acids: Chemistry and Biology, vol. 2, p. 9, Academic Press, New York, 1955.
108. Lippman, M., Halterman, R., Perry, S., Leventhal, B., and Thompson, E. B. Glucocorticoid binding proteins

in human leukemic lymphoblasts, *Nature (New Biol.)* 242:157, 1973.

109. Loeb, L. A., Agarwal, S. S., and Woodside, A. M. Induction of DNA polymerase in human lymphocytes by phytohemagglutinin, *Proc. Natl. Acad. Sci. U.S.A.* 61:827, 1968.

110. Loeb, L. A., Ewald, J. L., and Agarwal, S. S. DNA polymerase and DNA replication during lymphocyte transformation, *Cancer Res.* 30:2514, 1970.

111. Lopes, J., Nachbar, M., Zucker-Franklin, D., and Silber, R. Lymphocyte plasma membranes: analysis of proteins and glycoproteins by SDS-gel electrophoresis, *Blood* 41:131, 1973.

112. Lucas, D. O., Shohet, S. B., and Merler, E. Changes in phospholipid metabolism which occur as a consequence of mitogenic stimulation of lymphocytes, *J. Immunol.* 106:768, 1971.

113. Lucas, Z. J. Pyrimidine nucleotide synthesis: regulatory control during transformation of lymphocytes in vitro, *Science* 156:1237, 1967.

114. McCaffrey, R. P., et al. Terminal deoxynucleotidyl transferase (TT): a thymus-specific enzyme in acute lymphoblastic leukemia (ALL) cells, prog. 66th ann. mtg. Am. Soc. Clin. Invest., p. 51a, 1974.

115. McCarthy, B. J. Arrangement of base sequences in deoxyribonucleic acid, *Bact. Rev.* 31:215, 1967.

116. MacHaffie, R. A., and Wang, C. H. The effect of phytohemagglutinin upon glucose catabolism in lymphocytes, *Blood* 29:640, 1967.

117. McIntyre, O. R., and Ebaugh, F. G., Jr. The effect of phytohemagglutinin on leucocyte cultures as measured by P^{32} incorporation in the DNA, RNA, and acid soluble fractions, *Blood* 19:443, 1962.

118. MacManus, J. P., and Whitfield, J. F. Stimulation of DNA synthesis and mitotic activity of thymic lymphocytes by cyclic adenosine 3', 5'-monophosphate, *Exp. Cell Res.* 58:188, 1969.

119. Makman, M. H., Dvorkin, B., and White, A. Influence of cortisol on the utilization of precursors of nucleic acids and protein by lymphoid cells in vitro, *J. Biol. Chem.* 243:1485, 1968.

120. Makman, M. H., Dvorkin, B., and White, A. Evidence for induction by cortisol *in vitro* of a protein inhibitor of transport and phosphorylation processes in rat thymocytes, *Proc. Natl. Acad. Sci. U.S.A.* 68:1269, 1971.

121. Makman, M. H., Nakagawa, S., and White, A. Studies of the mode of action of adrenal steroids on lymphocytes, *Recent Prog. Horm. Res.* 23:195, 1967.

122. Makman, M. H., Nakagawa, S., Dvorkin, B., and White, A. Inhibitory effects of cortisol and antibiotics on substrate entry and ribonucleic acid synthesis in rat thymocytes *in vitro*, *J. Biol. Chem.* 245:2556, 1970.

123. Manner, G., and Gould, B. S. Ribosomal aggregates in gamma-globulin synthesis in the rat, *Nature* 205:670, 1965.

124. Mashburn, L. T., and Wriston, J. C., Jr. Tumor inhibitory effect of L-asparaginase from Escherichia coli, *Arch. Biochem. Biophys.* 105:450, 1964.

125. Mendelsohn, J., Skinner, A., and Kornfeld, S. The rapid induction by phytohemagglutinin of increased alpha-aminoisobutyric acid uptake by lymphocytes, *J. Clin. Invest.* 50:818, 1971.

126. Morita, Y., and Munck, A. Effect of glucocorticoid *in vivo* and *in vitro* on net glucose uptake and amino acid incorporation by rat thymus cells, *Biochim. Biophys. Acta* 93:150, 1964.

127. Mueller, G. C., and Le Mahieu, M. Induction of ribonucleic acid synthesis in human leucocytes by phytohemagglutinin, *Biochim. Biophys. Acta* 114:100, 1966.

128. Munck, A. Steroid concentration and tissue integrity as factors determining the physiological significance of effects of adrenal steroids *in vitro*, *Endocrinology* 77:356, 1965.

129. Munck, A. Metabolic site and time course of cortisol action on glucose uptake, lactic acid output and glucose 6-phosphate levels of rat thymus cells in vitro, *J. Biol. Chem.* 243:1039, 1968.

130. Munck, A., and Brinck-Johnsen, T. Specific and nonspecific physicochemical interactions of glucocorticoids and related steroids with rat thymus cells *in vitro*, *J. Biol. Chem.* 243:5556, 1968.

131. Neiman, P. E., and Henry, P. H. Ribonucleic acid-deoxyribonucleic acid hybridization and hybridization competition studies of the rapidly labeled ribonucleic acid from normal and chronic lymphocytic leukemia lymphocytes, *Biochemistry* 8:275, 1969.

132. Neiman, P. E., and Henry, P. H. An analysis of the rapidly synthesized ribonucleic acid of the normal human lymphocyte by agarose-polyacrylamide gel electrophoresis, *Biochemistry* 10:1733, 1971.

133. Nowell, P. C. Phytohemagglutinin: an initiator of mitosis in cultures of normal human leukocytes, *Cancer Res.* 20:462, 1960.

134. Oppenheim, J. J. Relationship of in vitro lymphocyte transformation to delayed hypersensitivity in guinea pigs and man, *Fed. Proc.* 27:21, 1968.

135. Oppenheim, J. J., Whang, J., and Frei, E., III. Immunologic and cytogenetic studies of chronic lymphocytic leukemic cells, *Blood* 26:121, 1965.

136. Pachman, L. M., The carbohydrate metabolism and respiration of isolated small lymphocytes, *Blood* 30:691, 1967.

137. Parrott, D. M., and De Sousa, M. A. B. Changes in the thymus-dependent areas of lymph nodes after immunological stimulation, *Nature* 212:1316, 1966.

138. Pearmain, G., Lycette, R. R., and Fitzgerald, P. H. Tuberculin-induced mitosis in peripheral blood leucocytes, *Lancet* i:637, 1963.

139. Penner, P. E., Cohen, L. H., and Loeb, L. A. RNA-dependent DNA polymerase: presence in normal human cells, *Biochem. Biophys. Res. Commun.* 42:1228, 1971.

140. Pogo, B. G. T., Allfrey, V. G., and Mirsky, A. E. RNA synthesis and histone acetylation during the course of gene activation in lymphocytes, *Proc. Natl. Acad. Sci. U.S.A.* 55:805, 1966.

141. Quaglino, D., and Hayhoe, F. G. J. Metabolic changes in short-term "in vitro" cultures of normal and leukaemic cells; studies with cytochemistry and autoradiography, *in* F. G. J. Hayhoe (ed.), Current Re-

search in Leukaemia, p. 124, Cambridge University Press, Cambridge, England, 1965.

142. Quaglino, D., Hayhoe, F. G. J., and Flemans, R. J. Cytochemical observations on the effect of phytohaemaglutinin in short-term tissue cultures, *Nature* 196:338, 1962.

143. Quaglino, D., Torelli, U., Sauli, S., and Mauri, C. Cytochemical and autoradiographic investigations on normal and myelomatous plasma cells, *Acta Haematol.* 38:79, 1967.

144. Quastel, M. R., and Kaplan, J. G. Inhibition by oubain of human lymphocyte transformation induced by phytohemagglutinin in vitro, *Nature* 219:198, 1968.

145. Quastel, M. R., and Kaplan, J. G. Significance of the early stimulation by phytohemagglutinin of potassium transport in lymphocytes in vitro, *J. Cell Biol.* 47:164a, 1970.

146. Rabinowitz, Y. Separation of lymphocytes, polymorphonuclear leukocytes, and monocytes on glass columns, including tissue culture observations, *Blood* 23:811, 1964.

147. Rabinowitz, Y., and Dietz, A. A. Genetic control of lactate dehydrogenase and malate dehydrogenase isozymes in cultures of lymphocytes and granulocytes: effect of addition of phytohemagglutinin, actinomycin D or puromycin, *Biochim. Biophys. Acta* 139:254, 1967.

148. Rabinowitz, Y., and Dietz, A. A. Effect of phytohemagglutinin in cultures on the lactate dehydrogenases of lymphocytes from chronic lymphatic leukemia, *Blood* 31:166, 1968.

149. Rabinowitz, Y., Farmer, R., and Czebotar, V. Deoxycytidine pathway in separated normal and leukemic leukocytes with effects of cell culture, *Blood* 38:312, 1971.

150. Rabinowitz, Y., Wong, P., and Wilhite, B. A. Effect of phytohemagglutinin on enzymes of thymidine salvage pathway of cultured chronic lymphatic leukemic lymphocytes, *Blood* 35:236, 1970.

151. Rheingold, J. J., and Wislocki, G. B. Histochemical methods applied to hematology, *Blood* 3:641, 1948.

152. Rigby, P. G., and Ryan, W. L. The effect of cyclic AMP and related compounds on human lymphocyte transformation (HLT) stimulated by phytohemagglutinin (PHA), *Rev. Eur. Etud. Clin. Biol.* 15:774, 1970.

153. Robert, M. S., Smith, R. G., and Gallo, R. C. Viral and cellular DNA polymerase: comparison of activities with synthetic and natural RNA templates, *Science* 176:789, 1972.

154. Robineaux, R., Bona, C., Anteunis, A., and Orme-Roselli, L. La capacité endocytaire des lymphocytes ganglionnaires du cobaye, normaux et transformés in vitro, *Ann. Inst. Pasteur (Paris)* 117:790, 1969.

155. Rogers, J. C., Boldt, D., Kornfelds, S., Skinner, A., and Valeri, C. R. Excretion of deoxyribonucleic acid by lymphocytes stimulated with phytohemagglutinin or antigen, *Proc. Natl. Acad. Sci. U.S.A.* 69:1685, 1972.

156. Rosen, J. M., Milholland, R. J., and Rosen, F. A comparison of the effect of glucocorticoids on glucose uptake and hexokinase activity in lymphosarcoma P 1798, *Biochim. Biophys. Acta* 219:447, 1970.

157. Rosen, J. M., Fina, J. J., Milholland, R. J., and Rosen, F. Inhibition of glucose uptake in lymphoma P 1798 by cortisol and its relationship to the biosynthesis of deoxyribonucleic acid, *J. Biol. Chem.* 245:2074, 1970.

158. Rosen, J. M., Fina, J. J., Milholland, R. J., and Rosen, F. Inhibitory effect of cortisol *in vitro* on 2-deoxyglucose uptake and RNA and protein metabolism in lymphosarcoma P 1798, *Cancer Res.* 32:350, 1972.

159. Rosenau, W., Baxter, J. D., Rousseau, G. G., and Tomkins, G. M. Mechanism of resistance to steroids: glucocorticoid receptor defect in lymphoma cells, *Nature (New Biol.)* 237:20, 1972.

160. Rosenberg, S. A., and Levy, R. Synthesis of nuclear-associated proteins by lymphocytes within minutes after contact with phytohemagglutinin, *J. Immunol.* 108:1105, 1972.

161. Rousseau, G. G., et al. Steroid-induced nuclear binding of glucocorticoid receptors in intact hepatoma cells, *J. Mol. Biol.* 79:539, 1973.

162. Rubin, A. D., Havemann, K., and Dameshek, W. Studies in chronic lymphocytic leukemia: further studies of the proliferative abnormality of the blood lymphocyte, *Blood* 33:313, 1969.

163. Rühl, H., Kirchner, H., and Bochert, G. Kinetics of the Zn^{2+}- stimulation of human peripheral lymphocytes in vitro, *Proc. Soc. Exp. Biol. Med.* 137:1089, 1971.

164. Salmon, S. E., and Fudenberg, H. H. Abnormal nucleic acid metabolism of lymphocytes in plasma cell myeloma and macroglobulinemia, *Blood* 33:300, 1969.

165. Sarngadharan, M. G., Sarin, P. S., and Reitz, M. S. Reverse transcriptase activity of human acute leukaemic cells: purification of the enzyme, response to AMV 70S RNA, and characterization of the DNA product, *Nature (New Biol.)* 240:67 1972.

166. Scharff, M. D., and Uhr, J. W. Functional ribosomal unit of gammaglobulin synthesis, *Science* 148:646, 1965.

167. Schmid, J. R., Oechslin, R. J., and Moeschlin, S. Infectious mononucleosis, and autoradiographic study of DNA- and RNA-synthesis, *Scand. J. Haematol.* 2:18, 1965.

168. Schrek, R., and Rabinowitz, Y. Effects of phytohemagglutinin on rat and normal and leukemic human blood cells, *Proc. Soc. Exp. Biol. Med.* 113:191, 1963.

169. Schubert, D. Immunoglobulin assembly in a mouse myeloma, *Proc. Natl. Acad. Sci. U.S.A.* 60:683, 1968.

170. Schubert, D., and Cohn, M. Immunoglobulin biosynthesis. III. Blocks in defective synthesis, *J. Mol. Biol.* 38:273, 1968.

171. Schuler, D., Riss, S., and Siegler, J. About the glycolysis of lymphocytes and granulocytes in infancy and childhood, *Ann. Paediatr.* 198:285, 1962.

172. Scott, R. B. Glycogen in peripheral blood leukocytes. I. Characteristics of synthesis and turnover of glycogen in vitro, *J. Clin. Invest.* 47:344, 1968.

173. Scott, R. B., and Still, W. J. S. Glycogen in human peripheral blood leukocytes: the macromolecular state of leukocyte glycogen, *J. Clin. Invest.* 47:358, 1968.

174. Sell, S., Rowe, D. S., and Gell, P. G.

H. Studies on rabbit lymphocytes in vitro. III. Protein, RNA, and DNA synthesis by lymphocyte culture after stimulation with phytohemagglutinin, with staphylococcal filtrate, with antiallotype serum, and with heterologous antiserum to rabbit whole serum, *J. Exp. Med.* 122:823, 1965.

175. Shapiro, A. L., Scharff, M. D., Maizel, J. V., and Uhr, J. W. Synthesis of excess light chains of gamma globulin by rabbit lymph node cells, *Nature* 211:243, 1966.

176. Shapiro, A. L., Scharff, M. D., Maizel, J. V., and Uhr, J. W. Polyribosomal synthesis and assembly of the H and L chains of gamma globulin, *Proc. Natl. Acad. Sci. U.S.A.* 56:216, 1966.

177. Sherr, C. J., Schenkeim, J., and Uhr, J. W. Synthesis and intracellular transport of immunoglobulin in secretory and nonsecretory cells, *Ann. N.Y. Acad. Sci.* 190:250, 1971.

178. Sherr, C. J., and Uhr, J. W. Immunoglobulin synthesis and secretion. III. Incorporation of glucosamine into immunoglobulin on polyribosomes, *Proc. Natl. Acad. Sci. U.S.A.* 64:381, 1969.

179. Sherr, C. J., and Uhr, J. W. Immunoglobulin synthesis and secretion. V, *Proc. Natl. Acad. Sci. U.S.A.* 66:1183, 1970.

180. Shirakawa, S., and Saunders, G. F. In vivo methylation of DNA in human leukocytes, *Proc. Soc. Exp. Biol. Med.* 138:369, 1971.

181. Silber, R., Unger, K. W., and Ellman, L. RNA metabolism in normal and leukaemic leucocytes: further studies on RNA synthesis, *Br. J. Haematol.* 14:261, 1968.

182. Silber, R., Unger, K. W., and Grooms, R. RNA synthesis in normal leucocytes, leukaemia and macroglobulinemia, *Nature* 205:1211, 1965.

183. Sinks, L. F., and Hayhoe, F. G. J. Unstable rapidly labelled RNA in chronic lymphocytic leukaemic cells, *Nature* 213:1140, 1967.

184. Stähelin, H., Suter, E., and Karnovsky, M. L. Studies on the interaction between phagocytes and tubercle bacilli. I. Observations on the metabolism of guinea pig leuco-

cytes and the influence of phagocytosis, *J. Exp. Med.* 104:121, 1956.

185. Stevens, R. H., and Williamson, A. R. Specific IgG mRNA molecules from myeloma cells in heterogenous nuclear and cytoplasmic RNA containing poly-A, *Nature* 239:143, 1972.

186. Stevens, R. H., and Williamson, A. R. Isolation of messenger RNA coding for mouse heavy chain immunoglobulin, *Proc. Natl. Acad. Sci. U.S.A.* 70:1127, 1973.

187. Stevens, R. H., and Williamson, A. R. Translational control of immunoglobulin synthesis. I, Repression of heavy-chain synthesis, *J. Mol. Biol.* 78:505, 517; 1973.

188. Stevens, R. H., and Williamson, A. R. Isolation of nuclear pre-mRNA which codes for immunoglobulin heavy chain, *Nature (New Biol.)* 245:101, 1973.

189. Stjernholm, R. L. Carbohydrate metabolism in leukocytes. VII. Metabolism of glucose, acetate, and propionate by human plasma cells, *J. Bacteriol.* 93:1657, 1967.

190. Stjernholm, R. L., and Falor, W. H. Early biochemical changes in phytohemagglutinin-stimulated human lymphocytes of blood and lymph, *J. Reticuloendothel. Soc.* 7:471, 1970.

191. Stuart, J. J., and Ingram, M. The effect of cortisol on viability and glucose uptake in rat thymocytes *in vitro*, *Proc. Soc. Exp. Biol. Med.* 136:1146, 1971.

192. Sunaga, K., and Koide, S. S. Interaction of calf thymus histones and DNA with steroids, *Steroids* 9:451, 1967.

193. Tanaka, Y., Epstein, L. B., Brecher, G., and Stohlman, F., Jr. Transformation of lymphocytes in cultures of human peripheral blood, *Blood* 22:614, 1963.

194. Tawde, S., Scharff, M. D., and Uhr, J. W. Mechanisms of γ-globulin synthesis, *J. Immunol.* 96:1, 1966.

195. Taylor, R. B., Duffus, W. P. H., Raff, M. C., and de Petris, S.: Redistribution and pinocytosis of lymphocyte surface immunoglobulin molecules induced by anti-immunoglobulin antibody, *Nature (New Biol.)* 233:225, 1971.

196. Thomas, D. B., and Phillips, B.

Membrane antigens specific for human lymphoid cells in the dividing phase, *J. Exp. Med.* 138:64, 1973.

197. Torelli, U. L., Henry, P. H., and Weissman, S. M. Characteristics of the RNA synthesized in vitro by the normal human small lymphocyte and the changes induced by phytohemagglutinin stimulation, *J. Clin. Invest.* 47:1083, 1968.

198. Tormey, D. C., Kamin, R., and Fudenberg, H. H. Quantitative studies of phytohemagglutinin-induced DNA and RNA synthesis in normal and agammaglobulinemic leukocytes, *J. Exp. Med.* 125:863, 1967.

199. Turk, J. L., and Stone, S. H. Implications of the cellular changes in lymph nodes during the development and inhibition of delayed type hypersensitivity, *in* D. B. Amos and H. Koprowski (eds.), Cell-Bound Antibodies, p. 51, Wistar Institute Press, Philadelphia, 1963.

200. Valentine, W. N., Follette, J. H., and Lawrence, J. S. The glycogen content of human leukocytes in health and various disease states, *J. Clin. Invest.* 32:251, 1953.

201. Vannotti, A. Metabolic pattern of leucocytes within the circulation and outside it, *in* G. E. W. Wolstenholme and M. O'Connor (eds.), Ciba Foundation Study Group 10, Biological Activity of the Leucocyte, p. 79, Little, Brown and Co., Boston, 1961.

202. Warner, J. R., Soeiro, R., Birnboim, H. C., Girard, M., and Darnell, J. E. Rapidly labeled HeLa cell nuclear RNA. I. Identification by zone sedimentation of a heterogeneous fraction separate from ribosomal precursor RNA, *J. Mol. Biol.* 19:349, 1966.

203. Weissman, I. L. Thymus cell maturation, *J. Exp. Med.* 137:504, 1973.

204. Werthamer, S., Hicks, C., and Arnaral, L. Protein synthesis in human leukocytes and lymphocytes. I. Effect of steroid and sterols, *Blood* 34:348, 1969.

205. Williamson, A. R., and Askonas, B. A. Biosynthesis of immunoglobulins: the separate classes of polyribosomes synthesizing heavy and light chains, *J. Mol. Biol.* 23:201, 1967.

206. Wira, C., and Munck, A. In vitro binding of ^{3}H-cortisol to rat thymus nuclei, *Fed. Proc.* 28:702, 1969.

207. Wolff, J. S. III, Langstaff, J. A., Weinberg, G., and Abell, C. W. DNA dependent RNA polymerase activity of nuclei isolated from human peripheral blood lymphocytes, *Biochem. Biophys. Res. Commun.* 26:366, 1967.

208. Yahara, I., and Edelman, G. M. Restriction of the mobility of lymphocyte immunoglobulin receptors by concanavalin A, *Proc. Natl. Acad. Sci. U.S.A.* 69:608, 1972.

209. Zucker-Franklin, D. The ultrastructure of lymphocytes, *Semin. Hematol.* 6:4, 1969.

Chapter 15 Lymphocytes, Plasma Cells, and the Immune Response

The major emphasis of this chapter is on leukocyte behavior and function, rather than on the immunologic phenomena associated with leukocytes. Still, some discussion of the role of lymphoid cells in the immune response is necessary for a better understanding of the functions of normal lymphocytes and plasma cells and the aberrations of these functions in human disease. More comprehensive surveys of immune responses are available elsewhere (21, 61, 76, 99, 111, 122, 153, 159, 169, 209, 227, 231, 232).

The immunologic response to specific antigen is a complex process involving several types of cells and, presumably, genetic control at several levels. Administration of antigen to the experimental animal or man initiates a series of cell divisions and cellular differentiation within the lymphoid system, resulting in the production of large numbers of plasma cells that produce specific antibody and/or the appearance of sensitized lymphoid cells capable of diverse reactions with antigen. The latter response, usually termed the delayed hypersensitivity reaction or cell-mediated immune response (as distinct from antibody-mediated), is thought to be responsible for contact hypersensitivity, transplantation immunity, reaction to certain microbial parasites, and antitumor immunity (220).

The techniques for measuring antibody synthesis and antibody-mediated reactions are considerably more sophisticated than those for measuring delayed hypersensitivity. Consequently, more information is available on those factors initiating and controlling the humoral immune response than on the factors governing cell-mediated immune reactions.

In this chapter we shall be concerned with the following:
(a) The commitment of individual plasma cells and lymphocytes to the production of a single class of antibody molecules—molecules specific in allotype and antigen-binding affinity.
(b) The recognition of antigen by sensitized and nonsensitized cells.
(c) The interaction of various cell types in the production of specific antibody and cell-mediated immune reactions.
(d) The role of clonal proliferation of cell populations in the production of antibody of progressively higher affinity for antigen.
(e) The effect on the type of immune response of antigen dose, route of administration, administration with adjuvants, and time after antigen administration.
(f) Factors other than antigen controlling the production of specific antibody.

One Cell, One Antibody

The clonal selection theory of antibody synthesis originally presented by Burnet (25, 26), and now widely accepted, proposes that cells of the lymphoid system become committed to the synthesis of a specific antibody molecule in a random fashion *before* exposure to antigen. To account for the great variety of antibody molecules, it is proposed (95) that either there is a large number of separate gene lines, each of which codes for a particular sequence on the variable region of the immunoglobulin molecule, or alternatively, there is a high degree of lymphoid cell somatic variability introduced by somatic mutation or somatic recombination (116). Most evidence favors the alternative of a multiplicity of gene lines; perhaps 10^3 light-chain and 10^3 heavy-chain genes. In either case, precommitted cells bearing specifically reactive antibody on their surface are presumed to interact with antigen and as a result of this interaction are stimulated to proliferate and, in some cases, to synthesize antibody (Fig. 15.1). Such cells have been designated antigen-reactive cells (ARCs). Antigen-reactive cells constitute all or part of the population of lymphoid cells that bind antigen at their surface (antigen-binding cells, ABCs). Some antigen-reactive cells may give rise to progeny that produce antibody; others must interact with an antibody-producing cell, which subsequently undergoes proliferation.

A single cell thus stimulated, and its resulting progeny (clones), would produce a homogeneous population of antibody molecules. The heterogeneity of serum antibodies for a single antigen should, therefore, reflect heterogeneity of the antibody-synthesizing cellular population—in other words, several clones.

This theory and its various elaborations (203) require that an individual antibody-synthesizing cell synthesize a very limited spectrum, and probably only a single type, of

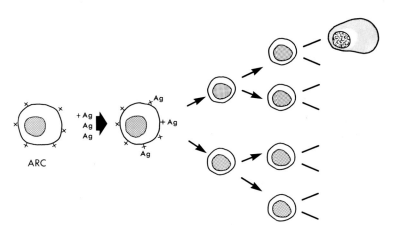

Figure 15.1 Schematic representation of the interaction of antigen (*Ag*) with an antigen-reactive cell (*ARC*). Cell surface receptors for interaction with antigen are denoted *X*. When the cell binds antigen, it is stimulated to proliferate. B cells ultimately give rise to an immunoglobulin-producing plasma cell. The antigen reactive cell may be a T cell, which secondarily interacts with B cells in the development of a humoral immune response.

antibody molecule. The antibody molecule would be of specific allotype, with a restricted affinity for antigen, and would belong to a specific class of immunoglobulins. These theoretical arguments are supported by strong experimental evidence showing that single plasma cells, and probably also single lymphocytes, synthesize antibody molecules of a unique specificity and characteristic affinity. Furthermore, these antibody-producing cells appear to arise as the result of stimulation by antigen of the proliferation of a specific clone of precursor cells. That is, during the primary and secondary immune response specific precursor cells proliferate in response to antigen. This proliferation leads to an enlarged population of lymphoid cells, which differentiate into antibody-secreting plasma cells.

Plasma Cells

Evidence from a number of laboratories supports the idea that individual plasma cells make antibody of a single immunoglobulin class (IgG, IgM, IgA, IgD, *or* IgE) and of a single subclass. Furthermore, the immunoglobulin produced by a single cell is of a single light-chain type (kappa or lambda; see Chapter 16). This evidence has been obtained in studies of human and animal materials (13–15, 30, 165, 170).

Although occasional studies (162) suggest that individual cells may convert from IgM production to IgG production in the course of the immune response, most investigations support the supposition that only a single immunoglobulin class is produced by a single cell. For example, Merchant and Brahmi (129), employing a modification of the Jerne hemolytic plaque technique, placed individual antibody-producing cells between two separate layers of agar containing sheep erythrocytes as the target antigen. One agar layer was assayed for the presence of IgG hemolysing antibody, the other for IgM antibody. In no instance was a single cell observed to produce more than one class of antibody.

A similar situation exists with regard to production of subclasses of immunoglobulin molecules. Single plasma cells from heterozygous rabbits have been demonstrated to produce immunoglobulins of only one of the two allotypes possible, never both (171). Interestingly, in at least some model systems immunization of a homozygous mother against the different immunoglobulin allotype of the father resulted in a relative suppression of the paternal allotype in the heterozygous offspring (52, 57, 117–119). This observation, as well as others (112), suggests that one can apply negative pressure for selection of immune cells of defined immunoglobulin subclass.

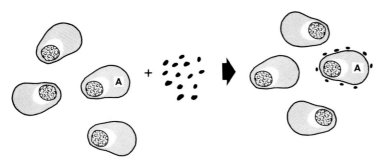

Figure 15.2 Schematic representation of a technique for identification of a cell producing specific antibody. The antibody-producing cell denoted *A* is synthesizing antibody against the bacterial particles. Some of these immunoglobulins are arrayed at the cell surface and are capable of binding the bacterial particles around the cell.

The accumulated evidence favors the concept that individual antibody-producing cells make antibody of a single immunologic specificity (78, 88, 120, 154, 155, 161, 172). For example, in a series of classic experiments, Nossal and his colleagues (154, 155, 161) immunized rats with two noncross-reacting strains of *Salmonella* and then immobilized individual antibody-producing cells in microdrops. Using aggregation between the *Salmonella* and the immune cell as a test of antibody production (Fig. 15.2), they demonstrated that virtually all the drops contained immune cells producing antibodies of a single specificity. The few apparent double-producers were probably artifacts.

A variety of other techniques and test antigens applied to this question have resulted in the same conclusion: *individual immune cells produce antibodies of a single specificity.* Rare exceptions have been reported (7). This general concept may be carried even further; individual antibody-producing cells make antibodies that are homogeneous with respect to antigen-binding properties (affinity) (59, 121), and the heterogeneity of antibody affinity for a single antigen probably reflects different clones of antibody-producing cells.

Lymphocytes

The morphologically identifiable protein-synthesizing apparatus of lymphocytes is considerably less well developed than that of antibody-secreting plasma cells, and the amount of immunoglobulin produced by lymphocytes is correspondingly less. As a result, the technical difficulties of identifying the class, subclass, and affinity of immunoglobulins produced by single lymphocytes has been much greater.

Blastogenic transformation and DNA synthesis are

triggered when antibody to specific immunoglobulin or anti-allotype sera are mixed with lymphocytes (77, 197). The mechanism of this induction is believed to be an antigen-antibody reaction (immunoglobulin–anti-immunoglobulin) on the surface membrane of the lymphocyte. Therefore specific antisera can be used to define the characteristics of the immunoglobulin that is bound to, and presumably produced by, the lymphocyte.

Using such antisera with blood lymphocytes from an allotypically heterozygous rabbit has produced evidence that the individual lymphocytes bear surface immunoglobulins of only a single allotype (75, 196).

Although evidence favors the commitment of individual antibody-producing lymphocytes and plasma cells to the synthesis of individual immunoglobulins, the mechanism of this commitment is unknown. A number of genetic and somatic mutation theories have been proposed, but at this point there is insufficient evidence to choose among them.

Antigen Recognition

The Humoral Immune Response

Even if we accept the thesis that individual immunocytes produce antibody of a very restricted type and specificity and that such cells may be stimulated to proliferation by contact with antigen, the question remains concerning what mechanisms enable cells to recognize and interact with antigen. The answer at this time must still contain a considerable amount of speculation as well as established facts.

The initiation by antigen of a cellular response involving proliferation, morphologic transformation, and antibody synthesis is believed to require, as an essential early event, a combination between the antigen and antibody molecules attached to the cell surface (Fig. 15.1). Certain small lymphocytes actively synthesize immunoglobulin-like molecules arrayed at the cell surface (39, 178, 198). These cells are believed to be principally the bone-marrow–derived B lymphocytes (9, 11, 42, 43, 92) that are the precursors of antibody-synthesizing cells. T lymphocytes may also have some antigen-binding immunoglobulins on their surface (5, 126, 145), although these molecules probably occur at a lesser density than those of B cells. The attached surface antibody on the B lymphocytes allows these cells to adhere to antigen-coated columns (124, 151, 234). The fact that these antigen-binding molecules are similar to serum immunoglobulin is demonstrated by the observation that antigen adherence to lymphoid cells is blocked by preincubating the cells with antibodies directed against serum immunoglobulins (28, 115).

A number of other studies support the concept of antigenic similarity between serum immunoglobulins and antigen-binding sites on the surface membranes of these lymphoid cells (128, 140, 230). A reasonable question to pose, therefore, is whether these antigen-binding sites are in fact identical to the antibody produced by the immunocyte.

Walters and Wigzell (229) answered this question by showing that the retention of antibody-forming cells and "immunologic memory cells" by antigen-coated columns could be blocked if the cells were preincubated with anti-immunoglobulin. The use of specific antisera to heavy- and light-chain antigens made is possible to demonstrate that the cell membrane receptors had the same heavy chain as the humoral antibody eventually produced by these cells and that light chains were involved in the receptor sites also. Furthermore, the membrane receptor molecules probably have the same number of antigen-binding sites as the corresponding humoral antibody produced by these cells (123).

One interpretation of these observations is that *membrane-bound antigen-binding receptors are expressions of the potential capacity of these cells to produce soluble immunoglobulins—that is, humoral antibody.*

Antigen Recognition and the Cellular Immune Response

Thus far we have been concerned with antigen recognition by cells capable of humoral antibody synthesis. What about those lymphoid cells involved in delayed hypersensitivity reactions? Here the facts are considerably less clear and the speculation considerably more abundant.

There are two alternatives open to an antigen-responsive lymphoid cell: humoral antibody synthesis or a cellular immune response. The decision between these alternatives may be explained in two ways: first, that antigen-responsive cells are precommitted to one or the other immune response; in other words, that lymphoid populations are already subdivided before exposure to antigen. The second possibility is that antigen-responsive cells can take either pathway, with the local environment determining the route. The "local environment" may be the geographic location, the presence of other cell types, the type and concentration of antigen, or perhaps other factors.

Arguments in favor of separate lymphocyte populations and precommitment include (a) the known precommitment of lymphocytes in other respects (class and allotype of immunoglobulin produced), and (b) the association of delayed hypersensitivity with thymus-dependent lympho-

cytes and of humoral antibody-synthesizing cells with bursal derivation or its mammalian equivalent (B cells) (45, 70, 108, 127, 166, 218).

Accepting these arguments that there is a population or populations of lymphocytes precommitted to a cellular immune response, what is the nature of the cellular receptor triggering the cellular response? Some interesting experiments investigating this point are those of Schlossman and his co-workers (190). They studied the immune response to alpha dinitrophenol-oligolysines, compounds in which a single DNP group is attached to the N-terminal alpha amino group. The compounds of this group differ from one another only in the length of the lysine chain. The observations of these investigators indicate that for the induction of delayed hypersensitivity reactions the same stearic requirements exist as for the initial induction of immunity. In contrast, the requirements for the interaction of the humoral antibody produced by sensitized cells with antigenic determinants are less rigorous. Their studies further suggest that the cellular receptor for antigen necessary for triggering cell-mediated immune reactions is not simply conventional antibody immunoglobulin; whether it represents "conventional" antibody of unusually restricted affinity is debatable. The nature of the cellular receptor for the initiation of cellular immune responses is not presently known.

Interactions between Immunocytes

The interaction of subpopulations of lymphoid cells and of lymphoid cells with macrophages is necessary for the full expression of immunologic reactivity (3, 27, 73, 80, 87, 127, 131, 132, 134, 156, 157, 236). Reduced to simplest terms, the synthesis of specific antibody by B cells and their progeny requires the helper function of T cells and, in some cases, of macrophages. This interaction is necessary for response to most antigens. However, B cells may react directly to some complex bacterial antigens without the cooperation of other cell types (48). Janossy and his colleagues have recently presented a clear analysis of the mechanism of T-independent stimulation of B cells by ligands (100).

Cellular interactions resulting in clonal proliferation, and ultimately in antibody synthesis, are summarized in Fig. 15.3. As shown, an antigen-reactive T cell is stimulated to proliferate by antigen, which results in a clone of reactive cells. Such cells act as "helpers," in association with macrophages, in presenting antigen to appropriate B cells in a form that is palatable. The B cells thereby are stimulated to proliferate and yield a clone of antibody-forming cells. Evidence for this sequence is cited in the sections that follow.

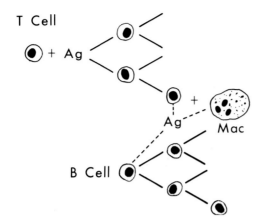

Figure 15.3 Cellular interactions in the synthesis of antibody. T cells interact with antigen (*Ag*) and are stimulated to proliferate. The progeny of this proliferation interact with antigen and macrophages (*Mac*) to stimulate the proliferation of the precursors of immunoglobulin-producing cells (B cells).

Subpopulations of Lymphocytes

Studies of the interaction of subpopulations of lymphocytes with antigen in the immune response have utilized both in vivo and in vitro model systems. Examples of in vivo models are animals depleted of specific lymphoid population by one or more precedures: thymectomy, anti-θ antisera, and/or whole body irradiation. Animals genetically deficient in thymic function also have been used (167). The effects of a specific lymphocyte population may be examined by using it to replete such depleted animals. For example, thymocytes may be injected into neonatally irradiated mice to produce nearly pure populations of T cells.

Similarly, in vitro systems for examination of the interaction of lymphocyte populations have used combinations of cells derived from single anatomic sites such as the thymus, peripheral blood, bone marrow, or thoracic duct. Many test systems have used the Jerne plaque assay to quantitate the number of antibody-producing cells (102). This assay utilizes the formation of a zone of hemolysis around lymphoid cells, which are suspended in agar containing foreign red blood cells. The erythrocytes serve as antigens to quantitate the number of antibody-forming cells. The cell that synthesizes antibody is generally designated as the plaque-forming cell (PFC).

As indicated previously, good evidence shows that there is a population of lymphoid cells that carry on their surfaces receptor molecules for interaction with antigen (1, 92, 145, 194). A reasonable assumption is that such cells are triggered to synthesize antibody of the same specific-

ity after exposure to antigen, and that such cells are the precursors of antibody-forming clones (3). It seems, however, that response to certain antigens (sheep erythrocytes, for instance) requires the presence of other lymphoid and nonlymphoid cell populations that do not themselves synthesize antibody. For example, the removal of the subpopulation of glass-adherent spleen cells reduces the number of hemolytic plaque-forming cells developing from the remaining nonadhering lymphoid population. The readdition of intact or irradiated adherent cells or peritoneal exudate cells restores the number of PFCs (90, 94). Such interacting cell populations can be separated also by centrifugation on albumin (135).

In vivo studies utilizing mice depleted of lymphoid cells by irradiation showed that the immune response to sheep red blood cells could not be restored by the administration of pure populations of either thymus-derived T cells or bone marrow (B) cells, but only by their combination (35, 44, 132, 136, 160). B cells provide the precursor of the antibody-synthesizing plaque-forming cells—whereas T cells and their progeny serve as helpers, but do not directly synthesize antibody.

The effect of anti-θ-serum on the in vivo response to antigen also points to the involvement of theta-positive T cells in the immune response (176, 189). The requirement for cell cooperation with B cells in the production of hemolytic antibody is generally agreed upon (51, 150, 189). The mechanism of this interaction is largely unknown, but it is the stimulus to interesting speculations (65–68).

A number of studies suggest that the helper T lymphocytes are antigen specific (90, 132, 136, 177, 221); that is, they also have antigen-binding receptors on their surfaces (145). One suggestion is that these T cells concentrate immunogenic molecules on their surface and present them to antibody-producing precursor cells (B cells). This is a reasonable working hypothesis until more information is available (33, 34, 40, 41, 79, 91, 130, 132, 133, 136, 137, 149, 160, 177, 201, 212).

In an alternative hypothesis, T cells synthesize and release immunoglobulin (IgT). IgT-antigen complexes bind to macrophages or macrophage-like cells, which then stimulate B-cell responses (65, 67, 68).

The following simplified hypothetical sequence of events in T-B interactions can be proposed (see Fig. 15.3). (*a*) The thymus conditions cells (T cells) that interact with antigen during the early phases of an immune response (*antigen-reactive T cells*, ARCs). (*b*) After contact with antigen, reactive T cells proliferate and produce cells capable of interacting with macrophages and bone-marrow–derived lymphoid cells (B cells). The progeny of the antigen-reactive T cells are sometimes called *inducer cells* (201). (*c*) The marrow-derived B cells and their progeny produce specific antibody (44).

This hypothetical sequence incorporates the following conclusions: (*a*) bone-marrow–derived cells cannot substitute for thymic antigen-reactive cells in the early events in immune response; (*b*) bone-marrow–derived cells are generally concerned with the latter stages of immunoglobulin synthesis and its specificity; and (*c*) the induction of antibody synthesis requires that antigen be available to interact with antigen-reactive cells and their viable progeny, the inducer cells.

An important basis of this hypothetical sequence is that *one* source of specificity in the production of antibody derives from the antigen-reactive cells of thymic origin and their progeny, the inducer cells. But is this the only source of specificity? Or are there other lymphocyte populations, such as marrow-derived B cells, which also demonstrate specificity in interaction with antigen?

Complex experiments using reconstitution of irradiated mice by thymocytes and small graded doses of antigen-primed marrow cells (130) indicate that mouse bone-marrow cells *also* contain some cells that are antigen specific, a conclusion supported by other investigations (32, 106). For example, under certain conditions humoral antibody responses in irradiated mice can be elicited by transplantation of marrow cells without the involvement of thymocytes (4).

Katz and Benacerraf (105) recently have reviewed the regulatory influence of activated T cells on the responses of B cells to antigens. It is probable that under some circumstances T cells may exert a suppressive effect also on B-cell function (181, 182) and limit the humoral immune response. This effect might also be mediated by IgT (68).

It is clear that our knowledge of T cell-B cell interactions is still very rudimentary. Evidence, which is accumulating rapidly, indicates that there are in fact several subpopulations of both these types of lymphoid cells. Greaves and his colleagues have recently summarized our knowledge of this complex and interesting field (86).

Lymphocyte-Macrophage Interactions

A number of observations indicate that phagocytic mononuclear cells may be involved in an initial interaction with antigen in the so-called afferent limb of the immune response. Such antigen-laden phagocytes (monocytes and macrophages) have to contact antigen and then interact with sensitized lymphocytes, thus stimulating the lymphoid cells to blastogenic transformation and proliferation. The lines of evidence supporting this concept are as

Table 15.1 Evidence for macrophage involvement in the blastogenic response of lymphocytes to antigen.

99–100 percent pure populations of lymphocytes show reduced blastogenic response to antigen.
Mononuclear phagocytes added to pure populations of lymphocytes restore response to antigen.
Antigen-coated monocytes induce lymphocyte transformation.
Antigen-containing macrophages can induce antibody formation in appropriate recipient animals.
Responding lymphocytes form an immunologic cluster around a central macrophage.

follows (Table 15.1). Pure populations of sensitized peripheral blood lymphocytes containing no mononuclear phagocytes show a greatly reduced blastogenic response to antigens in vitro; addition of these phagocytes restores the lymphocyte response to normal levels (93). Similar results are obtained when surface-adherent and nonadherent populations of mouse spleen are studied (147, 148). Most lymphocytes are nonadherent; monocytes and macrophages adhere to a charged surface.

Human monocytes and macrophages exposed to a specific antigen in vitro and then washed free of any unbound antigen can induce blastogenic transformation of autologous lymphocytes (37, 89). Macrophages are more efficient than monocytes in this process, probably because of their greater surface area and more effective binding of antigen.

Another argument in favor of an involvement of macrophages in the immune response is that normal, nonimmune lymphoid cells administered to an immunologically inert, X-irradiated recipient can induce antibody synthesis only if given in conjunction with living macrophages containing antigen (225).

After administration of a radioactive antigen to an intact animal, the label is found associated with medullary macrophages, as well as with the surface processes of dendritic reticular cells within the cortical areas of lymph nodes (156, 157).

Intimate contact between the surfaces of the mononuclear cells and the lymphocyte clearly seems necessary for maximal lymphocyte response in vitro (37, 89, 148). Separation of the two cell types by a cell-impermeable filter curtails the lymphocyte response. In vitro, the central mononuclear phagocyte and the surrounding lymphocyte form an "immunologic island" (Fig. 15.4). The formation of such clusters is required for continued division of antibody-forming cells. Close contact and cytoplasmic con-

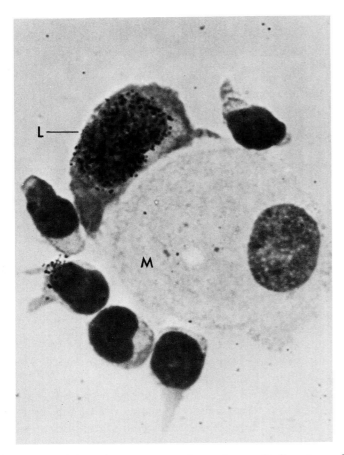

Figure 15.4 A lymphocyte-macrophage cluster. Radioautograph of thymidine-labeled transformed lymphocyte (*L*) and untransformed lymphocytes surrounding an antigen-sensitized macrophage (*M*). Silver grains are localized to the lymphocyte nuclei; Giemsa stain.

nections between lymphocytes and macrophages in vivo have been demonstrated (192, 200, 207).

A further requirement for lymphocyte stimulation by macrophages is that the mononuclear cell be viable and that an intact energy metabolism be present (37).

It is not known definitely whether the antigen is bound to the surface of the macrophage or is distributed internally, nor is it known whether the antigen is modified by the cell (107, 225). A portion of exogenous antigen does escape localization within phagocytic vacuoles and becomes associated with the rough-surfaced endoplasmic reticulum of the macrophage (29). Small amounts of antigen are retained in immunogenic form for long peroids of time within the macrophage, although the major portion is quickly degraded. Furthermore, immunogenic antigen may remain bound to the plasma membrane of macrophages (191, 226).

Perhaps the most important unanswered questions in this area are first, whether macrophages do in fact "process" the antigen in some way, and second, what the role of macrophage RNA is in the "instruction" of the lymphocytes.

RNA prepared from macrophages that have been exposed to specific antigen can induce autologous lymphocytes to produce the corresponding antibody (6, 19, 69, 73, 82–84, 173). It has been reported that antibody induction by macrophage RNA is biphasic, with an early IgM component and a later IgG component. Furthermore, the IgM antibody is said to have the allotype specificity of the macrophage from which the RNA is obtained, whereas the IgG antibody possesses the allotype of the lymph node donor (2).

An early and understandable conclusion from these observations was that macrophage RNA possessed an "informational macromolecule" capable of instructing the lymphocytes. Careful studies did, however, demonstrate that the macrophage RNA was contaminated with minute amounts of antigen (6, 18, 73, 82). This observation raised the possibility that macrophage RNA was acting as an adjuvant to enhance the antigenicity of small amounts of antigen. Later, more comprehensive studies have indicated that it is unlikely that macrophages process the antigen in any critical manner. These findings militate against the notion that the macrophage RNA is in any way instructional (184, 185, 226).

Notwithstanding these qualifications, it seems clear that under certain circumstances there is an intimate relation between mononuclear phagocytes and lymphocytes in the initiation of a response to antigen. Macrophages at the center of an immunologic cluster may retain certain types of antigen, making it available to the surrounding lymphocytes.

Cell Surface Receptors

Evidence that certain lymphoid cells are capable of binding antigen has already been cited (10, 42, 43, 92, 146). Both B and T cells have this functional attribute. It appears likely that the avidity or density of receptors is greater on the surface of B cells. All available evidence supports the concept that the antigen-binding receptors are immunoglobulin in nature (5, 85, 163, 237).

As shown in Fig. 15.5, lymphoid cells also have surface receptors that bind antigen-antibody–complement complexes (17, 164). The same receptors, or others, may bind antigen-antibody complexes without complement (10, 36). Still others may bind complement (164) or cleaved products of complement (186). Such receptors appear to be associated mainly with B cells (9, 11, 36). They are also

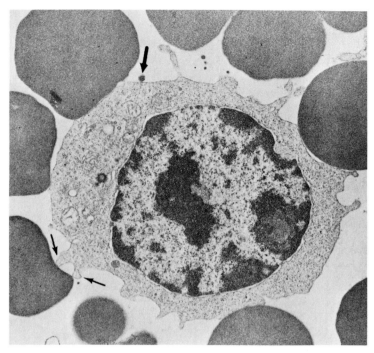

Figure 15.5 A rosette of sheep erythrocytes sensitized by antibody and complement on a spleen lymphocyte. Several broad contacts between sensitized erythrocytes and the lymphocyte are noted. A part of the sensitized erythrocyte projection in contact with the lymphocyte is indicated by a thick arrow, and a multiple contact is indicated by thin arrows. Magnification × 8,000. (From L-T. Chin, A. Eden, V. Nussenzweig, and L. Weiss, *Cell. Immunol.* 4:279, 1972. Reprinted by permission of authors and publisher.)

found on human leukemic cells and on lymphoblastoid cell lines (202). The receptors for antigen complexes will bind antibody alone through the Fc portion of the immunoglobulin molecule (9, 11, 36, 168) and will bind aggregated gamma globulin (47). Immune complexes

Table 15.2 Summary of cell surface receptors (see refs. 9–11, 17, 36, 47, 103, 113, 164, 202).

Cell type	Surface receptor for—		
	IgG	IgM-C	SRBC
B lymphocyte	+	+	0
T lymphocyte	0	0	+
Macrophage	+	+	0

Note: IgG = immunoglobulin G ± antigen; IgM-C = IgM-complement complexes (with C3 probably the key component); SRBC = sheep erythrocytes.

bound to the surface of B lymphocytes may be either shed externally or internalized into the cell (62).

T lymphocytes also bind sheep erythrocytes by nonimmune mechanisms to form rosettes (103, 113) and may have surface receptors for histamine (174). Monocytes and macrophages have similar receptors for immunoglobulin and complement. These are considered in detail in Chapter 25. The biological function of receptors on the cell surface is not definitely known. Presumably they are involved in the capture of antigen and immune complexes and in cellular interactions.

Table 15.2 summarizes some of the identified cell surface receptors.

Clonal Proliferation and Synthesis of High-affinity Antibody

The binding affinity of an antibody refers to the strength of its interaction with the corresponding antigenic determinant (203). A strong bond is formed between an antigenic determinant and a high-affinity antibody.

It has been observed consistently that the average binding affinity of antibodies increases with time during an immune response (60, 63, 101, 114, 203, 204, 211). An interesting and appealing hypothesis has been proposed as an explanation:

The increase in average binding affinity of antibodies during the immune response can be explained by the selective proliferation, stimulated by antigen, of those specific cells that are best able to bind antigen (processed antigen) because they bear antibody of higher affinity. These proliferating cells form an expanding and dynamically changing population of lymphoid cells from which plasma cells differentiate. As the antigen concentration decreases in the lymphoid tissues and as higher affinity antibody is produced by some cells, the cells bearing lower affinity antibody being less able to bind antigen competitively would tend to represent a progressively smaller fraction of this proliferating population (203).

Experiments by Nussenzweig and his colleagues (12, 165) and others (195) support this hypothesis. Davie and Paul have shown that during the course of the immune response the avidity of cellular immunoglobulin receptors for antigen increases. These receptors occur on the surface of B lymphocytes, suggesting that this cell type is primarily responsible for the "antigen-driven" increase in antibody avidity (42, 43). Therefore, a clear relationship seems likely between B lymphocyte proliferation and the production of humoral antibody of increasingly high avidity for antigen. This phenomenon is illustrated in Fig. 15.6.

Populations of T lymphocytes also show an increase in antigen sensitivity with time after immunization. This

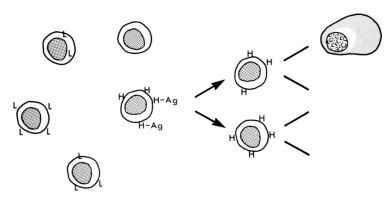

Figure 15.6 Schematic representation of the selection by antigen (*Ag*) of immunoglobulin-synthesizing cells producing high-affinity antibody. Immunoglobulin-synthesizing cells producing low-affinity antibody are represented by *L*; those synthesizing high-affinity antibody are denoted by *H*. When an immune complex is formed on the cell producing high-affinity antibody, it is stimulated to proliferate, ultimately giving rise to an immunoglobulin-producing plasma cell.

observation initially was thought to represent an increase in affinity for antigen of receptors on T lymphocytes. Recently, however, Cohen and Paul (38) demonstrated that the changing antigen sensitivity was the result of the changing antigen avidity of cytophilic antibody. Such antibody coats the small number of macrophages found in most T-cell populations.

Additional evidence indicates that the proliferative potential of B lymphocyte clones may be finite and that such clones eventually may undergo senescence (235).

The Influence of Antigen Dose and Immunizing Procedures on the Immune Response

Antigen Dose

Several studies have examined the effect of antigen dose on the amount and affinity of antibody produced by experimental animals (60, 81, 203, 204, 210). Early in the immune response, serum antibody concentration is higher when a larger dosage of antigen is given. Late in the immune response, higher concentrations of antibody occur when relatively low doses of antigen are administered. Interestingly, the dose of antigen that produces maximal concentrations of antibody late in the immune response is also the optimal dose for producing very high-affinity antibody (204).

These observations on the relation between antigen dose and the subsequently measured concentration and affinity of antibody can be explained by the clonal selection

hypothesis (203). With large doses of antigen, sufficient material is available to interact with lymphoid cells bearing antigen recognition sites of low affinity, as well as those bearing sites of high affinity. All cells with recognition sites thus are stimulated to proliferate and produce antibody, which is then heterogeneous with regard to affinity. Under these conditions there is little selection pressure favoring the cells with high-affinity antibody and little maturation in affinity occurs.

In contrast, when lower antigen doses are employed, there is more competition for the available antigen and cells with higher-affinity receptors are favored. These cells bind antigen, proliferate, and produce antibody of high affinity.

Tolerance

A detailed consideration of tolerance is beyond the scope of this book, and the interested reader should consult the excellent reviews available (22, 31, 56, 208). However, no consideration of the effect of antigen concentration on the cellular and humoral immune response would be complete without some understanding of immunologic tolerance, which may be defined as the specific depression of immunologic reactivity induced by previous exposure to antigen. The two general ways in which tolerance can be induced correspond to the concepts of high- and low-dose tolerance introduced by Mitchison (138). High-dose tolerance is induced by administration of antigen in amounts greatly in excess of those necessary for optimal immunization. Low-dose tolerance is induced by the repeated administration of subimmunogenic amounts of antigen, usually in gradually increasing doses (216).

High-dose tolerance is most readily induced during the neonatal period, whereas low-dose tolerance is best achieved with antigens in a nonphagocytizable form (53–55, 71, 158). For example, when all high-molecular-weight material is removed from BCG by ultracentrifugation, very small doses of the remaining nonaggregated material will readily induce tolerance in mice. A polysaccharide antigen, such as that from the *Pneumococcus*, which does not contain a nonphagocytizable tolerogenic fraction, does not exhibit two separate zones for tolerance induction (96, 97, 205).

Another factor influencing the development of tolerance is the proliferation of immunologically responsive cells. Those factors that depress immunocyte proliferation tend to promote the induction of tolerance; for example, high-dose irradiation (98) and antimetabolites. The maneuvers that nonspecifically stimulate proliferation tend to inhibit the induction of tolerance or may even abort an existing state of tolerance. Examples of non-specific stimuli are endotoxin (24), adjuvants (152), and appropriate doses of X rays (64, 125).

A number of investigators have observed that tolerance is generally of finite duration and that circulating antibodies may appear spontaneously as the tolerant state wanes (139, 206, 213, 217). Induction of tolerance appears to preferentially affect cells producing high-affinity antibody. Thus, in studies of newborn and adult animals made tolerant to DNP-protein complexes by low doses of antigen, the small amounts of antibody produced by partially tolerant animals were of low affinity (214, 215).

Available evidence suggests that the thymus-dependent antigen-reactive cells are the target for techniques used for tolerance induction (79, 133, 212). This concept cannot, however, be considered as definitive at the present time.

To explain the observations made in relation to the induction of tolerance, a number of hypotheses have been suggested. Of these, the most cogent are that (a) either the antigen-reactive cell, its progeny, or the antibody-producing cells become unresponsive to antigen or die under the conditions of tolerance induction; or (b) under the conditions of tolerance induction, the immunocytes are stimulated to differentiate without going through the period of significant clonal proliferation necessary to generate sufficient numbers of the antibody-forming cells. Another hypothesis suggests that T-cell products (IgT) operating in the absence of functionally normal macrophages can suppress B-cell function (66).

These observations and hypotheses on the induction of tolerance can be fitted together in the following way. When antigen is presented to an animal in a form and concentration in which it can be localized (perhaps on macrophages and reticulum cells) and then presented indirectly to immunologically reactive B cells, the latter cells are stimulated to proliferate and ultimately give rise to adequate numbers of antibody-forming cells. On the other hand, when antigen reacts directly with B lymphoid cells, tolerance may develop either as a result of cell destruction or of premature differentiation without sufficient preliminary proliferation. High-zone tolerance may result from overwhelming the antigen-localizing capacity and direct interaction of antigen with B lymphoid cells. Low-zone tolerance may result from very low doses of nonphagocytizable antibody being inefficiently bound to macrophages but still interacting with those lymphoid cells bearing surface-bound high-affinity antibody. Under all conditions, the injection of antigen may incite two competing processes—one inducing antibody formation; the other, a tolerance state. The outcome of this competition would reflect the various conditions operative at any particular time. At present, this construct must be considered purely theoretical (56, 66).

Route of Administration and the Effect of Adjuvant

In addition to the importance of the dose of antigen, its route of administration is critical in determining the type of immunologic response. For example, the intradermal or subcutaneous route is much more effective at inducing delayed hypersensitivity than is injection by other routes. This fact has been demonstrated with a variety of protein and carbohydrate antigen (8, 46, 104, 220). Direct injection of antigen into lymph nodes will induce delayed hypersensitivity (16, 74), as will intraperitoneal, or even intravenous, injection when combined with adjuvant (109, 224).

Delayed hypersensitivity is now generally induced with antigen suspended in Freund's complete adjuvant—a suspension of tubercle bacilli in mineral oil (49, 72). However, other materials such as finely divided alumina will function as adjuvant. With Freund's adjuvant administered to guinea pigs, tuberculin sensitivity may develop as early as the third or fourth day. Rist (183) and Saenz (187) originally observed that the sensitizing action of killed microorganisms is greatly enhanced by the addition of mineral oil. They suggested that the oil might act as a solvent for lipopolysaccarides and in addition as a nonmetabolizable depot of antigen. The wax-D component of the tubercle bacillus appears also to be important for adjuvant effects (179). Injection of Freund's adjuvant into primitive species, such as the lamprey eel and the guitar fish, leads to the development of progressively growing granulomatous lesions that eventually overwhelm and kill the host.

The precise mode of action of adjuvants is not understood. The slow release of antigen and the inflammatory response with accumulation of mononuclear cells and macrophages is thought to be important, but there is no definitive proof of this assumption.

In summary, those factors that are known to favor the cellular immune response in preference to a humoral immune response include minute amounts of antigen, an intradermal route of administration, and the use of adjuvants. Another circumstance favoring the induction of delayed hypersensitivity is the presentation of a new determinant attached to a tolerant cell (110, 144). It has also been suggested (143) from studies of the efficacy of antigen-loaded allogeneic macrophages (20) that the homograft rejection reaction may function in the manner of a nonspecific adjuvant.

Other Factors Controlling the
Production of Specific Antibody

In addition to the parameters we have considered, many other factors are involved in control of the immune response. A relatively new field of investigation, of unusual interest and importance, is that of a genetic control. It is outside the scope of this text, however, and the interested reader is referred to the excellent reviews available elsewhere (116, 199). In this section we shall be concerned with the control of antibody synthesis by humoral antibody.

A variety of evidence supports the notion that passively administered humoral antibody will specifically inhibit the production of new antibody against concomitantly administered antigens (23, 223), a phenomenon known as immunologic suppression. A striking feature of this phenomenon is the high degree of specificity of the suppression. On this basis it has been suggested that the passively administered antibody combines with the antigenic determinants and prevents their contact or interaction with potential antibody-forming cells. The administration of antibody thus produces a block in the "afferent" arm of the immune response. The degree of afferent suppression of antibody synthesis is a function of the amount and affinity of the antibody administered (50, 223, 228).

Suppression of immunity is readily achieved when passively administered antibody is given shortly before, simultaneously with, or shortly after antigen. When administration is delayed, suppression is only partial and large amounts of passively administered antibody are required (233). Similarly, suppression of a secondary immune response is more difficult to achieve than suppression of a primary response (222).

These observations of immunologic suppression are consistent with the idea that passively administered antibody competes with cell-bound antibody for the available antigen. It is possible that this conclusion may encompass a concept of feedback inhibition of antibody synthesis by circulating antibody. Thus, Uhr and Baumann and others have suggested that circulating antibody may serve to limit antibody synthesis (222, 223). One would predict that two factors might be important in such feedback control: the concentration and the antigen-binding affinity of the circulating antibody. It has been suggested that circulating antibody influences the maturation of the immune response by competing most effectively with cells synthesizing antibody of low affinity, thereby favoring those cells synthesizing high-affinity antibody.

Summary

We have reviewed evidence on (*a*) the commitment of individual antibody-producing cells to a restricted class of immunoglobulin molecules; (*b*) the mechanism of antigen recognition by immunologically reactive cells; (*c*) the interaction of various cell-types—antigen-reactive, antibody-producing, lymphocyte, and macrophage; (*d*) the role of clonal proliferation in the production of high-affinity antibody; (*e*) the effect of the antigen dosage schedule and mode of administration, and (*f*) the control of antibody synthesis by humoral antibody. The accumulated evidence is all consistent with the clonal selection hypothesis of antibody synthesis.

The observations summarized may be organized in the following *hypothetical* scheme: administration of antigen leads to its interaction with phagocytic mononuclear cells and either directly or indirectly with antigen-reactive cells bearing on their surface pre-existing antibody or antibody-like molecules. Following the interaction of antigen with cells bearing surface antibody, the cell itself, or one of its contacts, is stimulated to proliferate and synthesize antibody, giving rise to a clone of potential antibody-forming cells. In the process those cells bearing surface antibody of the highest affinity are in the most favorable position to trap antigen and proliferate. The subsequent increase in antigen-binding affinity during the maturation of the immune response then reflects the more advantageous position of those clones stimulated to proliferate.

Chapter 15 References

1. Ada, G. L., and Byrt, P. Specific inactivation of antigen-reactive cells with I-labelled antigen, *Nature* 222:1291, 1969.

2. Adler, F. L., Fishman, M., and Dray, S. Antibody formation initiated in vitro. III. Antibody formation and allotypic specificity directed by ribonucleic acid from peritoneal exudate cells, *J. Immunol.* 97:554, 1966.

3. Anderson, R. E., Sprent, J., and Miller, J. F. A. P. Cell-to-cell interaction in the immune response, *J. Exp. Med.* 135:711, 1972.

4. Armstrong, W. D., Diener, E., and Shellam, G. R. Antigen-reactive cells in normal, immunized, and tolerant mice, *J. Exp. Med.* 129:393, 1969.

5. Ashman, R. F., and Raff, M. C. Direct demonstration of theta-positive antigen-binding cells with antigen-induced movement of thymus-dependent cell receptors, *J. Exp. Med.* 137:69, 1973.

6. Askonas, B. A., and Rhodes, J. M. Immunogenicity of antigen-containing ribonucleic acid preparations from macrophages, *Nature* 205:470, 1965.

7. Attardi, G., Cohn, M., Horibata, K., and Lennox, E. S. Antibody formation by rabbit lymph node cells. IV. The detailed methods for measuring antibody synthesis by individual cells, the kinetics of antibody formation by rabbits and the properties of cell suspensions, *J. Immunol.* 92:372, 1964.

8. Baker, A. B. Complement fixation as related to resistance and allergy in experimental tuberculosis, *Am. Rev. Tuberc.* 31:54, 1935.

9. Basten, A., Miller, J. F. A. P., Sprent, J., and Pye, J. A receptor for antibody on B lymphocytes. I. Method of detection and functional significance, *J. Exp. Med.* 135:610, 1972.

10. Basten, A., Miller, J. F. A. P., Warner, N. L., and Pye, J. Specific inactivation of thymus-derived (T) and non-thymus-derived (B) lymphocytes by 125 I-labelled antigen, *Nature (New Biol.)* 231:104, 1971.

11. Basten, A., Warner, N. L., and Mandel, T. A receptor for antibody on B lymphocytes. II. Immunochemical and electron microscopy characteristics, *J. Exp. Med.* 135:627, 1972.

12. Benacerraf, B., Nussenzweig, V., Maurer, P. H., and Stylos, W. Relationship between the net electrical charge of antigens and specific antibodies. An example of selection by antigen of cells producing highest affinity antibody, *Isr. J. Med. Sci.* 5:171, 1969.

13. Bernier, G. M., Ballieux, R. E., Tominaga, K. T., and Putman, F. W. Heavy chain subclasses of human γ globulin. Serum distribution and cellular localization, *J. Exp. Med.* 125:303, 1967.

14. Bernier, G. M., and Cebra, J. J. Polypeptide chains of human gamma-globulin cellular localization by fluorescent antibody, *Science* 144:1590, 1964.

15. Bernier, G. M., and Cebra, J. J. Frequency distribution of α, γ, κ and λ polypeptide chains in human lymphoid tissues, *J. Immunol.* 95:256, 1965.

16. Bessau, G. Immunbiologie der Tuberkulose. Tuberkulinempfindlichkeit und spezifischer Tuberkuloseschutz, *Klin. Wochenschr.* 4:337, 1925.

17. Bianco, C., Patrick, R., and Nussenzweig, V. A population of lymphocytes bearing a membrane receptor for antigen-antibody-complement complexes. I. Separation and characterization, *J. Exp. Med.* 132:702, 1970.

18. Bishop, D. C., and Gottlieb, A. A. Distribution of antigen-ribonucleoprotein complexes within rat peritoneal exudate cells, *J. Immunol.* 107:269, 1971.

19. Bishop, D. C., Pisciotta, A. V., and Abramoff, P. Synthesis of normal and "immunogenic RNA" in peritoneal macrophage cells, *J. Immunol.* 99:751, 1967.

20. Bloch, H., and Nordin, A. A. Production of tuberculin sensitivity, *Nature* 187:434, 1960.

21. Bloom, B. R., and Glade, P. R. (eds.) In Vitro Methods in Cell-Mediated Immunity, Academic Press, New York, 1971.

22. Brent, L. Tissue transplantation immunity, *Prog. Allergy*, 5:271, 1958.

23. Brody, N. I., Walker, J. G., and Siskind, G. W. Studies on the control of antibody synthesis, interaction of antigenic competition and suppression of antibody formation by passive antibody on the immune response, *J. Exp. Med.* 126:81, 1967.

24. Brooke, M. S. Conversion of immunological paralysis to immunity by endotoxin, *Nature* 206:635, 1965.

25. Burnet, F. M. The Clonal Selection Theory of Acquired Immunity, Vanderbilt University Press, Nashville, Tenn., 1959.

26. Burnet, F. M. The impact on ideas of immunology, *Cold Spring Harbor Symp. Quant. Biol.* 32:1, 1967.

27. Bush, M. E., Alkan, S. S., Nitecki, D. E., and Goodman, J. W. Antigen recognition and the immune response. "Self-help" with symmetrical bifunctional antigen molecules, *J. Exp. Med.* 136:1478, 1972.

28. Byrt, P., and Ada, G. L. An in vitro reaction between labelled flagellin or haemolyanin and lymphocyte-like cells from normal animals, *Immunology* 17:503, 1969.

29. Catanzaro, P. J., Graham, R. C., Jr., and Schwartz, H. J. Ultrastructural identification of possible sites of antigen processing in macrophages, *J. Immunol.* 103:618, 1969.

30. Cebra, J. J., Colberg, J. E., and Dray, S. Rabbit lymphoid cells differentiated with respect to α-, λ-, and μ-heavy polypeptide chains and to allotypic markers Aa1 and Aa2, *J. Exp. Med.* 123:547, 1966.

31. Chase, M. W. Immunologic tolerance, *Am. Rev. Microbiol.* 13:349, 1959.

32. Chiller, J. M., Habicht, G. S., and Wiegle, W. O. Cellular sites of immunologic unresponsiveness, *Proc. Natl. Acad. Sci. U.S.A.* 65:551, 1970.

33. Claman, H. N., and Chaperon, E. A. Immunologic complementation between thymus and marrow cells—a model for the two-cell theory of immunocompetence, *Transplant. Rev.* 1:92, 1969.

34. Claman, H. N., Chaperon, E. A., and Triplett, R. F. Immunocompetence of transferred thymus-marrow cell combinations, *J. Immunol.* 97:828, 1966.

35. Claman, H. N., Chaperon, E. A., and Triplett, R. F. Thymus-marrow cell combinations. Synergism in antibody production, *Proc. Soc. Exp. Biol. Med.* 122:1167, 1966.

36. Cline, M. J., Sprent, J., Warner, N. L., and Harris, A. W. Receptors for immunoglobulin on B lymphocytes and cells of a cultured plasma cell tumor, *J. Immunol.* 108:1126, 1972.

37. Cline, M. J., and Swett, V. C. The interaction of human monocytes and lymphocytes, *J. Exp. Med.* 128:1309, 1968.

38. Cohen, B. E., and Paul, W. E. Macrophage control of time-dependent changes in antigen sensitivity of immune T lymphocyte populations, *J. Immunol.* 112:359, 1974.

39. Coombs, R. R. A., Feinstein, A., and Wilson, A. B. Immunoglobulin determinants on the surface of human lymphocytes, *Lancet* 2:1157, 1969.

40. Cudkowicz, G., Shearer, G. M., and Ito, T. Cellular differentiation of the immune system of mice. VI. Strain differences in class differentiation and other properties of marrow cells, *J. Exp. Med.* 132:623, 1970.

41. Cudkowicz, G., Shearer, G. M., and Priore, R. L. Cellular differentiation of the immune system of mice. V. Class differentiation in marrow precursors of plaque-forming cells, *J. Exp. Med.* 130:481, 1969.

42. Davie, J. M., and Paul, W. E. Receptors on immunocompetent cells. IV, *J. Exp. Med.* 135:643, 1972.

43. Davie, J. M., and Paul, W. E. Receptors on immunocompetent cells. V, *J. Exp. Med.* 135:660, 1972.

44. Davies, A. J. S., Leuchars, E., Wallis, V., Marchant, R., and Elliot, E. V. The failure of thymus-derived cells to produce antibody, *Transplantation* 5:222, 1967.

45. Denman, A. M., Denman, E. J., and Embling, P. H. Changes in the lifespan of circulating small lymphocytes in mice after treatment with anti-lymphocyte globulin, *Lancet* 1:321, 1968.

46. Derick, C. L., Hitchcock, C. H., and Swift, H. F. Reactions of rabbits to non-hemolytic streptococci. III. A study of modes of sensitization, *J. Exp. Med.* 52:1, 1930.

47. Dickler, H. B., and Kunkel, H. G. Interaction of aggregated γ-globulin with B lymphocytes, *J. Exp. Med.* 136:191, 1972.

48. Diener, E., O'Callaghan, F., and Kraft, N. Immune response in vitro to salmonella H-antigens, not affected by anti-theta serum, *J. Immunol.* 107:1775, 1971.

49. Dienes, L., and Schoenheit, E. W. Local hypersensitiveness. I. Sensitization of tuberculous guinea pigs with egg-white and timothy pollen, *J. Immunol.* 14:9, 1927.

50. Dixon, F. J., Jacot-Guillarnod, H., and McConahey, P. J. The effect of passively administered antibody on antibody synthesis, *J. Exp. Med.* 125:1119, 1967.

51. Doria, G., Martinozzi, M., Agarossi, G., and DiPietro, S. In vitro primary immune response resulting from the interaction between bone marrow-derived and thymus cells, *Experientia* 26:410, 1970.

52. Dray, S. Effect of maternal isoantibodies on the quantitative expression of two allelic genes controlling γ-globulin allotypic specificities, *Nature* 195:677, 1962.

53. Dresser, D. W. Acquired immunological tolerance to a fraction of bovine gamma globulin, *Immunology* 4:13, 1961.

54. Dresser, D. W. Specific inhibition of antibody production. I. Protein-overloading paralysis, *Immunology* 5:161, 1962.

55. Dresser, D. W. Specific inhibition of antibody production. II. Paralysis induced in adult mice by small quantities of protein antigen, *Immunology* 5:378, 1962.

56. Dresser, D. W., and Mitchison, N. A. The mechanism of immunological paralysis, *Adv. Immunol.* 8:129, 1968.

57. Dubiski, S. Synthesis of allotypically defined immunoglobulins in rabbits, *Cold Spring Harbor Symp. Quant. Biol.* 32:311, 1967.

58. Dupuy, J. M., Perey, D. Y. E., and Good, R. A. Passive transfer with plasma, of delayed allergy in guinea pigs, *Lancet* 1:551, 1969.

59. Eisen, H. N., Simms, E. S., and Potter, M. Mouse myeloma proteins with antihapten antibody activity. The protein produced by plasma cell tumor MOPC-315, *Biochemistry* 7:4126, 1968.

60. Eisen, H. N., and Siskind, G. W. Variations in affinities of antibodies during the immune response, *Biochemistry* 3:996, 1964.

61. Elves, M. W. The Lymphocytes, J. B. Lippincott, Philadelphia, 1966.

62. Engers, H. D., and Unanue, E. R. The fate of anti-Ig-surface Ig complexes on B lymphocytes, *J. Immunol.* 110:465, 1973.

63. Farr, R. S. A quantitative immunochemical measure of the primary interaction between I*BSA and antibody, *J. Infect. Dis.* 103:239, 1958.

64. Fefer, A., and Nossal, G. J. V. Abolition of neonatally-induced homograft tolerance in mice by sublethal X-irradiation, *Transplant. Bull.* 29:73, 1962.

65. Feldmann, M. Cell interactions in the immune response in vitro. V., *J. Exp. Med.* 136:737, 1972.

66. Feldmann, M. Antigen specific T cell factors and their role in the regulation of TB interaction, *in* E. E. Sercarz, A. R. Williamson, and C. F. Fox (eds.), The Immune System. Genes, Receptors, Signals, p. 497, Academic Press, New York, 1974.

67. Feldmann, M., and Basten, A. Cell interactions in the immune response in vitro. IV., *J. Exp. Med.* 136:722, 1972.

68. Feldmann, M., and Nossal, G. J. V. Tolerance, enhancement and the regulation of interactions between T cells, B cells and macrophages, *Transplant. Rev.* 13:3, 1972.

69. Fishman, M., and Adler, F. L. Antibody formation initiated in vitro. II. Antibody synthesis in X-irradiated recipients of diffusion chambers containing nucleic acid derived from macrophages incubated with antigen, *J. Exp. Med.* 117:595, 1963.

70. Ford, W. L. The mechanism of lymphopenia produced by chronic irradiation of the rat spleen, *Br. J. Exp. Pathol.* 49:502, 1968.

71. Frei, P. C., Benacerraf, B., and Thorbecke, G. J. Phagocytosis of the antigen, a crucial step in the induction of the primary response, *Proc. Natl. Acad. Sci. U.S.A.* 53:20, 1965.

72. Freund, J., Casals, J., and Hosmer,

E. P. Sensitization and antibody formation after injection of tubercle bacilli and paraffin oil, *Proc. Soc. Exp. Biol. Med.* 37:509, 1938.

73. Friedman, H. P., Stavitsky, A. B., and Solomon, J. M. Induction in vitro of antibodies to phage T2: antigens in the RNA extract employed, *Science* 149:1106, 1965.

74. Gastinel, P., Coutel, Y., and Civatte, A. Contribution à l'etude de la tuberculose expérimentale du cobaye par inoculation intraganglionnaire, *Ann. Inst. Pasteur* 81:314, 1951.

75. Gell, P. G. H. Restrictions on antibody production by single cells, *Cold Spring Harbor Symp. Quant. Biol.* 32:441, 1967.

76. Gell, P. G. H. Features of cellular versus humoral immunity, *in* M. Landy and H. S. Lawrence (eds.), Mediators of Cellular Immunity, p. 80, Academic Press, New York, 1969.

77. Gell, P. G. H., and Sell, S. Studies on rabbit lymphocytes in vitro. II. Induction of blast transformation with antisera to six IgG allotypes and summation with mixtures of antisera to different allotypes, *J. Exp. Med.* 122:813, 1965.

78. Gershon, H., Bauminger, S., Sela, M., and Feldman, M. Studies on the competence of single cells to produce antibodies of two specificities, *J. Exp. Med.* 128:223, 1968.

79. Gershon, R. K., Wallis, V., Davies, A. J. S., and Leuchars, E.: Inactivation of thymus cells after multiple injections of antigen, *Nature* 218:380, 1968.

80. Gisler, R. H., and Dukor, P. A three-cell mosaic culture: in vitro immune response by a combination of pure B- and T-cells with peritoneal macrophages, *Cell. Immunol.* 4:341, 1972.

81. Goidl, E. A., Paul, W. E., Siskind, G. W., and Benacerraf, B.: The effect of antigen dose and time after immunization on the amount and affinity of anti-hapten antibody, *J. Immunol.* 100:371, 1968.

82. Gottlieb, A. A. Macrophage ribonucleoprotein: nature of the antigenic fragment, *Science* 165:592, 1969.

83. Gottlieb, A. A., Glisin, V. R., and Doty, P. Studies on macrophage RNA involved in antibody production, *Proc. Natl. Acad. Sci. U.S.A.* 57:1849, 1967.

84. Gottlieb, A. A., and Straus, D. S. Physical studies on the light density ribonucleoprotein complex of macrophage cells, *J. Biol. Chem.* 244:3324, 1969.

85. Greaves, M. F., and Hogg, N. M. Immunoglobulin determinants on the surface of antigen binding T- and B-lymphocytes in mice, *Prog. Immunol.* 1:111, 1971.

86. Greaves, M. F., Owen, J. J. T., and Raff, M. C. T and B lymphocytes, Elsevier/Excerpta Medica, North-Holland Publishing Co., Amsterdam, 1973.

87. Greaves, M. F., Torrigiani, G., and Roitt, I. M. Blocking of the lymphocyte receptor site for cell mediated hypersensitivity and transplantation reactions by anti-light chain sera, *Nature* 222:885, 1969.

88. Green, I., Vassalli, P., Nussenzweig, V., and Benacerraf, B. Specificity of the antibodies produced by single cells following immunization with antigens bearing two types of antigenic determinants, *J. Exp. Med.* 125:511, 1967.

89. Hanifin, J. M., and Cline, M. J. Human monocytes and macrophages. Interaction with antigen and lymphocytes, *J. Cell Biol.* 46:97, 1970.

90. Hartmann, K. U. Induction of a hemolysin response in vitro. Interaction of cells of bone marrow origin and thymic origin, *J. Exp. Med.* 132:1267, 1970.

91. Haskill, J. S., Byrt, P., and Marbrook, J. In vitro and in vivo studies of the immune response to sheep erythrocytes using partially purified cell preparations, *J. Exp. Med.* 131:57, 1970.

92. Haskill, J. S., Elliott, B. E., Kerbel, R., Axelrad, M. A., and Eidinger, D. Classification of thymus-derived and marrow-derived lymphocytes by demonstration of their antigen-binding characteristics, *J. Exp. Med.* 135:1410, 1972.

93. Hersh, E. M., and Harris, J. E. Macrophage-lymphocyte interaction in the antigen-induced blastogenic response of human peripheral blood leukocytes, *J. Immunol.* 100:1184, 1968.

94. Hoffman, M. Peritoneal macrophages in the immune response to SRBC in vitro, *Immunology* 18:791, 1970.

95. Hood, L., Gray, W. R., Sanders, B. G., and Dreyer, W. J. Light chain evolution, *Cold Spring Harbor Symp. Quant. Biol.* 32:133, 1967.

96. Howard, J. G., Elson, J., Christie, G. H., and Kinsky, R. G. Studies on immunological paralysis. II. The detection and significance of antibody-forming cells in the spleen during immunological paralysis with type III pneumococcal polysaccharide, *Clin. Exp. Immunol.* 4:41, 1969.

97. Howard, J. G., and Siskind, G. W. Studies on immunological paralysis. I. A consideration of macrophage involvement in the induction of paralysis and immunity by type II pneumococcal polysaccharide, *Clin. Exp. Immunol.* 4:29, 1969.

98. Humphrey, J. H. The suppression of immune responses by nonspecific agents, *in* M. Samter (ed.), Immunological Diseases, p. 100, Little, Brown and Co., Boston, 1965.

99. Humphrey, J. H., and White, R. G. Immunology for Students of Medicine, 3rd ed., F. A. Davis Co., Philadelphia, 1970.

100. Janossy, G., Humphrey, J. H., Pepys, M. B., and Greaves, M. F. Complement independence of stimulation of mouse splenic B lymphocytes by mitogens, *Nature (New Biol.)* 245:108, 1973.

101. Jerne, N. K. A study of avidity. Based on rabbit skin responses to diphtheria toxin-antitoxin mixtures, *Acta Pathol. Microbiol. Scand.*, suppl. 87.

102. Jerne, N. K., Nordin, A. A., and Henry, C. The agar plaque technique for recognizing antibody-producing cells, *in* D. B. Amos and H. Koprowski (eds.), Cell-Bound Antibodies, p. 109, Wistar Institute Press, Philadelphia, 1963.

103. Jondal, M., Holm, G., and Wigzell, H. Surface markers on human T and B lymphocytes. I. A large population of lymphocytes forming non-immune rosettes with sheep red blood cells, *J. Exp. Med.* 136:207, 1972.

104. Julianelle, L. A. Reactions of rabbits to intracutaneous injections

of pneumococci and their products. IV. The development of skin reactivity to derivatives of pneumococcus, *J. Exp. Med.* 51:625, 1930.

105. Katz, D. H., and Benacerraf, B. The regulatory influence of activated T cells on B cell responses to antigen, *Adv. Immunol.* 15:1, 1972.

106. Kennedy, J. C., Treadwell, P. E., and Lennox, E. S. Antigen-specific synergism in the immune response of irradiated mice given marrow cells and peritoneal cavity cells or extracts, *J. Exp. Med.* 132:353, 1970.

107. Kölsch, E., and Mitchison, N. A. The subcellular distribution of antigen in macrophages, *J. Exp. Med.* 128:1059, 1968.

108. Lance, E. M., and Batchelor, V. R. Selective suppression of cellular immunity by antilymphocyte serum, *Transplantation* 6:490, 1968.

109. Landsteiner, K., and Chase, M. W. Studies on the sensitization of animals with simple chemical compounds. IX. Skin sensitization induced by injection of conjugates, *J. Exp. Med.* 73:431, 1941.

110. Lawrence, H. S. Homograft sensitivity. An expression of the immunologic origins and consequences of individuality, *Physiol. Rev.* 39:811, 1959.

111. Lawrence, H. S., and Landy, M. (eds.), Perspectives in Immunology, Mediators of Cellular Immunity, Academic Press, New York, 1969.

112. Lawton, A. R. III, Asofsky, R., Hylton, M. B., and Cooper, M. D. Suppression of immunoglobulin class synthesis in mice. I. Effects of treatment with antibody to μ-chain, *J. Exp. Med.* 135:277, 1972.

113. Lay, W. H., Mendes, N. F., Bianco, C., and Nussenzweig, V. Binding of sheep red blood cells to a large population of human lymphocytes, *Nature* 230:531, 1971.

114. Little, J. R., and Eisen, H. N. Preparation and characterization of antibodies specific for the 2,4,6-trinitrophenic group, *Biochemistry* 5:3385, 1966.

115. McConnell, I., Munro, A., Gurner, B. W., and Coombs, R. R. A. Studies on actively allergized cells. I. The cytodynamics and morphology of rosette-forming lymph node cells in mice and inhibition of rosette-formation with antibody to mouse immunoglobulins, *Int. Arch. Allergy Appl. Immunol.* 35:209, 1969.

116. McDevitt, H. O., and Benacerraf, B. Genetic control of specific immune responses, *Adv. Immunol.* 11:31, 1969.

117. Mage, R. G. Quantitative studies on the regulation of expression of genes for immunoglobulin allotypes in heterozygous rabbits, *Cold Spring Harbor Symp. Quant. Biol.* 32:203, 1967.

118. Mage, R. G., and Dray, S. Persistence of altered expression of allelic γG-immunoglobulin allotypes in an "allotype suppressed" rabbit after immunization, *Nature* 212:699, 1966.

119. Mage, R. G., Young, G. O., and Dray, S. An effect upon the regulation of gene expression: allotype suppression at the *a* locus in heterozygous offspring of immunized rabbits, *J. Immunol.* 98:502, 1967.

120. Mäkelä, O. The specificity of antibodies produced by single cells, *Cold Spring Harbor Symp. Quant. Biol.* 32:423, 1967.

121. Mäkelä, O. Cellular heterogeneity in the production of an anti-hapten antibody, *J. Exp. Med.* 126:159, 1967.

122. Mäkelä, O., Cross, A. M., and Kosunen, T. U. (eds.), Cell Interactions and Receptor Antibodies in Immune Responses, Academic Press, New York, 1971.

123. Mäkelä, O., Cross, A. M., and Ruoslahti, E. Similarities between the cellular receptor antibody and the secreted antibody, *in* R. T. Smith and R. A. Good (eds.), Cellular Recognition, p. 287, Appleton-Century-Crofts, New York, 1969.

124. Mäkelä, O., and Nossal, G. J. V. Bacterial adherence: a method for detecting antibody production by single cells, *J. Immunol.* 87:447, 1961.

125. Mäkelä, O., and Nossal, G. J. V. Accelerated breakdown of immunological tolerance following whole body irradiation, *J. Immunol.* 88:613, 1962.

126. Marchalonis, J. J., Atwell, J. L., and Cone, R. E. Isolation of surface immunoglobulin from lymphocytes from human and murine thymus, *Nature (New Biol.)* 235:240, 1972.

127. Martin, W. J., and Miller, J. F. A. P. Cell to cell interaction in the immune response, *J. Exp. Med.* 128:855, 1968.

128. Mason, S., and Warner, N. L. The immunoglobulin nature of the antigen recognition site on cells mediating transplantation immunity and delayed hypersensitivity, *J. Immunol.* 104:762, 1970.

129. Merchant, B., and Brahmi, Z. Duplicate plating of immune cell products: analysis of globulin class secretion by single cells, *Science* 167:69, 1970.

130. Miller, H. C., and Cudkowicz, G. Antigen-specific cells in mouse bone marrow. I. Lasting effects of priming on immunocyte production by transferred marrow, *J. Exp. Med.* 132:1122, 1970.

131. Miller, J. F. A. P. Interaction between thymus-dependent (T) cells and bone marrow derived (B) cells in antibody responses, *in* O. Mäkelä, A. Cross, and T. U. Kosunen (eds.), Cell Interactions and Receptor Antibodies in Immune Response, p. 293, Academic Press, New York, 1971.

132. Miller, J. F. A. P., and Mitchell, G. F. Cell to cell interaction in the immune response, *J. Exp. Med.* 128:801, 1968.

133. Miller, J. F. A. P., and Mitchell, F. G. Cell to cell interaction in the immune response. V. Target cells for tolerance induction, *J. Exp. Med.* 131:674, 1970.

134. Miller, J. F. A. P., and Sprent, J. Cell-to-cell interaction in the immune response. VI., *J. Exp. Med.* 134:66, 1971.

135. Mishell, R. I., Dutton, R. W., and Raidt, D. J. Cell components in the immune response. I. Gradient separation of immune cells, *Cell. Immunol.* 1:175, 1970.

136. Mitchell, G. F., and Miller, J. F. A. P. Cell-to-cell interaction in the immune response, *J. Exp. Med.* 121:821, 1968.

137. Mitchell, G. F., and Miller, J. F. A. P. Immunological activity of thymus and thoracic-duct lymphocytes, *Proc. Natl. Acad. Sci. U.S.A.* 59:296, 1968.

138. Mitchison, N. A. Induction of im-

munological paralysis in two zones of dosage, *Proc. R. Soc. Lond. (Biol.)* 161:275, 1964.

139. Mitchison, N. A. Recovery from immunological paralysis in relation to age and residual antigen, *Immunology* 9:129, 1965.

140. Mitchison, N. A. Antigen recognition responsible for the induction in vitro of the secondary response, *Cold Spring Harbor Symp. Quant. Biol.* 32:431, 1967.

141. Mitchison, N. A. Recognition of antigen, *in* K. B. Warren (ed.), Differentiation and Immunology, p. 29, Academic Press, New York, 1968.

142. Mitchison, N. A. Cell populations involved in immune responses, *in* M. Landy and W. Braun (eds.), Immunological Tolerance: A Reassessment of Mechanisms of the Immune Responses, p. 115, Academic Press, New York, 1969.

143. Mitchison, N. A. Features of cellular versus humoral immunity, *in* H. S. Lawrence and M. Landy (eds.), Mediators of Cellular Immunity, p. 73, Academic Press, New York, 1969.

144. Mitchison, N. A., and Dube, O. L. Studies on the immunological response to foreign tumor transplants in the mouse. II. The relation between hemagglutinating antibody and graft resistance in the normal mouse and mice pretreated with tissue preparations, *J. Exp. Med.* 102:179, 1955.

145. Modabber, F., Morikawa, S., and Coons, A. H. Antigen-binding cells in normal mouse thymus, *Science* 170:1102, 1970.

146. Moller, G. (ed.). Antigen-binding lymphocyte receptors, *Transplant. Rev.* 5:3, 1970.

147. Mosier, D. E. A requirement for two cell types for antibody formation in vitro, *Science* 158:1573, 1967.

148. Mosier, D. E. Cell interactions in the primary immune response in vitro: a requirement for specific cell clusters, *J. Exp. Med.* 129:351, 1969.

149. Mosier, D. E., Fitch, F. W., Rowley, D. A., and Davies, A. J. S. Cellular deficit in thymectomized mice, *Nature* 225:276, 1970.

150. Munro, A., and Hunter, P. In vitro reconstitution of the immune response of thymus-derived mice to sheep red blood cells, *Nature* 225:277, 1970.

151. Naor, D., and Sulitzneau, D. Binding of radioiodinated bovine serum albumin to mouse spleen cells, *Nature* 214:687, 1967.

152. Neeper, C. A., and Seastone, C. V. Mechanisms of immunologic paralysis by pneumococcal polysaccharide. II. The influence of non-specific factors on the immunity of paralyzed mice to pneumococcal infection, *J. Immunol.* 91:378, 1963.

153. Nelson, D. S. Macrophages and Immunity, John Wiley & Sons, New York, 1969.

154. Nossal, G. J. V. Antibody production by single cells, *Br. J. Exp. Pathol.* 39:544, 1958.

155. Nossal, G. J. V. Antibody production by single cells. IV. Further studies on multiply immunized animals, *Br. J. Exp. Pathol.* 41:89, 1960.

156. Nossal, G. J. V., Abbot, A., and Mitchell, J. Antigens in immunity. XIV. Electron microscopic radioautographic studies of antigen capture in the lymph node medulla, *J. Exp. Med.* 127:263, 1968.

157. Nossal, G. J. V., Abbot, A., Mitchell, J., and Lummus, Z. Antigen in immunity. XV. Ultrastructural features of antigen capture in primary and secondary lymphoid follicles, *J. Exp. Med.* 127:277, 1968.

158. Nossal, G. J. V., and Ada, G. L. Recognition of foreignness in immune and tolerant animals, *Nature* 201:580, 1964.

159. Nossal, G. J. V., and Ada, G. L. Antigens, Lymphoid Cells, and the Immune Response, Academic Press, New York, 1971.

160. Nossal, G. J. V., Cunningham, A., Mitchell, G. F., and Miller, J. F. A. P. Cell-to-cell interaction in the immune response. III., *J. Exp. Med.* 128:839, 1968.

161. Nossal, G. J. V., and Mäkelä, O. Kinetic studies on the incidence of cells appearing to form two antibodies, *J. Immunol.* 88:604, 1962.

162. Nossal, G. J. V., Szenberg, A., Ada, G. L., and Austin, C. M. Single cell studies on 19s antibody production, *J. Exp. Med.* 119:485, 1964.

163. Nossal, G. J. V., Warner, N. L., Lewis, H., and Sprent, J. Quantitative features of a sandwich radioimmunolabeling technique for lymphocyte surface receptors, *J. Exp. Med.* 135:405, 1972.

164. Nussenzweig, V., et al. Receptors for C3 on B lymphocytes: possible role in the immune response, *in* B. Amos (ed.), Progress in Immunology, p. 78, Academic Press, New York, 1971.

165. Nussenzweig, V., Green, I., Vassalli, P., and Benacerraf, B. Changes in the proportion of guinea pig γ_1 and γ_2 antibodies during immunization and the cellular localization of these immunoglobulins, *Immunology* 14:601, 1968.

166. Ormai, S., and Clercq, E. Polymethacrylic acid: effects on lymphocyte output of the thoracic duct in rats, *Science* 163:471, 1969.

167. Pantelouris, E. M. Observations on the immunobiology of "nude" mice, *Immunology* 20:247, 1971.

168. Paraskevas, F., Orr, K. B., Anderson, E. D., Lee, S. T., and Israels, L. G. The biological significance of Fc receptor on mouse B-lymphocytes, *J. Immunol.* 108:1729, 1972.

169. Pearsall, N. N., and Weiser, R. S. The Macrophage, Lea & Febiger, Philadelphia, 1970.

170. Pernis, B., and Chiappino, G. Identification in human lymphoid tissues of cells that produce group 1 or group 2 gamma-globulins, *Immunology* 7:500, 1964.

171. Pernis, B., Chiappino, G., Kelus, A. S., and Gell, P. G. H. Cellular localization of immunoglobulins with different allotypic specificities in rabbit lymphoid tissues, *J. Exp. Med.* 122:853, 1965.

172. Peterson, H. H., and Ingraham, J. S. Limitation of single cells to the production of a single antibody in response to a coupled antigen, *Fed. Proc.* 26:641, 1967.

173. Pinchuck, P., Fishman, M., Adler, F. L., and Maurer, P. H. Antibody formation: initiation in "nonresponder" mice by macrophage synthetic polypeptide RNA, *Science* 160:194, 1968.

174. Plant, M., Lichtenstein, L. M., Gillespie, E., et al. Studies on the mechanism of lymphocyte-mediated

cytolysis. IV. Specificity of the histamine receptor on effector T cells, *J. Immunol.* 111:389, 1973.

175. Plotz, P. H. Specific inhibition of an antibody response by affinity labelling, *Nature* 223:1373, 1969.

176. Raff, M. C. Theta isoantigen as a marker of thymus-derived lymphocytes in mice, *Nature* 224:378, 1969.

177. Raff, M. C. Role of thymus-derived lymphocytes in the secondary humoral immune response in mice, *Nature* 226:1257, 1970.

178. Raff, M. C., Sternberg, M., and Taylor, R. B. Immunoglobulin determinants on the surface of mouse lymphoid cells, *Nature* 225:553, 1970.

179. Raffel, S., Arnaud, L. E., Dukes, C. D., and Huang, J. S. The role of the "wax" of the tubercle bacillus in establishing delayed hypersensitivity. II. Hypersensitivity to a protein antigen, egg albumin, *J. Exp. Med.* 90:53, 1949.

180. Rajewsky, K., Schirrmacher, V., Nase, S., and Jerne, N. K. The requirement of more than one antigenic determinant for immunogenicity, *J. Exp. Med.* 129:1131, 1969.

181. Rich, R. R., and Pierce, C. W. Biological expressions of lymphocyte activation. I., *J. Exp. Med.* 137:205, 1973.

182. Rich, R. R., and Pierce, C. W. Biological expressions of lymphocyte activation. II., *J. Exp. Med.* 137:649, 1973.

183. Rist, N. Les lésions métastatiques produites par les bacilles tuberculeux morts enrobés dans les paraffines, *Ann. Inst. Pasteur.* 61:121, 1938.

184. Roelants, G. E., and Goodman, J. W. Immunochemical studies on the poly-γ-D-glutamyl capsule of *Bacillus anthracis* IV. The association with peritoneal exudate cell ribonucleic acid of the polypeptide in immunogenic and nonimmunogenic forms, *Biochemistry* 7:1432, 1968.

185. Roelants, G. E., and Goodman, J. W. The chemical nature of macrophage RNA-antigen complexes and their relevance to immune induction, *J. Exp. Med.* 130:557, 1969.

186. Ross, G. D., et al. Two different complement receptors on human

lymphocytes, *J. Exp. Med.* 138:798, 1973.

187. Saenz, A. Influence de la désensibilisation sur la dispersion des germes de surinfection chez des cobayes rendus hyperallergiques au moyen de bacilles tuberculeux morts enrobés dans l'huile de vaseline, *C. R. Soc. Biol.* 130:219, 1939.

188. Sahiar, K., and Schwartz, R. S. Inhibition of 19S antibody synthesis by 7S antibody, *Science* 145:395, 1964.

189. Schimpl, A., and Wecker, E. Inhibition of in vitro immune response by treatment of spleen cell suspensions with anti-θ-serum, *Nature* 226:1258, 1970.

190. Schlossman, S. F. Features of cellular versus humoral immunity, *in* H. S. Lawrence and M. Landy (eds.), Mediators of Cellular Immunity, p. 101, Academic Press, New York, 1969.

191. Schmidtke, J. R., and Unanue, E. R. Macrophage-antigen interaction: uptake, metabolism, and immunogenicity of foreign albumin, *J. Immunol.* 107:331, 1971.

192. Schoenberg, M. D., Mumaw, V. R., Moore, R. D., and Weisberger, A. S. Cytoplasmic interaction between macrophages and lymphocytic cells in antibody synthesis, *Science* 143:964, 1964.

193. Schwartz, R. S. Specificity of immunosuppression by antimetabolites, *Fed. Proc.* 25:165, 1966.

194. Segal, S., Globerson, A., Feldman, M., Hainovich, J., and Givol, D. Specific blocking in vitro of antibody synthesis by affinity labelling reagents, *Nature* 223:1374, 1969.

195. Sela, M., and Mozes, E. Dependence of the chemical nature of antibodies on the net electrical charge of antigens, *Proc. Natl. Acad. Sci. U.S.A.* 55:445, 1966.

196. Sell, S. Studies on rabbit lymphocytes in vitro. VIII. The relationship between heterozygosity and homozygosity of lymphocyte donor and per cent blast transformation induced by antiallotype sera, *J. Exp. Med.* 127:1139, 1968.

197. Sell, S., and Gell, P. G. H. Studies on rabbit lymphocytes in vitro. I. Stimulation of blast transformation with an antiallotype serum, *J. Exp. Med.* 122:423, 1965.

198. Sell, S., and Gell, P. G. H. Studies

on rabbit lymphocytes in vitro. IV. Blast transformation of the lymphocytes from newborn rabbits induced by antiallotype serum to a paternal IgG allotype not present in the serum of the lymphocyte donors, *J. Exp. Med.* 122:923, 1965.

199. Sercarz, E. E., Williamson, A. R., and Fox, C. F. The Immune System. Genes, Receptors, Signals, Academic Press, New York, 1974.

200. Sharp, J. A., and Burwell, R. G. Interaction ("peripolesis") of macrophages and lymphocytes after skin homografting or challenge with soluble antigens, *Nature* 188:474, 1960.

201. Shearer, G. M., and Cudkowicz, G. Distinct events in the immune response elicited by transferred marrow and thymus cells. I. Antigen requirements and proliferation of thymic antigen-reactive cells, *J. Exp. Med.* 130:1243, 1969.

202. Shevach, E. M., Herberman, R., Frank, M. M., and Green, I. Receptors for complement and immunoglobulin on human leukemic cells and human lymphoblastoid cell lines, *J. Clin. Invest.* 51:1933, 1972.

203. Siskind, G. W., and Benacerraf, B. Cell selection by antigen in the immune response, *Adv. Immunol.* 10:1, 1969.

204. Siskind, G. W., Dunn, P., and Walker, J. G. Studies on the control of antibody synthesis. II. Effect of antigen dose and of suppression by passive antibody on the affinity of antibody synthesized, *J. Exp. Med.* 127:55, 1968.

205. Siskind, G. W., and Howard, J. G. Studies on the induction of immunological unresponsiveness to pneumococcal polysaccharide in mice, *J. Exp. Med.* 124:417, 1966.

206. Siskind, G. W., Paterson, P. Y., and Thomas, L. Induction of unresponsiveness and immunity in newborn and adult mice with pneumococcal polysaccharide, *J. Immunol.* 90:929, 1963.

207. Smith, C. W., Goldman, A. S., and Yates, R. D. Interactions of lymphocytes and macrophages from human colostrum, *Exp. Cell Res.* 69:409, 1971.

208. Smith, R. T. Immunological toler-

ance of nonliving antigens, *Adv. Immunol.* 1:67, 1961.

209. Smith, R. T., and Landy, M. (eds.). Immune Surveillance, Academic Press, New York, 1970.

210. Sterzl, J. Immunological tolerance as the result of terminal differentiation of immunologically competent cells, *Nature* 209:416, 1966.

211. Talmage, D. W., and Maurer, P. H. I^{131}-labelled antigen precipitation as a measure of quantity and quality of antibody, *J. Infect. Dis.* 92:288, 1953.

212. Taylor, R. B. Cellular cooperation in the antibody response of mice to two serum albumins: specific function of thymus cells, *Transplant. Rev.* 1:114, 1969.

213. Terres, G., and Hughes, W. L. Acquired immune tolerance in mice to crystalline bovine serum albumin, *J. Immunol.* 83:459, 1959.

214. Theis, G. A., and Siskind, G. W. Selection of cell populations in induction of tolerance: affinity of antibody formed in partially tolerant rabbits, *J. Immunol.* 100:138, 1968.

215. Theis, G. A., Thorbecke, G. J., and Siskind, G. W. Antibody affinity in immunological tolerance, *Fed. Proc.* 27:685, 1968.

216. Thorbecke, G. J., and Benacerraf, B. Tolerance in adult rabbits by repeated non-immunogenic doses of bovine serum albumin, *Immunology* 13:141, 1967.

217. Thorbecke, G. J., Siskind, G. W., and Goldberger, N. The induction in mice of sensitization and immunological unresponsiveness by neonatal injection of bovine γ-globulin, *J. Immunol.* 87:147, 1961.

218. Turk, J. L. Delayed Hypersensi-tivity, p. 105, John Wiley & Sons, New York, 1967.

219. Turk, J. L., and Willoughby, D. A. Central and peripheral effects of anti-lymphocyte sera, *Lancet* 1:249, 1967.

220. Uhr, J. W. Delayed hypersensitivity, *Physiol. Rev.* 46:359, 1966.

221. Uhr, J. W. Models for receptor sites on thymic lymphocytes, *in* H. S. Lawrence and M. Landy (eds.), Mediators of Cellular Immunity, p. 413, Academic Press, New York, 1969.

222. Uhr, J. W., and Baumann, J. B. Antibody formation. II. The specific anamnestic antibody response, *J. Exp. Med.* 113:959, 1961.

223. Uhr, J. W., and Möller, G. Regulatory effect of antibody on the immune response, *Adv. Immunol.* 8:81, 1968.

224. Uhr, J. W., Salvin, S. B., and Pappenheimer, A. M., Jr. Delayed hypersensitivity. II. Induction of hypersensitivity in guinea pigs by means of antigen-antibody complexes, *J. Exp. Med.* 105:11, 1957.

225. Unanue, E. R., and Askonas, B. A. Persistence of immunogenicity of antigen after uptake by macrophages, *J. Exp. Med.* 127:915, 1968.

226. Unanue, E. R., and Cerottini, J. C. The immunogenicity of antigen bound to the plasma membrane of macrophages, *J. Exp. Med.* 131:711, 1970.

227. Van Furth, R. (ed.). Mononuclear Phagocytes, F. A. Davis Co., Philadelphia, 1970.

228. Walker, J. G., and Siskind, G. W. Effect of antibody affinity upon its ability to suppress antibody formation, *Immunology* 14:21, 1968.

229. Walters, C. S., and Wigzell, H. Demonstration of heavy and light chain antigenic determinants on the cell-bound receptor for antigen. Similarities between membrane-attached and humoral antibodies produced by the same cell, *J. Exp. Med.* 132:1233, 1970.

230. Warner, N. L., Byrt, P., and Ada, G. L. Blocking of the lymphocyte antigen receptor site with anti-immunoglobulin sera in vitro, *Nature* 226:942, 1970.

231. Weiser, R. S., Myrvik, Q. N., and Pearsall, N. N. Fundamentals of Immunology, Lea & Febiger, Philadelphia, 1970.

232. Weiss, L. The Cells and Tissues of the Immune System. Structure, Functions, Interactions, Prentice-Hall, Englewood Cliffs, N.J., 1972.

233. Wigzell, H. Antibody synthesis at the cellular level. Antibody-induced suppression of 7S antibody synthesis, *J. Exp. Med.* 124:953, 1966.

234. Wigzell, H., and Anderson, B. Cell separation on antigen-coated columns. Elimination of high rate antibody-forming cells and immunological memory cells, *J. Exp. Med.* 129:23, 1969.

235. Williamson, A. R., and Askonas, B. A. Senescence of an antibody-forming cell clone, *Nature* 238:337, 1972.

236. Zaalberg, O. B., Van der Meul, V. A., and Van Twisk, M. J. Antibody production by isolated spleen cells: a study of the cluster and the plaque techniques, *J. Immunol.* 100:451, 1968.

237. Zucker-Franklin, D., and Berney, S. Electron microscope study of surface immunoglobulin-bearing human tonsil cells, *J. Exp. Med.* 135:533, 1972.

Chapter 16   Plasma Cells, Lymphocytes, and Immunoglobulins

The response of the immune system to antigenic challenge is complex, involving cell activation, cell proliferation, and specific antibody synthesis. In the preceding chapter we considered general aspects of this response, including antigen recognition, cellular interactions, and clonal proliferation and its relation to the production of high-affinity antibody. In this chapter we shall consider the characteristics of the antibody molecules and some of the details of their synthesis.

The principal source of immunoglobulins is the plasma cell, although lymphocytes also may manufacture small amounts of these proteins. Unless otherwise indicated, we shall be considering normal plasma cell products and synthetic mechanisms. In Chapter 20 the characteristics of malignant plasma cells and their products will be described.

Immunoglobulin Structure

The immunoglobulin G (IgG) molecule may be taken as the prototype immunoglobulin. Other immunoglobulins are basically similar to IgG, although they may differ in the number of subunits or in the structure of the component chains. The IgG antibody molecule is composed of four polypeptide chains and attached carbohydrates, as shown schematically in Fig. 16.1. Two of the polypeptide chains are of molecular weight about 52,000 each and are designated *heavy chains*. Each is made up of about 450 amino acids. The two *light chains* of the molecule each are composed of about 214 amino acids and have a molecular weight of 22,000. On the basis of structure, the light chains are divided into two major classes—kappa and lambda. As shown in Fig. 16.1, the chains are linked together by disulfide bridges and hydrogen bonding. The carbohydrate components are attached primarily to the heavy chains. The entire immunoglobulin molecule, including carbohydrate, has a molecular weight of between 150,000 and 180,000, depending on the size of the heavy chains and attached polysaccharide.

A more detailed view of the structure of IgG, shown in Fig. 16.2, is based on data provided by Edelman and his associates (30), and shows the locations of the carbohydrate moieties as well as those of the inter- and intrachain disulfide bridges. The approximate region between amino acids 220 and 240 is called the *hinge region* and contains the interchain disulfide bond (5, 37, 38).

The three-dimensional configuration of the immunoglobulin molecule is determined by the amino acid sequence and the constraints placed by the intra- and interchain disulfide bonds. From X-ray crystallographic studies, a three-dimensional picture of the molecule has gradually emerged (6, 124).

Structure-function Relationships

The various functional activities of the antibody molecule are spatially separated. These are depicted schematically in Fig. 16.3. Antigen-binding activity occurs at two distinct sites, which accounts for the bivalent nature of the interaction of antibody with antigen. The antigen-binding region may be isolated by treatment of the immunoglobulin molecule with papain (24, 30, 45, 78, 88,

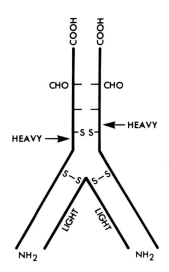

Figure 16.1 Simplified scheme of the basic immunoglobulin structure. The molecule is composed of two heavy and two light polypeptide chains held together by disulfide bonds. Carbohydrate is attached to the heavy chains.

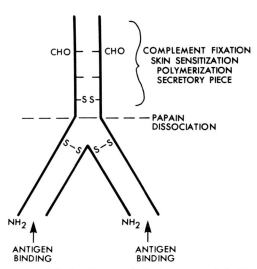

Figure 16.3 Simplified scheme of the immunoglobulin molecule, showing the spatial separation of the antigen-binding sites from the sites of other biological functions. Papain cleaves the molecule in the region shown in the diagram. The two cleaved portions of the molecule containing the antigen-binding sites are the Fab pieces. The rest of the molecule is the Fc piece.

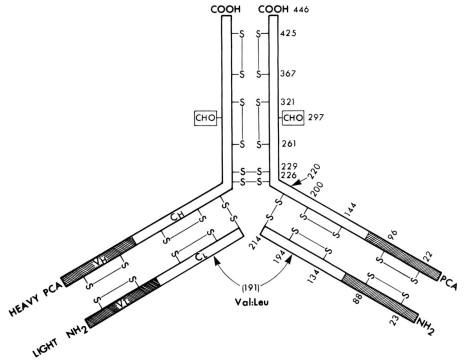

Figure 16.2 More detailed scheme of immunoglobulin structure, showing the variable (V) region of the heavy and light chains. The numbers denote positions of amino acids in the polypeptide chains. The positions of the inter- and intrachain disulfide bridges are shown. *CHO* denotes the position of the carbohydrate moieties. For more detailed information, see references 6, 30, 37, 38, 92, 124.

89, 92); this causes hydrolysis in the hinge region. In combination with agents that dissociate disulfide bonds, it also releases a portion of the molecule known as the *Fab piece.* Two such pieces are released, each consisting of the N-terminal half of one heavy chain plus an entire light chain. Each Fab piece contains an antigen-binding site and acts as a univalent antibody molecule.

The nonantigen-binding properties of the immunoglobulin molecules are located at the other end. These properties include complement fixation, skin sensitization, polymerization, and attachment of the secretory piece. The portion of the immunoglobulin molecule associated with these functional characteristics is also released by papain digestion and is designated the *Fc piece.* It includes the C-terminal ends of both heavy chains.

In general, the biologic properties of the immunoglobulin molecules are associated with the Fc piece, whereas the antigen-binding properties are associated with the Fab piece.

Variable and Common Regions of the Immunoglobulin Chains

Each immunoglobulin polypeptide chain can be viewed as having subunits of about 110 amino acids and an internal disulfide bridge (see Fig. 16.2). There are two such regions on each light chain and four on each heavy chain. Beginning at the N-terminal end of each polypeptide chain, the first region of 110 amino acids is the *variable* (V) region. Thus, the entire immunoglobulin molecule will have variable regions associated with each of two heavy (H) chains and with each of two light (L) chains. The variable regions of the H and L chains are involved in antigen binding (111). If one examines IgG immunoglobulins of a single light-chain class (for example, kappa), the principal differences in the amino acid composition among molecules would be found in the variable regions.

The remainder of each chain is usually termed the *common* (C) region. The common region contains disulfide bridges linking the heavy and light chains.

Light-chain Variable Regions Three levels of variability can be found in the V region of light chains (amino acids 1 to 110): (a) the composition in certain portions of the molecule is constant; for example, glycine occurs in positions 8 to 10 (141); (b) three or more subclasses of human light chains (I, II, III, and so forth) can be identified based on distinctive amino acids and specific locations in the sequence and on regular deletions from the common sequence (51, 52, 62, 65, 77, 85); and (c) in the rest of the amino acid sequence—particularly in regions 24 to 34, 52 to 55, and 89 to 97—variations in amino acid composition

give each light chain its distinctive characteristics (141). Variation in these regions probably confers on each light chain an immunologic specificity; that is, these hypervariable regions probably are involved in antigen binding (42).

Light-chain Common Regions Common regions of either kappa or lambda structure are found in light chains. Each of these has a characteristic and largely invariant amino acid sequence (positions 110 to 214). At position 191 of the C region of kappa light chain, leucine or valine may be present. If leucine is present, the chain is said to have the Inv-1 antigen; if valine is present, the chain has the Inv-3 antigen (7, 49, 76, 123). These differences probably represent allelic forms of the gene controlling the composition of the C region of the kappa light chain.

The characteristic amino acid sequence of the C region of lambda chains may be altered in several positions (51, 78). For example, in position 190, lysine (OZ antigen positive) or arginine (OZ antigen negative) may be present (3, 31, 32).

Common Regions of Heavy Chains The common region of the heavy chains includes the amino acid sequence of approximately 120 to 440. Many forms of this region exist, each of which is characteristic for a given subclass of heavy chain, such as gamma 1, gamma 2, mu, and the like (27, 36, 91, 137). Thus all IgG molecules of gamma 1 subclass probably have roughly similar sequences of amino acids of the C region of the heavy chains.

The C regions of the two heavy chains of an IgG molecule are linked together by disulfide bonds in the region of amino acids 220 to 240—the hinge region. As noted above, this region is susceptible to attack by papain (88).

Variable Regions of Heavy Chains At the present time the variable region of the heavy chains has been studied less intensively than the corresponding region of the light chains. As noted above, three hypervariable subregions have been delineated in the variable region of light chains. Recently, three hypervariable subregions have been identified in the variable region of IgG heavy chains isolated from patients with myeloma. These include amino acid sequences 31 to 37, 86 to 91, and 101 to 109 (20, 61, 135). Based on studies with animal immunoglobulins, antigen binding characteristics probably are determined by these hypervariable regions.

Gene Control of Immunoglobulin Structure

The C regions of immunoglobulin polypeptide chains appear to be under the control of three separate and independent genes. One gene controls the C region of heavy chains; the other genes control the C regions of kappa and lambda light chains (53, 78, 141). At least one gene with two allelic forms (Inv-1 and Inv-3) controls the kappa C region. The several genes that control human heavy-chain C regions on gamma 1, gamma 2, and gamma 3 molecules are linked (84), as are genes for gamma and alpha chains in the mouse (48). It is still not known whether genes for all human heavy-chain C regions are linked.

There appear to be three separate pools of V-region genes: one for kappa chains, one for lambda chains, and one for all classes of heavy chains (53, 78, 141). Each of these pools probably consists of many hundreds or thousands of genes.

The human X chromosome may contain the quantitative genes for immunoglobulin M (44).

From the foregoing, it follows that the assembly of a complete immunoglobulin polypeptide chain requires expression of two sets of genes—one for the C region and one for the V region. The mechanism by which this cooperative expression is achieved is not certain. Recent theories suggest a coordination in the chain before transcription of the DNA sequence into RNA; that is, prior to initiation of specific immunoglobulin synthesis.

A single plasma cell and its progeny manufacture and secrete an immunoglobulin that is unique in composition (17). This composition reflects the expression of the genes for the V and C portions of the light chains and the heavy chains. The heterogeneous population of immunoglobulins found in the body reflects the heterogeneity of the plasma cell clones producing them.

Informative reviews of immunoglobulin structure and gene expression have recently been published (53, 54, 78, 93, 94, 113).

Classes of Immunoglobulins

The Family of Immunoglobulin Molecules

Five major classes of normal human immunoglobulins have been identified thus far: IgG, IgA, IgM, IgD, and IgE. For each normal immunoglobulin there is a paraprotein counterpart secreted by a neoplastic lymphoid cell or plasmacyte (see Chapter 20). These major classes may be distinguished on the basis of physical and chemical characteristics and immunochemical features, as well as metabolic and functional properties.

Physicochemical and immunochemical properties of the five classes of immunoglobulins are listed in Table 16.1; concentrations and metabolic characteristics of these molecules are given in Table 16.2, and their biologic properties are listed in Table 16.3 (24, 57, 62, 64, 75, 97, 100, 127).

The IgG molecules are the most abundant immunoglobulins in normal human serum, having a sedimentation rate $(S^0_{20,w})$ of 6.6. As a consequence of their relatively small size they are distributed in the extravascular space, as well as in the circulation. Selectively transported through the placenta, they are catabolized relatively slowly, with a half-life of about 21 days. IgG molecules contain most of the antibody made in the secondary immune response to a protein antigen.

IgA molecules are part of the secretory immunoglobulin system of man and other mammals. They may be 7 S, 9 S, 11 S, or 13 S. The molecules are found in colostrum, tears, saliva, nasal and gastric secretions, and in the fluid of the lower gastrointestinal tract (22). The immunoglobulin in these secretions is found in association with a "secretory piece" (127). IgA, which will be considered in more detail below, is found distributed approximately equally between

Table 16.1 Physicochemical and immunochemical properties of immunoglobulin molecules.

Properties	IgG	IgA	IgM	IgD	IgE
Physicochemical					
Sedimentation rate $s^0_{20,w}$	6.6 S	7 S (9 S, 11 S, 13 S)	18 S	6.5 S	7.9 S
Molecular weight	150,000–180,000	150,000–165,000 (7 S)	900,000–1,000,000	150,000	185,000
Electrophoretic mobility	$\gamma(\beta)$	β	γ-β	γ-β	γ-β
Carbohydrate total (%)	2.9	7.5	11.8		12.1
Glucosamine (%)	1.30	2.3	4.4		4.6
Sialic acid (%)	0.30	1.8	1.3		1.1
Immunochemical					
Heavy chains	γ	α	μ	δ	ϵ
Light chains					
Kappa/lambda ratio	2 : 1	1 : 1	3 : 1	1 : 4	
Inv (kappa)	+	+	+	+	

Table 16.2 Serum concentration and metabolism of immunoglobulins.

Property	IgG	IgA	IgM	IgD	IgE
Serum concentration (mg/ml)	12.4	2.5	1.2	0.03	0.0003
% intravascular	45	42	76	75	
Metabolism					
Half-life (days)	21	5.8	5.1	2.8	2.2
% catabolized/day	6	28	18	37	89
Synthetic rate (mg/kg/day)	30	25	6	0.4	

the intra- and extravascular space. Its half-life is relatively short—5.8 days.

IgM is a large molecule, 18S to 19S, formed by the polymerization of five 7S subunits (Fig. 16.4) through disulfide bridges on the heavy (μ) chains (75). They are catabolized relatively rapidly, with a $T_{1/2}$ of 5.1 days. Because of their large size, IgM molecules are restricted to the vascular space. Low molecular weight (7S) IgM may be found in the sera of patients with Waldenström's macroglobulinemia and a variety of other disorders (18). The structure and function of IgM molecules have been excellently reviewed by Metzger (74).

IgD (6.5S) is about the size of IgG and is found only in small amounts in normal serum (97, 100). About 75 percent of the protein is found in the vascular space, and the turnover rate is very rapid, with a $T_{1/2}$ of 2.8 days. Although the normal functions of IgD are largely unknown, IgD molecules with antibody activity have been identified (41).

IgE molecules are present in human serum in minute amounts only. These molecules with sedimentation rates of 7.9S have a very short $T_{1/2}$ of 2.2 days. They are extremely potent in sensitizing skin, lungs, and certain other tissues to allergic reactions. The IgE immune system is often referred to as the *reaginic* immune system.

Table 16.3 Functional characteristics of different classes of immunoglobulins.

Characteristic	IgG	IgA	IgM	IgD	IgE
Agglutination efficiency	+	*	++++	*	
C' fixation	+	0	++	*	0
External secretions	+	+++	+	*	++
Placental transport	+++	0	0	0	0
Skin sensitization	+	0	0	0	+++

* = uncertain.

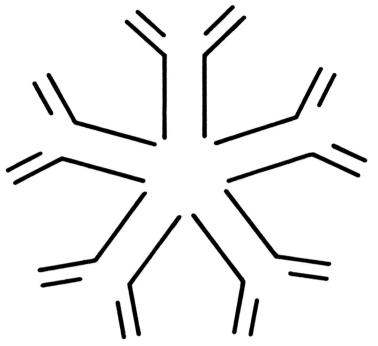

Figure 16.4 Schematic representation of the IgM molecule, consisting of five 7S subunits held together through disulfide bridges.

IgM molecules often are potent at complement fixation. Some IgG molecules share this property, but it is lacking in IgA molecules. Some IgG molecules also have skin-sensitizing activity. Placental transport appears to be restricted to IgG immunoglobulins.

Serologically identified subclasses have been identified within several of the major immunoglobulin classes. The best studied in this regard is the IgG class, but IgM and IgA subclasses have been identified as well (37, 39).

Subclasses of IgG

At least four subclasses of IgG molecules have been identified on the basis of serologic specificity. All four normally are present in serum. As shown in Table 16.4, these subclasses differ in heavy-chain structure, in the ratio of kappa-to-lambda light chains, in metabolic properties, and in functional attributes (24, 81, 122, 142).

IgG_1 is the predominant subclass and accounts for between 65 and 75 percent of IgG molecules. Its heavy chain is designated gamma 1. It is found in a variety of antibodies and fixes complement. IgG_2 and IgG_4 bind complement poorly. Antibodies to some carbohydrates are predominantly of IgG_2 specificity. IgG_3 is unique in its rapid catabolic rate and its tendency to aggregate.

The four types of heavy chains that specify each of

Table 16.4 Properties of subclasses of IgG.

Property	IgG$_1$	IgG$_2$	IgG$_3$	IgG$_4$
% of total IgG	65	23	8	4
Subclass-specific antigens	γ1	γ2	γ3	γ4
Kappa/lambda ratio	2:1	1:1	1:1	5:1
Gm determinants	1,2,4,17	23	5,13,14,21	
Metabolism				
Half-life (days)	21	20	7	21
% IV catabolized/day	7	7	17	7
Functional characteristics				
Complement binding	+	±	+	0
Heterologous skin				
sensitization	+	0	+	+

these subclasses of IgG molecules are controlled by separate but closely associated genes. Within each subclass there are allelic genes that are expressed in Gm allotypes.

IgA

Immunoglobulin A was first isolated and described in detail by Heremans and his colleagues in 1959 (47). While catabolized significantly more rapidly than IgG, IgA is synthesized at approximately the same rate—mainly by plasma cells scattered in the gastrointestinal and respiratory tracts. Peripheral lymph nodes and spleen contain only one IgA-producing cell for every five or six IgG-producing cells (125, 128).

IgA is the predominant immunoglobulin in colostrum, tears, saliva, and other fluids of the gastrointestinal and respiratory tracts. It is therefore the major antibody class in fluids covering the mucous membrane in contact with the external environment. This secretory IgA is mostly 11 S in sedimentation, thus differing from 7 S serum IgA in size as well as in amino acid composition and antigenic characteristics. These distinctive properties result from an associated nonimmunoglobulin glycoprotein, designated the *secretory piece* or *T component*. The 11 S secretory molecule probably consists of two 7 S IgA molecules plus the T component of 60,000 molecular weight. The total molecular weight is 390,000 (128). The T component is synthesized in epithelial cells, whereas the IgA itself is produced in plasma cells; it may be made in genetically deficient individuals who fail to synthesize IgA (16, 125). The T component may confer on the IgA molecule increased resistance to proteolysis in the digestive fluids.

Secretory IgA has hemagglutinating activity and perhaps antibacterial and antiviral activity (1, 98, 112). Its antibacterial action is uncertain, since IgA does not fix complement. Secretory IgA may opsonize bacteria (136)

and prevent the adherence of bacteria to epithelial cells, thereby preventing colonization (138).

Human infants are born lacking IgA. They are exposed to considerable quantities of IgA in colostrum, but absorb relatively little. Adult levels in the serum are reached between ages four and twelve years. Some people never develop appreciable serum levels of IgA (50). Such deficient individuals may be entirely normal (43) or may suffer from diarrhea and malabsorption (26) or recurrent sinopulmonary infection (115). IgA deficiency may also be associated with a variety of immunologic disorders, including ataxia telangiectasia (see Chapter 18).

Tomasi recently has reviewed the current status of investigations in the field of secretory immunoglobulins (126).

IgE

Prausnitz and Küstner first identified reaginic activity in human serum and correlated it with atopic allergic disease. They were the first to demonstrate that skin-sensitizing activity could be transferred by serum from sensitive to normal subjects. The basis of this Prausnitz-Küstner reaction is reaginic antibody. A variety of observations in the past decade has suggested that reaginic antibody is distinct from typical IgG antibody (55, 57). The work of Ishizaka and his colleagues demonstrated that the principal constituent of reaginic skin-sensitizing antibody is IgE (56, 57).

The analysis of the physical characteristics of IgE has been aided greatly by the identification of a few patients with multiple myeloma whose tumors secreted an IgE paraprotein (64, 87) and of patients with allergy (57). IgE antibodies are divalent. They have little or no capacity to fix complement. If IgE is heated at 56° for four hours, it retains its ability to combine with antigen but loses its capacity to sensitize cells.

IgE appears to sensitize tissues by fixation to cells through the Fc portion of the molecule. When the cells so sensitized are mast cells or basophils, histamine is released by the further addition of specific antigen or antibody to IgE. Lung tissue sensitized with IgE may release a second pharmacologic mediator slow-reacting substance of anaphylaxis (SRS-A). An intact Fab is necessary for release of both histamine and SRS-A (58, 59).

Cells that stain with fluoresceinated antibody to IgE have been found in tonsils, in bronchial and peribronchial lymph nodes, in Peyer's patches, and in mucosal lymph tissues of the stomach, nose, and rectum of the monkey (121). Few cells are found in the spleen or subcutaneous lymph nodes. This distribution suggests a local synthesis of IgE in the respiratory tract in respiratory allergic diseases. The distribution of IgE-producing cells is strikingly similar to that of IgA-producing cells. IgE has been demonstrated in nasal washings and sputa from asthmatic patients.

Immunoglobulin Synthesis

Heavy chains, as well as light chains, are synthesized as entire subunits rather than assembled from smaller polypeptide subunits (19, 63). Synthesis appears to occur primarily on membrane-bound, rather than free, polyribosomes (108, 119).

The synthesis of immunoglobulin molecules is illustrated in Fig. 16.5. Nascent light chains released from the polyribosomes enter an intracellular pool of free light chains. These then link with heavy chains to form covalently associated immunoglobulin molecules $(HL)_2$ (106, 139). In investigations of the mechanisms of immunoglobulin assembly, a variety of intermediates has been proposed, including HL, H_2, and L_2 (10, 103, 143). Schubert (103) demonstrated that in at least one myeloma cell line an HL intermediate was associated with heavy-

chain polyribosomes and that L chains were synthesized in a twofold excess over H chains. This observation indicated that the association of L with H chains occurred at least in part while the latter was still associated with polyribosomes.

Assembly of the immunoglobulin molecule takes place as indicated in Fig. 16.5: (a) H and L chains are made on different-sized polyribosomes; (b) nascent L chains are released and enter a pool; (c) free L chains complement with H-chain monomers bound to polyribosomes forming the dimer HL; (d) the HL dimer complements with another dimer to form $(HL)_2$ either on the heavy-chain polyribosomes or after release into the cytosol; (e) polyribosome-bound $(HL)_2$ is released; and (f) $(HL)_2$ is secreted. In both myelomas and lymph nodes there is a synthesis of L chains in excess of H chains (4, 104–106). The excess L chains are either degraded within the cell or secreted.

This concept of construction of the H and L chains is strengthened by the existence of mouse myeloma mutants, which are blocked at the step of complementation between HL dimers (90) or after dimerization of H and L chains (103, 104). Some tumors secrete $(HL)_2$, HL, and L_2, as well as L chains (23, 66, 101); others may secrete H_2 and H_2L (4). A variety of disorders of assembly of immunoglobulin molecules, therefore, may be seen in naturally occurring multiple myeloma and in animal model systems.

Recently, Baumal and his colleagues (10, 11) have shown that the predominant intermediates (HL, H_2L, or H_2) vary depending on which of the subclasses of immunoglobulin chain (IgG_1, IgG_{2a}, IgG_{2b}) is being synthesized. They also showed that *most* of the covalent and noncovalent assembly of IgG occurs after release of newly synthesized H and L chains from the polyribosomes. Furthermore, assembly was not complete until ten or more minutes after synthesis of the polypeptide chain.

The first sugar of the carbohydrate moiety of IgG, N-acetylglucosamine, is incorporated into nascent polypeptide chains while they are still on the polyribosomes (82, 110, 118). The enzymes that catalyze this addition have been partially purified (102). Recent studies of IgA synthesis in mouse myeloma tumors suggest that the pathway of assembly of the IgA monomer is $H + H \rightarrow H_2$; $H_2 + L + L \rightarrow H_2L_2$. Final assembly of the monomers into IgA polymers, $H_2L_2 \rightarrow (H_2L_2)_N$, occurs close to the time of secretion (8).

Studies from a number of laboratories suggest that newly synthesized H and L chains are released from the polyribosomes into the cisternae of the endoplasmic reticulum (16) and then are transported to the outside of the cell near the Golgi apparatus (21, 102, 108, 120)

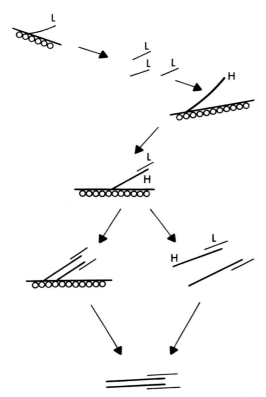

Figure 16.5 Synthesis of immunoglobulins on polyribosomes (ooooo). Light (L) and heavy (H) chains are synthesized on different polyribosomes. L chains unite with H chains while the latter are still attached to polyribosomes.

(see Fig. 14.1). In cell-free systems for the synthesis of immunoglobulins, an intact endoplasmic reticulum is also necessary (129, 130). It was noted earlier that most of the IgG synthesis in mammalian cells is thought to occur on membrane-bound polyribosomes. As a generalization, proteins made for secretion are made on polyribosomes attached to the endoplasmic reticulum (bound), whereas nonexportable proteins are formed on polyribosomes in the cell sap (free polyribosomes) (83, 95).

A recent review by Buxbaum of the biosynthesis of immunoglobulins is recommended for the interested reader (19).

Surface-bound Immunoglobulin

At some point between intracellular assembly of immunoglobulins and their appearance in the extracellular fluid, these molecules must venture to the cell surface. Based on current knowledge, it is likely that surface-bound immunoglobulins are quantitatively greater on B lymphocytes than on T cells.

A variety of test systems has been used to demonstrate the presence of IgG on the surface of IgG secreting cells. For example, bacteria adhere to plasma cells forming antibacterial antibody (see Fig. 15.2) and may be used to detect such cells in a heterogeneous population (70, 99). Immunofluorescent techniques may be used to detect surface-bound immunoglobulin (2). Radioactively labeled antibody to IgG and antibody labeled with ferritin have been used in similar fashion (96). Finally, the surface protein may be radioactively labeled and isolated enzymatically (12, 72).

By means of these techniques immunoglobulins have indeed been found on the surface of murine myeloma cells (12, 96); on the surface of human and animal B lymphocytes, both normal (28, 29, 40) and abnormal (2); and on some established lines of human lymphoma cells (33, 107).

Thymocytes and T lymphocytes may also have surface immunoglobulins (71, 73, 79), which are probably identical to antigen-binding sites (46). The density of immunoglobulins on the surface of these cells is probably less than that on B lymphocytes (86).

Electron microscopic studies of human lymphoid cells bearing surface immunoglobulins have been reported recently (144).

Immunoglobulin Catabolism

The total circulating pool of IgG is about 500 mg/kg of body weight, and the total pool is about 1,150 mg/kg. Therefore, about half of IgG molecules are intravascular and the remainder are extravascular. IgG has the longest

survival of any serum protein: a $T_{1/2}$ of 21 to 23 days, with a fractional catabolic rate of 6.7 percent per day. The fractional catabolic rates of IgM, IgA, IgD, and IgE are 18, 28, 37, and 89 percent of the intravascular pool per day (114, 117, 133).

In addition to the differences in catabolic rates among these major classes of immunoglobulins, different subclasses of IgG have different catabolic rates. For example, IgG_1, IgG_2, and IgG_4 have half-lives of about 23 days, whereas IgG_3 has a shorter survival with a half-life between 6.6 and 7.7 days (80, 116).

A number of factors may control the rate of immunoglobulin catabolism. Disorders with an increase in catabolic rate are listed in Table 16.5. Some factors, such as metabolic rate and renal function, influence the catabolism of several immunoglobulins and other serum proteins (35, 134); other factors influence the catabolism of only a single class of immunoglobulin. For example, the rate of catabolism of IgG varies with the serum concentration of this molecule. The lower the concentration, the slower the catabolic rate and the longer the survival (Fig. 16.6). The circulating half-life may be as long as 70 days in severe IgG-deficient states (114, 132, 133). By contrast, in multiple myeloma with high concentrations of circulating IgG, the half-life of the molecule may be very short (69). A limit of a $T_{1/2}$ of about 11 days is reached when the serum IgG concentration reaches about 30 mg/ml (about 2.5 times normal). The survival of IgG molecules is related to the serum concentration of IgG or of the Fc piece of the IgG molecule; it is not affected by the concentration of other immunoglobulins or the number of plasma cells synthesizing immunoglobulins (34). In a similar manner the survival of IgE molecules has been shortened in a patient with IgE myeloma and high serum concentration of this protein (87).

The catabolism of IgA and IgM appears to be indepen-

Table 16.5 Disorders associated with increased catabolism of immunoglobulin.

Disorder	Immunoglobulins affected
Hypermetabolism	All major classes
High serum IgG concentration	IgG
Familial idiopathic hyper- catabolic hypoproteinemia	IgG, albumin
Wiskott-Aldrich syndrome	IgG, IgA, albumin
Myotonic dystrophy	IgG
Antibodies to immunoglobulin	Class specific
IgG-IgM gelation	IgG
Excessive corticosteroids	IgG, others

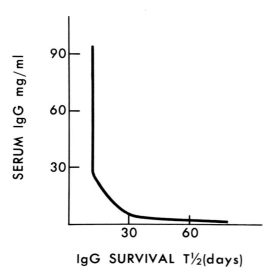

Figure 16.6 Inverse relation between serum concentration of IgG and survival of the molecule. The higher the concentration, the shorter the survival, up to a limiting half-life of about 11 days.

dent of their serum concentration (9). The mechanism by which IgG catabolism is related to its concentration is not known, although interesting hypotheses have been offered (15).

Disorders with increased catabolism of immunoglobulins may affect a single class or all classes of these proteins. For example, familial hypercatabolic hypoproteinemia is associated with increased catabolism of IgG and albumin and decreased serum levels of these proteins. The mechanism of hypercatabolism is unknown (131).

The Wiskott-Aldrich syndrome is associated with hypercatabolism of several serum proteins and abnormal humoral and cellular immune responses (13, 14, 25).

Myotonic dystrophy is a disorder characterized by an inherited muscular abnormality with myotonia, cataracts, frontal balding, and gonadal atrophy. The serum concentration of IgG usually is low and the IgG catabolic rate greatly increased (mean $T_{1/2} = 11.4$ days) (140), whereas metabolism of IgA, IgM, and IgD is normal. The IgG molecules of these patients do not appear to be intrinsically abnormal, since their survival is normal in healthy recipients. It therefore appears that host factors account for the abnormal metabolism of IgG in myotonic dystrophy.

Immunoglobulin catabolism may be accelerated if the host develops antibody to one of the classes of the immunoglobulins. For example, patients with selective absence of IgA may develop antibodies to the IgA molecule. These antibodies are of IgG type (117). Another example of immunoglobulin interaction that may result in shortened survival of one class of molecules has been described in a patient with Sjögren's syndrome (60). This patient had a high concentration of monoclonal IgM that formed a cryogel with IgG. Neither immunoglobulin alone would gel, only the combination.

Many other factors undoubtedly influence immunoglobulin metabolism. A few years ago, Levy and Waldmann (68) demonstrated that adrenocorticosteroids may increase the catabolic rate of certain subclasses of IgG in the mouse. This observation may explain the hypoglobulinemia sometimes observed with prolonged steroid therapy in man.

Chapter 16 References

1. Adinolfi, M., Glynn, A. A., Lindsay, M., and Milne, C. M. Serological properties of γA antibodies to *Escherichia coli* present in human colostrum, *Immunology* 10:517, 1966.

2. Aisenberg, A. C., and Bloch, K. J. Immunoglobulins on the surface of neoplastic lymphocytes, *N. Engl. J. Med.* 287:272, 1972.

3. Appella, E., and Ein, D. Two types of lambda polypeptide chains in human immunoglobulins based on an amino acid substitution at position 190, *Proc. Natl. Acad. Sci. U.S.A.* 57:1449, 1967.

4. Askonas, B. A., and Williamson, A. R. Biosynthesis of immunoglobulins. Free light chain as an intermediate in the assembly of γG-molecules, *Nature* 211:369, 1966.

5. Askonas, B. A., and Williamson, A. R. Interchain disulphide-bond formation in the assembly of immunoglobulin G: heavy chain dimer as an intermediate, *Biochem. J.* 109:637, 1968.

6. Avey, H. P., Poljack, R. J., Rossi, G., and Nisonoff, A. Crystallographic data for the Fab fragment of a human myeloma immunoglobulin, *Nature* 220:1248, 1968.

7. Baglioni, C., Zonta, L. A., Cioli, D., and Carbonara, A. Allelic antigenic factor Inv(a) of the light chains of human immunoglobulins: chemical basis, *Science* 152:1517, 1966.

8. Bargellesi, A., Periman, P., and Scharff, M. D. Synthesis, assembly, and secretion of γglobulin by mouse myeloma cells. IV. Assembly of IgA, *J. Immunol.* 108:126, 1972.

9. Barth, W. F., Wochner, R. D., Waldmann, T. A., and Fahey, J. L. Metabolism of human gamma macroglobulins, *J. Clin. Invest.* 43:1036, 1964.

10. Baumal, R., Potter, M., and Scharff, M. D. Synthesis, assembly and secretion of gamma globulin in mouse myeloma cells. III., *J. Exp. Med.* 134:1316, 1971.

11. Baumal, R., and Scharff, M. D. Synthesis, assembly and secretion of IgA$_{2a}$ by the mouse plasma cell tumors MOPC 173 and MOPC 494, *Fed. Proc.* 29:577, 1970.

12. Baur, S., Schenkein, I., and Uhr, J. W. Cell surface immunoglobulin. I. Isolation and characterization of immunoglobulin from murine myeloma cells, *J. Immunol.* 108:748, 1972.

13. Blaese, R. M., Strober, W., Brown, R. S., and Waldmann, T. A. The Wiskott-Aldrich syndrome: a disorder with a possible defect in antigen processing or recognition, *Lancet* 1:1056, 1968.

14. Blaese, R. M., Strober, W., and Waldmann, T. A. Hypercatabolism of several serum proteins in the Wiskott-Aldrich syndrome, *J. Clin. Invest.* 48:8a, 1969.

15. Brambell, F. W. R., Hemmings, W. A., and Morris, I. G. A theoretical model of γ-globulin catabolism, *Nature* 203:1352, 1964.

16. Brandtzaeg, P. Hidden antigenic determinant in secretory immunoglobulin A, *Nature* 220:292, 1968.

17. Burnet, F. M. The impact on ideas of immunology, *Cold Spring Harbor Symp. Quant. Biol.* 32:1, 1967.

18. Bush, S. T., Swedlund, H. A., and Gleich, G. J. Low molecular weight IgM in human sera, *J. Lab. Clin. Med.* 73:194, 1969.

19. Buxbaum, J. N. The biosynthesis, assembly and secretion of immunoglobulins, *Semin. Hematol.* 10:33, 1973.

20. Capra, J. D. Hypervariable region of human immunoglobulin heavy chains, *Nature (New Biol.)* 230:61, 1971.

21. Choi, Y. S., Knopf, P. M., and Lennox, E. S. Intracellular transport and secretion of an immunoglobulin light chain, *Biochemistry* 101:668, 1971.

22. Claman, H. N., Merrill, D. A., and Hartley, T. F. Salivary immunoglobulins: normal adult values and dissociation between serum and salivary levels, *J. Allergy* 40:151, 1967.

23. Coffino, P., Laskov, R., and Scharff, M. D. Immunoglobulin production: method for quantitatively detecting variant myeloma cells, *Science* 167:186, 1970.

24. Cohen, S., and Milstein, C. Structure and biological properties of im-

munoglobulins, *Adv. Immunol.* 7:1, 1967.

25. Cooper, M. D., Chase, H. P., Lowman, J. T., Krivit, W., and Good, R. A. Wiskott-Aldrich syndrome: an immunologic deficiency disease involving the afferent limb of immunity, *Am. J. Med.* 44:499, 1968.

26. Crabbe, P. A., and Heremans, J. F. Selective IgA deficiency with steatorrhea, *Am. J. Med.* 42:319, 1967.

27. Cunningham, B. A., Pflumm, M. N., Rutishauser, U., and Edelman, G. M. Subgroups of amino acid sequences in the variable regions of immunoglobulin heavy chains, *Proc. Natl. Acad. Sci. U.S.A.* 64:997, 1969.

28. Davie, J. M., and Paul, W. E. Receptors on immunocompetent cells. IV. Direct measurement of avidity of cell receptors and cooperative binding of multivalent ligands, *J. Exp. Med.* 135:643, 1972.

29. Davie, J. M., and Paul, W. E. Receptors on immunocompetent cells. V. Cellular correlates of the "maturation" of the immune response, *J. Exp. Med.* 135:660, 1972.

30. Edelman, G. M., Cunningham, B. A., Gall, W. E., Gottlieb, P. D., Rutishauser, U., and Waxdal, M. J. The covalent structure of an entire γG immunoglobulin molecule, *Proc. Natl. Acad. Sci. U.S.A.* 63:78, 1969.

31. Ein, D. Nonallelic behavior of the Oz group in human lambda immunoglobulin chains, *Proc. Natl. Acad. Sci. U.S.A.* 60:982, 1968.

32. Ein, D., and Fahey, J. L. Two types of lambda polypeptide chains in human immunoglobulins, *Science* 156:947, 1967.

33. Eskeland, T., and Klein, E. Isolation of 7S IgM and kappa chains from the surface membrane of tissue culture cells derived from a Burkitt lymphoma, *J. Immunol.* 107:1368, 1971.

34. Fahey, J. L., and Robinson, A. G. Factors controlling serum γ-globulin concentration, *J. Exp. Med.* 118:845, 1963.

35. Farthring, C. P., Gerwing, J., and Shewell, J. The catabolism of ^{131}I-labeled homologous γ-globulin in normal, hyperthyroid and hypo-

thyroid rats, *J. Endocrinol.* 21:83, 1960.

36. Frangione, B., Milstein, C., and Pink, J. R. L. Structural studies of immunoglobulin G, *Nature* 221:145, 1969.

37. Frangione, B., Prelli, F., Mihaesco, C., Wolfenstein, C., Mihaesco, E., and Franklin, E. C. Structural studies of immunoglobulin G, M and A heavy chains, *Ann. N.Y. Acad. Sci.* 190:71, 1971.

38. Frangione, B., and Wolfenstein-Todel, C. Partial duplication in the "hinge" region of IgA$_1$ myeloma proteins, *Proc. Natl. Acad. Sci. U.S.A.* 69:3673, 1972.

39. Franklin, E. C., and Frangione, B. Two serologically distinguishable subclasses of μ-chains of human macroglobulins, *J. Immunol.* 99:810, 1967.

40. Froland, S., Natvig, J. B., and Berdal, P. Surface-bound immunoglobulin as a marker of B lymphocytes in man, *Nature (New Biol.)* 234:251, 1971.

41. Gleich, G. J., Bieger, R. C., and Stankievic, R. Antigen combining activity associated with immunoglobulin D, *Science* 165:606, 1969.

42. Goetzl, E. J., and Metzger, H. Affinity labelling of a mouse myeloma protein which binds nitrophenyl ligands. Sequence and position of a labelled tryptic peptide, *Biochemistry* 9:3862, 1970.

43. Goldberg, L. S., Barnett, E. V., and Fudenberg, H. H. Selective absence of IgA: a family study, *J. Lab. Clin. Med.* 72:204, 1968.

44. Grundbacher, F. J. Human X chromosome carries quantitative genes for immunoglobulin M, *Science* 176:311, 1972.

45. Haber, E. Immunochemistry, *Ann. Rev. Biochem.* 37:497, 1968.

46. Haskill, J. S., Elliott, B. E., Kerbel, R. Axelrad, M. A., and Eidinger, D. Classification of thymus-derived and marrow-derived lymphocytes by demonstration of their antigen-binding characteristics, *J. Exp. Med.* 135:1410, 1972.

47. Heremans, J. F., Heremans, M-Th., and Schultze, H. E. Isolation and description of a few properties of the B$_2$A-globulin of human serum, *Clin. Chim. Acta* 4:96, 1959.

48. Hertzenberg, L. A., and Warner, N. L. Genetic control of mouse im-munoglobulins, *in* B. Cinader (ed.), Regulation of the Antibody Response, p. 322, Charles C Thomas, Springfield, Ill., 1968.

49. Hilschmann, N., and Craig, L. C. Amino acid sequence studies with Bence-Jones proteins, *Proc. Natl. Acad. Sci. U.S.A.* 53:1403, 1965.

50. Hong, R., and Ammann, A. J. Selective absence of IgA, *Am. J. Pathol.* 69:491, 1972.

51. Hood, L., and Ein, D. Immunoglobulin lambda chain structure: two genes, one polypeptide chain, *Nature* 220:764, 1968.

52. Hood, L., Gray, W. R., Sanders, B. G., and Dreyer, W. J. Light chain evolution, *Cold Spring Harbor Symp. Quant. Biol.* 32:133, 1967.

53. Hood, L., and Talmage, D. W. Mechanism of antibody diversity: germ line basis for variability, *Science* 168:325, 1970.

54. Hood, L. Waterfield, M. D., Morris, J., and Todd, C. W. Light chain structure and theories of antibody diversity, *Ann. N.Y. Acad. Sci.* 190:26, 1971.

55. Ishizaka, K. The identification and significance of gamma E, p. 70, *Hosp. Practice*, Sept. 1969.

56. Ishizaka, K., and Ishizaka, T. Human reaginic antibodies and immunoglobulin E, *J. Allergy* 42:330, 1968.

57. Ishizaka, K., and Ishizaka, T. Mechanisms of reaginic hypersensitivity: a review, *Clin. Allergy* 1:9, 1971.

58. Ishizaka, T., Ishizaka, K., Johansson, S. G. O., and Bennich, H. Histamine release from human leukocytes by anti-γE antibodies, *J. Immunol.* 102:884, 1969.

59. Ishizaka, T., Ishizaka, K., Orange, R. P., and Austen, K. F. Release of histamine and slow reacting substance of anaphylaxis (SRS-A) by γE system from sensitized monkey lung, *J. Allergy*, 43:168, 1969.

60. Johnson, J. S., and Waldmann, T. A. Accelerated catabolism of IgG secondary to its interaction with autoreactive monoclonal IgM, *Fed. Proc.* 28:501, 1969.

61. Kehoe, J. M., and Capra, J. D. Localization of two additional hypervariable regions in immunoglobulin heavy chains, *Proc. Natl. Acad. Sci. U.S.A.* 68:2019, 1971.

62. Killander, J. (ed.). Nobel Symposium on Gamma Globulins, Interscience Publishers, New York, 1967.

63. Knopf, P. M., Parkhouse, R. M. E., and Lennox, E. S. Biosynthetic units of an immunoglobulin heavy chain, *Proc. Natl. Acad. Sci. U.S.A.* 58:2288, 1967.

64. Kochwa, S., Terry, W. D., Capra, J. D., and Yang, N. L. Structural studies of immunoglobulin E. I. Physicochemical studies of the IgE molecule, *Ann. N.Y. Acad. Sci.* 190:49, 1971.

65. Langer, B., Steinmetz-Kayne, M., and Hilschmann, N. Die vollständige Aminosauresequenz des Bence Jones Protein Neu (λ-typ). Subgruppen in variablen Teil bei Immunoglobulin-L-ketten vom λ-typ, *Hoppe-Seylers Z. Physiol. Chem.* 349:945, 1968.

66. Laskov, R., and Scharff, M. D. Synthesis, assembly and secretion of gamma globulin by mouse myeloma cells. I., *J. Exp. Med.* 131:515, 1970.

67. Lawrence, H. S., and Zweiman, B. Transfer factor deficiency response — a mechanism of anergy in Boeck's sarcoid, *Trans. Assoc. Am. Physicians* 81:240, 1968.

68. Levy, A. L., and Waldmann, T. A. The effect of hydrocortisone on immunoglobulin metabolism, *J. Clin. Invest.* 49:1679, 1970.

69. Lippincott, S. W., Korman, S., Fong, C., Stickley, E., Wolins, W., and Hughes, W. L. Turnover of labeled normal gamma globulin in multiple myeloma, *J. Clin. Invest.* 39:565, 1960.

70. Mäkelä, O., and Nossal, G. J. V. Bacterial adherence: a method for detecting antibody production by single cells, *J. Immunol.* 87:447, 1961.

71. Marchalonis, J. J., Atwell, J. L., and Cone, R. E. Isolation of surface immunoglobulin from lymphocytes from human and murine thymus, *Nature (New Biol.)* 235:240, 1972.

72. Marchalonis, J. J., Cone, R. E., and Santer, V. Enzymic iodination. A probe for accessible surface proteins of normal and neoplastic lymphocytes, *Biochem. J.* 124:921, 1971.

73. Mason, S., and Warner, N. L. The immunoglobulin nature of the antigen recognition site on cells mediating transplantation immunity

and delayed hypersensitivity, *J. Immunol.* 104:762, 1970.

74. Metzger, H. Structure and function of γM macroglobulins, *Adv. Immunol.* 10:57, 1969.

75. Miller, F., and Metzger, H. Characterization of a human macroglobulin. II. Distribution of the disulfide bonds, *J. Biol. Chem.* 240:4740, 1965.

76. Milstein, C. The disulphide bridges of immunoglobulin κ-chains, *Biochem. J.* 101:338, 1966.

77. Milstein, C. Linked groups of residues in immunoglobulin κ chains, *Nature* 216:330, 1967.

78. Milstein, C., and Pink, J. R. L. Structure and evolution of immunoglobulins, *Proc. Biophys.* 21:209, 1970.

79. Modabber, F., Morikawa, S., and Coons, A. H. Antigen-binding cells in normal mouse thymus, *Science* 170:1102, 1970.

80. Morell, A., Terry, W. D., and Waldmann, T. A. Relation between metabolic properties and serum concentration of IgG-subclasses in man, *Clin. Res.* 17:356, 1969.

81. Morell, A., Terry, W. D., and Waldmann, T. A. Metabolic properties of IgG subclasses in man, *J. Clin. Invest.* 49:673, 1970.

82. Moroz, C., and Uhr, J. W. Synthesis of the carbohydrate moiety of γ-globulin, *Cold Spring Harbor Symp. Quant. Biol.* 32:263, 1967.

83. Nathans, D. Puromycin inhibition of protein synthesis: incorporation of puromycin into peptide chains, *Proc. Natl. Acad. Sci. U.S.A.* 51:585, 1964.

84. Natvig, J. B., Kunkel, H. G., Yount, W. J., and Nielsen, J. C. Further studies of the γG-heavy chain gene complexes, with particular reference to the genetic markers Gm(g) and Gm(a), *J. Exp. Med.* 128:763, 1968.

85. Niall, H. D., and Edman, P. Two structurally distinct classes of kappa-chains in human immunoglobulins, *Nature* 216:262, 1967.

86. Nossal, G. J. V., Warner, N. L., Lewis, H., and Sprent, J. Quantitative features of a sandwich radioimmunolabeling technique for lymphocyte surface receptors, *J. Exp. Med.* 135:405, 1972.

87. Ogawa, M., McIntyre, O. R., Ishi-

zaka, K., Ishizaka, T., Terry, W. D., and Waldmann, T. A. Biologic properties of E myeloma proteins, *Am. J. Med.* 51:193, 1971.

88. Porter, R. R. The hydrolysis of rabbit γ-globulin and antibodies with crystalline papain, *Biochem. J.* 73:119, 1959.

89. Porter, R. R. The combining sites of antibodies, pp. 157–174, Harvey Lectures 1969–1970.

90. Potter, M., and Kuff, E. L. Disorders in the differentiation of protein secretion in neoplastic plasma cells, *J. Mol. Biol.* 9:537, 1964.

91. Press, E. M., and Hogg, N. M. Comparative study of two immunoglobulin G Fd-fragments, *Nature* 223:807, 1969.

92. Putnam, F. W. Immunoglobulin structure: variability and homology, *Science* 163:633, 1969.

93. Putnam, F. W., Shimizu, A., Paul, C., Shinoda, T., and Kohler, H. The amino acid sequence of human macroglobulins, *Ann. N.Y. Acad. Sci.* 190:83, 1971.

94. Putnam, F. W., Shimizu, A., Paul, C., and Shinoda, T. Variation and homology in immunoglobulin heavy chains, *Fed. Proc.* 31:193, 1972.

95. Redman, C. M. Biosynthesis of serum proteins and ferritin by free and attached ribosomes of rat liver, *J. Biol. Chem.* 244:4308, 1969.

96. Reif, A. E. Binding of rabbit antibodies to a mouse myeloma protein by the myeloma cells *in vitro*, *Proc. Soc. Exp. Biol. Med.* 133:744, 1970.

97. Rogentine, G. N., Rowe, D. S., Bradley, J., Waldmann, T. A., and Fahey, J. L. Metabolism of human immunoglobulin D (IgD), *J. Clin. Invest.* 45:1467, 1966.

98. Rossen, R. D., Butler, W. T., Cate, T. R., Szwed, C. F., and Couch, R. B. Protein composition of nasal secretion during respiratory virus infection, *Proc. Soc. Exp. Biol. Med.* 119:1169, 1965.

99. Rotman, B., and Cox, D. R. Specific detection of antigen-binding cells by localized growth of bacteria, *Proc. Natl. Acad. Sci. U.S.A.* 68:2377, 1971.

100. Rowe, D. S., and Fahey, J. L. A new class of human immunoglobulins. II. Normal serum IgD, *J. Exp. Med.* 121:185, 1965.

101. Scharff, M. D., Shapiro, A. L., and Ginsberg, B. The synthesis, assembly and secretion of gamma globulin polypeptide chains by cells of a mouse plasma-cell tumor, *Cold Spring Harbor Symp. Quant. Biol.* 32:235, 1967.

102. Schenkein, I., and Uhr, J. W. Immunoglobulin synthesis and secretion. I. Biosynthetic studies of the addition of the carbohydrate moieties, *J. Cell Biol.* 46:42, 1970.

103. Schubert, D. Immunoglobulin assembly in a mouse myeloma, *Proc. Natl. Acad. Sci. U.S.A.* 60:683, 1968.

104. Schubert, D., and Cohn, M. Immunoglobulin biosynthesis. III. Blocks in defective synthesis, *J. Mol. Biol.* 38:273, 1968.

105. Shapiro, A. L., Scharff, M. D., Maizel, J. V., Jr., and Uhr, J. W. Synthesis of excess light chains of gamma globulin by rabbit lymph node cells, *Nature* 211:243, 1966.

106. Shapiro, A. L., Scharff, M. D., Maizel, J. V., Jr., and Uhr, J. W. Polyribosomal synthesis and assembly of the H and L chains of gamma globulin, *Proc. Natl. Acad. Sci. U.S.A.* 56:216, 1966.

107. Sherr, C. J., Baur, S., Grundke, I., Zeligs, J., Zeligs, B., and Uhr, J. W. Cell surface immunoglobulin. III. Isolation and characterization of immunoglobulin from nonsecretory human lymphoid cells, *J. Exp. Med.* 135:1392, 1972.

108. Sherr, C. J., Schenkein, I., and Uhr, J. W. Synthesis and intracellular transport of immunoglobulin in secretory and nonsecretory cells, *Ann. N.Y. Acad. Sci.* 190:250, 1971.

109. Sherr, C. J., and Uhr, J. W. Immunoglobulin synthesis and secretion, III. Incorporation of glucosamine into immunoglobulin on polyribosomes, *Proc. Natl. Acad. Sci. U.S.A.* 64:381, 1969.

110. Sherr, C. J., and Uhr, J. W. Immunoglobulin synthesis and secretion. V. Incorporation of leucine and glucosamine into immunoglobulin on free and bound polyribosomes, *Proc. Natl. Acad. Sci. U.S.A.* 66:1183, 1970.

111. Singer, S. J., and Thorpe, N. O. On the location and structure of the active sites of antibody molecules, *Proc. Natl. Acad. Sci. U.S.A.* 60:1371, 1968.

112. Smith, C. B., Bellanti, J. A., and Chanock, R. M. Immunoglobulins in serum and nasal secretions following infection with type I parainfluenza virus and injection of inactivated vaccines, *J. Immunol.* 99:133, 1967.

113. Solomon, A., and McLaughlin, C. L. Immunoglobulin structure determined from products of plasma cell neoplasms, *Semin. Hematol.* 10:3, 1973.

114. Solomon, A., Waldmann, T. A., and Fahey, J. L. Clinical and experimental metabolism of normal 6.6S γ-globulin in normal subjects and in patients with macroglobulinemia and multiple myeloma, *J. Lab. Clin. Med.* 62:1, 1963.

115. South, M. A., Wollheim, F. A., Warwick, W. J., Cooper, M. D., and Good, R. A. Local deficiency of immune globulin A in the saliva of patients with chronic sinopulmonary disease, *J. Pediatr.* 67:940, 1965.

116. Spiegelberg, H. L., Fishkin, B. G., and Grey, H. Catabolism of γG-myeloma proteins of different subclasses in man, *Fed. Proc.* 27:731, 1968.

117. Strober, W., Wochner, R. D., Barlow, M. H., McFarlin, D. E., and Waldmann, T. A. Immunoglobulin metabolism in ataxia telangiectasia, *J. Clin. Invest.* 47:1905, 1968.

118. Sutherland, E. W. III, Zimmerman, D. H., and Kern, M. Synthesis and secretion of gamma globulin by lymph node cells: the acquisition of carbohydrate residues of immunoglobulin in relation to interchain disulfide bond formation, *Proc. Natl. Acad. Sci. U.S.A.* 69:167, 1972.

119. Swenson, R. M., and Kern, M. The synthesis and secretion of γ-globulins by lymph node cells. I. The microsomal compartmentalization of γ-globulins, *Proc. Natl. Acad. Sci. U.S.A.* 57:417, 1967.

120. Swenson, R. M., and Kern, M. The synthesis and secretion of γ-globulin by lymph node cells. III. The slow acquisition of the carbohydrate moiety of γ-globulin and its relationship to secretion, *Proc. Natl. Acad. Sci. U.S.A.* 59:546, 1968.

121. Tada, T., and Ishizaka, K. Distribution of γE-forming cells in lymphoid tissues of the human and monkey, *J. Immunol.* 104:377, 1970.

122. Terry, W. D., Fahey, J. L., and Steinberg, A. G. GM and INV factors in subclasses of human IgG, *J. Exp. Med.* 122:1087, 1965.

123. Terry, W. D., Hood, L. E., and Steinberg, A. G. Genetics of immunoglobulin κ-chains: chemical analysis of normal human light chains of differing Inv types, *Proc. Natl. Acad. Sci. U.S.A.* 63:71, 1969.

124. Terry, W. D., Matthews, B. W., and Davies, D. R. Crystallographic studies of a human immunoglobulin, *Nature* 220:239, 1968.

125. Tomasi, T. B., Jr. Human immunoglobulin A, *N. Engl. J. Med.* 279:1327, 1969.

126. Tomasi, T. B., Jr. Secretory immunoglobulins, *N. Engl. J. Med.* 287:500, 1972.

127. Tomasi, T. B., and Bienenstock, J. Secretory immunoglobulins, *Adv. Immunol.* 9:2, 1968.

128. Tomasi, T. B., and Czerwinski, D. S. Secretory IgA system, *in* D. Bergsma and R. A. Good (eds.), Immunological Deficiency Diseases in Man, p. 270, National Foundation, New York, 1968.

129. Vassalli, P. Studies on cell-free synthesis of rat immunoglobulins. I. A cell-free system for protein synthesis prepared from lymph-node microsomal vesicles, *Proc. Natl. Acad. Sci. U.S.A.* 58:2117, 1967.

130. Vassalli, P., Lisowska-Bernstein, B., and Lamm, M. E. Cell-free synthesis of rat immunoglobulin. III. Analysis of the cell-free made chains and of their mode of assembly, *J. Mol. Biol.* 56:1, 1971.

131. Waldmann, T. A., Miller, E. J., and Terry, W. D. Hypercatabolism of IgG and albumin: a new familial disorder, *Clin. Res.* 16:45, 1968.

132. Waldmann, T. A., and Schwab, P. J. IgG (7S gamma globulin) metabolism in hypogammaglobulinemia: studies in patients with defective gamma globulin synthesis, gastrointestinal protein loss, or both, *J. Clin. Invest.* 44:1523, 1965.

133. Waldmann, T. A., and Strober, W. Metabolism of immunoglobulins, *Prog. Allergy* 13:1, 1969.

134. Waldmann, T. A., Strober, W., and Mogielnicki, R. P. The renal handling of low molecular weight proteins, *J. Clin. Invest.* 51:2162, 1972.

135. Wang, A. C., Fudenberg, H. H., and Pink, J. R. Heavy-chain variable regions in normal and pathological immunoglobulins, *Proc. Natl. Acad. Sci. U.S.A.* 68:1143, 1971.

136. Wernet, P., Breu, H., Knop, J., and Rowley, D. Antibacterial action of specific IgA and transport of IgM, IgA, and IgG from serum into the small intestine, *J. Infect. Dis.* 124:223, 1971.

137. Wikler, M., Køhler, H., Shinoda, T., and Putnam, F. W. Macroglobulin structure: homology of mu and gamma heavy chains of human immunoglobulins, *Science* 163:75, 1969.

138. Williams, R. C., and Gibbons, R. J. Inhibition of bacterial adherence by secretory immunoglobulin A: a mechanism of antigen disposal, *Science* 177:697, 1972.

139. Williamson, A. R., and Askonas, B. A. Biosynthesis of immunoglobulins: the separate classes of polyribosomes synthesizing heavy and light chains, *J. Mol. Biol.* 23:201, 1967.

140. Wochner, R. D., Drews, G., Strober, W., and Waldmann, T. A. Accelerated breakdown of immunoglobulin G (IgG) in myotonic dystrophy: a hereditary error of immunoglobulin catabolism, *J. Clin. Invest.* 45:321, 1966.

141. Wu, T. T., and Kabat, E. A. An analysis of the sequences of the variable regions of Bence Jones proteins and myeloma light chains and their implications for antibody complementarity, *J. Exp. Med.* 132:211, 1970.

142. Yount, W. J., Dorner, M. M., Kunkel, H. G., and Kabat, E. A. Studies on human antibodies. VI. Selective variations in subgroup composition and genetic markers, *J. Exp. Med.* 127:633, 1968.

143. Zolla, S., Buxbaum, J., Franklin, E. C., and Scharff, M. D. Synthesis and assembly of immunoglobulins by malignant human plasmacytes. I. Myelomas producing γ-chains and light chains, *J. Exp. Med.* 132:148, 1970.

144. Zucker-Franklin, D., and Berney, S. Electron microscope study of surface immunoglobulin-bearing human tonsil cells, *J. Exp. Med.* 135:533, 1972.

Chapter 17 Lymphoid Cell Effector Substances and Cell-mediated Cytotoxic Reactions

The field of cellular immunity encompasses a number of areas of study, including classic delayed hypersensitivity reactions, homograft rejection, graft-versus-host reactions, and antitumor immunity. These and related topics are the subject of this chapter.

Until recently the study of delayed hypersensitivity reactions was made difficult by the lack of a measurable effector substance; that is, an immunologic reagent equivalent to that of immunoglobulin in humoral immune reactions. The limitation of using cutaneous inflammation as the final measurement of complex cellular events is apparent. For a long time the notion that cellular immune reactions could be categorized with immunologic reactions rested solely on the observed requirement for prior specific sensitization (45, 140, 301).

In the early 1940s Landsteiner and Chase discovered the cellular transfer of delayed hypersensitivity (164, 165). This feat marked a turning point in the analysis of cell-mediated immune reactions and the mechanisms of delayed hypersensitivity. Their investigations provided a means of separating these reactions from those mediated by humoral antibody. The transfer of tuberculin hypersensitivity by viable leukocytes from sensitive donors was observed in 1949 by Lawrence (166), paving the way for study of the first identified lymphocyte effector substance—transfer factor. Subsequently a number of substances were found to be released from, or produced by, sensitized lymphocytes incubated with specific antigen. These substances are recognized by their activity in a variety of experimental assay systems and have been termed "lymphokines" (66) or "effector substances." They are the products of both B and T cells (190). Thus far, the attempts to separate and identify their physical characteristics have been rudimentary. However, a start has been made and a number of activities produced by or liberated from sensitized human blood lymphocytes in response to antigen have been identified (59, 173). The best characterized of these are illustrated in Fig. 17.1 and described in more detail in Tables 17.1 and 17.2.

The list of effector substances must be regarded as tentative. Several "factors" regarded as independent may actually be the activities of a single substance assayed under different conditions. A brief description of these effector substances follows.

(a) Transfer factor (TF) was the first of the lymphocyte effector substances to be well characterized (166, 170). Its biological activity is demonstrable by the transfer of cutaneous reactivity to specific antigens.

(b) Migration inhibitory factor (MIF) is one of the better characterized lymphocyte effector substances. It is released by sensitive lymphocytes in the presence of specific antigen and has the property of inhibiting the migration of normal, nonsensitized macrophages (19, 57).

(c) Lymphotoxin (lymphocytotoxin, or LT) is another putative effector substance liberated from sensitized lymphocytes in the presence of antigen or mitogen and is assayed by its ability to kill or interfere with the growth of a wide variety of target cells in vitro.

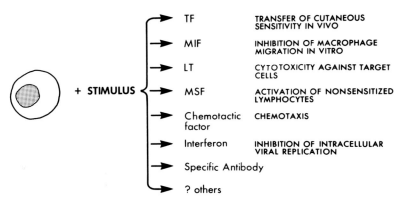

Figure 17.1 Schematic showing incubation of lymphocytes with nonspecific mitogen or appropriate antigen to stimulate the release of a number of biologically active effector substances. *TF* = transfer factor; *MIF* = migration inhibitory factor; *LT* = lymphocytotoxin; and *MSF* = mitosis-stimulating factor.

(d) Mitosis stimulating factor (MSF) is a factor which, under appropriate conditions of stimulation of sensitized human or guinea pig lymphocytes, can be detected in the supernatant medium and can induce blastogenic transformation and mitosis of nonsensitized lymphocytes. This activity may reflect the ac-

tion of multiple mitogenically active substances, since relatively little progress has been made in purification of this factor.

(e) Chemotactic factor is a recently described effector substance released by sensitized lymphocytes. In contrast to MIF, which seems to inhibit macrophage migration, chemotactic factor appears to orient the movement of macrophages.

(f) Interferon is one of the better characterized of the effector substances. It is released by sensitized lymphocytes under antigenic stimulation or from nonsensitized lymphocytes by nonspecific mitogens; its activity is assayed by tests of inhibition of viral replication within tissue culture lines.

(g) Immunoglobulin is a specific antibody molecule that must be listed among the effector molecules produced by lymphocytes; immunoglobulins are, of course, the best known and studied of the effector substances.

In the subsequent sections of this chapter we shall consider in detail the information available on each of these lymphokines.

Lymphocyte Effector Substances

Transfer Factor

Beginning with the demonstration in 1949 of the transfer of delayed hypersensitivity to tuberculin in man by viable leukocytes from sensitized donors, Lawrence and his colleagues for more than two decades have studied the factor or factors responsible for the transfer (166, 170, 171).

Table 17.1 Effector substances (lymphokines) produced by lymphocytes.

Transfer factor
Factors affecting macrophages
　Migration inhibitory factor (MIF)
　Chemotactic factor
　Macrophage aggregation factor (MAF) (? same as MIF)
　Macrophage-activating factor
Cytotoxic factors
　Lymphocytotoxin (LT)
Mitogenic factors
　Mitosis-stimulating factor (MSF)
Chemotactic factors
　For neutrophils
　For eosinophils
　For lymphocytes
　For macrophages (as above)
Interferon
Immunoglobulin
Growth-inhibitory factors
　Proliferation inhibitory factor (PIF)
　Clonal inhibitory factor
Skin reactive factor (? same as MIF or chemotactic factor)

Table 17.2 Comparison of properties of four effector substances.

Property	Transfer factor	Migration inhibitory factor	Guinea pig lymphotoxin	Chemotactic factor
Molecular weight	< 10,000	35,000–55,000	25,000–55,000 (guinea pig) 90,000 (human)	35,000–55,000 150,000
Electrophoresis		Prealbumin	Albumin	Albumin
CsCl p25 (isopycnic centrifugation in CsCl)	?	1.43	1.34	?
Heat stability (56° for 30 min)	Sensitive	Stable	Sensitive	Stable
Protease	Stable	Sensitive	Stable	
Neuraminidase		Sensitive	Stable	Stable
DNase, RNase	Stable	Stable	Stable	Stable
Species specificity	Specific	Relatively specific		Nonspecific

Activities Transfer factor is assayed in vivo by its ability to confer upon a recipient delayed hypersensitivity to antigen to which the donor is specifically sensitive. For example, leukocyte transfer factor from a tuberculin-negative, histoplasmin-positive donor will induce cutaneous reactivity to histoplasmin but not to tuberculin in an unsensitized recipient. Leukocyte preparations from nonsensitive donors will not confer sensitivity.

Reactivity is systemic (that is, generalized rather than confined to the site of transfer factor administration), and its onset is rapid, occurring within a few hours. The duration of sensitivity is long, usually lasting from months to years. The capacity for transfer of delayed hypersensitivity is a function of the degree of sensitivity of the donor and the dosage of white cells used; however, exceedingly minute amounts of white cells (3×10^8 cells) (167) or white cell extracts suffice to transfer sensitivity from a strongly reactive donor.

Transfer factor injected in vivo also confers on the recipient's lymphocytes the ability to undergo blastogenic transformation and to make migration inhibitory factor (MIF) in vitro in response to specific antigen. Transfer factor does not cross species barriers in vivo and does not transfer the capacity for serum antibody response (174).

Tests in vitro have demonstrated that transfer factor effects can cross species lines. For example, dialyzable human transfer factor causes transformation of mouse lymphocytes (1) and of monkey lymphocytes (8). In vitro experiments therefore do not appear to display the species specificity required of an in vivo transfer reaction.

Accumulated evidence suggests that transfer factor can convert nonsensitized lymphocytes to a sensitized state that encompasses all the activities generally associated with delayed hypersensitivity reactivity: in vivo cutaneous reactivity (9), in vitro blastogenic transformation, clonal proliferation of lymphoid cells, and elaboration of MIF. However, attempts at inducing contact sensitivity, usually regarded as a form of delayed hypersensitivity reaction (46), generally have been unsuccessful or ambiguous.

Physical Characteristics Relatively early in the study of transfer factor it was apparent that extracts of leukocytes prepared by freezing and thawing or osmotic lysis were as effective as the intact cell in the transfer of delayed hypersensitivity (168, 169). These observations paved the way for physical characterization of the effector substance (see Table 17.2).

Transfer factor is a dialyzable substance with a molecular weight of less than 10,000. It is not itself immunogenic, in that it does not stimulate the formation of reacting antibodies. Transfer factor does not resemble the immunoglobulins (172), and immunoglobulin contamination is generally not detectable.

Lawrence has suggested that the main candidates for transfer factor activity are dialyzable polynucleotide and/or polypeptide chains (170, 171). Transfer factor is unaffected by DNase, RNase, DNase plus trypsin treatment, or storage in the frozen state for long periods of time. It is, however, inactivated if exposed to heat of 56° or higher for 30 minutes or more.

Detailed methods for the isolation and purification of transfer factor have been published (10, 28, 79, 80, 84, 93, 171). DNase-treated extracts of between 2 and 6×10^8 frozen and thawed leukocytes are dialyzed against distilled water overnight at refrigerator temperatures. The dialysates are filtered and stored in a frozen or lyophilized state until used. Dialysis separates transfer factor from leukocyte-bound transplantation antigens as well as most other lymphocyte effector substances.

In addition to being released by cell lysis, transfer factor may be liberated from sensitized lymphocytes in vitro by the addition of specific antigen. For example, when lymphocytes from a tuberculin-positive subject are incubated with tuberculin, transfer factor appears in the supernatant fluid and is no longer detectable in extracts prepared from the cells. The release of transfer factor by antigen is quite selective. For example, when purified protein derivative (PPD) is added to a mixed leukocyte population containing diphtheria-toxoid–sensitive as well as tuberculin-sensitive cells, only the tuberculin transfer factor is released into the supernatant fluid (175).

Mechanism of Action Marshall, Valentine, and Lawrence studied clonal proliferation of lymphocytes with cinematographic techniques (177, 200). They observed that when tuberculin was added to cultures of peripheral blood lymphocytes from a sensitive subject, less than 2 percent of the population was stimulated to transform, divide, and undergo clonal proliferation. By the seventh day of culture, 20 to 30 percent of the cells were transformed, all having arisen from the few percent initially stimulated to division. Using this technique, they cultured nonsensitive lymphocytes with transfer factor from a sensitive donor and observed precisely the same series of events: clonal proliferation of a small portion of the population, and no recruitment of nonproliferating cells. These observations are taken as evidence in support of Burnet's clonal selection hypothesis, that a small portion of the circulating lymphocyte population is capable of response and clonal proliferation in the presence of specific antigen.

It is not clear how a dialyzable leukocyte extract rapidly

confers upon a recipient's lymphocytes the specific immunologic reactivity of the donor and subsequently initiates a state of prolonged sensitivity. A number of possible interpretations of this phenomenon have been suggested (170, 171): (a) transfer factor is, or contains, a sensitizing antigen or "superantigen"; (b) TF is an immunoglobulin either of a known type or of as yet undiscovered nature; (c) TF is an informational molecule capable of replication or self-perpetuation; and (d) TF is a derepressor of a select population of nonsensitized lymphocytes.

To counter the argument that transfer factor is an antigen or a superantigen operating by enhancing a state of latent sensitivity in the recipient, Lawrence and his colleagues selected coccidioidin-negative recipients from an area where *Coccidioides immitis* does not occur. Such recipients became sensitive to coccidioidin after receiving transfer factor from sensitive donors (254).

Another argument against transfer factor operating as an antigen is the observation that it can confer specific homograft sensitivity to foreign histocompatibility antigens to which the recipients have not been previously exposed (169–171, 176).

The argument against transfer factor being an antibody or immunoglobulin of known type is simply that such immunoglobulins have not been detected in transfer factor preparations using sensitive assay techniques (174).

Summarizing these and other observations, Lawrence concluded that transfer factor, first, initiates de novo sensitivity rather than enhancing latent sensitivity and, second, exhibits a high degree of immunologic specificity (171).

If transfer factor is neither modified immunoglobulin nor antigen, how then does it operate? "Since the polynucleotides present in the [leukocyte] dialysates are rather small to code for the amounts and the specificity of information required, the interpretation of transfer factor as an informational molecule is difficult to sustain." (171) Certainly a molecular weight of 10,000 (10) is too small to code for an intact immunoglobulin or even for a significant portion of the light chain. Although there has been considerable speculation that transfer factor acts as an immunogen or some type of superantigen (cf. 302), one must conclude that at this point the precise composition and mechanism of action of transfer factor are undefined.

Transfer Factor and Cellular Immune Deficiencies

Agammaglobulinemia. In an extensive series of studies Good and his colleagues demonstrated the transfer of delayed hypersensitivity by leukocytes to several antigens in patients with agammaglobulinemia (94–96). Although the elements involved in sensitization were not clearly

identified as transfer factor by the means currently used to characterize this activity (cf. 93), the pattern of recipient response was consistent with a transfer factor effect (cf. 170, 171, 248).

Sarcoidosis. Patients with Boeck's sarcoid often show a loss of delayed hypersensitivity to a variety of antigens despite unimpaired antibody production. Loss of delayed hypersensitivity is partial rather than complete, and reactivity may be normal during periods of disease remission (45, 95, 141).

Patients with sarcoidosis also respond abnormally to transfer factor. When leukocytes from tuberculin-positive donors are administered intradermally to normal tuberculin-negative recipients, subsequent challenge with antigen results in intense reaction at the local site of leukocyte deposition and also in remote unprepared skin sites (166, 170). Application of this technique to patients with sarcoidosis reveals that only local sensitivity is transferred; systemic sensitivity does not appear (305).

The simplest interpretation of this phenomenon is that sarcoidosis patients do not respond to transfer factor, and the local reaction merely reflects the interaction of locally deposited donor cells or transfer factor with antigen. In contrast, patients with sarcoidosis usually demonstrate a brisk reaction to Kveim antigen—an antigen prepared from spleen containing sarcoid granulomata. Furthermore, the granulomatous delayed reaction to Kveim antigen may be transferred from patients with active sarcoidosis to normal subjects (13, 178). It appears that patients with this disorder are reacting to Kveim antigen and producing an appropriate transfer factor at a time when other delayed hypersensitivity reactions are completely or partially suspended.

Hodgkin's disease and other malignancies. Patients with active Hodgkin's disease may be anergic and fail to respond to the transfer of leukocytes with the development of appropriate sensitivity (95, 147). Like the patients with sarcoidosis, the patients with advanced Hodgkin's disease usually have normal immunoglobulin production despite impaired delayed hypersensitivity. Selective abnormality of delayed hypersensitivity is not a general feature of hematologic malignancies other than Hodgkin's disease, although the same phenomenon has been observed in some patients with advanced cancer. In these patients leukocytes or dialyzable transfer factor either fail to produce systemic reactivity or produce only weak reactivity (117, 278).

Immunologic reconstitution. A number of attempts have been made to reconstitute a normal immunologic response in patients with congenital or acquired impairment of the immunologic apparatus (see Chapter 18). Sensitized leukocytes or, more rarely, dialyzable extracts of leukocytes have been used in patients with a variety of diseases, including progressive or generalized vaccinia (148, 227), chronic cutaneous moniliasis (39, 306), lepromatous leprosy (41, 64; cf. 300, 312), and ataxia telangiectasia (243, 244).

In those rare patients experiencing a successful induction of delayed hypersensitivity reactivity by leukocyte transfusion, the evidence that transfer factor was the responsible substance is questionable. The few reports that have claimed successful restoration of immunologic competence with materials that meet the available criteria for transfer factor have usually been greeted with skepticism. The therapeutic potential of using transfer factor to attempt such restoration is still largely unexplored. Transfer factor has the theoretical advantage of being nonantigenic and therefore amenable to repeated administration without the induction of graft-versus-host reactions. The latter reactions constitute both a theoretical and real limitation to the administration of sensitized leukocytes (166).

Migration Inhibitory Factor (MIF)

In 1962 George and Vaughan placed peritoneal exudate cells from antigen-sensitized guinea pigs in capillary tubes and demonstrated that migration of these cells out of the tubes and into a lucite chamber was inhibited in the presence of antigen (84). Migration of cells from unsensitized animals was not inhibited (cf. 54–59). The principal migratory cell in the peritoneal exudate population is the macrophage. Inhibited cells gather in dense clumps, whereas normal cells migrate out from the open end of the capillary tube in a lacy and fanlike pattern (Fig. 17.2). The initial studies with this interesting technique used PPD as the sensitizing antigen (60). Later studies used purified proteins such as diphtheria toxoid or ovalbumin to sensitize guinea pigs (57).

Experiments were designed to elucidate the role of circulating antibody in migration inhibition: cells from animals producing antibodies but not exhibiting delayed hypersensitivity were not inhibited by antigens, whereas cells from animals both producing antibody and exhibiting delayed hypersensitivity were inhibited by antigen (57). Furthermore, attempts at passively sensitizing cells with high-titer antisera in order to make them susceptible to antigen-induced inhibition of migration were uniformly unsuccessful.

Further evidence that the migration inhibition test is correlated with delayed hypersensitivity rather than humoral antibody production has been obtained from experiments with a series of well-defined antigens (270): oligo-

peptides of L-lysine coupled to dinitrophenol (DNP) hapten. These studies indicated that only DNP-oligopeptides, which are immunogenic and can elicit delayed hypersensitivity in vivo, are capable of specific inhibition of cell migration in vitro.

One can conclude on the basis of these observations that: (a) *the migration inhibition test is associated with delayed hypersensitivity;* (b) *the specificity of the reaction to antigen in vitro is the same as that of the cutaneous reaction* (21, 63); and (c) *there is no evidence that circulating antibody plays a critical role in inhibition of migration.*

The in vitro inhibition of migration by specific antigen may have an in vivo counterpart. Nelson and Boyden (220) demonstrated that the injection of antigen into the peritoneal cavity of guinea pigs with delayed hypersensitivity causes a marked decrease in the number of macrophages found in exudates. The antigen possibly interacts with the cells of the peritoneal cavity to produce clumping and adherence to the peritoneal lining, just as the antigen induces clumping in vitro.

The Effector Cells   Early in the study of the migration inhibition test it was demonstrated that when cells from sensitized and nonsensitized animals were mixed, as few as 2.5 percent sensitive cells were sufficient to cause inhibition of the entire population by antigens (62). Since

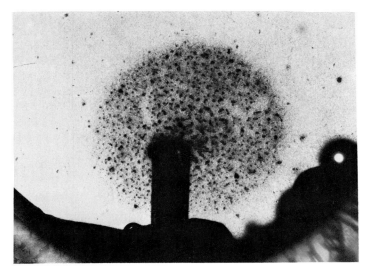

Figure 17.2 The capillary migration test for MIF (migration inhibitory factor). Leukocyte populations comprising antigen-sensitive lymphocytes and macrophages are centrifuged down in a capillary tube. In the absence of antigen, the macrophages migrate from the tube in the fanlike pattern shown in the figure. If antigen is added, migration of cells is inhibited and they cluster around the opening of the tube.

peritoneal exudate cells are a heterogeneous mixture of leukocytes containing primarily macrophages (about 80 percent), lymphocytes (about 20 percent), and a few percent neutrophils, eosinophils, and mast cells, studies had to be undertaken to determine which of these was responsible for the inhibition reaction. When lymphocytes from lymph nodes or spleens of sensitized animals were mixed with peritoneal exudate cells from nonimmunized animals, the migration of the resulting population was inhibited by specific antigen (55–57). Neither sensitive lymph node cells alone nor unsensitized peritoneal exudate cells alone were inhibited. Further studies in which lymphocytes and macrophages separately were isolated from peritoneal exudates indicated that nonimmune peritoneal exudate cells are inhibited by antigen when a small percentage of sensitive lymphocytes are present in the mixture. Furthermore, peritoneal exudates from which the lymphocytes have been removed are no longer inhibited by antigen (20).

These observations suggest that *two different cell types are required for the demonstration of antigen-dependent inhibition of migration: the first is the sensitized lymphocyte, the second is the migrating macrophage.*

Migration inhibitory factor has been identified also in experimental systems using human leukocytes isolated from lymph nodes (142, 292–295). A positive correlation between skin test reactivity to antigen and specific inhibition of cell migration in vitro was obtained from 27 subjects. In addition, inhibition has been described with the use of sensitized human leukocytes, specific antigen, and normal unsensitized guinea pig macrophages (296).

Recently several investigators have demonstrated that lymphocytes can be stimulated to produce MIF by plant lectin such as conconavalin A (59, 245, 271). Of even more interest is the recent observation that MIF may not be a product of lymphocytes solely, but may be produced by established lines of both lymphoid and nonlymphoid cells (232, 298). Its production apparently does not require lymphoid cell proliferation (23).

Metabolic Requirements and the Cell Surface   In vitro studies have shown that antigen-sensitized cells need to be viable in order to exert their influence on unsensitized migrative cells (62). Freezing and thawing or heating to 56° for 30 minutes ablates the activity of the sensitized cells. Protein synthesis is thought to be necessary for the antigen-induced inhibition of migration to be manifest. Exposure of cells to proteolytic enzymes such as trypsin and chymotrypsin also alters their ability to respond to antigen (61). The proteolytic enzymes probably are acting on some membrane proteins that have a fairly high turn-

over rate; 24 hours after exposure to trypsin the sensitive cells regain the ability to be inhibited by specific antigen.

MIF as a Soluble Effector Substance   Shortly after the demonstration that the migration of sensitized peritoneal exudate population was inhibited by specific antigen, attempts were made to reproduce the phenomenon with cell-free media that might contain soluble substances released by the effector cells. Normal peritoneal exudate cells were inhibited from migration by the addition of cell-free supernatant from sensitized lymph node cells incubated for 24 hours with specific antigen.

Although many explanations of this observation are possible, the simplest interpretation is that sensitized lymphocytes are stimulated by antigen to release substances that inhibit the migration of normal peritoneal exudate cells (20). Again, protein synthesis appears necessary for the production or release of MIF.

These early studies of soluble migration inhibitory factor suffer from certain inherent limitations. First, large amounts of antigen are present in the supernatant medium that contains the active factor (58). Second, the supernatant obtained in such experiments rapidly loses inhibitory activity when diluted even slightly—a phenomenon presenting considerable difficulty in attempts at fractionation and purification.

Certain characteristics of migration inhibitory factor have been defined (279). The active material in the supernatant is stable to heating at 56° for 30 minutes and is nondialyzable. The activity is destroyed by trypsin and chymotrypsin but not by DNase or RNase, suggesting a factor that contains protein as part of the active moiety (57, 255). Guinea pig MIF activity is also destroyed by neuraminidase (59). Preliminary efforts at fractionation suggest that the molecular weight of the active material is approximately 35,000 to 55,000 (24, 255). It is separable from albumin and chemotactic factor by electrophoresis on polyacrylamide gels (57, 58, 256). It is probably a glycoprotein (59). The characteristics of human and guinea pig MIF differ considerably (258). The interaction of sensitized lymphocytes with specific antigen releases a factor that causes nonsensitized peritoneal exudate cells to aggregate. Macrophage aggregation factor (MAF) (see Table 17.1) correlates in similar fashion with a state of delayed hypersensitivity (185) and may be identical to MIF (217).

Mechanism of Action of Migration Inhibitory Factor   At the present time, little is known about the mechanism of action of migration inhibitory factor. The appellation "migration inhibitory factor" suggests that the substance acts by an inhibitory process rather than by stimulating some activity. This is not necessarily the case. In fact, as we shall see in Chapter 24, some evidence exists that antigen added to sensitized peritoneal exudate cells may increase the number of glass-adherent macrophages and may stimulate macrophage maturation in vitro (59, 311). MIF appears to make macrophages "sticky" and to enhance their phagocytic capacity and oxidative metabolism (211, 216, 218). Macrophages treated in vitro with MIF come to resemble the "angry" macrophages that arise in vivo in response to certain microbial challenges (193). The effect of MIF on macrophages is inhibited by certain glucocorticoids (7).

Lymphotoxin (Lymphocytotoxin)

When lymphoid cells are stimulated to blastogenic transformation by specific antigen or nonspecific mitogen, they cause destruction of allogeneic target cells in vitro (136). Once activated in vitro, aggressor lymphocytes can injure all adjacent target cells, whether or not these target cells possess the inciting antigens (265–267). Target cell injury usually requires direct contact with activated lymphocytes, but can also occur to some extent in the absence of such contact. Injury occurring in the absence of direct contact is presumed to result from an effector substance or substances released by the aggressor lymphocytes (99, 163, 266). For example, studies of both immune and phytohemagglutinin-stimulated normal mouse lymphocytes have indicated that destruction of target L cells was associated with release of a soluble, nonspecific cell toxin by the activated lymphocytes. This substance was designated lymphotoxin, or LT (100), and the following questions were asked about its generation (99): "i) what cells release lymphotoxin; ii) what treatments or agents will trigger its release; and iii) is the release of lymphotoxin a general biological phenomenon shared by the lymphoid cells of many animal species?"

Only viable and metabolically intact lymphoid cells have been demonstrated to release lymphotoxin in vitro (320). Other cell types appear to be inactive in this regard, as are thymic lymphocytes or lymphocytes from patients with chronic lymphocytic leukemia or Hodgkin's disease (99).

Lymphocytes from a variety of mammalian species, including the cat, rat, rabbit, and man, can be stimulated by phytohemagglutinin to produce lymphotoxin (321). They can be stimulated by a variety of other agents as well, including pokeweed mitogen, streptolysin O, and the mixed leukocyte reaction. The degree of lymphocyte stimulation by nonspecific mitogens correlates with the amount of lymphotoxin released. Specific antigens, such as PPD and histoplasmin, and cell-bound antigens stimu-

late release of lymphotoxin by specifically immune lymphocytes. Interference with lymphocyte energy metabolism, or with protein synthesis, blocks lymphotoxin release, as does hydrocortisone at 100-fold physiologic concentration. Blocking of DNA and RNA synthesis reduces but does not stop lymphotoxin release (99).

Physical Characteristics   The physical characteristics of murine, guinea pig, and human lymphotoxin have been partially defined and are indicated in Table 17.2 (59, 99, 102, 156–158). Within a given species, the lymphotoxin induced by a variety of stimulants is physically identical.

Human lymphotoxin is stable over the pH range of 5 to 8, but is sensitive to heating at 85° and to phenol. It is resistant to treatment with DNase, RNase, and trypsin. Its molecular weight is approximately 90,000 (102). Lebowitz and Lawrence (179) studied a lymphocytotoxin released by tuberculin-sensitive human lymphocytes incubated for 36 hours with tuberculin. They found the active moiety to be nondialyzable, resistant to freezing and thawing, but inactivated by heating at 56° for 30 minutes. Human lymphotoxin recently has been extensively purified (268). Mouse lymphotoxin appears to be antigenically distinct from human lymphotoxin (101). Guinea pig lymphotoxin migrates with albumin in acrylamide gel electrophoresis and is therefore distinct from MIF (53). The characteristics of guinea pig lymphotoxin are summarized in Table 17.2.

Mechanism of Action   The rate and extent of target cell destruction by lymphotoxin is dependent upon the concentration of the effector substance (163, 322). The higher the concentration, the more rapid and extensive the cytotoxic effects. At lower concentrations the target cells may be affected for a time but can subsequently recover. Target cells sublethally injured by lymphotoxin appear to recuperate by active, energy-dependent processes. Thus, inhibition of the energy metabolism or macromolecular biosynthesis of target cells greatly enhances their susceptibility to lymphotoxin.

A variety of cell types is injured by lymphotoxin in vitro including human, primate, rabbit, hamster, mouse, and chicken tissue culture cells and erythrocytes. When cells are exposed to lymphotoxin, the first morphologic evidence of cell injury is cytoplasmic vacuolization. The cytoplasmic membrane then forms blebs, and cell processes shed into the supernatant medium. The target cell becomes round and disintegrates.

On the basis of electron microscopic and other observations, it has been suggested that lymphotoxin interacts with the target cell plasma membrane (99, 320).

In addition to lymphotoxin, other growth inhibitory factors have been described (see Table 17.1). These include proliferation inhibitory factor (PIF) (6) and clonal inhibitory factor. It is not yet certain whether these are distinctive substances or merely additional biological properties of already identified lymphocyte mediators.

Mitosis Stimulating Factor

Valentine and Lawrence observed that when cell-free media, obtained from tuberculin-sensitive lymphocytes incubated with PPD, are added to nonsensitized lymphocytes, the latter undergo blastogenic transformation and repeated division (307, 308). The material in the supernatant that is responsible for activation of normal lymphocytes is destroyed by heating at 56° for 30 minutes and is nondialyzable. This latter characteristic distinguishes it from transfer factor and from migration inhibitory factor (see Table 17.2). Furthermore, the activity is not sedimented at $100,000 \times g$, a property that separates it from blastogenic transformation antigens found in mixed leukocyte cultures (144, 145). Mitosis stimulating factor is destroyed by treatment with proteases. Its molecular weight has been tentatively placed at 25,000.

The mitosis stimulating factor is released relatively slowly when sensitized lymphocytes are incubated with antigen. The stimulating material requires 18 to 24 hours' incubation for its production. In contrast, transfer factor is liberated within an hour.

There may well be several blastogenic factors produced by lymphocytes (144).

These preliminary observations open up new areas of investigation, in that the complex relation between antigen-released transfer factor, migration inhibitory factor, and mitosis stimulating factor are still to be resolved.

Chemotactic Factor

Bloom and Bennett (19, 21) demonstrated that material purified by Sephadex chromatography and containing MIF produced a skin reaction resembling a delayed type hypersensitivity reaction. This observation raised the question of how macrophages initially accumulated at the site of migration inhibitory factor injection, and stimulated a search for a chemotactic activity. The assay system utilizes two small chambers separated by a cell-permeable Millipore filter. Peritoneal exudate cells are placed in the upper chamber and the material to be assayed for chemotactic activity is placed in the lower chamber. Cells migrating from the upper to the lower chamber are enumerated after removing and staining the filter.

Ward and David found that the supernatants of antigen-stimulated, sensitized peritoneal exudate cells contained a chemotactic factor as well as a migration inhibitory factor (58, 313). This activity has subsequently been characterized in more detail, as indicated in Table 17.2 (314). The major chemotactic factor thus far analyzed is that which has activity for macrophages. This chemotactic "factor" resembles MIF in that its production is antigen specific. It is nondialyzable and heat-stable at 56° for 30 minutes (315) and elutes from Sephadex G-100 with an albumin marker. Its molecular weight is approximately 60,000, although larger molecules have also been found (59). Another characteristic of chemotactic factor is that it is species nonspecific.

Chemotactic activity can be distinguished from MIF activity by electrophoresis on polyacrylamide gels (316).

In addition to chemotactic factor with activity for macrophages, other factors may exist with activity for eosinophils, neutrophils, and lymphocytes (59, 314).

Interferon

Since the discovery of interferon in 1957, a vast amount of complex literature has been written on this subject (cf. 12, 77, 78, 85, 109, 127, 128, 330). We are concerned here with a brief survey of the biological role and nature of interferon and particularly its production by mammalian leukocytes.

The appearance of interferon activity in the circulation of an animal suffering from a viral infection generally coincides with clinical improvement (12). Detectable circulating antibody does not appear until several days later. The notion that the correlation between improvement and interferon appearance is meaningful is supported by many observations of the effectiveness of interferon against viral growth both in vivo and in vitro (77). It has been concluded, therefore, that interferon is a defense system against many viruses and is independent of the usual humoral immune mechanisms. This conclusion has been accepted with the proviso that the concentrations of circulating or secreted interferons may not be a valid index of the in situ concentration within infected cells.

Existing evidence suggests that interferon is a protein newly synthesized after viral infection, although some release of preformed interferon has not been excluded. Interferon may stimulate the host cell to form another protein, which is thought to combine with host ribosomes and cause them to translate host messenger RNA selectively and to reject foreign viral RNA messengers (11, 184, 198, 199, 290). However, this thesis has not yet been sufficiently proven.

Interferon is active against a broad range of viruses, although viruses vary considerably in their sensitivity. Interferon has been demonstrated in a variety of vertebrate species from fish to man (78), although the protein effector produced by any one species appears to be relatively specific for that species. For instance, human interferon protects human cells but does not protect chick cells or mouse cells. However, this specificity is not absolute (40). Interferon may also have some antitumor activity, perhaps by acting through an antiviral mechanism (107, 109, 180).

The chemical nature of interferon is still largely unknown. Certainly a protein moiety destroyed by protease digestion is necessary for biological activity. Some investigators have suggested that a carbohydrate component may be important, at least in some species (228).

In general, interferons are resistant to low pH and to moderate heat. Purified chick interferon is heterogeneous as to size and charge, and contains no detectable sugar moiety (74). Interferons have been grouped into discrete classes on the basis of molecular weight (20,000 to 30,000; 40,000 to 60,000; and 90,000 to 160,000), but the biological activity of these classes does not appear to differ (27, 146, 277, 331).

A variety of agents induces interferon production: all major groups of animal virus, fungal viruses, intracellular parasites including rickettsia bacteria and protozoa, and nonliving material including phytohemagglutinin, bacterial endotoxin, fungal cell wall carbohydrate, double-stranded RNA, and synthetic polyanions (77, 109).

The major sites of interferon synthesis in vivo may vary with the inducing agent. Studies indicate that the components of the reticuloendothelial system, including bone marrow, spleen, and circulating leukocytes, can make interferon in response to virus infection and bacterial endotoxin (129, 160, 161, 276, 286, 319). Whole-body irradiation of mice at sublethal doses reduces the interferon response to viruses by 90 percent. Administration of compatible bone marrow restores the response, suggesting that a major source of interferon is hematopoietic tissues (cited by ref. 77). Leukemic transformation can suppress interferon production (65).

Peritoneal exudate cells and circulating leukocytes can produce interferon in response to carboxylate copolymers, fungal polysaccharides, and endotoxin (26, 43, 159, 160, 277, 284). In addition, mammalian leukocytes, including human cells, have been demonstrated to produce interferon in vitro in response to viral infection (68).

The possibility that leukocytes may respond to virus infection with the production of interferon was first suggested by Gresser (108). He observed that as early as six hours after infection of human leukocytes with Sendai virus, high titers of interferon were detectable in the cul-

ture fluid. The interferon induced by Sendai virus infection of human leukocytes subsequently was found to have a molecular weight of approximately 25,000.

Glasgow and his colleagues investigated the role of interferon produced by leukocytes in response to experimental vaccinia infection of mice (85, 86). They demonstrated that populations of peritoneal exudate cells, comprised of 42 to 68 percent neutrophils and 32 to 58 percent mononuclear cells, produced interferon that inhibited viral multiplication. They also inoculated mice with leukocytes previously exposed to inactivated vaccinia viruses and demonstrated protection against subsequent challenge by active virus.

After these initial studies, attention focused on the lymphocyte as an important source of leukocyte interferon production. It was soon demonstrated that normal lymphocytes released interferon in response to phytohemagglutinin, streptolysin O, and pokeweed mitogen (81, 112, 318). Then came the critical observation that specific antigen could induce interferon production in sensitized lymphoid cells in vitro (106).

In 1970 Stinebring and Absher (282) demonstrated that mice infected with a strain of BCG produced interferon, which reached a peak six hours after intravenous challenge with tuberculin. Gresser (108) studied leukocytes from three patients with congenital agammaglobulinemia and one with thymic dysgenesis and lymphopenia and found no impairment of interferon synthesis consistent with the absence of increased susceptibility to virus infection (see Chapter 18).

An intriguing question is whether there is an immunologic recall phenomenon for interferon production by lymphocytes similar to that for antibody synthesis. Glasgow demonstrated that peritoneal exudates containing mixed cell populations, when obtained from a virus-immune animal, produced more interferon in response to specific virus challenge than cells from nonimmune animals (86). Our own laboratory has been concerned with the interaction between different types of leukocytes in the production of interferon in response to viral and nonviral inducers (71, 72). In cultures containing 96 to 100 percent pure populations of human macrophages, no interferon production was detectable in response to phytohemagglutinin or specific antigen. Cultures of lymphocytes of 99.5 to 100 percent purity produced low levels of interferon. When macrophages and lymphocytes were combined, the interferon response to phytohemagglutinin or to specific antigen (PPD) was greatly augmented. Syngeneic fibroblasts, HeLa cells, or mouse macrophages could not substitute for human macrophages in producing this augmentation of lymphocyte response. For macrophage augmentation, direct contact between lymphocytes and macrophages is necessary— a situation similar to that for lymphocyte-macrophage interaction in antibody synthesis or blastogenic transformation. These observations suggest that lymphocyte-macrophage interaction is necessary for a variety of immune reactions and for the elaboration of certain lymphocyte effector substances.

Other Factors

A variety of other, as yet poorly characterized, lymphocyte factors exist. In 1969 Lebowitz and Lawrence described a cloning inhibition factor (179), which may be identical to lymphotoxin.

Lymphoid-cell–mediated Cytotoxic Reactions

Lymphoid cells may function in certain tissue-damaging immune reactions, of which some confer benefit to the host and others are detrimental. Lymphoid-cell–mediated tissue injury is believed to be crucial in certain delayed hypersensitivity reactions, in naturally occurring and experimental autoimmune diseases, in a variety of allograft phenomena, and in some forms of tumor rejection (67, 110, 236, 237, 327). The cells destroyed in these processes are designated *target cells.* The cells inflicting destruction are designated *effector cells.* Effector cells may include a variety of lymphocyte populations, but they are primarily T cells as well as monocytes, macrophages, and perhaps neutrophils.

The cell that initiates cytotoxic reactions occurring in delayed hypersensitivity or allograft rejections has been assumed to be a sensitized lymphoid cell bearing recognition sites for antigens contained on or bound to the cells that are destroyed (91, 92). Although this seems often to be the case, uninstructed "normal" lymphoid cells can be recruited into the cytotoxic process too by a variety of pathways and thus amplify the destruction. The mechanisms by which lymphoid cells exert their cytotoxic effects are not yet completely understood, but almost certainly involve many of the effector substances already described. In this and subsequent sections of this chapter, we shall consider *cell-mediated cytotoxic reactions;* that is, reactions in which lymphoid cells function as effectors in close geographic proximity to the target cells. The prototype of such a reaction is the delayed hypersensitivity response. We shall draw a rather artificial distinction between cell-mediated reactions and those brought about primarily by humoral antibody and complement functioning in the absence of lymphoid cells. Under many circumstances cell-mediated cytotoxic reactions obviously occur simultaneously with and in the same location as those mediated by antibody and complement.

Cytotoxic Effects of Sensitized Lymphoid Cells on Antigenic Target Cells

A variety of cells may serve as the target cells of cytotoxic reactions. They may have major transplantation antigens different from those of the host or may bear tumor-specific antigens as a result of natural or experimental carcinogenesis from oncogenic viruses or chemicals (cf. 110, 123). The target cells may be coated with foreign antigens from parasites or other foreign materials.

The direct cytotoxic effect of sensitized lymphoid cells on antigenic target cells has been demonstrated in a number of in vitro model systems in which the effector cells are brought into intimate contact with the target cells. One of the first demonstrations of this phenomenon was that of Govaerts in 1960 (97). He showed that thoracic duct lymphocytes from a dog sensitized by a renal allograft aggregated around and subsequently destroyed cells from the donor kidney. Destruction occurred over a 24- to 48-hour period in vitro and was immunologically specific for renal cells of the donor. Subsequently other studies showed lymphoid-cell–mediated destruction of a number of allografted normal and malignant tissues (cf. 123, 237).

Aggregation Direct contact between the effector cells and the target cells seems to be a requisite for most cell-mediated cytotoxicity reactions. When the target tissues are grown as monolayers, the aggregation of sensitized lymphoid cells on and around these tissues is readily apparent (31, 162, 288). Aggregation usually precedes morphologic evidence of target cell injury and death. It also precedes more sensitive evidence of target cell injury, such as release of surface-bound radioisotopes (133). Under experimental conditions in which lymphoid cells are prevented from intimate contact with the target cells, destruction does not take place.

Although mixed aggregations of lymphoid cells and target cells are a necessary feature of cytotoxic reactions, they are not necessarily sufficient to produce destruction of target cells. The lymphoid cells must be "activated" in some manner, either by specific antigen or nonspecific mitogen. For example, polylysine produces aggregation of lymphoid cells but does not activate them, and use of this compound does not result in target cell lysis (131, 259).

Morphologic studies indicate that the aggregated lymphoid cells are highly motile (5). Adhesion of lymphocytes to the target cells by their uropods (191, 192) is relatively rare, as is the movement of lymphocytes into and out of the target cells (251).

Kinetics of Injury   The destruction of target cells by sensitized lymphoid cells occurs more slowly than cell destruction by soluble antibody and complement. Obviously the rate at which the reaction proceeds will depend on many variables, including the nature of the target cells, the source and numbers of the effector cells, and the assay system. In general, however, lymphoid-mediated cytotoxic reactions against antigen-bearing target cells are rarely detectable morphologically before 18 hours and require roughly 48 hours for completion (261). Similar kinetics are observed when the release of ^{14}C-thymidine from labeled target tissues is monitored, whereas release of membrane-bound chromium^{51} from damaged target cells can be detected as early as 1 to 3 hours (34, 35, 132). Similarly, colony inhibition assays based on the inhibition of the target cells' ability to form clones in tissue culture show a rapid destructive effect of sensitized lymphoid cells (37).

Effector Cells   When compared on the basis of equal numbers of cells, preparations from lymph nodes, spleen, peripheral blood, and thoracic duct fluid vary in their cytotoxic activity against target cells; thymus cells are inactive or only weakly active in cell-mediated cytotoxic reactions (34–36,122, 207, 325). In most of the experimental models, lymphoid cells appear to be the principal effector cells. The major role is played by the T cell, but B lymphocytes and perhaps other thymus-independent lymphoid cells ("killer" cells) may also exert a cytotoxic effect under some circumstances (210, 242, 309). It is now clear that under at least some experimental conditions, splenic lymphoid cells alone cannot mount an immunologically specific cytotoxic attack and that the addition of peritoneal exudate cells is required for target cell destruction. These peritoneal-derived cells are surface adherent and radiation resistant—characteristics of macrophages (73). Evidence has existed for several years that macrophages from sensitized donors can exert a cytotoxic effect by both phagocytic and nonphagocytic mechanisms (14, 103, 104).

The contribution of neutrophils to cell-mediated cytotoxic reactions usually has been considered negligible. In part, this view derives from the type of experimental studies of these reactions, where efforts have been directed at using purified populations of lymphoid cells. Whether in vivo neutrophils participate in the early stages of such reactions is largely unknown (cf. 87).

Effector Cell/Target Cell Ratios   In most experimental studies, a considerable excess of lymphoid cells over target cells has been necessary for the demonstration of a cytotoxic effect (35–37). Recently, Brunner and his collaborators (36) observed that at lymphoid/target cell ratios as low as 1:1, up to 20 percent of the targets were injured or destroyed within six hours—a time period not allowing significant lymphoid cell replication. These data suggest that one sensitized lymphoid cell can injure more than one target cell. The same investigators also showed that the number of effector cells required for a demonstrable cytotoxic effect was influenced by the type of target cell involved. For example, in an in vitro immunologic system involving the same H-2 antigens on a variety of cells, mastocytoma cells were destroyed more slowly than embryonic fibroblasts or spleen cells.

Immunologic Specificity   It is useful to regard lymphoid-cell–mediated cytotoxicity reactions as a two-step phenomenon: *in the first step, contact between a target and effector cell is established by means of antigenic determinants on the target cells and antibody-like receptors on some cells of the effector population; in the second step, viable and metabolically intact lymphoid cells induce lysis of the target cells,* probably by means of effector substances that operate over a short range.

Only the first step of this process appears to involve immunologic specificity, that is, recognition of and interaction with specific antigenic determinants on the target cell. Thus if lymphoid cells are nonspecifically activated and brought into contact with target cells, they will exert a cytolytic effect also. In this latter circumstance, however, there is no specificity in the interaction between effector and target cells.

It is not definitely known whether the sensitized lymphoid cells that react with antigen bound to the target cells in the first step are the same cells that execute the lytic reaction in the second step. Evidence from cinematographic studies suggests that this is indeed the case.

Generally, a common feature of the lymphoid-cell–mediated cytotoxic reaction is the presence on the target cell of antigenic determinants to which the host organism is sensitized. These antigens may be either constituents of the target cell surface or foreign antigens that are adsorbed to or exist in close proximity to the target cell surface (for example, tuberculin injected into a tuberculin-sensitive subject).

Various experimental models have been used to demonstrate the immunologic specificity of the cell-mediated cytotoxic reaction. Lymphoid cells from animals immunized against a given variety of tumor will destroy cells derived from this tumor, but not cells derived from antigenically different tumors (91, 123, 264). Similarly, lymphoid cells from BALB/c mice immunized against cells from the C3H mouse will kill C3H cells, but not cells originating from mouse strains of other genotypes (262). In all cases examined, mouse lymphoid-cell–mediated cytotoxic reactions are specific for those target cells bearing the same H-2 antigens as the cells used as immunogens (32). Results are similar for the human HL-A system (187).

A number of lines of evidence indicate a high degree of specificity for cell-mediated cytotoxic reactions. For example, Brondz (32) demonstrated that for mouse lymphoid cells to be cytotoxic they had to be obtained from donors sensitized to all, or nearly all, defined H-2 antigenic determinants on the target cells. Lymphoid cells from donors sensitized to only half of the antigens failed to kill the target cells.

Presumably, the factors that influence the initial recognition of the target cell antigens by the effector populations (step one of the reaction) also influence the immunologic specificity of cell-mediated cytotoxic reactions. One factor may be antigenic density on the target cell surface (36, 209). Another factor influencing specificity may be circulating antibody. The role played by humoral antibody in the recognition system of the cell-mediated cytotoxic reaction is uncertain. Most evidence favors a recognition system independent of humoral antibody. For example, attempts at eluting antibody from effector lymphoid cells have been largely unsuccessful (33, 289, 325). Similarly, efforts at imparting cytotoxic activity to lymphoid cells by exposure to antibody in vitro have usually failed (31, 207, 235, 259, 325). Furthermore, washed lymphoid cells in the complete absence of serum may retain cytotoxic activity (260, 261).

Under a variety of circumstances, humoral antibody directed against target cell antigens can block the cytotoxic effect of specifically sensitized lymphoid cells. For example, antibodies directed against H-2 antigens of mouse cells block the cytotoxic activity of lymphoid cells from immunized allogeneic mice (197, 207). This interference by humoral antibody is thought to have relevance for host immunologic defenses against certain tumors (cf. 119, 150, 151, 155). Such blocking antibodies may interfere with the cytolytic effect of cellular defense units and result in intensified tumor growth, a phenomenon known as *enhancement*.

Although we have marshalled evidence against the participation of antibody in cell-mediated cytolytic reactions, it would be erroneous to conclude that antibodies rarely or never participate in cytotoxic reactions or are only inhibitory for such reactions. Those reactions that we regard as primarily cell mediated probably represent a complex balance between cellular elements and humoral factors. Two examples will be cited. Hellström and his colleagues (118, 121) described tumor-specific immune systems in which humoral antibody did not block the tumorolytic effect of lymphoid cells. The antibodies were obtained from sera of animals in which the tumors had regressed. These antisera were often directly cytotoxic against the tumor when complement was present. Another example of the coordination of cellular and humoral factors is the induction of cytotoxicity of lymphoid cells from nonimmune donors by antibody to target cell antigens. Under certain experimental conditions antigenic target cells, when treated with heat-inactivated antisera, will be destroyed when exposed to an excess of lymphoid cells obtained from nonimmunized donors. The antisera themselves can be used at dilutions too high to exert a cytotoxic effect directly in the absence of lymphoid cells (38, 134, 188, 196, 197, 236, 238, 241, 289, 317). Lymphoid cells obtained from peripheral blood, thoracic duct, spleen, and lymph nodes generally have been effective in this passive sensitization system, whereas thymus and leukemic lymphocytes have been noncytotoxic. The lymphocytes must be viable and metabolically intact. Aggregation of lymphoid cells around the target cells occurs in a manner similar to that in which sensitized lymphocytes aggregate.

The mechanism of recognition by nonimmune lymphoid cells of antigen-bearing target cells sensitized by antibody is not certain. It is known that monocytes have receptor sites for IgG globulin and specifically for the Fc portion of the molecule (183) and that some lymphocytes have similar receptors (50), which might permit the approximation of IgG antibody-coated target cells and effector cells.

A number of model systems have been described in which the immunologic recognition of target cell antigens is induced by in vitro "sensitization" of lymphoid cells (83, 137, 143, 269). The culture conditions necessary for the demonstration of in vitro sensitization are complex (cf. 123). Perlmann and his colleagues have recently reviewed induction and inhibition of cytotoxicity by humoral antibody (242).

In summary, lymphoid-cell–mediated cytotoxic reactions may be viewed as a two-step phenomenon. Immunologically specific target cell antigen recognition resides in the first step, in which contact is established between effector and target cells. Recognition is thought to result from antibody-like receptors on some cells in the lymphoid population. In certain circumstances, however, humoral antibody can induce in vitro cytotoxicity of unsensitized lymphoid cells that presumably lack antigen-specific receptors. It is likely that reactions that are primarily cell mediated occur together with humoral antibody-dependent reactions in such phenomena as delayed hypersensitivity reactions and in tumor and allograft rejection.

Cytotoxic Mechanisms
One characteristic feature of cell-mediated cytotoxicity is the clustering of lymphoid cells around the target cells. With time-lapse cinematographic techniques it has been demonstrated that after random movement some sensitized lymphoid cells attach to target tumor cells, after which the latter appear to swell and lyse (259).

With very rare exceptions, it has been shown that the lymphoid cells must be alive in order to exert their cytotoxic effects (31, 33, 325). Low temperature prevents cytotoxicity, but not aggregation (326). Inhibitors of electron transport (241), of RNA and protein synthesis (34), as well as cation chelators (125, 201), interfere with lymphoid-mediated cytotoxic reactions to a greater or lesser extent (cf. 130). High doses of X-ray (15,000 r), which impair cell viability, also are inhibitory (263). In short-term experiments, lymphoid cell DNA synthesis and cell division are not required; however, this observation does not exclude the possibility that the division of sensitized and recruited nonsensitized lymphoid cells plays a role during the relatively slow pace of development of cell-mediated cytotoxic reactions in vivo.

Although most of the evidence presently available suggests that the lysis of target cells requires direct contact with viable and metabolically intact effector lymphoid cells, it is quite possible that toxic substances such as lymphotoxin are released locally and contribute to target cell damage. Such damage would lack immunologic specificity, since cells free of antigenic determinants might also be injured. Recent data suggest that lymphocyte cyclic AMP (adenosine monophosphate) may play a role in modulating cytolytic activity (124, 126, 285).

Complement-independent Mechanisms The subcellular mechanisms of cell-mediated cytotoxic reactions are almost completely unknown. Addition of complement generally does not enhance the cytotoxic effect of lymphoid cells on antigenic target cells. This observation has been interpreted as indicating that cell-mediated cytotoxic mechanisms are different from those of humoral antibodies and complement. In some experimental model systems, target cell destruction can be induced by lym-

phoid cells in the complete absence of complement or, for that matter, any serum component. *Therefore, cell-mediated cytotoxic mechanisms independent of complement must exist.* However, those experimental models in which lymphoid cells function in the absence of serum are highly artificial and do not necessarily mirror the events that might occur in vivo. It is known that under appropriate circumstances lymphoid cells can destroy a target cell that bears a partially activated complement sequence on its surface.

Complement-dependent Mechanisms Cytolysis produced by humoral antibody is rapid and requires activation of the complement sequence. The complement-fixing humoral antibody initiates a series of enzymatic cleavage reactions that culminates in activation of a variety of complement components (cf. 214). Activation of the terminal complement components C8 and C9 is critical for cell lysis by humoral antibody.

The complement system has a number of biologic functions in addition to that of cell lysis (214). For example, activation of the first four components of the complement sequence on a cell surface results in aggregation of certain lymphoid cells and macrophages having receptor sites for activated C3. This phenomenon is known as *immune adherence* (138, 219, 221, 223). Activation of these same complement components in the presence of mixed mononuclear cell populations may result in target cell lysis, a phenomenon that can be illustrated by the following experiment (240). Anti-Forsmann macroglobulin antibodies were themselves incapable of lysing chromium[51]-labeled chicken erythrocytes. Addition of the first three components of complement (C1, C2, and C4), together or in the presence of peripheral blood lymphoid cells, produced no lysis. However, lysis occurred when C3 was added to the target cells containing the first three components, provided mononuclear cells (lymphocytes and monocytes) were present. The reaction required viable, metabolically intact mononuclear cells and took 10 to 20 hours to reach completion.

When the target-cell–bound complement sequence is further activated to the C7 stage (but C8 and C9 are excluded), addition of viable mononuclear cells results in lysis within a few hours (237, 240). Both lymphocyte- and monocyte-enriched populations are active in this process. Lysis occurs more rapidly than if the sequence is activated only to the C3 stage, but not so rapidly as if C8 and C9 are added.

The complement sequence activated on target cell surfaces by a number of different pathways may interact with mononuclear cells, including monocytes and lymphocytes, and result in cell lysis. *The lymphoid-complement system may therefore function as a cytotoxic mechanism in addition to the complement-independent system.*

Studies with Mitogens The nonspecific aggregation of lymphoid cells to target cells by phytohemagglutinin has been shown to result in target cell destruction (47, 130, 132, 197, 207, 208, 260). The same effect is produced by a number of mitogenic agents capable of stimulating lymphocyte DNA synthesis, "blastogenic transformation," and mitosis. Removal of the hemagglutinating activity of phytohemagglutinin by absorption does not abolish mitogenic activity, nor does it remove the cytotoxicity-promoting activity (224, 257).

Generally, lymphoid cells that are difficult to stimulate by phytohemagglutinin are only weakly cytotoxic (cf. 181). Examples of cells difficult to stimulate include thymocytes, blood lymphocytes from patients with chronic lymphocytic leukemia and Hodgkin's disease in relapse, and Burkitt lymphoma cells (131, 135, 239). There is evidence that those cytotoxic lymphocytes responding to phytohemagglutinin are all thymus-dependent T cells (cf. 105, 202, 203, 303).

Specific Antigen Antigen-induced blastogenic transformation generally occurs more slowly and is of lesser magnitude than that induced by PHA (cf. 181, 182). Nevertheless, lymphoid cells from sensitive donors become cytotoxic to allogeneic tissue culture cells when incubated with specific antigen in vitro (133, 265–267).

Stimulation of blastogenic transformation by antigens is thought to reflect a state of delayed hypersensitivity (cf. 204, 231). Thus, *a positive correlative relation between delayed hypersensitivity in vivo and antigen-induced lymphoid cytotoxicity in vitro* appears to be a valid operational concept, although exceptions are known.

One cannot state categorically that whenever lymphoid cells are blastogenically transformed, they become cytotoxic for neighboring cells. The cytotoxic phenomenon has complexities that defy simple explanation. For example, the plant lectin conconavalin A is a strong stimulant to lymphocyte DNA synthesis and mitosis (90, 287); it does not, however, induce cytotoxically active cells. Another example of the dissociation of lymphoid blastogenic transformation and cytotoxicity can be achieved with xenogenic antilymphocyte sera (15). Thus, although the cells must be activated, blast transformation and DNA synthesis per se do not seem to be sufficient to induce cytotoxicity activity.

Relevance of Cytotoxic Reactions to Disease

Lymphoid-cell–mediated cytotoxic reactions can be induced in a variety of ways. Sensitized lymphocytes with appropriate receptors can recognize and destroy antigen-bearing target cells. Sensitized lymphoid cells activated by antigens other than those of the target cell surface can nonspecifically injure surrounding tissue cells. Cell-mediated cytotoxicity can be induced by minute amounts of humoral antibody interacting with target cell and nonsensitized effector cells. Finally, partially activated complement on the surface of target cells can interact with lymphoid cells, with resultant cytotoxic reactions. As discussed in preceding sections, each of these mechanisms has been defined by an appropriate in vitro model. The relevance of these mechanisms to human physiology and disease is indicated in Table 17.3 and is discussed in the succeeding sections of this chapter (246, 272).

Delayed Hypersensitivity, Exemplified by the Tuberculin Reaction

The delayed hypersensitivity reaction invoked in sensitive subjects by tuberculin has been regarded as the experimental prototype of the cell-mediated cytotoxic reaction. The histologic picture of the delayed hypersensitivity

Table 17.3 Relevance of experimental models of cytotoxicity to disease.

In vitro cytotoxic reaction	Possible in vivo counterpart
Lymphoid cells sensitized to target-cell antigens	Allograft rejection; tumor immunity; late phases of graft-vs-host reaction
Lymphoid cells sensitized to antigens adsorbed to target cells	Delayed hypersensitivity reactions to bacterial components
Nonimmune lymphoid cells sensitized by humoral antibody to target-cell antigens	Allograft rejection; tumor immunity
Lymphoid cells activated by nonspecific mitogens	Perhaps tissue injury in certain bacterial infections
Lymphoid cells and mononuclear phagocytes sensitized by activated complement on target cells	Diseases in which complement-fixing antibodies interact with tissue cells
Lymphoid cells stimulated in the mixed leukocyte culture reaction (allogeneic stimulation)	Lymphocyte transfer reactions; graft-vs-host reaction; perhaps allograft rejection

reaction induced by the injection of mycobacterial antigen intradermally into a sensitized animal is characterized by an early cellular response comprised chiefly of neutrophils. After 24 to 48 hours mononuclear cells predominate and accumulate around small blood vessels in dermis, subcutaneous fat, and connective tissue (299, 310). Focal necrosis of fat and muscle may also occur.

This delayed hypersensitivity reaction may be transferred to nonsensitized recipients by lymphoid cells but not by serum from immune donors (22). In this experimental model involving donated lymphoid cells, most of the infiltrating mononuclear cells at the site of the delayed hypersensitivity reaction originate from the nonsensitized host, and only 1 to 2 percent are of immune donor origin (75, 186). The mechanism of activation and recruitment of these nonsensitized lymphoid cells is not known, but it is assumed to involve the release of effector substances from sensitized cells.

The precise sequence of events in the delayed hypersensitivity reaction is by no means clear; however, the major protagonists in the drama and their roles are known. The following scheme may be taken as a rough program of events (cf. Fig. 17.3).

(a) Antigen is retained at the site of injection.
(b) Sensitized lymphocytes attracted to this site or entering by chance initiate the chain of events by interacting with antigen through specific surface receptors.
(c) As a result of this interaction, sensitized lymphoid cells may exert a *direct* cytotoxic effect on antigen-coated tissue cells, or may undergo blastogenic trans-

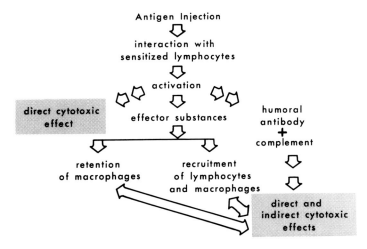

Figure 17.3 Scheme of cellular events in delayed hypersensitivity reactions.

formation (225) and nonspecifically injure surrounding tissue cells, whether these are antigen coated or not.
(d) Antigen adsorbed to macrophages at the site of reaction, as well as substances elaborated by sensitized lymphocytes, may recruit a fraction of nonsensitized lymphoid cells, which in turn may exert a cytotoxic effect on tissue cells.
(e) If humoral antibodies are in the circulation or produced locally, they may amplify the reaction by activation of nonsensitized lymphocytes.
(f) Humoral antibody may partially activate the complement sequence on cell surfaces, with subsequent interaction with lymphocytes producing a cytotoxic effect.

Although the role of complement in the delayed hypersensitivity reaction is not firmly established (3, 4, 301, 304), there is evidence that decomplementation of animals reduces reactivity (222, 324). Similarly, the part played by the variously described vascular permeability factors released by lymphoid cells is not clear (280). A detailed hypothesis regarding the subcellular events leading to the initiation of the delayed hypersensitivity reaction has been developed by Uhr (302).

Some of the pathologic features of active tuberculosis in the intact animal may reflect delayed hypersensitivity reactions, and the intense cell-mediated reactions to mycobacterial antigens may result in the typical granulomatous lesions. Cellular immunity is thought to be an important defense factor against certain intracellular parasites such as mycobacteria (194). However, direct destruction of microorganisms by lymphoid cells from sensitized donors has never been convincingly demonstrated. Rather, the immune lymphoid cells appear to exert their antiparasitic effect via interaction with macrophages (see Chapter 25) (225).

Allograft Rejection

After transplantation of tissue to a nonsensitized allogeneic recipient, a series of morphologic changes occurs within the recipient's lymphoid system. Among the first of these is the appearance of large pyroninophilic cells within the paracortical (thymus-dependent) areas of the regional lymph node (98). These cells are presumed to originate from small lymphocytes stimulated by contact with foreign transplantation antigens on the grafted tissue. Within six days, sensitized lymphocytes appear in the circulation of murine species. Mononuclear cells infiltrate the graft. As in delayed hypersensitivity reactions, most of these infiltrating cells are of host origin rather than from the sensitized donor (18, 215); that is, nonsensitized mononuclear cells are recruited. It may be that recruitment is controlled by transfer of specific information from sensitized to nonsensitized cells (2, 25).

By the eighth day after homotransplantation, the lymph nodes draining a graft demonstrate large numbers of basophilic replicating cells, whereas the lymphatics afferent to the node show no such cells (113, 250).

A variety of observations suggests that under some circumstances humoral antibody also may be involved in graft rejection (49, 51, 115, 281). Thus, allograft rejection in vivo may be mediated by a synergistic interaction of lymphoid cells and humoral antibody. The antibody may work directly on the graft, or small amounts may induce lymphoid-cell–mediated cytotoxic reaction.

Although all the events and their sequence in rejection of an allograft have not been clarified, one can propose the following working hypothesis on the basis of known observations (Fig. 17.4): as a consequence of exposure to allograft antigens, a small population of lymphoid cells in the draining lymph node is stimulated to transform into large, pyroninophilic cells and to divide. A portion of such cells finds its way into the graft and there may recruit nonsensitized lymphoid cells and mononuclear phagocytes. In response to the foreign antigen, antibody may be produced in the draining lymph nodes or locally within the graft. Such antibody interacting with antigen and complement may produce local vascular injury and accumulation of neutrophils, as well as induce a cytotoxic reaction of unsensitized lymphoid cells against the graft. The final cytotoxic injury of the allogeneic cells may be compounded of vascular impairment, direct cytotoxicity of antigenically stimulated sensitized lymphocytes, and nonsensitized lymphocytes interacting with antibody or cell-bound complement.

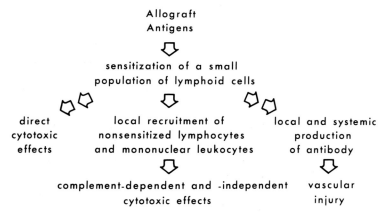

Figure 17.4 Scheme of cellular events in the cellular reaction to allograft antigens.

Graft-vs-Host Reactions

Administration of immunocompetent lymphocytes to an allogeneic host results in proliferation of donor cells mainly in the white pulp of the host spleen and in the cortical areas of host lymph nodes (98). There they differentiate into large pyroninophilic cells that divide and give rise to small lymphocytes. In mature, immunologically intact recipients these foreign cells are probably soon eliminated. If, however, the recipient is immunologically deficient or does not recognize the grafted cells as foreign (for example, an F_1 hybrid receiving parental lymphocytes), then the donor lymphocytes may continue to proliferate and produce the symptoms of graft-vs-host (GVH) reaction. In animals, this acute allogeneic disease usually is rapidly fatal and is characterized by skin rashes, diarrhea, and runting of young animals. Autotransplanted skin in such animals may show infiltration with lymphocytes, plasma cells, and macrophages (17).

Brent and Medawar (29, 30) produced tuberculin-like reactions by the intracutaneous inoculation of allogeneic lymphocytes into irradiated guinea pigs (600 r). The first phase of the reaction starts at about 6 hours after inoculation and is maximal by 48 hours. Evidence indicates that this phase is mediated by the interaction of donor lymphocytes with host leukocytes (cf. 252, 253), perhaps producing a local mixed leukocyte reaction with secondary skin injury (cf. 114). The second phase reaches maximal development after about five days and then gradually subsides. The second flare-up phase is regarded as a manifestation of sensitized donor cells after contact with foreign host antigens. It is inhibited by treatment with X-ray and antimitotic agents and probably requires donor cell replication. The final fadeout is ascribed to immunologic recovery of the host and rejection of the lymphocyte graft. This experimental model is known as the normal lymphocyte transfer (NLT). A similar sequence of events occurs with subcapsular injection of allogeneic lymphocytes and subsequent destruction of renal parenchyma (69, 70).

Antitumor Immunity

Over a decade ago Thomas suggested that cell-mediated immune reactions developed in the course of evolution as a defense against mutant cells and neoplasia (291). He argued that delayed hypersensitivity reactions were an inefficient means of eradicating microbial parasites and were, in fact, often damaging to host tissues. Furthermore, sensitivity to homografted foreign tissues was unlikely to have its basis in a defense mechanism developed in the course of evolution. However, both these reactions utilize mechanisms that could have evolved to recognize and destroy cells with foreign antigens, specifically those acquired as a result of neoplastic transformation.

The term *immunologic surveillance* was coined by Burnet (42) and focused attention on a basic function of the immunologic apparatus. The fundamental concept of this thesis is that lymphoid cells recognize newly acquired cell surface antigens, which arise as a consequence of viral or chemical carcinogenesis or a mutational event. Subsequent to this recognition, a variety of cell-mediated cytotoxic reactions and effector substances are mobilized to destroy the neoplastic cells. Implicit in this thesis is the concept that efficient operation of the surveillance apparatus affords a measure of protection against neoplasia and that the congenital or acquired defects in its operation enhance the risk of developing clinically apparent malignant disease. A considerable body of evidence supports this notion of immunologic surveillance. Easily understood arguments in its favor include the fact that there is an increased incidence of neoplastic disease occurring in genetic defects of the immune system in man (see Chapter 18) (95, 244) and in immunosuppressed animals treated with thymectomy plus antilymphocyte serum (82).

Renal transplant recipients who have received donor kidneys containing tumor will tolerate the graft and develop metastases as long as immunosuppressive therapy is continued, but will reject the kidney, the tumor, and its metastases when such therapy is stopped (328). In addition, there are now several reports of the development of neoplasms at the site of injection of antilymphocyte serum in patients receiving immunosuppressive drugs (233, 234).

The basic features of the tumor immune mechanisms resemble those of allograft rejection. The principal defense units appear to be cellular rather than humoral antibody, although both may interact (195). A complicating feature of antitumor immunity, basically irrelevant to nonmalignant allografts, is the growth potential of the neoplastic tissues. In addition, hosts with certain types of widespread neoplasia may show evidence of impaired immunologic capacity. For these reasons, immunologic defenses may be of more importance when tumors are small than when they are large and widespread.

A presumed requirement for the establishment of an immunologic reaction against an autochthonous or transplanted tumor is the presence of antigens on the tumor but not on the normal tissues of the host. That such tumor-specific antigens do in fact exist has been demonstrated in a variety of virus- and chemical-induced animal tumors (150, 151, 249). In fact, virtually all virus-induced animal neoplasms that have been studied contain tumor-specific transplantation antigens (TSTAs). This appellation derives from the fact that these antigens were first studied by transplantation techniques. They may be defined as macromolecules present on the surface of malignant cells and absent from the normal tissue cells of the same individual (151). In addition to their identification in experimental animal tumors, tumor-specific transplantation antigens have been demonstrated in certain human malignant conditions, including Burkitt's lymphoma (152) and melanoma (213). Related antigens have been found in association with colon carcinoma (88).

Tumors of known viral etiology have distinctive antigenic behavior. All neoplasms induced by the same virus have common TSTAs, which are different from those of tumors induced by other viruses. The first such virus-induced TSTA identified was in the polyoma virus system (110, 111). Subsequently TSTAs have been identified in both DNA and RNA virus-induced neoplasms.

In addition to surface antigens, tumor cells may have other types of specific antigens. For example, virus-induced neoplasms contain specific nuclear antigens (T, CS, or neoantigens) that are detectable by complement fixation or immunofluorescent techniques (111, 139, 247). Because these T antigens are not on the cell surface, they are not readily accessible to immunologic attack.

The various test systems used to assay for cellular immunity against TSTAs include: (a) adoptive transfer of immunity (16, 206); (b) neutralization tests (149, 154, 229, 230, 329); (c) tissue culture assays (103, 260); (d) blastogenic transformation of sensitized lymphocytes exposed to human tumor antigens in vitro (283); (e) demonstration of cutaneous delayed hypersensitivity reactions to tumor-specific transplantation antigens (48); and (f) the macrophage inhibition test of delayed hypersensitivity.

Studies of neutralization and colony inhibition tests have shown fairly conclusively that the antitumor immune defense is mediated primarily by lymphoid cells rather than by humoral antibody. This seems to be the situation for both chemically induced (154, 229, 230) and virus-induced (273–275) neoplasms as well as those induced by plastic film (153).

Although lymphocytes appear to be the primary defensive unit, for several reasons the contribution of cytotoxic antibodies in tumor rejection cannot be excluded. For example, SV-40 virus-induced hamster tumor cells placed in cell-impermeable but antibody-permeable Millipore filters are inhibited when implanted in specifically immune animals (52). Antibodies that inhibit Moloney sarcoma cells both in vivo and in vitro have been detected in the sera of mice in which the sarcomas have regressed (121). Cytophilic antibodies may render nonimmune macrophages capable of tumor cell destruction (297). Finally, cytotoxic antibodies against autochthonous tumor cells have been demonstrated in tumor-bearing patients (120, 122).

Notwithstanding these several studies of humoral antibodies, *the weight of evidence favors the lymphocyte as the primary defense unit in antitumor immunity.*

An important feature of certain tumor transplantation antigens is their stability in the face of selection pressures. For example, Sjögren (274) applied strong selection pressure against a polyoma virus-induced transplantation antigen by serial passage of antigenic tumors in preimmunized hosts. He found no qualitative or quantitative changes in antigenicity. Similar results have been observed in the Moloney tumor system (76). If the tumor-specific transplantation antigens are maintained despite potent immunologic pressure, it may mean that the specific antigenicity is closely linked with neoplastic behavior. Both are likely to be expressions of altered membrane topography and function.

Human neoplasms with antibodies reacting against tumor antigens include neuroblastoma (120), malignant melanoma (213), osteogenic sarcoma (212), and possibly carcinoma of the colon and lung (88, 89, 122).

Summary

In the preceding sections we have tried to draw a parallel between in vitro experimental models of lymphoid-cell–mediated cytotoxic reactions and certain natural or induced disease states in animals and man. Three groups of cellular immune reactions have been discussed:

(a) Specific cytotoxic reactions in which sensitized lymphocytes respond to foreign antigen present on or adsorbed by the target cell surface. Prototypes of such specific reactions are allograft rejection, antitumor immunity, and the tuberculin reaction.
(b) Cytotoxic reaction in which lymphoid cells and mononuclear cells are activated by antibody or complement components bound to the target cell. This reaction is nonspecific in the sense that nonsensitized lymphocytes may participate, although it is likely that in vivo both sensitized and nonsensitized effector cells are involved. Prototype reactions include certain instances of allograft rejection and complement-fixing antigen-antibody reactions.
(c) Cytotoxic reactions induced by lymphocytes nonspecifically activated by a variety of agents. Although many agents are stimulatory in vitro (for example, phytohemagglutinin, streptolysin S), it is not certain that such reactions exist under naturally occurring conditions in vivo.

From the preceding discussions it is apparent that in vivo lymphoid-cell–mediated cytotoxic reactions do not occur as an isolated entity but function in conjunction with complement, humoral antibody, and other types of circulating and tissue-phase leukocytes. Viable and metabolically intact lymphoid cells are necessary for such cytotoxic reactions. It is also apparent that lymphoid cells are a rich pharmacopoeia of pharmacologically active effector substances and that our knowledge of the numbers and operation of these substances is still in a rudimentary stage.

Chapter 17 References

1. Adler, W. H., and Smith, R. T. *In vitro* stimulation of mouse spleen cell suspensions, *Fed. Proc.* 28:813, 1969.

2. Alexander, P., Delorme, E. J., Hamilton, L. D. G., and Hall, J. G. Effect of nucleic acids from immune lymphocytes on rat sarcomata, *Nature* 213:569, 1967.

3. Asherson, G. L. The passive transfer of delayed hypersensitivity in the guinea-pig. II. The ability of passively transferred antibody to cause local inflammation and retention of antigen and the role of these phenomena in the passive transfer of delayed hypersensitivity, *Immunology* 13:441, 1967.

4. Asherson, G. L., and Loewi, G. The passive transfer of delayed hypersensitivity in the guinea-pig, *Immunology* 11:277, 1966.

5. Ax, W., Malchow, H., Zeiss, I., and Fischer, H. The behaviour of lymphocytes in the process of target cell destruction *in vitro*, *Exp. Cell Res.* 53:108, 1968.

6. Badger, A. M., Cooperband, S. R., and Green, J. A. Direct observations on the effect of "proliferation inhibitory factor" on the clonal growth of target cells, *J. Immunol.* 107:1259, 1971.

7. Balow, J. E., and Rosenthal, A. Glucocorticoid suppression of macrophage migration inhibitory factor, *J. Exp. Med.* 137:1031, 1973.

8. Baram, P., and Condoulis, W. V. The in vitro transfer of delayed type hypersensitivity to rhesus lymphocytes with "transfer factor" prepared from keyhole limpet hemocyanin sensitive rhesus peripheral white blood cells, *Fed. Proc.* 28:629, 1969.

9. Baram, P., and Mosko, M. M. A dialysable fraction from tuberculin-sensitive human white blood cells capable of inducing tuberculin-delayed hypersensitivity in negative recipients, *Immunology* 8:461, 1965.

10. Baram, P., Yuan, L., and Mosko, M. M. Studies on the transfer of human delayed-type hypersensitivity. I. Partial purification and characterization of two active components, *J. Immunol.* 97:407, 1966.

11. Baron, S., Buckler, C. E., Levy, H. B., and Friedman, R. M. Some factors affecting the interferon-induced antiviral state, *Proc. Soc. Exp. Biol. Med.* 125:1320, 1967.

12. Baron, S., and Levy, H. B. Interferon, *Ann. Rev. Microbiol.* 20:291, 1966.

13. Behrend, H., Havemann, K., and Rupec, M. Die passive Übertragung der Kveim-Reaktion mit Blutlymphocyten, *Klin. Wochenschr.* 18:1010, 1968.

14. Bennett, B., Old, L. J., and Boyse, E. A. Opsonization of cells by iso-antibody *in vitro*, *Nature* 198:10, 1963.

15. Biberfeld, P., Holm, G., and Perlmann, P. Inhibition of lymphocyte peripolesis and cytotoxic action in vitro by antilymphocyte serum (ALS), *Exp. Cell Res.* 54:136, 1969.

16. Billingham, R. E., Brent, L., and Medawar, P. B. Quantitative studies on tissue transplantation immunity; origin, strength and duration of actively and adoptively acquired immunity, *Proc. R. Soc. Lond. (Biol.)* 143:58, 1954.

17. Billingham, R. E., Defendi, V., Silvers, W. K., and Steinmuller, D. Quantitative studies on the induction of tolerance of skin homografts and on runt disease in neonatal rats, *J. Natl. Cancer Inst.* 28:365, 1962.

18. Billingham, R. E., Silvers, W. K., and Wilson, D. B. Further studies on adoptive transfer of sensitivity to skin homografts, *J. Exp. Med.* 118:397, 1963.

19. Bloom, B. R. IV. Biological activities of lymphocyte products, *in* H. S. Lawrence and M. Landy (eds.), Mediators of Cellular Immunity, p. 254, Academic Press, New York, 1969.

20. Bloom, B. R., and Bennett, B. Mechanism of a reaction in vitro associated with delayed-type hypersensitivity, *Science* 153:80, 1966.

21. Bloom, B. R., and Bennett, B. Migration inhibitory factor associated with delayed-type hypersensitivity, *Fed. Proc.* 27:13, 1968.

22. Bloom, B. R., and Chase, M. W. Transfer of delayed-type hypersensitivity. A critical review and experimental study in the guinea pig, *Prog. Allergy* 10:151, 1967.

23. Bloom, B. R., Gaffney, J., and Jimenez, L. Dissociation of MIF production and cell proliferation, *J. Immunol.* 109:1395, 1972.

24. Bloom, B. R., and Jimenez, L. Migration inhibitory factor and the cellular basis of delayed-type hypersensitivity reactions, *Am. J. Pathol.* 60:453, 1970.

25. Bondevik, H., and Mannick, J. A. RNA-mediated transfer of lymphocyte vs target cell activity, *Proc. Soc. Exp. Biol. Med.* 129:264, 1968.

26. Borecký, L., Lackovič, V., Blaškovič, D., Masler, L., and Šikl, D.: An interferon-like substance induced by mannans, *Acta Virol.* 11:264, 1967.

27. Boxaca, M., and Paucker, K. Neutralization of different murine interferons by antibody, *J. Immunol.* 98:1130, 1967.

28. Brandriss, M. W. Attempt to transfer contact hypersensitivity in man with dialysate of peripheral leukocytes, *J. Clin. Invest.* 47:2152, 1968.

29. Brent, L., and Medawar, P. Tissue transplantation: A new approach to the "typing" problem, *Br. Med. J.* 2:269, 1963.

30. Brent, L., and Medawar, P. Quantitative studies on tissue transplantation immunity. VII. The normal lymphocyte transfer reaction, *Proc. R. Soc. Lond. (Biol.)* 165:281, 1966.

31. Brondz, B. D. Interaction of immune lymphocytes in vitro with normal and neoplastic tissue cells, *Folia Biol.* 10:164, 1964.

32. Brondz, B. D. Complex specificity of immune lymphocytes in allogeneic cell cultures, *Folia Biol.* 14:115, 1968.

33. Brondz, B. D., and Bartova, L. M. Study of the influence of certain factors on the activity of lymphocytes in 6 allogeneic macrophage cultures, *Folia Biol.* 12:431, 1966.

34. Brunner, K. T., Mauel, J., Cerottini, J. C., and Chapuis, B. Quantitative assay of the lytic action of immune lymphoid cells on ^{51}Cr-labelled allogeneic target cells in vitro; inhibition by isoantibody and by drugs, *Immunology* 14:181, 1968.

35. Brunner, K. T., Mauel, J., Cerottini, J. C., Rudolf, H., and Chapuis, B. In vitro studies of cellular and humoral immunity induced by tumor allografts, *in* P. A. Miescher and P.

Grabar (eds.), Mechanisms of Inflammation Induced by Immune Reactions, p. 342, Schwabe & Co., Basel, 1968.

36. Brunner, K. T., Mauel, J., Rudolf, H., and Chapuis, B. Studies of allograft immunity in mice. I. Induction, development and in vitro assay of cellular immunity, *Immunology* 18:501, 1970.

37. Brunner, K. T., Mauel, J., and Schindler, R. *In vitro* studies of cell-bound immunity; cloning assay of the cytotoxic action of sensitized lymphoid cells on allogeneic target cells, *Immunology* 11:499, 1966.

38. Bubeník, J., Perlmann, P., and Hašek, M. Induction of cytotoxicity of lymphocytes from tolerant donors by antibodies to target cell alloantigens, *Transplantation* 10:290, 1970.

39. Buckley, R. H., Lucas, Z. J., Hattler, B. G., Jr., Zmijewski, C. M., and Amos, D. B. Defective cellular immunity associated with chronic mucocutaneous moniliasis and recurrent staphylococcal botryomycosis: immunological reconstitution by allogeneic bone marrow, *Clin. Exp. Immunol.* 3:153, 1968.

40. Bucknall, R. A. "Species specificity" of interferons: a misnomer?, *Nature* 216:1022, 1967.

41. Bullock, W. E., Fields, J. P., and Brandriss, M. W. An evaluation of transfer factor as immunotherapy for patients with lepromatous leprosy, *N. Engl. J. Med.* 287:1053, 1972.

42. Burnet, F. M. Immunologic aspects of malignant disease, *Lancet* i:1171, 1967.

43. Cantell, K., Strander, H., Saxén, L., and Meyer, B. Interferon response of human leukocytes during intrauterine and postnatal life, *J. Immunol.* 100:1304, 1968.

44. Chase, M. W. The allergic state, *in* R. J. Dubos and J. G. Hirsch (eds.), Bacterial and Mycotic Infections of Man, 4th ed., p. 238, J. B. Lippincott, Philadelphia, 1965.

45. Chase, M. W. Delayed-type hypersensitivity and the immunology of Hodgkin's disease, with a parallel examination of sarcoidosis, *Cancer Res.* 26:1097, 1966.

46. Chase, M. W. Hypersensitivity to

simple chemicals, *Harvey Lect.* 61:169, 1967.

47. Chu, E. H. Y., Stjernswärd, J., Clifford, P., and Klein, G. Reactivity of human lymphocytes against autochthonous and allogeneic normal and tumor cells *in vitro, J. Natl. Cancer Inst.* 39:595, 1967.

48. Churchill, W. H., Rapp, H. J., Kronman, B. S., and Borsos, T. Detection of antigens of a new diethylnitrosamine-induced transplantable hepatoma by delayed hypersensitivity, *J. Natl. Cancer Inst.* 41:13, 1968.

49. Clark, D. S., Foker, J. E., Good, R. A., and Varco, R. L. Humoral factors in canine renal allograft rejection, *Lancet* i:8, 1968.

50. Cline, M. J., Sprent, J., Warner, N. L., and Harris, A. W. Receptors for immunoglobulin on B lymphocytes and cells of a cultured plasma cell tumor, *J. Immunol.* 108:1126, 1972.

51. Cochrum, K. C., Davis, W. C., Kountz, S. L., and Fudenberg, H. H. Renal autograft rejection initiated by passive transfer of immune plasma, *Transplant. Proc.* 1:301, 1969.

52. Coggin, J. H., Jr., and Ambrose, K. R. A rapid *in vivo* assay for SV40 tumor immunity in hamsters, *Proc. Soc. Exp. Biol. Med.* 130:246, 1969.

53. Coyne, J. A., Remold, H. G., and David, J. R. Guinea pig macrophage inhibitory factor and lymphotoxin: are they different?, *Fed. Proc.* 30:647, 1971.

54. David, J. R. Suppression of delayed hypersensitivity in vitro by inhibition of protein synthesis, *J. Exp. Med.* 122:1125, 1965.

55. David, J. R. Delayed hypersensitivity in vitro: its mediation by cell-free substances formed by lymphoid cell-antigen interaction, *Proc. Natl. Acad. Sci. U.S.A.* 56:72, 1966.

56. David, J. R. Delayed hypersensitivity *in vitro, in* H. O. Schild (ed.), Proceedings of the Third Pharmacological Meeting, Immunopharmacology, vol. 11, p. 117, Pergamon Press, New York, 1968.

57. David, J. R. Macrophage migration, *Fed. Proc.* 27:6, 1968.

58. David, J. R. Biological activities of lymphocyte products, *in* H. S. Lawrence and M. Landy (eds.),

Mediators of Cellular Immunity, p. 262, Academic Press, New York, 1969.

59. David, J. R. Mediators produced by sensitized lymphocytes, *Fed. Proc.* 30:1730, 1971.

60. David, J. R., Al-Askari, S., Lawrence, H. S., and Thomas, L. Delayed hypersensitivity *in vitro.* I. The specificity of inhibition of cell migration by antigens, *J. Immunol.* 93:264, 1964.

61. David, J. R., Lawrence, H. S., and Thomas, L. The in vitro desensitization of sensitive cells by trypsin, *J. Exp. Med.* 120:1189, 1964.

62. David, J. R., Lawrence, H. S., and Thomas, L. Delayed hypersensitivity *in vitro.* II. Effect of sensitive cells on normal cells in the presence of antigen, *J. Immunol.* 93:274, 1964.

63. David, J. R., Lawrence, H. S., and Thomas, L. Delayed hypersensitivity *in vitro.* III. The specificity of hapten-protein conjugates in the inhibition of cell migration, *J. Immunol.* 93:279, 1964.

64. de Bonaparte, Y., Morgenfeld, M. C., and Paradisi, E. R. Medical letter, *N. Engl. J. Med.* 279:49, 1968.

65. De Maeyer-Guignard, J. Mouse leukemia: depression of serum interferon production, *Science* 177:797, 1972.

66. Dumonde, D. C., Wolstencroft, R. A., Panayi, G. S., Matthew, M., Morley, J., and Howson, W. T. "Lymphokines": non-antibody mediators of cellular immunity generated by lymphocyte activation, *Nature* 224:38, 1969.

67. Dutton, R. W. *In vitro* studies of immunological responses of lymphoid cells, *Adv. Immunol.* 6:253, 1967.

68. Edelman, R., and Wheelock, E. F. Enhancement of replication of vesicular stomatitis virus in human lymphocyte cultures treated with heterologous anti-lymphocyte serum, *Lancet* i:771, 1968.

69. Elkins, W. L. The interaction of donor and host lymphoid cells in the pathogenesis of renal cortical destruction induced by a local graft versus host reaction, *J. Exp. Med.* 123:103, 1966.

70. Elkins, W. L., and Guttman, R. D.

Pathogenesis of a local graft versus host reaction: immunogenicity of circulating host leukocytes, *Science* 159:1250, 1968.

71. Epstein, L. B., Cline, M. J., and Merigan, T. C. The interaction of human macrophages and lymphocytes in the phytohemagglutinin-stimulated production of interferon, *J. Clin. Invest.* 50:744, 1971.

72. Epstein, L. B., Cline, M. J., and Merigan, T. C. PPD-stimulated interferon: in vitro macrophage-lymphocyte interaction in the production of a mediator of cellular immunity, *Cell. Immunol.* 2:602, 1971.

73. Evans, R., and Alexander, P. Cooperation of immune lymphoid cells with macrophages in tumour immunity, *Nature* 228:620, 1970.

74. Fantes, K. H. Purification and physiochemical properties of interferons, *in* G. Rita (ed.), The Interferons. An International Symposium, p. 213, Academic Press, New York, 1968.

75. Feldman, J. D., and Najarian, J. S. Dynamics and quantitative analysis of passively transferred tuberculin hypersensitivity, *J. Immunol.* 91:306, 1963.

76. Fenyö, E. M., Biberfeld, P., and Klein, E. Studies on the relations between virus release and cellular immunosensitivity in Moloney lymphomas, *J. Natl. Cancer Inst.* 42:837, 1969.

77. Finkelstein, M. S., and Merigan, T. C. Interferon—1968. How much do we understand?, *Calif. Med.* 109:24, 1968.

78. Finter, N. Interferons, W. B. Saunders Co., Philadelphia, 1966.

79. Fireman, P., Boesman, M., Haddad, Z. H., and Gitlin, D. Passive transfer of tuberculin reactivity in vitro, *Science* 155:337, 1967.

80. Fireman, P., Boesman, M., Haddad, Z. H., and Gitlin, D. In vitro passive transfer of tuberculin reactivity, *Fed. Proc.* 27:29, 1968.

81. Friedman, R. M., and Cooper, H. L. Stimulation of interferon production in human lymphocytes by mitogens, *Proc. Soc. Exp. Biol. Med.* 125:901, 1967.

82. Gaugas, J. M., Chesterman, F. C., Hirsch, M. S., Rees, R. J. W., Harvey, J. J., and Gilchrist, C. Un

expected high incidence of tumours in thymectomized mice treated with anti-lymphocytic globulin and Mycobacterium leprae, *Nature* 221:1033, 1969.

83. Gell, P. G. H. Cellular hypersensitivity, *Int. Arch. Allergy Appl. Immunol.* 18:39, 1961.

84. George, M., and Vaughan, J. H. *In vitro* cell migration as a model for delayed hypersensitivity, *Proc. Soc. Exp. Biol. Med.* 111:514, 1962.

85. Glasgow, L. A. Interferon: a review, *J. Pediatr.* 67:104, 1965.

86. Glasgow, L. A. Leukocytes and interferon in the host response to viral infections. II. Enhanced interferon response of leukocytes from immune animals, *J. Bacteriol.* 91:2185, 1966.

87. Godleski, J. J., Lee, R. E., and Leighton, J. Studies on the role of polymorphonuclear leukocytes in neoplastic disease with the chick embryo and Walker Carcinosarcoma 256 *in vivo* and *in vitro*, *Cancer Res.* 30:1986, 1970.

88. Gold, P., and Freedman, S. O. Specific carcinoembryonic antigens of the human digestive system, *J. Exp. Med.* 122:467, 1965.

89. Gold, P., Gold, M., and Freedman, S. O. Cellular location of carcinoembryonic antigens of the human digestive system, *Cancer Res.* 28:1331, 1968.

90. Goldstein, I. J., and Iyer, R. N. Interaction of concanavalin A, a phytohemagglutinin, with model substrates, *Biochim. Biophys. Acta* 121:197, 1966.

91. Golstein, P., Svedmyr, E. A. J., and Wigzell, H. Cells mediating specific in vitro cytotoxicity. I. Detection of receptor-bearing lymphocytes, *J. Exp. Med.* 134:1385, 1971.

92. Golstein, P., Wigzell, H., Blomgren, H., and Svedmyr, E. A. J. Cells mediating specific in vitro cytotoxicity. II. Probable autonomy of thymus-processed lymphocytes (T cells) for the killing of allogeneic target cells, *J. Exp. Med.* 135:890, 1972.

93. Good, R. A. Transfer factor, *in* H. S. Lawrence and M. Landy (eds.), Mediators of Cellular Immunity, p. 191, Academic Press, New York, 1969.

94. Good, R. A., Cooper, M. D., Pe

terson, R. D. A., Kellum, M. J., Sutherland, D. E. R., and Gabrielsen, A. E. The role of the thymus in immune process, *Ann. N.Y. Acad. Sci.* 135:451, 1966.

95. Good, R. A., Kelly, W. D., Rotstein, J., and Varco, R. L. Immunological deficiency diseases. Agammaglobulinemia, hypogammaglobulinemia, Hodgkin's disease and sarcoidosis, *Prog. Allergy* 6:187, 1962.

96. Good, R. A., Varco, R. L., Aust, J. B., and Zak, S. J. Transplantation studies in patients with agammaglobulinemia, *Ann. N.Y. Acad. Sci.* 64:882, 1957.

97. Govaerts, A. Cellular antibodies in kidney homotransplantation, *J. Immunol.* 85:516, 1960.

98. Gowans, J. L., and McGregor, D. D. The immunological activities of lymphocytes, *Prog. Allergy* 9:1, 1965.

99. Granger, G. A. Cytotoxicity or stimulation by effector molecules, *in* H. S. Lawrence and M. Landy (eds.), Mediators of Cellular Immunity, p. 327, Academic Press, New York, 1969.

100. Granger, G. A., and Kolb, W. P. Lymphocyte *in vitro* cytotoxicity: mechanisms of immune and non-immune small lymphocyte mediated target L cell destruction, *J. Immunol.* 101:111, 1968.

101. Granger, G. A., Kolb, W. P., Williams, T. W., and Kramer, J. J. Inhibition of mouse lymphocyte-target L cell *in vitro* destruction with antiserum from lymphotoxin immunized animals, *Fed. Proc.* 28:630, 1969.

102. Granger, G. A., Laserna, E. C., Kolb, W. P., and Chapman, F. Human lymphotoxin: purification and some properties (phytohemagglutinin/human lymphocytes), *Proc. Natl. Acad. Sci. U.S.A.* 70:27, 1973.

103. Granger, G. A., and Weiser, R. S. Homograft target cells: specific destruction in vitro by contact interaction with immune macrophages, *Science* 145:1427, 1964.

104. Granger, G. A., and Weiser, R. S. Homograft target cells: contact destruction in vitro by immune macrophages, *Science* 151:97, 1966.

105. Greaves, M. F., Roitt, I. M., and Rose, M. E. Effect of bursectomy

and thymectomy on the responses of chicken peripheral blood lymphocytes to phytohaemagglutinin, *Nature* 220:293, 1968.

106. Green, J. A., Cooperband, S. R., and Kibrick, S. Immune specific induction of interferon production in cultures of human blood lymphocytes, *Science* 164:1415, 1969.

107. Gresser, I., Brouty-Boyé, D., Thomas, M-T., and Macieira-Coelho, A. Interferon and cell division. I. Inhibition of the multiplication of mouse leukemia L 1210 cells *in vitro* by interferon preparations, *Proc. Natl. Acad. Sci. U.S.A.* 66:1052, 1970.

108. Gresser, I., and Lang, D. J. Relationships between viruses and leucocytes, *Prog. Med. Virol.* 8:62, 1966.

109. Grossberg, S. E. The interferons and their inducers: molecular and therapeutic considerations, *N. Engl. J. Med.* 287:13, 1972.

110. Habel, K. Resistance of polyoma virus immune animals to transplanted polyoma tumours, *Proc. Soc. Exp. Biol. Med.* 106:722, 1961.

111. Habel, K. Specific complement-fixing antigens in polyoma tumors and transformed cells, *Virology* 25:55, 1965.

112. Haber, J., Rosenau, W., and Goldberg, M. Separate factors in phytohaemagglutinin induced lymphotoxin, interferon and nucleic acid synthesis, *Nature (New Biol.)* 238:60, 1972.

113. Hall, J. G. Studies of the cells in the afferent and efferent lymph of lymph nodes draining the site of skin homografts, *J. Exp. Med.* 125:737, 1967.

114. Hardy, D. A., and Ling, N. R. Effects of some cellular antigens on lymphocytes and the nature of the mixed lymphocyte reaction, *Nature* 221:545, 1969.

115. Hăsek, M., Skamene, E., Karakoz, I., Chutná, J., Nouza, K., Bubeník, J., Sovoká, V., Němec, M., and Jonák, J. Studies on the mechanism of rejection of tolerated skin homografts and abrogation of immunological tolerance by hyperimmune serum, *Folia Biol.* 14:411, 1968.

116. Hathaway, W. E., Githens, J. H., Blackburn, W. R., Fulginiti, V., and Kempe, C. H. Aplastic anemia, histiocytosis and erythrodermia in immunologically deficient children. Probable human runt disease, *N. Engl. J. Med.* 273:953, 1965.

117. Hattler, B. G., Jr., and Amos, D. B. Reactions obtained with transferred lymphocytes in patients with advanced cancer, *J. Natl. Cancer Inst.* 35:927, 1965.

118. Hellström, I., Hellström, K. E., Evans, C. A., Heppner, G. H., Pierce, G. E., and Yang, J. P. S. Serum-mediated protection of neoplastic cells from inhibition by lymphocytes immune to their tumor-specific antigens, *Proc. Natl. Acad. Sci., U.S.A.* 62:362, 1969.

119. Hellström, I., Hellström, K. E., and Pierce, G. E. *In vitro* studies of immune reactions against autochthonous and syngeneic mouse tumors induced by methylcholanthrene and plastic discs, *Int. J. Cancer* 3:467, 1968.

120. Hellström, I., Hellström, K. E., Pierce, G. E., and Bill, A. H. Demonstration of cell-bound and humoral immunity against neuroblastoma cells, *Proc. Natl. Acad. Sci. U.S.A.* 60:1231, 1968.

121. Hellström, I., Hellström, K. E., Pierce, G. E., and Fefer, A. Studies on immunity to autochthonous mouse tumors, *Proc. Transplant. Soc.* 1:90, 1969.

122. Hellström, I., Hellström, K. E., Pierce, G. E., and Yang, J. P. S. Cellular and humoral immunity to different types of human neoplasms, *Nature* 220:1352, 1968.

123. Hellström, K. E., and Hellström, I. Cellular immunity against tumor antigens, *Adv. Cancer Res.* 12:167, 1969.

124. Henney, C. S., Bourne, H. R., and Lichtenstein, L. M. The role of cyclic 3′, 5′ adenosine monophosphate in the specific cytolytic activity of lymphocytes, *J. Immunol.* 108:1526, 1972.

125. Henney, C. S., and Bubbers, J. E. Studies on the mechanism of lymphocyte-mediated cytolysis. I. The role of divalent cations in cytolysis by T lymphocytes, *J. Immunol.* 110:63, 1973.

126. Henney, C. S., and Lichtenstein, L. M. The role of cyclic AMP in the cytolytic activity of lymphocytes, *J. Immunol.* 107:610, 1971.

127. Hilleman, M. R. Immunologic, chemotherapeutic and interferon approaches to control of viral disease, *Am. J. Med.* 38:751, 1965.

128. Hilleman, M. R. Prospects for the use of double-stranded ribonucleic acid (Poly I:C) inducers in man, *J. Infect. Dis.* 121:196, 1970.

129. Ho, M., Postic, B., and Ke, Y. The systemic induction of interferon, *in* G. E. W. Wolstenholme and M. O'Connor (eds.), Ciba Foundation Symposium, Interferon, p. 19, Churchill, London, 1968.

130. Holm, G. The *in vitro* cytotoxicity of human lymphocytes: the effect of metabolic inhibitors, *Exp. Cell Res.* 48:334, 1967.

131. Holm, G., and Perlmann, P. Phytohaemagglutinin-induced cytotoxic action of unsensitized immunologically competent cells on allogeneic and xenogeneic tissue culture cells, *Nature* 207:818, 1965.

132. Holm, G., and Perlmann, P. Quantitative studies on phytohemagglutinin-induced cytotoxicity by human leukocytes against homologous cells in tissue culture, *Immunology* 12:525, 1967.

133. Holm, G., and Perlmann, P. Cytotoxic potential of stimulated human lymphocytes, *J. Exp. Med.* 125:721, 1967.

134. Holm, G., and Perlmann, P. Cytotoxicity of lymphocytes and its suppression, *Antibiot. Chemother.* 15:295, 1969.

135. Holm, G., Perlmann, P., and Johansson, B. Impaired phytohaemagglutinin-induced cytotoxicity in vitro of lymphocytes from patients with Hodgkin's disease or chronic lymphatic leukaemia, *Clin. Exp. Immunol.* 2:351, 1967.

136. Holm, G., Perlmann, P., and Werner, B. Phytohaemagglutinin-induced cytotoxic action of normal lymphoid cells on cells in tissue culture, *Nature* 203:841, 1964.

137. Holtzer, J. D., and Winkler, K. C. Quantitation of the cytotoxic effect of reticulo-lymphocytic cells in monolayer culture, *J. Pathol. Bacteriol.* 95:141, 1968.

138. Huber, H., Polley, M. J., Linscott, W. D., Fudenberg, H. H., and Müller-Eberhard, H. J. Human monocytes: distinct receptor sites for the third component of complement and for immunoglobulin G, *Science* 162:1281, 1968.

139. Huebner, R. J., Rowe, W. P.,

Turner, H. C., and Lane, W. T. Specific adenovirus complement-fixing antigens in virus-free hamster and rat tumors, *Proc. Natl. Acad. Sci. U.S.A.* 50:379, 1963.

140. Humphrey, J. H. Cell-mediated immunity—general perspectives, *Br. Med. Bull.* 23:93, 1967.

141. Israel, H. L. Sarcoidosis, *in* M. Samter and H. L. Alexander (eds.), Immunological Diseases, p. 406, Little, Brown and Co., Boston, 1965.

142. Jureziz, R. E., Thor, D. E., and Dray, S. Transfer with RNA extracts of the cell migration inhibition correlate of delayed hypersensitivity in the guinea pig, *J. Immunol.* 101:823, 1968.

143. Karush, F., and Eisen, H. N. A theory of delayed hypersensitivity. The main features of this phenomenon are explicable in terms of high-affinity humoral antibody, *Science* 136:1032, 1962.

144. Kasakura, S. Blastogenic factor from unstimulated leukocyte cultures: further evidence for heterogeneity, and mechanism of production, *J. Immunol.* 109:1352, 1972.

145. Kasakura, S., and Lowenstein, L. A factor stimulating DNA synthesis derived from the medium of leucocyte cultures, *Nature* 208:794, 1965.

146. Ke, Y. H., Ho, M., and Merigan, T. C. Heterogeneity of rabbit serum interferons, *Nature* 211:541, 1966.

147. Kelly, W. D., Lamb, D. L., Varco, R. L., and Good, R. A. An investigation of Hodgkin's disease with respect to the problem of homotransplantation, *Ann. N.Y. Acad. Sci.* 87:187, 1960.

148. Kempe, C. H. Studies on smallpox and complications of smallpox vaccination, *Pediatrics* 26:176, 1960.

149. Klein, E., and Sjögren, H. O. Humoral and cellular factors in homograft and isograft immunity against sarcoma cells, *Cancer Res.* 20:452, 1960.

150. Klein, G. Tumor antigens, *Ann. Rev. Microbiol.* 20:223, 1966.

151. Klein, G. Experimental studies in tumor immunology, *Fed. Proc.* 28:1739, 1969.

152. Klein, G. Clifford, P., Klein, E., Smith, R. T., Minowada, J., Kourilsky, F. M., and Burchenal, J. H. Membrane immunofluorescence reactions of Burkitt lymphoma cells from biopsy specimens and tissue cultures, *J. Natl. Cancer Inst.* 39:1027, 1967.

153. Klein, G., Sjögren, H. O., and Klein, E. Demonstration of host resistance against sarcomas induced by implantation of cellophane films in isologous (syngeneic) recipients, *Cancer Res.* 23:84, 1963.

154. Klein, G., Sjögren, H. O., Klein, E., and Hellström, K. E. Demonstration of resistance against methylcholanthrene-induced sarcomas in the primary autochthonous host, *Cancer Res.* 20:1561, 1960.

155. Klein, W. J., Jr. Lymphocyte-mediated cytotoxicity in vitro. Effect of enhancing antisera, *J. Exp. Med.* 134:1238, 1972.

156. Kolb, W. P., and Granger, G. A. A cell free cytotoxic factor produced by lymphoid cells during mutual *in vitro* aggressor lymphoid cell-target cell destruction, *Fed. Proc.* 27:687, 1968.

157. Kolb, W. P., and Granger, G. A. Lymphocyte in vitro cytotoxicity: characterization of human lymphotoxin, *Proc. Natl. Acad. Sci. U.S.A.* 61:1250, 1968.

158. Kolb, W. P., and Granger, G. A. Lymphocyte *in vitro* cytotoxicity: characterization of mouse lymphotoxin, *Cell. Immunol.* 1:122, 1970.

159. Kono, Y. Interferon-like inhibitor produced in bovine leukocyte cultures after inoculation with endotoxin (brief report), *Arch. Ges. Virusforsch.* 21:276, 1967.

160. Kono, Y. Rapid production of interferon in bovine leucocyte cultures, *Proc. Soc. Exp. Biol. Med.* 124:155, 1967.

161. Kono, Y., and Ho, M. The role of the reticuloendothelial system in interferon formation in the rabbit, *Virology* 25:162, 1965.

162. Koprowski, H., and Fernandes, M. V. Autosensitization reaction in vitro. Contactual agglutination of sensitized lymph node cells in brain tissue culture accompanied by destruction of glial elements, *J. Exp. Med.* 116:467, 1962.

163. Kramer, J. J., and Granger, G. A. An improved *in vitro* assay for lymphotoxin, *Cell. Immunol.* 3:144, 1972.

164. Landsteiner, K., and Chase, M. W. Studies on the sensitization of animals with simple chemical compounds. VII. Skin sensitization by intraperitoneal injections, *J. Exp. Med.* 71:237, 1940.

165. Landsteiner, K., and Chase, M. W. Experiments on transfer of cutaneous sensitivity to simple compounds, *Proc. Soc. Exp. Biol. Med.* 49:688, 1942.

166. Lawrence, H. S. Cellular transfer of cutaneous hypersensitivity to tuberculin in man, *Proc. Soc. Exp. Biol. Med.* 71:516, 1949.

167. Lawrence, H. S. The cellular transfer in humans of delayed cutaneous reactivity to hemolytic streptococci, *J. Immunol.* 68:159, 1952.

168. Lawrence, H. S. The transfer of generalized cutaneous hypersensitivity of the delayed tuberculin type in man by means of the constituents of disrupted leucocytes, *J. Clin. Invest.* 33:951, 1954.

169. Lawrence, H. S. The transfer in humans of delayed skin sensitivity to streptoccal M substance and to tuberculin with disrupted leucocytes, *J. Clin. Invest.* 34:219, 1955.

170. Lawrence, H. S. Transfer factor, *Adv. Immunol.* 11:195, 1969.

171. Lawrence, H. S. Transfer factor, *in* H. S. Lawrence and M. Landy (eds.), Mediators of Cellular Immunity, p. 145, Academic Press, New York, 1969.

172. Lawrence, H. S., Al-Askari, S., David, J., Franklin, E. C., and Zweiman, B. Transfer of immunological information in humans with dialysates of leucocyte extracts, *Trans. Assoc. Am. Physicians* 76:84, 1963.

173. Lawrence, H. S., and Landy, M. (eds.) Mediators of Cellular Immunity, Academic Press, New York, 1969.

174. Lawrence, H. S., and Pappenheimer, A. M., Jr. Transfer of delayed hypersensitivity to diphtheria toxin in man, *J. Exp. Med.* 104:321, 1956.

175. Lawrence, H. S., and Pappenheimer, A. M., Jr. Effect of specific antigen on release from human leucocytes of the factor concerned in transfer of delayed hypersensitivity, *J. Clin. Invest.* 36:908, 1957.

176. Lawrence, H. S., Rapaport, F. T., Converse, J. M., and Tillett, W. S. Transfer of delayed hypersensitivity to skin homografts with leukocyte

extracts in man, *J. Clin. Invest.* 39:185, 1960.

177. Lawrence, H. S., and Valentine, F. T. Transfer factor in delayed hypersensitivity, *Ann. N.Y. Acad. Sci.* 169:269, 1970.

178. Lebacq, E., and Verhaegen, H. Transfert passif du test de Kveim à des sujets normaux au moyen de leucocytes de maladies porteurs de sarcoïdose, *Rev. Fr. Etudes Clin. Biol.* 8:377, 1963.

179. Lebowitz, A., and Lawrence, H. S. Target cell destruction by antigen-stimulated human lymphocytes, *Fed. Proc.* 28:630, 1969.

180. Lieberman, M., Merigan, T. C., and Kaplan, H. S. Inhibition of radiogenic lymphoma development in mice by interferon, *Proc. Soc. Exp. Biol. Med.* 138:575, 1971.

181. Ling, N. R. Lymphocyte Stimulation, North-Holland Publishing Co., Amsterdam, 1971.

182. Ling, N. R., and Holt, P. J. L. The activation and reactivation of peripheral lymphocytes in culture, *J. Cell Sci.* 2:57, 1967.

183. LoBuglio, A. F., Cotran, R. S., and Jandl, J. H. Red cells coated with immunoglobulin G: binding and sphering by mononuclear cells in man, *Science* 158:1582, 1967.

184. Lockart, R. Z., Jr. Analysis of additional interference occurring after the removal of interferon, *J. Virol.* 1:1158, 1967.

185. Lolekha, S., Dray, S., and Gotoff, S. P. Macrophage aggregation *in vitro*: a correlate of delayed hypersensitivity, *J. Immunol.* 104:296, 1970.

186. Lubaroff, D. M., and Waksman, B. H. Delayed hypersensitivity: bone marrow as the source of cells in delayed skin reactions, *Science* 157:322, 1967.

187. Lundgren, G. Doctoral thesis, Balder, Stockholm, 1969, as cited by P. Perlmann and G. Holm, *Adv. Immunol.* 11:117, 1969.

188. Lundgren, G., Collste, L., and Möller, G. Cytotoxicity of human lymphocytes: antagonism between inducing processes, *Nature* 220:289, 1968.

189. McBride, R. A. Graft-*versus*-host reaction in lymphoid proliferation, *Cancer Res.* 26:1135, 1966.

190. MacDermott, R. P., et al. Reevaluation of in vitro cellular immunity using purified human T and B cells:

some unexpected findings, Prog. 66th Ann. Mtg. Am. Soc. Clin. Invest., p. 49a, 1974.

191. McFarland, W., and Heilman, D. H. Lymphocyte foot appendage: its role in lymphocyte function and in immunological reactions, *Nature* 205:887, 1965.

192. McFarland, W., Heilman, D. H., and Moorhead, J. F. Functional anatomy of the lymphocyte in immunological reactions in vitro, *J. Exp. Med.* 124:851, 1966.

193. Mackaness, G. B. The mechanism of macrophage activation, *in* S. Mudd (ed.), Infectious Agents and Host Reactions, p. 61, W. B. Saunders Co., Philadelphia, 1970.

194. Mackaness, G. B., and Blanden, R. V. Cellular immunity, *Prog. Allergy* 11:89, 1967.

195. Mackler, B. F. Role of soluble lymphocyte mediators in malignant-tumour destruction, *Lancet* ii:297, 1971.

196. MacLennan, I. C. M., and Harding, B., as cited by P. Perlmann and G. Holm, *Adv. Immunol.* 11:117, 1969.

197. MacLennan, I. C. M., and Loewi, G. Effect of specific antibody to target cells on their specific and non-specific interactions with lymphocytes, *Nature* 219:1069, 1968.

198. Marcus, P. I., Engelhardt, D. L., Hunt, J. M., and Sekellick, M. J. Interferon action: inhibition of vesicular stomatitis virus RNA synthesis induced by virion-bound polymerase, *Science* 174:593, 1971.

199. Marcus, P. I., and Salb, J. M. Molecular basis of interferon action: inhibition of viral RNA translation, *Virology* 30:502, 1966.

200. Marshall, W. H., Valentine, F. T., and Lawrence, H. S. Cellular immunity in vitro. Clonal proliferation of antigen-stimulated lymphocytes, *J. Exp. Med.* 130:327, 1969.

201. Mauel, J., Rudolf, H., Chapuis, B., and Brunner, K. T. Studies of allograft immunity in mice. II. Mechanism of target cell inactivation in vitro by sensitized lymphocytes, *Immunology* 18:517, 1970.

202. Meuwissen, H. J., Van Alten, P., Bach, F. H., and Good, R. A. Influence of thymus and bursa on *in vitro* lymphocyte function, *in* D. Bergsma (ed.), Immunologic Defi-

ciency Diseases in Man, p. 253, National Foundation, New York, 1968.

203. Miller, J. F. A. P., and Osoba, D. Current concepts of the immunological function of the thymus, *Physiol. Rev.* 47:437, 1967.

204. Mills, J. A. The immunologic significance of antigen induced lymphocyte transformation *in vitro*, *J. Immunol.* 97:239, 1966.

205. Mitchell, G. F., and Miller, J. F. A. P. Immunological activity of thymus and thoracic duct lymphocytes *Proc. Natl. Acad. Sci. U.S.A.* 59:296, 1968.

206. Mitchison, N. A., and Dube, O. L. Studies on the immunological response to foreign tumor transplants in the mouse. II. The relation between hemagglutinating antibody and graft resistance in the normal mouse and mice pretreated with tissue preparations, *J. Exp. Med.* 102:179, 1955.

207. Möller, E. Antagonistic effects of humoral isoantibodies on the in vitro cytotoxicity of immune lymphoid cells, *J. Exp. Med.* 122:11, 1965.

208. Möller, G., and Möller, E. Plaque-formation by non-immune and X-irradiated lymphoid cells on monolayers of mouse embryo cells, *Nature* 208:260, 1965.

209. Möller, E., and Möller, G. Quantitative studies of the sensitivity of normal and neoplastic mouse cells to the cytotoxic action of isoantibodies, *J. Exp. Med.* 115:527, 1962.

210. Möller, G., and Svehag, S-E. Specificity of lymphocyte-mediated cytotoxicity induced by *in vitro* antibody-coated target cells, *Cell. Immunol.* 4:1, 1972.

211. Mooney, J. J., and Waksman, B. H. Activation of normal rabbit macrophage monolayers by supernatants of antigen-stimulated lymphocytes, *J. Immunol.* 105:1138, 1970.

212. Morton, D. L., and Malmgren, R. A. Human osteosarcomas: immunologic evidence suggesting an associated infectious agent, *Science* 162:1279, 1968.

213. Morton, D. L., Malmgren, R. A., Holmes, E. C., and Ketcham, A. S. Demonstration of antibodies against human malignant melanoma by immunofluorescence, *Surgery* 64:233, 1968.

214. Müller-Eberhard, H. J. Chemistry and reaction mechanisms of complement, *Adv. Immunol.* 8:1, 1968.
215. Najarian, J. S., and Feldman, J. D. Passive transfer of transplantation immunity. I. Tritiated lymphoid cells. II. Lymphoid cells in millipore chambers, *J. Exp. Med.* 115:1083, 1962.
216. Nathan, C. F., and David, J. R. Alterations of macrophage functions by mediators from lymphocytes, *J. Exp. Med.* 133:1356, 1971.
217. Nathan, C. F., Remold, H. G., and David, J. R. Characterization of a lymphocyte factor which alters macrophage functions, *J. Exp. Med.* 137:275, 1973.
218. Nathan, C. F., Rosenberg, S. A., Karnovsky, M. L., and David, J. R. Effects of MIF-rich supernatants on macrophages, in J. E. Harris (ed.), Proc. Fifth Leukocyte Culture Conf., p. 629, Academic Press, New York, 1970.
219. Nelson, D. S. Immune adherence, *Adv. Immunol.* 3:131, 1963.
220. Nelson, D. S., and Boyden, S. V. The loss of macrophages from peritoneal exudates following the injection of antigens into guinea-pig with delayed-type hypersensitivity, *Immunology* 6:264, 1963.
221. Nelson, R. A., Jr. The immune-adherence phenomenon. An immunologically specific reaction between microorganisms and erythrocytes leading to enhanced phagocytosis, *Science* 118:733, 1953.
222. Neveu, T., and Biozzi, G. The effect of decomplementation on delayed-type hypersensitive reactions to a conjugated antigen in rats, *Immunology* 9:303, 1965.
223. Nishioka, K., and Linscott, W. D. Components of guinea pig complement. I. Separation of a serum fraction essential for immune hemolysis and immune adherence, *J. Exp. Med.* 118:767, 1963.
224. Nordman, C. T., de la Chapelle, A., and Gräsbeck, R. The interrelations of erythroagglutinating, leucoagglutinating and leucocyte-mitogenic activities in *Phaseolus vulgaris* phytohaemagglutinin, *Acta Med. Scand.* 412:49, 1964 (suppl.).
225. North, R. J., Mackaness, G. B., and Elliott, R. W. The histogenesis of immunologically committed lymphocytes, *Cell. Immunol.* 3:680, 1972.
226. Nussenzweig, V., and Benacerraf, B. Antihapten antibody specificity and L chain type, *J. Exp. Med.* 126:727, 1967.
227. O'Connell, C. J., Karzon, D. T., Barron, A. L., Plaut, M. E., and Ali, V. M. Progressive vaccinia with normal antibodies. A case possibly due to deficient cellular immunity, *Ann. Intern. Med.* 60:282, 1964.
228. Okazaki, H. Purification and properties of an inhibitory factor of virus infection, *Jap. J. Exp. Med.* 37:159, 1967.
229. Old, L. J., Boyse, E. A., Bennett, B., and Lilly, F. Peritoneal cells as an immune population in transplantation studies, in B. Amos and H. Koprowski (eds.), Cell-bound Antibodies, p. 89, Wistar Institute Press, Philadelphia, 1963.
230. Old, L. J., Boyse, E. A., Clarke, D. A., and Carswell, E. A. Antigenic properties of chemically induced tumors, *Ann. N.Y. Acad. Sci.* 101:80, 1962.
231. Oppenheim, J. J., Wolstencroft, R. A., and Gell, P. G. H. Delayed hypersensitivity in the guinea-pig to a protein-hapten conjugate and its relationship to in vitro transformation of lymph nodes, spleen, thymus and peripheral blood lymphocytes, *Immunology* 12:89, 1967.
232. Papageorgiou, P. S., Henley, W. L., and Glade, P. R. Production and characterization of migration inhibitory factor(s) (MIF) of established lymphoid and non-lymphoid cell lines, *J. Immunol.* 108:494, 1972.
233. Penn, I. Malignant tumors in organ transplant recipients, in Recent Results in Cancer Research, no. 35, Springer-Verlag, Berlin, 1970.
234. Penn, I., and Starzl, T. E. Malignant tumors arising de novo in immunosuppressed organ transplant recipients, *Transplantation* 14:407, 1972.
235. Perlmann, P., and Broberger, O. In vitro studies of ulcerative colitis. II. Cytotoxic action of white blood cells from patients on human fetal colon cells, *J. Exp. Med.* 117:717, 1963.
236. Perlmann, P., and Holm, G. Studies on the mechanism of lymphocyte cytotoxicity, in P. Miescher and P. Grabar (eds.), Mechanisms of Inflammation Induced by Immune Reactions, p. 325, Schwabe & Co., Basel, 1968.
237. Perlmann, P., and Holm, G. Cytotoxic effects of lymphoid cells in vitro, *Adv. Immunol.* 11:117, 1969.
238. Perlmann, P., Perlmann, H., and Biberfeld, P. Specifically cytotoxic lymphocytes produced by preincubation with antibody-complexed target cells, *J. Immunol.* 108:558, 1972.
239. Perlmann, P., Perlmann, H., and Holm, G. Cytotoxic action of stimulated lymphocytes on allogenic and autologous erythrocytes, *Science* 160:306, 1968.
240. Perlmann, P., Perlmann, H., Müller-Eberhard, H. J., and Manni, J. A. Cytotoxic effects of leukocytes triggered by complement bound to target cells, *Science* 163:937, 1969.
241. Perlmann, P., Perlmann, H., Wasserman, J., and Packalén, T. Lysis of chicken erythrocytes sensitized with PPD by lymphoid cells from guinea pigs immunized with tubercle bacilli, *Int. Arch. Allergy Appl. Immunol.* 38:204, 1970.
242. Perlmann, P., Perlmann, H., and Wigzell, H. Lymphocyte mediated cytotoxicity in vitro. Induction and inhibition by humoral antibody and nature of effector cells, *Transplant. Rev.* 13:91, 1972.
243. Peterson, R. D. A., Cooper, M. D., and Good, R. A. The pathogenesis of immunologic deficiency diseases, *Am. J. Med.* 38:579, 1965.
244. Peterson, R. D. A., Cooper, M. D., and Good, R. A. Lymphoid tissue abnormalities associated with ataxia-telangiectasia, *Am. J. Med.* 41:342, 1966.
245. Pick, E., Brostoff, J., Krejci, J., and Turk, J. L. Interaction between "sensitized lymphocytes" and antigen in vitro. II. Mitogen-induced release of skin reactive and macrophage migration inhibitory factors, *Cell. Immunol.* 1:92, 1970.
246. Pick, E., and Turk, J. L. The biological activities of soluble lymphocyte products, *Clin. Exp. Immunol.* 10:1, 1972.
247. Pope, J. H., and Rowe, W. P. Detection of specific antigen in SV40-transformed cells by immunofluorescence, *J. Exp. Med.* 120:121, 1964.
248. Porter, H. M. The demonstration of

delayed-type reactivity in congenital agammaglobulinemia, *Ann. N.Y. Acad. Sci.* 64:932, 1957.

249. Prehn, R. T. Cancer antigens in tumors induced by chemicals, *Fed. Proc.* 24:1018, 1965.

250. Prendergast, R. A. Cellular specificity in the homograft reaction, *J. Exp. Med.* 119:377, 1964.

251. Pulvertaft, R. J. V. Cellular associations in normal and abnormal lymphocytes, *Proc. R. Soc. Med.* 52:315, 1959.

252. Ramseier, H., and Billingham, R. E. Studies on delayed cutaneous inflammatory reactions elicited by inoculation of homologous cells into hamsters' skins, *J. Exp. Med.* 123:629, 1966.

253. Ramseier, H., and Streilein, J. W. Homograft sensitivity reactions in irradiated hamsters, *Lancet* i:622, 1965.

254. Rapaport, F. T., Lawrence, H. S., Millar, J. W., Pappagianis, D., and Smith, C. E. Transfer of delayed hypersensitivity to coccidioidin in man, *J. Immunol.* 84:358, 1960.

255. Remold, H. G., and David, J. R. Cellular hypersensitivity: characterization of migration inhibitory factor (MIF) by enzymatic treatment, *Fed. Proc.* 29:305, 1970.

256. Remold, H. G., Katz, A. B., Haber, E., and David, J. R. Studies on migration inhibitory factor (MIF): recovery of MIF activity after purification by gel filtration and disc electrophoresis, *Cell. Immunol.* 1:133, 1970.

257. Robbins, J. H. Human peripheral blood in tissue culture and the action of phytohemagglutinin, *Experientia* 20:164, 1963.

258. Rocklin, R. E., Remold, H. G., and David, J. R. Characterization of human migration inhibitory factor (MIF) from antigen-stimulated lymphocytes, *Cell. Immunol.* 5:436, 1972.

259. Rosenau, W. Interaction of lymphoid cells with target cells in tissue culture, *in* B. Amos and H. Koprowski (eds.), Cell-bound Antibodies, p. 75, Wistar Institute Press, Philadelphia, 1963.

260. Rosenau, W. Target cell destruction, *Fed. Proc.* 27:34, 1968.

261. Rosenau, W., and Moon, H. D. Lysis of homologous cells by sensitized lymphocytes in tissue culture, *J. Natl. Cancer Inst.* 27:471, 1961.

262. Rosenau, W., and Moon, H. D. The specificity of the cytologic effect of sensitized lymphoid cells *in vitro,* *J. Immunol.* 93:910, 1964.

263. Rosenau, W., and Moon, H. D. Studies on the mechanism of the cytolytic effect of sensitized lymphocytes, *J. Immunol.* 96:80, 1966.

264. Rosenau, W., and Morton, D. L. Tumor-specific inhibition of growth of methylcholanthrene-induced sarcomas *in vivo* and *in vitro* by sensitized isologous lymphoid cells, *J. Natl. Cancer Inst.* 36:825, 1966.

265. Ruddle, N. H., and Waksman, B. H. Cytotoxicity mediated by soluble antigen and lymphocytes in delayed hypersensitivity. I. Characterization of the phenomenon, *J. Exp. Med.* 128:1237, 1968.

266. Ruddle, N. H., and Waksman, B. H. Cytotoxicity mediated by soluble antigen and lymphocytes in delayed hypersensitivity. II. Correlation of the in vitro response with skin reactivity, *J. Exp. Med.* 128:1255, 1968.

267. Ruddle, N. H., and Waksman, B. H. Cytotoxicity mediated by soluble antigen and lymphocytes in delayed hypersensitivity. III. Analysis of mechanism, *J. Exp. Med.* 128:1267, 1968.

268. Russell, S. W., Rosenau, W., Goldberg, M. L., and Kunitomi, G. Purification of human lymphotoxin, *J. Immunol.* 109:784, 1972.

269. Schlossman, S. F. The immune response. Some unifying concepts, *N. Engl. J. Med.* 277:1355, 1967.

270. Schlossman, S. F., Ben-Efraim, S., Yaron, A., and Sober, H. A. Immunochemical studies on the antigenic determinants required to elicit delayed and immediate hypersensitivity reactions, *J. Exp. Med.* 123:1083, 1966.

271. Schwartz, H. J., Pelley, R. P., and Leon, M. A. Release of migration inhibitory factor from non-immune lymphoid cells by concanavalin A, *Fed. Proc.* 29:360, 1970.

272. Shacks, S. J., and Granger, G. A. Studies on in vitro models of cellular immunity, *J. Reticuloendothel. Soc.* 10:28, 1971.

273. Sjögren, H. O. Studies on specific transplantation resistance to polyoma-virus-induced tumors. III. Transplantation resistance to genetically compatible polyoma tumors induced by polyoma tumor homografts, *J. Natl. Cancer Inst.* 32:645, 1964.

274. Sjögren, H. O. Studies on specific transplantation resistance to polyoma-virus-induced tumors. IV. Stability of the polyoma cell antigen, *J. Natl. Cancer Inst.* 32:661, 1964.

275. Slettenmark, B., and Klein, E. Cytotoxic and neutralization tests with serum and lymph node cells of isologous mice with induced resistance against gross lymphomas, *Cancer Res.* 22:947, 1962.

276. Smith, T. J., and Wagner, R. R. Rabbit macrophage interferons. I. Conditions for biosynthesis by virus-infected and uninfected cells, *J. Exp. Med.* 125:559, 1967.

277. Smith, T. J., and Wagner, R. R. Rabbit macrophage interferons. II. Some physicochemical properties and estimations of molecular weights, *J. Exp. Med.* 125:579, 1967.

278. Solowey, A. C., Rapaport, F. T., and Lawrence, H. S. Cellular studies in neoplastic diseases, *in* E. S. Curtoni, P. L. Mattiuz, and R. M. Tosi (eds.), Histocompatibility Testing, p. 75, Williams & Wilkins Co., Baltimore, 1967.

279. Sorg, C., and Bloom, B. R. Products of activated lymphocytes. I. The use of radiolabeling techniques in the characterization and partial purification of the migration inhibitory factor of the guinea pig, *J. Exp. Med.* 137:148, 1973.

280. Spector, W. G., and Willoughby, D. A. Mediators of delayed hypersensitivity reactions, *in* P. A. Miescher and P. Grabar (eds.), Mechanisms of Inflammation Induced by Immune Reactions, p. 281, Schwabe & Co., Basel, 1968.

281. Spong, F. W., Feldman, J. D., and Lee, S. Transplantation antibody associated with first-set renal homografts, *J. Immunol.* 101:418, 1968.

282. Stinebring, W. R., and Absher, P. M. Production of interferon following an immune response, *Ann. N.Y. Acad. Sci.* 173:714, 1970.

283. Stjernsward, J., Clifford, P., Singh, S., and Svedmyr, E. Indications of cellular immunological reactions

against autochthonous tumour in cancer patients studied *in vitro, East Afr. Med. J.* 45:484, 1968.

284. Strander, H., and Cantell, K. Production of interferon by human leucocytes in vitro, *Ann. Med. Exp. Biol. Fenn.* 44:265, 1966.

285. Strom, T. B., Carpenter, C. B., Garovoy, M. R., et al. The modulating influence of cyclic nucleotides upon lymphocyte-mediated cytotoxicity, *J. Exp. Med.* 138:381, 1973.

286. Subrahmanyan, T. P., and Mims, C. A. A study of the production, source, and action of interferon appearing in mice after the intravenous injection of influenza virus, *Br. J. Exp. Pathol.* 48:568, 1967.

287. Sumner, J. B., and O'Kane, D. J. The chemical nature of yeast saccharase, *Enzymologia* 12:251, 1948.

288. Taylor, H. E., and Culling, C. F. A. Cytopathic effect *in vitro* of sensitized homologous and heterologous spleen cells on fibroblasts, *Lab. Invest.* 12:884, 1963.

289. Taylor, H. E., and Culling, C. F. A. Production of complement by spleen cells *in vitro* and its possible role in an allograft rejection model, *Nature* 220:506, 1968.

290. Taylor, J. Inhibition of interferon action by actinomycin, *Biochem. Biophys. Res. Commun.* 14:447, 1964.

291. Thomas, L. Mechanisms involved in tissue damage by the endotoxins of gram negative bacteria, *in* H. S. Lawrence (ed.), Cellular and Humoral Aspects of the Hypersensitivity States, p. 451, Paul B. Hoeber, New York, 1959.

292. Thor, D. E. Delayed hypersensitivity in man: a correlate in vitro and transfer by an RNA extract, *Science* 157:1567, 1967.

293. Thor, D. E. Human delayed hypersensitivity: an in vitro correlate and transfer by an RNA extract, *Fed. Proc.* 27:16, 1968.

294. Thor, D. E., and Dray, S. A correlate of human delayed hypersensitivity: specific inhibition of capillary tube migration of sensitized human lymph node cells by tuberculin and histoplasmin, *J. Immunol.* 101:51, 1968.

295. Thor, D. E., and Dray, S. The cell-migration-inhibition correlate of delayed hypersensitivity. Conversion of human nonsensitive lymph node cells to sensitive cells with an RNA extract, *J. Immunol.* 101:469, 1968.

296. Thor, D. E., Jureziz, R. E., Veach, S. R., Miller, E., and Dray, S. Cell migration inhibition factor released by antigen from human peripheral lymphocytes, *Nature* 219:755, 1968.

297. Tsoi, M-S., and Weiser, R. S. Mechanisms of immunity to sarcoma 1 allografts in the C57BL/Ks mouse. III. The additive and synergistic actions of macrophages and immune serum, *J. Natl. Cancer Inst.* 40:37, 1968.

298. Tubergen, D. G., Feldman, J. D., Pollock, E. M., and Lerner, R. A. Production of macrophage migration inhibition factor by continuous cell lines, *J. Exp. Med.* 135:255, 1972.

299. Turk, J. L. Delayed Hypersensitivity, North-Holland Publishing Co., Amsterdam, 1967.

300. Turk, J. L., and Waters, M. F. R. Immunological basis for depression of cellular immunity and the delayed allergic response in patients with lepromatous leprosy, *Lancet* ii:436, 1968.

301. Uhr, J. W. Delayed hypersensitivity, *Physiol. Rev.* 46:359, 1966.

302. Uhr, J. W. Transfer factor, *in* H. S. Lawrence and M. Landy (eds.), Mediators of Cellular Immunity, p. 209, Academic Press, New York, 1969.

303. Uhr, J. W. Models for receptor sites on thymic lymphocytes, *in* H. S. Lawrence and M. Landy (eds.), Mediators of Cellular Immunity, p. 419, Academic Press, New York, 1969.

304. Uhr, J. W., Salvin, S. B., and Pappenheimer, A. M., Jr. Delayed hypersensitivity. II. Induction of hypersensitivity in guinea pigs by means of antigen-antibody complexes, *J. Exp. Med.* 105:11, 1957.

305. Urbach, F., Sones, M., and Israel, H. L. Passive transfer of tuberculin sensitivity to patients with sarcoidosis, *N. Engl. J. Med.* 247:794, 1952.

306. Valdimarsson, H., Wood, C. B. S., Hobbs, J. R., and Holt, P. J. L. Immunological features in a case of chronic granulomatous candidiasis and its treatment with transfer factor, *Clin. Exp. Immunol.* 11:151, 1972.

307. Valentine, F. T., and Lawrence, H. S. Transfer of cellular hypersensitivity in vitro, *J. Clin. Invest.* 47:98a, 1968.

308. Valentine, F. T., and Lawrence, H. S. Lymphocyte stimulation: transfer of cellular hypersensitivity to antigen in vitro, *Science* 165:1014, 1969.

309. Van Boxel, J. A., Stobo, J. D., Paul, W. E., and Green, I. Antibody-dependent lymphoid cell-mediated cytotoxicity: no requirement for thymus-derived lymphocytes, *Science* 175:194, 1972.

310. Waksman, B. H. A comparative histopathological study of delayed hypersensitive reactions, *in* G. E. W. Wolstenholme and M. O'Connor (eds.), Ciba Foundation Symposium, Cellular Aspects of Immunity, p. 280, Little, Brown and Co., Boston, 1960.

311. Waksman, B. H. Biological activities of lymphocyte products, *in* H. S. Lawrence and M. Landy (eds.), Mediators of Cellular Immunity, p. 278, Academic Press, New York, 1969.

312. Waldorf, D. S., Sheagren, J. N., Trautman, J. R., and Block, J. B. Impaired delayed hypersensitivity in patients with lepromatous leprosy, *Lancet* ii:773, 1966.

313. Ward, P. A., and David, J. R. A leukotactic factor produced by sensitized lymphocytes, *Fed. Proc.* 28:630, 1969.

314. Ward, P. A., Offen, C. D., and Montgomery, J. R. Chemoattractants of leukocytes, with special reference to lymphocytes, *Fed. Proc.* 30:1721, 1971.

315. Ward, P. A., Remold, H. G., and David, J. R. Leukotactic factor produced by sensitized lymphocytes, *Science* 163:1079, 1969.

316. Ward, P. A., Remold, H. G., and David, J. R. The production by antigen-stimulated lymphocytes of a leukotactic factor distinct from migration inhibitory factor, *Cell. Immunol.* 1:162, 1970.

317. Wasserman, J., Packalen, T., Perlmann, P., and Perlmann, H. Cyto-

toxic lymphoid cells and antibodies from guinea pigs immunized with tubercle bacilli, *Int. Arch. Allergy Appl. Immunol.* 36:115, 1969.

318. Wheelock, E. F. Interferon-like virus-inhibitor induced in human leukocytes by phytohemagglutinin, *Science* 149:310, 1965.

319. Wheelock, E. F. Virus replication and high-titered interferon production in human leukocyte cultures inoculated with Newcastle disease virus, *J. Bacteriol.* 92:1415, 1966.

320. Williams, T. W., and Granger, G. A. Lymphocyte cytotoxicity *in vitro*: activation and release of a cytotoxic factor, *Nature* 218:1253, 1968.

321. Williams, T. W., and Granger, G. A. Lymphocyte *in vitro* cytotoxicity: lymphotoxins of several mammalian species, *Nature* 219:1076, 1968.

322. Williams, T. W., and Granger, G. A. Lymphocyte *in vitro* cytotox-icity: mechanism of lymphotoxin-induced target cell destruction, *J. Immunol.* 102:911, 1969.

323. Williamson, A. R., and Askonas, B. A. Senescence of an antibody-forming cell clone, *Nature* 238:337, 1972.

324. Willoughby, D. A., Polák, L., and Turk, J. L. Suppression of contact hypersensitivity and acute inflammation by anti-complement serum, *Nature* 219:192, 1968.

325. Wilson, D. B. Quantitative studies on the behavior of sensitized lymphocytes in vitro. I. Relationship of the degree of destruction of homologous target cells to the number of lymphocytes and to the time of contact in culture and consideration of the effects of isoimmune serum, *J. Exp. Med.* 122:143, 1965.

326. Wilson, D. B. Lymphocytes as mediators of cellular immunity: destruction of homologous target cells in culture, *Transplantation* 5:986, 1967.

327. Wilson, D. B., and Billingham, R. E. Lymphocytes and transplantation immunity, *Adv. Immunol.* 7:189, 1967.

328. Wilson, R. E., Hager, E. B., Hampers, C. L., Corson, J. M., Merrill, J. P., and Murray, J. E. Immunologic rejection of human cancer transplanted with a renal allograft, *N. Engl. J. Med.* 278:479, 1968.

329. Winn, H. J. Immune mechanisms in homotransplantation. I. The role of serum antibody and complement in the neutralization of lymphoma cells, *J. Immunol.* 84:530, 1960.

330. Wolstenholme, G. E. W., and O'Connor, M. (eds.). Ciba Foundation Symposium, Interferon, Churchill, London, 1968.

331. Youngner, J. S., Taube, S. E., and Stinebring, W. R. Inhibition of viral replication by interferons with different molecular weights, *Proc. Soc. Exp. Biol. Med.* 123:795, 1966.

B The Abnormal Lymphocyte and Plasma Cell

Chapter 18   Abnormalities of Production and Function

In 1952 Bruton described a boy with recurrent serious bacterial infections and undetectable levels of serum gamma globulin (27). This report drew attention to a hitherto unrecognized class of diseases — the genetic and acquired abnormalities of function of the immune system or, as they have been called, the *immunodeficiency diseases.* The first described disorder was appropriately called *agammaglobulinemia* (27). Since that time several hundreds of patients with abnormalities of the serum concentration of one or more serum immunoglobulins have been described. The terms *hypogammaglobulinemia* and *dysgammaglobulinemia* were coined to describe situations where serum immunoglobulin levels were reduced but still detectable, or in which a selective abnormality in one or two of the immunoglobulin classes occurred.

These patients presented a great variety of clinical signs and symptoms and often demonstrated enhanced susceptibility to infection. It soon became clear that the concept of a spectrum of immunologic deficiency diseases had to be extended to encompass disorders with normal or nearly normal serum immunoglobulin concentrations, but with major abnormalities of the cellular immune responses (145).

The immunologic deficiency diseases may be classified in a variety of ways. Obviously the first classifications were based on the serologic and clinical features of patients with immune disorders (16, 78). The anatomical features of the various disorders subsequently were incorporated as additional parameters in the classification schemes. Studies of affected individuals and their families permitted classification based on the mode of inheritance of those disorders that were clearly genetic in origin. The recent expansion of knowledge concerning the development of the immune system and the various cells involved in the immune response led to classifications based on abnormalities of lymphoid cell morphogenesis, as described in Chapter 12. The classification followed in this chapter is based upon quantitative or qualitative abnormalities of immunocyte number or function and takes into account such factors as anatomic pathology, genetic etiology, and developmental abnormalities.

An approach to the classification of immunologic deficiency diseases is given in Table 18.1 and in Fig. 18.1. Let us utilize these aids to consider how defects in the immune system may arise and how they are expressed.

Pathogenetic Mechanisms of Immunologic Deficiency

Historically, the first patient with immunologic deficiency disease was recognized because of increased susceptibility to infection and a notable reduction in serum gamma globulin concentrations (27). A markedly decreased number of plasma cells in the bone marrow and lymphoid organs was soon recognized as a consistent feature of this so-called Bruton-type agammaglobulinemia (infantile sex-linked agammaglobulinemia) (145, 158, 170). In a number of related immunologic deficiency syndromes characterized by agammaglobulinemia, hypogammaglobulinemia, or selective absence of a single class of immunoglobulins, a similar reduction in the number of plasma cells has been noted. In view of abundant evidence

Table 18.1 Classification of immunodeficiency diseases.

Disease	Plasma cell number	Circulating lymphocyte concentration	Serum immunoglobulins	Humoral immunity	Cellular immunity	Inheritance	Presumed defect
Bruton's agamma-globulinemia	↓	Nl	↓	↓	Nl	Sex-linked recessive	B-cell development
Transient hypogamma-globulinemia of infancy	↓	Usually Nl	↓ (IgG)	↓	Nl	?Familial	Delayed B-cell maturation
Swiss-type agamma-globulinemia	↓	↓	↓	↓	↓	Autosomal recessive	Failure of all lymphoid development
Agammaglobulinemia with thymoma (Good's syndrome)	↓	↓	↓	↓	Usually ↓	Acquired	Related to thymoma
Selective IgA deficiency	↓ (IgA)	Nl	↓ (IgA)	Nl	Nl	?Familial	Failure of development of IgA-producing cells
Primary lymphopenic agammaglobulinemia (Gitlin's syndrome)	Variable	Usually ↓	Variable ↓	↓ to some antigens	↓ to most antigens	Sex-linked or autosomal recessive	?
Autosomal recessive alymphopenia with normal immunoglobulins (Nezelof's syndrome)	Nl	↓	Nl	Probable ↓	↓	Autosomal recessive	Abnormal development of T cells
Wiskott-Aldrich syndrome	Nl	↓	Variable, often ↓ IgM	↓ to some antigens	↓	Sex-linked recessive	?Antigen recognition or processing
Lymphocyte loss syndromes	Usually Nl	↓	↓	↓ to some antigens	↓	Acquired	Loss of recirculating lymphocytes and immunoglobulins; generally from gastrointestinal tract
Thymic aplasia (DiGeorge's syndrome)	Nl	Nl	Nl	↓	↓	—	Failure of thymic development
Ataxia telangiectasia	Usually Nl	Variable ↓	Variable ↓	↓ to some antigens	↓ to some antigens	Autosomal recessive	?
Immunoglobulin deficiency of variable onset (primary acquired agammaglobulinemia)	Usually Nl	Usually Nl	Variable ↓	↓ to most antigens	↓ to some antigens	Sometimes familial	?
Lymphoreticular neoplasms							
(a) Hodgkin's disease	Usually Nl	Variable ↓	Variable ↓ or Nl	Usually Nl	Sometimes ↓	Acquired	Failure of T-cell development
(b) Chronic lymphocytic leukemia	?	↑ (B cells)	Variable ↓	Variable ↓	Variable ↓	Acquired	Abnormal B-cell proliferation
(c) Multiple myeloma	↑ (abnormal)	Usually Nl	↑ paraprotein ↓ normal	↓	Usually Nl	Acquired	Proliferating malignant B-cell clone
Disease of restricted abnormality of cellular immunity (lepromatous leprosy, sarcoidosis, chronic mucocutaneous candidiasis)	Nl	Usually Nl	Nl or ↑	Nl	↓ to restricted antigens	Familial (CMC); others acquired	?Antigen overload

↓ = deficiency; ↑ = excess; Nl = normal level.

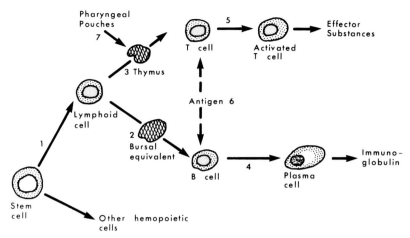

Figure 18.1 Summary of the development of lymphoid cells. A hematopoietic stem cell is committed to lymphoid differentiation (step 1) or to other cell lines as a consequence of microenvironmental or hormonal factors. Under the influence of the bursa or bursal equivalent (step 2) or of the thymus (step 3), lymphocytes acquire the characteristics of B cells or T cells respectively. B cells are the precursors of immunoglobulin-producing plasma cells (step 4) and T cells participate in cellular immune responses involving a variety of mediators (step 5). The interaction of B and T cells with antigen (step 6) is necessary for full expression of the humoral immune response. Normal development of the immune system involves formation of the thymus gland from the pharyngeal pouches of the embryo (step 7).

that documents the plasma cell as the chief cellular component of the immunoglobulin-producing system (see Chapters 12 to 16), it is not surprising that disorders characterized by a morphologically apparent reduction in the numbers of tissue plasma cells are also characterized by reduced concentrations of immunoglobulins.

Therefore, the first generalizations one can make in the classification of immunologic deficiency diseases are the following: *(a) those disorders characterized by a general absence of plasma cells have an associated reduction in serum immunoglobulin concentration; (b) those disorders characterized by selective absence of a class of plasma cells have reduced levels of the corresponding class of immunoglobulin.* In these disease syndromes the faulty mechanism may be placed at step 2 or step 4 of Fig. 18.2.

The evidence that plasma cells arise from lymphoid cell precursors is reasonably strong. Therefore one would predict that diseases having an abnormality or absence of lymphocyte formation might also have an associated decrease in the number of plasma cells and diminished immunoglobulin synthesis. Such an immunodeficiency disease might arise from a block at step 1. An example of

such a disease is the Swiss type of agammaglobulinemia (autosomal recessive alymphocytic agammaglobulinemia) (91, 188).

One could also predict that there might be diseases in which lymphocyte numbers were normal but their differentiation into plasma cells impaired (step 4), resulting in a reduction in the number of plasma cells and in immunoblobulin synthesis. The Bruton type of agammaglobulinemia may be an example of this type of disorder.

Another type of abnormality of lymphoid cell morphogenesis may be seen in diseases such as Nezelof's syndrome (autosomal recessive lymphopenia with normal immunoglobulins) (62, 138). The numbers of circulating lymphocytes in this disorder are low, but plasma cells are present and serum immunoglobulin concentrations are normal. Such a disease may originate from abnormalities of selected populations of T lymphocytes (step 3 or 5) and may not involve B lymphocytes.

As a second series of generalizations one may suggest that: *(a) diseases with a total absence of lymphocyte formation will also have absent plasma cell formation, cellular immune deficiencies, and decreased serum im-*

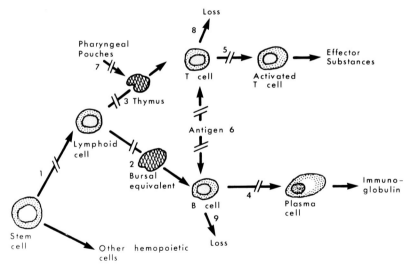

Figure 18.2 Summary of abnormalities of lymphoid cell differentiation. They may result from an absence of stem cells or a block at step 1. (The Swiss type of agammaglobulinemia may be an example of the latter disorder.) Abnormalities of B-cell differentiation may involve blocks at step 2 or step 4. (An example of this type of disorder may be Bruton-type agammaglobulinemia.) Abnormalities of T-cell function may result from blocks at step 7 (DiGeorge's syndrome), at step 3 (?Nezelof's syndrome), or at step 5. Abnormal T-cell development also impairs the humoral immune response of step 6 (as in DiGeorge's syndrome and neonatal thymectomy).

munoglobulins; (b) diseases may exist in which lympho-cytes are apparently normal in numbers but plasma cells are diminished, possibly as a consequence of failure of normal differentiation of the B lymphocyte im-munoglobulin-producing system; and (c) diseases may exist in which selected populations of lymphocytes are abnormal, such diseases being characterized by reduced or normal numbers of lymphocytes and by impaired cel-lular immunity.

The humoral antibody response to antigen is a complex phenomenon involving both a fully differentiated im-mune system and the interaction of several cell types (step 6). An impairment of humoral antibody response is easily understood in disorders having an absence of or markedly reduced serum immunoglobulins—for example, in Bruton's disease. Diseases with a selective absence of a single class of immunoglobulins may have selective abnormalities of humoral antibody response. Examples of this phenomenon are selective immunoglobulin defi-ciency and immune deficiency with thrombocytopenia (15, 16, 33, 34, 36, 45, 56, 69, 93, 112, 155, 159, 178).

Diseases also exist in which plasma cells are present and immunoglobulins are normal in concentration, but the humoral antibody response is abnormal as a con-sequence of the faulty differentiation and integration of the cellular components of the immune response (step 6). For instance, in certain species neonatal thymectomy re-sults in impaired humoral antibody response to certain antigens, despite normal concentrations of serum im-munoglobulins (12, 43, 77, 129, 132, 207). The human disease that is a counterpart of these experimental models is thymic aplasia (DiGeorge's syndrome) (49, 64, 86, 97, 119, 185). On the basis of these observations one can conclude that: (a) diseases characterized by severe defi-ciency of all classes of immunoglobulins always have an associated impairment of humoral antibody response; (b) diseases characterized by a selective deficiency of one or more classes of immunoglobulins may demonstrate selec-tive abnormalities of the humoral antibody response or may have no demonstrable abnormality; and (c) diseases with normal serum immunoglobulin concentrations but faulty cellular integration may show impairment of the humoral antibody response to specific antigens.

The factors governing the induction and manifestation of cellular immune responses differ in many respects from the factors governing humoral antibody synthesis. How-ever, the two types of immunologic response are closely integrated, both in the initial development and differen-tiation of the immune system and in the interaction of cellular and humoral components in the expression of the fully differentiated system (see Chapters 15 and 17). For ex-

ample, normal development of the thymus and T cells is critically important to the development of the cellular im-mune response, but it also plays a role in the full develop-ment of the humoral antibody response (77, 129, 131, 132). In the chicken, the bursa of Fabricius is concerned primarily, but not exclusively, with the humoral antibody-producing system (71, 145). The equivalent of the bursa of Fabricius has not been determined with certainty in mammals. However, a variety of observations suggests that the immunoglobulin-producing system is identified primarily with the bone-marrow–derived B lymphoid cell. Because of the relative separation of these classes of im-munocytes, one can readily understand diseases with normal or only slightly impaired humoral antibody response and a markedly defective cellular immune response. Examples may include autosomal recessive lym-phopenia with normal immunoglobulin (62, 138) and Hodgkin's disease (6, 78, 107). Conversely, disorders such as Bruton's disease and transient hypogammaglobu-linemia of infancy (103) predominantly show an impair-ment of humoral immune response and little deficiency in cellular response.

Finally, in some disorders both humoral and cellular responses are abnormal; for example, agammaglobu-linemia with thymoma (82, 105, 170).

To summarize: *it is possible to have selective abnor-mality of the cellular immune response, selective abnor-mality of the humoral immune response, or any combina-tion of the two.*

Thus far, we have been concerned with identifying how immunologic deficiency diseases can arise from abnormal-ities of immunocyte number, differentiation, function, or cellular interaction. The abnormalities themselves can arise in three ways: (a) from a noninherited aberration in fetal development with faulty development of an impor-tant lymphoid organ, such as the thymus in DiGeorge's syndrome; (b) from specific genetic defects; or (c) as a result of postnatal diseases that affect the lymphoid system—diseases such as malignancies and perhaps viral infections.

Immunologic Deficiency Diseases with Reduced Numbers of Plasma Cells

We shall first consider immunodeficiency diseases having reduced numbers of plasma cells in lymphoid tissues. Since these cells are the principal source of im-munoglobulins, the diseases share the feature of defective humoral antibody response.

Bruton's Disease

The congenital sex-linked type of agammaglobulinemia first described by Bruton (27) is a severe immunologic deficiency syndrome. Affected infants generally develop symptoms related to their deficiency at about five or six months of age. By this age the maternal antibodies transmitted via the placental circulation have largely disappeared (26, 141). Manifestations of immune deficiency generally are related to infections with pyogenic bacterial pathogens such as the *Streptococcus, Pneumococcus, Hemophilus,* and *Meningococcus.* These infections include pyoderma, pneumonia, otitis media, conjunctivitis, and meningitis. Infection with less common agents such as *Pneumocystis carinii* and pathogenic fungi also occurs (8, 32, 100, 165). Fatal hepatitis has been recorded (80).

Patients with sex-linked agammaglobulinemia (as well as other immunologic deficiencies) who survive early childhood as a result of the administration of antibiotics and gamma globulin may have an increased risk of developing hematologic malignancy in later life (17, 66, 143, 154, 197). The concept of immune surveillance against malignant transformation was summarized in Chapter 17. Schwartz (168) has recently proposed a mechanism for the development of neoplasia in immunodeficiency disease.

The salient features of the Bruton type of agamma-

globulinemia (42, 76, 78, 82, 113, 145, 150, 158, 170) are a sex-linked recessive mode of inheritance; a striking reduction in all three of the major classes of immunoglobulin; a markedly deficient or absent humoral antibody response to antigen; an intact cellular immune response; a normal number of circulating lymphocytes, but reduced numbers of plasma cells in lymphoid tissue, and reduced numbers of circulating B cells with surface immunoglobulin markers; a generally normal structure of the thymus gland; and an absence of germinal centers in both unstimulated and antigen-stimulated lymph nodes and spleen and appendiceal lymphoid tissue. Paracortical regions of lymph nodes for the most part are normal (Fig. 18.3).

Additional features of this disorder include an absence of pharyngeal lymphoid tissue apparent on roentgenogram (122) and, occasionally, neutropenia (81).

The pathogenic mechanisms of this immunologic deficiency disease are not known. An analogy has been drawn between this disorder and the defect in bursectomized chickens or bursectomized irradiated chickens (41, 71, 145, 199). Both the affected children and the experimental chickens have defects in humoral antibody synthesis, but not in cellular immune responses, and have similar anatomic abnormalities of the lymphoid tissue. However, since the mammalian equivalent (if one exists) of the bursa of Fabricius is not known, this analogy cannot at present be taken literally. Possible sites of abnormal cell differentiation are steps 2 and 4 of Fig. 18.2.

Transient Hypogammaglobulinemia of Infancy

Another immunodeficiency disease with reduced numbers of tissue plasma cells is hypogammaglobulinemia of infancy.

During the first five or six months of life, maternal immunoglobulins gradually disappear from the circulation of the newborn (26, 111, 141). It is not until after this time that defects in immunoglobulin production appear. Such defects may be transient and disappear with maturation if the affected child survives the stress of repeated infection. The following are the major features of transient hypogammaglobulinemia of infancy (103): it has a familial occurrence with a possible genetic basis; IgG is the principal serum immuglobulin reduced in concentration; the humoral antibody response to most antigens is depressed; cellular immune responses are intact; the number of circulating lymphocytes is usually normal, but tissue plasma cells are decreased; and germinal centers are rare or absent in peripheral lymphoid tissues.

As might be anticipated, children afflicted with this disorder suffer repeated pyogenic infections until the im-

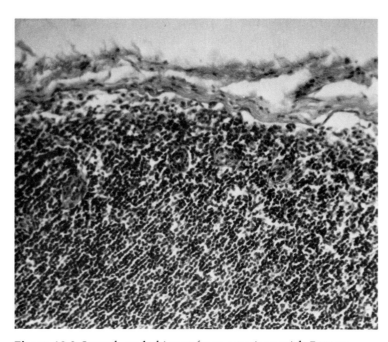

Figure 18.3 Lymph node biopsy from a patient with Bruton-type agammaglobulinemia. Note the absence of well-developed germinal centers. Hematoxylin and eosin stain. (Photograph courtesy of Dr. A. Ammann.)

munologic responses reach normal levels. A simplistic interpretation of these observations is that the syndrome reflects delayed maturation of the humoral antibody-producing component of the immune system (step 4, Fig. 18.2).

Swiss-Type Agammaglobulinemia

The Swiss type of agammaglobulinemia (autosomal recessive alymphocytic agammaglobulinemia) is a severe form of immunologic deficiency disease, which was initially defined by Swiss investigators (16, 70, 89–91, 188) and subsequently described in many countries (63–69). It is a "combined" immunodeficiency disease with abnormalities of both the cellular and humoral immune systems. Afflicted patients are usually recognized by failure of growth and serious infections in the first weeks of life—a feature that distinguishes this disorder from most other types of congenital agammaglobulinemia (69, 82). In addition, these patients are prone to infections with *Candida albicans* (90) and viruses that are relatively rare pathogens in patients with sex-linked agammaglobulinemia. Ulcerative colitis and malabsorption syndrome also have been reported in the Swiss type of agammaglobulinemia. Death tends to occur early in infancy.

Familial occurrence is well documented in this disorder (68, 145, 188), and consanguinity has been reported in some families. The principal features of this disease syndrome are an autosomal recessive mode of inheritance (145, 170); severe generalized immunoglobulin deficiency after the neonatal period (16, 50, 70, 90, 91, 157, 188, 193); deficient humoral antibody response to all antigens; impaired delayed hypersensitivity response to antigens, including 2,4-dinitrochlorobenzene (145, 157); striking lymphopenia in the blood, bone marrow, and lymphoid organs (68); absent plasma cells in lymphoid organs and bone marrow; thymus gland aplasia (weights from a few milligrams to 3 gm, in contrast to normal weights of 12 to 25 gm) (90, 145) (Figs. 18.4 and 18.5); and poor development of peripheral lymphoid tissue, with lymphocytes absent or reduced in numbers in tonsils, lymph nodes, spleen, and lamina propria of the small bowel (Figs. 18.6 to 18.8).

In patients studied at necropsy, the thymus gland may resemble the primitive epithelial anlage soon after its development from the gut wall. Thymic lymphocytes are absent, although a few may be present but fail to form a normal cortical structure. Hassall's corpuscles are usually absent (see Fig. 18.5). In some patients the thymus has not descended into a normal intrathoracic position, but has remained in an embryonic location in the neck (79, 90, 145). These observations suggest that the basic lesion of autosomal recessive agammaglobulinemia may be a fail-

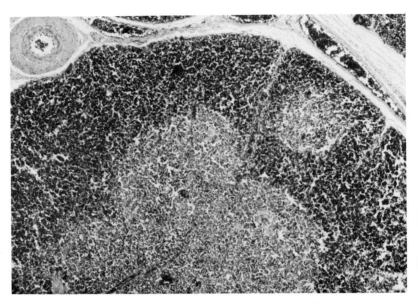

Figure 18.4 Section of thymus gland of a normal human newborn. Hematoxylin and eosin stain. Compare this with the schematic representation of the gland in Figs. 12.20 and 12.22.

ure of normal thymus development and perhaps other lymphoid tissue from the gut endothelium (step 1 or steps 2 and 3 of Fig. 18.2). Failure of development of the primordial lymphoid structure would result in a failure of development of peripheral lymphoid tissues and defective humoral and cellular immune responses. The failure of

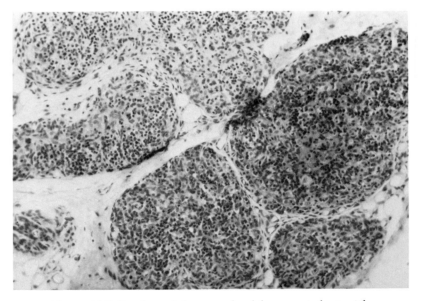

Figure 18.5 Section of thymus gland from an infant with Swiss-type agammaglobulinemia. Note poor development of lymphoid architecture. Hematoxylin and eosin stain. (Photograph courtesy of Dr. A. Ammann.)

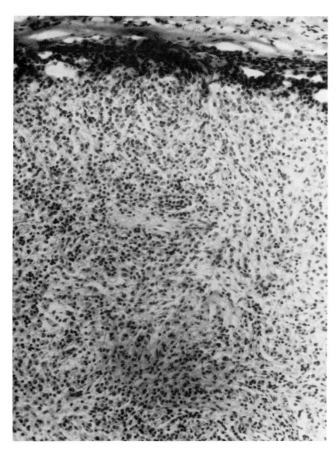

Figure 18.6 Section of lymph node from an infant with Swiss-type agammaglobulinemia. Lymphoid cells are absent and the normal architecture has not developed. Hematoxylin and eosin stain. (Photograph courtesy of Dr. A. Ammann.)

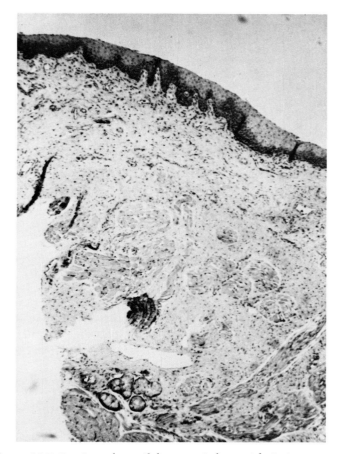

Figure 18.7 Section of tonsil from an infant with Swiss-type agammaglobulinemia. Note marked reduction in lymphoid cells.

development of the cellular immune response would lead to enhanced susceptibility to infection even during the first few months of postnatal life. The hypothesis that this disorder arises from faulty differentiation of a hematopoietic stem cell (step 1) is supported by the observation that immunologic reconstitution can be achieved by administration of genetically compatible bone marrow (128, 164). Transplantation has also achieved striking successes in other immunodeficiency diseases (10, 14, 23, 28, 48, 66, 117, 179, 208).

Agammaglobulinemia with Thymoma

Agammaglobulinemia with thymoma (Good's syndrome) is characterized by (82, 105): reduction in all classes of immunoglobulins; deficient humoral antibody response to all antigens; deficient cellular immune responses to most antigens; circulating lymphocyte levels low and often declining progressively with age; reduced or absent plasma cells in tissues; reduced or absent germinal

centers of lymphoid tissues, and possible deficiency in paracortical tissue; enlarged thymus gland, usually with a thymoma composed mainly of stromal epithelial spindle cells; and associated hematopoietic disorders.

In the category of agammaglobulinemic syndromes previously referred to as "primary acquired agammaglobulinemia" (that is, agammaglobulinemia with apparent onset in late childhood or adult life and without definable underlying predisposing disease), about 10 percent of patients have an associated thymoma (63, 73, 75, 102, 114, 124, 145, 187). The thymomas have been of the epithelial type, generally with a spindle-cell appearance. Both benign and malignant tumors have been described. In some cases lymphocytes and Hassall's corpuscles were absent; in others, scattered or abundant lymphocytes were observed.

The relation between the presence of the thymoma and the development of agammaglobulinemia is not clear. Certainly patients have been described with similar thy-

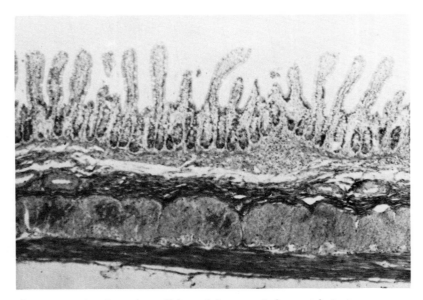

Figure 18.8 Section of small bowel from an infant with Swiss-type agammaglobulinemia. Lymphoid follicles are absent. Hematoxylin and eosin stain. (Photograph courtesy of Dr. A. Ammann.)

momas and unimpaired immunologic function (60, 161). In addition, complete removal of the adult thymus has relatively little effect on immune function (13, 125, 130). It may be that the thymomas associated with agammaglobulinemia elaborate a humoral substance that effects the immune response, or that these thymomas arise much earlier in life and therefore compromise normal thymic function earlier than would be suspected from the clinical course of the illness. The site of the disturbance in immunologic development is not known with certainty, although step 1 of Fig. 18.2 and the stem cell itself are possibilities.

Patients affected with thymoma and agammaglobulinemia usually die from pyogenic pathogen infections. Resistance to viruses and fungi may be compromised as well. No clear-cut genetic factors have been documented in the pathogenesis of this syndrome.

An interesting variety of hematologic abnormalities has been described in association with agammaglobulinemia and thymoma, including decreased numbers of eosinophils (75), anemia (114, 124, 152), leukopenia and specifically neutropenia (63, 114, 124, 152), rarely leukocytosis (114), and thrombocytopenia and purpura (145). Similar hematologic syndromes without the immunologic impairment have been described in association with thymoma (161).

Selective IgA Deficiency

The synthesis of IgA by a distinctive class of plasma cells has been discussed in Chapter 16. Selective IgA deficiency is associated with absence of IgA-producing plasma cells, particularly in the lamina propria. The major features of this syndrome are as follows (15, 34, 45, 85, 155, 201): levels of serum IgA are low, with generally normal levels of the other major immunoglobulins; humoral antibody response is normal except for the production of IgA antibodies; cellular immune responses are intact; and the thymus glands and lymph nodes are normal in architecture.

The importance of genetic factors in IgA deficiency is unknown, although some cases are clearly familial (74). Affected patients may be entirely healthy or may suffer from bronchitis, sinusitis, enteropathy with malabsorption syndrome, and steatorrhea and "autoimmune" diseases (34, 45, 94). These clinical manifestations presumably are related to the absence of IgA in exocrine secretion as well as in serum. They may also be related to low levels of IgE, often found in association with IgA deficiency (149).

The clinical picture of selective IgA deficiency and malabsorption syndrome may resemble that of nontropical sprue and may improve on a gluten-free diet, although the IgA levels are unaffected by this therapy (45, 189).

Despite the many described complications, it is quite common for patients with selective IgA deficiency to be entirely healthy. Asymptomatic IgA deficiency may be a fairly common phenomenon—involving between 1 in 400 and 1 in 700 of the general population (15).

The total immunglobulin levels in the secretions of patients with selective IgA deficiency may be nearly normal because of the increase in the amounts of IgG and IgM in these secretions (155, 176, 190).

In addition to patients with selective IgA deficiency, patients having other forms of immunologic deficiency disease with deficiencies of the major serum immunoglobulins have reductions in the immunoglobulin concentrations in their secretion (176). In such patients immunofluorescent studies show a paucity of lymphoid cells in the respiratory and gastrointestinal tracts. The relative roles of circulating antibody and antibody produced locally within the respiratory and gastrointestinal tract in resistance to respiratory and enteric pathogens are complex and still poorly defined (29, 189). A high percentage of patients with acquired agammaglobulinemia manifest diarrhea and malabsorption syndromes. Histologic examination of the small bowel often reveals blunted villi, absence of plasma cells in the lamina propria, and occasional lymphocytic infiltration. Immunofluorescent studies show absence of IgA-containing plasma cells (53, 54). Recently Moroz and his colleagues have described a new hereditary immunoglobulin A abnormality—absence of assembly of light and heavy chains of IgA (137).

Other Disorders

Several other disorders have been described in which tissue plasma cells sometimes are reduced in association with immunologic deficiency. These include ataxia telangiectasia, primary lymphopenic immunoglobulin deficiency (Gitlin's syndrome), so-called primary acquired agammaglobulinemia (nonsex-linked primary immunoglobulin deficiency of variable expression), and perhaps certain malignant hematologic disorders such as chronic lymphocytic leukemia and multiple myeloma. Since a decrease in the number of normal plasma cells is not an invariant feature of these disorders, they will be considered under subsequent classification headings.

Immunologic Deficiency Diseases with Reduced Numbers of Circulating Lymphocytes

One can catalogue immunologic deficiency diseases associated with lymphopenia into those in which there is deficient production of lymphocytes and those in which there is excessive loss or destruction of lymphocytes (steps 8 and 9, Fig. 18.2). Almost all disorders with very low lymphocyte levels have demonstrable deficiencies in cellular immune responses; they may or may not have associated defects in humoral antibody synthesis.

The Swiss type of agammaglobulinemia and agammaglobulinemia with thymoma could also be included in this category of immunologic deficiency disease with low levels of circulating lymphocytes. However, deficient plasma cell and immunoglobulin synthesis also is a prominent feature of these two disorders; for convenience they have been classed with the first category of immunologic deficiency diseases having reduced numbers of plasma cells.

Primary Lymphopenic Agammaglobulinemia

This disorder, also known as Gitlin's syndrome or thymic alymphoplasia, was first described by Gitlin and Craig in 1963 (68) and subsequently elaborated upon by other investigators (25, 59, 87, 133, 162, 167). Circulating lymphocyte counts are variable but usually low. The principal features of this disorder are the following: (a) genetic factors operative in some cases with a sex-linked or autosomal recessive mode of inheritance; (b) a variable deficiency of one or more immunoglobulin classes, with oc-

casional increases seen in some classes; (c) deficient humoral antibody response to some, but not all, antigens; (d) impaired cellular immune responses to most antigens; (e) circulating lymphocytes that are usually low, with a variable number of tissue plasma cells; (f) hypoplasia of the thymus involving both lymphoid cells and Hassall's corpuscles; and (g) a general deficiency of lymphocytes in peripheral lymphoid tissue, often with scattered foci preserved.

Thymic hypoplasia and reduction of peripheral lymphocytes are the "invariant" features of this disorder. The variable expression of points (a) through (d) above distinguish this disease from the Swiss type of agammaglobulinemia—the immunologic deficiency disease with which it is most likely to be confused.

As with other severe immunologic deficiency diseases involving both cellular and humoral immunity, affected patients are apt to die early in childhood, usually of pyogenic bacterial infection but occasionally of fungal, viral, or *Pneumocystis carinii* infection (68,95).

The variable nature of the defect in this disorder quite possibly means that there is a family of related diseases rather than a single entity. Pathogenetic mechanisms are unknown.

Nezelof's Syndrome

In 1964 Nezelof and his colleagues described a hereditary syndrome of thymic hypoplasia associated with normal immunoglobulins (138). It is known also as autosomal recessive alymphopenia with normal serum immunoglobulins. An identical or related condition was described in 1966 by Fulginiti and his collaborators (62). The following are the major features of this condition: an autosomal recessive mode of inheritance; normal serum levels of immunoglobulins; antibodies present in serum, but a probable deficiency in the humoral antibody response; impaired cellular immune responses; low levels of circulating lymphocytes; apparently normal numbers of plasma cells in the tissues; a hypoplastic thymus gland, which lacks lymphoid cells and Hassall's corpuscles; and reduction of lymphocytes in peripheral lymphoid tissue. Germinal centers may be present.

As might be predicted from the character of the thymus and peripheral lymphoid tissues and the presence of plasma cells, children affected by this disorder have a major impairment of cellular, but not of humoral, immune responses. They suffer from repeated bacterial, viral, fungal, and sometimes *Pneumocystis* infection. The normal immunoglobulin levels and numbers of plasma cells distinguish this syndrome from the Swiss type of agammaglobulinemia and from primary lymphopenic immunoglobulin deficiency.

Possible sites of abnormal immune system function in Nezelof's syndrome are at steps 3 and 5 of Fig. 18.2.

Wiskott-Aldrich Syndrome

Clinically, the Wiskott-Aldrich syndrome (immune deficiency with eczema and thrombocytopenia) is characterized by eczema, symptomatic thrombocytopenia caused by failure of thrombopoiesis, susceptibility to infection with a variety of pathogens (bacteria, fungi, viruses), and a high incidence of lymphoreticular malignancies (7, 19, 83, 118, 203). Affected children generally die within the first decade of life. The following are the principal immunologic features of this disorder (7, 20, 41, 99, 112, 134, 170, 177, 180, 201): sex-linked recessive mode of inheritance; immunoglobulin deficiency, variable as to class and degree (high concentrations of IgA and low IgM are probably most frequent); failure to make humoral antibody to some antigens; deficient cellular immune responses to most antigens; circulating lymphocyte levels that are usually low and decline progressively with time; normal numbers of plasma cells; a morphologically normal thymus gland; and a deficiency in the paracortical areas of lymph nodes.

The low levels of IgM observed in this disorder are probably correlated with the frequently observed absence of isohemagglutinins and a failure of humoral antibody response to carbohydrate antigens. The relation between immune deficiency, thrombocytopenia, and eczema is not understood. Possible sites for the defect in the immune system include steps 1, 3, 5, and 6 of Fig. 18.2. Other suggested sites of abnormality include antigen recognition or processing in the afferent limb of the immune response (197), although macrophage function appears to be normal (19).

Lymphocyte Loss

Several diseases have been described in which lymphocytes, as well as immunoglobulins and other proteins, are lost from the gastrointestinal tract (steps 8 and 9). A variety of causes of these protein-losing enteropathies has been identified and is shown in Table 18.2. Intestinal lymphangiectasia may be taken as a prototype of disease in which lymphocyte and immunoglobulin loss is associated with immunologic impairment (135, 184, 194).

Intestinal lymphangiectasia is a chronic disorder of the lymphatics associated with severe protein-losing enteropathy, hypoproteinemia, and severe edema. Malabsorption of fats occurs, but usually is not severe. The underlying pathology appears to be a structural abnormality of the lymphatic channels occurring as either an acquired

Table 18.2 Causes of gastrointestinal loss of protein and lymphocytes.

Disease	References
Intestinal lymphangiectasia	135, 181, 184, 194, 196
Whipple's disease	115
Regional enteritis	11
Constrictive pericarditis	46, 144
Tricuspid regurgitation	182

or a congenital malformation. Histologically the lymphatic channels of the small bowel are dilated.

The major immunologic features of this disorder are as follows: decreased serum immunoglobulins because of increased catabolism (loss); decreased humoral antibody response to some antigens; markedly impaired cellular immune responses; decreased circulating levels of lymphocytes; and a reduction in lymphocyte numbers in the peripheral tissue.

The defect in humoral antibody response in patients with this disorder is probably related to the reduction in serum immunoglobulins. This reduction mainly reflects increased catabolism/loss, since synthetic rates are normal or slightly increased, although a normal compensatory increase in synthesis does not occur.

The lymphocyte depletion secondary to gastrointestinal loss of cells is reflected in diminished delayed hypersensitivity reactivity and delayed allograft rejection. It is primarily the long-lived recirculating T cells that are lost in the gastrointestinal fluids in protein-losing enteropathies (200). Increased susceptibility to infection (usually pyogenic) occurs in a minority of patients with intestinal lymphangiectasia.

Lymphocytopenia is observed in other protein-losing enteropathies or cardioenteropathies, including Whipple's disease, regional enteritis, constrictive pericarditis, and severe tricuspid regurgitation, but not in sprue or allergic enteropathy. Those diseases with associated lymphocyte loss have structural dilation of the intestinal lymphatics (115, 144, 163, 183, 184, 194, 196, 198). Lymph fluid can sometimes be demonstrated to leak directly into the intestine (135, 181). In those protein-losing enteropathies that are reversible, such as Whipple's disease, constrictive pericarditis, and tricuspid regurgitation, the hypoproteinemia and lymphopenia also are reversible.

The best experimental model of the patient with lymphopenic gastroenteropathy is the animal with chronic thoracic duct drainage (121). The loss of proteins and cells in these experimental animals as a rule is more severe than in the clinical disease.

*Other Causes of Lymphopenia
and Immunologic Deficiency*

Those immunologic deficiency diseases classified as "secondary acquired agammaglobulinemia" (145) usually result either from involvement of the immune system by a hematologic malignancy or gastrointestinal loss of proteins and lymphocytes. In advanced active Hodgkin's disease lymphopenia, impaired cellular immune responses and enhanced susceptibility to infection may be associated phenomena (6). Chronic lymphocytic leukemia may be regarded as a disease where a deficiency of normal lymphocytes occurs in the presence of an increase in functionally abnormal lymphocytes (see Chapter 19). The hematologic malignancies that may produce immunologic impairment are considered in later sections of this chapter and later in this book.

Recently two nonrelated patients with moderate to severe lymphopenia, severly impaired cellular immunity, and adenosine-deaminase deficiency were reported (67). The enzyme deficiency may be related to the immunologic abnormality in these patients.

Seeger and his colleagues (169) have described a new familial lymphopenic immunodeficiency disease which they have designated *progressive lymphoid system deterioration*. It is characterized by rapidly developing lymphoid and hematopoietic cell depletion with death early in life.

Immunologic Deficiency States with Normal or Variable Numbers of Immunocytes

Thymic Aplasia

Infants with thymic aplasia (DiGeorge's syndrome) have agenesis of the thymus gland in association with absence of the parathyroid glands (49, 64, 85, 97, 119, 185). Other anomalies occur in this disorder, especially those of the cardiovascular system. Affected children suffer from hypocalcemia and recurrent or chronic infections and usually die in infancy. The basic defect appears to be primary failure of development of the third and fourth branchial arches that contain the primordia of the thymus and parathyroid glands. The principal immunologic features of the syndrome are normal serum immunoglobulin levels; deficient humoral antibody response; marked deficiency of cellular responses; circulating lymphocytes that are usually normal in numbers but occasionally reduced; presence of plasma cells in the tissues; thymic aplasia; and lymph nodes with germinal centers but with decreased lymphocytes in the paracortical areas (Fig. 18.9).

There is no evidence that this syndrome is genetic in

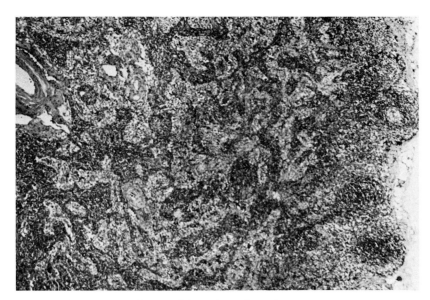

Figure 18.9 Abnormal lymph node architecture in a patient with DiGeorge's syndrome.

origin. Of considerable interest is the fact that despite evidence for complete absence of the thymus throughout gestation, circulating lymphocytes usually are normal in number. These lymphocytes almost certainly are of extrathymic origin. They have the appearance of normal small and medium-sized lymphocytes, but demonstrate a reduced responsiveness to phytohemagglutinin, antileukocyte serum, and allogeneic lymphocytes (119).

Ataxia Telangiectasia

Patients with ataxia telangiectasia are characterized by cerebellar ataxia and ocular telangiectasia (22, 35, 52, 186), repeated sinopulmonary infections, immunologic abnormalities (58, 120, 146, 186, 210) and, occasionally, reticuloendothelial neoplasms (22, 197). The following are the major immunologic features of this disorder (9, 52, 54, 55, 104, 120, 145–147, 160, 173, 183, 210): autosomal recessive inheritance; a deficiency of immunoglobulins, with the class involved and degree of change being variable from patient to patient (IgA and IgE are often low); a deficient humoral antibody response to some, but not all, antigens; a deficient cellular immune response to some, but not all, antigens; circulating lymphocyte levels that are variable but usually low; plasma cells that are usually present but occasionally absent; abnormal thymic architecture with a lack of cortical and medullary organization and Hassall's corpuscles; an occasional absent thymus at necropsy; and variable lymph node architecture (germinal centers occasionally decreased, lymphocytes deficient in the paracortical areas, occasional reticular hyperplasia).

Among the striking features of ataxia telangiectasia is the variability of the dysgammaglobulinemia; 43 of 58 reported cases had low or absent IgA, 14 had normal levels, and 1 had increased levels (52, 58, 146, 186, 210). Within this group, 10 patients had increased IgM and 2 had decreased levels of this immunoglobulin. Similarly, IgG levels are variable. The metabolism of immunoglobulins is variable in this disorder (120, 183). The synthesis of IgG may be normal, increased, or decreased. Patients with ataxia telangiectasia and low serum concentration of IgA may have markedly reduced synthetic rates of this protein—0.3 to 10 percent of normal. Administration of IgA to patients with ataxia telangiectasia may result in the formation of antibody to IgA.

Children with ataxia telangiectasia usually die before adolescence, generally of pulmonary infections. As with some of the other immune deficiency diseases, a high incidence of lymphoreticular malignancies has been reported among patients with this disorder (145, 147).

The pathogenetic mechanisms underlying cerebellar ataxia, telangiectasia, and immunologic impairment are unknown. It has been difficult to deduce a single biochemical abnormality or event in intrauterine development that could account for all the abnormalities observed. It has been suggested that the primary defect may lie in the area of thymic development (197).

Immunoglobulin Deficiency of Variable Onset

Primary immunoglobulin deficiency of variable onset has also been called, at one time or another, *primary acquired agammaglobulinemia,* and *primary immunoglobulin aberration.* This is a "wastebasket" categorization undoubtedly embracing a number of disorders of differing pathogenesis and clinical expression. For instance, it may include the primary dysgammaglobulinemias (that is, abnormality of one or more, but not all, immunoglobulin classes) of both childhood and adult life and also the congenital, nonsex-linked hypogammaglobulinemias. Some of the immunologic deficiency diseases in this category originally thought to be primary "acquired" were found often to have a genetic basis, frequently with consanguinity and related immune disorders within the family (51, 61, 204–206). Some disorders that are now catalogued for convenience within this group of immunologic deficiency diseases may soon warrant classification as distinctive disease entities. For example, the syndrome of IgM deficiency and susceptibility to fulminant meningococcal septicemia may be a distinct entity (92).

Undoubtedly, the acquisition of more information will result in better classifications of these diseases. For the moment, these are the chief immunologic characteristics of this group (16, 33, 36, 40, 69, 93, 145, 151, 158, 159, 166, 178): immunoglobulin deficiency that is variable as to degree and class of protein involved; deficiency of humoral antibody response to most antigens; deficient cellular immune responses to some, but not all, antigens; circulating lymphocyte and tissue plasma cells usually normal, but sometimes reduced in numbers; thymus gland usually morphologically normal (but data inadequate for full evaluation); and variable abnormality of germinal centers and paracortical areas of lymph node, with occasional reticulum cell hyperplasia.

Despite the heterogeneity of immunologic findings, certain features bind this group of affected patients together, including susceptibility to infection, high frequency of lymphoreticular malignancies and "autoimmune" diseases, and amyloidosis. Gastrointestinal disturbances are common and may include diarrhea, malabsorption, and protein-losing enteropathy (195). In some patients, jejunal villous atrophy is present; in others, nodular hyperplasia of intestinal lymphoid tissue occurs (98).

Viral Infection

Viral infection is a recently identified etiologic mechanism in some forms of immunodeficiency disease. Many infants affected by congenital rubella infection have increased levels of IgM during the period of virus excretion. In some, hypogammaglobulinemia may persist, although lymphocyte abnormalities and clinical manifestations may disappear with the passage of time (175). Lymphocytes of affected children often are unresponsive to phytohemaglutinin (139) or specific viral antigen (202). The lymphocyte defect appears to be a direct effect of virus infection (136).

Exposure of lymphocytes from adults to either rubella virus or Newcastle disease virus interferes with their capacity to respond to phytohemagglutinin (127, 136). Other viral diseases, such as rubeola and varicella, usually do not interfere with lymphocyte responsiveness. When there is virus-induced impairment of lymphocyte responsiveness to phytohemagglutinin, cellular immune responses appear to be diminished as well.

Alteration of lymphocyte responsiveness may occur in other types of infections. The number of cells undergoing mitosis is said to be reduced in the blood of patients with infectious hepatitis and in normal leukocytes incubated in hepatitis serum (126). Mycoplasma organisms also inhibit leukocyte mitosis (44). Lymphopenia occurring during the course of generalized viral or mycoplasma infections may be a result of antibody-associated lymphotoxin (96).

Hodgkin's Disease and Other Neoplasms

Patients with advanced Hodgkin's disease often exhibit the following abnormalities of immunologic function (see also Chapter 22): reduced response to a variety of antigens that induce delayed hypersensitivity reactions (1), delayed homograft rejection (108), and increased susceptibility to certain infections (2). These are the major features of the immunologic response in such patients (4, 78, 88, 108): serum immunoglobulin levels are generally normal; humoral antibody response is usually normal; cellular immune responses are deficient; the levels of circulating lymphocytes are usually normal, but may be reduced; tissue plasma cells are present; and the thymus gland and lymph nodes are abnormal when involved by the malignant process.

The blastogenic response of the peripheral blood lymphocytes from patients with active Hodgkin's disease is generally reduced both to specific antigens, such as vaccinia, and to phytohemagglutinin (4, 88). These lymphocytes may be morphologically abnormal, with unusual cytoplasmic processes (18). They are also said to be abnormal in the lymphocyte transfer reaction (3). Under conditions in which transfer factor induced tuberbulin sensitivity in normal subjects, it failed to do so in patients with Hodgkin's disease (78, 108). Immunologic abnormalities occurring in Hodgkin's disease are considered in more detail in Chapter 22 and in the recent review of Young and his colleagues (209).

The immunologic defect in chronic lymphocytic leukemia appears to be quite different from that in Hodgkin's disease and is manifested mainly by an inability to produce humoral antibody in response to new antigens. One-to two-thirds of patients with chronic lymphocytic leukemia have hypogammaglobulinemia (57, 106). In vivo cellular immune responses appear to be relatively intact in this disorder; however, in vitro a number of defects in lymphocyte response are demonstrable (24, 140, 171). These abnormalities probably result from a dilution of normal T lymphocytes by neoplastic B cells (5, 148, 172). Immunologic abnormalities occurring in chronic lymphocytic leukemia will be considered in more detail in Chapter 19.

Another type of acquired immunologic deficiency is that associated with multiple myeloma. In this disorder neoplastic plasma cells produce large amounts of homogeneous immunoglobulins that generally lack definable antibody activity, or have antibody activity against a very restricted class of antigens. In this disease normal immunoglobulin synthesis may be compromised and the catabolism of normal immunoglobulins may be increased with consequent impairment of immunologic defenses against infectious agents (142). Abnormalities of the immune response in multiple myeloma are considered in greater detail in Chapter 20.

Lepromatous Leprosy, Sarcoidosis, and Chronic Mucocutaneous Candidiasis

In the lepromatous form of leprosy there is very little inflammatory reaction to the invading microorganisms. The bacilli appear to proliferate unchecked, and macrophages laden with organisms are readily detected in the tissues and blood. There is a specific loss of skin sensitivity to *Mycobacterium leprae* and some other antigens, whereas humoral antibody production in general is intact. In contrast, tuberculoid leprosy is characterized by a generally benign, self-limited course with relatively few demonstrable organisms in the tissues. In the tubercular form of the disease, delayed reactivity to lepromin antigen is relatively intact (30, 31, 72, 153, 191).

The situation in lepromatous leprosy appears to be roughly equivalent to that in widely disseminated tuberculosis or systemic fungal infection; that is, anergy to the antigens of the invading parasite (72). In the case of lepromatous leprosy, delayed hypersensitivity sometimes is restored by the administration of leukocytes or transfer factor from lepromin-positive donors (31, 47).

Active sarcoidosis also may be characterized by impairment of delayed hypersensitivity reactions to a variety of bacterial, fungal, and simple chemical antigens, despite an intact humoral antibody-producing system (37, 101). Affected patients show diminished responsiveness to transfer factor (116, 192).

Lepromatous leprosy and sarcoidosis are examples of diseases with acquired defects of cellular immune responses (either specific or generalized) and preserved humoral immune responses. The mechanisms operative in producing these conditions are not known. Recent studies have demonstrated an absolute decrease in the number of circulating T lymphocytes and an increase in the number of B cells. Such lymphoid populations have a diminished response to phytohemagglutinin.

Chronic mucocutaneous candidiasis is a rare disorder and is either sporadic or familial. It is characterized by chronic recurrent *Candida* infections of the skin, nails, mucous membranes, and, in extremely rare cases, the parenchymal tissues. Associated conditions include polyendocrinopathy, dental dysplasia, and steatorrhea (21,

174). Clinical manifestations in different patients are variable. A number of investigators have observed negative delayed skin tests to *Candida albicans* (39, 123). The response of patients' lymphocytes to *Candida* antigen in vitro has been variable (39, 109). However, several investigators claim that these lymphocytes may fail to synthesize mediators such as migration inhibitory factor (MIF) (see Chapter 17) even though they may proliferate in response to antigen (38, 110, 156).

The site of the cellular defect in chronic mucocutaneous candidiasis is not known, but it may involve the production of specific mediators by T cells. The abnormalities of skin test and in vitro lymphocyte response are correctable by the administration of normal compatible allogeneic lymphocytes.

Summary and Prospects for Immunologic Reconstitution

Knowledge of the morphogenesis and cellular interactions of the immune system enables one to identify a number of functional abnormalities that are expressed as immunodeficiency disease. These abnormalities may involve stem cell differentiation into lymphoid cells, thymic development or function, B-cell development or function, B-cell and T-cell interactions and, possibly, the production of effector substances (see Fig. 18.2). Additionally, immunologic deficiency may result simply from excessive lymphocyte or immunoglobulin loss in the gastrointestinal tract.

It is convenient to divide the immunodeficiency disorders into the following categories: those characterized by lymphopenia; those with normal lymphocyte numbers but reduced plasma cells in the tissues (B-cell diseases); and those with normal or variable numbers of immunocytes but abnormal immunologic function.

In recent years a number of attempts have been made to achieve immunologic reconstitution in patients with immunodeficiency disease. Transfer factor has been tried in the Wiskott-Aldrich syndrome, lepromatous leprosy, and chronic mucocutaneous candidiasis. The success of these attempts has been variable. A more exciting approach has been transplantation of compatible allogeneic lymphoid cells, bone marrow, or thymus (DiGeorge's syndrome). These attempts have met with quite striking success when graft-vs-host disease has been controlled (10, 14, 23, 28, 48, 64, 117, 179, 208).

Chapter 18 References

1. Aisenberg, A. C. Studies on delayed hypersensitivity in Hodgkin's disease, *J. Clin. Invest.* 41:1964, 1962.
2. Aisenberg, A. C. Hodgkin's disease—prognosis, treatment and etiologic and immunologic considerations, *N. Engl. J. Med.* 270:508, 565, 617; 1964.
3. Aisenberg, A. C. Studies of lymphocyte transfer reactions in Hodgkin's disease, *J. Clin. Invest.* 44:555, 1965.
4. Aisenberg, A. C. Quantitative estimation of the reactivity of normal and Hodgkin's disease lymphocytes with Thymidine-2-^{14}C, *Nature* 205:1233, 1965.
5. Aisenberg, A. C., and Bloch, K. J. Immunoglobulins on the surface of neoplastic lymphocytes, *N. Engl. J. Med.* 287:272, 1972.
6. Aisenberg, A. C., and Leskowitz, S. Antibody formation in Hodgkin's disease, *N. Engl. J. Med.* 268:1269, 1963.
7. Aldrich, R. A., Steinberg, A. G., and Campbell, D. C. Pedigree demonstrating a sex-linked recessive condition characterized by draining ears, eczematoid dermatitis and bloody diarrhea, *Pediatrics* 13:133, 1954.
8. Allibone, E. C., Goldie, W., and Marmion, B. P. *Pneumocystis carinii* pneumonia and progressive vaccinia in siblings, *Arch. Dis. Child.* 39:26, 1964.
9. Amman, P., Lòpez, V., Bütler, R., and Rossi, E. Das Ataxie-Teleangiektasie-Syndrom (Louis-Bar-Syndrom) aus immunologischer Sicht, *Helv. Paediatr. Acta* 20:137, 1965.
10. Ammann, A. J., Meuwissen, H. J., Good, R. A., et al. Successful bone marrow transplantation in a patient with humoral and cellular immunity deficiency, *Clin. Exp. Immunol.* 7:343, 1970.
11. Ammann, R. W. Pathogenesis and etiology of regional enteritis, *in* H. L. Bockus (ed.), Gastroenterology, vol. 2, p. 242, W. B. Saunders Co., Philadelphia, 1964.
12. Archer, O. K., Kelly, W. D., Papermaster, B. W., and Good, R. A. Further morphological and immunological studies on the role of the thymus in immunobiology, *Fed. Proc.* 22:599, 1963.
13. Auerbach, R. Thymus: its role in lymphoid recovery after irradiation, *Science* 139:1061, 1963.
14. Bach, F. H., Albertini, R. J., Joo, P., et al. Bone-marrow transplantation in a patient with the Wiskott-Aldrich syndrome, *Lancet* ii:1364, 1968.
15. Bachmann, R. Studies on serum gamma A globulin level. III. Frequency of a-gamma-A globulinemia, *Scand J. Clin. Lab. Invest.* 17:316, 1965.
16. Barandun, S., Stampfli, K., Spengler, G. A., and Riva, G. Die Klinik des Antikörpermangel-syndroms, *Helv. Med. Acta* 26:163, 1959.
17. Bernuth, G. V., Minielly, J. A., Logan, G. B., and Gleich, G. J. Hodgkin's disease and thymic alymphoplasia in a 5-month-old infant, *Pediatrics* 45:792, 1970.
18. Bird, G. W. G. Cytoplasmic budding of lymphocytes in Hodgkin's disease, *Lancet* ii:1172, 1962.
19. Blaese, R. M., Oppenheim, J. J., Seeger, R. C., and Waldmann, T. A. Lymphocyte-macrophage interaction in antigen induced in vitro lymphocyte transformation in patients with the Wiskott-Aldrich syndrome and other diseases with anergy, *Cell. Immunol.* 4:228, 1972.
20. Blaese, R. M., Strober, W., Brown, R. S., et al. The Wiskott-Aldrich syndrome, *Lancet* i:1056, 1968.
21. Blizzard, R. M., and Gibbs, J. H. Candidiasis: studies pertaining to its association with endocrinopathies and pernicious anemia, *Pediatrics* 42:231, 1968.
22. Boder, E., and Sedgwick, R. P. Ataxia-telangiectasia, a familial syndrome of progressive cerebellar ataxia, oculocutaneous telangiectasia and frequent pulmonary infection, *Pediatrics* 21:526, 1958.
23. Bortin, M. M. A compendium of reported human bone marrow transplants, *Transplantation* 9:571, 1970.
24. Bouroncle, B. A., Clausen, K. P., and Aschenbrand, J. F. Studies of the delayed response of phytohemagglutinin (PHA) stimulated lymphocytes in 25 chronic lymphatic leukemia patients before and during therapy, *Blood* 34:166, 1969.
25. Breton, A., Walbaum, R., Boniface, L., Goudemand, M., and Dupont, A. Lymphocytophtisie avec dysgammaglobulinémie chez un nourrisson, *Arch. Fr. Pediatr.* 20:131, 1963.
26. Bridges, R. A., Condie, R. M., Zak, S. J., and Good, R. A. The morphologic basis of antibody formation development during the neonatal period, *J. Lab. Clin. Med.* 53:331, 1959.
27. Bruton, O. C. Agammaglobulinemia, *Pediatrics* 9:722, 1952.
28. Buckley, R. H., Amos, D. B., Kremer, W. B., and Stickel, D. L. Incompatible bone-marrow transplantation in lymphopenic immunologic deficiency: circumvention of fatal graft-versus-host disease by immunologic enhancement, *N. Engl. J. Med.* 285:1035, 1971.
29. Buescher, E. L., and Bellanti, J. A. Respiratory antibody to Franciscella tularensis in man, *Bacteriol. Rev.* 30:539, 1966.
30. Bullock, W. E. Studies of immune mechanisms in leprosy. I. Depression of delayed allergic response to skin test antigens, *N. Engl. J. Med.* 278:298, 1968.
31. Bullock, W. E., Fields, J. P., and Brandriss, M. W. An evaluation of transfer factor as immunotherapy for patients with lepromatous leprosy, *N. Engl. J. Med.* 287:1053, 1972.
32. Burke, B. A., Krovetz, L. J., and Good, R. A. Occurrence of Pneumocystis carinii pneumonia in children with agammaglobulinemia, *Pediatrics* 28:196, 1961.
33. Caramia, G., and Benatti, C. L'agammaglobulinemia "7 S" o disagammaglobulinemia, *Minerva Pediatr.* 16:492, 1964.
34. Cattan, D., Debray, C., Crabbe, P., Seligmann, M., Marche, C., and Danon, F. Duodénojéjunite infectieuse chronique avec atrophie villositaire subtotale et stéatorrhée réversible par antibiothérapie prolongée. Carence isolée en γA-immunoglobuline sérique et salivaire. Etude histologique et immunohistochimique des muqueuses

digestives, *Bull. Mem. Soc. Med. Hosp. Paris*, 117:177, 1966.

35. Centerwall, W. R., and Miller, M. M. Ataxia, telangiectasia, and sinopulmonary infections. A syndrome of slowly progressive deterioration in childhood, *Am. J. Dis. Child.* 95:385, 1958.

36. Chaptal, J., Jean, R., Bonnet, H. Robinet, M., and Rieu, D. Nouvelle forme de carence dissociée en immunoglobulines (hypo-γ, hypo-β 2M, hyper-β 2A globulinémie), *Arch. Fr. Pediatr.* 23:553, 1966.

37. Chase, M. W. Delayed-type hypersensitivity and the immunology of Hodgkin's disease, with a parallel examination of sarcoidosis, *Cancer Res.* 26:1097, 1966.

38. Chilgren, R. A., Meuwissen, H. J., Quie, P. G., Good, R. A., and Hong, R. The cellular immune defect in chronic mucocutaneous candidiasis, *Lancet* i:1286, 1969.

39. Chilgren, R. A., Quie, P. G., Meuwissen, H. J., and Hong, R. Chronic mucocutaneous candidiasis, deficiency of delayed hypersensitivity and selective local antibody defect, *Lancet* ii:688, 1967.

40. Comings, D. E. Congenital hypogammaglobulinemia, *Arch. Intern. Med.* 115:79, 1965.

41. Cooper, M. D., Chase, H. P., Lowman, J. T., Krivit, W., and Good, R. A. Wiskott-Aldrich syndrome — an immunologic deficiency disease involving the afferent limb of immunity, *Ann. J. Med.* 44:499, 1968.

42. Cooper, M. D., Lawton, A. R., and Bockman, D. E. Agammaglobulinaemia with B lymphocytes. Specific defect of plasma-cell differentiation, *Lancet* ii:791, 1971.

43. Cooper, M. D., Peterson, R. D. A., and Good, R. A. Delineation of the thymic and bursal lymphoid systems in the chicken, *Nature* 205:143, 1965.

44. Copperman, R., and Morton, H. E. Reversible inhibition of mitosis in lymphocyte cultures by non-viable mycoplasma, *Proc. Soc. Exp. Biol. Med.* 123:790, 1966.

45. Crabbé, P. A., and Heremans, J. F. Selective IgA deficiency with steatorrhea, *Am. J. Med.* 42:319, 1967.

46. Davidson, J. D., Waldmann, T. A., Goodman, D. S., and Gordon, R. S., Jr. Protein-losing gastroenteropathy in congestive heart failure, *Lancet* i:899, 1961.

47. de Bonaparte, Y., Morgenfeld, M. C., and Paradisi, E. R. Medical letter re. Bullock's studies of immune mechanisms in leprosy, *N. Engl. J. Med.* 279:49, 1968.

48. De Koning, J., Dooren, L. J., Van Bekkum, D. W., et al. Transplantation of bone-marrow cells and fetal thymus in an infant with lymphopenic immunological deficiency, *Lancet* i:1223, 1969.

49. DiGeorge, A. M. Congenital absence of the thymus and its immunological consequences, concurrence with congenital hypoparathyroidism, *in* R. A. Good and D. Bergsma (eds.), Immunologic Deficiency Diseases in Man, p. 116, National Foundation Press, New York, 1968.

50. Donohue, W. L. Alymphocytosis, *Pediatrics* 11:129, 1953.

51. Douglas, S. D., Goldberg, L. S., and Fudenberg, H. H. Clinical, serologic, and leukocyte function studies on patients with idiopathic "acquired" agammaglobulinemia and their families, *Am. J. Med.* 48:48, 1970.

52. Dunn, H. G., Meuwissen, H., Livingstone, C. S., and Pump, K. K. Ataxia-telangiectasia, *Can. Med. Assoc. J.* 91:1106, 1964.

53. Eidelman, S., and Davis, S. D. Immunoglobulin content of intestinal plasma cells in ataxia telangiectasia, *J. Clin. Invest.* 46:1051, 1967.

54. Eidelman, S., Davis, S. D., Lagunoff, D., and Rubin, C. E. The relationship between intestinal plasma cells and serum immunoglobulin A (IgA) in man, *J. Clin. Invest.* 45:1003, 1966.

55. Eisen, A. H., Karpati, G., Laszlo, T., Andermann, F., Robb, J. P., and Bacal, H. L. Immunologic deficiency in ataxia telangiectasia, *N. Engl. J. Med.* 272:18, 1965.

56. Fahey, J. L. Heterogeneity of γ-globulins, *Adv. Immunol.* 2:41, 1962.

57. Fairley, G. H., and Scott, R. B. Hypogammaglobulinaemia in chronic lymphatic leukaemia, *Br. Med. J.* 2:920, 1961.

58. Fireman, P., Boesman, M., and Gitlin, D. Ataxia telangiectasia, a dysgammaglobulinaemia with deficient γ1A (β2A)-globulin, *Lancet* i:1193, 1964.

59. Fireman, P., Johnson, H. A., and Gitlin, D. Presence of plasma cells and γ₁ M-globulin synthesis in a patient with thymic alymphoplasia, *Pediatrics* 37:485, 1966.

60. Fisher, E. R. Pathology of the thymus and its relation to human disease, *in* R. A. Good and A. E. Gabrielsen (eds.), The Thymus in Immunobiology, p. 676, Hoeber-Harper, New York, 1964.

61. Fudenberg, H. H., German, J. L. III, and Kunkel, H. G. The occurrence of rheumatoid factor and other abnormalities in families of patients with agammaglobulinemia, *Arthritis Rheum.* 5:565, 1962.

62. Fulginiti, V. A., Hathaway, W. E., Pearlman, D. S., Blackburn, W. R., Reiquam, C. W., Githens, J. H., Claman, H. N., and Kempe, C. H. Dissociation of delayed-hypersensitivity and antibody-synthesizing capacities in man, *Lancet* ii:5, 1966.

63. Gafni, J., Michaeli, D., and Heller, H. Idiopathic acquired agammaglobulinemia associated with thymoma. Report of two cases and review of the literature. *N. Engl. J. Med.* 263:536, 1960.

64. Gatti, R. A., Gershanik, J. J., Levkoff, A. H., Wertelecki, W., and Good, R. A. DiGeorge syndrome associated with combined immunodeficiency. *J. Pediatr.* 81:920, 1972.

65. Gatti, R. A., and Good, R. A. Occurrence of malignancy in immunodeficiency disease. A literature review, *Cancer* 28:89, 1971.

66. Gatti, R. A., and Good, R. A. Follow-up of correction of severe dual system immunodeficiency with bone marrow transplantation, *J. Pediatr.* 79:475, 1971.

67. Giblett, E. R., Anderson, J. E., Cohen, F., et al. Adenosine-deaminase deficiency in two patients with severely impaired cellular immunity, *Lancet* ii:1067, 1972.

68. Gitlin, D., and Craig, J. M. The thymus and other lymphoid tissues in congenital agammaglobulinemia. I. Thymic alymphoplasia and lymphocytic hypoplasia and their rela-

tion to infection, *Pediatrics* 32:517, 1963.

69. Gitlin, D., Janeway, C. A., Apt, L., and Craig, J. M. Agammaglobulinemia, *in* H. S. Lawrence (ed.), Cellular and Humoral Aspects of Hypersensitivity States, p. 375, Paul B. Hoeber, New York, 1959.

70. Glanzmann, E., and Riniker, P. Essentielle Lymphozytophthise. Ein neues Krankheitsbild aus der Säuglingspathologie, *Wien. Med. Wochenschr.* 100:35, 1950.

71. Glick, B., Chang, T. S., and Jaap, R. G. The bursa of Fabricius and antibody production, *Poultry Sci.* 35:224, 1956.

72. Godal, T., Myklestad, B., Samuel, D. R., and Myrvang, B. Characterization of the cellular immune defect in lepromatous leprosy: a specific lack of circulating *Mycobacterium leprae* reactive lymphocytes, *Clin. Exp. Immunol.* 9:821, 1971.

73. Godfrey, S. Thymoma with hypogammaglobulinaemia in an identical twin, *Br. Med. J.* 2:1159, 1964.

74. Goldberg, L. S., Barnett, E. V., and Fudenberg, H. H. Selective absence of IgA; a family study, *J. Lab. Clin. Med.* 72:204, 1968.

75. Good, R. A. Agammaglobulinemia: a provocative experiment of nature, *Bull. Univ. Minn. Hosp.* 26:1, 1954.

76. Good, R. A., Bridges, R. A., and Condie, R. M. Host-parasite relationships in patients with dysproteinemias, *Bact. Rev.* 24:115, 1960.

77. Good, R. A., and Gabrielsen, A. E. (eds.) The Thymus in Immunobiology, Hoeber-Harper, New York, 1964.

78. Good, R. A., Kelly, W. D., Rötstein, J., and Varco, R. L. Immunological deficiency diseases, *Prog. Allergy* 6:187, 1962.

79. Good, R. A., Martinez, C., Dalmasso, A. P., Papermaster, B. W., and Gabrielsen, A. E. Studies on the role of the thymus in developmental biology, with a consideration of the association of thymus abnormalities and clinical disease, *in* Third International Symposium, Immunopathology, p. 177, Benno Schwabe, Basel, 1963.

80. Good, R. A., and Page, A. R. Fatal complications of virus hepatitis in two patients with agammaglobulin-

emia, *Am. J. Med.* 29:804, 1960.

81. Good, R. A., and Varco, R. L. A clinical and experimental study of agammaglobulinemia, *J. Lancet* 75:245, 1955.

82. Good, R. A., and Zak, S. J. Disturbances in gamma globulin synthesis as "experiments of nature," *Pediatrics* 18:109, 1956.

83. Gordon, R. R. Aldrich's syndrome: familial thrombocytopenia, eczema and infection, *Arch. Dis. Child.* 35:259, 1960.

84. Hanson, L. A. Aspects of the absence of the IgA system, *in* R. A. Good and D. Bergsma (eds.), Immunologic Deficiency Diseases in Man, vol. 4, p. 292, National Foundation Press, New York, 1968.

85. Harrington, H. Absence of the thymus gland, *London Med. Gaz.* iii:314, 1829.

86. Hart, M. N., and Schwartz, D. C. Thymic agenesis. Report of a case, *Arch. Pathol.* 88:437, 1969.

87. Haworth, J. C., Hoogstraten, J., and Taylor, H. Thymic alymphoplasia, *Arch. Dis. Child.* 42:40, 1967.

88. Hersh, E. M., and Oppenheim, J. J. Impaired in vitro lymphocyte transformation in Hodgkin's disease, *N. Engl. J. Med.* 273:1006, 1965.

89. Hitzig, W. H. The Swiss type of agammaglobulinemia, *in* R. A. Good and D. Bergsma (eds.), Immunologic Deficiency Diseases in Man, vol. 4, p. 82, National Foundation Press, New York, 1968.

90. Hitzig, W. H., Biró, Z., Bosch, H., and Huser, H. Agammaglobulinämie und Alymphocytose mit Schwund des lymphatischen Gewebes, *Helv. Paediatr. Acta* 13:551, 1958.

91. Hitzig, W. H., and Willi, H. Hereditäre lymphoplasmocytäre Dysgenesie ("Allymphocytose mit Agammaglobulinämie"), *Schweiz. Med. Wochenschr.* 91:1625, 1961.

92. Hobbs, J. R., Milner, R. D. G., and Watt, P. J. Gamma-M deficiency predisposing to meningococcae septicaemia, *Br. Med. J.* 4:583, 1967.

93. Hobbs, J. R., Russell, A., and Worledge, S. M. Dysgammaglobulinaemia type IV C, *Clin. Exp. Immunol.* 2:589, 1967.

94. Hong, R., and Amman, A. J. Selec-

tive absence of IgA, *Am. J. Pathol.* 69:491, 1972.

95. Hoyer, J. R., Cooper, M. D., Gabrielsen, A. E., and Good, R. A. Lymphopenic forms of congenital immunologic deficiency diseases, *Medicine* 47:201, 1968.

96. Huang, S-W., Lattos, D. B., Nelson, D. B., Reeb, K., and Hong, R. Antibody-associated lymphotoxin in acute infection, *J. Clin. Invest.* 52:1033, 1973.

97. Huber, J., Cholnoky, P., and Zoethout, H. E. Congenital aplasia of parathyroid glands and thymus, *Arch. Dis. Child.* 42:190, 1967.

98. Hughes, W. S., Cerda, J. J., Holtzapple, P., and Brooks, F. P. Primary hypogammaglobulinemia and malabsorption, *Ann. Intern. Med.* 74:903, 1971.

99. Huntley, C. C., and Dees, S. C. Eczema associated with thrombocytopenic purpura and purulent otitis media. Report of five fatal cases, *Pediatrics* 19:351, 1957.

100. Hutchison, J. H. Congenital agammaglobulinaemia, *Lancet* ii:844, 1955.

101. Israel, H. L. Sarcoidosis, *in* M. Samter and H. L. Alexander (eds.), Immunological Diseases, p. 406, Little, Brown and Co., Boston, 1965.

102. Jacox, R. F., Mongan, E. S., Hanshaw, J. B., and Leddy, J. P. Hypogammaglobulinemia with thymoma and probable pulmonary infection with cytomegalovirus, *N. Engl. J. Med.* 271:1091, 1964.

103. Janeway, C. A., and Gitlin, D. Gamma globulins, *Adv. Pediatr.* 9:65, 1957.

104. Jeune, M., Larbre, F., Germain, D., and Freycon, F. Lymphocytophtisie, alymphocytose et hypogammaglobulinémie, *Arch. Fr. Pediatr.* 16:14, 1959.

105. Jeunet, F. S., and Good, R. A. Thymoma, immunologic deficiencies and hematological abnormalities, *in* R. A. Good and D. Bergsma (eds.), Immunologic Deficiency Diseases in Man, vol. 4, p. 192, National Foundation Press, New York, 1968.

106. Jim, R. T. S. Serum gamma globulin levels in chronic lymphocytic leukemia, *Am. J. Med. Sci.* 234:44, 1957.

107. Kelly, W. D., Good, R. A., and

Varco, R. L. Anergy and skin homograft survival in Hodgkin's disease, *Surg. Gynecol. Obstet.* 107:565, 1958.

108. Kelly, W. D., Lamb, D. L., Varco, R. L., and Good, R. A. An investigation of Hodgkin's disease with respect to the problem of homotransplantation, *Ann. N.Y. Acad. Sci.* 87:187, 1960.

109. Kirkpatrick, C. H., Chandler, J. W., Jr., and Schimke, R. N. Chronic mucocutaneous moniliasis with impaired delayed hypersensitivity, *Clin. Exp. Immunol.* 6:375, 1970

110. Kirkpatrick, C. H., Rich, R. R., Graw, R. G., Jr., et al. Treatment of chronic mucocutaneous moniliasis by immunologic reconstitution, *Clin. Exp. Immunol.* 9:733, 1971.

111. Knapp, E. L., and Routh, J. I. Electrophoretic studies of plasma proteins in normal children, *Pediatrics* 4:508, 1949.

112. Krivit, W., and Good, R. A. Aldrich's syndrome (thrombocytopenia, eczema, and infection in infants). Studies of the defense mechanisms, *Am. J. Dis. Child.* 97:137, 1959.

113. Kulneff, N., Pedersen, K. O., and Waldenström, J. Drei Fälle von Agammaglobulinämie. Ein klinischer, genetischer und physikalischchemischer Beitrag zur Kenntnis des Proteinstoffwechsels, *Schweiz. Med. Wochenschr.* 85:363, 1955.

114. Lambie, A. T., Burrows, B. A., and Sommers, S. C. Clinicopathologic conference. Refractory anemia, agammaglobulinemia, and mediastinal tumor, *Am. J. Clin. Pathol.* 27:444, 1957.

115. Laster, L., Waldmann, T. A., Fenster, L. F., and Singleton, J. W. Albumin metabolism in patients with Whipple's disease, *J. Clin. Invest.* 45:637, 1966.

116. Lawrence, H. S., and Zweiman, B. Transfer factor deficiency response—a mechanism of anergy in Boeck's sarcoid, *Trans. Assoc. Am. Physicians* 81:240, 1968.

117. Levey, R. H., Klemperer, M. R., Gelfand, E. W., et al. Bone-marrow transplantation in severe combined immunodeficiency syndrome, *Lancet* ii:571, 1971.

118. Lindberg, T., and Palmgren, B. Wiskott-Aldrich-Syndrom: Thrombozytopenie, Ekzem sowie Neigung zu Infektionen, *Arch. Kinderheilkd.* 166:164, 1962.

119. Lischner, H. W., Punnett, H. H., and DiGeorge, A. M. Lymphocytes in congenital absence of the thymus, *Nature* 214:580, 1967.

120. McFarlin, D. E., Strober, W., and Waldmann, T. A. Ataxia-telangiectasia, *Medicine* 51:281, 1972.

121. McGregor, D. D., and Gowans, J. L. Survival of homografts of skin in rats depleted of lymphocytes by chronic drainage from the thoracic duct, *Lancet* i:629, 1964.

122. Margulis, A. R., Feinberg, S. B., Lester, R. G., and Good, R. A. Roentgen manifestations of congenital agammaglobulinemia, *Radiology* 69:354, 1957.

123. Marmor, M. F., and Barnett, E. V. Cutaneous anergy without systemic disease, *Am. J. Med.* 44:979, 1968.

124. Martin, C. M., Gordon, R. S., and McCullough, N. B. Acquired hypogammaglobulinemia in an adult. Report of a case, with clinical and experimental studies, *N. Engl. J. Med.* 254:449, 1956.

125. Martinez, C., Kersey, J., Papermaster, B. W., and Good, R. A. Skin homograft survival in thymectomized mice, *Proc. Soc. Exp. Biol. Med.* 109:193, 1962.

126. Mella, B., and Lang, D. J. Leucocyte mitosis: suppression in vitro associated with acute infectious hepatitis, *Science* 155:80, 1967.

127. Mellman, W. J., Plotkin, S. A., Moorhead, P. S., and Hartnett, E. M. Rubella infection of human leucocytes, *Am. J. Dis. Child.* 110:473, 1965.

128. Meuwissen, H. J., Gatti, R. A., Terasaki, P., Hong, R., and Good, R. A. Treatment of lymphopenic hypogammaglobulinemia and bone-marrow aplasia by transplantation of allogeneic marrow. Crucial role of histocompatibility matching, *N. Engl. J. Med.* 281:691, 1969.

129. Miller, J. F. A. P. Immunological function of the thymus, *Lancet* ii:748, 1961.

130. Miller, J. F. A. P. Immunology. Immunological significance of the thymus of the adult mouse, *Nature* 195:1318, 1962.

131. Miller, J. F. A. P., and Mitchell, G. F. Thymus and antigen-reactive cells, *Transplant. Rev.* 1:3, 1969.

132. Miller, J. F. A. P., and Osoba, D. Current concepts of the immunological function of the thymus, *Physiol. Rev.* 47:437, 1967.

133. Miller, M. E., and Schieken, R. M. Thymic dysplasia. A separable entity from "Swiss agammaglobulinemia," *Am. J. Med. Sci.* 253:741, 1967.

134. Mills, S. D., and Winkleman, R. K. Eczema, thrombocytopenic purpura, and recurring infections, *Arch. Dermatol.* 79:466, 1959.

135. Mistilis, S. P., Skyring, A. P., and Stephen, D. D. Intestinal lymphangiectasia: mechanism of enteric loss of plasma-protein and fat, *Lancet* i:77, 1965.

136. Montgomery, J. R., South, M. A., Rawls, W. E., Melnick, J. L., Olson, G. B., Dent, P. B., and Good, R. A. Viral inhibition of lymphocyte response to phytohemagglutinin, *Science* 157:1068, 1967.

137. Moroz, C., Amir, J., and De Vries, A. A hereditary immunoglobulin A abnormality: absence of light–heavy-chain assembly, *J. Clin. Invest.* 50:2726, 1971.

138. Nezelof, C., Jammet, M. L., Lortholary, P., Labrune, B., and Lamy, M. L'hypoplasie héréditaire du thymus: sa place et sa responsabilité dans une observation d'aplasie lymphocytaire, normoplasmocytaire, et normoglobulinémique du nourrisson, *Arch. Fr. Pediatr.* 21:897, 1964.

139. Olson, G. B., South, M. A., and Good, R. A. Phytohaemagglutinin unresponsiveness of lymphocytes from babies with congenital rubella, *Nature* 214:695, 1967.

140. Oppenheim, J. J., Whang, J., and Frei, E. III. Immunologic and cytogenetic studies of chronic lymphocytic leukemic cells, *Blood* 26:121, 1965.

141. Orlandini, O., Sass-Kortsuk, A., and Ebbs, J. H. Serum gamma globulin levels in normal infants, *Pediatrics* 16:575, 1955.

142. Osserman, E. F., and Takatsuki, K. Plasma cell myeloma: gamma globulin synthesis and structure. A review of biochemical and clinical data, with the description of a newly-recognized and related syn-

drome, "H$^{\gamma-2}$-chain (Franklin's) disease," *Medicine* 42:357, 1963.

143. Page, A. R., Hansen, A. E., and Good, R. A. Occurrence of leukemia and lymphoma in patients with agammaglobulinemia, *Blood* 21:197, 1963.

144. Petersen, V. P., and Hastrup, J. Protein-losing enteropathy in constrictive pericarditis, *Acta Med. Scand.* 173:401, 1963.

145. Peterson, R. D. A., Cooper, M. D., and Good, R. A. The pathogenesis of immunologic deficiency diseases, *Am. J. Med.* 38:579, 1965.

146. Peterson, R. D. A., Cooper, M. D., and Good, R. A. Lymphoid tissue abnormalities associated with ataxia-telangiectasia, *Am. J. Med.* 41:342, 1966.

147. Peterson, R. D. A., Kelley, W., and Good, R. A. Ataxia-telangiectasia, *Lancet* i:1189, 1964.

148. Pincus, S., Bianco, C., and Nussenzweig, V. Increase proportion of complement-receptor lymphocytes in the peripheral blood of patients with chronic lymphocytic leukemia, *Blood* 40:303, 1972.

149. Polmar, S. H., Waldmann, T. A., Balestra, S. T., et al. Immunoglobulin E in immunologic deficiency diseases, *J. Clin. Invest.* 51:326, 1972.

150. Porter, H. M. Immunologic studies in congenital agammaglobulinemia, with emphasis on delayed hypersensitivity, *Pediatrics* 20:958, 1957.

151. Prasad, A. S., and Koza, D. W. Agammaglobulinemia, *Ann. Intern. Med.* 41:629, 1954.

152. Ramos, A. J. Presentation of case, *J.A.M.A.* 160:1317, 1956.

153. Rees, R. J. W. The significance of the lepromin reaction in man, *Prog. Allergy* 8:224, 1964.

154. Reisman, L. E., Mitani, M., and Zuelzer, W. W. Chromosome studies on leukemic children with and without congenital abnormalities, *J. Pediatr.* 63:739, 1963.

155. Rockey, J. H., Hanson, L. A., Heremans, J. F., and Kunkel, H. G. Beta-2A aglobulinemia in two healthy men, *J. Lab. Clin. Med.* 63:205, 1964.

156. Rocklin, R. E., Chilgren, R. A., Hong, R., and David, J. R. Transfer of cellular hypersensitivity in chronic mucocutaneous candidiasis

monitored in vivo and in vitro, *Cell. Immunol.* 1:290, 1970.

157. Rosen, F. S., Gitlin, D., and Janeway, C. A. Alymphocytosis, agammaglobulinaemia, homografts, and delayed hypersensitivity: study of a case, *Lancet* ii:380, 1962.

158. Rosen, F. S., and Janeway, C. A. The gamma globulins, *N. Engl. J. Med.* 275:709, 1966.

159. Rosen, F. S., Kevy, S., Merler, E., Janeway, C. A., and Gitlin, D. Recurrent bacterial infections and dysgammaglobulinemia, deficiency of 7S gamma-globulins in presence of elevated 19S gamma globulin: report of two cases, *Pediatrics* 28:182, 1961.

160. Rosenthal, I. M., Markowitz, A. S., and Medenis, R. Immunologic incompetence in ataxia-telaniectasia, *Am. J. Dis. Child.* 110:69, 1965.

161. Ross, J. F., Finch, S. C., Street, R. B., Jr., and Streider, J. W. The simultaneous occurrence of benign thymoma and refractory anemia, *Blood* 9:935, 1954.

162. Rothberg, R. M., and Ten Bensel, R. W. Thymic alymphoplasia with immunoglobulin synthesis, *Am. J. Dis. Child.* 113:639, 1967.

163. Rubin, C. E., Brandborg, L. L., Phelps, P. C., and Taylor, H. C. Studies of celiac disease. I. The apparent identical and specific nature of the duodenal and proximal jejunal lesion in celiac disease and idiopathic sprue, *Gastroenterology* 38:28, 1960.

164. Rubinstein, A., Speck, B., and Jeannet, M. Successful bone-marrow transplantation in a lymphopenic immunologic deficiency syndrome, *N. Engl. J. Med.* 285:1399, 1971.

165. Russell, J. G. B. Pneumocystis pneumonia associated with agammaglobulinaemia, *Arch. Dis. Child.* 34:338, 1959.

166. Sacrez, R., Willard, D., Beauvais, P., and Korn, R. Etude des troubles digestifs et respiratoires dans un cas de lymphocytophtisie du nourrisson, *Arch. Fr. Pediatr.* 20:401, 1963.

167. Schaller, J., Davis, S. D., Ching, Y., Lagunoff, D., Williams, C. P. S., and Wedgwood, R. J. Hypergammaglobulinaemia, antibody deficiency, autoimmune haemolytic

anaemia and nephritis in an infant with a familial lymphopenic immune defect, *Lancet* i:825, 1966.

168. Schwartz, R. S. Immunoregulation, oncogenic viruses, and malignant lymphomas, *Lancet* i:1266, 1972.

169. Seeger, R. C., Ammann, A. J., Good, R. A., and Hong, R. Progressive lymphoid system deterioration: a new familial lymphopenic immunological deficiency disease, *Clin. Exp. Immunol.* 6:169, 1970.

170. Seligmann, M., Fudenberg, H. H., and Good, R. A. A proposed classification of primary immunologic deficiencies, *Am. J. Med.* 45:817, 1968.

171. Sharman, C., Crossen, P. E., and Fitzgerald, P. H. Lymphocyte number and response to phytohaemagglutinin in chronic lymphocytic leukaemia, *Scand. J. Haematol.* 3:375, 1966.

172. Shevach, E. M., Herberman, R., Frank, M. M., et al. Receptors for complement and immunoglobulins on human leukemic cells and human lymphoblastoid cell lines, *J. Clin. Invest.* 51:1933, 1972.

173. Shuster, J., Hart, Z., Stimson, C. W., Brough, A. J., and Poulik, M. D. Ataxia telangiectasia with cerebellar tumor, *Pediatrics* 37:776, 1966.

174. Sjöberg, K-H. Moniliasis—an internal disease?, *Acta Med. Scand.* 179:157, 1966.

175. Soothill, J. F., Hayes, K., and Dudgeon, J. A. The immunoglobulins in congenital rubella, *Lancet* i:1385, 1966.

176. South, M. A., Cooper, M. D., Wollheim, F. A., Hong, R., and Good, R. A. The IgA system. I. Studies of the transport and immunochemistry of IgA in the saliva, *J. Exp. Med.* 123:615, 1966.

177. St. Geme, J. W., Jr., Prince, J. T., Burke, B. A., Good, R. A., and Krivit, W. Impaired cellular resistance to herpes-simplex virus in Wiskott-Aldrich syndrome, *N. Engl. J. Med.* 273:229, 1965.

178. Stiehm, E. R., and Fudenberg, H. H. Clinical and immunological features of dysgammaglobulinemia type 1, *Am. J. Med.* 40:805, 1966.

179. Stiehm, E. R., Lawlor, G. J., Jr., Kaplan, M. S., et al. Immunologic reconstitution in severe combined

immunodeficiency without bone-marrow chromosomal chimerism, *N. Engl. J. Med.* 286:797, 1972.

180. Stiehm, E. R., and McIntosh, R. M. Wiskott-Aldrich syndrome: a review and report of a large family, *Clin. Exp. Immunol.* 2:179, 1967.

181. Stoelinga, G. B. A., Van Munster, P. J. J., and Slooff, J. P. Chylous effusions into the intestine in a patient with protein-losing gastroenteropathy, *Pediatrics* 31:1011, 1963.

182. Strober, W., Cohen, L. S., Waldmann, T. A., and Braunwald, E. Tricuspid regurgitation. A newly recognized cause of protein-losing enteropathy, lymphocytopenia and immunologic deficiency, *Am. J. Med.* 44:842, 1968.

183. Strober, W., Wochner, R. D., Barlow, M. H., McFarlin, D. E., and Waldmann, T. A. Immunoglobulin metabolism in ataxia telangiectasia, *J. Clin. Invest.* 47:1905, 1968.

184. Strober, W., Wochner, R. D., Carbone, P. P., and Waldmann, T. A. Intestinal lymphangiectasia: a protein-losing enteropathy with hypogammaglobulinemia, lymphocytopenia and impaired homograft rejection, *J. Clin. Invest.* 46:1643, 1967.

185. Taitz, L. S., Zarate-Salvador, C., and Schwartz, E. Congenital absence of the parathyroid and thymus glands in an infant. (III and IV pharyngeal pouch syndrome), *Pediatrics* 38:412, 1966.

186. Thieffry, S., Arthuis, M., Aicardi, J., and Lyon, G. L'ataxie-télangiectasie (7 observations personnelles), *Rev. Neurol.* 105:390, 1961.

187. Thomson, A. D., and Thackray, A. C. The histology of tumours of the thymus, *Br. J. Cancer* 11:348, 1957.

188. Tobler, R., and Cottier, H. Familiäre Lymphopenie mit Agammaglobulinämie und schwerer Moniliasis. Die "essentielle Lymphocytophtisie" als besondere Form der frühkindlichen Agammaglobulinämie, *Helv. Paediatr. Acta* 13:313, 1958.

189. Tomasi, T. B., Jr., and Bienenstock, J. Secretory immunoglobulins, *Adv. Immunol.* 9:2, 1968.

190. Tomasi, T. B., Jr., Tan, E. M., Solomon, A., and Prendergast, R. A. Characteristics of an immune system common to certain external secretions, *J. Exp. Med.* 121:101, 1965.

191. Turk, J. L., and Bryceson, A. D. M. Immunological phenomena in leprosy and related diseases, *Adv. Immunol.* 13:209, 1971.

192. Urbach, F., Sones, M., and Israel, H. L. Passive transfer of tuberculin sensitivity to patients with sarcoidosis, *N. Engl. J. Med.* 247:794, 1952.

193. Waldenström, J. Monoclonal and polyclonal gammopathies and the biological system of gamma globulins, *Prog. Allergy* 6:320, 1962.

194. Waldmann, T. A. Protein-losing enteropathy, *Gastroenterology* 50:422, 1966.

195. Waldmann, T. A., and Laster, L. Abnormalities of albumin metabolism in patients with hypogammaglobulinemia, *J. Clin. Invest.* 43:1025, 1964.

196. Waldmann, T. A., and Schwab, P. J. IgG (7S gamma globulin) metabolism in hypogammaglobulinemia: studies in patients with defective gamma globulin synthesis, gastrointestinal protein loss, or both, *J. Clin. Invest.* 44:1523, 1965.

197. Waldmann, T. A., Strober, W., and Blaese, R. M. Immunodeficiency disease and malignancy, *Ann. Intern. Med.* 77:605, 1972.

198. Waldmann, T. A., Wochner, R. D., Laster, L., and Gordon, R. S., Jr. Allergic gastroenteropathy. A cause of excessive gastrointestinal protein loss, *N. Engl. J. Med.* 276:761, 1967.

199. Warner, N. L., Szenberg, A., and Burnett, F. M. The immunological role of different lymphoid organs in the chicken. I. Dissociation of immunological responsiveness, *Aust. J. Exp. Biol. Med. Sci.* 40:373, 1962.

200. Weiden, P. L., Blaese, R. M.,

Strober, W., et al. Impaired lymphocyte transformation in intestinal lymphangiectasia: evidence for at least two functionally distinct lymphocyte populations in man, *J. Clin. Invest.* 51:1319, 1972.

201. West, C. D., Hong, R., and Holland, N. H. Immunoglobulin levels from newborn period to adulthood and in immunoglobulin deficiency states, *J. Clin. Invest.* 41:2054, 1962.

202. White, L. R., Leikin, S., Villavicencio, O., et al. Immune competence in congenital rubella: lymphocyte transformation, delayed hypersensitivity and response to vaccination, *J. Pediatr.* 73:229, 1968.

203. Wiskott, A. Familiärer angeborener Morbus Werlhofi, *Monatsschr. Kinderheilkd.* 68:212, 1937.

204. Wolf, J. K. Primary acquired agammaglobulinemia, with a family history of collagen disease and hematologic disorders, *N. Engl. J. Med.* 266:473, 1962.

205. Wollheim, F. Inherited "acquired" hypogammaglobulinaemia, *Lancet* i:316, 1961.

206. Wollheim, F. A., Belfrage, S., Cöster, C., and Lindholm, H. Primary "acquired" hypogammaglobulinemia. Clinical and genetic aspects of nine cases, *Acta Med. Scand.* 176:1, 1964.

207. Wortis, H. H. Immunological responses of "nude" mice, *Clin. Exp. Immunol.* 8:305, 1971.

208. Yamamura, M., Newton, R. C. F., James, D. C. O., et al. Uncomplicated HL-A matched sibling bone marrow graft for combined immune deficiency, *Br. Med. J.* 2:265, 1972.

209. Young, R. C., Corder, M. P., Haynes, H. A., et al. Delayed hypersensitivity in Hodgkin's disease, *Am. J. Med.* 52:63, 1972.

210. Young, R. R., Austen, K. F., and Moser, H. W. Abnormalities of serum gamma 1A globulin and ataxia telangiectasia, *Medicine* 43:423, 1964.

Chapter 19 Chronic Lymphocytic Leukemia

Shortly after the initial description of leukemia by Virchow and Bennett in 1845, Virchow also described the entity we now identify as chronic lymphocytic leukemia (147). Chronic lymphocytic leukemia (or chronic lymphatic leukemia, CLL) may be defined as a disease of adult life in which there is a great increase in the numbers of mature lymphocytes in the circulation and in the lymphoid organs of the body. The manifestations of the disease are related to the proliferation of neoplastic cells: direct organ infiltration; loss of normal hematopoietic cells; immunologic abnormalities with increased susceptibility to infection and, in some patients, "autoimmune" phenomena such as hemolytic anemia and thrombocytopenia.

Chronic lymphocytic leukemia as a rule is easy to diagnose, since few other conditions in adult life produce such striking lymphocytosis and lymphadenopathy. Occasionally patients with CLL are encountered who have only slight increases in the number of lymphocytes and little or no palpable lymphadenopathy; in such patients the correct diagnosis becomes apparent with the passage of time. Difficulty may occasionally be encountered in differentiating chronic lymphocytic leukemia from lymphosarcoma that has infiltrated the bone marrow and "spilled over" into the circulating blood (162).

In Chapter 12 the morphogenesis of the normal lymphoid series was reviewed. In that and subsequent chapters, the complex interrelations between B cells and T cells were analyzed and the various morphologic forms of these cells were illustrated.

It is not surprising that a neoplastic counterpart exists for each of the maturational stages of the various lymphoid cells. Thus in the catalogue of human diseases one encounters B-cell malignancies and T-cell malignancies. Each of these may be further categorized by the maturational status of the predominant cell. This status may range from morphologically and functionally undifferentiated cells (as in acute lymphocytic leukemia) to highly differentiated lymphocytes and plasma cells.

In this chapter, and Chapters 20 and 22, the chronic lymphoproliferative syndromes are discussed. These include chronic lymphocytic leukemia, multiple myeloma, macroglobulinemia and the other monoclonal gammopathies, and the lymphocytic lymphomas. For convenience, Hodgkin's disease is listed among the lymphoproliferative disorders, although it is not certain that the lymphocyte is the neoplastic cell in this disease. Further knowledge may dictate a reclassification of Hodgkin's disease.

Another neoplastic disease of uncertain classification is leukemic reticuloendotheliosis or "hairy cell" leukemia. It is characterized by a chronic course, marked splenomegaly, and characteristic cells in the bone marrow, spleen, and lymph nodes. It is uncertain whether the malignant cells belong to the reticulum cell, histiocyte, or lymphoid cell series (17, 41, 45, 117, 124, 161). Recent evidence favors an origin in the lymphoid or reticulum cell series (see Chapter 27 for a more detailed discussion).

Many analogies exist between the chronic myeloproliferative (Chapter 10) and the chronic lymphoproliferative disorders. In both classes of disease the individual syndromes reflect the proliferation of one or more cell lines arising from a common pluripotent progenitor (see Figs. I.1 and 10.1).

Cytologic and Histologic Features

In chronic lymphocytic leukemia the peripheral smear is characterized by its monotony. The predominant feature is a great increase in the numbers of small lymphocytes, which may be more or less normal in appearance. Another feature of the peripheral blood smear is the frequent occurrence of broken lymphocytes or "basket cells."

As described in Chapters 12 and 13, a variety of small, intermediate, and large lymphocytes may be encountered in the blood, bone marrow, lymphoid tissues, and thoracic duct lymph of normal man. A similar variety of morphologic types of lymphocytes may be encountered in the blood of patients with chronic lymphocytic leukemia, although extremely immature forms such as those seen in acute lymphocytic leukemia (13) are rarely seen. In a given patient a single morphologic type of cell generally predominates throughout the course of his illness, giving the peripheral blood smear its monotonous appearance.

In 1924 Minot and Isaacs described large atypical lymphocytes from patients with chronic lymphocytic leukemia and related these cells to more rapidly progressive disease (91). Linman (84, 162) has suggested that the cells of chronic lymphocytic leukemia can be separated into two major types: small lymphocytes with exaggerated clumping of basichromatin, and large cells with prominent nucleoli. This is probably an oversimplified statement of a complex situation. Usually there is some heterogeneity among the cells of an individual patient and wide differences among patients. Examples of chronic lymphocytic leukemic cells are shown in Figs. 19.1 to 19.5. In this series of photographs the cells appear to be progressively less mature when judged by the usual morphologic criteria.

In chronic lymphocytic leukemia the white blood count may be greatly in excess of 100,000 per cubic millimeter of blood, with lymphocytes comprising 90 to 99 percent of the cells. These lymphocytes have a high ratio of nucleus to cytoplasm (Figs. 19.1 to 19.4). They may have only a thin rim of blue cytoplasm or they may appear to be entirely lacking cytoplasm (Figs. 19.1 and 19.3). Intracytoplasmic reddish granules are rare (see Fig. 19.6). The nuclear chromatin may be very dense (Fig. 19.1) or it may be more transparent than that seen in normal lymphocytes (Fig. 19.4). Folded or indented nuclei are not uncommon (Figs. 19.3 and 19.4), and nucleoli occasionally

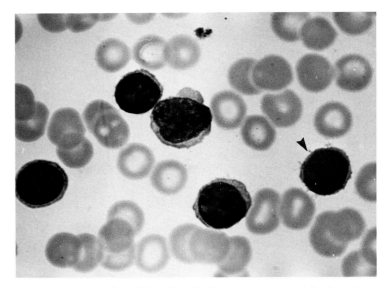

Figure 19.1 Peripheral blood cells from a patient with chronic lymphocytic leukemia. These cells resemble normal small lymphocytes except for the cell (*arrow*) with cytoplasmic projections. Giemsa stain.

are seen. The cells tend to lack the morphologic features of extreme immaturity that characterize the lymphoblast (see Chapters 12 and 21).

The cells infiltrating the lymph nodes, spleen, and bone marrow appear to be histologically similar to those in the blood. Generally, the normal architecture of these organs is destroyed and replaced by dense accumulations of small

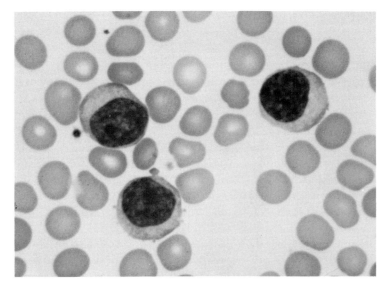

Figure 19.2 Cells from a patient with chronic lymphocytic leukemia. They resemble normal medium-sized lymphocytes. Giemsa stain.

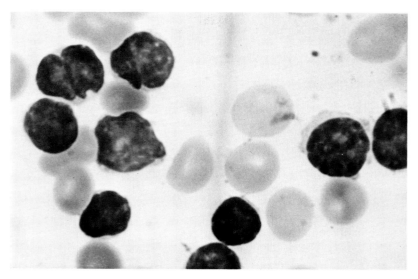

Figure 19.3 Peripheral blood cells from a patient with chronic lymphocytic leukemia demonstrating morphologic heterogeneity. Binucleate and immature cells are present. Giemsa stain.

lymphocytes. A variety of other tissues may be infiltrated with small round cells, including the tonsils, salivary and lacrimal glands (66, 116), skin (68, 159), gastrointestinal tract (26, 111), thymus (9), lungs and pleura (55), and eye (152, 159).

Incidence, Age, and Sex Distribution
The limitations in determining the precise incidence of a

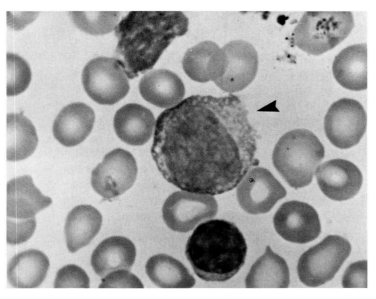

Figure 19.5 A very immature lymphoid cell (*arrow*) in the blood of a patient with chronic lymphocytic leukemia.

given morphologic type of leukemia are discussed in detail in Chapter 10.

In a number of reported series of patients between 1920 and 1967, chronic lymphocytic leukemia accounted for between 22 and 32 percent (mean, 29 percent) of all leukemias (7, 8, 12, 50, 115, 157). Chronic lymphocytic leukemia is said to be relatively common among Jews (102) and very uncommon among the Oriental populations of

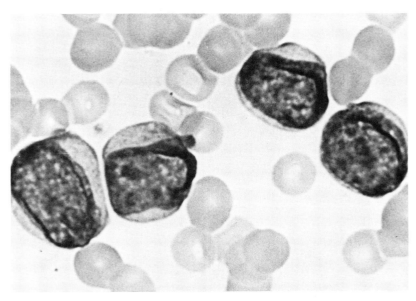

Figure 19.4 Morphologically immature cells from the blood of a patient with chronic lymphocytic leukemia. Note the prominent nucleoli.

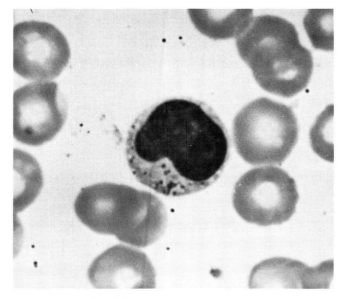

Figure 19.6 Peripheral blood lymphocyte with prominent cytoplasmic granules. Giemsa stain.

China and Japan (61, 137, 142, 150) and the New Zealand Maoris (57).

In the United States the case incidence of leukemia is approximately 60 per million population per year, with chronic lymphocytic leukemia constituting between 20 and 30 percent of the total (7, 114, 135). In Japan the overall incidence of leukemia is about 30 cases per million per year (18), and chronic lymphocytic leukemia constitutes only 2 to 3 percent of the total (149). This low incidence of chronic lymphocytic leukemia is also found among Japanese-Americans.

Chronic lymphocytic leukemia is a disease of late life. In different series the peak incidence has varied between ages 45 and 54 (91), 50 and 69 (115), and 55 years (27, 83, 86, 136, 154). In these series, as well as others (60, 136), males have predominated, the ratio of males to females being in the range of 2. Documented cases of chronic lymphocytic leukemia occurring in childhood are exceedingly rare (21, 27).

Chronic lymphocytic leukemia is almost always a disease of sporadic occurrence. Rarely has clustering of cases in families been reported (47, 58, 109, 160).

No obvious etiologic factors contributing to an increased incidence of chronic lymphocytic leukemia have been identified thus far. The studies of the Atomic Bomb Casualty Commission have not indicated a higher incidence in persons exposed to high levels of ionizing irradiation (44).

Clinical Features

General Manifestations

The onset of chronic lymphocytic leukemia is insidious. The patient may notice painless lumps in the cervical region, axillae, or groin. Less commonly, his complaints are of fatigue, anorexia, weight loss, palpitations, and weakness from anemia, or of abdominal fullness from an enlarging spleen. Even more rarely, the initial symptoms are referable to infiltration of an organ such as the skin. Not infrequently, the patient is entirely asymptomatic at the time of diagnosis, and an abnormality is detected on routine examination of the blood. Hypermetabolism is unusual in chronic lymphocytic leukemia unless this disease is badly neglected and reaches an advanced stage (79). Symptoms associated with hemolytic anemia and hemorrhagic manifestations resulting from thrombocytopenia may occur at any time during the course of the disease—but particularly in advanced, rather than early, stages. The frequency of symptoms and signs at the time of diagnosis is listed in Table 19.1.

Table 19.1 Frequency of symptoms and signs at time of diagnosis of chronic lymphocytic leukemia.

Symptoms and signs	Percentage of patients displaying symptoms
Weakness	36
Lymphoid masses	24
Weight loss	21
Infection and fever	17
Increased sweating	9
Dyspnea	9
Hemorrhagic manifestations	2
Lymphadenopathy	68
Splenomegaly	53
Hepatomegaly	25
Cutaneous bleeding	4

Source: Modified from reference 162.

Hematologic Abnormalities

In addition to obvious lymphocytosis in the peripheral blood, abnormalities of erythrocytes, granulocytes, and platelets are common in chronic lymphocytic leukemia. Anemia develops at some time in the course of the disease in most patients. It usually is of only moderate severity, but occasionally may be extremely severe. It is normocytic and normochromic unless overt hemolytic anemia develops, in which instance macrocytosis and immature forms of the erythroid series may be seen in the peripheral blood. In those cases with neither an overt antibody-induced hemolytic anemia nor splenic sequestration of erythrocytes, the mechanism of anemia is not apparent. Anemia in such patients appears to arise from a combination of modest shortening of red cell survival and inadequate marrow erythropoietic response (5, 104, 151). In various series acquired hemolytic anemia has occurred in between 10 and 25 percent of patients with chronic lymphocytic leukemia (99, 162). The antibodies associated with the autoimmune hemolytic process are usually of the "warm" type (20, 38, 51, 108, 145). The development of hemolytic anemia in the course of chronic lymphocytic leukemia does not necessarily carry a poor prognosis (157); it generally is responsive to therapy with corticosteroids.

The white blood count varies from slightly elevated levels to several hundred thousand per cubic millimeter. In a series of 130 patients the mean count at the time of diagnosis was 93,000/mm^3 and one-third of the patients had white blood counts in excess of 100,000/mm^3 (12). The absolute numbers of granulocytes tend to be reduced.

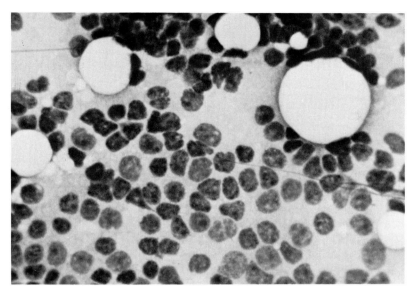

Figure 19.7 Bone marrow aspirate from a patient with chronic lymphocytic leukemia infiltrated by mature lymphoid cells.

The platelet count is either normal or reduced, almost never elevated. When thrombocytopenia is severe, hemorrhagic manifestations may dominate the clinical picture. Thrombocytopenia in chronic lymphocytic leukemia is generally responsive to corticosteroid therapy.

The bone marrow in patients with chronic lymphocytic leukemia is crowded with lymphocytes that constitute between 30 and 99 percent of the nucleated cell population (Fig. 19.7). With the exception of invasive lymphosarcoma, no other disorders have such bone marrow findings. Occasionally one can aspirate a lymphoid follicle from an otherwise normal bone marrow such that the smear contains abundant lymphocytes. However, examination of other smears, or of bone marrow biopsies, leads to the correct diagnosis. In aplastic anemia there may be a relative increase in marrow lymphocytes, but not an absolute increase.

Serum proteins often show pronounced changes in chronic lymphocytic leukemia. Hypoglobulinemia is not uncommon, particularly in the late stages of the disease. In one series about half of the patients had hypoglobulinemia (162). In a small number of patients the serum globulin concentration may be increased, particularly in the alpha-2 and beta-globulin region.

Organ Infiltration

In chronic lymphocytic leukemia, lymphadenopathy appears early and is often generalized and of striking magnitude. The nodes are usually firm, nontender, and matted.

Rarely, peripheral adenopathy is minimal or absent despite blood and bone marrow lymphocytosis (67). Adenopathy is apt to be present at the time of diagnosis. It may be sufficiently disfiguring to constitute the patient's major complaint. Splenomegaly is generally present from the time of onset of symptoms or at initial diagnosis. The degree of splenomegaly is not so marked as in chronic myelocytic leukemia, and infarcts of the spleen are relatively rare. However, discomfort from a large spleen may be a prominent feature of the disease.

Other collections of lymphoid tissues, such as the tonsils, may be clinically enlarged. Mikulicz's syndrome may be present as a result of salivary gland infiltration (66, 116).

Chronic lymphocytic leukemia probably has more associated skin manifestations than any other leukemia. Recent studies have suggested that these skin manifestations may indicate the presence of a T-cell malignancy rather than the more typical B-cell disease. This concept is discussed more completely in Chapter 22 in relation to Sézary's syndrome.

Skin manifestations may occur very early in chronic lymphocytic leukemia (159). Epstein and MacEachern (39) found that in a series of 60 patients, 8.3 percent had cutaneous involvement. A variety of dermal manifestations has been described (49). The process may begin with localized small, reddish papules containing lymphocytes (leukemia cutis). These may enlarge, spread, and coalesce until in time large areas of skin are involved (59). Other cutaneous manifestations include erythema with exfoliative dermatitis eventuating in thickened, reddened, scaling skin (the "red-man syndrome") (11, 48, 59, 68, 70, 128). Herpes zoster is frequent in chronic lymphocytic leukemia, probably occurring in 3 to 10 percent of all patients sometime during the course of their disease (35, 129).

Patients may react to smallpox vaccination with progressive localized inflammatory reaction or disseminated vaccinia (146). Reaction to mosquito bite may be exuberant.

Direct infiltration of the gastrointestinal tract is not uncommon in chronic lymphocytic leukemia, but only rarely is it of sufficient magnitude to produce clinical symptoms (14, 103, 113). In contrast, clinically apparent infiltration of the liver is common, although hepatocellular or obstructive jaundice is relatively uncommon.

Pulmonary and/or pleural involvement in chronic lymphocytic leukemia has been reported to occur in between 8 and 30 percent or more of patients (43, 55, 56, 162). Often diagnostic difficulties arise in distinguishing direct leukemia infiltration from infection or local intrapulmonic hemorrhage. Leukemic cells may be found in pleural effusions.

Leukemic infiltrates may occur in the genitourinary system and be manifest clinically as hematuria, prostatic symptoms, menometrorrhagia, enlarged kidneys, uric acid nephropathy (rarely), and priapism (130, 148).

Skeletal involvement probably occurs in less than 10 percent of patients with chronic lymphocytic leukemia (28). The incidence of skeletal involvement probably depends on the criteria used to diagnose chronic lymphocytic leukemia as opposed to lymphosarcoma. The latter disease more frequently involves bone.

Infectious Complications

Patients with chronic lymphocytic leukemia often suffer from repeated and severe bacterial and viral infections (90, 133). The frequency of herpes zoster infection and the frequent severity of vaccinia infection have already been commented upon. Bacterial infections are also frequent, often from unusual pathogens, and are poorly controlled by the patient's defense mechanisms. Increased susceptibility to both viral and bacterial infections is usually ascribed to impaired immunologic function. Additionally, host defenses against bacteria and fungi may be reduced by the granulocytopenia that is a frequent feature of chronic lymphocytic leukemia. The capacity of patients with this disease to produce circulating antibody is decreased (25, 71, 80, 92, 133) and the concentration of serum gamma globulin frequently is low (25, 76, 120). Cutaneous tests of delayed hypersensitivity have frequently been normal in chronic lymphocytic leukemia (25, 90, 139). There is usually not a good correlation between the immunologic deficit and the duration or extent of disease (25, 133).

Recently we have observed decreased production of interferon by chronic lymphocytic leukemic lymphocytes responding to mitogens (40). Impaired interferon synthesis may contribute to the propensity to viral infections.

Unusual Clinical Variants of Chronic Lymphocytic Leukemia

Chronic lymphocytic leukemia may involve various structures of the eye or the lacrimal gland, producing impairment of vision (152, 159). Hemorrhage or infiltration of the middle or inner ear may produce tinnitus and deafness (127). Direct central nervous system infiltration with malignant cells is relatively uncommon in chronic lymphocytic leukemia compared with acute leukemia (125). However, multifocal demyelinating disease (progressive multifocal leukencephalopathy) probably occurs more commonly in chronic lymphocytic leukemia than in

any other leukemia (138). Serious intracranial hemorrhage can of course occur at any time that thrombocytopenia develops.

A variety of disease syndromes resembling chronic lymphocytic leukemia but associated with a paraprotein are known (3) and will be described in Chapter 20.

Course of the Disease and Prognosis

Chronic lymphocytic leukemia differs clinically from the other varieties of leukemia in several respects. As stated previously, onset is insidious and the diagnosis is often made on incidental examination. There is no well-recognized preleukemia state such as is sometimes observed in the acute leukemias, and, although some authors disagree (59), there is almost never a terminal transition to an acute form of leukemia (87).

The course of chronic lymphocytic leukemia is highly variable. Many patients have few or no symptoms for many years and may live for 20 to 30 years with their disease. A minority of patients die within a few weeks or months of onset (162). In some patients, symptoms of lymphoid tumors predominate; in others, symptoms are related to immunologic abnormalities—hemolytic anemia and infectious complications. In a third group, symptoms of bone marrow failure predominate. Because of this variability, figures for median survival in this disease have little relevance to the individual patient. In Table 19.2 are listed survival figures obtained from various series. It is not clear why survival appears to be so much better in the series reported after 1951; different diagnostic criteria (exclusion of leukolymphosarcoma) and better supportive and specific therapy may be factors. Clearly, at the present time chronic lymphocytic leukemia tends to be an indolent malignant disease. It probably has a prolonged presymptomatic phase, so that median survival from onset is most likely in excess of 10 years (12), with many patients living in excess of 15 years (12, 54, 91, 157, 162) and even longer (89). Because chronic lymphocytic leukemia is a

Table 19.2 Median survival in chronic lymphocytic leukemia derived from several studies. Survival is measured in years from onset of symptoms or diagnosis.

Year of study or publication	Median survival (years)	References
1939	3.29	158
1925–1951	2.65	144
1966	6–9	12
1969	>6	162

disease of middle and old age, it is obvious that many patients will die from causes unrelated to this disorder.

It has been suggested on the basis of the variability of the course of the disease that there may be a benign and a malignant form of chronic lymphocytic leukemia with differing life expectancies (59). Data obtained from large series do not support the notion that there is a bimodal curve of survival (12, 162).

No single factor has prognostic value for survival in chronic lymphocytic leukemia, with the exception of the platelet count. The development of significant thrombocytopenia is a poor prognostic sign. The lymphocyte count generally increases with time and may do so in an exponential manner (121). Spontaneous remissions of disease rarely have been documented (22).

The Malignant Lymphocyte and Its Relation to Clinical Disease

As pointed out in Chapters 12 and 13, mammalian small lymphocytes may be divided into two major populations: thymus-derived (T) and bone-marrow–derived (B) lymphocytes. Evidence now accumulating favors the concept that increased numbers of lymphocytes in the peripheral blood of patients with chronic lymphocytic leukemia are mainly B lymphocytes. This evidence is based on the distribution of immunoglobulins on the cell surface (1, 77, 107, 112, 134, 153) and on the presence of complement receptors (107). In the study of Wilson and Nossal (153) 34 percent of the peripheral blood lymphocytes of the normal subjects appeared to be B lymphocytes, whereas more than 85 percent of the cells of three patients with chronic lymphocytic leukemia carried surface immunoglobulins. Occasionally, patients with chronic lymphocytic leukemia have unreleased intracellular monoclonal immunoglobulin (75).

The capacity of the lymphoid population to respond by blastogenic transformation to phytohemagglutinin appears to be a function of the content of T cells (36). The reduced or delayed response to phytohemagglutinin by chronic lymphocytic leukemic cells is well documented (16, 95, 156). There appears to be an inverse correlation between a high white blood count and the blastogenic response to phytohemagglutinin (65, 95, 131). Correspondingly, the cytotoxic effect of chronic lymphocytic leukemic lymphocytes against allogeneic tissues induced by phytohemagglutinin is reduced to below normal, as explained in Chapter 17 (69). The reduced responsiveness of chronic lymphocytic leukemia cells to mitogen may be explained by the finding that they have fewer surface binding sites for the mitogen than do normal lymphocytes (110).

Rubin and his colleagues (118) have analyzed the late-transforming population of leukemic lymphocytes in chronic lymphocytic leukemia, which they believe to be an aberrant population not detectable in normal subjects. Some findings suggest that normal and malignant lymphocytes may coexist in chronic lymphocytic leukemia (94, 123, 143). The malignant cells as a rule have a normal karyotype (95), although Goh (52) observed that aneuploid karyotypes (pseudodiploid) in cultures of phytohemagglutinin stimulated chronic lymphocytic leukemia lymphocytes after three to six days in culture.

Another characteristic of B lymphocytes is that relative to T cells they are sticky and are selectively removed by adherence to glass wool columns (53). Thompson and his colleagues (143) demonstrated that some chronic lymphocytic leukemic populations are abnormally adherent to polystyrene bead columns. Cells passing through the columns had greater responsiveness to phytohemagglutinin than did the unfractionated population.

Taken together, this series of observations suggests that two lymphocyte populations may be found in chronic lymphocytic leukemia: an abnormal, high-adherence, phytohemagglutinin-unresponsive population displaying B-cell characteristics, and a smaller, normal, nonadherent, phytohemagglutinin-responsive population with T-cell characteristics. Questions unanswered at present include: (a) is there a residual, normal B-cell population; (b) how is the abnormal B-cell population related to the impairment of humoral antibody production and hypogammaglobulinemia; and (c) is there an impairment in B lymphocyte-to-plasma cell transformation (4, 33, 34).

The molecular mechanisms of the B-lymphocyte abnormality in chronic lymphocytic leukemia are totally obscured. One report in the literature suggests that these cells may synthesize a species of RNA that is either of a low concentration or entirely absent in normal lymphocytes (93). Chronic lymphocytic leukemic cells may have other metabolic abnormalities: low levels of the lysosomal enzymes β-glucuronidase and acid phosphatase (19) and low or absent membrane 5'-nucleotidase (85). Rates of DNA repair are increased (72). The number of lysosomes in chronic lymphocytic leukemia cells is less than that found in normal small lymphocytes (37).

Life-span and Blood Clearance Rate

Based on the stability of the white blood count and lymphadenopathy, and the low cell turnover rate as reflected in uric acid excretion, one would predict that the leukemic leukocytes in most patients are long-lived. In other patients with more active disease it is difficult to estimate the life-span on these clinical grounds. If one defines life-span of a replicating or potentially replicating cell population as being equivalent to the generation time (that is, the time between two divisions), then there are no available data for the in vivo life-span of chronic lymphocytic leukemic cells (30). Data are available on the time interval between DNA synthesis and appearance of cells in the blood, and on cell life-span measured from DNA labeling studies. Many such investigations were performed when ^{32}P was used more extensively in treatment of this disorder. In the early days of such therapy, Osgood and his colleagues concluded that some chronic lymphocytic leukemic cells had an average life-span of 84 days (96–101). Christensen and Ottesen (23), measuring lymphocyte DNA-^{32}P, found a prolonged lymphocyte turnover time in three patients with chronic lymphocytic leukemia. Hamilton, in a series of studies (62–64), concluded that there were two populations of leukemic cells in the blood: the short-lived ones with an average life-span of 85 days and the long-lived ones with an average survival of approximately 300 days.

More recent studies using ^{51}Cr as the lymphocyte label have suggested that chronic lymphocytic leukemia is characterized by overproduction of a population of abnormally short-lived lymphocytes (126).

The clearance of lymphocytes from the blood of patients with chronic lymphocytic leukemia has been measured using a variety of radioisotope labels. The data have indicated an initially rapid clearance (approximately 18 to 20 hours) and a subsequent half-disappearance time of one to two weeks (compare a $T_{1/2}$ of seven hours for normal neutrophils) (2, 30, 46, 106, 141). The chronic lymphocytic leukemic lymphocyte, in leaving the blood, probably recirculates slowly through the lymph and lymphoid organs and again into the circulation (10, 88, 126, 163).

Rate of Cell Production; Generative Cycle

A high proportion of chronic lymphocytic leukemic cells do not label with tritiated thymidine and therefore are either in a prolonged G_1 phase of the cell cycle (G_0) or are end cells. The labeling index of normal lymphocytes is 0.05 to 0.1 percent (119, 155); in chronic lymphocytic leukemia it is 0 to 0.7 percent, with a mean of 0.2 percent (15, 119). This higher-than-normal labeling of cells by a pulse of tritiated thymidine, combined with a large increase in the numbers of lymphocytes, means that the total number of cells in DNA synthesis at a given time is quite high in chronic lymphocytic leukemia. However, the precise lymphocyte production rate is not known, although various estimates have been made (30). Evidence from

some studies (163) lends support to the notion that chronic lymphocytic leukemia is often a disease of lymphocyte accumulation rather than of high production rate (34). Other studies clearly indicate that the disease is characterized by overproduction of cells (126).

Compartment Size

Based on studies with lymphocytes radioactively labeled in vitro and reinfused, as well as on studies with extracorporeal irradiation, it has been suggested that in chronic lymphocytic leukemia there is a pool of lymphocytes that communicates rapidly with the peripheral blood. This pool has been designated the readily accessible compartment, or RAC (30, 140, 141). When labeled cells are infused, blood radioactivity declines, reaches a plateau by approximately 10 hours, and remains stable for about 24 hours. Based on such data, the following divergent estimates of RAC size have been made: (a) equal to the size of the blood pool (46); (b) 6 to 9 times the size of the blood pool (6, 32, 105); and (c) 0.33 to 4.6 times the size of the blood pool, with an average of 2.3 times (121). Similar calculations of the last estimate have been derived from extracorporeal irradiation of the blood (30). Clearly, however, precise data on compartment size do not exist.

Given the inadequacy of presently available data on lymphocyte kinetics in chronic lymphocytic leukemia, one can tentatively conclude that the cell production rate varies from slightly to greatly increased above normal. This phenomenon, combined with the generally long life-span of the leukemic cell, accounts for the great increase in lymphoid cells in the blood and tissues of patients with chronic lymphocytic leukemia.

Principles of Therapy

Given the fact that many patients with chronic lymphocytic leukemia have a benign and prolonged clinical course (12, 73, 74), treatment is often directed at improving the quality of survival by treating the complications of leukemia (24, 82). The major complications are collections of lymphoid tissues producing disfigurement or obstruction, systemic debilitating symptoms, hemolytic anemia, thrombocytopenia, and recurrent infections.

The major types of treatment available include external irradiation (78), alkylating agents (42), and adrenocorticosteroids (132). Internal irradiation from administration of radioisotopes such as ^{32}P no longer is widely used (97).

Local collections of lymphoid tissue producing obstruction or discomfort often respond best to local irradiation. Systemic symptoms and generalized adenopathy are best treated with an alkylating agent, unless marrow impairment limits such usage. Symptomatic hemolytic anemia and thrombocytopenia may be responsive to corticosteroids (132). The steroids are also used for their lymphocytolytic effects (122), when myelosuppression must be avoided. Unfortunately, more effective and novel approaches to the treatment of chronic lymphocytic leukemia are rare. Additional methods that have been tried include extracorporeal irradiation, antilymphocyte serum, and leukapheresis (29, 31, 81). Recently, the use of combinations of lympholytic drugs has met with some success in inducing complete remission in a minority of patients with chronic lymphocytic leukemia (74), and chemotherapists are tending to use more aggressive therapy aimed at prolonging life as well as improving its quality (24).

Summary

Chronic lymphocytic leukemia is one of the chronic lymphoproliferative disorders. The disease is characterized by overproduction and accumulation of moderately long-lived lymphocytes. Almost always these are B cells. The normal population of B and T cells is reduced as a result of an expanded neoplastic B-cell population. Consequent immunologic impairment is frequent.

The major clinical manifestations reflect the marked accumulation of lymphoid cells: loss of normal hematopoietic cells, local accumulations of lymphoid tissues, and susceptibility to infection. Autoimmune phenomena are common, although their mechanism is obscure.

Chapter 19 References

1. Aisenberg, A. C., and Bloch, K. J. Immunoglobulins on the surface of neoplastic lymphocytes, *N. Engl. J. Med.* 287:272, 1972.

2. Bainbridge, D. R., Brent, L., and Gowland, G. Distribution of allogenic ^{51}Cr-labelled lymph node cells in mice, *Transplantation* 4:138, 1966.

3. Ballard, H. S., Hamilton, L. M., Marcus, A. J., et al. A new variant of heavy chain-disease (μ-chain disease), *N. Engl. J. Med.* 282:1060, 1970.

4. Bergsagel, D. The chronic leukemias. A review of disease manifestations and the aims of therapy, *Can. Med. Assoc. J.* 96:1615, 1967.

5. Berlin, N. I., Lawrence, J. H., and Lee, H. C. The pathogenesis of the anemia of chronic leukemia: measurement of the life span of the red blood cell with glycine-2-C^{14}, *J. Lab. Clin. Med.* 44:860, 1954.

6. Bernard, J., and Binet, J. L. Lymphe et circulation des lymphocytes chez l'homme, *Nouv. Rev. Fr. Hematol.* 6:585, 1966.

7. Best, W. R., and Limarzi, L. R. Age, sex, race, and hematologic classification of 916 leukemia cases, *J. Lab. Clin. Med.* 40:778, 1952.

8. Bethell, F. H. Leukemia; the relative incidence of its various forms and their response to radiation therapy, *Ann. Intern. Med.* 18:757, 1943.

9. Bichel, J. Mediastinal tumors in leukosis, *Acta Radiol.* 28:81, 1947.

10. Binet, J. L., Villeneuve, B., Becart, R., Logeais, Y., Laudat, P., and Mathey, J. Temps de passage dans le canal thoracique des lymphocytes du sang de la leucémie lymphoïde chronique, *Nouv. Rev. Fr. Hematol.* 7:621, 1967.

11. Bluefarb, S. M. Leukemia Cutis, Charles C Thomas, Springfield, Ill., 1960.

12. Boggs, D. R., Sofferman, S. A., Wintrobe, M. M., et al. Factors influencing the duration of survival of patients with chronic lymphocytic leukemia, *Am. J. Med.* 40:243, 1966.

13. Boggs, D. R., Wintrobe, M. M., and Cartwright, G. E. The acute leukemias, *Medicine* 41:163, 1962.

14. Boikan, W. S. Leukemic changes of the gastro-intestinal tract, *Arch. Intern. Med.* 47:42, 1931.

15. Bond, V. P., Fliedner, T. M., Cronkite, E. P., Rubini, J. R., Brecher, G., and Schork, P. K. Proliferative potentials of bone marrow and blood cells studied by in vitro uptake of H^3-thymidine, *Acta Haematol.* 21:1, 1959.

16. Bouroncle, B. A., Clausen, K. P., and Aschenbrand, J. F. Studies of the delayed response of phytohemagglutinin (PHA) stimulated lymphocytes in 25 chronic lymphatic leukemia patients before and during therapy, *Blood* 34:166, 1969.

17. Bouroncle, B. A., Wiseman, B. K., and Doan, C. A. Leukemic reticuloendotheliosis, *Blood* 13:609, 1958.

18. Brill, A. B., Tomonaga, M., and Heyssel, R. M. Leukemia in man following exposure to ionizing radiation. A summary of the findings in Hiroshima and Nagasaki, and a comparison with other human experience, *Ann. Intern. Med.* 56:590, 1962.

19. Brittinger, G., König, E., Cohnen, G., and Aberle, H. G. Lysosomale Enzyme in Lymphozyten, I. Lymphoretikuläre Erkrankungen: Vergleich des Enzymgehaltes (saure Phosphatase, β-glucuronidase) unstimulierter Blutlymphozyten mit der Blastentransformation nach Phytohämagglutinin-Stimulierung in vitro, *Acta Haematol.* 44:205, 1970.

20. Brody, J. I., and Beizer, L. H. The cross-reactivity of lymphocyte and red cell antibodies, *J. Lab. Clin. Med.* 63:819, 1964.

21. Casey, T. P. Chronic lymphocytic leukaemia in a child presenting at the age of two years and eight months, *Aust. Ann. Med.* 17:70, 1968.

22. Chervenick, P. A., Boggs, D. R., and Wintrobe, M. M. Spontaneous remission in chronic lymphocytic leukemia, *Ann. Intern. Med.* 67:1239, 1967.

23. Christensen, B., and Ottesen, J. The age of leukocytes in the blood stream of patients with chronic lymphatic leukemia, *Acta Haematol.* 13:289, 1955.

24. Cline, M. J., and Haskell, C. M.

Cancer Chemotherapy, 2nd ed., W. B. Saunders, Philadelphia, 1975.

25. Cone, L., and Uhr, J. W. Immunological deficiency disorders associated with chronic lymphocytic leukemia and multiple myeloma, *J. Clin. Invest.* 43:2241, 1964.

26. Cornes, J. S., and Jones, T. G. Leukaemic lesions of the gastrointestinal tract, *J. Clin. Pathol.* 15:305, 1962.

27. Court Brown, W. M., and Doll, R. Leukaemia in childhood and young adult life. Trends in mortality in relation to aetiology, *Br. Med. J.* 2:981, 1961.

28. Craver, L. F., and Copeland, M. M. Changes of the bones in the leukemias, *Arch. Surg.* 30:639, 1935.

29. Cronkite, E. P. Extracorporeal irradiation of the blood in the treatment of leukemia and for immunosuppression, *Ann. Intern. Med.* 67:415, 1967.

30. Cronkite, E. P., and Schiffer, L. M. Kinetics of normal lymphopoiesis and chronic lymphocytic leukemia, *in* A. S. Gordon (ed.), Regulation of Hematopoiesis, vol. 2, p. 1455, Appleton-Century-Crofts, New York, 1970.

31. Curtis, J. E., Hersh, E. M., and Freireich, E. J. Leukapheresis therapy of chronic lymphocytic leukemia, *Blood*, 39:163, 1972.

32. Cuttner, J., Cronkite, E. P., Kesse, M., and Fliedner, T. M. Behavior of autotransfused in vitro H^3-cytidine (H^3-CDR)-labeled lymphocytes in chronic lymphocytic leukemia (CLL), *J. Clin. Invest.* 43:1236, 1964.

33. Dameshek, W. Chronic lymphocytic leukemia—an accumulative disease of immunologically incompetent lymphocytes, *Blood* 29:566, 1967.

34. Dameshek, W. The immunoproliferative disorders, *in* A. S. Gordon (ed.), Regulation of Hematopoiesis, vol. 2, p. 1527, Appleton-Century-Crofts, New York, 1970.

35. Dayan, A. D., Morgan, H. G., Hope-Stone, H. F., and Boucher, B. J. Disseminated herpes zoster in the reticuloses, *Am. J. Roentgenol.* 92:116, 1964.

36. Doenhoff, M. J., Davies, A. J., Leu-

chars, E., et al. The thymus and circulating lymphocytes of mice, *Proc. Soc. Lond. (Biol.)* 176:69, 1971.

37. Douglas, S. D., Cohnen, G., König, E., and Brittinger, G. Lymphocyte lysosomes and lysosomal enzymes in chronic lymphocytic leukemia, *Blood* 41:511, 1973.

38. Dreyfus, B., Le Bolloc'h-Combrisson, A., Malassenet, R., and Jacob, S. Sur l'anémie des leucémies lymphoïdes, *Nouv. Rev. Fr. Hematol.* 1:771, 1961.

39. Epstein, E., and MacEachern, K. Dermatologic manifestations of the lymphoblastoma-leukemia group, *Arch. Intern. Med.* 60:867, 1937.

40. Epstein, L. B., and Cline, M. J. Chronic lymphocytic leukemia: studies on mitogen-stimulated lymphocyte interferon production. *Clin. Exp. Immunol.* 16:553, 1974.

41. Ewald, O. Die leukämische Reticuloendotheliose, *Dtsch. Arch. Klin. Med.* 142:222, 1923.

42. Ezdinli, E. Z., and Stutzman, L. Chlorambucil therapy for lymphomas and chronic lymphocytic leukemia, *J.A.M.A.* 191:444, 1965.

43. Falconer, E. H., and Leonard, M. E. Pulmonary involvement in lymphosarcoma and lymphatic leukemia, *Am. J. Med. Sci.* 195:294, 1938.

44. Finch, S. C., Hoshino, T., Itoga, T., et al. Chronic lymphocytic leukemia in Hiroshima and Nagasaki, Japan, *Blood* 33:79, 1969.

45. Flandrin, G., Daniel, M. T., Fourcade, M., et al. Leucémie à "tricholeucocyte" (hairy cell leukemia), étude clinique et cytologique de 55 observations, *Nouv. Rev. Fr. Hematol.* 13:609, 1973.

46. Fliedner, T. M. Experimental studies on PHA-stimulated lymphocytes and auto-transfusion of ^{3}H-cytidine labelled lymphocytes in chronic lymphocytic leukaemia, *in* J. M. Yoffey (ed.), The Lymphocyte in Immunology and Haemopoiesis, p. 198, Edward Arnold, London, 1967.

47. Fraumeni, J. F., Jr., Vogel, C. L., and DeVita, V. T. Familial chronic lymphocytic leukemia, *Ann. Intern. Med.* 71:279, 1969.

48. Gate, J., and Cuilleret, P. A propos des manifestations cutanées des leucémies, *J. Med. Lyon* 18:299, 1937.

49. Gates, O. Cutaneous tumors of leukemia and lymphoma, *Arch. Dermatol.* 37:1015, 1938.

50. Gauld, W. R., Innes, J., and Robson, H. N. A survey of 647 cases of leukaemia 1938–51, *Br. Med. J.* 1:585, 1953.

51. Geller, W. Chronic lymphocytic leukemia with hemolytic anemia. A long survival, *Arch. Intern. Med.* 114:444, 1964.

52. Goh, K-O. Pseudodiploid chromosomal pattern in chronic lymphocytic leukemia, *J. Lab. Clin. Med.* 69:938, 1967.

53. Greaves, M. F., and Hogg, N. M. Antigen binding sites on mouse lymphoid cells, *in* O. Mäkelä, A. Cross, and T. V. Kosunen (eds.), Proceedings of the Third Sigrid Jusélius Symposium, Cell interactions and receptor antibodies in immune responses, p. 145, Academic Press, New York, 1970.

54. Green, R. A. and Dixon, H. Expectancy for life in chronic lymphatic leukemia, *Blood* 25:23, 1965.

55. Green, R. A., and Nichols, N. J. Pulmonary involvement in leukemia, *Ann. Rev. Resp. Dis.* 80:833, 1959.

56. Green, R. A., Nichols, N. J., and King, E. J. Alveolar-capillary block due to leukemic infiltration of the lung, *Am. Rev. Resp. Dis.* 80:895, 1959.

57. Gunz, F. W. Incidence of some aetiological factors in human leukaemia, *Br. Med. J.* 1:326, 1961.

58. Gunz, F. W., and Dameshek, W. Chronic lymphocytic leukemia in a family, including twin brothers and a son, *J.A.M.A.* 164:1323, 1957.

59. Gunz, F. W., and Dameshek, W. Leukemia, 2nd ed., p. 237, Grune & Stratton, New York, 1964.

60. Gunz, F. W., and Hough, R. F. Acute leukemia over the age of fifty: a study of its incidence and history, *Blood* 11:882, 1956.

61. Haenszel, W., and Kurihara, M. Studies of Japanese migrants. I. Mortality from cancer and other diseases among Japanese in the United States, *J. Natl. Cancer Inst.* 40:43, 1968.

62. Hamilton, L. D. Nucleic acid turnover studies in human leukaemic cells and the function of lymphocytes, *Nature* 178:597, 1956.

63. Hamilton, L. D. *In* J. W. Rebuck, F. A. Bethell, and R. W. Monto (eds.), The Leukemias: Etiology, Pathophysiology and Treatment, p. 381, Academic Press, New York, 1957.

64. Hamilton, L. D. Carbon^{14}-labeling of DNA in studying hemopoietic cells, *in* F. Stohlman, Jr. (ed.), The Kinetics of Cellular Proliferation, p. 151, Grune & Stratton, New York, 1959.

65. Havemann, K., and Rubin, A. D. The delayed response of chronic lymphocytic leukemia lymphocytes to phytohemagglutinin in vitro, *Proc. Soc. Exp. Biol. Med.* 127:668, 1968.

66. Hird, A. J. Mikulicz's syndrome, *Br. Med. J.* 2:416, 1949.

67. Hirschfeld, H. Über chronische Leukämien ohne Milz- und Lymphknoten vergrösserung, *Med. Klin.* 28:1160, 1932.

68. Hitch, J. M., and Smith, D. C. Lymphatic leukemia. Report of a case apparently limited to the skin, superficial lymphatic glands and blood stream, *Arch. Dermatol.* 36:1, 1937.

69. Holm, G., Perlmann, P., and Johansson, B. Impaired phytohemagglutinin-induced cytotoxicity in vitro of lymphocytes from patients with Hodgkin's disease or chronic lymphatic leukemia, *Clin. Exp. Immunol.* 2:351, 1967.

70. Holten, C. Leukemic erythrodermia, a survey and a report of a case treated with ACTH, *Acta Med. Scand.* 266:557, 1952 (suppl.).

71. Howell, K. M. The failure of antibody formation in leukemia, *Arch. Intern. Med.* 26:706, 1920.

72. Huang, A. T., Kremer, W. B., Laszlo, J., and Setlow, R. B. DNA repair in human leukaemic lymphocytes, *Nature (New Biol.)* 240:114, 1972.

73. Huguley, C. M. Long-term study of chronic lymphocytic leukemia: interim report after 45 months, *Cancer Chemother. Rep.* 16:241, 1962.

74. Huguley, C. M., Jr. Chronic myelocytic and chronic lymphocytic leukemia, *Cancer* 30:41, 1973.

75. Hurez, D., Flandrin, G.,

Preud'homme, J. L., et al. Unreleased intracellular monoclonal macroglobulin in chronic lymphocytic leukemia, *Clin. Exp. Immunol.* 10:223, 1972.

76. Jim, R. T. S. Serum gamma globulin levels in chronic lymphocytic leukemia, *Am. J. Med. Sci.* 234:44, 1957.

77. Johansson, B., and Klein, E. Cell surface localized IgM-kappa immunoglobulin reactivity in a case of chronic lymphocytic leukemia, *Clin. Exp. Immunol.* 6:421, 1970.

78. Johnson, R. E., Kagan, A. R., Gralnick, H. R., and Fass, L. Radiation-induced remissions in chronic lymphocytic leukemia, *Cancer* 20:1382, 1967.

79. Krantz, C. I., and Riddle, M. C. The basal metabolism in chronic lymphatic leukemia, *Am. J. Med. Sci.* 175:229, 1928.

80. Larson, D. L., and Tomlinson, L. J. Quantitative antibody studies in man. III. Antibody response in leukemia and other malignant lymphomata, *J. Clin. Invest.* 32:317, 1953.

81. Laszlo, J., Buckley, C. E. III, and Amos, D. B. Infusion of isologous immune plasma in chronic lymphocytic leukemia, *Blood* 31:104, 1968.

82. Lawrence, J. H. The treatment of chronic leukemia, *Med. Clin. North Am.* 38:525, 1954.

83. Leavell, B. S. Chronic leukemia. A study of the incidence and factors influencing the duration of life, *Am J. Med. Sci.* 196:329, 1938.

84. Linman, J. W. Principles of Hematology, Macmillan, New York, 1966.

85. Lopes, J., Zucker-Franklin, D., and Silber, R. Heterogeneity of 5'-nucleotidase activity in lymphocytes in chronic lymphocytic leukemia, *J. Clin. Invest.* 52:1297, 1973.

86. MacMahon, B., and Clark, D. Incidence of the common forms of human leukemia, *Blood* 11:871, 1956.

87. McPhedran, P., and Heath, C. W., Jr. Acute leukemia occurring during chronic lymphocytic leukemia, *Blood* 35:7, 1970.

88. Manaster, J., Frühling, J., and Strykmans, P. Kinetics of lymphocytes in chronic lymphocytic leu-

kemia. I. Equilibrium between blood and a "readily accessible pool," *Blood* 41:425, 1973.

89. Marlow, A. A., and Bartlett, G. R. Survival for twenty-nine years in chronic lymphocytic leukemia, *J.A.M.A.* 152:1033, 1953.

90. Miller, D. G., and Karnofsky, D. A. Immunologic factors and resistance to infection in chronic lymphatic leukemia, *Am. J. Med.* 31:748, 1961.

91. Minot, G. P., and Isaacs, R. Lymphatic leukemia. Age incidence duration, and benefit derived from irradiation, *Boston Med. Sci. J.* 191:1, 1924.

92. Moreschi, C. Über antigene und pyrogene Wirkung des Typhusbacillus bei leukämischen Kranken, *Z. Immunitaetsforsch.* 21:410, 1914.

93. Neiman, P. E., and Henry, P. H. Ribonucleic acid–deoxyribonucleic acid hybridization and hybridization-competition studies of the rapidly labeled ribonucleic acid from normal and chronic lymphocytic leukemia lymphocytes, *Biochemistry* 8:275, 1969.

94. Nowell, P. C. Differentiation of human leukemic leukocytes in tissue culture, *Exp. Cell Res.* 19:267, 1960.

95. Oppenheim, J. J., Whang, J., and Frei, E. III. Immunologic and cytogenetic studies of chronic lymphocytic leukemic cells, *Blood* 26:121, 1965.

96. Osgood, E. E. The threshold dose of P[32] for leukemic cells of the lymphocytic and granulocytic series, *Blood* 16:1104, 1960.

97. Osgood, E. E. Treatment of chronic leukemia, *J. Nucl. Med.* 5:139, 1964.

98. Osgood, E. E. The relative dosage required of total body X-ray vs. intravenous ^{32}P for equal effectiveness against leukemic cells of the lymphocytic series or granulocytic series in chronic leukemia, *J. Nucl. Med.* 6:421, 1965.

99. Osgood, E. E., and Seaman, A. J. Treatment of chronic leukemias. Results of therapy by titrated, regularly spaced total body radioactive phosphorous, or roentgen irradiation, *J.A.M.A.* 150:1372, 1952.

100. Osgood, E. E., Seaman, A. J., and

Tivey, H. Comparative survival times of X-ray treated versus P[32] treated patients with chronic leukemias under the program of titrated, regularly spaced total-body irradiation, *Radiology* 64:373, 1955.

101. Osgood, E. E., Tivey, H., Davison, K. B., Seaman, A. J., and Li, G. J. The relative rates of formation of new leukocytes in patients with acute and chronic leukemias, *Cancer* 5:331, 1952.

102. Panton, P. N., and Valentine, F. C. O. Chronic lymphoid leukaemia, *Lancet* i:914, 1929.

103. Pearson, B., Stasney, J., and Pizzolato, P. Gastrointestinal involvement in lymphatic leukemia, *Arch. Pathol.* 35:21, 1943.

104. Pengelly, C. D. R., and Wilkinson, J. F. The frequency and mechanism of haemolysis in the leukaemias, reticuloses and myeloproliferative diseases, *Br. J. Haematol.* 8:343, 1962.

105. Perry, S., Irvin, G. L. III, and Whang, J. Studies of lymphocyte kinetics in man, *Blood* 29:22, 1967.

106. Pfisterer, H., Bolland, H., Nennhuber, J., and Stich, W. Lymphocytenabban nach in-vitro-Markierung mit Na$_2$^{51}CrO$_4$. I. Methode und Ergebnisse bei Normalpersonen, *Klin. Wochenschr.* 45:995, 1967.

107. Pincus, S., Bianco, C., and Nussenzweig, V. Increased proportion of complement-receptor lymphocytes in the peripheral blood of patients with chronic lymphocytic leukemia, *Blood* 40:303, 1972.

108. Pisciotta, A. V., Jermain, L. F., and Hinz, J. E. Chronic lymphocytic leukemia, hypogammaglobulinemia and autoimmune hemolytic anemia — an experiment of nature, *Blood* 15:748, 1960.

109. Portmann, U. V., and Robinson, W. H. Lymphatic leukemia occurring simultaneously in Negro brother and sister, *Cleve. Clin. Q.* 18:33, 1951.

110. Presant, C. A., and Kornfeld, S. Characterization of the cell surface receptor for the *Agaricus bisporus* hemagglutinin, *J. Biol. Chem.* 247:6937, 1972.

111. Prolla, J. C., and Kirsner, J. B. The gastrointestinal lesions and compli-

cations of the leukemias, *Ann. Intern. Med.* 61:1084, 1964.

112. Rabellino, E., Colon, S., Grey, H. M., and Unanue, E. R. Immunoglobulins on the surface of lymphocytes. I. Distribution and quantitation, *J. Exp. Med.* 133:156, 1971.

113. Rigler, L. G. Leukemia of the stomach producing hypertrophy of the gastric mucosa, *J.A.M.A.* 107:2025, 1936.

114. Rosenthal, N. The lymphomas and leukemias, *Bull. N.Y. Acad. Med.* 30:583, 1954.

115. Rosenthal, N., and Harris, W. Leukemia. Its diagnosis and treatment, *J.A.M.A.* 104:702, 1935.

116. Rowe, S. N. Mikulicz's syndrome with chronic lymphatic leukemia, *N. Engl. J. Med.* 202:863, 1930.

117. Rubin, A. D., Douglas, S. D., Chessin, L. N., et al. Chronic reticulolymphocytic leukemia, *Am. J. Med.* 47:149, 1969.

118. Rubin, A. D., Havemann, K., and Dameshek, W. Studies in chronic lymphocytic leukemia. Further studies of the proliferative abnormality of the blood lymphocyte, *Blood* 33:313, 1969.

119. Rubini, J. R., Bond, V. P., Keller, S., Fliedner, T. M., and Cronkite, E. P. DNA synthesis in circulating blood leukocytes labeled in vitro with H[3] thymidine, *J. Lab. Clin. Med.* 58:751, 1961.

120. Rundles, R. W., Coonrad, E. V., and Arends, T. Serum proteins in leukemia, *Am. J. Med.* 16:842, 1954.

121. Schiffer, L. M. Kinetics of chronic lymphocytic leukemia, *Ser. Haematol.* 1:3, 1968.

122. Schrek, R. Prednisone sensitivity and cytology of viable lymphocytes as tests for chronic lymphocytic leukemia, *J. Natl. Cancer Inst.* 33:837, 1964.

123. Schrek, R. Effect of phytohemagglutinin on lymphocytes from patients with chronic lymphocytic leukemia, *Arch. Pathol.* 83:58, 1967.

124. Schrek, R., and Donnelly, W. J. "Hairy" cells in blood in lymphoreticular neoplastic disease and "flagellated" cells of normal lymph nodes, *Blood* 27:199, 1966.

125. Schwab, R. S., and Weiss, S. Neurologic aspect of leukemia, *Am. J. Med. Sci.* 189:766, 1935.

126. Scott, J. L., McMillan, R., Marino, J. V., et al. Leukocyte labeling with [51]chromium. IV. The kinetics of chronic lymphocytic leukemic lymphocytes, *Blood* 41:155, 1973.

127. Shanbrom, E., and Finch, S. C. The auditory manifestations of leukemia, *Yale J. Biol. Med.* 31:144, 1958.

128. Shanbrom, E., and Kahn, D. Treatment of leukemia cutis with Demecolcin, *Ann. Intern. Med.* 47:565, 1957.

129. Shanbrom, E., Miller, S., and Haar, H. Herpes zoster in hematologic neoplasias: some unusual manifestations, *Ann. Intern. Med.* 53:523, 1960.

130. Shapiro, J. H., Ramsay, C. G., Jacobson, H. G., Botstein, C. C., and Allen, L. B. Renal involvement in lymphomas and leukemias in adults, *Am. J. Roentgenol.* 88:928, 1962.

131. Sharman, C., Crossen, P. E., and Fitzgerald, P. H. Lymphocyte number and response to phytohaemagglutinin in chronic lymphocytic leukaemia, *Scand. J. Haematol.* 3:375, 1966.

132. Shaw, R. K., Boggs, D. R., Silberman, H. R., et al. A study of prednisone therapy in chronic lymphocytic leukemia, *Blood* 17:182, 1961.

133. Shaw, R. K., Szwed, C., Boggs, D. R., Fahey, J. L., Frei, E. III, Morrison, E., and Utz, J. P. Infection and immunity in chronic lymphocytic leukemia, *Arch. Intern. Med.* 106:467, 1960.

134. Shevach, E. M., Herberman, R., Frank, M. M., et al. Receptors for complement and immunoglobulins on human leukemic cells and human lymphoblastoid cell lines, *J. Clin. Invest.* 51:1933, 1972.

135. Shimkin, M. B. Mortality from leukemia and the lymphomas in the United States, *in* Proc. Third National Cancer Conf., p. 305, J. B. Lippincott, Philadelphia, 1957.

136. Shimkin, M. B., Lucia, E. L., Opperman, K. C., and Mettier, S. P. Lymphocytic leukemia: an analysis of frequency, distribution and mortality at the University of California Hospital, 1913–1947, *Ann. Intern. Med.* 39:1254, 1953.

137. Shimkin, M. B., and Loveland, D. B. A note on mortality from lymphatic leukemia in Oriental populations of the United States, *Blood* 17:763, 1961.

138. Sibley, W. A., and Weisberger, A. S. Demyelinating disease of the brain in chronic lymphocytic leukemia, *Arch. Neurol.* 5:300, 1961.

139. Sokal, J. E., and Primikirios, N. The delayed skin test response in Hodgkin's disease and lymphosarcoma. Effect of disease activity, *Cancer* 14:597, 1961.

140. Stryckmans, P. A., Chanana, A. D., Cronkite, E. P., Greenberg, M. L., and Schiffer, L. M. In-vivo behavior of in-vitro irradiated lymphocytes in chronic lymphocytic leukemia (CLL), *Clin. Res.* 14:328, 1966.

141. Stryckmans, P. A., Chanana, A. D., Cronkite, E. P., Greenberg, M. L., and Schiffer, L. M. Studies on lymphocytes. IX. The survival of autotransfused labeled lymphocytes in chronic lymphocytic leukemia, *Eur. J. Cancer* 4:241, 1968.

142. Takeda, K. Geographical pathology of leukaemia in Japan, *Acta Un. Int. Contra Cancr.* 16:1629, 1960.

143. Thompson, A. E. R., Robinson, M. A., and Wetherley-Mein, G. Heterogeneity of lymphocytes in chronic lymphocytic leukemia, *Lancet* ii:200, 1966.

144. Tivey, H. The prognosis for survival in chronic granulocytic and lymphocytic leukemia, *Am. J. Roentgenol.* 72:68, 1954.

145. Troup, S. B., Swisher, S. N., and Young, L. E. The anemia of leukemia, *Am. J. Med.* 28:751, 1960.

146. Ultmann, J. E. Generalized vaccinia in a patient with chronic lymphocytic leukemia and hypogammaglobulinemia, *Ann. Intern. Med.* 61:728, 1964.

147. Virchow, R. Cellular Pathology (F. Chance, trans.), Great Books of St. John's reprint, Edwards Bros., Ann Arbor, Mich., 1940.

148. Voigt, K-G., and Helbig, W. Pathologie der Nieren bei Leukämien, *Folia Haematol.* 81:121, 1963.

149. Wakisaka, G., Uchino, H., Nakamura, T., Shirakawa, S., Adachi, A., Sakurai, M., and Miyamoto, K. Present status of leukemia in Japan with special reference to epidemiology and studies on the effect of

chemotherapy, *Acta Haematol.* 31:214, 1964.

150. Wells, R., and Lau, K. S. Incidence of leukaemia in Singapore and rarity of chronic lymphocytic leukaemia in Chinese, *Br. Med. J.* 1:759, 1960.

151. Wetherley-Mein, G., Epstein, I. S., Foster, W. D., and Grimes, A. J. Mechanisms of anaemia in leukaemia, *Br. J. Haematol.* 4:281, 1958.

152. Weve, H. Lymphomatosis iridis bei Leukämie, *Arch. Augenheilkd.* 105:710, 1932.

153. Wilson, J. D., and Nossal, G. J. V. Identification of human T and B lymphocytes in normal peripheral blood and in chronic lymphocytic leukaemia. *Lancet* ii:788, 1971.

154. Windeyer, B. W., and Stewart, J. W. The leukaemias, *in* S. Cade (ed.), Malignant Disease and Its Treatment by Radium, 2nd ed., vol. 4, p. 347, John Wright and Sons, Bristol, England, 1952.

155. Winkelstein, A., and Craddock, C. G. Comparative response of normal human thymus and lymph node cells to phythohemagglutinin in culture, *Blood* 29:594, 1967.

156. Winter, G. C. B., Osmond, D. G., Yoffey, J. M., and Mahy, D. J. Leucocyte cultures with phytohaemagglutinin in chronic lymphatic leukaemia, *Lancet* ii:563, 1964.

157. Wintrobe, M. M. Clinical Hematology, 6th ed., p. 985, Lea & Febiger, Philadelphia, 1967.

158. Wintrobe, M. M., and Hasenbush, L. L. Chronic leukemia. The early phase of chronic leukemia, the results of treatment and the effects of complicating infections; a study of eighty-six adults, *Arch. Intern. Med.* 64:701, 1939.

159. Wintrobe, M. M., and Mitchell, D. M. Atypical manifestations of leukaemia, *Q. J. Med.* 9:67, 1940.

160. Wisniewski, D., and Weinreich, J. Lymphatische Leukämie bei Vater und Sohn, *Blut* 12:241, 1966.

161. Yam, L. T., Castoldi, G. L., Garvey, M. D., and Mitus, W. J. Functional cytogenetic and cytochemical study of the leukemic reticulum cells, *Blood* 32:90, 1968.

162. Zacharski, L. R., and Linman, J. W. Chronic lymphocytic leukemia versus chronic lymphosarcoma cell leukemia. Analysis of 496 cases, *Am. J. Med.* 47:75, 1969.

163. Zimmerman, T. S., Godwin, H. A., and Perry, S. Studies of leukocyte kinetics in chronic lymphocytic leukemia, *Blood* 31:277, 1968.

Chapter 20 Multiple Myeloma, Macroglobulinemia, and Other Monoclonal Gammopathies

Various disorders are characterized by proliferation of either normal or neoplastic plasma cells (154). In this chapter we shall consider multiple myeloma and related neoplastic conditions that share two features: the proliferation of malignant lymphoid cells or plasma cells, and the production of a homogeneous immunoglobulin. These conditions are sometimes referred to as *gammopathies*, or *monoclonal gammopathies*, because of the associated overproduction of a single class of immunoglobulin. These disorders are part of the lymphoproliferative spectrum of diseases.

Chapters 12 and 13 reviewed the morphogenesis of the lymphoid series and presented data supporting the rationale for dividing the lymphoid cells into two major categories: B cells and T cells. In Chapter 15 evidence was presented in support of the concept that B cells are the precursors of immunoglobulin-producing cells. Normal B cells comprise a cytologic spectrum from undistinguished small lymphocytes to well-differentiated plasma cells (see Chapter 12 figures). The B-cell neoplasias comprise a similar spectrum encompassing small lymphocytes, medium lymphocytes, "activated" lymphocytes, and plasma cells at various levels of morphologic maturity. The preceding chapter reviewed chronic lymphocytic leukemia—a B-cell disorder characterized primarily by small and medium-sized lymphocytes. We shall now examine B-cell disorders in which production of immunoglobulins is a prominent feature of the clinical picture. Generally, the neoplastic cells involved in these disorders have at least some cytologic features of more mature B cells (plasma cells). As illustrated in Figs. 20.1 to 20.4, a variety of morphologic forms of neoplastic B cells may be encountered in the bone marrow of patients with monoclonal gammopathies. The relation between these cells and their normal counterparts is apparent.

Multiple Myeloma

Incidence, Age, and Sex Distribution

Multiple myeloma is a disease of old age, with median onset between the ages of sixty and seventy; cases with onset before age forty are exceedingly rare (127, 307). There are good arguments that well-documented multiple myeloma does not occur before age thirty (307).

Most series of patients with multiple myeloma published before 1961 showed a preponderance (3:1 or 3:2) of males to females with the diagnosis of multiple myeloma (18, 281). In more recent series the reverse has been true (91, 307).

The reported incidence of new cases of multiple myeloma in England and Scandinavia has varied between 2.4 and 4 per 100,000 population per year (91, 201, 307). In the United States the disease is somewhat more common in blacks than in Caucasians (194). Rare reports document familial occurrence of multiple myeloma (6, 217). Whether the disease is the same (that is, the same paraprotein) in all affected members of involved families is not known.

Studies of the Atomic Bomb Casualty Commission indicate a striking increase in the incidence of multiple

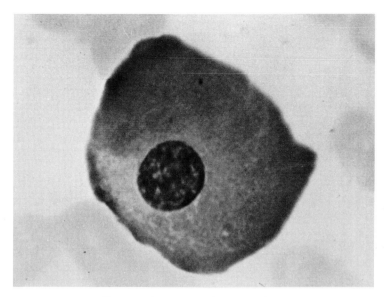

Figure 20.1 A "flame" plasma cell from the bone marrow of a patient with multiple myeloma. Note the densely clumped nuclear chromatin, the eccentric nucleus, and the perinuclear clear zone. Giemsa stain.

myeloma in persons exposed to high levels of irradiation (10), and Lewis has suggested that there may be a higher incidence of multiple myeloma in American radiologists than might be anticipated from chance alone (180). With the exception of ionizing irradiation, no known factors predispose man to this disease.

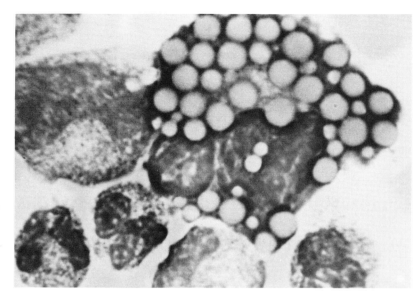

Figure 20.3 A large plasma cell filled with glycoprotein inclusions. With Giemsa stain the inclusions were clear light pink. Such inclusions are sometimes called Mott bodies. More distinctly red inclusions are called Russell bodies. Macrophages with glycoprotein or lipoprotein inclusions may have a similar appearance.

Clinical Features

General Manifestations A reading of the original description in 1850 of a patient with multiple myeloma is a rewarding experience for any student of hematology. "A case of mollities and fragilitas ossium, accompanied with

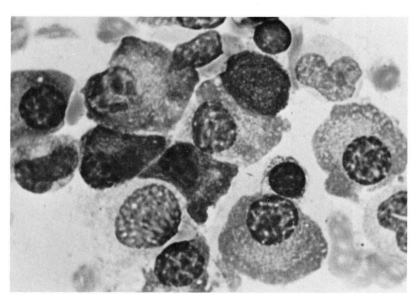

Figure 20.2 Plasma cells in the bone marrow of a patient with multiple myeloma. Heterogeneity of cellular morphology is apparent. Giemsa stain.

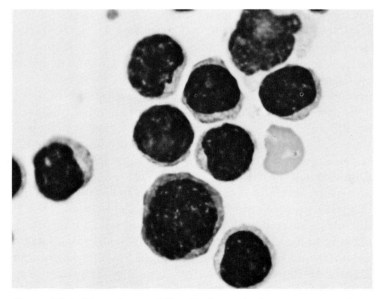

Figure 20.4 "Lymphocytoid" cells from the bone marrow of a patient with Waldenström's macroglobulinemia.

urine strongly charged with animal matter" (190) is a classic description of a patient with multiple myeloma who suffered from painful bones, fractures, and anemia. Sir Henry Bence Jones, who acted as a consultant in this intriguing case, documented "animal matter" in the urine by means of a simple test and as a consequence managed to gain most of the recognition for the early description of multiple myeloma.

The major clinical features reported in that original description still hold today: bone pain as a consequence of widespread osteolytic lesions and fractures, and pallor reflecting anemia. The principal clinical manifestations of multiple myeloma are summarized in Table 20.1.

The major proliferation of neoplastic plasma cells takes place within the bones and bone marrow. The principal clinical manifestations appear to be a direct or indirect consequence of this proliferation: osteoporosis, osteolytic lesions with little osteoblastic reaction, and, occasionally, hypercalcemia, which is thought to be a consequence of bone resorption. Neoplastic infiltration is also associated with loss of normal erythropoietic and sometimes granulopoietic elements of the bone marrow, with resultant anemia and neutropenia.

Other clinical manifestations appear to be related to the production of large amounts of a homogeneous gamma globulin by the malignant plasma cell. Renal tubular dysfunction and, ultimately, renal failure may result from the hypergammaglobulinemia and excessive production of light chains.

Suppression of normal antibody immunoglobulin production may occur as a consequence of the excessive con-

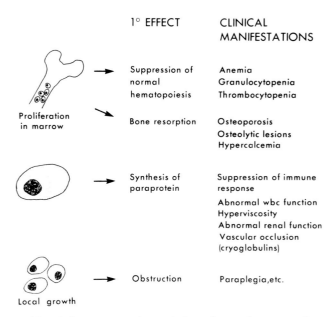

Figure 20.5 Schematic outline of the relation between clinical manifestations of multiple myeloma and neoplastic plasma cell proliferation and synthesis of paraprotein.

centration of circulating paraprotein. The subsequent immunologic impairment, coupled with the frequently occurring neutropenia, results in a greatly increased susceptibility to infection. Infection is therefore a prominent feature of multiple myeloma.

Rarely, the paraprotein is of such a high concentration and of such physical structure that it contributes to a greatly increased serum viscosity. This may result in symptoms of hyperviscosity, including neurologic and ophthalmologic disturbances. Hyperviscosity syndrome is relatively rare in multiple myeloma and will be considered in more detail in the section of this chapter entitled "Macroglobulinemia."

Abnormal protein production occasionally results in amyloidosis with organ infiltration and, often, renal failure. Finally, the clinical manifestations of multiple myeloma may result from direct local proliferation of plasma cells and formation of a plasmacytoma that may produce local compressive symptoms. For example, an extradural plasmacytoma may produce spinal cord compression and paraplegia.

The pathophysiologic mechanisms by which multiple myeloma can cause derangement of normal functions and produce clinical manifestations are illustrated in Fig. 20.5 (cf. 262). The abnormalities observed on physical examination can be anticipated from the foregoing discussion. The patient is often pale; he may sit or lie in positions in which he can guard against inadvertent movement of a

Table 20.1 Clinical manifestations of multiple myeloma.

Common manifestations
  Bone pain, fractures
  Pallor, tachycardia, other symptoms of anemia
  Recurrent infections, especially pulmonary
  Renal failure
  Hypercalcemia with neurologic abnormalities and
    gastrointestinal disturbances
Uncommon manifestations
  Hyperviscosity syndrome with neurologic and ocular
    disturbances
  Local plasmacytoma producing compression or obstruction
    of a vital organ
  Amyloidosis
Rare manifestations
  Hepatic functional abnormality
  Splenomegaly and lymphadenopathy
  Skin involvements

painful back or extremity; there may be obvious musculoskeletal abnormalities, such as stooped posture, joint tenderness, muscular spasm, and, occasionally, local masses of tumor tissue; the rib cage may be soft.

Hepatomegaly is reported to occur in nearly 60 percent and splenomegaly in about 25 percent of patients with multiple myeloma (58, 59, 295). These rates are high relative to my own experience. Lymphadenopathy also is unusual (307).

Skin involvement in multiple myeloma, although well documented (42), is extremely uncommon. In my own experience of over a hundred cases I have not seen skin involvement unless thrombocytopenic purpura, amyloidosis, or cold precipitable proteins were present as part of the disease. However, pyoderma gangrenosum has been described in association with multiple myeloma and other paraproteinemias (77, 247).

Having looked at the general clinical manifestations of multiple myeloma, we shall now consider individual organ systems predominantly involved by the disease.

Involvement of the Skeletal System   When Wright described the roentgenographic appearance of a patient with multiple myeloma in 1900, he was probably the first physician to do so (319). The first comprehensive monograph was that of Geschickter and Copeland in 1928 (127). Subsequently, several excellent articles and monographs have documented the variety of skeletal manifestations of multiple myeloma (140, 213, 225).

Roentgenograms may show both axial and appendicular skeletal involvement in multiple myeloma, although as a rule axial involvement predominates (127). Two types of lesions are seen on X ray: discrete osteolytic foci with little reaction in the surrounding bone (Fig. 20.6), and generalized osteoporosis.

The finding of osteolytic lesions by roentgenogram is usually clear cut, and the only diagnostic challenge is differentiation from metastatic carcinoma. The finding of generalized osteoporosis, or marked osteoporosis of the vertebral bodies, is more difficult to interpret, since osteoporosis from other causes is a common finding in the age group in which multiple myeloma occurs. However, widespread osteolytic lesions are a more usual finding. Early in the disease these are often confined to the axial skeleton. In late-stage disease the extremities are commonly involved. Occasionally, patients have no obvious skeletal lesions early in their disease (307).

In multiple myeloma a common finding on roentgenogram of the skull is multiple round osteolytic lesions of variable size and with little surrounding bone reaction (Fig. 20.6). In some cases, when only a few lesions are

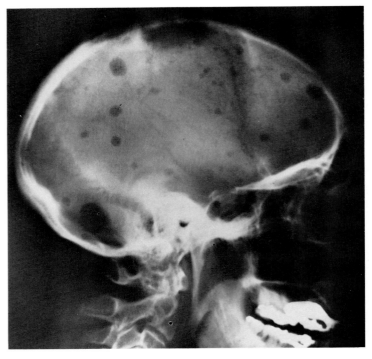

Figure 20.6 Roentgenogram of the skull demonstrating osteolytic lesions.

present and located near the midline, distinction from Pacchionian granulations may be difficult. The base of the skull is rarely involved, perhaps because of the absence of myeloid marrow in that area. The mandible occasionally shows evidence of the disease process.

Involvement of the thoracic cage by multiple myeloma is common. The most frequent lesions are fractures of the ribs. Small subpleural tumors arising from the ribs are not uncommon. A plasmacytoma occasionally has the roentgenographic appearance of a primary lung tumor. Clavicular and scapular involvement occurs, and spontaneous fracture of the sternum should always arouse suspicion of multiple myeloma (281).

The vertebral column is a common site of involvement by multiple myeloma, and back pain is the most frequent presenting complaint. Lesions vary from osteoporosis to focal lytic lesions to total vertebral collapse (140). Occasionally a plasmacytoma may grow as an extradural mass and cause spinal cord compression. The last thoracic and first lumbar vertebrae are the most common sites of first fractures (307). The lack of new bone proliferation observed in histologic sections and by roentgenograms is reflected in a serum alkaline phosphatase level that generally is normal in patients with multiple myeloma (91, 281).

The etiology of the bone pain experienced with multiple myeloma is uncertain, although bone infarction has been suspected as a cause (56). The mechanism of bone resorption also is unknown, but recent observations suggest that myeloma cells may produce a bone-resorbing material (216).

Renal Involvement   Proteinuria is an extremely common manifestation of multiple myeloma. In Drivsholm's series, 60 percent of the patients had proteinuria at the time of diagnosis, and 85 percent had proteinuria at some time during their illness (91). Snapper observed proteinuria in 90 percent of his cases and documented the following frequency of abnormalities in the urinary sediment: pyuria, 80 percent; hematuria, 45 percent; and casts, 20 percent (281).

One of the first comprehensive descriptions of the pathology of myeloma kidney was that of Thannhauser and Krauss in 1920 (294). They noted tubules distended by hyaline material, with atrophy of the tubular cells and the presence of peritubular fibrosis. They did not document the characteristic giant cells encountered in such kidneys. The presence of intratubular casts has also been documented by nephron dissection (224). Protein droplets have been observed within tubular cells (11).

The pathogenetic mechanisms of renal failure in multiple myeloma are not clear. It is known that the kidney may be involved in the catabolism of light chains. These proteins are probably pinocytosed by the renal tubular cells and subsequently degraded. This catabolic mechanism may be overwhelmed by the overproduction of light chains (Bence Jones protein). Excessive Bence Jones proteinuria has been assumed to be in some manner detrimental to renal tubular function (91, 225). Another mechanism of renal damage in multiple myeloma is hypercalcemia and hypercalciuria. Renal calcinosis is not uncommon in patients with this disease (281). Arends and Mandema (12) consider hypercalcemia to be the critical pathogenetic mechanism in the production of the myeloma kidney. The kidney parenchyma occasionally may be infiltrated directly by myeloma cells, but these tend to be small accumulations unlikely to affect renal function. The kidney may also be infiltrated with amyloid.

Renal involvement by multiple myeloma may be expressed clinically as renal tubular dysfunction, which may be limited to abnormality of acidification (212) or which may be sufficiently flagrant to possess all the features of the Fanconi's syndrome (101, 278). Glomerular damage also may occur (14). Ultimately, renal failure supervenes with a typical clinical picture of azotemia. Hypertension is very rarely associated with a renal failure in multiple myeloma.

Hematologic Manifestations   In multiple myeloma the bone marrow is almost always infiltrated by plasma cells. This is apparent both in aspirates and in biopsies of the marrow (51).

Red cells.   Anemia occurs sometime in the course of disease in well over 80 percent of patients with multiple myeloma (62, 91, 281). The anemia is generally normochromic and normocytic, and the reticulocyte count is not elevated. The precise mechanism of anemia is not known. As a general rule, the red cell life-span is moderately shortened without a compensatory erythropoiesis by the bone marrow (62). Melena and subsequent iron deficiency contribute to the anemia of some patients. Severe hemolysis or hypersplenism is very rare (307). The occurrence of renal failure may contribute to the anemia. The precise pathogenetic mechanisms of both the shortened red cell life-span and the inadequate erythropoietic response are obscure.

Red cell morphology usually is distorted by the striking rouleau formation in the smear of the peripheral blood. Cryoglobulins rarely interfere with enumeration of red cells. A rare occurrence in myeloma is the development of sideroblastic anemia, which may presage the appearance of acute myeloblastic leukemia (164).

Leukocytes.   Leukocyte number and differential count are often normal in multiple myeloma. However, Snapper observed leukopenia at some time in the course of disease in 40 percent of patients (281). Sometimes profound granulocytopenia is present before the initiation of any therapy (300, 307), probably as a result of plasma cell infiltration of the bone marrow (Figs. 20.2 and 20.7) and resultant inadequate granulopoiesis. With the advent of aggressive chemotherapy in the past few years, leukopenia induced by drugs has become almost a constant feature of the clinical picture. In a small series of cases we observed that leukopenia, like anemia, was sometimes responsive to androgen therapy (62). Patients with multiple myeloma may respond to infection with the appropriate leukocytosis and granulocytosis, or their granulocytic response may be impaired. One report suggests that phagocytic function may be weakened as a consequence of the abnormal protein (234).

The occurrence of plasma cells in the blood of patients with multiple myeloma is a point of some controversy. Snapper observed that 22 percent of his patients had plasmacytosis, and DiGuglielmo is said to have found plasmacytosis in 60 percent of all patients with multiple

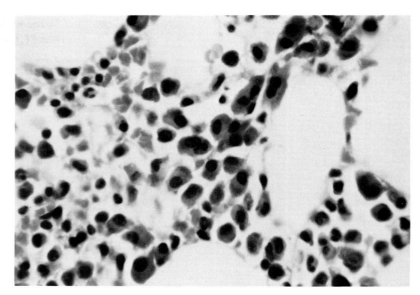

Figure 20.7 Section of a bone marrow clot demonstrating extensive infiltration by neoplastic plasma cells. Hematoxylin and eosin stain.

myeloma. Such observations must be accepted with caution. Plasma cells in small numbers may be encountered in the blood of normal subjects, and the numbers may increase in certain immunologic reactions. It is in fact very unusual to encounter myeloma patients with plasmacytosis of noteworthy degree. The rare syndrome of plasmacytosis sufficient to be considered plasma cell leukemia does occur, however, and will be considered separately. Multiple myeloma and chronic lymphocytic leukemia rarely occur simultaneously (307). Since both of these diseases probably arise from proliferation of a single clone of neoplastic B cells, simultaneous occurrence must indeed be a rare phenomenon.

Platelets and the coagulation mechanism. In some series thrombocytopenia with a platelet count of less than 100,000 occurs in about 1 in 4 patients with untreated myeloma (91, 281) and at a much lower frequency in other series (32, 307). Thrombocytopenia often results from vigorous chemotherapy. The high levels of paraprotein may interfere with platelet function even when the platelet count is normal (233).

In addition to thrombocytopenia and thrombocytopathy as causes of hemorrhagic manifestations in multiple myeloma, a variety of coagulation defects may occur and lead to bleeding diathesis. Three types of coagulopathy have been identified (220, 281): antithrombin activity, decreased antihemophilic globulin, and circulating fibrinolysin. Antithrombin activity is more common in IgG myeloma than in IgA myeloma. Such coagulation abnormalities do not necessarily lead to bleeding diathesis.

Neurologic Involvement A variety of neurologic syndromes may be associated with multiple myeloma (Table 20.2). Of these, the most serious is paraplegia secondary to extradural spinal cord compression and/or vertebral collapse (268). Despite the frequency of involvement of the skull in multiple myeloma, intracranial extension of the tumor is very rare and infiltration of the dura and brain is exceedingly unusual (60). However, cranial nerve palsies are not uncommon; the sixth intracranial nerve is the one usually affected by plasmacytoma near the base of the brain.

Peripheral neuropathy also may occur in multiple myeloma. There may be a variety of pathogenetic mechanisms including nerve compression, amyloid infiltration, and, rarely, a peculiar leukoencephalopathy of the type observed in various lymphoproliferative malignancies (40, 84, 163). Another unusual neurologic syndrome is polyradiculitis of the Guillain-Barré type occurring in association with serum paraprotein, high cerebrospinal fluid protein concentrations, plasmacytosis in the marrow, and osteolytic and osteosclerotic lesions (221, 256, 307).

Encephalopathy with loss of higher cortical function and even frank coma has been associated with very high levels of serum and cerebrospinal fluid protein (320). This is more common in macroglobulinemia than in multiple myeloma. The pathogenesis of this interesting syndrome is unknown, although it has often been ascribed to abnormalities of cerebral perfusion consequent to the paraprotein.

Immunologic Impairment and Microbial Defense Patients with multiple myeloma often have reduced levels of normal immunoglobulins at a time when they have greatly increased concentrations of serum paraprotein. Their ability to synthesize humoral antibody in response to antigenic stimulation also is impaired (105, 174, 183). Cellular immune responses (delayed hypersensitivity reactions) tend to be unimpaired in multiple myeloma (183).

The reason for the reduced levels of normal immunoglobulins is not certain. The catabolic rate of

Table 20.2 Neurologic involvement in multiple myeloma.

Spinal cord and cranial nerve compression
Amyloidosis and peripheral neuropathy
Leukoencephalopathy of unknown etiology
Polyradiculitis of unknown etiology
Coma related to increased viscosity
Hypercalcemia

normal globulins, as well as of paraproteins, probably is increased in multiple myeloma (184, 285). Furthermore, the rate of synthesis of normal immunoglobulins may be reduced in the presence of high concentrations of paraprotein.

In addition to immunologic impairment, the high levels of paraprotein present in multiple myeloma can interfere with granulocyte phagocytic function (234). However, granulocytopenia probably is a more frequent and more important abnormality of the host defense against microbial agents. Taken together, the multiple aberrations summarized in Table 20.3 lead to an enhanced susceptibility to infection in multiple myeloma. An increased frequency of bacterial infection is well recognized in this disorder (105). Infection, particularly of the lungs, is often a terminal event. Ventilatory insufficiency as a result of thoracic cage involvement may be a contributing factor.

Less Usual Clinical Variants

Plasma Cell Leukemia   Plasma cell leukemia was reviewed in 1946–47 and again in 1969 (185, 214, 243). It is exceedingly rare and probably accounts for less than 2 percent of plasmacytic dyscrasias (38, 79, 226). The age incidence is approximately the same as that of typical myeloma (52, 243).

The clinical manifestations of plasma cell leukemia have been well described (9, 38, 243, 260, 296). The clinical course may vary: the pattern of fulminant acute leukemia may already be established at the time of initial diagnosis, or a leukemic picture may gradually emerge in the setting of otherwise classical multiple myeloma (243). Until quite recently, the proliferating plasma cells seen in plasmacytic leukemia were thought to be so poorly differentiated that they could produce little or no paraprotein (M protein) (cf. 102, 296). When the more usual multiple myeloma undergoes transition to plasma cell leukemia, the same M protein may be produced. Even

the very unusual paraproteins such as IgD (33) and IgE (157, 158, 243) have been described in plasma cell leukemia.

In an analysis of 57 patients with plasmacytic leukemia, the peripheral white blood count varied between 4,000 and 262,000/mm³ (mean, 51,000), with the percentage of plasma cells varying between 6 and 99 percent (mean, 56 percent) (243). As anticipated, examination of the bone marrow revealed plasma cell infiltration varying from complete replacement of the nucleated cells to as little as 10 percent. The morphology of the leukemic cell has been as varied as that observed in classical multiple myeloma: from very immature (89) to of variable maturity (206). Occasionally, the cells are described as "lymphoid" (122, 266). As a generalization, no correlation has been established among cytology, the type of paraprotein produced, or the clinical course of the disease. The same lack of correlation has been observed in classical multiple myeloma (52, 226). As is true in other acute leukemias, cells of the leukemic form of plasma cell dyscrasias have a high rate of RNA and protein synthesis (215).

Plasma cell leukemia tends to be a more aggressive disease than classical multiple myeloma. Hemorrhagic manifestations, hepatosplenomegaly, and lymphadenopathy appear to be more common in the leukemic patient. In the leukemic form of the disease the average duration of survival from the onset of subjective complaints is 4.8 months (243). In typical multiple myeloma, average survival is 20 to 24 months (226). In the leukemic form, survival does not correlate with the number of plasma cells in the peripheral blood or marrow, or with the type of M protein produced.

As a general rule, plasma cell leukemia is unresponsive to conventional therapy, although rare exceptions have been noted (30, 31).

Amyloidosis   Amyloidosis is a relatively rare complication of multiple myeloma (226). There are subtle differences in the clinical manifestations of amyloid disease among patients with primary amyloidosis, myeloma-associated amyloidosis, and secondary amyloidosis (45, 47, 66, 292). Regardless of the classification of amyloidosis, renal disease is a major feature of the illness of most affected patients (26, 45). However, minor differences occur among these disease categories. For example, in one series mesenchymal involvement, especially cardiac, occurred in 90 percent of patients with primary and myeloma-associated disease and in only 61 percent of those with secondary amyloidosis. Tongue involvement and carpal tunnel syndrome also were more common in myeloma-associated and primary amyloidosis. Occasionally patients

Table 20.3 Impaired antimicrobial defense mechanisms in multiple myeloma.

Abnormality	Mechanism
1. Reduced levels of normal immunoglobulin	1. Impaired synthesis; hypercatabolism
2. Defective humoral antibody response to antigen	2. ?Inhibition by paraprotein
3. Granulocytopenia	3. Marrow infiltration; chemotherapy
4. Defective phagocytosis	4. Paraprotein interference
5. Impaired ventilation	5. Thoracic cage involvement

Table 20.4 Clinical manifestations of amyloidosis associated with multiple myeloma.

Cardiac
    Congestive heart failure
    Cardiomegaly without heart failure
    Conduction defects
Renal
    Proteinuria
    Nephrotic syndrome
    Renal failure
Parenchymal organs
    Hepatosplenomegaly
    Gastrointestinal infiltration
    Macroglossia
Miscellaneous
    Cutaneous nodules
    Carpal tunnel syndrome
    Purpura

SOURCE: See references 161, 170, and 182.

present with the symptoms of amyloidosis rather than those of multiple myeloma, but manifestations of amyloidosis and myeloma are apt to become clinically apparent at about the same time. The major clinical manifestations of amyloidosis associated with multiple myeloma are summarized in Table 20.4.

If a nephrotic syndrome develops, the degree of proteinuria is of the same magnitude in myeloma-associated and other forms of amyloidosis. It is worth noting that the kidneys may be large, normal, or contracted in amyloid renal disease. Cardiac and renal involvement appear to be the principal causes of death in patients with myeloma and amyloidosis. Gastrointestinal involvement is manifested by bleeding. Hepatosplenomegaly developing in a patient with multiple myeloma should suggest the possibility of amyloidosis.

The appearance of amyloidosis is a poor prognostic sign in multiple myeloma. Few patients live longer than one year after biopsy establishes the diagnosis of amyloidosis (45). Rectal biopsy is the easiest means of obtaining a tissue diagnosis, especially if it is combined with Congo red staining and polarized light microscopy (209).

The origin of the amyloid deposition in primary, secondary, or myeloma-associated amyloidosis is still not known with certainty (25, 26, 54, 55, 65, 66, 98, 124, 178, 239). Some patients with primary amyloidosis produce a paraprotein; others do not (26, 70, 230).

Amyloid is a fibrillar protein. Under the electron microscope all types of amyloid have a similar ultrastructural appearance. Certain amyloid fibrils from patients with primary and myeloma-associated amyloidosis have as

their major subunit the variable region of homogeneous light chains (129, 166, 293). In contrast, a component that constitutes up to 50 percent of the protein in amyloid fibrils from patients with secondary amyloidosis—and one type of familial amyloidosis—is unrelated to any known immunoglobulin (96, 151, 178, 179, 239). The possibility remains that this nonimmunoglobulin amyloid protein is the product of enzymatic digestion of a larger immunoglobulin molecule (128). Recently a third class of amyloid fibril protein was obtained from a patient with primary amyloidosis (150). Glenner and his colleagues have recently reviewed the nature and pathogenesis of amyloidosis (130).

Extraosseous Multiple Myeloma   Multiple myeloma is primarily a disease of the bone and bone marrow; however, in about 70 percent of cases soft-tissue infiltration by plasma cells, particularly of liver, spleen, and lymph nodes, is found at necropsy (59, 139). Sometimes discrete extraosseous tumor masses occur and give rise to symptoms that may dominate the clinical picture (94, 139, 141, 257).

Anatomic sites in which extraosseous plasmacytomas may cause symptoms by compression, obstruction, or hemorrhage include the gastrointestinal tract from the stomach to the rectum (276), the liver (83, 92, 288), brain (168), breast (250), upper airway (53, 90, 141), lymph nodes (218, 257, 277), retroperitoneal space (28, 94, 306), intrathoracic space (144) including lungs and pleural space (106, 120, 123, 162), subcutaneous tissue (94), skin (90, 92, 139), and buccal mucosa (181).

The course of solitary extramedullary plasmacytoma may be identical to that of typical multiple myeloma, or it may be more prolonged (94, 141, 218, 277).

Other Variants   Several additional variants of myeloma have been reported. Hyperviscosity syndrome occurs, although it is distinctly rare relative to the incidence in macroglobulinemia (34, 316). Hemorrhagic ascites is also a rare complication of multiple myeloma (238).

Paraprotein Synthesis

It is believed that an individual plasma cell normally produces an immunoglobulin of only a single class, although the possibility that a cell may switch from IgM to IgG synthesis has not been completely excluded (see Chapter 12). As seen in Fig. 20.8, antibody produced by a single cell runs as a narrow band on electrophoresis (199). Myeloma proteins found in the blood and urine of patients with myelomatosis are of a single class also.

One of the basic abnormalities of diseases such as multiple myeloma, macroglobulinemia, and related disorders is the excessive proliferation of a clone of plasma cells. The consequence of this proliferation is the synthesis of large quantities of a homogeneous protein. Since all the cells of the clone are the progeny of a single cell, they would be expected to produce identical proteins unless some of the cells of the clone had undergone somatic mutation in the course of proliferation. Myeloma is therefore characterized by the presence of a "monoclonal gam-

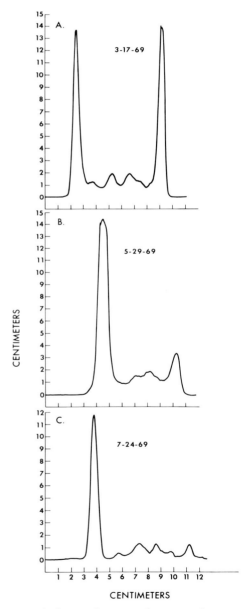

Figure 20.8 Serial electrophoresis of serum of a patient with multiple myeloma showing a gradual diminution of the M component in the course of chemotherapy.

mopathy." In contrast, diseases such as cirrhosis, chronic infections, and collagen diseases are characterized by diffuse hyperglobulinemia or "polyclonal gammopathy"; that is, an increase in all gamma globulin fractions (298).

As discussed in Chapter 16, immunoglobulins are composed of two heavy and two light chains or are polymers or aggregates of such molecules. The light chains are of either κ or λ subclass. Light chains of a single class are paired with heavy chains of a single class. For example, an IgG molecule may be either $\gamma 2\kappa 2$ or $\gamma 2\lambda 2$. Similarly, an IgA molecule may be either $\alpha 2\kappa 2$ or $\alpha 2\lambda 2$. With five known classes of heavy chains and two light chains, ten different serum immunoglobulins may be formed. A number of structural variants of each class of polypeptide chain have been recognized. For example, more than twenty variants of the Gm locus of the gamma chain have been recognized (203), and at least three variants of the Inv locus of the light chain (21). Other structural features of the heavy chains permit further subclassification. It is obvious from the foregoing that a given immunoglobulin may be described in detail by the class and subclass of its light and heavy chains. As a general rule, most or all of the molecules of a given paraprotein have identical features. For practical purposes, a paraprotein may be defined as an immunoglobulin of narrow electrophoretic mobility whose heavy and/or light chains have been shown immunochemically to be of only one type.

Occasionally in multiple myeloma and related disorders more than one M component is observed in a single patient (136). This phenomenon presumably arises from the coexistence of two or more lines of malignant cells (76, 100, 167, 249, 264, 267). Each of these is presumed to produce a single type of protein. The paraproteins observed in multiple myeloma are thought to be related to the normally occurring antibody immunoglobulin. In fact, antibody activity against specific antigenic determinants has been documented for several human and mouse myeloma proteins (204, 301).

The incidence of serum paraproteins in a "normal" population of 7,000 has been recorded by Hällén (134) as 1 percent in individuals over fifty years of age and 3 percent in those over seventy. Most of these do not appear to be of pathological significance (19). In a large hospital population the incidence of paraprotein was about the same, but almost two-thirds of the patients had reticuloendothelial malignancy (146, 148). Features suggesting the presence of malignancy included Bence Jones proteinemia, a reduction in the concentration of normal immunoglobulin, high levels of paraprotein, and a progressive increase in the concentration of paraprotein.

In normal antibody-forming cells and well-differentiated plasmacytoma cells, heavy-chain synthesis and light-chain synthesis are well balanced, and less than 1 percent of synthesized protein leaves the cell as free light chains (17, 228, 229). In myelomatosis and some related disorders, immunoglobulin synthesis may be unbalanced so that free light chains appear in the serum or urine. In some cases no heavy chains are synthesized or released, and Bence Jones proteins are the only detectable paraproteins. Thus patients with multiple myeloma may synthesize either an intact paraprotein molecule or a portion of the molecule, or both the intact molecule and free light chains in some combination. Almost invariably, the Bence Jones protein produced in a given patient with multiple myeloma is of a single light-chain type—κ or λ. The Bence Jones protein has been shown to be synthesized by the malignant plasma cell in vitro (16, 205), as are other paraproteins (299).

When both serum and urine are examined electrophoretically, a paraprotein can be demonstrated in 87 to 99 percent of patients with multiple myeloma (52, 147, 227). The amount of paraprotein produced may be enormous and reach levels of 12 or more gm/100 ml of serum, but is more usually in the range of 3 to 4 gm. A few patients apparently do not produce a detectable paraprotein (69, 147).

A variety of techniques is available for demonstrating the presence of a paraprotein. Filter paper electrophoresis is the simplest and cheapest, but has certain limitations in defining the type of paraprotein (168) (Fig. 20.8). A more sophisticated and more difficult technique is electrophoresis on either cellulose acetate or polyacrylamide (143, 145). Since electrophoretic mobility alone usually is insufficient to define precisely the type of paraprotein, immunoelectrophoresis is used instead. These newer methods have largely replaced the older, more cumbersome technique of ultracentrifugation of serum and urine. By the coordinated use of the ultracentrifuge and electrophoresis, it has been possible to show that IgA paraproteins often form polymers or complexes (197, 307). Data concerning the various classes of paraprotein observed in multiple myeloma and macroglobulinemia are summarized in Table 20.5.

The relative amounts of the different classes of immunoglobulins in normal serum are 70(IgG), 25(IgA), 5(IgM), 0.2(IgD), and 0.1(IgE). The order of frequency with which specific types of paraproteins occur in patients with myeloma and macroglobulinemia is roughly the same (Table 20.6). IgG myeloma is 2 to 3 times more common than IgA myeloma and is about 15 times more common that IgM macroglobulinemia (147, 228). IgD myeloma (149, 255) and IgE myeloma (153, 156, 157) are extremely rare. Bence Jones proteinemia or proteinuria, with absence of other paraproteins, occurs in about 20 percent of patients with multiple myeloma (147, 283, 314).

The presence or absence of a paraprotein or the subclass of paraprotein does not appear to have important prognostic significance for survival or response to therapy in patients with myeloma (52). Within a given class there is no significant correlation among the amount of M component and the percentage of plasma cells in the marrow, the degree of uremia, or the degree of hypercalcemia. Hobbs (147) has suggested that Bence Jones myeloma occurring in relatively young patients may carry a graver prognosis and that IgG myeloma may be associated with more profound reductions in normal immunoglobulins and more frequent infections. However, these differences among myeloma types are not dramatic.

The reported incidence of IgD paraproteins among M components has varied between 1 and 3 percent. Lambda light chains predominate over κ light chains in IgD myelomatosis (80, 104, 110, 173, 322). In the other types of

Table 20.5 Characteristics of different classes of immunoglobulins observed in multiple myeloma and macroglobulinemia.

Present nomenclature	IgG (γG)	IgA (γA)	IgD (γD)	IgE (γE)	IgM (γM)
Electrophoretic mobility	$\beta_1-\gamma_3$	$\alpha_2-\gamma_2$	$\gamma-\beta$	$\gamma-\beta$	$\beta-\gamma$
Molecular weight	150,000	150,000–500,000	150,000	185,000	900,000–1,000,000
Sediment constant	6.6–7 S	7 S (7–14 S)	7 S	7.9 S	19–20 S
Carbohydrate content (%)	2.5–2.9	7–7.5	—	11–12	>10
Light chains	κ or λ	κ or λ	κ or λ	κ or λ	κ or λ
Gm factors	+	−	−	−	−
Inv factors	+	+	+	+	+
Normal serum concentration (gm/100 ml)	0.8–1.5	0.06–0.19	0.003	—	0.039–0.117

Table 20.6 Frequency distribution of immunological classes of paraproteins among patients with myeloma. Figures are approximate and depend on sensitivity of methods used to detect paraprotein.

Class	Percent of total (approximate)
IgG	50–55
IgA	20–25
Bence Jones protein only	20
IgD	1–3
IgE	<0.1
Biclonal	1–2
None detectable	1–8

SOURCE: References 148, 149, 228, and 314.

myelomatosis, κ chains predominate over λ chains (173, 317). In contrast to the situation in IgA and IgG myeloma, concentrations of the paraprotein rarely reach high levels in IgD myeloma, probably because of the rapid rate of catabolism of this paraprotein (248). Bence Jones proteinuria is almost always found in IgD myeloma (104, 149). The rare reported cases with IgE myeloma appear to have had either the typical clinical features of other types of myeloma (157) or plasma cell leukemia (222, 263).

In a few of the patients in one series of 212 cases of myelomatosis, no paraprotein could be detected in serum or concentrated urine even by sophisticated techniques (147). Severe reduction of normal immunoglobulins was observed in this group of patients (186). The lack of a detectable paraprotein may mean a particularly poor prognosis (146).

The data on the distribution of the various types of myeloma are summarized in Table 20.6.

A variety of clinical manifestations of myeloma may be related directly or indirectly to the presence of a paraprotein. These include increased catabolism and decreased synthesis of normal immunoglobulins (285, 308), renal dysfunction, hyperviscosity syndrome with certain IgG paraproteins (193), chemotactic defects (235), low serum sodium (121), and cryoglobulinemia and cold sensitivity.

Course and Prognosis of Disease

When multiple myeloma is untreated or when it does not respond to chemotherapy, the course of disease is unremitting progression. The number of symptomatic bone lesions increases; pain becomes constant and exceedingly severe. Ultimately the patient becomes bedridden and the rate of bone resorption is accelerated. At this stage hypercalcemia or renal failure are often preterminal events. If the patient does not succumb to these, infection may be the final event. In some patients this inexorable progression is modified by chemotherapy, which temporarily arrests plasma cell proliferation and reduces the body burden of neoplastic plasma cells and the associated paraproteinemia.

Indirect evidence indicates that the body may carry a considerable burden of neoplastic plasma cells (perhaps 10^{10} or 10^{11} cells) without myeloma being clinically apparent and without the paraprotein being detected by currently available techniques (262, 290). As the tumor mass increases further, clinical symptoms, paraprotein concentration, and tumor cell numbers increase in a roughly parallel manner until a plateau in cell numbers occurs at approximately 10^{12} cells. Thereafter tumor cell numbers do not increase much further, although clinical symptoms may progress until death occurs.

If the disease responds to chemotherapy, tumor cell numbers decrease. A slower but parallel fall occurs in paraprotein concentration. The concentration of M protein therefore is an indirect indicator of tumor cell mass and responsiveness to therapy. The rate of plasma cell proliferation probably is highest when the tumor mass is small, and the proliferative rate probably diminishes as the tumor cell mass increases above 10^{10} cells. Such a tumor growth pattern is said to follow Gompertzian kinetics (290).

In a series of 238 multiple myeloma patients reported in 1960, median survival from the time of diagnosis was only 3.5 months, although 16 percent of patients survived longer than 18 months and 8 percent for 3 years. Median survival was 8.5 months from onset of symptoms (107). In another series in 1964, 10 percent of patients lived 56 months from diagnosis (289). Survival was quite prolonged in some affected individuals, even before the modern age of chemotherapy (195).

In a more recent series (52) of 112 patients with myelomatosis, median survival from diagnosis was about 17 months. One-third died within a year, and about 6 percent survived longer than 3 years. Clinical factors associated with longer survival include good initial performance, hemoglobin greater than 9 gm/100 ml, a serum calcium less than 12 gm/100 ml, and a blood urea nitrogen less than 30 mg/100 ml. In this series response to therapy was not influenced by the type of paraprotein. Response to chemotherapy was correlated with a better survival.

Principles of Therapy

In multiple myeloma one treats both the neoplastic proliferation of plasma cells and the secondary manifestations of this proliferation (for example, hypercalcemia, hyperviscosity, and infection). In this disorder supportive therapy is a critical adjunct to successful chemotherapy.

Specific Therapy   In multiple myeloma, as in other malignant diseases, it is important to have objective criteria of the response to therapy. The relief of pain and an increase in the patient's activity, although difficult to quantitate, are most important. Objective criteria include decreases in serum myeloma protein concentration (Fig. 20.8) and urinary Bence Jones protein; control of anemia, renal insufficiency, and hypercalcemia; and reduction of bone marrow plasmacytosis. Although arrest of lytic bone lesions often occurs with chemotherapy, recalcification is rare (7).

Among the cytotoxic drugs, only alkylating agents have been consistently useful in the treatment of the malignant plasma cell disorders. Melphalan, a phenylalanine derivative of nitrogen mustard, and cyclophosphamide have been most widely used and can be expected to produce an objective beneficial response in approximately 30 percent of patients with multiple myeloma (35).

Melphalan. Continuous daily therapy, initial loading doses followed by smaller maintenance levels, and intermittent intensive courses have all been used (36, 48, 61). In general, the level of the white blood count has been used as the guide to treatment and is maintained in the range 3,000 to 4,000/mm³; the white blood count should not be permitted to fall below 2,000/mm³. In occasional patients, thrombocytopenia rather than leukopenia is the dose-limiting sign of toxicity and may necessitate discontinuing the treatment.

It is clear that patients whose disease responds to alkylating agents live longer than nonresponders (7).

Cyclophosphamide. Cyclophosphamide is about as effective as melphalan in inducing remission and prolonging life in patients with multiple myeloma. It can be expected to induce remission in 30 to 50 percent of patients. Cyclophosphamide is given in dosages of 1 to 3 mg/kg/day until the white blood count falls below 4,000 to 5,000/mm³. Thereafter the dosage is adjusted downward to keep the white count above 2,000 and preferably between 3,000 and 4,000/mm³. In addition to myelosuppression, the complications of cyclophosphamide treatment include alopecia and hemorrhagic cystitis.

Melphalan and cyclophosphamide have been reported to produce beneficial results in some of the unusual variants of multiple myeloma, including extraosseous tumors, acute renal failure, and plasmacytic leukemia (61). High-dose, intermittent cyclophosphamide may be effective when the disease has become resistant to melphalan therapy (35).

Adrenocorticosteroids are used in the treatment of hypercalcemic complications of multiple myeloma and in the primary treatment of this disorder (109).

One report indicates that sodium fluoride may increase bone density in some patients with multiple myeloma. The general efficacy of this agent, however, still has not been established. Recently, combination therapy with melphalan-prednisone-procarbazine (8) and melphalan-prednisone (73, 126) has produced excellent response rates.

A question frequently asked by the physician is when chemotherapy should be started in treating the patient with multiple myeloma. Most authorities agree that treatment should be started when the diagnosis is established. The disease is almost always inexorably progressive, and spontaneous remission or regression is virtually unknown. Treatment should be started early.

Supportive Therapy Supportive treatment of the complications of myeloma is a necessary adjunct to specific chemotherapy. Each of the complications of disease requires a rational approach.

Hypercalcemia. Hypercalcemia is a frequent manifestation of multiple myeloma, which, if uncontrolled, leads to gastrointestinal and neurologic disturbances, renal failure, and untimely death. Often hypercalcemia can be controlled by adequate hydration, ambulation, and diminished calcium intake. Usually, however, adrenocorticosteroids and intravenous diuretics are required to control severe hypercalcemia. Steroids appear to work by reducing calcium resorption from bone. Occasionally they fail and oral phosphate solutions may be required. Phosphates, however, are not without their own hazards and must be used with caution. The intravenous use of phosphates is extremely hazardous and is not recommended.

Renal failure. In general, this complication of myeloma responds poorly to either supportive therapy or specific chemotherapy. In occasional patients, however, gratifying results can be achieved by high fluid intake, treatment of complicating renal infection, and specific chemotherapy.

Lytic bone lesions. Symptomatic bone lesions, such as collapsed vertebrae, are best treated by local radiation therapy. Although recalcification is infrequently achieved, symptomatic relief is often possible. Spinal cord compression is treated by radiotherapeutic and neurosurgical decompression, and sometimes chemotherapy. Supportive bracing of an involved spine may be necessary for ambulation.

Anemia. The complex anemia of multiple myeloma is best treated by androgens. Some patients cannot tolerate such therapy because of virilization, fluid retention, or change in personality. Fluoxymesterone may produce cholestatic jaundice.

Infection. Bacterial infection should be treated promptly with antibiotics after the appropriate cultures have been obtained and before the organisms have had time to grow out. Because of the poor immune response, live vaccines such as vaccinia should be avoided. Catastrophic complications result from casual vaccinations. The role of prophylactic gamma globulin or normal plasma in preventing infections in these patients remains uncertain.

Hyperviscosity syndrome. This relatively rare complication of multiple myeloma is manifested by visual disturbances and occasionally neurological disturbances accompanied by alteration of consciousness. If the problem is acute, vigorous plasmapheresis can be tried, although it is not usually so successful in reducing viscosity in multiple myeloma as in macroglobulinemia. In the slowly evolving clinical condition, specific antineoplastic chemotherapy is a more reliable method of reducing serum protein concentration and viscosity.

Macroglobulinemia

Definition and Classification

In 1944 Waldenström described a disorder occurring in adult life that was characterized by insidious onset, anemia, bleeding diathesis, and an elevated erythrocyte sedimentation rate, and associated with an increase in serum globulin and infiltration of the bone marrow by "lymphocytoid-plasma" cells (302). The increased serum globulin was subsequently characterized as an IgM macroglobulin (303). This disease syndrome has come to be known as *primary* or *Waldenström's macroglobulinemia.* Many of the clinical features are traceable to the effects of high concentrations of a large asymmetrical protein in the vascular space. This immunoglobulin conforms to the definition of a paraprotein: it is electrophoretically homogeneous and has only one class of light chain. Rarely, antigenic heterogeneity among macroglobulins has been observed (137, 319) and rarely, more than one paraprotein has been detected in a single patient (4).

Macroglobulinemia of significant degree has also been observed without the typical cytologic features of lymphocytoid plasma cells in the bone marrow. It has been seen in association with lymphomas, chronic lymphocytic leukemia, and carcinoma (20, 148, 210). It is difficult to know how to classify this latter group and how to determine whether it is secondary macroglobulinemia or primary macroglobulinemia occurring in fortuitous association with another malignancy. Macroglobulinemia has been observed in a small number of patients with otherwise typical features of myelomatosis (147); this group also is difficult to classify.

One definition of macroglobulinemia is that of Waldenström himself: the concentration of macroglobulin in the serum exceeds 10 percent of the total serum globulin. Another definition is a serum concentration of IgM greater than 1 gm/100 ml—a value ten times the normal.

The Sia water test often is used as crude screening for the presence of high concentrations of macroglobulins, which form a precipitate when serum is added to distilled water (246). The test is not specific for macroglobulinemia and is positive in a variety of disorders with increased concentrations of IgM. Increased levels of polyclonal serum macroglobulins (that is, not homogeneous paraproteins) have been observed in rheumatoid arthritis, chronic infections, cirrhosis, kala-azar, toxoplasmosis, and a variety of neoplastic disorders.

Paraprotein Synthesis

The paraprotein found in patients with macroglobulinemia is almost certainly synthesized by the lymphocytoid cells found in the bone marrow, the lymph nodes, and, occasionally, the blood (63, 241, 299). The paraprotein usually migrates as a homogeneous beta or fast gamma globulin on paper electrophoresis (Fig. 20.9). It can be identified by ultracentrifugation of serum or by immunoelectrophoresis. Macroglobulins (Chapter 16) are composed of five subunits of two heavy chains plus two light chains (87, 208). Each of the subunits has a molecular weight of approximately 200,000 and the weight of the

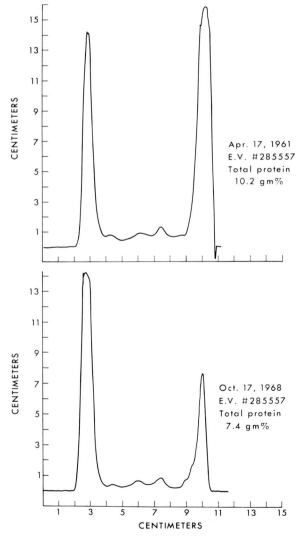

Figure 20.9 Two patterns of electrophoresis of serum of a patient with Waldenström's macroglobulinemia. The pattern at the bottom shows a reduction in the macroglobulin spike after chemotherapy.

entire molecule is 1,000,000 (169). At high concentrations, macroglobulins undergo polymerization and may form polymers with a molecular weight of several million. Because of their large size, macroglobulins are confined to the vascular space and are not distributed in extracellular fluid as are IgG paraproteins. Their large size and asymmetric structure alter the flow properties of the blood, increasing its viscosity. Thus the pathogenesis of the hyperviscosity syndrome may be related to the abnormal paraprotein. The M protein may coat the formed elements of the blood, including red cells, leukocytes, and platelets, and thus interfere with their function and survival (64, 232–234, 258). In some cases macroglobulin paraproteins precipitate at or near ambient temperatures. These proteins are called cryoglobulins; they produce a characteristic clinical picture of skin and mucous membrane ulcerative lesions, presumably because of precipitation and interference with vascular perfusion at these sites.

Several studies of macroglobulinemia suggest that antibody synthesis (23, 105), and particularly IgM antibody synthesis (236), is impaired. This phenomenon may contribute to the increased frequency of infection observed in macroglobulinemia. Normal and pathologic IgM molecules are catabolized normally in macroglobulinemia (27). IgG is catabolized normally or slowly in this disorder (285).

A patient has been described with malignant disease of the plasma cell–lymphoid series who had in his serum a paraprotein with antigenic determinants common to the 19 S macroglobulins, but differing from macroglobulins in its smaller size and physicochemical properties (284). The disease picture was different from typical multiple myeloma or macroglobulinemia. The anomalous protein in this patient may be related to low-molecular-weight IgM antibodies, which have been described in normal human sera, in several disease states, and in the serum of other species (165, 198, 254, 265).

The monoclonal paraprotein of some patients with Waldenström's macroglobulinemia may have anti-antibody activity (310).

Incidence and Age Distribution

Waldenström's macroglobulinemia occurs in the elderly, rarely before the age of sixty (93, 152, 192, 200). There is evidence indicating that macroglobulinemia may occur with increased frequency in some families (108, 271).

Bachmann (20), in a 1965 study of 554 patients whose serum contained M components, observed definite myelomatosis in 50 of these patients. Of the 554 paraproteins, 95 were IgM. Fifty-seven patients had Waldenström's ma-

croglobulinemia, lymphoma, chronic lymphocytic leukemia, and related disorders. The remaining IgM paraproteins were observed in patients with carcinoma and a variety of other conditions.

Clinical and Laboratory Features

General Manifestations The most common presenting complaints of patients with macroglobulinemia are weakness, fatigue, and weight loss. Less common presenting manifestations are bleeding, impaired vision, organomegaly, and manifestations associated with neuropathy. Weakness and fatigue are related at least in part to the anemia that frequently complicates macroglobulinemia.

Between 30 and 50 percent of patients have lymphadenopathy, hepatomegaly, or splenomegaly—alone or in combination (49, 68, 160, 200). Visual disturbances and/or abnormal funduscopic examination also occur in about 30 to 50 percent of patients. These findings include tortuosity and engorgement of the retinal vasculature, "sausage linking" of retinal veins, hemorrhage, and sometimes frank retinal vein thromboses (3, 15, 78, 135, 200, 270, 287) (Fig. 20.10). Such changes are thought to be the result

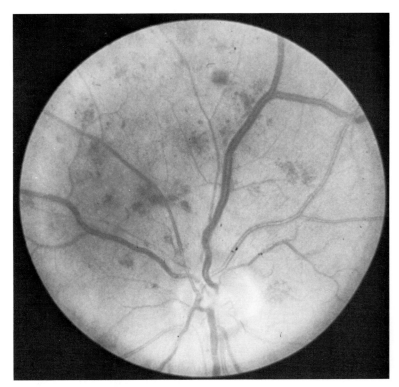

Figure 20.10 Retina of a patient with Waldenström's macroglobulinemia and hyperviscosity syndrome.

of increased blood viscosity and altered flow. They are corrected by reduction in the amount of paraprotein.

The diagnosis of macroglobulinemia is generally suspected with the finding of an elevated erythrocyte sedimentation rate, hyperglobulinemia (49, 93, 138, 200) or a homogeneous beta or gamma globulin spike on conventional paper electrophoresis. Confirmation of the diagnosis requires ultracentrifugation of the serum or immunoelectrophoresis. Macroglobulins normally constitute up to 5 percent of serum immunoglobulin (133, 246). Concentrations between 5 and 15 percent have been observed in systemic lupus erythematosus (304), nephrosis (304), and rheumatoid arthritis (291), as well as in macroglobulinemia. A concentration exceeding 15 percent is probably found only in macroglobulinemia (133, 246). In most series, Bence Jones proteinemia occurs in 10 to 20 percent of patients with Waldenström's macroglobulinemia, but in considerably higher frequency when very sensitive tests are applied (81).

Infection occurs with moderate frequency in macroglobulinemia, but is not so prominent a feature of this disease as it is of multiple myeloma (44, 105, 152, 311). Susceptibility to infection probably results from a combination of impaired antibody globulin synthesis and paraprotein interference with phagocytic leukocyte function. White cell levels are usually normal in macroglobulinemia (152, 200), but occasionally are low (68).

Although lytic bone lesions have been described in macroglobulinemia (5, 309, 313), they are relatively rare (152, 200). Another unusual feature of this disease is a leukemic blood picture (63).

Clinical and pathological renal manifestations of macroglobulinemia other than proteinuria are relatively uncommon (13, 171, 192). However, glomerular abnormalities with amyloid or IgM deposits are well documented (211). Tubular protein casts and macrophage reactions of the type seen in multiple myeloma are rarely observed in macroglobulinemia. In both paraprotein disorders, amyloidosis can occur (46, 66–68, 111, 196, 230).

Pulmonary manifestations may result from direct cellular infiltration, as well as hyperviscosity (132, 244).

Hyperviscosity Syndrome   The usual features of the hyperviscosity syndrome seen commonly in macroglobulinemia, and rarely in multiple myeloma, include blurred vision, retinal hemorrhage, dilated retinal veins, central nervous system abnormalities, tinnitus, mucous membrane bleeding, and, occasionally, gastrointestinal hemorrhage. These manifestations are correlated with increased blood viscosity and probably result from sludging and stagnation of blood in capillaries and small venules. Refractory congestive heart failure may also be a feature of the hyperviscosity syndrome.

Relative serum viscosity is measured by the ratio of the rate of descent of water or saline to that of serum through a small glass orifice in an instrument called a viscometer. Normally this ratio is about 1 in 1.5 (103). In patients with IgG myeloma the ratio may be increased to 1 in 2 to 4. It may be even higher in IgA myeloma, particularly if high-molecular-weight IgA polymers are present. The highest levels of serum viscosity are seen in macroglobulinemia, where values up to 1 in 40 have been observed.

Despite a number of theoretical limitations on the use of capillary viscometers (223, 253), useful information can be obtained from them. Manifestations of the hyperviscosity syndrome are rarely observed when the relative serum viscosity is less than 6. Visual and retinal hemorrhagic manifestations generally appear when the relative viscosity is 8 to 10. The viscosity at which symptoms appear varies from patient to patient. However, for a given patient the level at which symptoms appear is fairly constant. Serum viscosity appears to be determined by the concentration and physical characteristics of the constituent globulins, including their size, shape, and flexibility (286). Macroglobulins are large and asymmetrical and are often associated with the hyperviscosity syndrome (103, 286). IgG immunoglobulins may also occasionally produce the hyperviscosity syndrome in myelomatosis. Generally they produce hyperviscosity under unusual circumstances: (a) when they occur as high-molecular-weight polymers, (b) when their configuration is normal but their concentration is very high, and (c) when they occur as highly asymmetric molecules (193, 280).

There is a roughly linear relationship in the paraproteinemias between protein concentration and relative serum viscosity (286). This observation explains why reduction in the concentration of paraprotein, for example by plasmapheresis (269, 279), results in an amelioration of symptoms. The effects of plasmapheresis may be observed within hours or days.

In an animal tumor model system of macroglobulinemia, viscosity is a function both of the plasma concentration of macroglobulins and of the hematocrit. Aggregation of erythrocytes and high concentrations of macroglobulins appear to contribute to blood viscosity (253). Plasma colloids, including macroglobulins, may adsorb to the red cell surface—forming a "sticky" and viscous coat. Such colloids may increase viscosity of flow at a low shear rate (57, 297, 312) and interfere with blood flow in the microcirculation (252). Rosenblum (251) has suggested that erythrocyte aggregation may be more detrimental to the microcirculation than increased blood viscosity per se.

Anemia Anemia occurs in over 80 percent of patients with macroglobulinemia (49, 64, 152, 200). The etiology of this anemia is complex. When the disease is active and the paraprotein concentration is high, shortened erythrocyte survival is the rule. Overt hemolysis may be observed (1). Correction of the marked degree of paraproteinemia may restore red cell life-span toward normal.

The degree of hemolysis generally is not so marked that a normal bone marrow could not compensate by enhanced erythropoiesis. However, the erythropoietic response in patients with macroglobulinemia is often inadequate and may be totally impaired (64). The reason for this defective erythropoiesis is unknown.

A factor contributing to anemia in many patients with macroglobulinemia is blood loss, particularly gastrointestinal blood loss with subsequent development of iron deficiency.

The hematocrit and hemoglobin concentration in macroglobulinemia may not adequately reflect the total body red cell mass. The plasma volume is usually expanded in some degree, often to a high degree, as a consequence of the intravascular sequestration of osmotically active paraprotein. Consequently, the red cells are diluted in the large vessels by the increased plasma volume, and the reduction in hematocrit, hemoglobin, and red cell count is greater than the reduction in red cell mass. Plasmapheresis will partially correct the striking anemia observed in many patients (64).

Hemostasis A bleeding diathesis has been described in about 60 percent of patients with macroglobulinemia (68, 93, 152, 160, 200). Thrombocytopenia, severe enough to cause bleeding, is found in about half the patients with bleeding diathesis (64, 152). In those patients whose platelet count is normal, bleeding tedency can be explained on two bases: abnormal platelet function and abnormal coagulation. Bleeding appears to be more common with higher concentrations of paraprotein (235).

High concentrations of macroglobulins have been thought to coat platelets and prevent the release of platelet factor 3 (231, 232). They are associated with abnormal platelet adhesiveness and prolonged bleeding time—tests of platelet plug formation (235).

Various coagulation defects have been described in macroglobulinemia, including abnormalities of fibrinogen, prothrombin, and factors V and VII (142, 152, 155, 188). Patients with both macroglobulinemia and IgA myelomatosis tend to have lower than normal levels of plasma-

clotting factors. In a large series of studies, Perkins and his colleagues (235) observed that elevated levels of paraprotein correlated with abnormal values in the thrombin time, prothrombin time, and thromboplastin generation tests. These observations raised the possibility of direct interaction of paraprotein with coagulation factors. However, abnormalities in these tests did not correlate with the presence of clinical bleeding. Rather, a bleeding tendency correlated best with abnormalities of platelet function. The same authors also reviewed the extensive literature on hemostasis in paraproteinemic disorders.

Most investigators agree that plasmapheresis is an effective means of correcting abnormalities of hemostasis in macroglobulinemia provided it is not so vigorous that secondary depletion of coagulation factors occurs (71, 131, 235, 269, 282).

Neurologic Manifestations The combination of neurologic abnormality and hyperglobulinemia has been called the Bing-Neel syndrome (37, 39, 40). In a survey of 182 patients with macroglobulinemia, 46 had coexisting neurologic manifestations (187). Such neurologic complications have been classified into five groups (1, 82, 85, 93, 187): (*a*) acute focal brain syndromes, including stroke; (*b*) diffuse brain syndromes and encephalopathies; (*c*) peripheral neuropathies; (*d*) subarachnoid hemorrhage; and (*e*) mixed neurologic syndromes. Some of these neurologic manifestations are attributable to impaired perfusion and are wholly or partially reversible. Others are irreversible, presumably because of structural damage to the nervous system. The complexity of the mechanisms of the neural injury is appreciated in studies of the peripheral neuropathy that occurs in between 8 and 20 percent of patients with macroglobulinemia (103, 187). A wide variety of nerve lesions has been described, including lymphocytic infiltration (1), perineural deposition of amorphous periodic acid-Schiff-positive material (82), intraneural and perivascular amyloid deposits (219), and demyelination (85). The most frequently cited possible mechanisms of neuropathy in paraproteinemias are sludging of the blood in vasa nervorum and direct cellular infiltration (24, 125). Macroglobulinemia must be considered in the differential diagnosis of sudden deafness (259). Another unusual neurologic manifestation is cerebellar ataxia.

Cryoglobulinemia A plasma protein that precipitates at temperatures below 37° C was discovered fortuitously in a patient with myelomatosis, extensive purpura, retinal vein thrombosis, and Raynaud's phenomenon (315). Such proteins—called cryoglobulins (177)—precipitate from the blood and form a gelatinous mass as the blood cools. They are found in a variety of conditions, including systemic lupus erythematosus, kala-azar, rheumatoid arthritis, and cirrhosis, but most commonly in the paraproteinemias (191, 202). The cryoprecipitin usually consists of IgG or IgM paraprotein, or a complex of IgM with normal IgG (74, 75). The presence of significant concentrations of cryoglobulins is often associated with a characteristic clinical syndrome of cutaneous purpura, cold intolerance with Raynaud's phenomenon, and at the extreme, necrosis at the tips of the fingers, nose, and toes. Perforation of the nasal septum is often seen. These manifestations presumably relate to cooling of blood in these peripheral sites, with subsequent protein precipitation and sludging of flow. Cryoglobulins may also activate the complement sequence (75).

Course and Prognosis

Macroglobulinemia is generally a benign disease, compatible with long survival provided management of high levels of plasma paraprotein is not neglected. Kappeler and his colleagues (160) recorded an average life expectancy of 38 to 40 months from the time symptoms first appear. In a study of 10 patients, Cohen and his co-workers (68) found an average survival of 34 months from diagnosis and 55 months from clinical onset of symptoms. Similarly, Imhof and his colleagues (152) found that the usual clinical course lasted 2 to 10 years and observed 5 cases in which patients survived more than 14 years. These observations are quite impressive in view of the fact that the onset of macroglobulinemia is apt to be late in life. When death occurs from macroglobulinemia, it is usually caused by either untreated hyperviscosity syndrome with bleeding or infection. Rarely, it results from anemia and congestive heart failure or untreated "coma paraproteinicium."

Principles of Therapy

The signs and symptoms of the hyperviscosity syndrome may be temporarily controlled by intensive plasmapheresis (61, 269, 270, 282). In acute situations, plasmapheresis is the therapy of choice. The underlying principle is that the offending paraprotein can be removed more rapidly than it can be replaced by synthesis. For long-term control of excessive paraproteinemia and associated symptomatology, chemotherapy is more reliable. Alkylating agents that interact with the neoplastic plasmacytoid cells as a rule have been successful (44, 61, 189).

Other Monoclonal Gammopathies

In recent years it has come to be recognized that monoclonal gammopathy can occur in settings other than clas-

Table 20.7 Lymphoproliferative neoplasms and nonneoplastic diseases sometimes associated with paraproteins.

Neoplastic-lymphoproliferative	Nonneoplastic
Multiple myeloma	Primary generalized amyloidosis
Macroglobulinemia	Collagen diseases
Plasma cell leukemia	Lichen myxedematosus
γ-heavy chain disease	Hepatobiliary and gastrointestinal diseases
α-heavy chain disease	Chronic cold agglutinin syndrome
μ-heavy chain disease	Idiopathic cryoglobulinemia
Lymphomas	Benign monoclonal gammopathy
Leukemias	Aplastic anemia
	Myelofibrosis

sical myelomatosis and macroglobulinemia. The occurrence of paraproteins has been observed in association with four different clinical settings: (a) lymphoproliferative disorders — for example, heavy-chain disease and chronic lymphocytic leukemia; (b) nonhematologic malignancy; (c) nonmalignant diseases; and (d) an apparently benign condition known as benign monoclonal gammopathy. Examples of lymphoproliferative disorders and nonmalignant conditions sometimes associated with monoclonal gammopathies are listed in Table 20.7.

Lymphoproliferative Disorders

Heavy-(Gamma-)chain Disease   Paraproteinemia has been recognized in a variety of lymphoproliferative disorders other than classic myeloma and macroglobulinemia. In some of these disorders fragments, rather than intact immunoglobulins, are synthesized by the neoplastic cells. The best delineated of these gammopathies are the heavy-chain diseases (113). In myeloma and macroglobulinemia, synthesis of heavy (H) chains is nearly balanced with that of light (L) chains, so that a homogeneous intact immunoglobulin is produced; occasionally there is some excess of H or L chains in the serum or urine because of a slight imbalance in the synthetic rate. In the heavy-chain diseases, however, the synthesis and assembly of immunoglobulin chains is more disordered. Gamma, alpha, or mu heavy chains are either synthesized in great excess or not properly assembled with L chains. The result is paraproteinemia and paraproteinuria with a single class of heavy chains or fragments of heavy chains.

The initial description of heavy-(gamma-)chain disease was published in 1963 (118, 119). Since then, at least 13 patients have been described (99, 116, 229). The syndrome of heavy-chain disease consists of lymphadenopathy, hepatosplenomegaly, and recurrent fevers. Bony lesions and pathologic fractures are rare. Amyloidosis has been described in at least one patient with heavy-(gamma-)chain disease. The clinical and pathological picture generally has looked like malignant lymphoma.

The patients usually have been males over age forty, although the disorder has been described in females (175). Edema and erythema of the uvula and soft palate have been noted in several patients. There may be increased susceptibility to bacterial infection. Characteristic findings include moderate anemia, relative lymphocytosis, and eosinophilia. Thrombocytopenia was present in three of the seven patients initially described. In the lymph nodes and bone marrow the dominant cell types are atypical plasma cells, and lymphocytes, reticulum cells, and eosinophils. Undifferentiated cells are also seen. Proteinuria is the rule. The paraprotein detected in serum and urine has the chemical and immunologic properties of gamma chains and has no resemblance to lambda or kappa chains.

Evidence that the heavy chains result from imbalanced synthesis rather than immunoglobulin degradation has been provided by a number of investigators (50, 97, 115, 118). In several instances the heavy gamma chains have been incomplete, lacking a component equivalent to part of the Fc fragment (99, 114). Thus an IgG globulin fragment resembling the Fc piece produced by papain digestion of IgG (237) is found in the urine (118, 229).

Heavy-(Alpha-)chain Disease In 1968–69, Seligmann described four patients with alpha-chain disease (272, 274, 275). Each of these, as well as the next two patients described with this disorder, had a malignant lymphoma of the intestine associated with malabsorption syndrome and a paraprotein abnormality (273).

Most of the patients described have been Arabs, although the disorder does occur in other Mediterranean peoples (43). Again, evidence favors the view that the alpha-chain fragments observed in the serum and urine of these patients are synthetic products of the tumor, rather than degradation products of intact immunoglobulin (274). The pathologic protein is devoid of light chains and is closely related to the alpha polypeptide chains of the IgA$_1$ subclass. The characteristic feature of these proteins is their tendency to polymerize, which explains their low output in the urine (275).

Gastrointestinal involvement may be rationalized on the basis that plasma cells in this location produce mainly IgA immunoglobulin (245).

The major clinical-pathological features of the reported cases of alpha-chain disease are chronic diarrhea with malabsorption occurring in young patients age twenty to twenty-five (273). The small intestinal lamina propria is densely infiltrated with lymphoid cells, and the villae are atrophic. Plasma cells predominate, but lymphocytes and reticulum cells are frequent. Diffuse mesentery lymphadenopathy was present in two patients. These are the general features of the so-called "Mediterranean lymphoma" (95, 245). The pleomorphism of the cellular infiltrate is reminiscent of heavy gamma chains and primary macroglobulinemia.

Heavy-(Mu-)chain Disease In 1970 Ballard and his colleagues described a new variant of heavy-chain disease: mu-chain disease (22). A paraprotein was found in the serum of a patient with a malignant lymphoproliferative disorder resembling chronic lymphocytic leukemia. The anomalous protein appeared to be a fragment of the heavy chain of immunoglobulin M. Clinical features included a white count of 55,200/mm^3 (90 percent lymphocytes), hepatosplenomegaly without significant lymphadenopathy, and amyloidosis with carpal tunnel syndrome. Electrophoresis of the serum revealed a rapidly migrating IgM component that had only mu-chain determinants and no light-chain determinants. An M component in the urine appeared to be composed of kappa light chains. The heavy-chain fragments of molecular weight 55,000 probably did not pass through the glomerular membrane because of their tendency to polymerize and form high-molecular-weight complexes. Since the description of this initial case of heavy-(mu-)chain disease, more detailed analyses in other patients, with similar clinical features, have been reported (112, 113, 116, 117, 159, 176, 323).

Other Lymphoproliferative Disorders In addition to their association with myelomatosis, macroglobulinemia, and heavy-chain diseases, paraproteins have been observed in a variety of less well-defined lymphoproliferative disorders, including "malignant disease of the plasma cell lymphatic system" (284), "diffuse lymphoma" (210), "lymphosarcoma," "reticulosarcoma," giant follicular lymphoma, and chronic lymphocytic leukemia (148), poorly differentiated lymphoproliferative disorder with red cell hypoplasia and cold hemoglobinuria (240), and primary amyloidosis with "plasma cell dyscrasia" (2).

Other Disease States

Paraproteins have been observed in a variety of disease states other than lymphoproliferative disorders: carcinoma; myelosclerosis; lichen myxedematosus; a variety of gastrointestinal diseases, including ulcerative colitis and cirrhosis; Henoch-Schoenlein purpura and aplastic anemia; and a variety of collagen diseases, including rheumatoid arthritis, systemic lupus erythematosus, idiopathic cryoglobulinemia, and cold agglutinin syndrome (41, 72, 134, 147, 207, 242). Monoclonal IgG gammopathy recently has been described in three patients with hyperparathyroidism (88).

A variety of transient paraproteinemias, usually appearing and disappearing over the course of a few weeks or months, must also be included in this category. Again, these have been associated with a variety of diseases (321). The relation between the paraproteins and these disorders is obscure. It is not known whether appearance of the paraproteins is a fortuitous occurrence in the setting of common diseases or whether it represents reaction to a disease process on the part of the reticuloendothelial system. The evidence that nonlymphoreticular malignancies are causally associated with paraproteins is not convincing.

A summary of some lymphoproliferative and non-neoplastic diseases in which paraproteins have been reported is given in Table 20.7.

Benign Monoclonal Gammopathies

Between 1944 and 1964, Waldenström drew attention to a syndrome that has been designated benign monoclonal gammopathy (benign essential monoclonal hyperglobulinemia) (302–306). In this condition a serum paraprotein is observed in a patient who has no apparent underlying disease. The concentration of paraprotein usually is only moderately high, and the level tends to be remarkably stable for many years. A moderate anemia is not uncommon. The condition tends to remain benign and there is usually no transition to a malignant lymphoproliferative disorder for a period of at least two to three years (19, 86, 134, 306). Parameters that suggest an underlying malignancy rather than a benign condition include a paraprotein concentration above 3 gm percent, a rapid increase in the concentration of serum paraprotein, and the development of severe anemia. Available data suggest that benign monoclonal gammopathy may be a good deal more common than multiple myeloma and macroglobulinemia (19).

Benign monoclonal gammopathy should be distinguished from hyperglobulinemic purpura (Waldenström), which is characterized by recurrent episodes of purpura and polyclonal hypergammaglobulinemia (29, 303).

Summary

Multiple myeloma and macroglobulinemia are disorders in which a clone of neoplastic B cells proliferates. In multiple myeloma the clinical manifestations reflect both the proliferation of malignant cells within the bone marrow and the immunoglobulin tumor product. In macroglobulinemia the monoclonal large asymmetrical immunoglobulin within the vascular space usually produces the major clinical features of the disease. A variety of other lymphoproliferative disorders occurs in which intact immunoglobulin or fragments of the molecule are secreted by the malignant cells. In addition, benign monoclonal gammopathies exist.

Chapter 20 References

1. Aarseth, S., Ofstad, E., and Torvick, A. Macroglobulinaemia Waldenström. A case with haemolytic syndrome and involvement of the nervous system, *Acta Med. Scand.* 169:691, 1961.
2. Abruzzo, J. L., Amante, C. M., and Heimer, R. Primary amyloidosis with "monoclonal" immunoglobulin A proteinemia, *Am. J. Med.* 45:460, 1967.
3. Ackerman, A. L. The ocular manifestations of Waldenström's macroglobulinaemia and its treatment, *Arch. Ophthalmol.* 67:701, 1962.
4. Adelson, H. T. Macroglobulinaemia of Waldenström apparently associated with two paraproteins, *N. Engl. J. Med.* 265:20, 1961.
5. Adner, P. L., Wallenius, G., and Werner, I. Macroglobulinaemia and myelomatosis, *Acta Med. Scand.* 168:431, 1960.
6. Alexander, L. L., and Benninghoff, D. L. Familial multiple myeloma. II. Final pathological findings in two brothers and a sister, *J. Natl. Med. Assoc.* 59:278, 1967.
7. Alexanian, R., Bergsagel, D. E., Migliore, P. J. Melphalan therapy for plasma cell myeloma, *Blood* 31:1, 1968.
8. Alexanian, R., Bonnet, J., Gehan, E., Haut, A., Hewlett, J., Lane, M., Monto, R., and Wilson, H. Combination chemotherapy for multiple myeloma, *Cancer* 30:382, 1972.
9. Anderson, J., and Osgood, E. E. Acute plasmacytic leukemia responsive to cyclophosphamide, *J.A.M.A.* 193:844, 1965.
10. Anderson, R. E., and Ishida, K. Malignant lymphoma in survivors of the atomic bomb in Hiroshima, *Ann. Intern. Med.* 61:853, 1964.
11. Apitz, K. Die Paraproteinosen (über die Störung des Eiweisstoffwechsels bei Plasmocytom), *Virchows Arch. (Pathol. Anat.)* 306:631, 1940.
12. Arends, A., and Mandema, E. Observations on the pathogenesis of the so-called myeloma kidney, *in* Aa. Videbaek (ed.), Proc. VI Congress European Soc. Haematol. (Copenhagen, 1957), p. 137, S. Karger, Basel, 1958.
13. Argani, I., and Kipkie, G. F. Macroglobulinemic nephropathy. Acute renal failure in macroglobulinemia of Waldenstrom, *Am. J. Med.* 36:151, 1964.
14. Armstrong, J. B. A study of renal function in patients with multiple myeloma, *Am. J. Med. Sci.* 219:488, 1950.
15. Ashton, N., Kok, D'A., and Foulds, W. S. Ocular pathology in macroglobulinemia, *J. Pathol. Bacteriol.* 86:453, 1963.
16. Askonas, B. A., and Fahey, J. L. Formation of Bence-Jones protein and myeloma protein *in vitro* by the plasma-cell tumour MPC-2, *Biochem. J.* 80:261, 1961.
17. Askonas, B. A., and Williamson, A. R. Balanced synthesis of light and heavy chains of immunoglobulin G, *Nature* 216:264, 1967.
18. Atkinson, F. R. B. Multiple myelomata, *Med. Press* 195:312, 327; 1937.
19. Axelsson, U., and Hällén, J. Review of fifty-four subjects with monoclonal gammopathy, *Br. J. Haematol.* 15:417, 1968.
20. Bachmann, R. The diagnostic significance of the serum concentration of pathological proteins, (M-components), *Acta Med. Scand.* 178:801, 1965.
21. Baglioni, C., Zonta, L. A., and Cioli, D. Allelic antigenic factor Inv(a) of the light chains of human immunoglobulins: chemical basis, *Science* 152:1517, 1966.
22. Ballard, H. S., Hamilton, L. M., Marcus, A. J., and Illes, C. H. A new variant of heavy-chain disease (μ-chain disease), *N. Engl. J. Med.* 282:1060, 1970.
23. Barandun, S., Huser, H. J., and Hässig, A. Klinische Erscheinungsformen des Antikörpermangelsyndroms, *Schweiz. Med. Wochenschr.* 88:78, 182; 1958.
24. Barron, K. D., Rowland, L. P., and Zimmerman, H. M. Neuropathy with malignant tumor metastases, *J. Nerv. Ment. Dis.* 131:10, 1960.
25. Barth, W. F., Glenner, G. G., Waldmann, T. A., and Zelis, R. F. Primary amyloidosis: NIH Clinical Staff Conference, *Ann. Intern. Med.* 69:787, 1968.
26. Barth, W. F., Willerson, J. T., Waldmann, T. A., and Decker, J. L. Primary amyloidosis. Clinical, immunochemical, and immunoglobulin metabolism studies in fifteen patients, *Am. J. Med.* 47:259, 1969.
27. Barth, W. F., Wochner, R. D., Waldmann, T. A., and Fahey, J. L. Metabolism of human gamma macroglobulins, *J. Clin. Invest.* 43:1036, 1964.
28. Batts, M., Jr. Multiple myeloma. Review of forty cases, *Arch. Surg.* 39:807, 1939.
29. Baughan, M. A., Daniels, J. C., Levin, W. C., and Ritzmann, S. E. Hyperglobulinemic purpura (Waldenström)—a report of 4 cases and review of literature, *Tex. Rep. Biol. Med.* 29:149, 1971.
30. Bayrd, E. D. Sustained remission in multiple myeloma, *Blood* 10:662, 1955.
31. Bayrd, E. D., and Hall, B. E. Unusual remission after radiophosphorus therapy in a case of "acute plasma cell leukemia," *Blood* 3:1019, 1948.
32. Bayrd, E. D., and Heck, F. J. Multiple myeloma: a review of eighty-three proved cases, *J.A.M.A.* 133:147, 1947.
33. Ben Bassat, I., Frand, U. I., Isersky, C., and Ramot, B. Plasma cell leukemia with IgD paraprotein, *Arch. Intern. Med.* 121:361, 1968.
34. Benninger, G. W., and Kreps, S. I. Aggregation phenomenon in an IgG multiple myeloma resulting in the hyperviscosity syndrome, *Am. J. Med.* 51:287, 1971.
35. Bergsagel, D. E., Cowan, D. H., and Hasselback, R. Plasma cell myeloma: response of melphalan-resistant patients to high-dose intermittent cyclophosphamide, *Can. Med. Assoc. J.* 107:851, 1972.
36. Bergsagel, D. E., and Pruzanski, W. Recognizing and treating plasma cell neoplasia, *Postgrad. Med.* 43:200, 1968.
37. Bichel, J., Bing, J., and Harboe, N. Another case of hyperglobulinemia and affection of the central nervous system, *Acta Med. Scand.* 138:1, 1950.
38. Bichel, J., Effersoe, P., Gormsen, H., and Harboe, N. Leukemic myelomatosis (plasma cell leukemia). A review with report of four cases, *Acta Radiol.* 37:196, 1952.
39. Bing, J., Fog, M., and Neel, A. V. Report of a third case of hyperglob-

ulinemia with affection of the central nervous system on a toxi-infectious basis and some remarks on the differential diagnosis, *Acta Med. Scand.* 91:409, 1937.

40. Bing, J., and Neel, A. V. Two cases of hyperglobulinaemia with affection of the central nervous system on a toxi-infectious basis (myelitis, polyradiculitis, spinal-fluid · changes), *Acta Med. Scand.* 88:492, 1936.

41. Birch, C. A., Cooke, K. B., Drew, C. E., London, D. R., Mackenzie, D. H., and Milne, M. D. Hyperglobulinaemic purpura due to a thymic tumour, *Lancet* i:693, 1964.

42. Bluefarb, S. M. Cutaneous manifestations of multiple myeloma, *Arch. Dermatol.* 72:506, 1955.

43. Bonomo, L., Dammacco, F., Marano, R., and Bonomo, G. M. Abdominal lymphoma and alpha chain disease, *Am. J. Med.* 52:73, 1972.

44. Bouroncle, B. A., Datta, P., and Frajole, W. J. Waldenström's macroglobulinemia: report of three patients treated with cyclophosphamide, *J.A.M.A.* 189:729, 1964.

45. Brandt, K., Cathcart, E. S., and Cohen, A. S. A clinical analysis of the course and prognosis of forty-two patients with amyloidosis, *Am. J. Med.* 44:955, 1968.

46. Braunsteiner, H., Oswald, E., Pakesch, F., and Reimer, E. Lymphoreticulosen mit Makroglobulinaemia, *Wien. Z. Inn. Med.* 37:349, 1956.

47. Briggs, G. W. Amyloidosis, *Ann. Intern. Med.* 55:943, 1961.

48. Brook, J., Bateman, J. R., Gocka, E. F., Nakamura, E., and Steinfeld, J. L. Long-term low dose melphalan treatment of multiple myeloma, *Arch. Intern. Med.* 131:545, 1973.

49. Butler, E. A., Flynn, F. V., Harris, H., and Robson, E B. The laboratory diagnosis of macroglobulinaemia with special references to starch-gel electrophoresis, *Lancet* ii:289, 1961.

50. Buxbaum, J. N., and Preud'homme, J. L. Alpha and gamma heavy chain diseases in man: intracellular origin of the aberrant polypeptides, *J. Immunol.* 109:1131, 1972.

51. Canale, D. D., Jr., and Collins, R. D. Use of bone marrow particle sections in the diagnosis of multiple myeloma, *Am. J. Clin. Pathol.* 61:382, 1974.

52. Carbone, P. P., Kellerhouse, L. E., and Gehan, E. A. Plasmacytic myeloma. A study of the relationship of survival to various clinical manifestations and anomalous protein type in 112 patients, *Am. J. Med.* 42:937, 1967.

53. Carson, C. P., Ackerman, L. V., and Maltby, J. D. Plasma cell myeloma. A clinical, pathologic, and roentgenologic review of 90 cases, *Am. J. Clin. Pathol.* 25:849, 1955.

54. Cathcart, E. S., and Cohen, A. S. The relation between isolated human amyloid fibrils and human γ-globulin and its subunits, *J. Immunol.* 96:239, 1966.

55. Cathcart, E. S., Ritchie, R. F., Cohen, A. S., and Brandt, K. Immunoglobulins and amyloidosis. An immunologic study of sixty-two patients with biopsy-proved disease, *Am. J. Med.* 52:93, 1972.

56. Charkes, N. D., Durant, J., and Barry, W. E. Bone pain in multiple myeloma. Studies with radioactive [87]Sr, *Arch. Intern. Med.* 130:53, 1972.

57. Charm, S. E., McComis, W., and Kurland, G. Rheology and structure of blood suspensions, *J. Appl. Physiol.* 19:127, 1964.

58. Churg, J., and Gordan, A. J. Multiple myeloma with unusual visceral involvement, *Arch. Pathol.* 34:546, 1942.

59. Churg, J., and Gordan, A. J. Multiple myeloma. Lesions of the extra-osseous hematopoietic system, *Am. J. Clin. Pathol.* 20:934, 1950.

60. Clarke, E. Cranial and intracranial myelomas, *Brain* 77:61, 1954.

61. Cline, M. J., and Haskell, C. M., Cancer Chemotherapy, 2nd ed., J. B. Saunders, Philadelphia, 1975.

62. Cline, M. J., and Berlin, N. I. Studies of the anemia of multiple myeloma, *Am. J. Med.* 33:510, 1962.

63. Cline, M. J., and Mackenzie, M. R. Synthesis of macroglobulins *in vitro*, *Nature* 213:90, 1967.

64. Cline, M. J., Solomon, A., Berlin, N. I., and Fahey, J. L. Anemia in macroglobulinemia, *Am. J. Med.* 34:213, 1963.

65. Cohen, A. S. The constitution and genesis of amyloid, *in* G. W. Richter and M. A. Epstein (eds.), International Review of Experimental Pathology, vol. 4, p. 159, Academic Press, New York, 1965.

66. Cohen, A. S. Medical progress. Amyloidosis, *N. Engl. J. Med.* 277:522, 574, 628; 1967.

67. Cohen, A. S. Studies on the amyloid fibril, *in* B. M. Wagner and D. E. Smith (eds.), International Academy of Pathology Monographs, The Connective Tissue, p. 8, Williams & Wilkins Co., Baltimore, 1967.

68. Cohen, R. J., Bohannon, R. A., and Wallerstein, R. O. Waldenström's macroglobulinemia, *Am. J. Med.* 41:274, 1966.

69. Coltman, C. A., Jr. Multiple myeloma without a paraprotein, *Arch. Intern. Med.* 120:687, 1967.

70. Conn, H. O., and Quintiliani, R. Severe diarrhea controlled by gamma globulin in a patient with agammaglobulinemia, amyloidosis, and thymoma, *Ann. Intern. Med.* 65:528, 1966.

71. Conway, N., and Walker, J. M. Treatment of macroglobulinemia, *Br. Med. J.* 2:1296, 1962.

72. Cooke, K. B. Essential paraproteinaemia, *Proc. R. Soc. Med.* 62:777, 1969.

73. Costa, G. Melphalan and prednisone: an effective combination for the treatment of multiple myeloma, *Am. J. Med.* 54:589, 1973.

74. Costanzi, J. J., Coltman, C. A., Jr., Clark, D. A., Tennenbaum, J. I., and Criscuolo, D. Cryoglobulinemia associated with a macroglobulin. Studies of a 17.5S cryoprecipitating factor, *Am. J. Med.* 39:163, 1965.

75. Costanzi, J. J., Coltman, C. A., Jr., and Donaldson, V. H. Activation of complement by a monoclonal cryoglobulin associated with cold urticaria, *J. Lab. Clin. Med.* 74:902, 1969.

76. Costea, N., Yakulis, V. J., Libnoch, J. A., Pilz, C. G., and Heller, P. Two myeloma globulins (IgG and IgA) in one subject and one cell line, *Am. J. Med.* 42:630, 1967.

77. Cowan, M. A. Ulceration of the skin in multiple myeloma, *Br. J. Dermatol.* 73:415, 1961.

78. Coyle, J. T., Frank, P. E., Leonard, A. L., and Weiner, A. Macroglobulinemia and its effects on the eye, *Arch. Ophthalmol.* 65:75, 1961.

79. Creyssel, R., Fine, J. M., Groulade, J., and Betuel, H. Étude immuno chimique de 463 sérums contenant une paraprotéine, *in* H. Peters (ed.), Protides of the biological fluids. Proc. Colloquium II (1963), p. 97, Elsevier Publishing Co., Amsterdam, 1964.

80. Dammacco, F., and Bonomo, L. IgD-myelomatosis. Report of a case, *Scand. J. Haematol.* 5:161, 1968.

81. Dammacco, F., and Waldenström, J. Serum and urine light chain levels in benign monoclonal gammapathies, multiple myeloma, and Waldenström's macroglobulinaemia, *Clin. Exp. Immunol.* 3:911, 1968.

82. Darnley, J. D. Polyneuropathy in Waldenström's macroglobulinemia, *Neurology* 12:617, 1962.

83. Davis, H., Caron, G. A., and McKinney, M. B. Multiple myeloma presenting clinically as obstructive jaundice, *Postgrad. Med. J.* 35:668, 1959.

84. Davison, C., and Balser, B. H. Myeloma and its neural complications, *Arch. Surg.* 35:913, 1937.

85. Dayan, A. D., and Lewis, P. D. Demyelinating neuropathy in macroglobulinemia, *Neurology* 16:1141, 1966.

86. Derycke, C., Fine, J. M., and Boffa, G. A. Dysglobulinémies "essentielles" chez les sujets ages, *Nouv. Rev. Fr. Hematol.* 5:729, 1965.

87. Deutsch, H. F., and Morton, J. I. Human serum macroglobulins and dissociation units. I. Physicochemical properties, *J. Biol. Chem.* 231:1107, 1958.

88. Dexter, R. N., Mullinax, F., Estep, H. L., and Williams, R. C. Monoclonal IgG gammopathy and hyperparathyroidism, *Ann. Intern. Med.* 77:759, 1972.

89. Djaldetti, M., and Joshua, H. Acute plasma cell leukemia. A case report, *Isr. Med. J.* 20:109, 1961.

90. Dolin, S., and DeWar, J. P. Extramedullary plasmacytoma, *Am. J. Pathol.* 32:83, 1956.

91. Drivsholm, A. Myelomatosis. A clinical and biochemical study of 105 cases, *Acta Med. Scand.* 176:509, 1964.

92. Durant, J. R., Barry, W. E., and Learner, N. The changing face of multiple myeloma, *Lancet* i:119, 1966.

93. Dutcher, T. F., and Fahey, J. L. The histopathology of the macroglobulinemia of Waldenström, *J. Natl. Cancer Inst.* 22:887, 1959.

94. Edwards, G. A., and Zawadzki, Z. A. Extraosseous lesions in plasma cell myeloma. A report of six cases, *Am. J. Med.* 43:194, 1957.

95. Eidelman, S., Parkins, R. A., and Rubin, C. E. Abdominal lymphoma presenting as malabsorption. A clinico-pathological study of nine cases in Israel and a review of the literature, *Medicine* 45:111, 1966.

96. Ein, D., Buell, D. N., and Fahey, J. L. Biosynthetic and structural studies of a heavy chain disease protein, *J. Clin. Invest.* 48:785, 1969.

97. Ein, D., and Waldmann, T. A. Metabolic studies of a heavy chain disease protein, *J. Immunol.* 103:345, 1969.

98. Ein, D., Kimura, S., and Glenner, G. G. An amyloid fibril protein of unknown origin: partial amino acid sequence analysis, *Biochem. Biophys. Res. Commun.* 46:498, 1972.

99. Ellman, L. L., and Bloch, K. J. Heavy-chain disease. Report of a seventh case, *N. Engl. J. Med.* 278:1195, 1968.

100. Engle, R. L., Jr., and Nachman, R. L. Two Bence Jones proteins of different immunologic types in the same patient with multiple myeloma, *Blood* 27:74, 1966.

101. Engle, R. L., Jr., and Wallis, L. A. Multiple myeloma and the adult Fanconi syndrome. I. Report of a case with crystal-like deposits in the tumor cells and in the epithelial cells of the kidney, *Am. J. Med.* 22:5, 1957.

102. Engle, R. L., Jr., and Wallis, L. A. Paraimmunoglobulinopathies, *in* Tice's Practice of Medicine, vol. 1, p. 301, Harper & Row, Hagerstown, Md., 1973.

103. Fahey, J. L., Barth, W. F., and Solomon, A. Serum hyperviscosity syndrome, *J.A.M.A.* 192:464, 1965.

104. Fahey, J. L., Carbone, P. P., Rowe, D. S., and Bachmann, R. Plasma cell myeloma with D-myeloma protein (IgD myeloma), *Am. J. Med.* 45:373, 1968.

105. Fahey, J. L., Scoggins, R., Utz, J. P., and Szwed, C. F. Infection, antibody response, and gammaglobulin components in multiple myeloma and macroglobulinemia, *Am. J. Med.* 35:698, 1963.

106. Favis, E. A., Kerman, H. D., and Schildecker, W. Multiple myeloma manifested as a problem in the diagnosis of pulmonary disease, *Am. J. Med.* 28:323, 1960.

107. Feinleib, M., and MacMahon, B. Duration of survival in multiple myeloma, *J. Natl. Cancer Inst.* 24:1259, 1960.

108. Fine, J. M., Massari, R., Boffa, G. A., et al. Macroglobulinémie monoclonale à caractère familial présente chez trois sujets d'une même fratrie, *Transfusion* 9:333, 1966.

109. Finkel, H. E., Yount, W. J., Salmon, S. E., and Schilling, A. Current concepts in the therapy of multiple myeloma, *Med. Clin. North Am.* 50:1569, 1966.

110. Fishkin, B. G., Glassy, F. J., Hattersley, P. G., Horose, F. M., and Spiegelberg, H. L. IgD multiple myeloma. A report of five cases, *Am. J. Clin. Pathol.* 53:209, 1970.

111. Forget, B. G., Squires, J. W., and Sheldon, H. Waldenström's macroglobulinemia with generalized amyloidosis, *Arch. Intern. Med.* 118:363, 1966.

112. Forte, F. A., Prelli, F., Yount, W. J., Jerry, L. M., Kochwa, S., Franklin, E. C., and Kunkel, H. G. Heavy chain disease of the μ (γM) type: report of the first case, *Blood* 36:137, 1970.

113. Frangione, B., and Franklin, E. C. Heavy chain diseases: clinical features and molecular significance of the disordered immunoglobulin structure, *Semin. Hematol.* 10:53, 1973.

114. Frangione, B., and Milstein, C. Partial deletion in the heavy chain disease protein ZUC, *Nature* 224:597, 1969.

115. Franklin, E. C. Structural studies of human 7S γ-globulin (G immunoglobulin): further observations of a naturally occurring protein related to the crystallizable (fast) fragment, *J. Exp. Med.* 120:691, 1964.

116. Franklin, E. C. Heavy-chain dis-

eases, *N. Engl. J. Med.* 282:1098, 1970.

117. Franklin, E. C., Frangione, B., Prelli, F., Buxbaum, J., and Scharff, M. A possible molecular defect in μ chain disease, *Clin. Res.* 18:533, 1970.

118. Franklin, E. C., Lowenstein, J., Bigelow, B., and Metzger, M. Heavy chain disease—a new disorder of serum γ-globulins: report of the first case, *Am. J. Med.* 37:332, 1964.

119. Franklin, E. C., Meltzer, M., Guggenheim, F., and Lowenstein, J. An unusual micro-gamma-globulin in the serum and urine of a patient, *Fed. Proc.* 22:264, 1963.

120. Freeman, Z. Myelomatosis with extensive pulmonary involvement, *Thorax* 16:378, 1961.

121. Frick, P. G., Schmid, J. R., Kistler, J. J., and Hitzig, W. H. Hyponatremia associated with hyperproteinemia in multiple myeloma, *Helv. Med. Acta* 33:317, 1967.

122. Fritze, E., and Van de Loo, J. Makroglobulinämie Waldenström mit plasmazellulärer Leukämie, *Med. Klin.* 60:173, 1965.

123. Gabriel, S. Multiple myeloma presenting as pulmonary infiltration: report of a case, *Dis. Chest* 47:123, 1965.

124. Gafni, J., Merker, H-J., Shibolet, S., Sohar, E., and Heller, H. On the origin of amyloid. Study of an amyloid tumor in multiple myeloma, *Ann. Intern. Med.* 65:1031, 1966.

125. Garcin, R., Mallarmé, J., and Rondot, P. Névrites dysglobulinémiques, *Presse Med.* 70:111, 1962.

126. George, R. P., Poth, J. L., Gordan, D., and Schrier, S. L. Multiple myeloma—intermittent combination chemotherapy compared to continuous therapy, *Cancer* 29:1665, 1972.

127. Geschickter, C. F., and Copeland, M. M. Multiple myeloma, *Arch. Surg.* 16:807, 1928.

128. Glenner, G. G., Ein, D., Eanes, E. D., Bladen, H. A., Terry, W., and Page, D. L. Creation of "amyloid" fibrils from Bence Jones proteins in vitro, *Science* 174:712, 1971.

129. Glenner, G. G., Terry W., Harada, M., Isersky, C., and Page D. Amyloid fibril proteins: proof of homology with immunoglobulin light chains by sequence analyses, *Science* 172:1150, 1971.

130. Glenner, G. G., Terry, W., and Isersky, C. Amyloidosis: its nature and pathogenesis, *Semin. Hematol.* 10:65, 1973.

131. Godal, H. C., and Borchgrevink, C. F. The effect of plasmapheresis on the hemostatic function in patients with macroglobulinemia Waldenstrom and multiple myeloma, *Scand. J. Clin. Lab. Invest.* 84:133, 1965 (suppl.).

132. Greenberg, S. D., Heisler, J. G., Gyorkey, F., and Jenkins, D. E. Pulmonary lymphoma versus pseudolymphoma, *South. Med. J.* 65:775, 1972.

133. Gross, P. A. M., Gitlin, D., and Janeway, C. A. The gamma globulins and their clinical significance. III. Hypergammaglobulinemia, *N. Engl. J. Med.* 260:121, 1959.

134. Hällén, J. Discrete gammaglobulin (M-) components in serum. Clinical study of 150 subjects without myelomatosis, *Acta Med. Scand.* 462:1, 1966 (suppl.).

135. Hanlon, D. G., Bayrd, E. D., and Kearns, T. P. Macroglobulinemia—report of four cases, *J.A.M.A.* 167:1817, 1958.

136. Hannestad, K., and Christensen, T. B. Multiple M-components in a single individual, *Immunochemistry* 8:917, 1971.

137. Harboe, M., Deverill, J., and Godal, H. C. Antigenic heterogeneity of Waldenström type γM-globulins. *Scand. J. Haematol.* 2:137, 1965.

138. Harders, H. Waldenström's macroglobulinaemia: the causes of some of its more important clinical manifestations, *Ger. Med. Mon.* 2:137, 1957.

139. Hayes, D. W., Bennett, W. A., and Heck, F. J. Extramedullary lesions in multiple myeloma. Review of literature and pathologic studies, *Arch. Pathol.* 53:262, 1952.

140. Heiser, S., and Schwartzman, J. J. Variation in the roentgen appearance of the skeletal system in myeloma, *Radiology* 58:178, 1952.

141. Hellwig, C. A. Extramedullary plasma cell tumors as observed in various locations, *Arch. Pathol.* 36:95, 1943.

142. Henstell, H. H., and Kligerman, M. A new theory of interference with the clotting mechanism: the complexing of euglobulin with Factor V, Factor VII and prothrombin, *Ann. Intern. Med.* 49:371, 1958.

143. Heremans, J. F., and Heremans, M-Th. Immunoelectrophoresis, *Acta Med. Scand.* 367:27, 1961 (suppl.).

144. Herskovic, T., Andersen, H. A., and Bayrd, E. D. Intrathoracic plasmacytomas. Presentation of 21 cases and review of literature, *Dis. Chest* 47:1, 1965.

145. Hobbs, J. R. A staining method for proteins and dextran on cellulose acetate, *Nature* 207:292, 1965.

146. Hobbs, J. R. Paraproteins, benign or malignant? *Br. Med. J.* 3:699, 1967.

147. Hobbs, J. R. Immunochemical classes of myelomatosis. Including data from a therapeutic trial conducted by a medical research council working party, *Br. J. Haematol.* 16:599, 1969.

148. Hobbs, J. R. Paraproteins, *Proc. R. Soc. Med.* 62:773, 1969.

149. Hobbs, J. R., Slot, G. M. J., Campbell, C. H., Clein, G. P., Scott, J. T., Crowther, D., and Swan, H. T. Six cases of gamma-D myelomatosis, *Lancet* ii:614, 1966.

150. Husby, G., Natvig, J. G., and Sletten, K. New third class of amyloid fibril protein, *J. Exp. Med.* 139:773, 1974.

151. Husby, G., Sletten, K., Michaelsen, T. E., and Natvig, J. B. Alternative, non-immunoglobulin origin of amyloid fibrils, *Nature (New Biol.)* 238:187, 1972.

152. Imhof, J. W., Baars, H., and Verloop, M. C. Clinical and haematological aspects of macroglobulinemia Waldenström, *Acta Med. Scand.* 163:349, 1959.

153. Ishizaka, K., and Ishizaka, T. Physicochemical properties of reaginic antibody. I. Association of reaginic antibody with an immunoglobulin other than A- or G-globulin, *J. Allergy* 37:169, 1966.

154. Isobe, T., and Osserman, E. F. Pathologic conditions associated with plasma cell dyscrasias: a study of 806 cases, *Ann. N.Y. Acad. Sci.* 190:507, 1971.

155. Jim, R. T. S., and Steinkamp, R. C. Macroglobulinemia and its relationship to other paraproteins. With a case report, *J. Lab. Clin. Med.* 47:540, 1956.

156. Johansson, S. G. O. Immuno-globulin ND (IgE). Clinical and Immunological Studies, Söder-ström and Finn, Uppsala, 1968.

157. Johansson, S. G. O., and Bennich, H. Immunological studies of an atypical (myeloma) immuno-globulin, *Immunology* 13:381, 1967.

158. Johansson, S. G. O., and Bennich, H. Studies on a new class of human immunoglobulins. I. Im-munological properties, *in* J. Kil-lander (ed.), Gamma Globulins. Structure and Control of Bio-synthesis, Proc. Third Nobel Sym-posium, pp. 193–197, Almqvist & Wiksell, Stockholm, 1967.

159. Josephson, A. S., Price, E., and Biro, L. A low molecular weight frag-ment related to IgM in the serum of a patient with an IgA plasma cell dyscrasia, *Clin. Res.* 17:604, 1969.

160. Kappeler, R., Krebs, A., and Riva, G. Klinik der Makroglobulinämie Waldenström. Beschreibung von 21 Fällen und Übersicht der Literatur, *Helv. Med. Acta* 25:54, 1958.

161. Kark, R. M., Pirani, C. L., Pollak, V. E., Muehrcke, R. C., and Blainey, J. D. The nephrotic syn-drome in adults: a common dis-order with many causes, *Ann. In-tern. Med.* 49:751, 1958.

162. Kennedy, J. D., and Kneafsey, D. V. Two cases of plasmacytoma of the lower respiratory tract, *Thorax* 14:353, 1959.

163. Kenny, J. J., and Moloney, W. C. Multiple myeloma: diagnosis and management in a series of 57 cases, *Ann. Intern. Med.* 46:1079, 1957.

164. Khaleeli, M., Keane, W. M., and Lee, G. R. Sideroblastic anemia in multiple myeloma: a preleukemic change, *Blood* 41:17, 1973.

165. Killander, J. Separation of human immunoglobulins by gel filtration and zone electrophoresis, *Acta Soc. Med. Upsalien.* 68:230, 1963.

166. Kimura, S., Guyer, R., Terry, W. D., and Glenner, G. G. Chemical evi-dence for λ-type amyloid fibril pro-teins, *J. Immunol.* 109:891, 1972.

167. Kistner, S., and Norberg, R. The simultaneous occurrence of two different myeloma proteins, *Scand. J. Clin. Lab. Invest.* 17:321, 1965.

168. Kramer, W. Plasmocytoma of the brain in Kahler's disease (multiple myeloma), *Acta Neuropathol.* 2:438, 1963.

169. Kunkel, H. G. Macroblobulins and high molecular weight antibodies, *in* F. W. Putnam (ed.), The Plasma Proteins, vol. 1, pp. 279–307, Aca-demic Press, New York, 1960.

170. Kyle, R. A., and Bayrd, E. D. "Pri-mary" systemic amyloidosis and myeloma. Discussion of rela-tionship and review of 81 cases, *Arch. Intern. Med.* 107:344, 1961.

171. Lamm, M. E. Macroglobulinemia: report of two cases, *Am. J. Clin. Pathol.* 35:53, 1961.

172. Laurell, C. B., Laurell, S., and Skoog, N. Buffer composition in paper electrophoresis. Consider-ations on its influence, with special reference to the interaction between small ions and proteins, *Clin. Chem.* 2:99, 1956.

173. Laurell, C. B., and Snigurowicz, O. The frequency of kappa and lambda chains in pathologic serum γG, γA, γD, and γμ immunoglobulins, *Scand. J. Haematol.* 4:46, 1967.

174. Lawson, H. A., Stuart, C. A., Paull, A. M., Phillips, A. M., and Phillips R. W. Observations on the antibody content of the blood in patients with multiple myeloma, *N. Engl. J. Med.* 252:13, 1955.

175. Lebreton, J. P., Rivat, C., Rivat, L., Guillemot, L., and Ropartz, C. Une immunoglobulinopathie méconnue: la maladie des chaines lourdes, *Presse Med.* 75:2251, 1967.

176. Lee, S. L., Rosner, F., Ruberman, W., and Glasberg, S. Mu-chain dis-ease, *Ann. Intern. Med.* 75:407, 1971.

177. Lerner, A. B., and Watson, C. J. Studies on cryoglobulins. I. Unusual purpura associated with presence of a high concentration of cryoglobulin (cold precipitable serum globulin), 416—studies of cryoglobulins. II. The spontaneous precipitation of protein from serum at 5°C in various disease states. *Am. J. Med. Sci.* 214:410, 416; 1947.

178. Levin, M., Franklin, E. C., Frangione, B., and Pras, M. The amino acid sequence of a major nonimmunoglobulin component of some amyloid fibrils, *J. Clin. In-vest.* 51:2773, 1972.

179. Levin, M., Pras, M., and Franklin, E. C. Immunologic studies of the major nonimmunoglobulin protein of amyloid, *J. Exp. Med.* 138:373, 1973.

180. Lewis, E. B. Leukemia, multiple myeloma, and aplastic anemia in American radiologists, *Science* 142:1492, 1963.

181. Lightstone, A. C., and Cohen, H. J. Plasmacytic mucosal infiltrates in multiple myeloma, *Arch. Der-matol.* 82:921, 1960.

182. Lindemann, R. D., Scheer, R. L., and Raisz, L. G. Renal amyloidosis, *Ann. Intern. Med.* 54:883, 1961.

183. Linton, A. L., Dunnigan, M. G., and Thomson, J. A. Immune responses in myeloma, *Br. Med. J.* 2:86, 1963.

184. Lippincott, S. W., Korman, S., Fong, C., Stickley, E., Wolins, W., and Hughes, W. L. Turnover of labeled normal gamma globulin in multiple myeloma, *J. Clin. Invest.* 39:565, 1960.

185. Lob, M., Jéquier-Doge, E., and Rey-mond, A. Un nouveau cas de leu-cémie plasmocellulaire, *Schweiz. Med. Wochenschr.* 77:500, 1947.

186. Löffler, H., Knopp, A., and Krecke, H-J. Cases of multiple myeloma (plasmacytoma) "without parapro-tein," *Ger. Med. Mon.* 12:226, 1967.

187. Logothetis, J., Silverstein, P., and Coe, J. Neurologic aspects of Wal-denström's macroglobulinemia. Re-port of a case, *Arch. Neurol.* 3:564, 1960.

188. Long, L. A., Riopelle, J. L., Fran-coeur, M., Pare, A., Poirier, P., Georgesco, M., and Colpron, G. Macroglobulinemia. Effect of ma-croglobulins on prothrombin con-version accelerators, *Can. Med. Assoc. J.* 73:726, 1955.

189. McCallister, B. D., Bayrd, E. D., Harrison, E. G., and McGuckin, W. F. Primary macroglobulinemia. Re-view with a report on thirty-one cases and notes on the value of continuous chlorambucil therapy, *Am. J. Med.* 43:394, 1967.

190. Macintyre, W. A case of mollities and fragilitas ossium, accompanied with urine strongly charged with animal matter, *Med. Chir. Trans.* 33:211, 1850.

191. Mackay, I. R., Eriksen, N., Mo-tulsky, A. G., and Volwiler, W. Cryo- and macroglobulinemia. Elec-

trophoretic, ultracentrifugal and clinical studies, *Am. J. Med.* 20:564, 1956.

192. MacKenzie, M. R. Macroglobulinemia, *Calif. Med.* 108:136, 1968.
193. MacKenzie, M. R., Fudenberg, H. H., and O'Reilly, R. A. The hyperviscosity syndrome. I. In IgG myeloma. The role of protein concentration and molecular shape, *J. Clin. Invest.* 49:15, 1970.
194. MacMahon, B., and Clarke, D. W. The incidence of multiple myeloma, *J. Chronic Dis.* 4:508, 1956.
195. Magnus-Levy, A. Multiple myeloma (XII), *Acta Med. Scand.* 95:218, 1938.
196. Mandema, E., Van der Schaaf, P. C., and Huisman, T. H. J. Investigations on the amino acid composition of a macroglobulin and of a cryoglobulin, *J. Lab. Clin. Med.* 45:261, 1955.
197. Mannik, M. Binding of albumin to γA-myeloma proteins and Waldenström macroglobulins by disulfide bonds, *J. Immunol.* 99:899, 1967.
198. Marchalonis, J., and Edelman, G. M. Phylogenetic origins of antibody structure. I. Multichain structure of immunoglobulins in the smooth dogfish (mustelus canis), *J. Exp. Med.* 122:601, 1965.
199. Marchalonis, J. J., and Nossal, G. J. V. Electrophoretic analysis of antibody produced by single cells, *Proc. Natl. Acad. Sci. U.S.A.* 61:860, 1968.
200. Martin, N. H. Macroglobulinaemia. A clinical and pathological study, *Q. J. Med.* 29:179, 1960.
201. Martin, N. H. The incidence of myelomatosis, *Lancet* i:237, 1961.
202. Meltzer, M., and Franklin, E. C. Cryoglobulinemia—a study of twenty-nine patients, *Am. J. Med.* 40:828, 1966.
203. Merler, E., and Rosen, F. S. The gamma globulins. I. The structure and synthesis of the immunoglobulins, *N. Engl. J. Med.* 275:480, 536; 1966.
204. Metzger, H. Myeloma proteins and antibodies, *Am. J. Med.* 47:837, 1969.
205. Meyer, F. *In vitro* incorporation of C14-lysine into Bence-Jones protein, *Proc. Soc. Exp. Biol. Med.* 110:106, 1962.
206. Meyer, L. M., and Rutzky, J. An unusual case of acute plasma-cell

leukemia treated with a folic acid antagonist and urethane, *Cancer* 4:1043, 1951.
207. Migliore, P. J., and Alexanian, R. Monoclonal gammopathy in human neoplasia, *Cancer* 21:1127, 1968.
208. Miller, F., and Metzger, H. Characterization of a human macroglobulin. I. The molecular weight of its subunit, *J. Biol. Chem.* 240:3325, 1965.
209. Missmahl, H. P. Rectal biopsy in the diagnosis of amyloidosis, *Ger. Med. Mon.* 9:101, 1964.
210. Moore, D. F., Migliore, P. J., Shullenberger, C. C., and Alexanian, R. Monoclonal macroglobulinemia in malignant lymphoma, *Ann. Intern. Med.* 72:43, 1970.
211. Morel-Maroger, L., Basch, A., Danon, F., Verroust, P., and Richet, G. Pathology of the kidney in Waldenström's macroglobulinemia. Study of sixteen cases, *N. Engl. J. Med.* 283:123, 1970.
212. Morris, R. C., Jr., and Fudenberg, H. H. Impaired renal acidification in patients with hypergammaglobulinemia, *Medicine* 46:57, 1967.
213. Moseley, J. E. Bone Changes in Hematologic Disorders (Roentgen Aspects), Grune & Stratton, New York, 1963.
214. Moss, W. T., and Ackerman, L. V. Plasma cell leukemia, *Blood* 1:396, 1946.
215. Mullinax, F., Mullinax, G. L., and Himrod, B. RNA metabolism and protein synthesis in plasma cell leukemia, *Am. J. Med.* 42:302, 1967.
216. Mundy, G. R., Luben, R. A., Raisz, L. G., et al. Bone-resorbing activity in supernatants from lymphoid cell lines, *N. Engl. J. Med.* 290:867, 1974.
217. Nadeau, L. A., Magalini, S. I., and Stefanini, M. Familial multiple myeloma, *Arch. Pathol.* 61:101, 1956.
218. Nelson, M. G., and Lyons, A. R. Plasmacytoma of lymph glands, *Cancer* 10:1275, 1957.
219. Nick, J., Contamin, F., Brion, S., Guillard, A., and Guiraudon. Macroglobulinemie de Waldenstróm avec neuropathie amyloïde. Observation anatomoclinique, *Rev. Neurol. (Paris)* 109:21, 1963.
220. Niléhn, J-E., and Nilsson, I. M.

Coagulation studies in different types of myeloma, *Acta Med. Scand.* 445:194, 1966 (suppl.).
221. Odelberg-Johnsson, O. Report of a case, osteosclerotic changes in myelomatosis, *Acta Radiol.* 52:139, 1959.
222. Ogawa, M., Kochwa, S., Smith, C., Ishizaka, K., and McIntyre, O. R. Clinical aspects of IgE myeloma, *N. Engl. J. Med.* 281:1217, 1969.
223. Oka, S. A review on rheometry for biological studies, *Biorheology* 1:57, 1962.
224. Oliver, J. New directions in renal morphology: a method, its results and future, *Harvey Lect.* 40:102, 1944–45.
225. Olmer, J., Mongin, M., Muratore, R., and Denizet, D. Myélomes, Macroglobulinémies et Dysglobulinémies Voisines, Masson et Cie., Paris, 1961.
226. Osserman, E. F. Plasma-cell myeloma. II. Clinical aspects (concluded), *N. Engl. J. Med.* 261:1006, 1959.
227. Osserman, E. F., Graff, A., Marshall, M., Lawlor, D., and Graff, S. Incorporation of N15-L-aspartic acid into the abnormal serum and urine proteins of multiple myeloma (studies of the interrelationship of these proteins), *J. Clin. Invest.* 36:352, 1957.
228. Osserman, E. F., and Takatsuki, K. Plasma cell myeloma: gamma globulin synthesis and structure, *Medicine* 42:357, 1963.
229. Osserman, E. F., and Takatsuki, K. Clinical and immunochemical studies of four cases of heavy (Hγ2) chain disease, *Am. J. Med.* 37:351, 1964.
230. Osserman, E. F., Takatsuki, K., and Talal, N. The pathogenesis of "amyloidosis," *Semin. Hematol.* 1:3, 1964.
231. Pachter, M. R., Johnson, S. A., and Basinski, D. H. The effect of macroglobulins and their dissociation units on release of platelet factor 3, *Thromb. Diath. Haemorrh.* 3:501, 1959.
232. Pachter, M. R., Johnson, S. A., Neblett, T. R., and Truant, J. P. Bleeding, platelets, and macroglobulinemia, *Am. J. Clin. Pathol.* 31:467, 1959.
233. Penny, R., Castaldi, P. A., and Whitsed, H. M. Inflammation and

haemostasis in paraproteinaemias, *Br. J. Haematol.* 20:35, 1971.

234. Penny, R., and Galton, D. A. G. Studies on neutrophil function: II. Pathological aspects, *Br. J. Haematol.* 12:633, 1966.

235. Perkins, H. A., MacKenzie, M. R., and Fudenberg, H. H. Hemostatic defects in dysproteinemias, *Blood* 35:695, 1970.

236. Pitts, N. C., and McDuffie, F. C. Defective synthesis of IgM antibodies in macroglobulinemia, *Blood* 30:767, 1967.

237. Porter, R. R. The structure of the heavy chain of immunoglobulin and its relevance to the nature of antibody-combining site, *Biochem. J.* 105:417, 1967.

238. Poth, J. L., and George, R. P. Hemorrhagic ascites: an unusual complication of multiple myeloma, *Calif. Med.* 115:61, 1971.

239. Pras, M., and Reshef, T. The acid soluble fraction of amyloid—a fibril forming protein, *Biochim. Biophys. Acta* 271:193, 1972.

240. Prasad, A. S., Berman, L., Tranchida, L., and Poulik, M. D. Red cell hypoplasia, cold hemoglobinuria and M-type gamma G serum paraprotein and Bence-Jones proteinuria in a patient with lymphoproliferative disorder, *Blood* 31:151, 1968.

241. Preud'homme, J. L., Hurez, D., and Seligmann, M. Immunofluorescence studies in Waldenström's macroglobulinemia, *Eur. J. Clin. Biol. Res.* 15:1127, 1970.

242. Pruzanski, W., and Ogryzlo, M. A. The changing pattern of diseases associated with M components, *Med. Clin. North Am.* 56:371, 1972.

243. Pruzanski, W., Platts, M. E., and Ogryzlo, M. A. Leukemic form of immunocytic dyscrasia (plasma cell leukemia). A study of ten cases and a review of the literature, *Am. J. Med.* 47:60, 1969.

244. Rabiner, S. F., Aprill, S. N., and Radner, D. B. Waldenström's macroglobulinemia. Report of a case with pulmonary involvement and improvement in pulmonary symptoms only following chlorambucil therapy, *Am. J. Med.* 53:685, 1972.

245. Rambaud, J. C., Bognel, C., Prost, A., Bernier, J. J., Le Quintrec, Y., Lambling, A., Danon, F., Hurez, D., and Seligmann, M. Clinicopatho-logical study of a patient with "Mediterranean" type of abdominal lymphoma and a new type of IgA abnormality ("alpha chain disease"), *Digestion* 1:321, 1968.

246. Ritzmann, S. E., Thurn, R. H., Truax, W. E., and Levin, W. C. The syndrome of macroglobulinemia. Review of the literature and a report of two cases of macrocryogelglobulinemia, *Arch. Intern. Med.* 105:939, 1960.

247. Röckl, H., Knedel, M., and Schröpl, F. On the presence of paraproteinemia in serpiginous ulcerous pyoderma (pyoderma gangraenosum—dermatitis ulcerosa). Über das Vokommen von Paraproteinämie bei Pyodermia ulcerosa serpiginosa (Pyoderma gangraenosum—Dermatitis ulcerosa), *Hautarzt* 15:165, 1964.

248. Rogentine, G. N., Rowe, D. S., Bradley, J., Waldmann, T. A., and Fahey, J. L. Metabolism of human immunoglobulin D (IgD), *J. Clin. Invest.* 45:1467, 1966.

249. Rosen, B. J., Smith, T. W., and Bloch, K. J. Multiple myeloma associated with two serum M components, γG type K and γA type L, *N. Engl. J. Med.* 277:902, 1967.

250. Rosenberg, B., Attie, J. N., and Mandelbaum, H. L. Breast tumors as the presenting signs of multiple myeloma, *N. Engl. J. Med.* 269:359, 1963.

251. Rosenblum, W. I. Vasoconstriction, blood viscosity, and erythrocyte aggregation in macroglobulinemic and polycythemic mice, *J. Lab. Clin. Med.* 73:359, 1969.

252. Rosenblum, W. I., and Asofsky, R. M. Malfunction of cerebral microcirculation in macroglobulinemic mice. Relationship to increased blood viscosity, *Arch. Neurol.* 18:151, 1968.

253. Rosenblum, W. I., and Asofsky, R. M. Factors affecting blood viscosity in macroglobulinemic mice, *J. Lab. Clin. Med.* 71:201, 1968.

254. Rothfield, N. F., Frangione, B., and Franklin, E. C. Slowly sedimenting mercaptoethanol-resistant antinuclear factors related antigenically to M immunoglobulins (γ₁M-globulin) in patients with systemic lupus erythematosus, *J. Clin. Invest.* 44:62, 1965.

255. Rowe, D. S., and Fahey, J. L. A new class of human immunoglobins. II. Normal serum IgD, *J. Exp. Med.* 121:185, 1965.

256. Rowland, L. P., and Schneck, S. A. Neuromuscular disorders associated with malignant neoplastic disease, *J. Chronic Dis.* 16:777, 1963.

257. Rowlands, B., and Shaw, N. Extramedullary plasmocytoma, *Br. Med. J.* 2:1302, 1954.

258. Rozenberg, M. C., and Dintenfass, L. Platelet aggregation in Waldenström's macroglobulinaemia, *Thromb. Diath. Haemorrh.* 14:202, 1965.

259. Ruben, R. J., Distenfeld, A., Berg, P., and Carr, R. Sudden sequential deafness as the presenting symptom of macroglobulinemia, *J.A.M.A.* 209:1364, 1969.

260. Rubinstein, M. A. Multiple myeloma as a form of leukemia, *Blood* 4:1049, 1949.

261. Rudders, R. A., Yakulis, V., and Heller, P. Double myeloma, *Am. J. Med.* 55:215, 1973.

262. Salmon, S. E. Immunoglobulin synthesis and tumor kinetics of multiple myeloma, *Semin. Hematol.* 10:135, 1973.

263. Salmon, S. E., McIntyre, O. R., and Ogawa, M. IgE myeloma: total body tumor cell number and synthesis of IgE and DNA, *Blood* 37:696, 1971.

264. Sanders, J. H., Fahey, J. L., Finegold, I., Ein, D., Reisfeld, R., and Berard, C. Multiple anomalous immunoglobulins, *Am. J. Med.* 47:43, 1969.

265. Sandor, G., Korach, S., and Mattern, P. 7 S globulin, immunologically identical to 19 S gamma-1 (beta-2)-M-globulin, a new protein of horse serum, *Nature* 204:795, 1964.

266. Sataline, L. Acute plasmacytic leukemia with hypercalcemia. Report of a case without bone lesions, *Ohio State Med. J.* 61:138, 1965.

267. Scheurlen, P. G. Multiple myeloma with several anomalous proteins, *Ger. Med. Mon.* 9:138, 1964.

268. Schneider, M., and Mazabraud, M. Les signes révélateurs du myélome et leur fréquence relative (the revealing signs of myeloma and their relative incidence), *Rev. Rhum. Mal. Osteoartic.* 26:660, 1959.

269. Schwab, P. J., and Fahey, J. L. Treatment of Waldenström's ma-

croglobulinemia by plasmapheresis, *N. Engl. J. Med.* 263:574, 1960.

270. Schwab, P. J., Okun, E., and Fahey, J. L. Reversal of retinopathy in Waldenström's macroglobulinemia by plasmapheresis. A report of two cases, *Arch. Ophthalmol.* 64:515, 1960.

271. Seligmann, M. A genetic predisposition to Waldenström's macroglobulinaemia, *Acta Med. Scand.* 445:140, 1966 (suppl.).

272. Seligmann, M., Danon, F., Hurez, D., Mihaesco, E., and Preud'homme, J-L. Alpha-chain disease: a new immunoglobulin abnormality, *Science* 162:1396, 1968.

273. Seligmann, M., Mihaesco, E., and Frangione, B. Studies on alpha chain disease, *Ann. N.Y. Acad. Sci.* 190:487, 1971.

274. Seligmann, M., Mihaesco, E., Hurez, D., Mihaesco, C., Preud'homme, J-L., and Rambaud, J-C. Immunochemical studies in four cases of alpha chain disease, *J. Clin. Invest.* 48:2374, 1969.

275. Seligmann, M., and Rambaud, J-C. IgA abnormalities in abdominal lymphoma (A-chain disease). *Isr. J. Med. Sci.* 5:151, 1969.

276. Sharma, K. D., and Shrivastav, J. D. Extramedullary plasmacytoma of the gastrointestinal tract with a case report of plasmoma of the rectum and a review of the literature, *Arch. Pathol.* 71:229, 1961.

277. Simon, M. A., and Eidlow, S. Plasmacytoma of lymph node: report of a case with multiple myeloma, *N. Engl. J. Med.* 243:335, 1950.

278. Sirota, J. H., and Hamerman, D. Renal function studies in an adult subject with the Fanconi syndrome, *Am. J. Med.* 16:138, 1954.

279. Skoog, W. A., Adams, W. S., and Coburn, J. W. Metabolic balance study of plasmapheresis in a case of Waldenström's macroglobulinemia, *Blood* 19:425, 1962.

280. Smith, E., Kochwa, S., and Wasserman, L. R. Aggregation of IgG globulin in vivo. I. The hyperviscosity syndrome in multiple myeloma, *Am. J. Med.* 39:35, 1965.

281. Snapper, I., Turner, L. B., and Moscovitz, H. L. Multiple Myeloma, Grune & Stratton, New York, 1953.

282. Solomon, A., and Fahey, J. L. Plasmapheresis therapy in macroglobu-

linemia, *Ann. Intern. Med.* 58:789, 1963.

283. Solomon, A., Killander, J., Grey, H. M., and Kunkel, H. G. Low-molecular-weight proteins related to Bence Jones proteins in multiple myeloma, *Science* 151:1237, 1966.

284. Solomon, A., and Kunkel, H. G. A "monoclonal" type, low molecular weight protein related to γM-macroglobulins, *Am. J. Med.* 42:958, 1967.

285. Solomon, A., Waldmann, T. A., and Fahey, J. L. Metabolism of 6.6 S γ-globulin in normal subjects and patients with macroglobulinemia and multiple myeloma, *J. Lab. Clin. Med.* 62:1, 1963.

286. Somer, T. The viscosity of blood, plasma, and serum in dys- and paraproteinemias, *Acta Med. Scand.* 456:1, 1966 (suppl.).

287. Spalter, H. F. Abnormal serum proteins and retinal vein thrombosis, *Arch. Ophthalmol.* 62:868, 1959.

288. Stark, E., and Amidon, E. L. Diffuse plasma cell myelomatosis, *Arch. Pathol.* 46:183, 1948.

289. Study Committee of the Midwest Cooperative Chemotherapy Group: Multiple myeloma. General aspects of diagnosis, course, and survival, *J.A.M.A.* 188:741, 1964.

290. Sullivan, P. W., and Salmon, S. E. Kinetics of tumor growth and regression in IgG multiple myeloma, *J. Clin. Invest.* 51:1697, 1972.

291. Svartz, N. Macroglobulins in rheumatoid arthritis. Preliminary report, *Acta Med. Scand.* 158:163, 1957.

292. Symmers, W. St.C. Primary amyloidosis: a review, *J. Clin. Pathol.* 9:187, 1956.

293. Terry, W. D., Page, D. L., Kimura, S., et al. Structural identity of Bence Jones and amyloid fibril proteins in a patient with plasma cell dyscrasia and amyloidosis, *J. Clin. Invest.* 52:1276, 1973.

294. Thannhauser, S. J., and Krauss, E. Über eine degenerative Erkrankung der Harukanälchen (Nephrose) bei Bence-jones'scher Albuminurie mit Nierenschwund (kleine, glatte, weisse Niere), *Deutsch. Arch. Klin. Med.* 133:183, 1920.

295. Thomas, F. B., Clausen, K. P., and Greenberger, N. J. Liver disease in multiple myeloma, *Arch. Intern. Med.* 132:195, 1973.

296. Thorling, E. B. Leukaemic myelomatosis (plasma-cell leukaemia), *Acta Haematol.* 28:222, 1962.

297. Thorsén, G., and Hint, H. Aggregation, sedimentation and intravascular sludging of erythrocytes, *Acta Chir. Scand.* 154:3, 1950 (suppl.).

298. Tomasi, T. B., Jr. Human gamma globulin, *Blood* 25:382, 1965.

299. Van Furth, R., Schmit, H. R. E., and Hijmans, W. The formation in vitro of paraproteins in multiple myeloma and Waldenström's macroglobulinemia, *Br. J. Haematol.* 12:202, 1966.

300. Vaughan, J., and Raphael, S. R. Case of multiple myeloma complicated by agranulocytosis, *Br. Med. J.* 1:27, 1956.

301. Videbaek, A., Mansa, B., and Kjems, E. A human IgA-myeloma protein with anti-streptococcal hyaluronidase (ASH) activity, *Scand. J. Haematol.* 10:181, 1973.

302. Waldenström, J. Incipient myelomatosis or "essential" hyperglobulinemia with fibrinogenopenia—a new syndrome? *Acta Med. Scand.* 117:216, 1944.

303. Waldenström, J. Zwei interessante Syndrome mit Hyperglobinämie (purpura Hyperglobulinaemica und Makroglobulinämie), *Schweiz. Med. Wochenschr.* 78:927, 1948.

304. Waldenström, J. Abnormal proteins in myeloma, *Adv. Intern. Med.* 5:398, 1952.

305. Waldenström, J. Stoffwechsel der Eiweisse und Aminosäuren. Thannhausers Lehrbuch des Stoffwechsels und der Stoffwechsel-Krankheiten, p. 455, George Thieme Verlag, Stuttgart, 1957.

306. Waldenström, J. The occurrence of benign essential monoclonal (M type), non-macromolecular hyperglobulinemia and its differential diagnosis, *Acta Med. Scand.* 176:345, 1964.

307. Waldenström, J. Diagnosis and Treatment of Multiple Myeloma, Grune & Stratton, New York, 1970.

308. Waldmann, T. A., and Strober, W. Metabolism of immunoglobulins, *Prog. Allergy* 13:1, 1969.

309. Wanner, J., and Siebenmann, R. Über eine subakut verlanfende osteolytische Form der Makroglobulinämie Waldenström mit Plasmazellenleukämie, *Schweiz. Med. Wochenschr.* 87:1243, 1957.

310. Warner, N. L., MacKenzie, M. R., and Fudenberg, H. H. Anti-antibody activity of a monoclonal macroglobulin, *Proc. Natl. Acad. Sci. U.S.A.* 68:2846, 1971.

311. Weissman, G., and Cohen, B. R. Macroglobulinemia: studies of serum and synovial fluid from a patient with multiple infections, *J. Mount Sinai Hosp.* 26:125, 1959.

312. Wells, R. E. Rheology of blood in the microvasculature, *N. Engl. J. Med.* 270:832, 1964.

313. Welton, J., Walker, S. R., Sharp, G. C., Herzenberg, L. A., Wistar, R., and Creger, W. P. Macroglobulinemia with bone destruction, *Am. J. Med.* 44:280, 1968.

314. Williams, R. C., Jr., Brunning, R. D., and Wollheim, F. A. Light-chain disease. An abortive variant of multiple myeloma, *Ann. Intern. Med.* 65:471, 1966.

315. Wintrobe, M. M., and Buell, M. V. Hyperproteinemia associated with multiple myeloma. With report of a case in which an extraordinary hyperproteinemia was associated with thrombosis of the retinal veins and symptoms suggesting Raynaud's disease, *Bull. Johns Hopkins Hosp.* 52:156, 1933.

316. Wolf, R. E., Alperin, J. B., Ritzmann, S. E., and Levin, W. C. IgG-K-multiple myeloma with hyperviscosity syndrome — response to plasmapheresis, *Arch. Intern. Med.* 129:114, 1972.

317. Wollheim, F. A., and Snigurowicz, J. Studies on the macroglobulins of human serum IV: The frequency of light chain types K and L in polyclonal and monoclonal γM, *Scand. J. Haematol.* 4:111, 1967.

318. Wollheim, F. A., and Williams, R. C., Jr. Studies on the macroglobulins of human serum II: Heterogeneity of antigenic determinants among M-components in Waldenström's macroglobulinemia, *Acta Med. Scand.* 445:115, 1966 (suppl.).

319. Wright, J. H. A case of multiple myeloma, *Trans. Assoc. Am. Physicians* 15:137, 1900.

320. Wuhrmann, F., and Märki, H. H. Dysproteinämien und Paraproteinämien, Schwabe & Co., Basel, 1963.

321. Young, V. H. Transient paraproteins, *Proc. R. Soc. Med.* 62:778, 1969.

322. Zawadzki, Z. A., and Rubini, J. R. D-myeloma. Report of two cases, *Arch. Intern. Med.* 119:387, 1967.

323. Zucker-Franklin, D., Franklin, E. C., and Hamilton, L. Cellular studies on μ chain disease, *Clin. Res.* 18:422, 1970.

Chapter 21 Acute Lymphocytic Leukemia and the Acute Lymphoproliferative Disorders

The first microscopic observations of leukemic cells were probably made by Donné, who in 1839 studied the blood of a patient in the Hôtel Dieu in Paris (89). It was not until about 1845, however, that leukemia was recognized as a distinct clinical entity and was described as "suppuration of the blood" (27, 414). By 1857 leukemia with an acute course had been described (137), and by 1889 the clinical manifestations were well known (110).

Acute Lymphocytic Leukemia

Definition and Relation to Other Acute Lymphoproliferative Disorders

Acute lymphocytic leukemia (or acute lymphoblastic leukemia, or ALL) may be defined as a malignant disease characterized by (a) widespread infiltration of the bone marrow and other organs by proliferating poorly differentiated cells of the lymphoid series; (b) reduction of the normal hematopoietic cells with resultant anemia, granulocytopenia, and thrombocytopenia; and (c) a rapidly fatal course from bleeding, infection, or anemia if the disease is untreated.

The neoplastic cells are characterized by unrestrained proliferation. "Unrestrained" takes cognizance of the observation that although most cells of the body proliferate at one time or another, they are subject to rigid control mechanisms that limit this normal proliferation. Leukemic blast cells behave as if they are not subject to these control mechanisms. The loss of responsiveness to controls in leukemia may be partial rather than complete and

under certain circumstances, such as in vitro culture, some leukemia cells may undergo relatively normal differentiation (290).

The proliferating cells are recognized as lymphoid on the basis of their morphology in Romanovsky-stained preparations, although some histochemical characteristics aid in their identification. In any large series of patients, a morphologic spectrum of cells is seen that varies from primitive, undifferentiated cells to cells clearly resembling the mature circulating lymphocyte (see Fig. 21.1). At the extreme primitive end of the spectrum the cells have no distinctive morphologic characteristics and cannot reliably be classified as lymphoid cells (Fig. 21.2). Patients with a predominance of such cells are often said to have "acute undifferentiated leukemia" or "stem cell leukemia." These poorly differentiated leukemias can be considered as behaving like acute lymphocytic leukemia because of their occurrence in childhood and their pattern of response to drug therapy. Consequently, most hematologists classify them with acute lymphocytic leukemia.

Another disorder that is occasionally confused with acute lymphocytic leukemia is so-called "hairy cell leukemia" (64, 157, 326, 362), which has been described in Chapter 19.

From what we know of the origin of hematopoietic cells from a common, pluripotent stem cell with few distinctive morphologic characteristics (Chapter 2), it is not surprising that we see a spectrum of leukemic disorders comprising cells in a variety of stages of differentiation.

Several hematopoietic disorders are characterized by

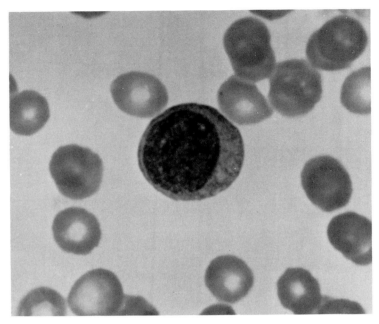

Figure 21.1 Lymphoblast from the peripheral blood of a patient with acute lymphocytic leukemia. Note the prominent nucleoli. The resemblance of this cell to the normal medium-sized lymphocyte is apparent.

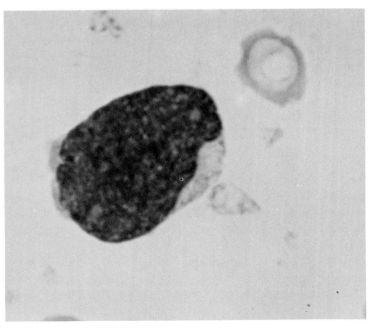

Figure 21.2 A large morphologically undifferentiated cell from the blood of a patient with acute lymphocytic leukemia.

proliferation of poorly differentiated hematopoietic cells. These disorders may resemble lymphoblastic leukemia in their hematologic and clinical manifestations. Clearly, the acute myeloproliferative disorders such as acute myelocytic leukemia and acute monocytic leukemia have a roughly similar natural history, although they are characterized by some distinctive morphologic, biochemical, epidemiologic, and clinical features.

Several hematopoietic disorders are characterized by the proliferation of lymphoid cells that are poorly differentiated or moderately well differentiated. These disorders tend to be relatively "acute" and have a natural history lasting a few weeks to a few years. They are grouped together as the *acute lymphoproliferative disorders* and include lymphocytic leukemia, certain lymphomas, infectious mononucleosis, and certain disorders characterized by transient lymphocytosis.

Some lymphosarcomas that invade the bone marrow and peripheral blood (to be discussed in the next chapter) may resemble acute lymphocytic leukemia morphologically and clinically. They comprise a similar spectrum of cellular differentiation. Such "leukolymphosarcomas" probably arise from a proliferating hematopoietic cell with approximately the same degree of differentiation as the cells of acute lymphocytic leukemia.

None of the other acute lymphoproliferative disorders is easily confused with lymphoblastic leukemia. Infectious mononucleosis and infectious lymphocytosis (321) are easily differentiated morphologically and clinically. There is no reason to believe that these disorders give rise to a sustained lymphoproliferative process.

The basic concept to be borne in mind is that lymphoblastic leukemia is a neoplastic disease characterized by proliferation of a spectrum of lymphoid cells of varying degrees of differentiation. The disease resembles other malignant disorders arising from poorly differentiated hematopoietic cell proliferation and is easily distinguished from benign, self-limited lymphoproliferative disorders.

Incidence and Etiologic Considerations

Many of the salient features regarding incidence and possible etiology of acute leukemia have already been considered in Chapter 11 in the discussion of myeloblastic leukemia. Here we shall consider only the distinctive features that characterize acute lymphocytic leukemia.

Incidence Acute lymphocytic leukemia is primarily a disease of children and young adults, although occurrence has been reported in all ages up to the ninth decade of life. The peak incidence occurs between ages four and five years (46, 87, 146, 245, 286, 287, 431). Surprisingly, congenital leukemia is probably more often myelogenous than lymphocytic in nature (28).

Acute lymphoblastic leukemia accounts for about 20 or 25 percent of all reported cases of leukemia (33, 87, 146, 431). The male/female ratio is near unity (87). Many series have shown a greater incidence of acute lymphoblastic leukemia in white persons than in blacks (325, 431). However, this has not been the experience of all investigators (271, 272). The role of social and economic factors involved in determining the reported frequency of diagnosis of this disease entity is difficult to assess (163, 272). Glass and his colleagues (162) make the point that "in a relatively rare disease such as leukemia, it is important to keep in mind the possibility that seemingly high concentrations of cases may be generated by over-zealous statistical manipulation."

In 1967 a downturn in childhood leukemia mortality of the white population of the United States was reported (127).

Hereditary and Familial Factors   The difficulties in assessing the role of hereditary and familial factors in the origin of acute lymphocytic leukemia are well described in recent reviews (126, 269, 442). An association between childhood leukemia and several congenital disorders has been proposed. These disorders, characterized either by chromosomal anomalies from meiotic accident or by an inherited pattern sometimes associated with an increased incidence of chromosomal breaks, include Down's syndrome, G-trisomy (74, 242, 254, 291, 419), D-trisomy (443), Bloom's syndrome (38, 332, 358), and ataxia telangiectasia (184). The acute leukemia occurring in these disease disorders is more often myelogenous than lymphocytic (126, 442). Often the leukemia occurring in mongolism is characterized as "acute stem cell leukemia" (335). Zuelzer and Cox (442) pointed out also that a leukemic blood picture in the neonate with mongolism may not in fact be a true leukemia, but may sometimes be a leukemoid reaction with immature granulocytes and normoblasts.

Some striking familial (5, 173, 183, 413, 442), as well as nonfamilial (120), clusters in acute leukemia have been described. However, such clusters are quite rare and their significance is unknown. Their existence may be ascribed to indeterminate genetic or environmental factors. About 25 instances of concordant leukemia in twins are known (442); of these, all but 4 were acute leukemia involving children. In large series there is a high relative risk of concordance among like-sex twins, an observation suggesting that monozygous twins have a higher concordance rate

(274). However, the absolute risk of concordance among monozygous twins is exceedingly low (80, 442). Pearson and his colleagues (318) concluded that this low risk argues against a major role for genetic factors in childhood leukemia. Most of the large-scale surveys have failed to provide firm evidence for genetic factors in the majority of cases of acute leukemia of childhood (16, 173, 175, 273, 296, 388, 413). A few exceptions have been reported, however (341).

Children born of leukemic mothers do not appear to have an increased incidence of leukemia (8).

Environmental Factors   In Chapter 11 we summarized the evidence linking acute myelocytic leukemia to environmental factors such as radiation and chemicals that produce marrow damage and chromosomal abnormalities (see 36, 37, 55, 126, 212, 261, 377, 420). These factors have shown more of an association with myelogenous leukemia than with acute lymphoblastic leukemia.

For more than sixty years certain viruses have been implicated as possible causative agents in certain types of leukemia (3). Without exception, the viruses identified have proven to be RNA viruses. Such leukemogenic viruses have been isolated from the cat, rat, mouse, and chicken (398). The leukemogenic effect of irradiation and certain chemicals may also be mediated by activation of a latent leukemia virus (22, 220, 339). There is an ongoing search for oncogenic viruses in man (230).

The evidence supporting a viral etiology for acute leukemia in man is provocative but not conclusive. Much of the attention has focused on the discovery of an enzyme, reverse transcriptase, in leukemic cells (12, 15, 85, 144, 168, 397, 399). This enzyme, an RNA-dependent DNA polymerase, appears to be a unique feature of the known oncogenic RNA viruses and perhaps of a few other RNA viruses that have low oncogenic potential in vitro. It apparently is absent in other RNA viruses (for example, polio), in DNA viruses, and in uninfected mammalian cells (15, 399). Consequently, the presence of the enzyme in the mammalian cell is prima facie evidence for the presence of an oncogenic RNA virus. However, such a marker does not tell us whether the RNA viruses are passengers in leukemic cells or are functioning as oncogenic agents. Current views on the status of RNA-dependent DNA polymerase in oncogenic viruses and cells have recently been summarized (143).

Spiegelman and his colleagues (20, 21, 185) have recently demonstrated that human leukemic cells may contain RNA homologous to that of the mouse leukemia agent. Human sarcoma may possess similar RNA. If confirmed, this observation would suggest remarkable parallelism of leukemia in mice and men.

Because the known animal leukemias are caused by RNA viruses, rather than DNA viruses, there has not been much emphasis on the DNA oncogenic viruses as a potential cause of human leukemia. Nevertheless, it is thought that the DNA-containing Epstein-Barr virus may be etiologic in human infectious mononucleosis and possibly in Burkitt's lymphoma (174). Again, the possibility has not been excluded that this is a passenger virus.

The DNA virus, SV-40, is oncogenic in certain animal systems (97). Considerable excitement ensued when it was learned that many of the early lots of polio vaccine administered to human children and neonates contained this virus. However, after more than eight years of observation no increased incidence of leukemia or other cancers in children receiving the contaminated vaccine has been reported (126, 128).

Certain features of animal leukemia should be borne in mind, since they may have relevance to human disease. Most animal leukemias are passed from parent to offspring in vertical fashion (172). As a consequence of this transmission, the infected animal may be immunologically tolerant of the viral antigen, meaning that in postnatal life it cannot be immunized against the virus by conventional means. Such an observation may have significance for the use of viral vaccines, should the human disease be shown to have a similar pattern of transmission. It has also been suggested that virogenic material may be integrated into the mammalian genome and may be ubiquitous. Activation of the viral genetic material and expression in malignant transformation of the cell would then be triggered by some external event such as irradiation. This "oncogene theory" (214) has important implications for our approach to prevention of leukemia. If the gene is truly ubiquitous, there is little reason to approach leukemia as one would approach a horizontally transmitted viral disease. The role of immunosuppression in the expression of oncogenic virus may well assume increasing importance (48, 197).

Hematologic Features

The basic hematologic features of lymphoblastic leukemia are similar to those of other acute leukemias. The classic picture is that of marked leukocytosis with primitive cells, anemia, granulocytopenia and thrombocytopenia in the peripheral blood, and a bone marrow packed with poorly differentiated blast cells (Fig. 21.3). A variant of this typical picture is *aleukemic leukemia*, in which the peripheral white blood count is normal or low and few blast cells appear in the circulation. Other

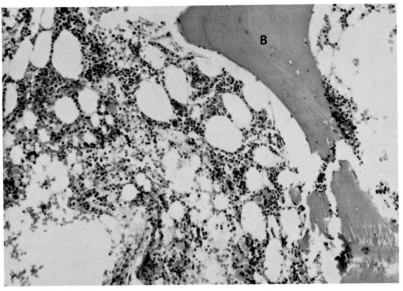

Fig. 21.3A

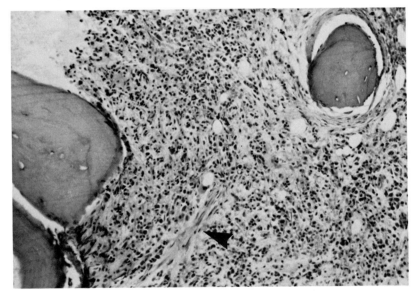

Fig. 21.3B

Figure 21.3 Bone marrow biopsies from a normal subject and one with acute lymphocytic leukemia. Hematoxylin and eosin stain. In Fig. 21.3A, the normal subject, the large cells are megakaryocytes and *B* is a bone spicule. In the leukemic patient, Fig. 21.3B, some fibrosis is evident (*arrow*) in addition to the dense lymphoid cell infiltration.

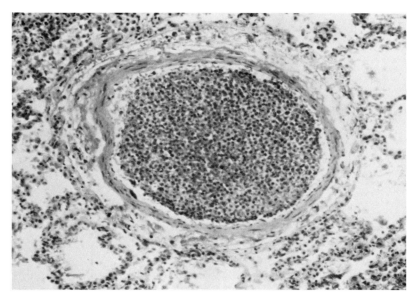

Figure 21.4 A pulmonary blood vessel plugged by leukemic leukocytes.

variants include those with initially normal platelet and/or granulocyte counts. Thus, the peripheral leukocyte count may vary from very low levels below 1,000/mm³ to very high levels greater than 400,000/mm³. Roughly 50 percent of children with acute leukemia present with an aleukemic picture (343). As a generalization, patients with low white counts do better than those with marked degrees of leukocytosis, probably because of the higher body burden of malignant cells in the latter group.

Intravascular clumping of blast cells may occur in patients with blast counts in excess of 100,000/mm³ (Fig. 21.4). This can lead to occlusion of microscopic blood vessels and poor perfusion of critical tissues such as the brain. In addition, perivascular infiltration of the central nervous system and associated hemorrhage is more common when the blast count is high (138). Intracerebral hemorrhage is the rule under these circumstances. This is probably the major factor linking extreme degrees of leukocytosis with poor prognosis (133, 135, 187, 434).

Anemia is the rule in untreated acute lymphocytic leukemia, occurring in well over 90 percent of patients (46). It is generally normocytic and normochromic. Occasionally hypochromic anemia, secondary to blood loss, or macrocytic anemia is observed. High degrees of reticulocytosis are unusual. The percentage of normoblasts in the bone marrow is reduced, and bizarre cells of the erythroid series are frequently encountered. The mechanisms of anemia are not always evident. In some patients there is obvious bleeding or, rarely, hemolysis. The type

of autoimmune hemolytic anemia seen in chronic lymphocytic leukemia is rarely observed in acute leukemia. Frequently, erythropoiesis is suppressed by the drugs used in therapy. It has long been suggested that the erythroid marrow may be crowded out by blast cells (see Fig. 21.3B) with resultant inadequate erythropoiesis. Whether this morphologically apparent crowding does, in fact, exert a physiologic effect is uncertain. Studies of erythropoiesis in acute leukemia have yielded variable results, from depression to higher than normal levels of red cell production (47, 215, 302, 319, 426, 440). Consequently, no facile generalization is possible, and each patient with acute leukemia must be studied in detail to ascertain the mechanism of anemia operative in his case.

Over the years it has been suggested that the anemia of acute leukemia may be an expression of defective proliferation and/or maturation of erythroid precursors, possibly at the level of the stem cell, which results in decreased or ineffective erythropoiesis (409, 428). Recent evidence suggests that in the acute leukemias the stem cell compartment available for erythroid differentiation may be decreased in size (69, 147). Erythropoietin production appears to be normal (440).

Thrombocytopenia is observed at some time during the course of illness in more than 90 percent of patients with acute lymphocytic leukemia (346). Severe thrombocytopenia is said to be somewhat more common in lymphoblastic leukemia than in myeloblastic leukemia (46, 431). When severe thrombocytopenia occurs, the platelets are often large and have bizarre shapes. Thrombocytopenia is thought to result from reduced numbers of megakaryocytes in the bone marrow, although in some cases excessive sequestration of platelets by the spleen may be a contributing factor. As a generalization, bleeding increases progressively as the platelet count falls below 50,000 (89, 129, 150, 292, 330). However, occasional patients with platelet counts of 1,000 or 2,000/mm³ have no significant hemorrhage.

Severe anemia and thrombocytopenia are thought to be factors associated with a poor prognosis (434); however, these are probably not significant when red cells and platelets are available for transfusion (100, 186). As indicated earlier, a low platelet count together with a high blast cell count does carry a very grave prognosis.

Bone marrow aspirate from the untreated patient with lymphoblastic leukemia as a rule is crowded with primitive cells (Fig. 21.5). The marrow fat spaces are obliterated (Fig. 21.6) and the normal erythropoietic, granulocytic, and megakaryocytic elements are relatively reduced. Bone marrow biopsy shows infiltration with a uniform round cell population (Fig. 21.3B). Under high magnification, the

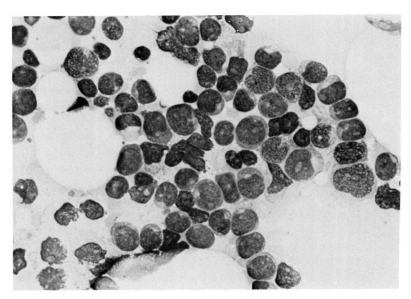

Figure 21.5 Immature lymphoid cells in bone marrow aspirate of a patient with acute lymphocytic leukemia. Giemsa stain.

Romanovsky-stained bone marrow aspirate may show the variety and degrees of cellular differentiation seen in the peripheral blood. After therapy, the marrow may be acellular or fibrotic (see Fig. 9.2). During periods of remission, significant levels of lymphocytosis (greater than 20 percent) in the bone marrow may be observed. In contrast to previously held concepts (35), this lymphocytosis is not a

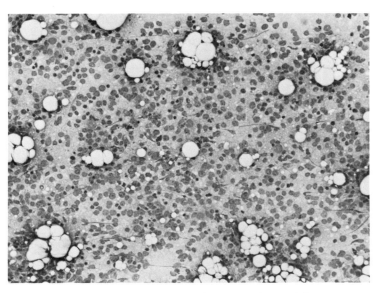

Figure 21.6 Bone marrow aspirate from a patient with acute lymphocytic leukemia. The marrow fat spaces are almost entirely obliterated.

poor prognostic sign (379). Extreme eosinophilia is a rare concomitant of acute lymphoblastic leukemia (384).

Morphology and Cytochemistry   In the beginning of this chapter it was pointed out that the cells of patients with lymphoblastic leukemia encompass a spectrum of various degrees of differentiation. This spectrum is illustrated in Figs. 21.1, 21.2, and 21.5. A "typical" blast cell of intermediate degree of differentiation (Fig. 21.1) has a high nucleus/cytoplasm ratio with a thin rim of blue cytoplasm usually containing no inclusions. The nucleus is round or oval and composed of coarsely granular or stippled chromatin that tends to be more condensed around the rim of the nucleus and nucleoli, giving the appearance of a distinct membrane. One or two nucleoli are present, although these are generally not so prominent as in the myeloblast. A small, clear zone may be seen surrounding the nucleus. The most undifferentiated lymphoid cells cannot be distinguished with certainty from primitive myeloblasts, in either the light or the electron microscope (compare Fig. 21.2 with Figs. 11.1 and 11.5).

A comparison of the cytochemical reactions of the lymphoblasts and the myeloblasts is given in Table 11.2 and in Table 27.2. The lymphoblast is peroxidase-negative and shows little sudanophilia. PAS-positive material, when present, is collected as coarse granules in a necklace about the nucleus (182, 288). Lymphoblasts are said to be unique in possessing nuclear aryl sulphatase activity (113, 249).

Recent evidence suggests that leukemic lymphoblasts share an enzymatic marker (terminal deoxynucleotidyl transferase) with T cells (266). Interestingly, this enzyme has also been observed in the primitive cells of the blast crisis of chronic myelocytic leukemia.

Proliferation   There is considerable variation from patient to patient in the proliferative activity of the leukemia population as measured by the percentage of cells incorporating tritiated thymidine (labeling index) and by the mitotic index (347, 357). In the same patient the labeling index tends to be higher in the bone marrow than in the peripheral blood (66, 232, 284), suggesting that the blood is not the most important proliferating compartment. There is a small but statistically significant diurnal variation in the bone marrow proliferative activity (357), similar in some respects to that observed in normal myeloid marrow (283). The leukemic marrow is composed of both dividing and nondividing cells (285). The latter are thought to be arrested in a prolonged G_1 phase of the cell cycle. The dividing compartment is composed primarily of the large blast cells; the nondividing compartment is composed primarily of smaller blast cells (66, 148, 357) (see Figs. 11.8 and 11.9). The labeling index changes with time in a given patient; this change can be related directly to the proportion of large dividing blast cells in the marrow (357).

The large, proliferating blasts are not thought to maintain themselves but, after one or two divisions, become much smaller and enter the nondividing compartment (148, 149, 285). An important question, therefore, is whether the smaller blast cells are end cells destined to die or whether they are capable of reentering the proliferative cycle. The answer seems to be that they retain the ability to reenter the proliferative pool—for example, when there is a reduction in the number of large blast cells by administration of chemotherapeutic drugs (140).

At the time of diagnosis, the labeling index varied between 1.8 and 15.5 (mean 6.7 percent) in 23 patients with lymphoblastic leukemia (357). At the time of relapse, the labeling indexes were generally higher, with a mean of 17.7 percent. The generation time (that is, the time for the cell to complete one reproductive cycle) was the same at the time of diagnosis and relapse in three patients. This generation time had a minimal value of approximately 60 hours. A number of the drugs used in chemotherapy have profound effects on the proliferative cycle of leukemic lymphoblasts. For example, L-asparaginase and hydrocortisone appear to arrest the entry of cells into DNA synthesis (S phase) as well as having a direct cytotoxic effect on the cells. Cyclophosphamide appears to arrest entry into S phase, to inhibit DNA synthesis, and to arrest cells in mitosis. Cytosine arabinoside and methotrexate inhibit DNA synthesis (247).

The recruitment of nondividing cells into the proliferating compartment when the large, proliferating blasts are killed by drugs has some interesting clinical implications (140). It suggests that cellular proliferation in leukemia may be subject to some regulation. Many tumors follow so-called Gompertzian kinetics in their growth pattern, which means that the fraction of cells proliferating may decrease as the tumor gets larger (see Fig. 11.7). The same may be true for lymphoblastic leukemia, with the result that when one decreases the tumor mass by drugs, the labeling index of proliferation of the remaining cells increases. When more cells are in the proliferative phase, the tumor is more susceptible to chemotherapeutic agents, which act primarily to inhibit DNA synthesis (see below).

Cytogenetics   The concept that malignancy might be related to a breakdown of the normal mitotic process, leading to an abnormal complement of chromosomes, was probably first suggested by Boveri in 1929 in his classic studies of sea urchin eggs (51). Ford and his colleagues in 1958 were the first to attempt chromosomal studies of human leukemia (125). They observed an abnormal chromosome pattern in an adequately studied bone marrow preparation from a case of "blast cell" leukemia. Shortly thereafter, Baikie and his associates (13) found chromosomal anomalies in four of five patients with acute leukemia, and Sandberg and his co-workers related such abnormalities to the existence of leukemic stem cell lines (351–353). Since then, many investigators have observed chromosomal anomalies in the acute leukemias (14, 223, 235, 335, 349, 418, 427). The important observations are these: (a) chromosomal abnormalities occur in roughly half the patients studied, and (b) chromosomal abnormalities vary from case to case, but appear to be characteristic for any given patient. The chromosomal abnormalities, such as aneuploidy, are observable when disease is in relapse, whereas the normal diploid complement is seen during hematologic remission. This important observation suggests that the anomaly is related to a leukemic stem cell line.

Chromosomal abnormalities in leukemia may also be related to chemotherapy (25, 301, 427). The abnormalities associated with chemotherapy commonly consist of breaks, chromosome contraction, precocious separation of the centromere, despiralization, and, more rarely, polyploidization. As noted earlier, congenital cytogenetic abnormalities of several varieties are associated with an increased incidence of leukemia: Bloom's syndrome, Down's syndrome, mongolism, trisomy-D syndrome, and congenital anemia (Fanconi's syndrome).

Many authors have noted that the most frequent abnormalities of acute leukemia occur in chromosome groups C, D, E, and, perhaps most commonly, G (181, 235, 427). The chromosomal anomalies in chronic myelocytic leukemia and Down's syndrome are also in the G group (242, 310, 407), suggesting that genes concerned with the regulation of white cell production are in this group.

One difference between the behavior of the chromosomal abnormality in lymphoblastic leukemia and in chronic myelocytic leukemia is apparent. In the lymphoblastic disease normal stem cells with normal karyotype are the rule during remission. In chronic myelocytic leukemia the Ph[1] chromosome abnormality tends to persist in the marrow during remission, suggesting that most of the proliferating cells still are abnormal.

In acute lymphocytic leukemia there is no correlation between the presence of a chromosomal abnormality and age, sex, clinical behavior of disease, or prognosis.

Antigenicity   Recent evidence indicates that the leukemia cell may bear on its surface certain unique antigens (11, 136, 177, 180, 255, 327, 345, 415, 423). The significance and origin of these neoantigens is not known. One may speculate that they are a reexpression of antigens expressed in fetal life in a manner analogous to carcinoembryonic antigen in carcinoma of the colon. Alternatively they may be related to a carrier state for virus. Vigorous work is under way to explore antigenic differences between normal and leukemic cells in immunotherapy.

Clinical Features and Natural History

The onset of lymphoblastic leukemia usually is acute, and most patients have symptoms for less than three months before the diagnosis is made (46). Initial symptoms are those related to anemia, bleeding diathesis, or bone or lymph node infiltration. The clinical features of lymphoblastic leukemia resemble those of other acute leukemias and may be conveniently divided into four categories:

Symptoms related to bone marrow infiltration
    Anemia
    Granulocytopenia → infection
    Thrombocytopenia → bleeding
Symptoms related to specific organ infiltration
    Central nervous system
    Lung
    Any organ
Metabolic derangements
    Hyperuricemia; uric acid nephropathy
    Hypercalcemia
Abnormalities related to chemotherapy
    Suppression of rapidly dividing tissues: hair loss, gastrointestinal ulcerations, bone marrow suppression
    Immunologic suppression
    Toxicities associated with specific drugs (hemorrhagic cystitis, neuropathy, hepatic toxicity, and so on)

Hematologic manifestations related to bone marrow infiltration have already been considered. These may be aggravated by cytotoxic chemotherapy (72). Bleeding, infection, hyperuricemia, and psychotherapeutic management are the major problems facing the physician in the care of the leukemic patient.

Infection   Infectious complications may be of bacterial, viral, fungal, or protozoan origin and are a major cause of death in lymphoblastic leukemia (40–45, 192, 231, 258, 367). These infections may be with common pathogens such as the *Pneumococcus* or the *Staphylococcus*, or may be with so-called "opportunistic pathogens." This term

has been used to designate organisms that are rarely pathogenic in normal subjects, but that take advantage of the impaired defenses of the diseased host. Examples are bacteria such as *Listeria*, fungi such as *Candida* and *Asperigilla*, protozoa such as *Pneumocystis carinii*, and viruses such as cytomegalovirus (58, 394). At the present time the most common life-threatening infections in patients with lymphoblastic leukemia result from gram-negative organsims.

The breaches in host antimicrobial defenses are multiple (Table 21.1). Far and away the most important abnormality is the reduction in the number of phagocytic leukocytes as a result of the underlying disease process and/or chemotherapy. Both neutrophils and monocytes may be reduced in numbers. As a rough rule of thumb, when the blood granulocyte count falls below 1,000/mm³, susceptibility to microbial infection increases, and when the granulocyte count falls below 600/mm³, infection is likely.

Even when normal numbers of phagocytes are present, their mobilization to sites of infection may be impaired by adrenal glucocorticoids, and their microbicidal activity may be abnormal as a consequence of the disease process, and drug and irradiation therapy (71, 252). Furthermore, the production of antibody opsonin necessary for phagocytosis may be depressed by chemotherapy. In a short-term study of patients with acute leukemia undergoing continuous therapy, it was noted that even though the serum IgG levels fell within two to four weeks, they returned to normal slowly with continuation of therapy (236, 270). Lymphocyte transformation may be impaired long after cessation of chemotherapy (216). Even when children with acute leukemia are in remission, they appear to be at risk of infection with opportunistic pathogenic microorganisms (375, 376), probably as a result of immunosuppressive therapy. A good review of the management of infections in patients with leukemia and lymphoma has recently been published (257). Transfusion of normal

Table 21.1 Impaired host defense mechanisms in lymphoblastic leukemia.

Granulocytes
    Granulocytopenia secondary to disease, drugs, or irradiation
    Impaired granulocyte mobilization with corticosteroids
Monocytes
    Monocytopenia secondary to disease or drugs
Immunocytes
    Abnormal function related to immunosuppressive drugs; steroids, antimetabolites, asparaginase
    ?Abnormal interferon production

granulocytes is an important new adjunct to the treatment of the granulocytopenic patient (166, 167).

Specific Organ Infiltration The clinical manifestations related to leukemic infiltration of specific organs are protean. In any large series of patients with lymphoblastic leukemia, symptomatic involvement of virtually every organ is eventually encountered.

Skin. Diverse skin lesions are observed in lymphoblastic leukemia, including localized leukemic infiltrates, petechiae and ecchymoses, infectious complications, and nonspecific, exfoliative dermatitis (39, 231, 365, 367, 431, 432). The mucous membrane of the nasopharynx may be involved.

Lymph nodes and spleen. Lymph node and splenic enlargement is very frequent in lymphoblastic leukemia, as shown in Fig. 21.7, and may be an early sign of the disease (46, 342). Generally, the nodes are firm, nontender, and diffusely involved by the disease process. Uncommonly, the mediastinal lymph nodes are strikingly enlarged, and patients have been initially investigated because of an abnormal chest roentgenogram with mediastinal enlargement (77). The tonsils may be infiltrated by the neoplastic process and may present a picture of necrotizing tonsilitis. The spleen is usually enlarged, but splenic infarcts are rare.

Cardiovascular-respiratory system. Tachycardia and dyspnea are, of course, common manifestations of the anemia complicating acute leukemia and may be the presenting complaints. Very rarely is the heart infiltrated to a degree sufficient to produce abnormalities of conduction (6, 53). Such abnormalities and congestive heart failure can more often be ascribed to drug treatment with daunomycin (29).

The lung is a more common site of clinically symptomatic infiltration in acute leukemia (169). Diverse manifestations have been observed, including localized infiltration, diffuse miliary lesions associated with alveolar-capillary block syndrome (170, 338), large lesions producing airway obstruction, and (rarely) pleural effusions. Local pulmonary infiltration is often difficult to distinguish from hemorrhage or an infectious process. The upper airway and nasopharynx may also be infiltrated or involved by bleeding or infection (104, 264). Gingivitis, oral ulcerations, petechial hemorrhage, and epistaxis are all common manifestations of disease.

Gastrointestinal tract and liver. The gastrointestinal tract may be involved by direct leukemic infiltration (79, 89, 237), by hemorrhage, by drug-induced ulceration, and by mucosal breaks with secondary bacterial or fungal infection. Any site may be involved, from the mouth to the anus. A particularly bad complication is perirectal abscess; its development is associated with a poor prognosis.

Microscopic leukemic infiltrates of the gastrointestinal tract are common, but associated clinical symptoms are rare. Manifestations related to drug therapy are much more common. Most cytotoxic drugs damage the rapidly proliferating gastrointestinal epithelial cells, with resultant ulceration, secondary infection, and hemorrhage. Similarly the liver often shows widespread infiltration by leukemic cells, even when disease is in apparent remission (369); however, manifestations of hepatic dysfunction related to this infiltration are relatively rare. Hepatocellular disease more commonly reflects injury with drugs such as 6-mercaptopurine (111, 371), large doses of methotrexate (73), or L-asparaginase (312, 396).

Portal hypertension with hypersplenism and bleeding

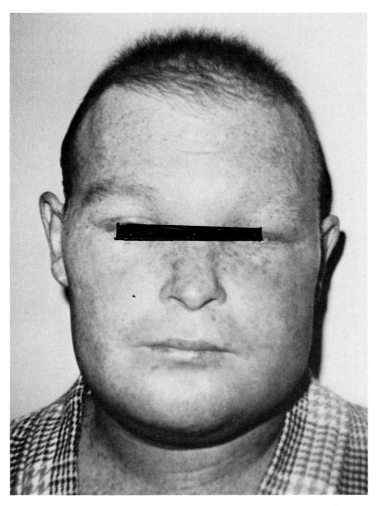

Figure 21.7 Prominent facial fullness resulting from lymph node infiltration by leukemic cells ("bull-neck" effect).

esophageal varices have been observed in a child receiving prolonged chemotherapy (248, 425).

Bones and joints. Spontaneous bone pains occur in 40 to 50 percent of children with acute leukemia, and roentgenographic abnormalities of bone occur in 50 to 70 percent (19, 81, 89, 373, 432). The correlation between bone pain and radiographically visible lesions is imperfect. A long interval may exist between the first appearance of bone pain and of a visible lesion. Many lesions are probably too small to be visualized.

The most common histologic changes in bone with leukemic involvement are thinning of the trabeculae and infiltration of the periosteum with leukemic cells. Less common changes include erosion of the cortex following endosteal infiltration, widening and/or plugging of the haversian canals, bone necrosis, and new bone formation in the periosteum (7, 195, 217, 226, 404). The pathologic bone changes and retardation of growth correlate with activity of disease and return toward normal with induction of remission (404). Osteosclerosis is a relatively rare finding; hypocalcemia has been reported (218).

Roentgenographic changes are most prominent around the ends of long bones in the region of rapid growth (430). These changes include transverse bands of decreased density at the end of the metaphysis; osteolytic lesions; subperiosteal new bone formation; and, rarely, osteosclerotic lesions (103, 297, 374, 430). These lesions occasionally may be associated with hypercalcemia, which is presumed to arise from excessive bone resorption.

The mechanism of bone destruction in lymphoblastic leukemia is not known. Whether crowding and pressure changes alone are sufficient explanation is uncertain. Likewise, the mechanism of bone pain is obscure. Bone necrosis with reticulin fibrosis of the marrow cavity has been suggested as a major cause of bone pain in lymphoblastic leukemia (244).

Joint, as well as bone, symptoms may be prominent in childhood acute leukemia, and the initial picture may simulate rheumatoid arthritis or rheumatic fever, with red, swollen joints (76, 89, 103, 328, 404). Infiltration of the synovia may be present, or bone involvement adjacent to the joint capsule may produce pain referable to the joint. Gouty arthritis secondary to hyperuricemia is another possible occurrence.

Genitourinary tract. Genitourinary manifestations of leukemia may include hematuria, cystitis, pyelonephritis, priapism, and renal failure. Failure may occur from hyperuricemia and uric acid nephropathy or, more rarely, as a consequence of leukemic ureteral obstruction, direct renal infiltration, or drug therapy.

Microscopic foci of leukemic cells in the kidney are frequent (194, 309, 369); however, infiltration of sufficient magnitude to produce renal enlargement is relatively uncommon (46, 165), and impairment of renal function as a consequence of infiltration is distinctly rare (159, 309).

A major cause of the renal failure occurring in acute leukemia is an increased concentration of uric acid in the blood and urine. Because of the insolubility of uric acid crystals, especially at low pH, these may precipitate in the renal tubule, producing a characteristic uric acid nephropathy and anuria (275, 378). Although this complication is usually seen with rapid lysis of leukemic cells following chemotherapy, it is occasionally observed in untreated patients when the turnover of nucleic acid purines is sufficiently high to increase the levels of uric acid in blood and urine (350). Adequate hydration and alkalinization of the urine generally are sufficient to prevent uric acid nephropathy; however, use of the xanthine oxidase inhibitor, allopurinol, is more reliable as a means of preventing complications from hyperuricemia (348, 416). With very high levels of uric acid or established anuria, osmotic diuresis and dialysis have been used (18, 105, 210, 275).

Testicular involvement by lymphoblastic leukemia is well documented. An important point is that the testis may be infiltrated at a time when the patient is in hematologic remission (160, 282).

Nervous system and special senses. Any part of the eye may be involved by hemorrhage or by direct infiltration of leukemic cells. When the disease is in relapse, the eye grounds characteristically reveal numerous round to flame-shaped hemorrhages with pale centers, and the choroid or retina may show patchy white infiltration that has a "hard" rather than a "cotton wool" appearance (49, 94, 164, 278, 314). The veins may be dilated, and perivenous sheathing is characteristic. These changes are not pathognomonic of leukemia, and some may be seen in severe anemia alone. Papilledema may result from direct infiltration of the optic nerve (196) or, more commonly, from increased intracranial pressure.

The middle and inner ears also may be involved by hemorrhage, infection, or direct leukemic infiltration (253).

Lymphoblastic leukemia has a variety of central nervous system manifestations (304, 364); of these, hemorrhage associated with thrombocytopenia and meningeal leukemia are most common (117, 293, 307, 370, 392). Meningeal leukemia probably begins in the arachnoid and subsequently extends into the brain parenchyma (329). It is thought to arise because most of the drugs used in leukemic treatment do not effectively cross the blood–brain barrier. Consequently, the meninges are thought to form a sanctuary where the leukemic cells can proliferate unimpeded by drugs. This is a popular, but not necessarily correct, theory. However, the incidence of meningeal leukemia has increased, and this complication can occur when the disease is in peripheral remission and no abnormal hematologic manifestations are apparent. The early symptoms of meningeal leukemia may include headache and nausea. If the early warning signals are neglected, further increase in intracranial pressure may lead to papilledema, convulsions, cranial nerve palsies (especially of the sixth nerve), and separation of the suture lines. In addition to meningeal leukemia, any portion of the central nervous system may be infiltrated by microscopic or macroscopic collections of leukemia cells (213, 253).

The cerebrospinal fluid findings in meningeal leukemia are characteristic: low sugar, elevated protein, and leukemic cells (306, 385). The appearance of cells that are readily identified in the fluid may precede symptomatic neurologic manifestations (380). It is important to make the diagnosis early, since this manifestation of leukemia yields readily to therapy.

Intracranial hemorrhage associated with thrombocytopenia is often subdural or subarachnoid (171). Hemorrhage associated with thrombocytopenia and very high white counts is often diffuse within the substance of the brain, perhaps as a result of leukemic infiltration (135, 138). Such hemorrhage can also occur in the absence of thrombocytopenia.

Neurologic manifestations of acute leukemia less common than hemorrhage or meningeal infiltration include: compression of the spinal cord or nerve roots by a leukemic mass (89, 364, 393), bacterial or viral infections, and the neurologic syndrome of multifocal leukencephalopathy (23, 340, 429).

Principles of Therapy

The basis of chemotherapy in acute leukemia is exploitation of the subtle differences in metabolism, growth kinetics, and regeneration potential between normal bone marrow and leukemia cells. Effective antileukemic drugs work at a few key points: they interact directly with the DNA macromolecule and thereby prevent its replication or transcription; they interfere with new DNA formation by blocking synthesis of critical precursors; they inhibit the mitotic apparatus; or they selectively reduce the availability of certain amino acids (Fig. 21.8). Adrenocorticosteroids may exert a lympholytic effect, but the precise mode of action is unknown. It has been suggested in Chapter 14 that the glucocorticoids interfere with glucose transport and/or phosphorylation in sensitive cells. Prop-

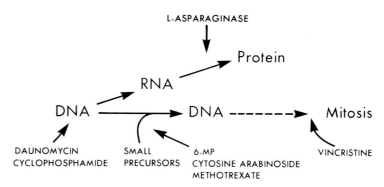

Figure 21.8 Known sites of action of antileukemic drugs. The drugs in common use act by interfering with DNA or protein synthesis or with cell mitosis. *6-MP* = 6-mercaptopurine.

erties of the currently available effective antileukemic agents are summarized in Table 21.2.

Anticancer drugs are conveniently divided into two classes: those that work during a specific part of the cell cycle (usually DNA synthesis) and those whose cytotoxic action is expressed against cells in any phase of the cell cycle. The former are called "cell cycle specific" and include antimetabolites and antimitotic agents; the latter are "cell cycle nonspecific" and include alkylating agents, antibiotics, and glucocorticoids. The cell cycle is illustrated in Fig. 21.9.

The strategy of modern chemotherapy in treating acute lymphocytic leukemia is to attack the disease with multiple active agents simultaneously, with the objective of rapidly reducing the numbers of leukemic cells and restoring bone marrow function to normal (30, 112, 186, 208, 375, 376). When the marrow status is normal and other evidence of disease is eliminated, the disease is said to be in remission. The induction and duration of remission correlate with survival in this disease. Consequently, the

Cell Cycle

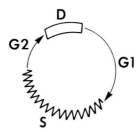

Figure 21.9 The life cycle of a dividing cell. D = division (mitosis). G_1 is the pre-DNA synthetic phase. DNA synthesis occurs during the S phase and ceases with initiation of the G_2 phase.

Table 21.2 Properties of antileukemic drugs. Reference numbers are given in parentheses.

Drug	Mechanism of action	Distribution	Duration in body	Metabolism; excretion	Toxicities
Daunomycin	Inhibits DNA and RNA synthesis (99)	Unknown	Unknown	Uncertain	Myelosuppression, cardiopathy
Cyclophosphamide	Alkylating agent, cross-linkage of DNA	Total body water	Plasma $T_{1/2}$ = 4 hrs	Activated in vivo (123); renal	Myelosuppression, cystitis, alopecia
Cytosine arabinoside	Inhibits DNA synthesis; inhibits de novo deoxycytidine riboside synthesis (82)	Total body water; enters cerebrospinal fluid (83)	Plasma $T_{1/2}$ < 20 min (83)	Metabolized; renal (83)	Myelosuppression (408)
6-mercaptopurine	Inhibits de novo purine and DNA synthesis (114)	Total body water (178)	Plasma $T_{1/2}$ = 1.5 hrs (178, 263)	Metabolized; renal (178, 263)	Myelosuppression, hepatic (111)
Methotrexate	Inhibits dihydrofolate reductase and DNA synthesis (32)	Total body water (188)	Plasma $T_{1/2}$ < 4 hrs (188); bound to tissue enzyme for weeks (32)	Renal (32, 260)	Myelosuppression, gastrointestinal, renal, hepatic (193)
Vincristine	Inhibits mitotic spindle formation (276, 277)	Unknown	Cleared from plasma in a few min	Biliary (222)	Neuropathy (227, 295, 354); alopecia
L-asparaginase	Depletion of asparagine (54)	Extracellular fluid (311)	Variable, plasma $T_{1/2}$ = 4–48 hrs (78)	Metabolized; immune clearance	Hepatitis, pancreatitis, serum sickness, inhibition of protein synthesis, coagulopathy (256, 360, 395)
Prednisone	Lymphoid cell lysis; ?inhibition of glucose transport (101, 243)	Total body water	≥24 hrs (65)	Metabolized; renal	Peptic ulceration, psychosis, diabetes, electrolyte disturbance

objective of treatment is to induce and maintain remission. From animal models, clinicians have extrapolated the notion that the greater the reduction in the numbers of leukemic cells by drugs, the longer the duration of remission once drugs are withdrawn. For example, there may be 1×10^{11} leukemic cells when the disease is full blown and clinically active, and the disease may be undetectable if there are less than 1×10^{10} cells. If the numbers of malignant cells can be reduced to 1×10^6, then the time required for reappearance of symptoms will be longer than if the number is only reduced to 1×10^8 or 1×10^9 cells. Obviously, the absolute time required will depend on the doubling time of the population of leukemic cells.

This doubling time is a complex variable, which probably changes as the number of cells changes (see Chapter 11). Nevertheless, the duration of the remission unmaintained by drugs is currently the best guide to the effectiveness of chemotherapy in reducing the numbers of leukemic cells (130, 134, 186, 206, 207, 209, 233).

As the mass of leukemic cells, both replicating and nonreplicating, increases to 10^{10} or 10^{11}, clinical manifestations appear and the normal marrow elements are crowded out. With progressive expansion of the leukemic mass to 10^{11} or 10^{12} cells, the fraction of the malignant cells in the nonreplicating pool increases. Therefore the initial therapy for the leukemic child presenting with flagrant disease should be with a combination of agents that work against both proliferating and nonproliferating cells. A frequently employed combination of drugs is prednisone (cycle nonspecific) and vincristine (cycle specific) (151, 187, 366, 389). In more aggressive attempts at remission induction, daunomycin (nonspecific) (391), 6-mercaptopurine (specific), or methotrexate (specific) are added to the two-drug combination (29, 30, 134, 281). The rate of remission induction for two drugs is roughly 85 percent; for three or four drugs, it is 88 to 100 percent. Particulars of the drug combinations and remission induction rates are given in Table 21.3.

Once remission is induced, various means of attacking residual leukemic cells have been tried: single agents used alone until relapse occurs; multiple agents used separately according to some prearranged program; multiple agents used simultaneously or in cycles; and immunotherapy (30, 50, 67, 122, 131, 132, 187, 207, 240, 324, 327, 382).

Evaluation of these approaches is very difficult, since no means of determining numbers of remaining malignant cells is available. It seems quite likely, however, that cyclic "reinduction schedules" in which combinations of effective agents are used cyclically at predetermined intervals will prove to be the most effective (30, 241, 324). The precise time that such therapy must be continued in order to achieve the best results is not known. From the current state of our knowledge, an estimate of two to three years after the induction of remission seems reasonable (187, 208, 241, 324, 375).

It is now quite clear that systemic chemotherapy alone may be inadequate for achieving complete remission or cure in lymphoblastic leukemia. The meninges and the testes may still harbor malignant cells despite a morphologically normal bone marrow (305). Consequently, the

most recent trend is "total therapy," comprising systemic drugs and irradiation of the neuraxis (9, 241, 324, 375).

Although such prolonged and arduous therapy carries a high emotional price for the patient and his family (34), it also carries the potential of cure of an otherwise fatal disease (9, 241, 324). For the drug regimens used in the intensive treatment of childhood leukemia the reader should consult recent publications (10, 30, 241, 324, 375).

A relatively new approach to the therapy of acute leukemia or bone marrow failure is transplantation of allogeneic bone marrow. The major problems associated with such an approach include eradication of all malignant cells, supportive care during periods of aplasia, engraftment, and graft-vs-host disease (166, 280, 355, 356, 383, 401–403). An additional problem is the emergence of leukemia in the engrafted cells (401).

Infectious Mononucleosis

Hematologic and Clinical Manifestations
Infectious mononucleosis is a benign, self-limited, lymphoproliferative disorder characterized by increased numbers of morphologically abnormal lymphocytes in the peripheral circulation, fever, lymphadenopathy, splenomegaly, and pharyngitis.

History Infectious mononucleosis was probably first described by Pfeiffer in 1889 in Germany under the appropriate name of *glandular fever* (323). In this country an epidemic was first reported in 1896 (424), and by 1909 the presence of circulating abnormal mononuclear cells was identified (56). Early in this century, sporadically occurring cases were often confused with acute leukemia (411, 431). In 1920 Sprunt and Evans classified these sporadic cases and coined the term *infectious mononucleosis*, pointing out the association with abnormal circulating cells (387). The realization that glandular fever and infectious mononucleosis were one and the same entity came shortly thereafter (262, 406). Definitive work on the morphology of the leukocytes was published by Downey and McKinlay in 1923 (102), and in 1932 the characteristic serologic abnormality was discovered by Paul and Bunnell (317).

Clinical Features Sporadic cases occur most commonly in adolescents and young adults (24, 31, 107); the epidemic disorder occurs most often in childhood (431). Although infectious mononucleosis occurs after the age of forty, it is exceedingly rare at this time of life (368).

The clinical illness can be conveniently divided into three phases: the prodromal period of nonspecific malaise,

Table 21.3 Drug combinations given as therapy in acute lymphocytic leukemia.

Drug combination	No. of patients	Percent remissions
Prednisone, vincristine	411	83–87
Prednisone, vincristine, daunomycin	> 100	89–100
Prednisone, vincristine, 6-mercaptopurine, methotrexate	35	94
Asparaginase, vincristine, prednisone	70	69–85
Cytosine arabinoside, asparaginase	17	81

which may last a week or more; the period of full-blown disease, which may last a few days to three weeks; and the period of convalescence (145).

The incubation period is unknown; suggestions that it may be as long as seven weeks have appeared in the literature (431). A typical case presents with pharyngitis, cervical and axillary lymphadenopathy, and fever. In about 10 percent of cases fever and headache are the major clinical manifestations. Icterus, anemia, or bleeding only rarely are the earliest signs (199, 200). Striking fatigue is characteristic of full-blown illness.

Lymph node enlargement is the rule. Cervical and axillary involvement is prominent. Signs of infectious lymphadenitis are usually absent (75). Hyperplasia of the pharyngeal lymphoid tissue in association with pharyngeal inflammation is common. Severe laryngeal or pharyngeal edema or obstruction by lymphoid tissue is rare (333, 438). Splenomegaly probably occurs in at least 50 percent of patients (431); it is usually of moderate degree but occasionally is impressive. Splenic rupture is a feared, but fortunately infrequent, complication (204, 219, 439). Rarely, infectious mononucleosis may simulate Hodgkin's disease (1). The fever of infectious mononucleosis occurs in some 90 to 97 percent of patients (75, 199, 431). It has no characteristic pattern. It is often below 103° F and rarely reaches levels in excess of 106° F.

In addition to these common manifestations, a series of less common physical signs and symptoms occur in infectious mononucleosis (88, 203). Custer and Smith (86) have documented pathologic changes in the tissue in a series of patients with infectious mononucleosis who died in accidents or of neurologic complications.

Skin and mucous membranes. A faint, generalized erythema may occur in infectious mononucleosis, and in about 10 percent of cases there is a distinct, fine, macular rash resembling rubella (107, 264). Hemorrhagic manifestations are well documented, although they are distinctly uncommon (68, 102, 316, 330). Edema of the eyelids is an interesting and not so rare complication (316). Crops of palatal petechiae occurring near the junction of the hard and soft palate may be seen in about 25 percent of patients.

Cardiopulmonary. Electrocardiographic changes consistent with myocarditis may be seen in about 15 percent of cases (107), and more rarely pericarditis and conduction defects have been described (107, 202, 344, 372). Pleural effusions and pulmonary parenchymal changes have been documented (108, 268). One case report describes the association between infectious mononucleosis and an anterior mediastinal mass (421).

Genitourinary. Orchitis has been described in mononucleosis (436). It is probable that infectious mononucleosis can cause a benign, self-limited glomerulonephritis associated with red cell casts and proteinuria (400). Heterophile-reactive antigen has been seen in kidney biopsies by indirect immunofluorescence (322).

Gastrointestinal. Hepatomegaly occurs in about one-third of cases. Liver involvement detected by elevation of serum enzymes such as glutamic oxalacetic transaminase is common in infectious mononucleosis (107, 140, 337). Definite jaundice is not uncommon. Liver biopsy may show sinusoidal mononuclear cell infiltration and hepatic cell damage (234, 279). Nonspecific abdominal pain, nausea, vomiting, and diarrhea may all occur in some patients. Pancreatitis probably occurs also, as evidenced by elevated serum amylase activity (300, 433).

Nervous system. Clinically symptomatic central nervous system involvement occurs in less than 1 percent of patients with infectious mononucleosis (422). Manifestations may include headache, blurred vision, psychotic behavior, convulsions, cranial nerve palsies, peripheral neuropathy, focal encephalomyelitis, and anterior horn disease (4, 118, 299, 361). Guillain-Barré syndrome is a dread, but fortunately rare, complication (93, 109).

From the foregoing it should be clear that the manifestations of infectious mononucleosis may be extremely diverse, although the typical syndrome of fever, malaise, glandular enlargement, and pharyngitis is the most common manifestation of this disorder.

Infectious mononucleosis can be confused with a number of other diseases: toxoplasmosis (336), adenovirus (176), and cytomegalovirus infection (238).

Hematologic Manifestations A characteristic feature of infectious mononucleosis is the presence of abnormal lymphocyte forms in the peripheral circulation. Most of the morphologic descriptions of these cells can be traced back to Downey and McKinlay (102), who identified three types of cells. The distinctions among these types do not seem to be very important either clinically or for our understanding of the disease process. In general, the cell is 1.5 to 3 times the size of a small lymphocyte, with a lower nucleus/cytoplasm ratio. The nucleus is oval, lobulated, or—less commonly—round. The chromatin is less condensed than that of the normal lymphocyte but is not so fine as that of a normal monocyte. Nucleoli may be present. Although the cytoplasm may be foamy, more often it has no distinctive features other than more dense staining at the periphery and scalloping where the membrane contacts other cells (Fig. 21.10).

A Swiss cheese appearance of the nucleus after sterile incubation of the cells in vitro is said to be characteristic of this disease (158).

These cells are probably of lymphoid origin. They have no distinctive histochemical pattern and are peroxidase-

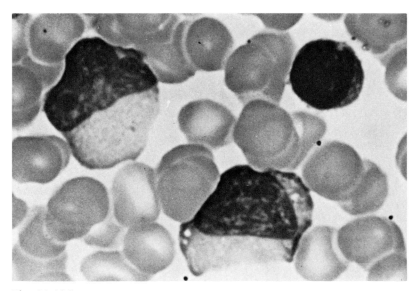

Fig. 21.10A

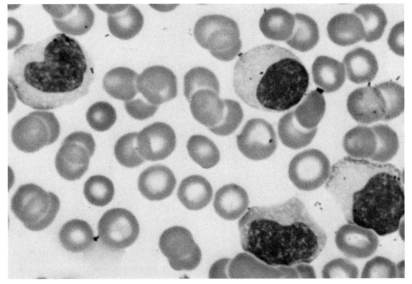

Fig. 21.10B

Figure 21.10 Atypical lymphoid cells from the blood of two patients with infectious mononucleosis. In Fig. 21.10A note the indentation and apparent condensation of the cytoplasm at the points of contact with erythrocytes. The cells in Fig. 21.10B show some of the same features but less prominently.

negative (142). Details of their ultrastructure have been described (315, 335, 363). They are nonphagocytic. Their most striking feature is an extremely high rate of DNA and RNA synthesis, which may rival that of leukemic lymphoblasts (70, 115, 141). Mitoses may be seen in the peripheral blood (52, 60). Continuously proliferating cell lines may be established from the peripheral blood of patients with infectious mononucleosis (161). They may produce immunoglobulins and interferon in vitro (228).

Cells resembling those of infectious mononucleosis may be encountered in other viral illnesses (191, 246, 386). Similar cells may be seen occasionally in severe pyogenic infections and hypersensitivity reactions (386). They are often called "Türk" cells after the nineteenth-century morphologist (410). Examples of Türk cells from patients with measles and hypersensitivity reaction respectively are shown in Figs. 21.11 and 21.12.

Although the white count in infectious mononucleosis ranges from extremes of less than 2,000/mm³ (90, 405, 406, 437) to greater than 40,000/mm³ (31), it is generally in the range of 12,000 to 18,000. The white count is often low during the first days of disease (145), then begins to rise on the fourth or fifth day of illness in parallel with clinical symptomatology. Numerous exceptions to this pattern are observed, however. The characteristic blood changes may occur as early as the second day or as late as the fourteenth day of illness.

The abnormal lymphocytes often constitute more than 60 percent of the circulating cells and may be as high as 97 percent (31). Neutrophils may increase in numbers early in the disease, but usually decrease and "shift to the left" in full-blown disease. During this phase the alkaline phosphatase of the neutrophil is often low (390). Eosinopenia is common, although eosinophilia has also been described (124, 229).

Anemia as a result of infectious mononucleosis is exceedingly rare. When it occurs it is usually of the Coombs'-positive, autoimmune, hemolytic type. Anti-i cold agglutinins have been described and may be responsible for hemolysis (57, 121, 221, 289).

Thrombocytopenia below 100,000/mm³ occurs only rarely in infectious mononucleosis (59, 68, 330, 431). Generalized hemorrhagic manifestations occur when thrombocytopenia develops. Occasionally the bleeding time may be prolonged despite a normal platelet count (31, 405).

Serologic Abnormalities

In 1932 Paul and Bunnell reported their observation that the serum of patients with infectious mononucleosis contained agglutinins against sheep erythrocytes in high

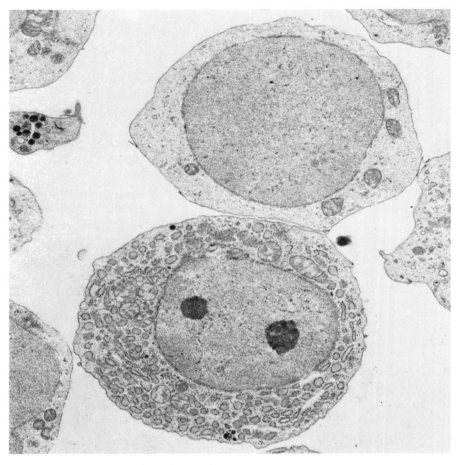

Figure 21.11 A lymphocyte (*top*) and a Türk cell (*bottom*) from a patient with measles. The Türk cell has well-developed rough endoplasmic reticulum in which sacs are dilated with protein secretion. (From A. I. Spriggs and D. W. Jerrome, *Br. J. Haematol.* 13:764, 1967. Reprinted by permission of authors and publisher.)

titer (317). This provided the basis for serologic diagnosis of this disease. Increased specificity for the "heterophile" test was provided by the observation that the agglutinin could be absorbed by beef red cells but not by guinea pig kidney. Agglutinins to sheep erythrocytes that occurred in other disorders such as serum sickness and transplantation reactions (331) could be absorbed by the guinea pig kidney (92).

For serologic diagnosis serial dilutions of heat-inactivated serum are incubated for two hours at room temperature with a 2-percent suspension of washed sheep erythrocytes. Agglutination is then read macroscopically or with the low-power objective of a microscope (90–92, 251). In normal subjects the titer may be 1:28 or 1:56; in patients with infectious mononucleosis it is greater than

1:224. The highest titers are found during the second or third week of illness and slowly decline over the next four to eight weeks. Rarely, a positive reaction may persist for four months. A positive test is found in more than 80 percent of patients with infectious mononucleosis sometime during the first three weeks of illness (31). If the reaction is equivocal or occurs in an unusual clinical setting, differential absorption with guinea pig kidney and beef red cells is usually tried.

A number of simple screening tests have been devised that provide essentially the same results as the classic agglutination test (205, 250, 265). A very simple, rapid slide test uses formalinized horse red cells as the immunologic indicator. Such cells are stable and are specifically agglutinated by the heterophile antibody in infectious mononucleosis. The diagnostic accuracy is said to be 99 percent.

Probably the most commonly employed serologic test at the present time is the "mono-spot" test (417). It appears to be specific for heterophile antibody and has few false negatives.

In addition to the heterophile reaction, other serologic abnormalities are encountered in infectious mononucleosis. Occasionally false positive serologic tests for syphilis (201), cryoglobulins (224) and antinuclear antibodies (225), or rheumatoid factors (61–63) are encountered. Increases in immunoglobulin levels may occur in the course of the disease (2, 24, 435). Polyclonal IgM antibodies are synthesized in plasmacytoid cells in the lymph nodes and bone marrow (61–63).

Etiology

The cause of infectious mononucleosis is not definitely known. Recently, however, strong evidence has been obtained for a herpes-like virus as an etiologic agent. The Epstein-Barr virus (EBV) (116) was originally observed in continuous cell cultures obtained from Burkitt's lymphoma (Chapter 22). Henle and her colleagues (190), using an immunofluorescent technique, demonstrated a relation between the development of antibody to EBV and infectious mononucleosis. This association was soon confirmed with observation of rising antibody titers in the course of the illness (119, 153, 198, 303). Rising antibody titers have been observed in both heterophile-positive and heterophile-negative infectious mononucleosis. Patients with infectious mononucleosis may continue to excrete EBV for prolonged periods of time.

The case for association between EBV and infectious mononucleosis was strengthened when viral antigen was found in continuous cultures derived from peripheral leukocytes of patients with symptomatic, heterophile-positive disease (98, 298). Virus-like particles are also seen in such cells, although it is uncertain whether these are indeed EBV, since similar particles are seen in cell cultures derived from leukemia or other neoplastic disease (441) and from normal healthy subjects (294). These particles may represent persistence of herpes-like virus after infection of cells of the reticuloendothelial system and may be necessary for cell growth in vitro (95, 156, 308). Such particles are found in Burkitt's lymphoma cell lines, and high titers of antibodies to EBV are found in typical patients with this African lymphoma (189). Antibodies to EBV are also found in wild chimpanzees in the area endemic to Burkitt's lymphoma (259).

Does EBV induce a lymphoproliferative disorder? Some evidence suggests that it does. Blastoid transformation, chromosome changes, and established long-term growth can be induced in leukocytes from EBV seronegative, normal subjects by partially purified EBV (156). Epstein-Barr virus can stimulate cellular DNA synthesis, a function normally associated with oncogenic viruses (154). Finally, human lymphoid cells transformed by EBV can induce tumors in newborn mice (95).

Infectious mononucleosis can occur in patients with acute leukemia and is associated with rising EBV antibody titer (96). EBV infection can be transmitted by blood and may be related to a mononucleosis-like picture seen in the postperfusion syndrome (155). At the present time the weight of evidence favors a herpes-like virus as etiologic in infectious mononucleosis; however, only further studies will clarify some of the complex interrelationships between viral infection and this hematologic disease (152, 179).

Acute Infectious Lymphocytosis

Acute infectious lymphocytosis is a benign, self-limited, lymphoproliferative disorder. In 1941 C. H. Smith wrote a description of infectious lymphocytosis distinguishing this entity from infectious mononucleosis (381). Since that time sporadic cases and clusters of cases have been reported (84, 211). A spectrum of clinical symptomatology has been reported, including asymptomatic illness (359), diarrhea (106), respiratory symptoms (17, 313), and aseptic meningitis (26, 412). The unifying thread has been the presence of increased numbers of small lymphocytes of normal appearance. Often eosinophils are increased in numbers. Lymphocyte counts may be 90,000/mm³ (211). Except where paralysis has occurred, clinical disease has generally been benign, with the increased lymphocyte count returning to normal within three to four weeks. Significant splenomegaly and lymphocytosis are rare. Olson

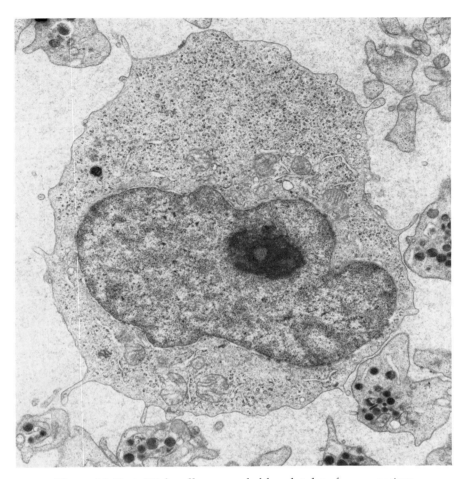

Figure 21.12 A Türk cell surrounded by platelets from a patient with hypersensitivity reaction. The nucleus is slightly lobed and has a prominent nucleolus. The cytoplasm contains a few mitochondria and a few cisternae of endoplasmic reticulum. Large areas are occupied by small groups of ribosomes. (From A. I. Spriggs and D. W. Jerrome, *Br. J. Haematol.* 13:764, 1967. Reprinted by permission of authors and publisher.)

and his colleagues suggested that the syndrome might be caused by adenovirus infection (313). Other viruses have been considered also. Most recently, a virus similar to Coxsackie A has been proposed as one of the etiologic agents (211). Parasitic agents have been suggested. For the moment, we cannot say whether there is one cause of this interesting disorder, or many.

Summary

The acute lymphoproliferative disorders are characterized by the proliferation and accumulation of lymphoid cell populations and by an acute clinical course. They may result from virus infection or antigenic stimulation, or they may be neoplastic in origin.

Acute lymphocytic leukemia is the most common malignant acute lymphoproliferative disorder. Only a small fraction of the neoplastic lymphocytes are in the proliferative cycle at any given time. However, virtually the entire population eventually enters the cycle. The consequence is accumulation of large numbers of immature cells, which may reach levels of 10^{11} or 10^{12} when the disease becomes clinically manifest. The resultant loss of normal hematopoietic cells and widespread organ infiltration account for most of the clinical manifestations of this acute leukemia. The objective of modern therapy is to reduce the number of malignant cells and possibly to eradicate all of them. Cures are achievable by chemotherapy.

Infectious mononucleosis is the most frequent recognized nonmalignant acute lymphoproliferative disorder. Its clinical and hematologic manifestations are exceedingly diverse. The etiology of infectious mononucleosis is still uncertain, although recent evidence points toward a pathogenetic role for a herpes-like virus.

Chapter 21 References

1. Agliozzo, C. M., and Reingold, I. M. Infectious mononucleosis simulating Hodgkin's disease. A patient with Reed-Sternberg cells, *Am. J. Clin. Pathol.* 56:730, 1971.
2. Allansmith, M., and Bergstresser, P. Sequence of immunoglobulin changes resulting from an attack of infectious mononucleosis, *Am. J. Med.* 44:124, 1968.
3. Allen, D. W., and Cole, P. Viruses and human cancer, *N. Engl. J. Med.* 286:70, 1972.
4. Ambler, M., Stoll, J., Tzamalouskas, A., and Albala, M. M. Focal encephalomyelitis in infectious mononucleosis. A report with pathological description, *Ann. Intern. Med.* 75:579, 1971.
5. Anderson, R. C. Familial leukemia. A report of leukemia in five siblings, with a brief review of the genetic aspects of this disease, *Am. J. Dis. Child.* 81:313, 1951.
6. Aronson, S. F., and Leroy, E. Electrocardiographic findings in leukemia, *Blood* 2:356, 1947.
7. Asceuzi, A., and Marinozzi, V. Some biophysical aspects of changes in bone in blood diseases, *Am. J. Clin. Pathol.* 30:187, 1958.
8. Ask-Upmark, E. Another follow-up study of children born of mothers with leukemia, *Acta Med. Scand.* 175:391, 1964.
9. Aur, R. J. A., Simone, J. V., Hustu, H. O., and Verzosa, M. S. A comparative study of central nervous system irradiation and intensive chemotherapy early in remission of childhood acute lymphocytic leukemia, *Cancer* 29:381, 1972.
10. Aur, R. J. A., Verzosa, M. S., Hustu, H. O., and Simone, J. V. Response to combination therapy after relapse in childhood acute lymphocytic leukemia, *Cancer* 30:334, 1972.
11. Bach, M. L., Bach, F. H., and Joo, P. Leukemia-associated antigens in the mixed leukocyte culture test, *Science* 166:1520, 1969.
12. Bader, J. P. The role of deoxyribonucleic acid in the synthesis of Rous sarcoma virus, *Virology* 22:462, 1964.
13. Baikie, A. G., Court Brown, W. M., Jacobs, P. A., and Milne, J. S. Chromosome studies in human leukaemia, *Lancet* ii:425, 1959.
14. Baikie, A. G., Jacobs, P. A., McBride, J. A., and Tough, I. M. Cytogenetic studies in acute leukaemia, *Lancet* ii:425, 1959.
15. Baltimore, D. Viral RNA-dependent DNA polymerase. RNA-dependent DNA polymerase in virions of RNA tumour viruses, *Nature* 226:1209, 1970.
16. Barber, R., and Spiers, P. Oxford survey of childhood cancers. Progress report II, Monthly Bulletin of the Ministry Health and Public Health Laboratory Service (London), 23:46, 1964.
17. Barnes, G. R., Jr., Yannet, H., and Lieberman, R. Clinical study of an institutional outbreak of acute infectious lymphocytosis, *Am. J. Med. Sci.* 218:646, 1949.
18. Barry, K. G., Hunter, R. H., Davis, T. E., and Crosby, W. H. Acute uric acid nephropathy. Treatment with mannitol diuresis and peritoneal dialysis, *Arch. Intern. Med.* 111:452, 1963.
19. Baty, J. M., and Vogt, E. C. Bone changes of leukemia in children, *Am. J. Roentgenol.* 34:310, 1935.
20. Baxt, W. G., and Spiegelman, S. Nuclear DNA sequences present in human leukemic cells and absent in normal leukocytes, *Proc. Natl. Acad. Sci. U.S.A.* 69:3737, 1972.
21. Baxt, W., Hehlman, R., and Speigelman, S. Human leukaemic cells contain reverse transcriptase associated with a high molecular weight virus-related RNA, *Nature (New Biol.)* 240:72, 1972.
22. Beard, J. W. Introduction to avian leukemia, *in* M. A. Rich (ed.), Experimental Leukemia, p. 205, Appleton-Century-Crofts, New York, 1968.
23. Behar, A. Progressive multifocal leukoencephalopathy in a case of acute lymphatic leukemia, *Isr. J. Med. Sci.* 1:650, 1965.
24. Belfrage, S. Infectious mononucleosis. An epidemiological and clinical study, *Acta Med. Scand.* 171:531, 1962.
25. Bell, W. R., Whang, J. J., Carbone, P. P., Brecher, G., and Block, J. B. Cytogenetic and morphologic abnormalities in human bone marrow cells during cytosine arabinoside therapy, *Blood* 27:771, 1966.
26. Beloff, J. S., and Gang, K. M. Acute poliomyelitis and acute infectious lymphocytosis. Their apparent simultaneous occurrence in a summer camp, *J. Pediatr.* 26:586, 1945.
27. Bennett, J. H. Case of hypertrophy of the spleen and liver, in which death took place from suppuration of the blood, *Edinburgh Med. Surg. J.* 64:413, 1845.
28. Bernard, J., Chavelet, F., and Jacquillat, C. Leucémies du nouveauné (à propos de 4 observations), *Nouv. Rev. Fr. Hematol.* 4:125, 1964.
29. Bernard, J., Boiron, M., Jacquillat, C., and Weil, M. Rubidomycin in 400 patients with leukemia and other malignancies, Abstracts of the Simultaneous Sessions, XII Congress, Int. Soc. Hematol., p. 5, 1968.
30. Bernard, J., Jacquillat, C., and Weil, M. Treatment of the acute leukemias, *Semin. Hematol.* 9:181, 1972.
31. Bernstein, A. Infectious mononucleosis, *Medicine* 19:85, 1940.
32. Bertino, J. R., and Johns, D. G. Folate antagonists, *Ann. Rev. Med.* 18:27, 1967.
33. Best, W. R., and Limarzi, L. R. Age, sex, race, and hematologic classification of 916 leukemia cases, *J. Lab. Clin. Med.* 40:778, 1952.
34. Binger, C. M., Ablin, A. R., Feverstein, R. C., Kushner, J. H., Zoger, S., and Mikkelsen, C. Childhood leukemia. Emotional impact on patient and family, *N. Engl. J. Med.* 280:414, 1969.
35. Bisel, H. F. Criteria for the evaluation of response to treatment in acute leukemia, *Blood* 11:676, 1956.
36. Bizzozero, O. J., Jr., Johnson, K. G., and Ciocco, A. Radiation-related leukemia in Hiroshima and Nagasaki, 1946–1964. I. Distribution, incidence and appearance time, *N. Engl. J. Med.* 274:1095, 1966.
37. Bloom, A. D., Neriishi, S., Awa, A. A., Honda, T., and Archer, P. G. Chromosome aberrations in leucocytes of older survivors in the atomic bombings of Hiroshima and Nagasaki, *Lancet* ii:802, 1967.
38. Bloom, D. Congenital telangiectatic erythema resembling lupus erythematosis in dwarfs, *Am. J. Dis. Child.* 88:754, 1954.

39. Bluefarb, S. M. Leukemia Cutis, Charles C Thomas, Springfield, Ill., 1960.

40. Bodey, G. P. Fungal infections complicating acute leukemia, *J. Chron. Dis.* 19:667, 1966.

41. Bodey, G. P., Buckley, M., Sathe, Y. S., and Freireich, E. J. Quantitative relationships between circulating leukocytes and infection in patients with acute leukemia, *Ann. Intern. Med.* 64:328, 1966.

42. Bodey, G. P., Hart, J., Frиereich, E. J., and Frei, E. III. Studies of a patient isolator unit and prophylactic antibiotics in cancer chemotherapy. General techniques and preliminary results, *Cancer* 22:1018, 1968.

43. Bodey, G. P., McKelvey, E., and Karon, M. Chickenpox in leukemic patients—factors in prognosis, *Pediatrics* 34:562, 1964.

44. Bodey, G. P., Nies, B. A., and Freireich, E. J. Multiple organism septicemia in acute leukemia. Analysis of 54 episodes, *Arch. Intern. Med.* 116:266, 1965.

45. Bodey, G. P., Nies, B. A., Mohberg, N. R., and Freireich, E. J. Use of gamma globulin in infection in acute-leukemia patients, *J.A.M.A.* 190:1099, 1964.

46. Boggs, D. R., Wintrobe, M. M., and Cartwright, G. E. The acute leukemias. Analysis of 322 cases and review of the literature, *Medicine* 41:163, 1962.

47. Boiron, M., Paoletti, C., Tubiana, M., et al. L'anémie des leucoses aiguës, *Sem. Hop. Paris* 31:1123, 1955.

48. Borella, L. The immunosuppressive effects of Rauscher leukemia virus (RLV) upon spleen cells cultured in cell-impermeable diffusion chambers, *J. Immunol.* 108:45, 1972.

49. Borgeson, E. J., and Wagener, H. P. Changes in the eye in leukemia, *Am. J. Med. Sci.* 177:663, 1929.

50. Bortin, M. M., Rimm, A. A., and Saltzstein, E. C. Graft versus leukemia: quantification of adoptive immunotherapy in murine leukemia, *Science* 179:811, 1973.

51. Boveri, T. The Origin of Malignant Tumors, Williams & Wilkins Co., Baltimore, 1929.

52. Bowcock, H. Mitotic leukoblasts in the peripheral blood in infectious mononucleosis, *Am. J. Med. Sci.* 198:384, 1939.

53. Bregani, P., and Perrotta, P. Il cuore nelle leucemie (aspetti clinici ed elettrocardiografici), *Folia Cardiol.* 19:193, 1960.

54. Broome, J. D. Studies on the mechanism of tumor inhibition by L-asparaginase. Effects of the enzyme on asparagine levels in the blood, normal tissues, and 6C3HED lymphomas of mice: differences in asparagine formation and utilization in asparaginase-sensitive and -resistant lymphoma cells, *J. Exp. Med.* 127:1055, 1968.

55. Bross, I. D. J., and Natarajan, N. Leukemia from low-level radiation, *N. Engl. J. Med.* 287:107, 1972.

56. Burns, J. E. Glandular fever. Report of an epidemic in the children's ward of the Union Protestant Infirmary, *Arch. Intern. Med.* 4:118, 1909.

57. Calvo, R., Stein, W., Kochwa, S., and Rosenfield, R. E. Acute hemolytic anemia due to anti-i. Frequent cold agglutinins in infectious mononucleosis, *J. Clin. Invest.* 44:1033, 1965.

58. Cangir, A., and Sullivan, M. P. The occurrence of cytomegalovirus infections in childhood leukemia. Report of three cases, *J.A.M.A.* 195:616, 1966.

59. Carter, R. L. Platelet levels in infectious mononucleosis, *Blood* 25:817, 1965.

60. Carter, R. L. The mitotic activity of circulating atypical mononuclear cells in infectious mononucleosis, *Blood* 26:579, 1965.

61. Carter, R. L. Infectious mononucleosis. Some observations on the cellular localization of immune globulin synthesis, *Am. J. Clin. Pathol.* 45:574, 1966.

62. Carter, R. L. Antibody formation in infectious mononucleosis. I. Some immunochemical properties of the Paul-Bunnell antibody, *Br. J. Haematol.* 12:259, 1966.

63. Carter, R. L. Antibody formation in infectious mononucleosis. II. Other 19S antibodies and false-positive serology, *Br. J. Haematol.* 12:268, 1966.

64. Catovsky, D., Pettit, J. E., Galetto, J., et al. The B-lymphocyte nature of the hairy cell of leukemic re-ticuloendotheliosis, *Br. J. Haematol.* 26:29, 1974.

65. Chard, R. J., Smith, E. K., and Hartmann, J. R. Metabolic studies of prednisone in previously untreated acute leukemia of childhood, *Proc. Am. Assoc. Cancer Res.* 7:13, 1966.

66. Cheung, W. H., Rai, K. R., and Sawitsky, A. Characteristics of cell proliferation in acute leukemia, *Cancer Res.* 32:939, 1972.

67. Chevalier, L., and Glidewell, O. Schedule of 6-mercaptopurine and effect of inducer drugs in prolongation of remission maintenance in acute leukemia, *Proc. Am. Assoc. Cancer Res.* 8:10, 1967.

68. Clarke, B. F., and Davies, S. H. Severe thrombocytopenia in infectious mononucleosis, *Am. J. Med. Sci.* 248:703, 1964.

69. Clarkson, B. Ohkita, T., Ota, K., and Fried, J. Studies of cellular proliferation in human leukemia. I. Estimation of growth rates of leukemic and normal hematopoietic cells in two adults with acute leukemia given single injections of tritiated thymidine, *J. Clin. Invest.* 46:506, 1967.

70. Cline, M. J. Isolation and characterization of RNA from human leukocytes, *J. Lab. Clin. Med.* 68:33, 1966.

71. Cline, M. J. A new white cell test which measures individual phagocyte function in a mixed leukocyte population, *J. Lab. Clin. Med.* 81:311, 1973.

72. Cline, M. J., and Haskell, C. M. Cancer Chemotherapy, 2nd ed., W. B. Saunders, Philadelphia, 1975.

73. Coe, R. A., and Bull, F. E. Cirrhosis associated with methotrexate treatment of psoriasis, *J.A.M.A.* 206:1515, 1968.

74. Conen, P. E., and Erkman, B. Combined mongolism and leukemia. Report of eight cases with chromosome studies, *Am. J. Dis. Child.* 112:429, 1966.

75. Contratto, A. W. Infectious mononucleosis. A study of one hundred and ninety-six cases, *Arch. Intern. Med.* 73:449, 1944.

76. Conybeare, E. T. A case of leukaemia simulating acute rheumatism and Still's disease, *Guys Hosp. Rep.* 86:343, 1936.

77. Cooke, J. V. Mediastinal tumor in

acute leukemia. A clinical and roentgenologic study, *Am. J. Dis. Child.* 44:1153, 1932.

78. Cooney, D. A., and Handschumacher, R. E. Investigation of L-asparagine metabolism in animals and human subjects, *Proc. Am. Assoc. Cancer Res.* 9:15, 1968.

79. Cornes, J. S., Jones, T. G., and Fisher, G. B. Gastroduodenal ulceration and massive hemorrhage in patients with leukemia, multiple myeloma, and malignant tumors of lymphoid tissue, *Gastroenterology* 41:337, 1961.

80. Court Brown, W. M., and Doll, R. Leukaemia in childhood and young adult life. Trends in mortality in relation to aetiology, *Br. Med. J.* 1:981, 1961.

81. Craver, L. F., and Copeland, M. M. Changes of the bones in the leukemias, *Arch. Surg.* 30:639, 1935.

82. Creasey, W. A., DeConti, R. C., and Kaplan, S. R. Biochemical studies with 1-beta-D-arabinofuranosylcytosine in human leukemic leukocytes and normal bone marrow cells, *Cancer Res.* 28:1074, 1968.

83. Creasey, W. A., Papac, R. J., Markiw, M. E., Calabresi, P., and Welch, A. D. Biochemical and pharmacological studies with 1-beta-D-arabinofuranosylcytosine in man, *Biochem. Pharmacol.* 15:1417, 1966.

84. Crisalli, M., and Terragna, A. La malattia di Smith (Linfocitosi infettiva acuta). Revisione della letteratura e presentazione di tre casi, *Minerva Pediatr.* 10:849, 1958.

85. Culliton, B. J. Reverse transcription: one year later, *Science* 172:926, 1971.

86. Custer, R. P., and Smith, E. B. The pathology of infectious mononucleosis, *Blood* 3:830, 1948.

87. Cutler, S. J., Axtell, L., and Heise, H. Childhood leukemia in Connecticut:1940–1962, *Blood* 30:1, 1967.

88. Dalrymple, W. Systemic effects of mononucleosis, *Postgrad. Med.* 43:158, 1968.

89. Dameshek, W., and Gunz, F. Leukemia, 2nd ed., pp. 1, 185, Grune & Stratton, New York, 1964.

90. Davidsohn, I. Serologic diagnosis of infectious mononucleosis, *J.A.M.A.* 108:289, 1937.

91. Davidsohn, I., and Lee, C. L. The laboratory in the diagnosis of infectious mononucleosis (with additional notes on epidemiology, etiology, and pathogenesis), *Med. Clin. North Am.* 46:225, 1962.

92. Davidsohn, I., Stern, K., and Kashiwagi, C. The differential test for infectious mononucleosis, *Am. J. Clin. Pathol.* 21:1101, 1951.

93. Davie, J. C., Ceballos, R., and Little, S. C. Infectious mononucleosis with fatal neuronitis, *Arch. Neurol.* 9:265, 1963.

94. Dawson, D. B. H. Changes in the fundus in diseases of the blood, *in* J. F. Wilkinson (ed.), Modern Trends in Blood Diseases, p. 212, Butterworth and Co., London, 1955.

95. Deal, D. R., Gerber, P., and Chisari, F. V. Heterotransplantation of two human lymphoid cell lines transformed in vitro by Epstein-Barr virus, *J. Natl. Cancer Inst.* 47:771, 1971.

96. Deardorff, W. L., Gerber, P., and Vogler, W. R. Infectious mononucleosis in acute leukemia with rising Epstein-Barr virus antibody titers, *Ann. Intern. Med.* 72:235, 1970.

97. Diamandopoulos, G. T. Leukemia, lymphoma, and osteosarcoma induced in the Syrian golden hamster by simian virus 40, *Science* 176:173, 1972.

98. Diehl, V., Henle, G., Henle, W., and Kohn, G. Demonstrations of a herpes group virus in cultures of peripheral leukocytes from patients with infectious mononucleosis, *J. Virol.* 2:663, 1968.

99. Di Marco, A. Mechanism of action of daunomycin, *Acta Genet. Med. (Roma)* 17:102, 1968.

100. Djerassi, I., and Farber, S. Control and prevention of hemorrhage: platelet transfusion, *Cancer Res.* 25:1499, 1965.

101. Dougherty, T. F., and White, A. Functional alterations in lymphoid tissue induced by adrenal cortical secretion, *Am. J. Anat.* 77:81, 1945.

102. Downey, H. and McKinlay, C. A. Acute lymphadenosis compared with acute lymphatic leukemia, *Arch. Intern. Med.* 32:82, 1923.

103. Dresner, E. The bone and joint lesions in acute leukaemia and their response to folic acid antagonists, *Q. J. Med.* 19:339, 1950.

104. Duffy, J. H., and Driscoll, E. J. Oral manifestations of leukemia, *Oral Surg.* 11:484, 1958.

105. Duke, M. Peritoneal dialysis in leukemia and uric acid nephropathy, *Am. J. Med. Sci.* 245:426, 1963.

106. Dunn, H. G. Acute infectious lymphocytosis. Report on a group of cases in a day nursery, *Br. Med. J.* 1:78, 1952.

107. Dunnet, W. N. Infectious mononucleosis, *Br. Med. J.* 1:1187, 1963.

108. Eaton, O. M., Little, P. F., and Silver, H. M. Infectious mononucleosis with pleural effusion, *Arch. Intern. Med.* 115:87, 1965.

109. Eaton, O. M., Stevens, H., and Silver, H. M. Respiratory failure in polyradiculoneuritis associated with infectious mononucleosis, *J.A.M.A.* 194:609, 1965.

110. Ebstein, W. Ueber die acute Leukämie und Pseudoleukämie, *Dtsch. Arch. Klin. Med.* 44:343, 1889.

111. Einhorn, M., and Davidsohn, I. Hepatotoxicity of mercaptopurine, *J.A.M.A.* 188:802, 1964.

112. Ekert, H., Colebatch, J. H., and Matthews, R. N. Short courses of cytosine arabinoside and L-asparaginase in children with acute leukemia, *Cancer* 30:643, 1972.

113. Ekert, H., and Denett, X. An evaluation of nuclear aryl sulphatase activity as an aid to the cytological diagnosis of acute leukemia, *Aust. Ann. Med.* 15:152, 1966.

114. Elion, G. B., and Hitchings, G. H. Metabolic basis for the actions of analogs of purines and pyrimidines, *Adv. Chemother.* 2:91, 1965.

115. Epstein, L. B., and Brecher, G. DNA and RNA synthesis of circulating atypical lymphocytes in infectious mononucleosis, *Blood* 25:197, 1965.

116. Epstein, M. A., Barr, Y. M., and Achong, B. G. Studies with Burkitt's lymphoma, *Wistar Inst. Symp. Monogr.* 4:69, 1965.

117. Evans, A. E. and Craig, M. Central nervous system involvement in children with acute leukemia. A study of 921 patients, *Cancer* 17:256, 1964.

118. Evans, A. S. Infectious Mononucleosis, *in* W. J. Williams, E. Beutler, A. J. Erslev, and R. W. Rundles (eds.), Hematology, p. 843, McGraw-Hill, New York, 1972.

119. Evans, A. S., Niederman, J. C., and McCollum, R. W. Seroepidemiologic studies of infectious mononucleosis with EB virus, *N. Engl. J. Med.* 279:1121, 1968.

120. Evatt, B. L., Chase, G. A., and Heath, C. W., Jr. Time-space clustering among cases of acute leukemia in two Georgia counties, *Blood* 41:265, 1973.

121. Fakete, A. M., and Kerpelman, E. J. Acute hemolytic anemia complicating infectious mononucleosis, *J.A.M.A.* 194:1326, 1965.

122. Fass, L., and Fefer, A. Studies of adoptive chemoimmunotherapy of a Friend virus–induced lymphoma, *Cancer Res.* 32:997, 1972.

123. Foley, G. E., Friedman, O. M., and Drolet, B. P. Studies on the mechanism of action of cytoxan. Evidence of activation in vivo and in vitro, *Cancer Res.* 21:57, 1961.

124. Foord, A. G., and Butt, E. M. The laboratory diagnosis of infectious mononucleosis, *Am. J. Clin. Pathol.* 9:448, 1939.

125. Ford, C. E., Jacobs, P. A., and Lajtha, L. G. Human somatic chromosomes, *Nature* 181:1565, 1958.

126. Fraumeni, J. F., Jr. Clinical epidemiology of leukemia, *Semin. Hematol.* 6:250, 1969.

127. Fraumeni, J. F., Jr., and Miller, R. W. Leukemia mortality: downturn rates in the United States, *Science* 155:1126, 1967.

128. Fraumeni, J. F., Jr., Ederer, F., and Miller, R. W. An evaluation of the carcinogenicity of simian virus 40 in man, *J.A.M.A.* 185:713, 1963.

129. Freeman, G. *in* Proc. Second Conf. on Folic Acid Antagonists in the Treatment of Leukemia, March 11, 1951, *Blood* 7:152, 1952.

130. Frei, E. III, and Freireich, E. J. Progress and perspectives in the chemotherapy of acute leukemia, *Adv. Chemother.* 2:269, 1965.

131. Frei, E. III, Freireich, E. J., Gehan, E., et al. Studies of sequential and combination antimetabolite therapy in acute leukemia: 6 mercaptopurine and methotrexate, from the acute leukemia group B, *Blood* 18:431, 1961.

132. Frei, E. III, Karon, M., Levin, R. H., et al. The effectiveness of combinations of anti-leukemic agents in inducing and maintaining remission in children with acute leukemia, *Blood* 26:642, 1965.

133. Freireich, E. J., Gehan, E. A., Sulman, D., Boggs, D. R., and Frei, E. III. The effect of chemotherapy on acute leukemia in the human, *J. Chronic Dis.* 14:593, 1961.

134. Freireich, E. J., Henderson, E. S., Karon, M. R., and Frei, E. III. The treatment of acute leukemia considered with respect to cell population kinetics, *in* The Proliferation and Spread of Neoplastic Cells, p. 441, Williams & Wilkins Co., Baltimore, 1968.

135. Freireich, E. J., Thomas, L. B., Frei, E. III, Fritz, R. D., and Forkner, C. E. A distinctive type of intracerebral hemorrhage associated with "blastic crisis" in patients with leukemia, *Cancer* 13:146, 1960.

136. Fridman, W. H., and Kourilsky, F. M. Stimulation of lymphocytes by autologous leukaemic cells in acute leukaemia, *Nature* 224:277, 1969.

137. Friedreich, N. Ein neuer Fall von Leukämie, *Virchows Arch. (Pathol. Anat.)* 12:37, 1857.

138. Fritz, R. D., Forkner, C. E., Jr., Freireich, E. J., Frei, E. III, and Thomas, L. B. The association of fatal intracranial hemorrhage and "blastic crisis" in patients with acute leukemia, *N. Engl. J. Med.* 261:59, 1959.

139. Futterweit, W. Serum alkaline phosphatase activity in infectious mononucleosis. A clinical study of fifty-five cases, *Arch. Intern. Med.* 108:253, 1961.

140. Gabutti, V., Pileri, A., Tarocco, R. P., and Gavosto, F. Proliferative potential of out-of-cycle leukaemic cells, *Nature* 224:375, 1969.

141. Gahrton, G., and Foley, G. E. Leukemia-like pattern of the DNA, and RNA and protein content of individual mononuclear cells in the peripheral blood of patients with infectious mononucleosis, *Cancer Res.* 29:1076, 1969.

142. Galbraith, P., Mitus, W. J., Gollerkeri, M., and Dameshek, W. The "infectious mononucleosis cell." A cytochemical study, *Blood* 22:630, 1963.

143. Gallo, R. C. RNA-dependent DNA polymerase in viruses and cells: views on the current state, *Blood* 39:117, 1972.

144. Gallo, R. C., Yang, S. S., and Ting, R. C. RNA-dependent DNA polymerase of human acute leukaemic cells, *Nature* 228:927, 1970.

145. Gardner, H. T., and Paul, J. R. Infectious mononucleosis at the New Haven Hospital, 1921 to 1946, *Yale J. Biol. Med.* 19:839, 1947.

146. Gauld, W. R., Innes, J., and Robson, H. N. A survey of 647 cases of leukaemia, 1938–1951, *Br. Med. J.* 1:585, 1953.

147. Gavosto, F., Gabutti, V., Masera, P., and Pileri, A. The problem of anaemia in the acute leukaemias. Kinetic study, *Eur. J. Cancer* 6:33, 1970.

148. Gavosto, F., Pileri, A., Bachi, C., and Pegoràro, L. Proliferation and maturation defect in acute leukaemia cells, *Nature* 203:92, 1964.

149. Gavosto, F., Pileri, A., Gabutti, V., and Masera, P. Non-self-maintaining kinetics of proliferating blasts in human acute leukaemia, *Nature* 216:188, 1967.

150. Gaydos, L. A., Freireich, E. J., and Mantel, N. The quantitative relation between platelet count and hemorrhage in patients with acute leukemia, *N. Engl. J. Med.* 266:905, 1962.

151. George, P., Hernandez, K., Hustu, O., Borella, L., Holton, C., and Pinkel, D. A study of "total therapy" of acute lymphocytic leukemia in children, *J. Pediatr.* 72:399, 1968.

152. Gerber, P. Activation of Epstein-Barr virus by 5-bromodeoxyuridine in "virus-free" human cells, *Proc. Natl. Acad. Sci. U.S.A.* 69:83, 1972.

153. Gerber, P., Hamre, D., Moy, R. A., and Rosenblum, E. N. Infectious mononucleosis: complement-fixing antibodies to herpes-like virus associated with Burkitt lymphoma, *Science* 161:173, 1968.

154. Gerber, P., and Hoyer, B. H. Induction of cellular DNA synthesis in human leukocytes by Epstein-Barr virus, *Nature* 231:46, 1971.

155. Gerber, P., Walsh, J., Rosenblum, E. N., and Purcell, R. H. Association of EB virus infection with the postperfusion syndrome, *Lancet* i:593, 1969.

156. Gerber, P., Whang-Peng, J., and

Monroe, J. R. Transformation and chromosome changes induced by Epstein-Barr virus in normal human leukocyte cultures, *Proc. Natl. Acad. Sci. U.S.A.* 63:740, 1969.

157. Ghadially, F. N., and Skinnider, L. F. Ultrastructure of hairy cell leukemia, *Cancer* 29:444, 1972.

158. Ghaemi, A., and Seaman, A. J. "Swiss cheese" nuclei—an incubation-induced lesion of infectious mononucleosis lymphocytes, *Am. J. Clin. Pathol.* 39:492, 1963.

159. Gilbert, E. F., Rice, E. C., and Lechaux, P. A. Renal function in children with leukemia. A clinical pathological study, *Am. J. Dis. Child.* 93:150, 1957.

160. Givler, R. L. Testicular involvement in leukemia and lymphoma, *Cancer* 69:1290, 1969.

161. Glade, P. R., Hirshaut, Y., Stites, D. P., et al. Infectious mononucleosis: in vitro evidence for limited lymphoproliferation, *Blood* 33:292, 1969.

162. Glass, A. G., Hill, J. A., and Miller, R. W. Significance of leukemia clusters, *J. Pediatr.* 73:101, 1968.

163. Glass, A. G., Mantel, N., Gunz, F. W., and Spears, G. F. S. Time-space clustering of childhood leukemia in New Zealand, *J. Natl. Cancer Inst.* 47:329, 1971.

164. Goldbach, L. J. Leukemic retinitis, *Arch. Ophthalmol.* 10:808, 1933.

165. Gowdey, J. F., and Neuhauser, E. B. D. The roentgen diagnosis of diffuse leukemic infiltration of the kidneys in children, *Am. J. Roentgenol.* 60:13, 1948.

166. Graw, R. G., Jr., Herzig, G., Perry, S., and Henderson, F. S. Normal granulocyte transfusion therapy, *N. Engl. J. Med.* 287:367, 1972.

167. Graw, R. G., Jr., Yankee, R. A., Rogentine, G. N., et al. Bone marrow transplantation from HL-A matched donors to patients with acute leukemia. Toxicity and antileukemic effect, *Transplantation* 14:79, 1972.

168. Green, M., Rokutanda, M., Fujinaga, K., et al. Mechanism of carcinogenesis by RNA tumor viruses, I. An RNA-dependent DNA polymerase in murine sarcoma viruses, *Proc. Natl. Acad. Sci. U.S.A.* 67:385, 1970.

169. Green, R. A., and Nichols, N. J. Pulmonary involvement in leukemia, *Am. Rev. Respir. Dis.* 80:833, 1959.

170. Green, R. A., Nichols, N. J., and King, E. J. Alveolar-capillary block due to leukemic infiltration of the lung, *Am. Rev. Respir. Dis.* 80:895, 1959.

171. Groch, S. N., Sayre, G. P., and Heck, F. J. Cerebral hemorrhage in leukemia, *Arch. Neurol.* 2:439, 1960.

172. Gross, L. Oncogenic Viruses, 2nd ed., Pergamon Press, New York, 1970.

173. Guasch, J. Hérédité des leucémies, *Sang* 25:384, 1954.

174. Gunvén, P., Klein, G., Henle, G., Henle, W., and Clifford, P. Epstein-Barr virus in Burkitt's lymphoma and nasopharyngeal cancer. Antibodies to EBV associated membrane and viral capsid antigens in Burkitt lymphoma patients, *Nature* 228:1053, 1970.

175. Gunz, F. W. Studies on the incidence and aetiology of leukemia in New Zealand, *N. Z. Med. J.* 65:857, 1966 (suppl.).

176. Gutekunst, R. R., and Heggie, A. D. Viremia and viruria in adenovirus infections. Detection in patients with rubella or rubelliform illness, *N. Engl. J. Med.* 264:374, 1961.

177. Gutterman, J. U., Mavligit, G., McCredie, K. B., Bodey, G. P., Sr., Freireich, E. J., and Hersh, E. M. Antigen solubilized from human leukemia: lymphocyte stimulation, *Science* 177:1114, 1972.

178. Hamilton, L., and Elion, G. B. The fate of 6-mercaptopurine in man, *Ann. N.Y. Acad. Sci.* 60:304, 1954.

179. Hampar, B., Derge, J. G., Martos, L. M., and Walker, J. L. Synthesis of Epstein-Barr virus after activation of the viral genome in "virus-negative" human lymphoblastoid (Raji) made resistant to 5 bromodeoxyuridine, *Proc. Natl. Acad. Sci. U.S.A.* 69:78, 1972.

180. Harris, R. Leukaemia antigens and immunity in man, *Nature* 241:95, 1973.

181. Hauschka, T. S. The chromosomes in ontogeny and oncogeny, *Cancer Res.* 21:957, 1961.

182. Hayhoe, F. G. J. Cytochemical as-

pects of leukemia and lymphoma, *Semin. Hematol.* 6:261, 1969.

183. Heath, C. W., Jr., and Moloney, W. C. Familial leukemia. Five cases of acute leukemia in three generations, *N. Engl. J. Med.* 272:882, 1965.

184. Hecht, F., Koler, R. D., Rigas, D. A., Dahnke, G. S., Case, M. P., Tisdale, V., and Miller, R. W. Leukaemia and lymphocytes in ataxia-telangiectasia, *Lancet* ii:1193, 1966.

185. Hehlmann, R., Kufe, D., and Spiegelman, S. RNA in human leukemic cells related to the RNA of a mouse leukemia virus, *Proc. Natl. Acad. Sci. U.S.A.* 69:435, 1972.

186. Henderson, E. S. Combination chemotherapy of acute lymphocytic leukemia of childhood, *Cancer Res.* 27:2570, 1967.

187. Henderson, E. S. Treatment of acute leukemia, *Semin. Hematol.* 6:271, 1969.

188. Henderson, E. S., Adamson, R. H., and Oliverio, V. T. The metabolic fate of tritiated methotrexate. II. Absorption and excretion in man, *Cancer Res.* 25:1018, 1965.

189. Henle, G., Henle, W., Clifford, P., et al. Antibodies to Epstein-Barr virus in Burkitt's lymphoma and control groups, *J. Natl. Cancer Inst.* 43:1147, 1969.

190. Henle, G., Henle, W., and Diehl, V. Relationship of Burkitt's tumor-associated herpes-type virus to infectious mononucleosis, *Proc. Natl. Acad. Sci. U.S.A.* 59:94, 1968.

191. Henson, D. Cytomegalic inclusion disease following multiple blood transfusions, *J.A.M.A.* 199:278, 1967.

192. Hersh, E. M., Bodey, G. P., Nies, B. A., and Freireich, E. J. Causes of death in acute leukemia. A ten year study of 414 patients from 1954–1963, *J.A.M.A.* 193:105, 1965.

193. Hersh, E. M., Wong, V. G., Henderson, E. S., and Freireich, E. J. Hepatotoxic effects of methotrexate, *Cancer* 19:600, 1966.

194. Heuchel, G., and Vom Dahl, D. Leukämie und Niere. Klinische Symptomatik und Funktion der Niere bei Leukämie, *Blut* 5:390, 1959.

195. Hilbish, T. F., Besse, B. E., Lusted, L. B., Daves, M. L., Thomas, L. B., and Forkner, C. A. Acute leukemia.

Skeletal manifestations in children and adults, *Arch. Intern. Med.* 104:741, 1959.

196. Hill, E. Papilledema and intracranial complications of leukemia, *Am. J. Ophthalmol.* 15:1127, 1932.

197. Hirsch, M. S., Black, P. H., and Proffitt, M. R. Immunosuppression and oncogenic virus infections, *Fed. Proc.* 30:1852, 1971.

198. Hirshaut, Y., Glade, P., Moses, H., Manaker, R., and Chessin, L. Association of herpes-like virus infection with infectious mononucleosis, *Am. J. Med.* 47:520, 1969.

199. Hoagland, R. J. Infectious mononucleosis, *Am. J. Med.* 13:158, 1952.

200. Hoagland, R. J. Diagnosis of infectious mononucleosis, *Blood* 16:1045, 1960.

201. Hoagland, R. J. False-positive serology in mononucleosis, *J.A.M.A.* 185:783, 1963.

202. Hoagland, R. J. Mononucleosis and heart disease, *Am. J. Med. Sci.* 248:1, 1964.

203. Hoagland, R. J. Infectious Mononucleosis, Grune & Stratton, New York, 1967.

204. Hoagland, R. J., and Henson, H. M. Splenic rupture in infectious mononucleosis, *Ann. Intern. Med.* 46:1184, 1957.

205. Hoff, G., and Bauer, S. A new rapid slide test for infectious mononucleosis, *J.A.M.A.* 194:351, 1965.

206. Holland, J. F. Progress in the treatment of acute leukemia, *in* W. Dameshek and R. M. Dutcher (eds.), Perspectives in Leukemia, p. 217, Grune & Stratton, New York, 1968.

207. Holland, J. F. Clinical studies of unmaintained remissions in acute lymphocytic leukemia, *in* The Proliferation and Spread of Neoplastic Cells, p. 453, Williams & Wilkins Co., Baltimore, 1968.

208. Holland, J. F., and Glidewell, O. Induction, consolidation, intensification, reinduction, and maintenance chemotherapy of acute lymphocytic leukemia, Abstracts of the Simultaneous Sessions, XII Congress, Int. Soc. Hematol., p. 9, 1968.

209. Holland, J. F., and Glidewell, O. Chemotherapy of acute lymphocytic leukemia of childhood, *Cancer* 30:1480, 1972.

210. Holland, P., and Holland, N. H.

Prevention and management of acute hyper-uricemia in childhood leukemia, *J. Pediatr.* 72:358, 1968.

211. Horwitz, M. S., and Moore, G. T. Acute infectious lymphocytosis. An etiologic and epidemiologic study of an outbreak, *N. Engl. J. Med.* 279:399, 1968.

212. Hoshino, T., Kato, H., Finch, S. C., and Hrubec, Z. Leukemia in offspring of atomic bomb survivors, *Blood* 30:719, 1967.

213. Howell, A., and Gough, J. Acute lymphatic leukaemia with facial diplegia and double abducens palsy, *Lancet* i:723, 1932.

214. Huebner, R. J., and Todaro, G. J. Oncogenes of RNA tumor viruses as determinants of cancer, *Proc. Natl. Acad. Sci. U.S.A.* 64:1087, 1969.

215. Huff, R. L., Hennessy, T. G., Austin, R. E., Garcia, J. F., Roberts, B. M., and Lawrence, J. H. Plasma and red cell iron turnover in normal subjects and in patients having various hematopoietic disorders, *J. Clin. Invest.* 29:1041, 1950.

216. Humphrey, G. B., Nesbit, M. E., Chary, K. K. N., and Krivit, W. Impaired lymphocyte transformation in leukemic patients after intensive therapy, *Cancer* 29:402, 1972.

217. Jaffe, H. L. Skeletal manifestations of leukemia and malignant lymphoma, *Bull. Hosp. Joint Dis.* 13:217, 1952.

218. Jaffe, N., Paed, D., Kim, B. S., and Vawter, G. F. Hypocalcemia—a complication of childhood leukemia, *Cancer* 29:392, 1972.

219. Janbon, M., and Bertrand, L. Sur la rupture de la rate dans la mononucléose infectieuse, *Sang* 31:235, 1960.

220. Jarrett, O. Evidence for the viral etiology of leukemia in the domestic mammals, *Adv. Cancer Res.* 13:39, 1970.

221. Jenkins, W. J., Koster, H. G., Marsh, W. L., and Carter, R. L. Infectious mononucleosis: an unsuspected source of anti-i, *Br. J. Haematol.* 11:480, 1965.

222. Johnson, I. S., Armstrong, J. G., Gorman, M., and Burnett, J. P., Jr. The vinca alkaloids: a new class of oncolytic agents, *Cancer Res.* 23:1390, 1963.

223. Johnston, A. W. The chromosomes in a child with mongolism and acute leukemia, *N. Engl. J. Med.* 264:591, 1961.

224. Kaplan, M. E. Cryoglobulinemia in infectious mononucleosis: quantitation and characterization of the cryoproteins, *J. Lab. Clin. Med.* 71:754, 1968.

225. Kaplan, M. E., and Tan, E. M. Antinuclear antibodies in infectious mononucleosis, *Lancet* i:561, 1968.

226. Karelitz, S. Unusual forms of periosteal elevation, *Am. J. Dis. Child.* 33:394, 1927.

227. Karon, M., Freireich, E. J., Frei, E. III, et al. The role of vincristine in the treatment of childhood acute leukemia, *Clin. Pharmacol. Ther.* 7:332, 1966.

228. Kasel, J. A., Haase, A. T., Glade, P. R., and Chessin, L. N. Interferon production in cell lines derived from patients with infectious mononucleosis, *Proc. Soc. Exp. Biol. Med.* 128:351, 1968.

229. Kauffman, R. E. Eosinophilia in infectious mononucleosis, *Am. J. Med. Sci.* 219:206, 1950.

230. Kawakami, T. G., Nuff, S. D., Buckley, P. M., Dungworth, D. L., Snyder, S. P., and Gilden, R. V. C-type virus associated with Gibbon lymposarcoma, *Nature (New Biol.)* 235:170, 1972.

231. Keidan, S. E., and Mainwaring, D. Association of Herpes zoster with leukemia and lymphoma in children, *Clin. Pediatr.* 4:13, 1965.

232. Killmann, S-A. Proliferative activity of blast cells in leukemia and myelofibrosis. Morphological differences between proliferating and non-proliferating blast cells, *Acta Med. Scand.* 178:263, 1965.

233. Killmann, S-A. Acute leukemia: development, remission/relapse pattern. Relationship between normal and leukemic hemopoiesis, and the 'sleeper-to-feeder' stem cell hypothesis, *Ser. Haematol.* 1:103, 1968.

234. Kilpatrick, Z. M. Structural and functional abnormalities of liver in infectious mononucleosis, *Arch. Intern. Med.* 117:47, 1966.

235. Kiossoglou, K. A., Mitus, W. J., and Dameshek, W. Chromosomal aberrations in acute leukemia, *Blood* 26:610, 1965.

236. Kiran, O., and Gross, S. The G-immunoglobulins in acute leukemia in children. Hematologic and immunologic relationships, *Blood* 33:198, 1969.

237. Kirshbaum, J. D., and Preuss, F. S. Leukemia. A clinical and pathologic study of one hundred and twenty-three fatal cases in a series of 14,400 necropsies, *Arch. Intern. Med.* 71:777, 1943.

238. Klemola, E., and Kääriäinen, L. Cytomegalovirus as a possible cause of disease resembling infectious mononucleosis, *Br. Med. J.* 2:1099, 1965.

239. Körver, H. Knochenveränderungen bei Leukämien im Kindesalter, *Monatsschr. Kinderheilkd.* 100:319, 1952.

240. Krivit, W., Brubaker, C., Thatcher, L. G., Pierce, M., Perrin, E., and Hartmann, J. R. Maintenance therapy in acute leukemia of childhood. Comparison of cyclic vs. sequential methods. *Cancer* 21:352, 1968.

241. Krivit, W., Gilchrist, G., and Beatty, E. C., Jr. The need for chemotherapy after prolonged complete remission of acute leukemia of childhood, *J. Pediatr.* 76:138, 1970.

242. Krivit, W., and Good, R. A. Simultaneous occurrence of mongolism and leukemia. Report of a nationwide survey, *Am. J. Dis. Child.* 94:289, 1957.

243. Kummer, D., and Ochs, H-D. Cytostatischer Wirkungsmechanismus von Cortisol und verwandten Steroiden, *Z. Ges. Exp. Med.* 147:291, 1968.

244. Kundel, D. W., Brecher, G., Bodey, G. P., and Brittin, G. M. Reticulin fibrosis and bone infarction in acute leukemia. Implications for prognosis, *Blood* 23:526, 1964.

245. Kyle, R. A., Nobrega, F. T., Kurland, L. T., and Elveback, L. R. The 30-year trend of leukemia in Olmsted County, Minnesota, 1935 through 1964, *Mayo Clin. Proc.* 43:342, 1968.

246. Lamb, S. G., and Stern, H. Cytomegalovirus mononucleosis with jaundice as presenting sign, *Lancet* ii:1003, 1966.

247. Lampkin, B. C., Nagao, T., and Mauer, A. M. Synchronization and recruitment in acute leukemia, *J. Clin. Invest.* 50:2204, 1971.

248. Lascari, A. D., Givler, R. L., Soper, R. T., and Hill, L. F. Portal hypertension in a case of acute leukemia treated with antimetabolites for ten years, *N. Engl. J. Med.* 279:303, 1968.

249. Lawrinson, W., and Gross, S. Nuclear arylsulfatase activity in primitive hemic cells, *Lab. Invest.* 13:1612, 1964.

250. Lee, C. L., Davidsohn, I., and Mih, N. L. A capillary screening test for infectious mononucleosis, *Am. J. Clin. Pathol.* 44:162, 1965.

251. Lee, C. L., Takahashi, T., and Davidsohn, I. Sheep erythrocyte agglutinins and beef erythrocyte hemolysins in infectious mononucleosis serum, *J. Immunol.* 91:783, 1963.

252. Lehrer, R. I., and Cline, M. J. Leukocyte candidacidal activity and resistance to systemic candidiasis in patients with cancer, *Cancer* 27:1211, 1971.

253. Leidler, F., and Russell, W. O. The brain in leukemia. A clinico-pathologic study of twenty cases with a review of the literature, *Arch. Pathol.* 40:14, 1945.

254. LeJeune, J., Berger, R., Haines, M., Lafourcade, J., Vialatte, J., Satge, P., and Turpin, R. Constitution d'un clone à 54 chromosomes au cours d'une leucoblastose congénitale chez une enfant mongolienne, *C. R. Acad. Sci. (D) (Paris)* 256:1195, 1963.

255. Leventhal, B. G., Halterman, R. H., Rosenberg, E. B., and Herberman, R. B. Immune reactivity of leukemia patients to autologous blast cells, *Cancer Res.* 32:1820, 1972.

256. Leventhal, B. G., and Henderson, E. S. Therapy of acute leukemia with drug combinations which include asparaginase, *Cancer* 28:825, 1971.

257. Levine, A. S., Graw, R. G., Jr., and Young, R. C. Management of infections in patients with leukemia and lymphoma: current concepts and experimental approaches, *Semin. Hematol.* 9:141, 1972.

258. Levitan, A. A., and Perry, S. The use of an isolator system in cancer chemotherapy, *Am. J. Med.* 44:234, 1968.

259. Levy, J. A., Levy, S. B., Hirshaut, Y., Kafuko, G., and Prince, A. Presence of EBV antibodies in sera from wild chimpanzees, *Nature* 233:559, 1971.

260. Liegler, D., Henderson, E., Hahn, M. A., and Oliverio, V. Renal clearance and in vivo protein binding of methotrexate in man and changes associated with salicylate administration, *Proc. Am. Assn. Cancer Res.* 8:41, 1967.

261. Lisco, H., and Conrad, R. A. Chromosome studies on Marshall Islanders exposed to fallout radiation, *Science* 157:445, 1967.

262. Longcope, W. T. Infectious mononucleosis (glandular fever), with a report of ten cases, *Am. J. Med. Sci.* 164:781, 1922.

263. Loo, T. L., Luce, J. K., Sullivan, M. P., and Frei, E. III. Clinical pharmacologic observations on 6-mercaptopurine and 6-methylthiopurine ribonucleoside, *Clin. Pharmacol. Ther.* 9:180, 1968.

264. Love, A. A. Manifestations of leukemia encountered in otolaryngologic and stomatologic practice, *Arch. Otolaryngol.* 23:173, 1936.

265. Lovric, V. A. A slide test for diagnosis of infectious mononucleosis using stable reagents, *Med. J. Aust.* 1:7, 1965.

266. McCaffrey, R. P., Silverstone, A. E., Harrison, T. A., et al. Terminal deoxynucleotidyl transferase (TT): a thymus specific enzyme in acute lymphoblastic leukemia (ALL) cells, Prog. 66th Ann. Mtg., Am. Soc. Clin. Invest., p. 51a, 1974.

267. McCarthy, J. T., and Hoagland, R. J. Cutaneous manifestations of infectious mononucleosis, *J.A.M.A.* 187:153, 1964.

268. McCort, J. J. Infectious mononucleosis, with special reference to roentgenologic manifestations, *Am. J. Roentgenol.* 62:645, 1949.

269. McCullough, J. J., Korobkin, M. T., and Krivit, W. Genetics in acute lymphatic leukemia in childhood, *Ann. N.Y. Acad. Sci.* 155:777, 1968.

270. McKelvey, E., and Carbone, P. P. Serum immune globulin concentrations in acute leukemia during intensive chemotherapy, *Cancer* 18:1292, 1965.

271. MacMahon, B., and Clark, D. Incidence of the common forms of human leukemia, *Blood* 11:871, 1956.

white, L. H., and Hauschka, T. S. Chromosomal dichotomy in blood and marrow of acute leukemia, *Cancer Res.* 22:748, 1962.

352. Sandberg, A. A., Ishihara, T., Miwa, T., and Hauschka, T. S. The in vivo chromosome constitution of marrow from 34 human leukemias and 60 nonleukemic controls, *Cancer Res.* 21:678, 1961.

353. Sandberg, A. A., Koepf, G. F., Crosswhite, L. H., and Hauschka, T. S. The chromosome constitution of human marrow in various developmental and blood disorders, *Am. J. Hum. Genet.* 12:231, 1960.

354. Sandler, S. G., Tobin, W., and Henderson, E. S. Vincristine-induced neuropathy: a clinical study of fifty leukemic patients, *Neurology* 19:367, 1969.

355. Santos, G. W. Application of marrow grafts in human disease: its problems and potential, *in* M. G. Hanna (ed.), Contemporary Topics in Immunobiology, p. 143, Plenum Publishing Co., New York, 1972.

356. Santos, G. W., Sensenbrenner, L. L., Burke, P. J., Colvin, M., Owens, A. H., Jr., Bias, W. B., and Slavin, R. E. Marrow transplantation in man following cyclophosphamide, *Transplant. Proc.* 3:400, 1971.

357. Saunders, E. F., Lampkin, B. C., and Mauer, A. M. Variation of proliferative activity in leukemic cell populations of patients with acute leukemia, *J. Clin. Invest.* 46:1356, 1967.

358. Sawistsky, A., Bloom, D., and German, J. Chromosomal breakage and acute leukemia in congenital telangiectatic erythema and stunted growth, *Ann. Intern. Med.* 65:487, 1966.

359. Scalettar, H. E., Maisel, J. E., and Bramson, M. Acute infectious lymphocytosis. Report of an outbreak, *Am. J. Dis. Child.* 88:15, 1954.

360. Schein, P. S., Rakieten, N., Gordon, B. M., Davis, R. D., and Rall, D. P. The toxicity of *Escherichia coli* L-asparaginase, *Cancer Res.* 29:426, 1969.

361. Schnell, R. G., Dyck, P. J., Bowie, E. J. W., Klass, D. W., and Taswell, H. F. Infectious mononucleosis: neurologic and EEG findings, *Medicine* 45:51, 1966.

362. Schrek, R., and Donnelly, W. J. "Hairy" cells in blood in lympho-

reticular neoplastic disease and "flagellated" cells of normal lymph nodes, *Blood* 27:199, 1966.

363. Schumacher, H. R., McFeely, A. E., and Maugel, T. K. The mononucleosis cell. III. Electron microscopy, *Blood* 33:833, 1969.

364. Schwab, R. S., and Weiss, S. Neurologic aspect of leukemia, *Am. J. Med. Sci.* 189:766, 1935.

365. Scutt, R. Bullous' lesions in leukaemia, *Br. Med. J.* 1:139, 1952.

366. Selawry, O. S., Hananian, J., Wolman, I. J., et al. New treatment schedule with improved survival in childhood leukemia. Intermittent parenteral vs. daily oral administration of methotrexate for maintenance of induced remission, *J.A.M.A.* 194:75, 1965.

367. Shanbrom, E., Miller, S., and Haar, H. Herpes zoster in hematologic neoplasias: some unusual manifestations, *Ann. Intern. Med.* 53:523, 1960.

368. Shapiro, C. M., and Horwitz, H. Infectious mononucleosis in the aged, *Ann. Intern. Med.* 51:1092, 1959.

369. Sharp, H. L., Nesbit, M. E., White, J. G., and Krivit, W. Renal and hepatic pathology following initial remission of acute leukemia induced by prednisone, *Cancer* 20:1395, 1967.

370. Shaw, R. K., Moore, E. W., Freireich, E. J., and Thomas, L. B. Meningeal leukemia. A syndrome resulting from increased intracranial pressure in patients with acute leukemia, *Neurology* 10:823, 1960.

371. Shorey, J., Schenker, S., Suki, W. N., and Combes, B. Hepatotoxicity of mercaptopurine, *Arch. Intern. Med.* 122:54, 1968.

372. Shugoll, G. I. Pericarditis associated with infectious mononucleosis, *Arch. Intern. Med.* 100:630, 1957.

373. Silverman, F. N. The skeletal lesions in leukemia. Clinical and roentgenographic observations in 103 infants and children, with a review of the literature, *Am. J. Roentgenol.* 59:819, 1948.

374. Silverman, F. N. Treatment of leukemia and allied disorders with folic acid antagonists; effect of aminopterin on skeletal lesions, *Radiology* 54:665, 1950.

375. Simone, J., Aur, R. J. A., Hustu, H. O., and Pinkel, D. "Total therapy"

studies of acute lymphocytic leukemia in children, *Cancer* 30:1488, 1972.

376. Simone, J. V., Holland, E., and Johnson, W. Fatalities during remission of childhood leukemia, *Blood* 39:759, 1972.

377. Simpson, C. L., Hempelman, L. H., and Fuller, L. M. Neoplasia in children treated with X-rays in infancy for thymic enlargement, *Radiology* 64:840, 1955.

378. Sinks, L. F., Newton, W. A., Jr., Nagi, N. A., and Stevenson, T. D. A syndrome associated with extreme hyperuricemia in leukemia, *J. Pediatr.* 68:578, 1966.

379. Skeel, R. T., Henderson, E. S., and Bennett, J. M. The significance of bone marrow lymphocytosis of acute leukemia patients in remission, *Blood* 32:767, 1968.

380. Skeel, R. T., Yankee, R. A., and Henderson, E. S. Meningeal leukemia. Two simple methods for rapid detection of malignant cells in spinal fluid, *J.A.M.A.* 205:863, 1968.

381. Smith, C. H. Infectious lymphocytosis, *Am. J. Dis. Child.* 62:231, 1941.

382. Smith, R. T. Possibilities and problems of immunologic intervention in cancer, *N. Engl. J. Med.* 287:440, 1972.

383. Speck, B., Dooren, L. J., De Koning, J., Van Bekkum, D. W., Eernisse, J. G., Elkerbout, F., Vossen, J. M., and Van Rood, J. J. Clinical experience with bone marrow transplantation's failure and success, *Transplant. Proc.* 3:409, 1971.

384. Spitzer, G., and Garson, O. M. Lymphoblastic leukemia with marked eosinophilia: a report of two cases, *Blood* 42:377, 1963.

385. Spriggs, A. I., and Boddington, M. M. Leukaemic cells in cerebrospinal fluid, *Br. J. Haematol.* 5:83, 1959.

386. Spriggs, A. I., and Jerrome, D. W. Electron-microscopy of Türk cells, *Br. J. Haematol.* 13:764, 1967.

387. Sprunt, T. P., and Evans, F. A. Mononuclear leucocytosis in reaction to acute infections ("infectious mononucleosis"), *Bull. Johns Hopkins Hosp.* 31:410, 1920.

388. Steinberg, A. G. The genetics of acute leukemia in children, *Cancer* 13:985, 1960.

389. Storrs, R. C., Wolman, I. J., Gussoff, B. D., and Hananian, J. Remission maintenance in acute lymphocytic leukemia with hydroxyurea, *Cancer Res.* 26:241, 1966.

390. Štrámková, L., Kouba, K., and Bendová, N. Alkaline phosphatase in neutrophil leukocytes of patients with infectious mononucleosis and the effect of corticosteroid therapy, *Blood* 26:479, 1965.

391. Stryckmans, P. A., Manaster, J., LaChapelle, F., and Socquet, M. Mode of action of chemotherapy in vivo on human acute leukemia. I. Daunomycin, *J. Clin. Invest.* 52:126, 1973.

392. Sullivan, M. P. Intracranial complications in leukemia of children, *Pediatrics* 20:757, 1957.

393. Sullivan, M. P. Leukemic infiltration of meninges and spinal nerve roots, *Pediatrics* 32:63, 1963.

394. Sullivan, M. P. Cytomegalovirus complement-fixation antibody levels of leukemic children, *J.A.M.A.* 206:569, 1968.

395. Sutow, W. W., Garcia, F., Starling, K. A., Williams, T. E., Lane, D. M., and Gehan, E. A. L-asparaginase therapy in children with advanced leukemia, *Cancer* 28:819, 1971.

396. Tallal, L., Tan, C., Oettger, H., Wollner, N., McCarthy, M., Helson, L., Burchenal, J., Karnofsky, D., and Murphy, M. L. E. coli L-asparaginase in the treatment of leukemia and solid tumors in 131 children, *Cancer* 25:306, 1970.

397. Temin, H. M. The participation of DNA in Rous sarcoma virus production, *Virology* 23:486, 1964.

398. Temin, H. M. Carcinogenesis by avian sarcoma viruses, *Cancer Res.* 28:1835, 1968.

399. Temin, H. M., and Mizutani, S. RNA-dependent DNA polymerase in virions of Rous sarcoma virus, *Nature* 226:1211, 1970.

400. Tennant, F. S., Jr. The glomerulonephritis of infectious mononucleosis, *Tex. Rep. Biol. Med.* 26:603, 1968.

401. Thomas, E. D., Buckner, C. D., Fefer, A., Neiman, P., Bryant, J. I., Clift, R. A., Johnson, F. L., Ramberg, R. E., and Storb, R. Leukaemic transformation of engrafted human marrow cells in vivo, *Lancet* i:1310, 1972.

402. Thomas, E. D., Buckner, C. D., Rudolph, R. H., et al. Allogenic marrow grafting for hematologic malignancy using HL-A matched donor-recipient sibling pairs, *Blood* 38:267, 1971.

403. Thomas, E. D., Storb, R., Fefer, A., et al. Aplastic anaemia treated by marrow transplantation, *Lancet* i:284, 1972.

404. Thomas, L. B., Forkner, C. E., Jr., Frei, E. III, Besse, B. E., Jr., and Stabenau, Jr. The skeletal lesions of acute leukemia, *Cancer* 14:608, 1961.

405. Tidy, H. L. Glandular fever and infectious mononucleosis, *Lancet* ii:180, 236; 1934.

406. Tidy, H. L., and Morley, E. B. Glandular fever, *Br. Med. J.* 1:452, 1921.

407. Tjio, J. H., Carbone, P. P., Whang, J., and Frei, E. III. The Philadelphia chromosome and chronic myelogenous leukemia, *J. Natl. Cancer Inst.* 36:567, 1966.

408. Traggis, D. G., Dohlwitz, A., Das, L., Jaffe, N., Moloney, W. C., and Hall, T. C. Cytosine arabinoside in acute leukemia of childhood, *Cancer* 28:815, 1971.

409. Troup, S. B., Swisher, S. N., and Young, L. E. The anemia of leukemia, *Am. J. Med.* 28:751, 1960.

410. Türk, W. Untersuchungen über das Verhalten des Blutes bei akuten Infektions-krankheiten, Braumüller, Vienna, 1898.

411. Türk, W. Septische Erkrankungen bei Verkümmerung des Granulozytensystems, *Wien. Klin. Wochenschr.* 20:157, 1907.

412. Van der Kley, T. M. Acute infectious lymphocytosis and poliomyelitis, *Maandschr. Kindergeneesk.* 22:321, 1954.

413. Videbeak, A. Heredity in Human Leukemia and its Relation to Cancer (A Genetic and Clinical Study of 209 Probands), H. K. Lewis, London, 1947.

414. Virchow, R. L. Weisses Blut und Milztumoren, *Med. Z. Vereins Heilkd. Preussen* 15:157, 1846.

415. Viza, D., Davies, D. A. L., and Harris, R. Solubilization and partial purification of human leukaemic specific antigens, *Nature* 227:1249, 1970.

416. Vogler, W. R., Bain, J. A., Huguley, C. M., Palmer, H. G., and Lowrey, M. E. Metabolic and therapeutic effects of allopurinol in patients with leukemia and gout, *Am. J. Med.* 40:548, 1966.

417. Wahren, B. Diagnosis of infectious mononucleosis by the monospot test, *Am. J. Clin. Pathol.* 52:303, 1969.

418. Wahrman, J., Schaap, T., and Robinson, E. Manifold chromosome abnormalities in leukaemia, *Lancet* i:1098, 1962.

419. Wald, N., Borges, W. H., Li, C. C., Turner, J. H., and Harnois, M. C. Leukaemia associated with mongolism, *Lancet* i:1228, 1961.

420. Warren, S., and Gates, O. The induction of leukemia and life shortening in mice by continuous low-level external gamma radiation, *Radiat. Res.* 47:480, 1971.

421. Waterhouse, B. E., and Lapidus, P. H. Infectious mononucleosis associated with a mass in the anterior mediastinum, *N. Engl. J. Med.* 277:1137, 1967.

422. Wechsler, H. F., Rosenblum, A. H., and Sills, C. T. Infectious mononucleosis: report of an epidemic in an army camp. Parts I and II, *Ann. Intern. Med.* 25:113, 1946.

423. Weksler, M. E., and Birnbaum, G. Lymphocyte transformation induced by autologous cells: stimulation by cultured lymphoblast lines, *J. Clin. Invest.* 51:3124, 1972.

424. West, J. P. An epidemic of glandular fever, *Arch. Pediatr.* 13:889, 1896.

425. Wetherley-Mein, G., and Cottom, D. G. Portal fibrosis in acute leukemia, *Br. J. Haematol.* 2:345, 1956.

426. Wetherley-Mein, G., Epstein, I. S., Foster, W. D., and Grimes, A. J. Mechanisms of anaemia in leukaemia, *Br. J. Haematol.* 4:281, 1958.

427. Whang-Peng, J., Freireich, E. J., Oppenheim, J. J., Frei, E. III, and Tjio, J. H. Cytogenetic studies in 45 patients with acute lymphocytic leukemia, *J. Natl. Cancer Inst.* 42:881, 1969.

428. Wickramasinghe, S. N., Chalmers, D. G., and Cooper, E. H. A study of ineffective erythropoiesis in sideroblastic anaemia and erythraemic myelosis, *Cell Tissue Kinet.* 1:43, 1968.

429. Williams, H. M., Diamond, H. D., and Craver, L. F. The pathogenesis and management of neurological

complications in patients with malignant lymphomas and leukemia, *Cancer* 11:76, 1958.

430. Willson, J. K. V. The bone lesions of childhood leukemia. A survey of 140 cases, *Radiology* 72:672, 1959.

431. Wintrobe, M. M. Clinical Hematology, 6th ed., p. 982, Lea & Febiger, Philadelphia, 1967.

432. Wintrobe, M. M., and Mitchell, D. M. Atypical manifestations of leukaemia, *Q. J. Med.* 9:67, 1940.

433. Wislocki, L. C. Acute pancreatitis in infectious mononucleosis, *N. Engl. J. Med.* 275:322, 1966.

434. Wolff, J. A., Brubaker, C. A., Murphy, M. L., Pierce, M. I., and Severo, N. Prednisone therapy of acute childhood leukemia: prognosis and duration of response in 330 treated patients, *J. Pediatr.* 70:626, 1967.

435. Wollheim, F. A., and Williams, R. C., Jr. Studies on the macroglobulins of human serum. I. Polyclonal immunoglobulin class M (IgM) increase in infectious mononucleosis, *N. Engl. J. Med.* 274:61, 1966.

436. Wolnisty, C. Orchitis as a complication of infectious mononucleosis. Report of a case, *N. Engl. J. Med.* 266:88, 1962.

437. Wulff, H. R. Acute agranulocytosis following infectious mononucleosis, *Scand. J. Haematol.* 2:179, 1965.

438. Yeager, H. P. Airway obstruction in infectious mononucleosis, *Arch. Otolaryngol.* 80:583, 1964.

439. York, W. H. Spontaneous rupture of the spleen. Report of a case secondary to infectious mononucleosis, *J.A.M.A* 179:170, 1962.

440. Zaizov, R., and Matoth, Y. The pathogenesis of anemia in acute leukemia, *Isr. J. Med. Sci.* 7:1025, 1971.

441. Zeve, V. H., Lucas, L. S., and Manaker, R. A. Continuous cell culture from a patient with chronic myelogenous leukemia. II. Detection of herpes-like virus by electron microscopy, *J. Natl. Cancer Inst.* 37:761, 1966.

442. Zuelzer, W. W., and Cox, D. E. Genetic aspects of leukemia, *Semin. Hematol.* 6:228, 1969.

443. Zuelzer, W. W., Thompson, R. I., and Mastrangelo, R. Evidence for a genetic factor related to leukemogenesis and congenital anomalies: chromosomal aberrations in pedigree of an infant with partial D trisomy and leukemia, *J. Pediatr.* 72:367, 1968.

Chapter 22   Lymphocytic Lymphoma, Hodgkin's Disease, and Other Chronic Lymphoproliferative Disorders

The major lymphoid tissues of the body include the lymph nodes and spleen, the structures that comprise Waldeyer's ring, and the lymphoid follicles of the gastrointestinal and respiratory systems. These tissues are composed of several types of cells, including lymphocytes, plasma cells, phagocytic macrophages (histiocytes), reticular cells, and fibroblasts. The term *lymphoreticular system* is often applied to these tissues, which together comprise a portion of the reticuloendothelial system. The lymphoreticular system is part of the body's bulwark against microorganisms and antigenically altered cells, utilizing both phagocytic and immunologic defense mechanisms.

The cellular components of this system respond to appropriate stimuli by proliferation. For example, the intradermal inoculation of *Mycobacteria* induces hyperplasia of the draining lymph node, with several cell types joining in the proliferative reaction. The response to other stimuli may be predominantly by a single cell type, with other cellular elements sharing little in the proliferative reaction. For instance, *Bacillus pertussis* may evoke primarily a lymphocytic reaction in the respiratory tract, whereas *Listeria monocytogenes* may stimulate macrophage proliferation and activation.

The proliferative responses of the lymphoreticular system that are *appropriate* must be differentiated from those that are *neoplastic.* The term "appropriate" is used in the sense that a stimulus is identifiable and the process of response self-limited. The term "reactive" is used in a similar manner. An example of an appropriate response is hyperplasia of the submaxillary lymph node in response to an abscessed tooth. The term "neoplastic" implies a malignant process involving alteration in the control mechanisms that limit cellular proliferation; it also implies a process that is progressive rather than limited and that usually has no identifiable inciting stimulus. An example of a neoplastic response is the generalized lymphoid proliferation seen in lymphosarcoma.

Neoplastic proliferation resembles reactive hyperplasia in that it may involve a single cell type or several cell types. For example, lymphosarcoma may involve proliferation of only a morphologically uniform population of small lymphocytes or it may involve mixed histiocytic-lymphocytic proliferation.

No absolute criteria are currently available for differentiating reactive reticuloendothelial hyperplasia from neoplastic proliferation. The principal criteria in current use for determining a neoplastic process relate to the morphologic features of the lymphoid tissues: destruction of the normal lymph node architecture, invasion of the fibrous capsule (Fig. 22.1), and a high mitotic index. These are by no means absolute criteria, and all may be found as part of an appropriate defense response to an inflammatory stimulus. As Butler says, "Every pattern of lymphoma may be simulated by a reactive process" (39).

The clinical course of an illness may also provide a clue to the nature of the lymphoreticular reaction. Again, this criterion is not absolute and patients may die of a "benign" process involving lymph nodes, as well as from a malignancy. The problem is even more complex: in cer-

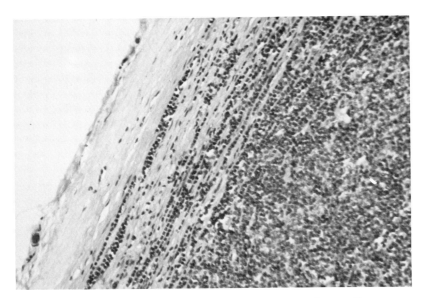

Figure 22.1 Section of lymph node from a patient with a well-differentiated lymphocytic lymphosarcoma demonstrating capsular infiltration.

tain diseases currently regarded as neoplastic, the proliferating malignant cell has not been identified with certainty. Hodgkin's disease is the prototype of such a malignant lymphoreticular disorder.

In time, the distinction between neoplastic and reactive lymphoreticular hyperplasia may prove to be merely semantic. As we shall discuss later on, the malignant disorders may prove to be "appropriate" responses to certain chemical, viral, or even immunologic stimuli.

In this chapter we shall first consider reactive hyperplasia of the lymphoreticular system, then some of the malignant processes that involve the lymphoid element: Hodgkin's disease and lymphomas with lymphocytic predominance. In Chapter 27 we shall discuss those neoplastic diseases in which histiocytic proliferation predominates. Other lymphoreticular disorders have been described earlier: chronic lymphocytic leukemia in Chapter 19, multiple myeloma in Chapter 20, and acute lymphocytic leukemia in Chapter 21.

Benign, Self-limited Lymphoreticular Proliferation

There is a large body of literature on neoplasia involving lymph nodes. In contrast, relatively few definitive articles have been written on the more common nonneoplastic disorders that give rise to lymphoid hyperplasia (123, 222, 276, 316). Butler (39) has summarized the characteristics of nonmalignant reactive hyperplasia of lymph nodes. These include proliferation of sinusoidal histiocytes, follic-

ular proliferation, and proliferation of "pulp" elements (histiocytes, lymphocytes, and endothelial cells).

A number of disorders may give rise to reactive hyperplasia. For convenience they may be divided into several groups, as in Table 22.1: infections, collagen disease, dermatopathies, drug-induced disorders, and inflammatory disorders of unknown etiology.

The mechanism of lymphoid hyperplasia is not always clearly known. Repeated antigenic stimuli may evoke a sequence of hyperplastic changes culminating as follicular hyperplasia (222). In several of the disorders listed in Table 22.1, the basis of lymph node hyperplasia is probably antigenic stimulation.

Some of the reactive lesions of lymph nodes may simulate lymphoma, including postvaccination lymphadenitis (153), dermatopathic lymphadenitis (166), Dilantin-induced adenopathy (288), and lymphadenopathy associated with rheumatoid arthritis and heroin use (128). For example, as many as 50 to 75 percent of patients with rheumatoid arthritis exhibit clinically significant lymphadenopathy at some time during their illness (234). Because of the associated fever, weight loss, and anemia, a clinical diagnosis of lymphoma may be considered. On biopsy, however, the lymph nodes show a characteristic benign follicular hyperplasia that is generally distinguishable from the nodular lymphomas (239, 264, 266).

In addition to the reactive hyperplasia cited above, other entities may simulate lymphoma on clinical grounds and by producing abnormal lymphangiograms. One is a benign condition known as *lymphangiopericytoma*, or *lymphangiomyomatosis*. This condition occurs

Table 22.1 Causes of reactive hyperplasia of the lymph nodes.

Infections	References
Bacterial: tuberculosis, syphilis	102, 154
Viral: postvaccination, herpes zoster, infectious mononucleosis	125, 153, 315
Protozoan: toxoplasmosis	270, 309, 319
Collagen disease	
Rheumatoid arthritis	234, 239
Systemic lupus erythematosus	
Dermatopathic disorders	166
Drugs	
Dilantin-associated lymphadenopathy	167, 288
Reactions of unknown origin	39, 316
Reactive follicular hyperplasia	
Reactive hyperplasia with prominent sinusoidal histiocytes	
Chronic nonspecific lymphadenitis	
"Allergic granulomatosis"	53, 250, 316

exclusively in women and is associated with chylothorax, pulmonary lymphangiectasia, and atypical lipid pneumonia. It is probably a hamartoma and may be related to the tuberous sclerosis disease complex (68, 97, 114). Other entities that may simulate lymphoma on clinical grounds include Boeck's sarcoid, carcinoma, and sarcoma involving lymph nodes. These conditions are readily distinguished from lymphoma by the histologic features of the involved lymph nodes.

Classification of the Lymphomas

Histopathologic Classification

Figure 22.2 illustrates an organizational framework for classification of the lymphomas. They may be subdivided into two broad histologic categories: those in which the nodular architecture of the normal node is more or less preserved, and those in which the nodular architecture is destroyed by diffuse infiltration of malignant cells.

A major consideration in histologic classification is whether one or more than one cell population is involved in the proliferative process. For example, some lymphomas involve the proliferation of a uniform population of small lymphocytes, whereas others are pleomorphic and involve lymphocytes, histiocytes, and plasma cells. Based on these histologic criteria, four major subdivisions of lymphomas may be recognized: nodular pleomorphic, nodular single-cell type, diffuse pleomorphic, and diffuse single-cell type.

Classification is further refined by consideration of the *type* of proliferating cell, by the degree of morphologic dif-

Table 22.2 Major histologic criteria used in classifying lymphomas.

Single-cell type or pleomorphic
Nodular or diffuse pattern
Lymphocytic or histiocytic
Degree of cellular differentiation
Presence of Reed-Sternberg cells

Table 22.3 Old and new histologic classifications of the non-Hodgkin's lymphomas.

Predominant cell type(s)	New classification	Old classification
Lymphocytic	Malignant lymphoma, lymphocytic type, well differentiated, nodular	Giant follicular lymphoma
Lymphocytic	Malignant lymphoma, lymphocytic type, well differentiated, diffuse	Small-cell lymphosarcoma; lymphocytic lympho-sarcoma
Lymphocytic	Malignant lymphoma, lymphocytic type, poorly differentiated	Large-cell lymphosarcoma; lymphoblastic lympho-sarcoma
Histiocytic-lymphocytic	Malignant lymphoma, mixed-cell type, poorly differentiated	
Primitive reticular	Malignant lymphoma, reticulum-cell type, undifferentiated	Reticulum-cell sarcoma: large-cell lympho-sarcoma
Histiocytic	Malignant lymphoma, reticulum-cell type, histiocytic	

ferentiation of the predominant cell, and by the presence or absence of the giant Reed-Sternberg cell. The major histologic features used in classifying lymphomas are summarized in Table 22.2. When a single cell type predominates, it is usually either lymphocytic or histiocytic. One may therefore recognize lymphomas of the following categories: diffuse-lymphocytic predominance, diffuse-histiocytic predominance, nodular-lymphocytic predominance, and nodular-histiocytic predominance.

In addition to being nodular and diffuse, histiocytic or lymphocytic, the lymphoma may be well or poorly differentiated. The degree of differentiation, based on morphologic criteria, is another important histologic feature used in classifying the lymphomas having a predominant single cell. These histologic classifications may be related to older classifications in the manner shown in Table 22.3.

Diffuse, well-differentiated lymphoma with lymphocytic predominance corresponds to the older classification of small-cell lymphosarcoma (proliferation of a uniform population of small lymphocytes, as in Fig. 22.3). The

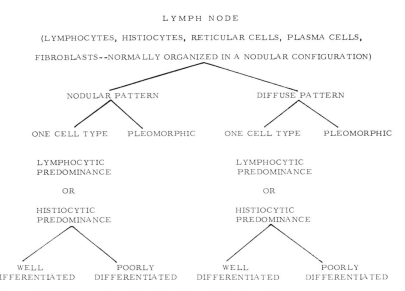

Figure 22.2 Scheme for classification of the lymphomas.

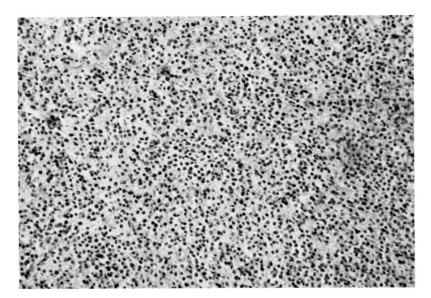

Figure 22.3 Lymph node showing well-differentiated lymphocytic lymphosarcoma, diffuse type. Note the uniform "round cell" infiltration and the lack of a nodular structure.

well-differentiated, nodular-lymphocytic predominant type corresponds to the former classification of giant follicular lymphosarcoma (Fig. 22.4). The lymphomas with histiocytic predominance correspond to reticulum cell sarcoma (Fig. 22.5). Histiocytic malignancies are considered in more detail in Chapter 27.

The presence of Reed-Sternberg cells is the criterion for diagnosing Hodgkin's disease. In fixed tissue sections

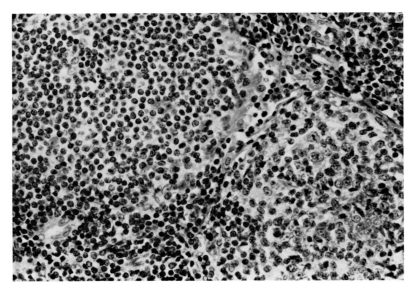

Figure 22.4 Lymph node showing nodular lymphocytic lymphoma of the well-differentiated type.

stained with hematoxylin and eosin, these cells are characterized by two or more large, vesicular nuclei with prominent nucleoli, giving the cell the appearance of two staring owl's eyes (Fig. 22.6). By electron microscopy these cells have a characteristic ultrastructure (88). They occur only rarely in other disorders (334). Reed-Sternberg cells can be demonstrated to contain IgG by immunohistochemical staining (127). The lymph nodes in Hodgkin's disease contain a pleomorphic cellular infiltrate, as well as the characteristic giant cells (186, 212).

In practice, the pathologist needs to review an entire lymph node — or sometimes several lymph nodes — in order to establish a precise histologic diagnosis. The use of aspirates or smears obtained from lymph nodes is interesting, but fails to provide the information on lymph node architecture that is critical in establishing a diagnosis (210). In the future it may be possible to classify the lymphomas in more detail according to morphology, function, and histochemical characteristics of explanted lymphoma cells (54, 294), and determine whether they are of B- or T-cell origin (260; cf. 69).

Correlation of Histology with Natural History

Lymphomas with a well-defined nodular pattern in general are more indolent in their growth characteristics than are lymphomas with a diffuse pattern. This situation has an obvious analogy to that existing with carcinomas. The epithelial malignancies, which retain a well-differentiated glandular pattern, often are less aggressive in their growth characteristics than are poorly differentiated carcinomas.

Predominant cell type is another useful histologic feature for predicting natural history. Lymphomas with histiocytic predominance tend to be more aggressive and less responsive to treatment than are those in which lymphocytes predominate.

The degree of morphologic differentiation of the predominant cell type is another useful index for determining natural history and therapeutic responsiveness. Well-differentiated lymphomas predictably run a longer course and are more responsive to treatment than those with little cellular differentiation.

Taken together, these histologic parameters indicate the following (178): in patients with lymphomas of the well-differentiated lymphocytic type, the course of the disease will be more benign than that of patients with lymphomas of histiocytic, mixed-cell type, or poorly differentiated lymphocytic types. Malignant lymphomas with a follicular pattern usually have a more benign course than those with a diffuse pattern.

When lymphomas have a follicular pattern, the differences in patient survival between those with lympho-

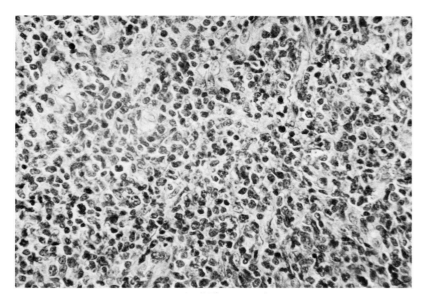

Figure 22.5 Lymph node showing diffuse histiocytic lymphoma of the poorly differentiated type. Note the large pale-staining "vesicular" nuclei, some with prominent nucleoli. The cytoplasmic boundaries are indistinct.

cytic predominance and those with histiocytic predominance are striking. When lymphomas have a diffuse pattern, the differences in survival between lymphocytic and histiocytic types are not so dramatic.

The correlation between histologic features and the course of Hodgkin's disease will be considered later in

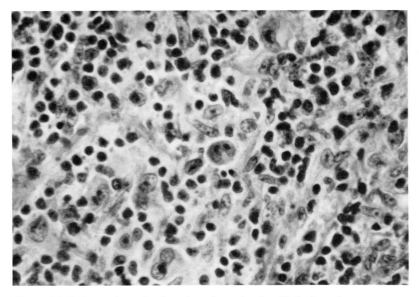

Figure 22.6 Lymph node showing the mixed cellularity of Hodgkin's disease. Note the binucleate Reed-Sternberg cell near the center of the field.

Table 22.4 Histologic classification of Hodgkin's disease.

Lukes and Butler "modern" (212, 213)	Jackson and Parker "traditional" (169)
Lymphocytic predominance (diffuse or nodular)	Paragranuloma
Nodular sclerosis Mixed cellularity Lymphocytic depletion (a) Diffuse fibrosis	Granuloma
(b) Reticular type	Sarcoma

this chapter. Old and new histologic classifications of Hodgkin's disease are listed in Table 22.4.

A number of excellent reviews of the histology of lymphomas, and of natural history correlated with morphology, are available (169, 212, 264–266, 285, 337).

Lymphomas with Lymphocytic Predominance

Incidence

It is estimated that 22,000 new cases of lymphoma are diagnosed annually in the United States and that 17,000 patients die with this disease. The precise incidence by histologic classification is not known. Such a figure would be difficult to obtain in view of the changing histologic criteria applied to the diagnosis of lymphoma over the past two decades. The lymphocytic lymphomas probably account for somewhat more than one-third of all lymphomas.

In 1949 there were 4.2 deaths from lymphoma per 100,000 population (133). Of these, 38.4 percent resulted from lymphosarcoma and follicular lymphoma (malignant lymphoma, lymphocytic type, well differentiated, nodular). Hodgkin's disease accounted for about 40 percent, and histiocytic lymphomas for the remainder. In a series of 618 cases at the Massachusetts General Hospital, 22 percent were lymphocytic lymphosarcoma and 14 percent were lymphoblastic (124). Roughly the same proportion of lymphocytic lymphomas was found in a 1961 series from Memorial Hospital in New York (283).

Lymphosarcoma (lymphocytic lymphoma) constitutes about the same proportion of all lymphoma cases in England, the United States, and Japan (5).

As a rule, Hodgkin's disease affects a younger group of patients than other lymphomas (165, 230, 268, 323). The lymphocytic and histiocytic lymphomas usually are diseases of middle and old age, with a median incidence between the fourth and sixth decades of life (305–307).

However, exceptions to this distribution are known, and both lymphocytic and histiocytic lymphoma have been observed in childhood (24, 177, 282). In most series males are more commonly affected by lymphocytic lymphoma than are females (283, 305–307). Familial occurrence is rare (354). Lymphomas occur in all races and, with the exception of Burkitt's lymphoma, no unusual geographic distribution is known.

Clinical and Laboratory Manifestations

Mechanisms The clinical manifestations of lymphocytic lymphomas are related to localized or generalized lymphocytic cell proliferation. This proliferation can produce symptomatic disease in the following ways: (*a*) by localized enlargement of lymph nodes that may be disfiguring or produce obstruction of a vital organ; for example, obstruction of a bronchus or of the common bile duct; (*b*) by infiltration of organs such as the kidney and spleen, producing organomegaly and malfunction (Fig. 22.7); (*c*) by infiltration of the bone marrow and interference with production of normal hematopoietic cells (Fig. 22.8); and (*d*) by replacement of the normal elements of the lymphoreticular system (Fig. 22.3), resulting in impaired defenses against microorganisms.

Presentation The majority of patients with lymphocytic lymphoma present with enlargement of a single peripheral lymph node or of multiple lymph nodes (283). Others present with enlargement of deep-seated lymph nodes,

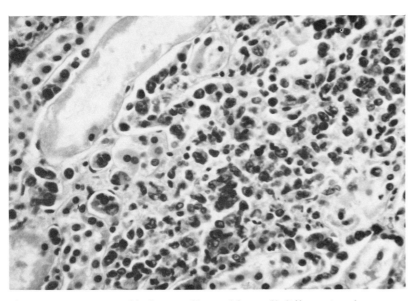

Figure 22.7 Section of kidney infiltrated by well-differentiated histiocytic lymphoma. Remnants of tubules can be seen throughout the photomicrograph.

with organomegaly, or with evidence of abnormal organ function. Weight loss is frequent. Fever and pruritus as initial manifestations are rare in patients with lymphocytic lymphoma (less than 5 percent), but are relatively common in patients with Hodgkin's disease.

Manifestations The major clinical manifestations of the various types of lymphoma are all similar. Where differences exist, they will be mentioned in the following discussion and emphasized in the sections on the histiocytic malignancies and Hodgkin's disease.

Lymph nodes and spleen. Superficial lymph node involvement occurs sometime during the course of illness in almost all patients with lymphoma. In addition, the mediastinal glands and the retroperitoneal lymph glands are often involved. Invasion of the latter is demonstrable by lymphangiography (Fig. 22.9) or displacement of the ureters demonstrated by intravenous pyelography. Retroperitoneal involvement is very common in well-differentiated nodular lymphocytic lymphoma (9, 124). Involvement of the cervical lymphatics may produce a "bullneck" appearance (see Fig. 21.7). Generally, lymphadenopathy is painless. The glands often have the consistency of hard rubber. They may be fixed or movable, single or matted. Superficial ulceration is rare. Splenomegaly occurs at some time during the course of disease in one-third or more of patients with lymphoma (124, 165, 283). Very large spleens are encountered during leukemic transition (283) and are frequent in nodular lymphoma (165).

Extranodal disease. A primary site of disease outside the lymph node system was noted in about one-fourth of the patients with "lymphosarcoma" observed by Rosenberg and his colleagues in 1961 at New York's Memorial Hospital (283). The most common extranodal primary site was the lymphatic tissues of Waldeyer's ring, which include the tonsils. Other frequently involved sites were the skin, stomach, and gastrointestinal tract and bone. Other parenchymal organs were less commonly involved.

Testicular tumors in older males are more likely to be of lymphomatous than of germinal cell origin.

Tonsils. Malignant lymphomas, particularly of the histiocytic variety, account for a large percentage of malignant tumors of the tonsils (170). These tumors involve the tonsils, soft palate, and uvula. Ulcerations may be present. Persistent pain and difficulty in swallowing are clinical clues to the presence of such tumors.

Skin. Various cutaneous manifestations are associated with lymphoma. These may result from tumorous infiltration of the skin, from dermatopathic changes related to

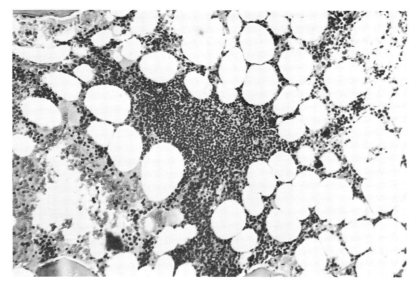

Fig. 22.8A

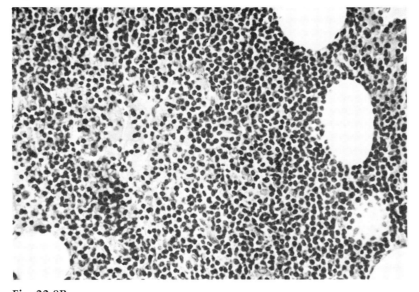

Fig. 22.8B

Figure 22.8 A lymphocytic ''nodule'' in a section of bone marrow biopsy is shown in Fig. 22.8A. The dense uniform cellular infiltration is apparent. The patient had a well-differentiated lymphocytic lymphoma. Hematoxylin and eosin stain. The same nodule is shown at a higher magnification in Fig. 22.8B.

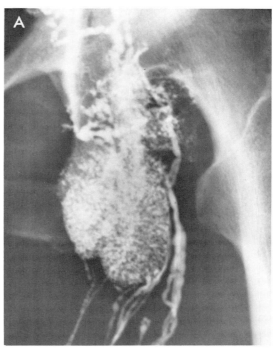

Fig. 22.9A

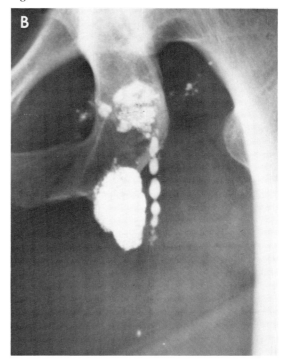

Fig. 22.9B

Figure 22.9 Lymphangiogram of a patient with Hodgkin's disease, showing a lymph node invaded by tumor (Fig. 22.9A). The same lymph node is shown after chemotherapy in Fig. 22.9B.

drug therapy, or from secondary viral or bacterial infection. Tumorous involvement can take many different clinical forms: erythema, macular or papular eruptions, bullae, eczematoid lesions, lichenification, and ulceration (17, 98, 108, 328). Firm intracutaneous bluish nodules are a relatively common lesion (98).

On physical examination the lesions are rarely specific for lymphomatous disease; the diagnosis generally is established by skin biopsy. Touch imprints of the cutaneous lesions may be helpful (108).

Varicella zoster eruptions are common complications of the lymphomas (283). These eruptions tend to be segmental, rarely disseminated (311). They heal slowly, and the pain, which can persist long after the cutaneous lesions have cleared, may be incapacitating.

Kaposi's sarcoma, usually beginning in the lower extremities, is an unusual disease entity that may be associated with malignant lymphoma (20).

Gastrointestinal tract. All the histologic forms of lymphoma may involve the digestive tract, but involvement by nodular lymphoma is relatively rare (9). Involvement may occur anywhere from the oropharynx to the anus. Lymphosarcoma accounts for about 2 percent of all gastric malignancies (218). Roentgenographically, lymphoma of the stomach may appear as a filling defect, a localized tumor, a diffusely infiltrating lesion simulating linitus plastica, or a pattern of giant rugae. Gastric emptying may be slowed. The symptoms experienced by the patient from gastric involvement may include anorexia, pain, vomiting, hematemesis, and melena (120, 269).

Involvement of the small bowel by lymphoma is approximately as frequent as involvement of the stomach. Sites of lymphoma, in order of frequency, are the ileum, cecum, rectum, jejunum, duodenum, and remainder of the colon (226, 283, 313). Although lymphoma is rare as compared with carcinoma of the large bowel, it makes up a significant (25 percent) proportion of small bowel malignancies (313, 360). Manifestations may include a palpable mass, pain, melena, and diarrhea (95). Intussusception may occur, or the clinical syndrome may suggest ulcerative colitis (107).

Lymphoma may present with malabsorption syndrome, which probably results from obstruction of the mesenteric lymph nodes and lacteals. In patients with malabsorption and abdominal lymphoma, diarrhea is a constant feature and steatorrhea a frequent one. Peroral jejunal biopsy often fails to reveal the diagnosis, whereas small bowel barium studies usually suggest it (240).

The radiologic manifestations of lymphomatous involvement of the intestinal tract are pleomorphic: single or multiple discrete tumors, polypoid lesions, stiff intestinal walls with diminished peristalsis, and anular lesions (76).

Involvement of the liver by lymphoma is frequent and may be manifest as diffuse enlargement, nodular involvement, invasion of the gallbladder, or obstruction of the extrahepatic biliary tract (163, 283, 323, 340). Jaundice often results, and the serum alkaline phosphatase is almost invariably elevated. Biliary obstruction as a cause of jaundice without concomitant infiltration of the liver is relatively rare (283). The pancreas may be massively involved by tumor.

Cardiorespiratory system. Although the heart itself frequently is involved by lymphoma, as evidenced by microscopic infiltration seen in tissue obtained in autopsy (46, 219, 277, 278), clinical manifestations are relatively rare.

Perhaps the most common clinical manifestation is pericardial effusion associated with lymphomatous infiltration. Such effusions may be serious and may even produce cardiac tamponade. Rare manifestations include arrhythmias and myocardial failure from direct cardiac infiltration. Acute myocardial infarction has been described (8), as has occlusion of major coronary vessels (173). Several fine reviews of heart involvement in leukemia and lymphoma have been published (173, 277, 278, 333).

Pulmonary involvement by lymphoma is much more common than cardiac involvement. In Rosenberg's series of 1,269 cases of lymphoma (283), intrathoracic lesions occurred sometime during the illness in between 51 percent (clinical) and 69 percent (postmortem). Mediastinal and bronchial lymphadenopathy were the most common lesions, followed by diffuse infiltration of lung parenchyma and, less commonly, by discrete lung nodules (Fig. 22.10). Endobronchial disease can also occur in Hodgkin's disease and other lymphomas (321). A problem frequently encountered in intrathoracic lymphoma is pleural effusion. When chylous pleural effusions are found in the absence of chest trauma, lymphoma should always be suspected (165).

Symptoms of pulmonary involvement by lymphomatous disease may include cough, dyspnea, chest pain, and hemoptysis. Depending on the type of involvement, the pattern of abnormalities in pulmonary function may suggest restrictive lung disease, abnormalities of perfusion-ventilation, alveolar-capillary block syndrome, or (more rarely) obstructive lung diseases. Roentgenographic manifestation may include well-defined lesions or hilar masses, hazy infiltrates, a diffuse alveolar pattern, or even consolidation of a lobe (66, 109, 126, 141, 162, 252, 287). Cavitation of lymphomatous pulmonary lesions is rare except in the case of Hodgkin's disease (356). The definitive

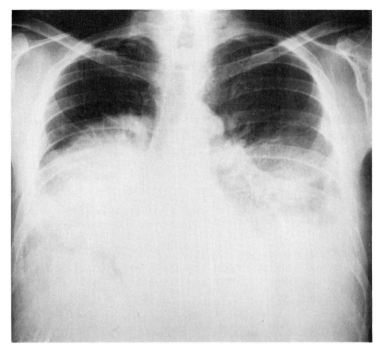

Figure 22.10 Chest roentgenogram of a patient with Hodgkin's disease showing pulmonary infiltration.

diagnosis of the cause of the pulmonary lesion often depends upon obtaining tissue either by percutaneous or transbronchoscopic lung biopsy or by open thoracotomy (140). Occasionally the diagnosis may be made by pleural biopsy or cytological examination of the pleural fluid (225).

Superior vena cava obstruction with characteristic venous engorgement, edema of the upper half of the body, dyspnea, and cyanosis is a serious complication of lymphoma and requires immediate therapeutic intervention. It occurs in about 2 percent of patients (276).

Bone. Radiologically apparent bone lesions are found in about 12 percent of patients with lymphocytic lymphoma. They occur in about 15 percent of patients with Hodgkin's disease and 20 percent of patients with histiocytic lymphoma (165, 283, 308, 344). The frequency of skeletal involvement demonstrable at autopsy is much higher than these figures (103, 329).

Clinical symptoms related to osseous involvement may include pain, neurologic deficits from compression fractures of the vertebral column, and the neurologic, gastrointestinal, and renal manifestations of hypercalcemia. Pain is the most frequent symptom. Lesions are most commonly found in the pelvis, vertebrae, ribs, and femoral bones (344), and they are generally osteolytic in lympho-

cytic lymphoma. Bone lesions are sometimes osteoblastic in histocytic lymphoma and Hodgkin's disease. Abnormal tumor vessels may be demonstrated to supply the osseous metastases (322).

Renal. In a large series of autopsy cases of malignant lymphoma, Richmond and his colleagues (274) found the kidney to be involved in 34 percent. In lymphocytic lymphoma with bone marrow involvement, the figure for kidney involvement was as high as 63 percent; in histiocytic lymphoma, it was 46 percent; in Hodgkin's disease, only 13 percent. A variety of renal lesions were observed: solitary and multiple nodules, diffuse infiltration (see Fig. 22.7), infiltration from perirenal disease, and single bulky tumors. Despite the frequency of kidney lesions at autopsy, involvement was suspected antemortem in only 14 percent of the patients. In these, clinical findings included a palpable mass and, rarely, renal failure.

Extrarenal involvement by lymphoma may produce ureteral obstruction, hydronephrosis, and renal failure (274, 304). Tumor involvement is usually demonstrable by ordinary roentgenogram, intravenous pyelography, or arteriography (300).

Renal involvement is usually a manifestation of widely disseminated lymphoma; only rarely does the disease arise in the kidney or have its predominant manifestation in this organ (73, 96, 130, 197, 224). Urate nephropathy is rare in lymphoma.

Nervous system. Nervous system involvement by lymphoma may take a variety of forms: (a) extradural spinal cord compression; (b) cranial bone involvement; (c) cranial and peripheral nerve infiltration; (d) dural involvement; (e) lymphomatous leptomeningitis; (f) direct infiltration of the brain substance; and (g) demyelination (25, 142, 172, 174, 223, 271, 273, 275, 286, 312, 349, 350). Of these, the most common acute complication seen by an oncology service is compression of the spinal cord by extradural or subdural tumor (85, 227, 351). Untreated, this complication inevitably results in paraplegia. Consequently, cord compression requires an immediate and vigorous therapeutic attack (61, 232).

Other organ systems. The thyroid gland may be infiltrated by lymphosarcoma and may even be the primary site of origin of the tumor (65, 124, 187). A number of authors have commented upon the similarity of changes in the thyroid gland of patients with lymphosarcoma and those of Hashimoto's thyroiditis (189).

The adrenal glands were involved in 25 percent of 277 autopsy patients with lymphoma (283). Rarely is the involvement of sufficient magnitude to produce adrenal insufficiency. Pituitary involvement is rare, also.

Orbital structures may be infiltrated by lymphosarcoma, producing proptosis and ocular dysfunction (91, 283). Generally, such involvement is a manifestation of disseminated disease; rarely is the orbit the primary site of involvement (352).

The blood. A variety of manifestations of lymphoma may be seen in the peripheral blood. Lymphocytopenia in the peripheral blood is fairly common in advanced disease that has been treated with vigorous chemotherapy and radiation therapy. Severe anemia is uncommon unless the bone marrow is depressed by chemotherapy or infiltrated by lymphoma (283, 354). Similarly, the development of severe leukopenia or thrombocytopenia should suggest marrow infiltration or drug toxicity.

In between 10 and 30 percent of cases, the bone marrow contains increased numbers of lymphoid cells, and in over 10 percent these constitute the predominant cellular element (168, 283) (see Fig. 22.8). Arbitrary criteria have been used to define leukemic transformation of lymphosarcoma (124): bone marrow replacement and a white blood count of over 30,000/mm³ with a predominance of lymphoid cells. Obviously, more subtle degrees of transition to leukemia may occur with spotty bone marrow infiltration and only a few abnormal circulating lymphocytes. The term *leukolymphosarcoma* has been applied to this disease complex. The morphology of the cells may vary from the mature lymphocytes characteristic of chronic lymphocytic leukemia to quite primitive, undifferentiated stem cells. Abnormal cytoplasmic ribosomal structures occasionally have been described in these malignant cells (4). Similarly, the clinical course may vary from that of chronic lymphocytic leukemia to that of acute leukemia. Leukolymphosarcoma occurs in about 10 percent of patients with lymphocytic lymphoma—more often in children than in adults (282, 283).

On occasion, paraproteins have been described in the blood of patients with lymphocytic lymphomas (49, 198).

Systemic Manifestations   Fever, pruritus, anorexia, and weight loss are relatively uncommon manifestations in the early stages of lymphocytic lymphoma (283, 323, 354), whereas they are relatively common in the early stages of disseminated Hodgkin's disease. Late in the course of lymphosarcoma these manifestations are frequent and may be quite prominent. However, only after a thorough attempt has been made to exclude infection should fever be ascribed to the underlying disease process (27, 190).

Infection is a frequent complication of all lymphomas (48, 229). It is particularly common during the late and preterminal phase of the disease. Bacterial, fungal, and viral infections all occur. Enhanced host susceptibility has been ascribed to altered immunologic reactivity, cytotoxic chemotherapy, and corticosteroid administration (119, 159, 229, 338). Chemotherapy probably exerts a deleterious effect on the host defense system by reducing the granulocyte reserve and by inducing immunosuppression; it apparently has little effect on reticuloendothelial phagocytic function per se (143).

Mode of Spread and Staging

Hodgkin's disease usually has a unifocal origin and spreads in a predictable manner (284). Consequently, for its proper management one must assess as accurately as possible the extent of spread of tumor. The process of determining extent of spread is called staging. Lymphocytic lymphomas may not have a clearly unifocal origin or predictable mode of spread. However, the observation that some apparently localized lymphocytic lymphomas (stages I and II) may be permanently cured by radiation therapy suggests that at least some of these tumors are not disseminated at the time of diagnosis (92, 281, 283).

Some forms of lymphosarcoma restricted to the spleen have been reported as curable (161). In a study of patients presenting with apparently localized tumors, Scheer observed no significant difference between lymphosarcoma and Hodgkin's disease in the mode of spread of disease (289). Peters, on the other hand, observed that prophylactic irradiation to uninvolved adjacent areas did not prolong survival of patients with lymphocytic and histiocytic lymphoma (257). In a study of 209 patients presenting with localized lymphoma, Han and Stutzman (148) determined the mode of spread (that is, the next area of disease involvement). New areas of involvement were limited to nodes adjacent to the original area in 68 percent of patients with Hodgkin's disease, but in only 36 percent of patients with lymphocytic and histiocytic lymphoma. This study suggests that in the majority of patients with non-Hodgkin's lymphoma, disease either is disseminated at the time of diagnosis or spreads in a noncontiguous manner.

Inasmuch as accurate staging is necessary for identification of the fraction of patients that have truly localized disease, recent studies of patients with lymphocytic lymphoma have addressed themselves to the evaluation of vigorous staging procedures (150, 342). These will be considered in the discussion on Hodgkin's disease.

Histiocytic Lymphomas

Histiocytic lymphoma (reticulum cell sarcoma) is logically considered with the other histiocytic malignancies and is discussed in Chapter 27. Still, the features of this disorder that contrast with those of lymphocytic lymphoma and Hodgkin's disease are worth considering briefly at this point:

(a) Histiocytic lymphomas are generally more agressive and less responsive to therapy than are the lymphocytic lymphomas.

(b) Histiocytic malignancies usually are widely disseminated at the time of initial diagnosis; Hodgkin's disease often is localized.

(c) Histiocytic lymphomas often have a primary site of involvement outside the lymph node system.

(d) Among the lymphomas, those of histiocytic type most frequently involve bone.

(e) Histiocytic lymphomas rarely involve the bone marrow and blood to produce a leukemic picture.

Hodgkin's Disease

Correlation of Histology with Natural History

Lymphoid tissues involved by Hodgkin's disease exhibit many histologic alterations, including fibrosis, proliferation or depletion of lymphocytes, cell necrosis, endothelial cell hyperplasia, and variable infiltration by neutrophils, plasma cells, and histiocytes. Reed-Sternberg cells are characteristic. These large cells, between 15 and 45 microns in diameter, have distinctive nuclear features: nuclei are multiple or multilobate with two or more large, acidophilic nucleoli; the nuclear membrane is thickened

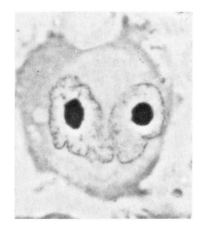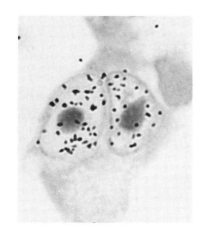
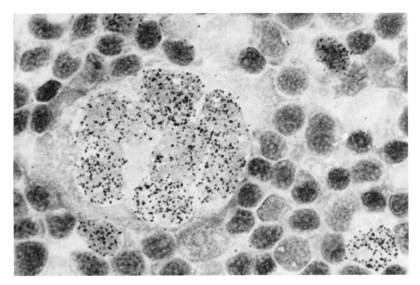

Figure 22.12 Bi- and multinucleate cells from long-term culture of tissues from a patient with Hodgkin's disease. A large multinucleate giant cell (*lower frame*) and a binucleate cell (*upper left*) are labeled by ³H-thymidine indicating DNA synthesis or repair. (Photographs courtesy of Dr. M. Kadin.)

and prominent (Figs. 22.6, 22.11, and 22.12). In vitro these cells are capable of DNA synthesis (169).

The "modern" and the "traditional" histologic classifications of Hodgkin's disease have been given in Table 22.4. A new histologic classification was proposed at a conference held in Rye, New York, in 1966 under the joint sponsorship of the National Cancer Institute and the American Cancer Society (212, 213). According to this classification, Hodgkin's disease may be subdivided into four histologic subtypes, examples of which are shown in Figs. 22.6 and 22.13 to 22.16: (a) lymphocytic predominance, (b) lymphocytic depletion, (c) mixed cellularity, and (d) nodular sclerosis. *Lymphocytic predominance* and *lymphocytic depletion* refer to the relative abundance of

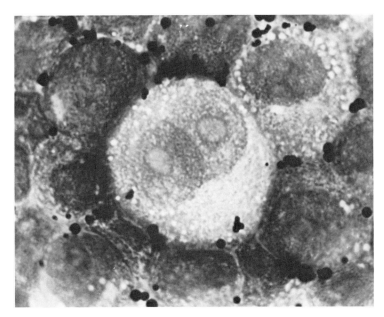

Figure 22.11 A cell resembling a Reed-Sternberg cell observed in long-term tissue culture of spleen cells from a patient with Hodgkin's disease. (Photograph courtesy of Dr. M. Kadin.)

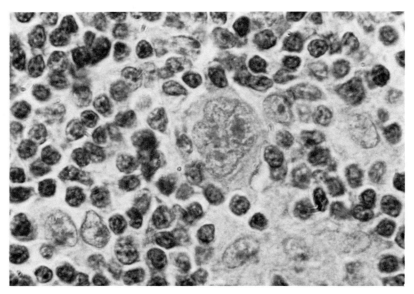

Figure 22.13 Lymph node showing Hodgkin's disease of the lymphocytic predominance type. Note the large multinucleate cell.

lymphocytic cells in the lymphoma. When lymphocytes are depleted, histiocytes tend to be prominent. *Mixed cellularity* is defined by a pleomorphic cellular infiltrate. *Nodular sclerosis* is defined by the presence of broad bands of collagen in the malignant lymph node.

More subtle histologic features are used to define further subclasses of Hodgkin's disease. For example, the lymphocytic depletion category may be accompanied by a disorderly diffuse fibrosis with infrequent Reed-Sternberg cells. In the reticular type of histologic pattern (sarcoma) there is diffuse overgrowth of neoplastic-appearing reticulum cells. In a variant of the nodular sclerosis type of disease that involves the thymus, Reed-Sternberg cells may be very rare (106, 184).

Classification of Hodgkin's disease into these various types is controversial. For example, three pathologists reviewed slides from 167 patients: all three agreed on histologic classifications 67 percent of the time, and two of the three agreed 92 percent of the time (186).

Nodular sclerosis is the most frequently encountered histologic type; lymphocyte predominance and lymphocyte depletion are relatively rare.

The following generalizations can be made about the relation between histologic type of disease and natural history (15, 31, 89, 115, 151, 186, 212, 238, 330, 335):

(a) Lymphocytic predominance carries the best prognosis for survival. Lymphocytic depletion and mixed cellu-

larity types have the worst prognosis. Nodular sclerosis is intermediate.

(b) Widespread disease (stages III and IV) and systemic symptoms are more frequently associated with lymphocytic depletion types of tumor. Localized disease (stages I and II) is more frequently associated with lymphocytic predominance and nodular sclerosis.

(c) Nodular sclerosis, when it is localized (stages I and II), occurs above the diaphragm; only very rarely does it involve the periaortic or iliac nodes.

(d) Hodgkin's disease seems to spread by contiguous involvement of adjacent lymph node groups (see below, Mode of Spread and Staging). When noncontiguous spread is encountered, it most often involves the lymphocytic depletion and mixed cellularity categories.

(e) Nodular sclerosis is about twice as frequent in females as in males. The other histologic types of tumor show a male predominance.

(f) Although there is considerable overlap in the age distribution of various histologic types of Hodgkin's disease, nodular sclerosis tends to involve the younger population (15 to 34 years of age).

Other histologic features of Hodgkin's disease may have prognostic implications. Recently Rappaport and Strum have pointed out that vascular invasion may indicate the occurrence of hematogenous dissemination (265).

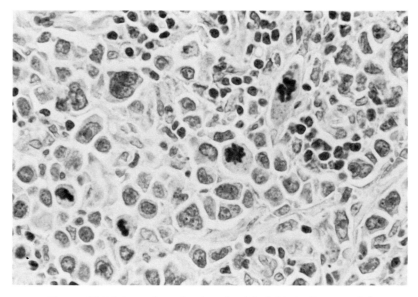

Figure 22.14 Lymph node showing Hodgkin's disease of the lymphocytic depletion type. Reed-Sternberg cells and mitotic figures are visible. Only a few small round cells (lymphocytes) are visible. The predominant cell resembles a poorly differentiated histiocyte. (Photograph courtesy of Dr. M. Kadin.)

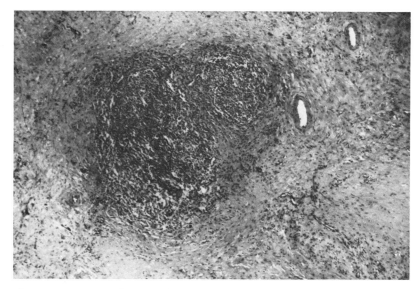

Figure 22.15 Lymph node showing Hodgkin's disease of the nodular sclerosis type. A nodule of small round cells is surrounded by "sclerotic" bands.

Mode of Spread and Staging

The stage of Hodgkin's disease in a given patient refers to the extent of the spread. Probably the most widely used staging classification in this country at the present time is that based on the 1966 Rye conference, later modified by investigators at Stanford University (285). The principal features of this classification system are given in Table 22.5.

There are two critical observations in the clinical approach to Hodgkin's disease: (*a*) in many instances the disease appears to progress in an orderly manner from one group of lymph nodes to another adjacent group—that is, the spread is contiguous; (*b*) in localized disease a sterilizing X-ray dose to the tumor kills or injures all tumor cells so that local recurrence is prevented. Detailed and accurate knowledge of the stage of disease is critically important, since *many patients with early lesions of localized disease can be cured by intensive local radiation therapy.*

Kaplan has commented recently on the evidence that Hodgkin's disease spreads by contiguous extension (182): "Analysis of the initial site of involvement in 340 consecutive, previously untreated cases of Hodgkin's disease revealed that over 90 percent of cases in stage II, III, and IV involved lymph node change that could be considered contiguous by the criterion of direct lymphocytic lymphatic communication. A similar pattern was also seen in cases in which post-treatment extensions occurred."

Table 22.5 Staging system for Hodgkin's disease.

Stage I	Involvement of a single lymph node region
Stage IE	Involvement of a single extralymphatic organ or site
Stage II$_n$	Involvement of two or more lymph node regions limited to one side of the diaphragm (*n* indicating the number of regions involved)
Stage IIE	Involvement of an extralymphatic organ or site and of one or more lymph node regions on the same side of the diaphragm
Stage III	Involvement of lymph node regions on both sides of the diaphragm
Stage IIIE	Same as III, but accompanied by localized involvement of extralymphatic organs
Stage IIIS	Same as III, but involving the spleen also
Stage IV	Disseminated disease in extralymphatic organs
A and B subclassification	The absence or presence respectively of unexplained fever, night sweats, or weight loss of more than 10 percent of body weight

SOURCE: Reference 285.

Other investigators have noted the same phenomenon (131, 256, 258, 262, 284).

A substantial number of patients (perhaps 10 percent) demonstrate noncontiguous distribution of disease in the lymphatic system. Often such a distribution involves

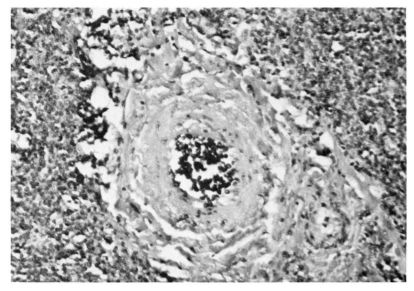

Figure 22.16 Section of lymph node from a patient with nodular sclerosis type of Hodgkin's disease.

"mediastinal skips," with disease in the cervical or supraclavicular area and in the periaortic lymph nodes, but not in the intermediate node areas (181, 284). It is thought that skipping may occur via retrograde flow in the thoracic duct.

In addition to orderly spread within the lymphatic system, other routes of dissemination have been defined. For example, the hilar lymph nodes may be the portal for the spread of Hodgkin's disease into the pulmonary parenchyma (182, 258). The upper periaortic nodes seem to be the gateway for spread to the spleen. Furthermore, Hodgkin's disease probably reaches the liver only after prior involvement of the spleen (136).

Subsequent to the Rye classification it has become clear that extralymphatic disease that is localized and related to adjacent lymph node disease does not adversely affect survival (45, 236); hence the introduction into the classification system of stages IIE and IIIE. For example, involvement of the supraclavicular and mediastinal lymph nodes with local extension from the hilum into the lung would be stage IIE. On the other hand, involvement of the liver or bone marrow always indicates stage IV disease.

Accurate clinical staging of Hodgkin's disease and other lymphomas requires meticulous investigation, including the following (280): history, physical examination, complete blood counts and erythrocyte sedimentation rate, roentgenograms of the chest (including tomography) and bones, intravenous pyelography, radioactive liver and spleen scans, liver function tests, bone marrow aspiration, and open biopsy (149). Relatively recent developments include the use of lymphangiography (202, 327, 342), peritoneoscopy (80), and diagnostic laparotomy including liver and lymph node biopsy and splenectomy (86, 150, 263). Scannings with radiostrontium and, more recently, with ⁶⁷gallium have been introduced as additional staging techniques. These procedures are still being evaluated (136, 152, 261). Difficulties are sometimes encountered in interpretation of the liver biopsy (134).

Testing for the presence of cutaneous anergy can also be helpful (3, 28); however, anergy occurs in a minority of patients with stage IV disease and thus is only a crude index of disease activity and extent of dissemination (362).

Incidence

Hodgkin's disease is universally distributed and does not have a known relation to occupation or social status. It is at least twice as common in males as in females and has a peak incidence in the third decade of life (216, 363). It has, however, been reported in children under three years of age (293) as well as in the very old. The age-incidence curves of Hodgkin's disease are bimodal, one mode falling in the 15 to 34 year age group and the other in old age (64, 217). More than 60 instances of familial disease have been reported (255).

In 1964 3,400 deaths caused by Hodgkin's disease were reported in the United States. This was approximately 1.2 percent of all deaths from cancer in this country. Hodgkin's disease is the most common form of lymphoma in Britain and the United States. By contrast, it is the least common form in Japan (5), where occurrence in young adults is negligible (216).

Clinical and Laboratory Manifestations; Prognosis

The common and uncommon clinical and laboratory manifestations of lymphocytic lymphomas have been discussed previously and resemble those of Hodgkin's disease. In the subsequent sections of this chapter we shall consider only those additional features that are unique to Hodgkin's disease or occur with unusual frequency in this disorder.

Prognostic Factors   As noted in Table 22.5 on the staging classification of Hodgkin's disease, particular attention is paid to the absence (A) or the presence (B) of documented symptoms, including weight loss, night sweats, and fever. Until recently the presence of generalized pruritus was also considered a sufficient criterion to indicate a B classification. The presence of these symptoms is important because they have prognostic implications. Disease with these symptoms has a worse prognosis than the same stage of disease without such symptoms. The lymphocytic depletion and mixed cellularity histologic types are more often associated with B symptoms than are the lymphocytic predominance and nodular sclerosis categories. Similarly, B symptoms are more likely to occur in stage III and IV disease than in stage I and II disease (335).

Other factors that are associated with a poor prognosis include the presence of lymphocytopenia, a high erythrocyte sedimentation rate, and severe anemia (326, 335). Lymphocytopenia is seen most frequently in the lymphocytic depletion category. The factors associated with more aggressive disease and an associated relatively poor prognosis are summarized in Table 22.6.

Clinical Manifestations in Lymph Nodes and Spleen   Enlarged lymph nodes are the most common early manifestation of Hodgkin's disease. Cervical glands are involved most frequently, followed by axillary and inguinal lymph nodes (323). Occasionally the mediastinal or retroperitoneal glands are involved first, and the patient comes to

Table 22.6 Factors indicating a relatively poor prognosis in Hodgkin's disease.

Lymphocyte depletion or mixed cellularity histologic types
Stage III or IV disease
B classification (objective symptoms)
High erythrocyte sedimentation rate
Lymphopenia
Severe anemia, in the absence of bleeding

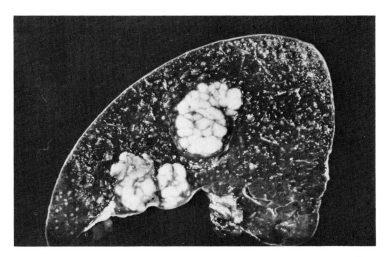

Figure 22.17 Nodules of tumor in the spleen of a patient with Hodgkin's disease.

the attention of a physician because of systemic symptoms or an abnormal chest roentgenogram. The nodes generally are painless, although Hodgkin's sarcomas (lymphocytic depletion, reticular type) occasionally may be painful (354). Splenic involvement by Hodgkin's disease is frequent and may be either diffuse or localized (Fig. 22.17).

Involvement of the tonsils and thyroid is rare in Hodgkin's disease relative to their involvement in other lymphomas (170, 348). Intrathoracic involvement occurs with about the same frequency in all types of lymphoma (283, 356). The roentgenographic picture may resemble primary lung cancer, metastatic cancer, or miliary tuberculosis. Pulmonary involvement occurs by extension of lymphatic disease and is rarely primary (329, 361). The diagnosis sometimes may be made from cytological analysis of the sputum, bronchial washings, or pleural fluid (325). Cardiac and pericardiac infiltration can occur in Hodgkin's disease as in other lymphomas. Panaortitis may be a complication of aggressive radiation therapy of these tumors (116).

Bone involvement by Hodgkin's disease is intermediate in frequency between that of lymphocytic and histiocytic lymphomas (344). In Hodgkin's disease the lesions are often osteoblastic; in lymphocytic lymphomas they are usually lytic. Osteoblastic involvement of a vertebra gives a characteristic "dead tooth" appearance. Involvement of the skull and extremities is rare (255).

Jaundice in Hodgkin's disease generally means hepatic infiltration by tumor, rarely extrahepatic obstruction (205, 206).

Neurologic manifestations in Hodgkin's disease have much the same characteristics as those associated with other lymphomas. Invasive disease of the brain has been described (122, 223, 295).

Fever in the absence of demonstrable infection is a frequent manifestation of Hodgkin's disease and is not usually observed in other lymphomas (137, 164, 204, 208). The occurrence of periodic pyrexia (Pel-Ebstein fever) (93) is more of historical interest than of clinical importance.

Despite the fact that pyrexia is part of the symptom complex of active Hodgkin's disease, a vigorous search for infectious agents should always be instituted when fever occurs. Infectious complications are frequent (47). Susceptibility to infection may result from immunologic abnormalities associated with underlying disease process or with drug-induced immunosuppression and granulocytopenia.

No characteristic feature of the peripheral blood is pathognomonic of Hodgkin's disease (30, 355). Anemia is frequent in stage III and IV disease. Frequently this anemia arises from shortened red cell survival and abnormal utilization of iron for erythropoiesis (62, 201). It is rarely Coombs positive. In active disease the "typical" leukocyte picture is granulocytosis, monocytosis, and lymphopenia. However, this typical picture is often absent. Extreme degrees of eosinophilia have been reported (11, 220). Only rarely are Reed-Sternberg cells seen in the circulation (290).

In one series Hodgkin's disease was identified in the bone marrow biopsy of 9 percent of untreated patients whose disease was more advanced than stage II (279, 280). A thorough search for bone marrow involvement should be made when there is an unexpected elevation of the serum alkaline phosphatase activity.

Relatively rare abnormalities of Hodgkin's disease include monoclonal light-chain excretion (207) and abnormalities of tryptophane metabolism and plasma pyridoxal phosphate (50). The more commonly abnormal laboratory values are those listed below, which include abnormalities of serum proteins (23):

Anemia
Granulocytosis
Eosinophilia
Lymphopenia
Monocytosis
Elevated erythrocyte sedimentation rate
Increased alpha globulins and other protein abnormalities
Increased serum alkaline phosphatase (indicating hepatic or bone involvement)
Increased serum copper

Immunologic Abnormalities

A number of investigations of the immunologic reactivity of patients with Hodgkin's disease have been conducted over the past 20 years. The following abnormalities were frequently observed: (a) impaired delayed hypersensitivity (51, 200, 291, 292); (b) delayed homograft rejection (188); and (c) defective lymphocyte transformation (147, 160, 171, 251). In contrast, primary (28) and secondary (51) antibody response is usually unimpaired. The described abnormalities are those of T-cell function, whereas B-cell function is intact (see Chapter 17). Interferon production (which may also be a T-cell function) may be abnormal in some patients with Hodgkin's disease and may contribute to difficulties in handling serious viral infections (6).

Listed below are the principal features that correlate with anergy in patients with Hodgkin's disease (362):

Advanced disease (stage III and IV)
B symptoms
Mixed cellularity and lymphocyte depletion
Lymphopenia

Anergy is relatively uncommon, occurring in only 12 percent of 103 patients in one study and in only 27 percent of patients with stage IV disease (362). Mumps antigen and dinitrochlorobenzene are the most useful skin tests for ruling out anergy. There is no correlation between skin test reactivity at the time of diagnosis and subsequent prognosis (362).

Recently, there has been some interest in the possibility of unique tumor-associated antigens occurring in Hodgkin's disease (247, 248). The significance of these "neo-antigens" is uncertain.

Course of the Disease

Only rarely do physicians in this country have an opportunity to see an unmodified natural history of Hodgkin's disease. Unmodified by therapy, the disease advances inexorably and ultimately kills the patient by one of a variety of mechanisms: infection, bleeding, or failure of a vital organ. Today, the patient may be cured if the disease is localized at the time of application of intensive radiation therapy, or the natural history may reflect both the progress of the disease and the effects of vigorous radiation therapy and chemotherapy.

With more effective therapy it has become necessary to establish a definition of cure in Hodgkin's disease. This is important for determining how long to continue therapy. Easson and Russell (92) have suggested: "We can speak of cure when in time—probably a decade or so after treatment—there remains a group of disease-free survivors whose progressive death rate from all causes is similar to that of a normal population of the same sex and age constitution." Some observations are pertinent: (a) for patients with stage I and II disease, at least 80 percent of those destined to relapse do so within four years, and more than 90 percent within ten years (118); (b) there is evidence that the curve of "relapse-free interval" may be qualitatively similar for stage I and II patients and for stage III and IV patients who have been treated intensively (118); and (c) a number of recent studies of long-term survival in Hodgkin's disease suggest that the chances of a permanent cure are excellent (52, 199, 310) if the patient is free of disease for ten years.

Associated Diseases

A variety of diseases has been reported to occur occasionally in association with Hodgkin's disease: acute leukemia, chronic lymphocytic leukemia (146), and Kaposi's sarcoma (132). The occurrence of Kaposi's sarcoma with Hodgkin's disease has been reported with such frequency that it is unlikely to be a chance association. The relation to leukemia is less clear cut. It is possible that leukemia sometimes may share a common etiology with Hodgkin's disease or that the treatment used in lymphoma is oncogenic (7).

Mycosis Fungoides and Sézary's Syndrome

Mycosis fungoides is a variety of lymphoma in which skin involvement is the most prominent manifestation. Recent students of this disorder believe that it originates in the skin and subsequently spreads to the lymph nodes and other organs, rather than the reverse (19, 341). Often there is a long, prodromal phase of nonspecific skin involvement before the frank appearance of malignant skin disease. In a large series of patients, the onset was variable: nonspecific dermatitis in 44 percent, psoriasiform dermatitis in 26 percent, and skin tumor in 14 percent (19, 99). The mean duration of the existence of skin lesions before the establishment of a diagnosis is 7.5 to 10 years, and cases are known in which this interval was 15 years.

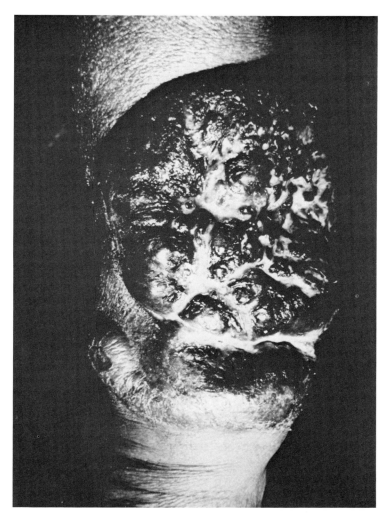

Figure 22.18 A large "fungating" skin lesion over the knee of a patient with advanced mycosis fungoides.

Once established, the skin lesions may be plaque-like (resembling psoriatic plaques), may be diffusely erythematous, or may be raised tumors with necrotic centers, as in Fig. 22.18. The raised tumors resemble those of serious mycotic infection, hence the name of the disease.

Early in mycosis fungoides the skin lesions are composed mainly of normal lymphoreticular cells; as the disease progresses, abnormal cells appear in greater number (345). The so-called mycosis cell has ultrastructural features that are distinct from the reticulum cell (111). The atypical cells may disappear with effective therapy. A characteristic histologic feature of the disorder is the Pautrier's microabscess.

Although this disease begins in the skin, lymph node involvement and systemic spread eventually occur in almost all untreated patients (121). Serial biopsies have

shown transition from reactive lymphadenopathy to obvious malignant lymphoma.

In addition to dramatic skin involvement, a variety of other clinical manifestations occurs (19, 99, 121). Eosinophilia is present in about one-half of infected patients, and hepatic involvement occurs in about 40 percent. Cardiac infiltration may occur in one-third of patients, and the roentgenographic appearance of the lung may resemble that of infiltration by metastatic tumor. Renal involvement and brain involvement (63) are rare complications.

Characteristic cells may circulate in the blood of patients with mycosis fungoides and the related Sézary's syndrome (29, 214) (Figs. 22.19 and 22.20). Similar cells occasionally are seen in the skin of patients with a variety of nonlyphomatous dermatoses (113).

Patients with mycosis fungoides appear to have a normal ability to produce circulating antibody and develop delayed hypersensitivity responses (18, 57). The skin lesions of mycosis fungoides may be altered by direct imposition of delayed hypersensitivity reactions (267).

In 1938 Sézary and Bouvrain described a syndrome comprised of edematous pigmented erythroderma, leonine facies, lymphadenopathy, and abnormal circulating cells that resemble the malignant histiocytes in the skin (302, 303) (Figs. 22.19 and 22.20). Later reports added further observations and described the abnormal circulating cells in detail (214, 331, 353). Clendenning suggested that Sézary's syndrome may be a leukemic phase of mycosis fungoides (56). Recent evidence suggests that the abnormal cells of mycosis fungoides and Sézary's syndrome are of T-cell origin (26, 94, 353).

Burkitt's Lymphoma

Burkitt's lymphoma was first described in 1958 as a common tumor of East African children (32). By 1960 the histopathology was well described (242) and the neoplasm was classified as a lymphoma with a distinctive morphologic pattern.

Histology

Biopsies of the Burkitt tumor show a microscopic appearance resembling a starry sky because of the presence of large, clear, mature histiocytes against a background of small, dark, immature lymphoid cells (44, 58, 87, 241, 332, 358) (Fig. 22.21). Such a "starry sky" appearance is striking, but not unique to Burkitt's lymphoma. It is described in other lymphocytic and histiocytic lymphomas of man (84, 244) and of animals (314). The lymphoid cells are poorly differentiated when seen by both light and electron microscopy (1). They are PAS-positive, but may stain with oil red-O (44). Mitoses are frequent. The Burkitt

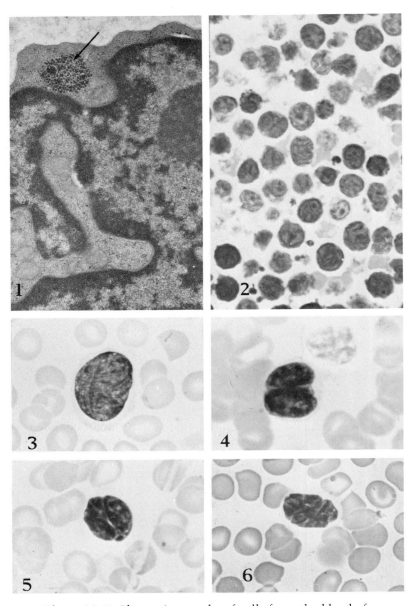

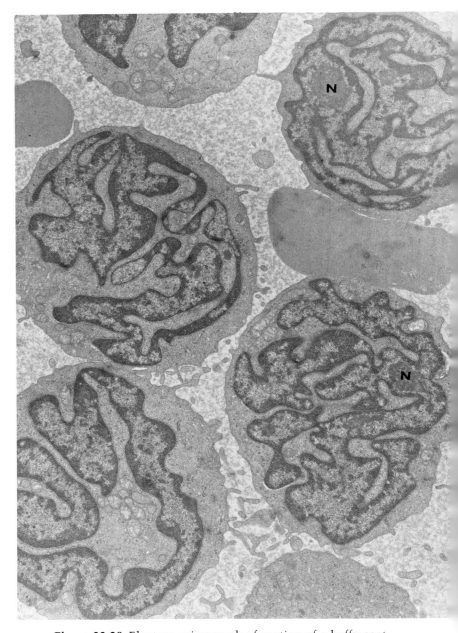

Figure 22.19 Photomicrographs of cells from the blood of a patient with Sézary's syndrome.

Panel 1: Portion of a Sézary cell from the peripheral blood. An aggregate of glycogen granules is seen in the cytoplasm (*arrow*). Uranyl and lead stained. Magnification approximately × 17,000.

Panel 2: Light micrograph. Portion of a buffy coat pellet prepared from the peripheral blood (1 μ semi-thin, plastic section, Azure II stained). Sézary cells with irregular, lobulated nuclei can be recognized. Magnification approximately × 1,000.

Panels 3–6: Peripheral blood films showing characteristic Sézary cells with nuclei that appear cerebriform with overlapping clefts and folds. Wright's stain. Magnification approximately × 1,100.

(From M. A. Lutzner and H. W. Jordan, *Blood* 31:719, 1968. Reprinted by permission of authors and publisher.)

Figure 22.20 Electron micrograph of portion of a buffy coat pellet from a patient with Sézary's syndrome. Four characteristic Sézary cells are shown. A nucleolus (*N*) is present in two of the cells. Nuclei are strikingly irregular, serpentine, indented, and lobulated. The nuclear pattern is heterochromatic, with nuclear particles concentrated at the nuclear membrane. Mitochondria can be seen in the cytoplasm. Uranyl and lead stained. Magnification approximately × 6,500. (From M. A. Lutzner and H. W. Jordan, *Blood* 31:719, 1968. Reprinted by permission of authors and publisher.)

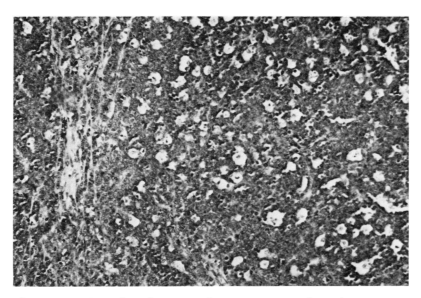

Figure 22.21 Lymph node section from a patient with Burkitt's lymphoma. Pale-staining histiocytes produce a starry sky appearance.

tumor cell may have a distinctive marker band in one chromosome (211).

Tumors histologically resembling Burkitt's lymphoma have been described in cats, dogs, and primates. The visceral lymphoma of cats most nearly resembles the African tumor in its clinical and pathological features (314, 317). A histologically similar tumor has been induced in Swiss mice by the inoculation of Rauscher virus (40).

Clinical Characteristics

In Africa Burkitt's tumor is predominantly, but not exclusively, a disease of childhood. Unlike other lymphomas, it commonly involves the jaw and long bones and paired abdominal and pelvic organs, while sparing the peripheral lymph nodes and spleen (58, 59, 241). The tumor may involve the thyroid and salivary glands. The involvement of the central nervous system may be prominent and is an indication for aggressive therapy (44). Unlike other childhood lymphomas, Burkitt's tumor rarely makes a leukemic transition (60, 324). Acute leukemia has occurred, however, in the sibling of a Burkitt's patient (320). When the tumor involves the bone marrow, the blood picture may be "leukoerythroblastic" (21, 359).

Burkitt's tumor is unusually responsive to chemotherapy, and long-enduring remissions may follow even a single course of cytotoxic drug (35, 37, 44). About 20 percent of patients have long-term remissions (233). Burkitt (36) and others have suggested that responsiveness to low-

dose chemotherapy may reflect host immune defenses against the tumor.

Immunologic responses in Burkitt's tumor patients are generally unimpaired, with the exception of a poor humoral response to primary antigens and a low serum IgM concentration in some patients with disseminated disease (44). Acute phase serum proteins are elevated in children with active tumor (215).

Geographic Distribution

Burkitt's lymphoma was originally described as occurring in a broad band across the tropical waist of Africa (16, 33, 34). Cases with similar histology and anatomic distribution have subsequently been reported from Papua-New Guinea (104, 332), Britain (13, 138, 299), Cuba (70), Puerto Rico (70), and Colombia (14).

A number of cases resembling Burkitt's lymphoma have been reported in the United States (44, 87, 203, 243, 364). In reviewing autopsy material obtained at Washington University between 1928 and 1964, Dorfman found several cases in children that had the typical histologic appearance and anatomical distribution characteristic of Burkitt's lymphoma (87).

In reviewing 148 cases of childhood lymphoma seen in the Armed Forces Institute of Pathology, O'Conor and his associates (243) found 20 tumors that resembled Burkitt's lymphoma biologically and morphologically. In a 1969 review of Burkitt's tumor at the National Institutes of Health, 21 cases were described (44). Despite the similarity of these tumors to the African lymphoma, it is not certain that they represent the same disease entity.

The typical lymphoma is found in high frequency in only certain areas of Africa and New Guinea (318). It is restricted to relatively low altitudes and is distributed in regions in which malaria is endemic. This association has led to two hypotheses; one suggests that a mosquito vector (144, 318) is the transmitter of disease, and the other suggests that immunologic suppression by malaria causes the expression of an oncogenic virus. Mosquitoes transmitted histiocytic lymphoma cells in one experimental animal model (12).

Serologic Abnormalities and Associated Virus

Continuously growing cell lines are readily established from Burkitt's lymphoma (221). In 1964 Epstein, Achong, and Barr (100, 101) examined cell cultures derived from two patients with Burkitt's tumor and detected virus particles morphologically resembling herpes virus. Particles of similar appearance subsequently were identified in other Burkitt's cell lines and occasionally in cell lines derived from patients with leukemia, infectious mononucleosis, Hodgkin's disease, and normal subjects (228, 231).

The virus particle identified in Burkitt's cells occurs in two forms: nonenveloped particles (75 mμ in diameter) distributed in nucleus and cytoplasm, and larger enveloped particles (110–115 mμ) located in the cytoplasm of lymphoblastoid cells. The larger particles appear to represent mature virus. The viral genome sometimes may be detected in Burkitt lymphoid cells even when serologic tests for viral antigens are negative (135). Viral DNA, although readily detectable in African Burkitt's lymphoma, was not found in similar disease in four American patients (249). The viruses appear to be immunologically distinct from any of the other known members of the herpes viruses of man and animals.

A number of techniques have been used to detect the prevalence and distribution of antibodies to this Epstein-Barr virus (EBV) in various populations: complement fixation (129, 157), membrane immunofluorescence (79, 192-195), blocking of immunofluorescence (196), cytotoxicity assay (105), and precipitin tests (245, 246). Of these, immunofluorescence has been applied most widely. Pearson and his colleagues (253) explored the relation between immunofluorescence of the Burkitt cell membrane and of the EBV. They concluded that antibodies directed against EBV antigen were different from antibodies reactive with the Burkitt cell membrane, although both types of antibody might be found in the same serum.

High levels of antibody to EBV are found associated with three diseases: Burkitt's lymphoma, infectious mononucleosis, and nasopharyngeal carcinoma (44, 79, 156).

In a prospective study, infectious mononucleosis was shown to occur only among individuals who had no antibody to EBV. During the incubation and early acute stages of the disease, antibodies regularly developed (158). High titers of antibody to EBV have been observed in occasional patients with Hodgkin's disease, systemic lupus erythematosus, sarcoidosis, and leprosy. In all these observations it has not been possible to discern whether the virus is playing an important role in the pathogenesis of disease or is merely a passenger. The case for an etiologic role for virus can be made most strongly in infectious mononucleosis.

There has been much speculation about the role of the immune system in the defense against Burkitt's lymphoma. That the role is significant has been deduced from the higher titers of reactive antibody, the frequency of cure by chemotherapy, and the observation of occasional spontaneous remissions (38). About one-half of patients with Burkitt's lymphoma in remission have delayed hypersensitivity reactions to autologous Burkitt's lymphoma protein extract (22).

Etiology of Lymphoma

Burkitt's lymphoma may be caused by a herpes-like virus; however, the case is by no means proven as it is a rather special malignancy in many ways. Relatively little is known about the etiology of the other more common lymphomas.

Epidemiologic Considerations

The suggestion that Hodgkin's disease incorporates more than one separate disease entity dates back almost to the original descriptions by Thomas Hodgkin and has been supported by more recent epidemiologic investigations demonstrating a bimodality of age-incidence curves (55, 90). The hypothesis has been most clearly delineated by Cole and his colleagues (64). With the possible exception of Burkitt's tumor, there is no evidence for horizontal transmission of the lymphomas—that is, these malignancies do not behave like communicable diseases. Only rarely do they show patterns of clustering in a geographic location or during a finite period of time (cf. 343). Lymphoreticular malignancies do occur in a higher frequency in association with certain congenital abnormalities of development of the lymphoreticular and hematopoietic systems than could be predicted by chance alone (67).

Recently RNA extracted from cells of Hodgkin's disease and other lymphomas has been shown to be homologous to those of a mouse leukemia virus (155). This observation has interesting implications for the etiology of the human disease, as does the recent demonstration of a C-type virus associated with a lymphosarcoma in the gibbon (185).

Immunologic Models

In addition to the known oncogenic agents—viruses, chemicals, and irradiation—it has long been suggested that immunologic mechanisms may be involved in the development of some neoplasms (71, 72, 110, 139, 183, 296, 336). Two examples can be used to illustrate this hypothesis. Schwartz and Beldotti (297) injected adult parental spleen cells into 4- to 6-week-old F_1 hybrid mice to produce a graft-vs-host reaction. A significant increase in lymphomas was observed in test animals as compared to controls. Walford (346, 347) injected adult spleen cells into newborn mice differing from the donor strain in only the weak histocompatibility H-1 locus. An increased frequency of lymphomas was observed in recipient animals.

Order and Hellman (248) have recently proposed a hypothesis for the pathogenesis of Hodgkin's disease in which T lymphocytes are presumed to undergo antigenic alteration in the course of viral infection. Normal, immunologically competent T cells of the same lymphoid organ react against the antigenically altered cells and initiate a chronic immune reaction that eventuates in neoplasia.

Lymphomas must now be considered a complication of renal allotransplantation. Three cases of reticulum cell sarcoma occurred in 151 renal allotransplant recipients in the course of 438 patient-years of survival. This incidence of 0.7 percent per year is more than 100 times greater than in the general population (254, 259). Reticulum cell sarcoma has developed at the site of antilymphocyte globulin injection in a renal transplant recipient (78). The presence of foreign transplantation antigens, together with immunosuppressive therapy, may be responsible for the strikingly increased incidence of lymphomas. The possible effects of immunosuppression on the development of neoplasia were discussed in more detail in Chapter 17.

Earlier we described how intense antigenic stimulation can produce a response in the lymphoreticular system that morphologically simulates lymphoma. We now come full circle and suggest that such stimulation, if sufficiently prolonged and intense, can induce lymphoma—particularly a lymphoma of the histiocytic cell type.

Principles of Therapy

Two observations are critical in the therapeutic approach to Hodgkin's disease and the lymphocytic lymphomas: (a)

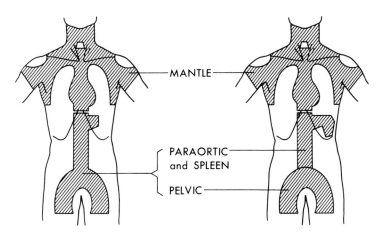

Figure 22.22 Schematic presentation of "mantle" and "inverted-Y" fields for lymphoid irradiation in lymphoma. The left-hand figure shows the fields excluding the spleen but including the splenic pedicle; the right-hand figure shows the fields for patients with intact spleens.

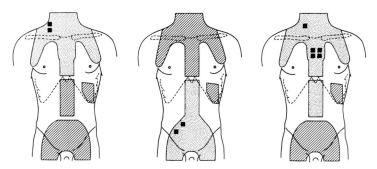

Figure 22.23 A schematic approach to the radiation therapy of patients with stage I and II Hodgkin's disease. The solid blocks (■) represent areas of identified disease. The stippled areas denote those usually treated by extended-field radiotherapy. The striped areas denote additional fields that would be included in total nodal irradiation.

in many instances the disease appears to progress in an orderly manner from one group of lymph nodes to another adjacent group; and (b) in localized disease, a sterilizing dose of X-ray to the tumor kills or injures all tumor cells so that local recurrence is prevented (175, 181, 237). Therefore, if one can identify all of the disease and if it is confined within the lymphatic system, it may be eradicated by intensive radiation therapy.

More than half the patients with Hodgkin's disease have localized tumor at the time of diagnosis and are potentially curable by radiation therapy. Localized disease at the time of diagnosis is much less common in the other malignant lymphomas; nevertheless, in some patients disease is localized and may also be cured by intensive radiation treatment. When disease is so widespread that radiation therapy with curative intent cannot be applied, then chemotherapy is indicated.

Radiation Therapy

Several radiation therapy centers have demonstrated that megavoltage radiation therapy of Hodgkin's disease produces a better survival rate than kilovoltage treatment (175, 176, 181, 237). The tumor recurrence rate is inversely related to the dosage of ionizing irradiation delivered: at 3,600 r tumor dose, the recurrence rate is 10 percent; at 4,000 r, it is less than 5 percent. Based on these observations the radiation therapist generally delivers about 4,000 r over a four-week period to the involved area or, more usually, to proximal extended fields (Figs. 22.22 and 22.23).

In patients with stage IA or IIA Hodgkin's disease there is only a slightly greater chance of increased survival time (and of time without clinically apparent disease) with extended-field therapy than with therapy of involved fields only. However, patients with stage IB or IIB disease receiving extended-field treatment do much better in survival rates and "disease-free" interval than those receiving limited therapy (237, 285).

The same difference probably exists in the response to limited vs extended-field radiation therapy in patients with IIIA Hodgkin's disease; however, data are still scanty (180, 181). Patients with a disease-free interval of two years have a 90-percent probability of a five-year survival (179). Stage IIIB and IV Hodgkin's disease should be treated with chemotherapy.

The five-year survival rate for all stages of Hodgkin's disease is about 73 percent (285); the comparable rate for other lymphomas is about 25 percent (283). In 1963 Peters reported the differences in survival among stage I, II, and III patients with non-Hodgkin's lymphoma as 50 percent, 23 percent, and 5 percent, respectively. She found that intensive radiation therapy of apparently uninvolved node areas did not improve survival (257). However, the dosage of radiation given to these patients was low by present-day standards. The guidelines for extent of radiation therapy as related to stage and histology of non-Hodgkin's lymphoma are not yet clearly defined.

Chemotherapy

In the past decade enormous strides have been made in the chemotherapeutic treatment of lymphomas. The beginnings of chemotherapy treatment can be traced to the introduction of nitrogen mustard into clinical medicine nearly 30 years ago (272). Appropriately used, this agent will produce remissions in 70 to 90 percent of patients with Hodgkin's disease; however, these are generally of short duration—about 10 weeks. When oral alkylating agents became available in the 1950s, Frei and Gamble (117) demonstrated that the disease-free interval could be prolonged if the drug was maintained during the period of remission. In the 1950s and 1960s adrenocorticosteroids also were shown to have some antitumor effect (145). From that time on, various new anticancer drugs have been introduced, some of which have clear efficacy against Hodgkin's disease and other lymphomas: vincristine, vinblastine, procarbazine, bis-chloronitrosourea, bleomycin, and adriamycin (61, 74, 75, 112, 191, 339).

The success of combination chemotherapy in the treatment of acute leukemia naturally led to applying this approach to the treatment of lymphoma. Studies in leukemia show that each chemotherapeutic agent has unique toxic properties and that a combination of agents does not necessarily result in additive toxicity; for example, methotrexate, 6-mercaptopurine, alkylating agents, and procarbazine are marrow-depressant; prednisone affects protein,

Table 22.7 Suggested conventional approach to the treatment of Hodgkin's disease and lymphocytic lymphoma.

Stage	Therapy
Hodgkin's disease	
IA, IIA	Extended-field radiation therapy
IIB, IIIA	Total nodal irradiation
IIIB, IVA, and IVB	Combination chemotherapy
Lymphocytic lymphoma	
I, II	Total nodal irradiation
III	Probably combination chemotherapy
IV	Combination chemotherapy

carbohydrate, and electrolyte metabolism; and vincristine has toxic effects mainly on peripheral nerves. The leukemia studies emphasize one other point: patients with partial remission tend to have shorter remission than those with complete remission.

One of the first drug combinations used in treatment of Hodgkin's disease was vinblastine and chlorambucil. This combination produced complete remissions in over half of treated patients, whereas either agent alone produced remissions in only about one-third of cases (337).

A major advance was made by the introduction of four-drug therapy for Hodgkin's disease (43, 83, 209). The agents (nitrogen mustard, vincristine, prednisone, and procarbazine) were administered during the first two weeks of monthly cycles. With such therapy, about 80 percent of previously untreated patients with Hodgkin's disease achieved a complete remission that was generally of long duration (83). The percentage of patients previously treated who achieved complete remission was smaller but still impressive (41, 42, 209).

Recently, combinations of cyclophosphamide, prednisone, and vincristine have been used in the management of patients with disseminated non-Hodgkin's lymphoma. Again, the multiple agents used together are clearly superior to single agents (10, 211, 235, 301).

A suggested approach to the treatment of Hodgkin's disease and lymphocytic lymphomas is outlined in Table 22.7 and in a recent review by DeVita and Canellos (81).

Summary

The lymphomas are classified on the basis of predominant cell type, degree of preservation of the nodal architecture, and identifying features such as Reed-Sternberg cells. The histologic categories of lymphoma correspond to clinical diseases with differing natural history and prognosis. In recent years aggressive radiation therapy and chemotherapy have been able to control and sometimes cure certain lymphomas.

Chapter 22 References

1. Achong, B. G., and Epstein, M. A. Fine structure of the Burkitt tumor, *J. Natl. Cancer Inst.* 36:877, 1966.
2. Adams, J. H., and Jackson, J. M. Intracerebral tumours of reticular tissue: the problem of microgliomatosis and reticulo-endothelial sarcomas of the brain, *J. Pathol. Bacteriol.* 91:369, 1966.
3. Aisenberg, A. C. Studies on delayed hypersensitivity in Hodgkin's disease, *J. Clin. Invest.* 41:1964, 1962.
4. Anday, G. J., Goodman, J. R., and Tishkoff, G. H. An unusual cytoplasmic ribosomal structure in pathologic lymphocytes, *Blood* 41:439, 1973.
5. Anderson, R. E., Ishida, K., Li, Y., Ishimaru, T., and Nishiyama, H. Geographic aspects of malignant lymphoma and multiple myeloma. Select comparisons involving Japan, England, and the United States, *Am. J. Pathol.* 61:85, 1970.
6. Armstrong, R. W., Gurwith, M. J., Waddell, D., and Merigan, T. C. Cutaneous interferon production in patients with Hodgkin's disease and other cancers infected with varicella or vaccinia, *N. Engl. J. Med.* 283:1182, 1970.
7. Arseneau, J. C., Sponzo, R. W., Levin, D. L., Schnipper, L. E., Bonner, H., Young, R. C., Canellos, G. P., Johnson, R. E., and DeVita, V. T. Nonlymphomatous malignant tumors complicating Hodgkin's disease, *N. Engl. J. Med.* 287:1119, 1972.
8. Bagby, G. C., Jr., Goldman, R. D., Newman, H. C., and Means, J. F. Acute myocardial infarction due to childhood lymphoma, *N. Engl. J. Med.* 287:338, 1972.
9. Baggenstoss, A. H., and Heck, F. J. Follicular lymphoblastoma (giant follicle hyperplasia of lymph nodes and spleen), *Am. J. Med. Sci.* 200:17, 1940.
10. Bagley, C. M., DeVita, V. T., Jr., Berard, C. W., and Canellos, G. P. Advanced lymphosarcoma: intensive cyclical combination chemotherapy with cycloposphamide, vincristine, and prednisone, *Ann. Intern. Med.* 76:227, 1972.
11. Baker, C., and Mann, W. N. Hodgkin's disease. A study of sixty-five cases, *Guys Hosp. Rep.* 89:83, 1939.
12. Banfield, W. G., Woke, P. A., and Mackay, C. M. Mosquito transmission of lymphomas, *Cancer* 19:1333, 1966.
13. Baskerville, A., Hunt, A. C., and Lucke, V. M. Burkitt's lymphoma in Great Britain, *Lancet* 2:547, 1966.
14. Beltran, G. Childhood lymphoma in Colombia, South America. With special mention of cases resembling Burkitt's tumor, *Cancer* 19:1124, 1966.
15. Berard, C. W., Thomas, L. B., Axtell, L. M., Kruse, M., Newell, G., and Kagan, R. The relationship of histopathological subtype to clinical stage of Hodgkin's disease at diagnosis, *Cancer Res.* 31:1776, 1971.
16. Berry, C. G. Lymphoma syndrome in Northern Nigeria, *Br. Med. J.* 3:668, 1964.
17. Bingham, C. T., and Quarrier, S. S. Reticulum cell sarcoma. Report of a case with pronounced cutaneous manifestations, *Arch. Dermatol.* 41:722, 1940.
18. Blaylock, W. K., Clendenning, W. E., Carbone, P. P., and Van Scott, E. J. Normal immunologic reactivity in patients with the lymphoma mycosis fungoides, *Cancer* 19:233, 1966.
19. Block, J. B., Edgcomb, J., Eisen, A., and Van Scott, E. J. Mycosis fungoides. Natural history and aspects of its relationship to other malignant lymphomas, *Am. J. Med.* 34:228, 1963.
20. Bluefarb, S. M., and Webster, J. R. Kaposi's sarcoma associated with lymphosarcoma, *Arch. Intern. Med.* 91:97, 1953.
21. Bluming A. Z., Ziegler, J. L., and Carbone, P. P. Bone marrow involvement in Burkitt's lymphoma: results of a prospective study, *Br. J. Haematol.* 22:369, 1972.
22. Bluming A. Z., Ziegler, J. L., Fass, L., et al. Delayed cutaneous sensitivity reactions to autologous Burkitt lymphoma protein extract. Results of a two and a half year study, *Clin. Exp. Immunol.* 9:713, 1971.
23. Boggs, D. R., and Fahey, J. L. Serum-protein changes in malignant disease. II. The chronic leukemias, Hodgkin's disease, and malignant melanoma, *J. Natl. Cancer Inst.* 25:1381, 1960.
24. Borella, L. Reticulum cell sarcoma in children, *Cancer* 17:26, 1964.
25. Brain, W. R. B., and Norris, F. H., Jr. The Remote Effects of Cancer on the Nervous System; the Proceedings of a Symposium, Grune & Stratton, New York, 1965.
26. Bronet, J-C., Flandrin, G., and Seligmann, M. Indications of the thymus-derived nature of the proliferating cells in six patients with Sézary's syndrome, *N. Engl. J. Med.* 289:341, 1973.
27. Browder, A. A., Huff, J. W., and Petersdorf, R. G. The significance of fever in neoplastic disease, *Ann. Intern. Med.* 55:932, 1961.
28. Brown, R. S., Haynes, H. A., Foley, H. T., Godwin, H. A., Berard, C. W., and Carbone, P. P. Hodgkin's disease. Immunologic, clinical, and histologic features of 50 untreated patients, *Ann. Intern. Med.* 67:291, 1967.
29. Brownlee, T. R., and Murad, T. M. Ultrastructure of mycosis fungoides, *Cancer* 26:686, 1970.
30. Bunting, C. H. The blood picture in Hodgkin's disease. Second paper, *Bull. Johns Hopkins Hosp.* 25:173, 1914.
31. Burke, W. A., Burford, T. H., and Dorfman, R. F. Hodgkin's disease of the mediastinum, *Ann. Thorac. Surg.* 3:287, 1967.
32. Burkitt, D. A sarcoma involving the jaws in African children, *Br. J. Surg.* 46:218, 1958.
33. Burkitt, D. Observations on the geography of malignant lymphoma, *East Afr. Med. J.* 38:511, 1961.
34. Burkitt, D. A tumour syndrome affecting children in tropical Africa, *Postgrad. Med. J.* 38:71, 1962.
35. Burkitt, D. African lymphoma. Observations on response to vincristine sulphate therapy, *Cancer* 19:1131, 1966.
36. Burkitt, D. Long-term remissions following one and two-dose chemotherapy for African lymphoma, *Cancer* 20:756, 1967.
37. Burkitt, D., Hutt, M. S. R., and Wright, D. H. The African lymphoma. Preliminary observations on

response to therapy, *Cancer* 18:399, 1965.

38. Burkitt, D., and Kyalwazi, S. K. Spontaneous remission of African lymphoma, *Br. J. Cancer* 21:14, 1967.

39. Butler, J. J. Non-neoplastic lesions of lymph nodes of man to be differentiated from lymphomas, *Natl. Cancer Inst. Monogr.* 32:233, 1969.

40. Butler, J. J., Szakacs, A., and Sinkovics, J. G. Virus-induced murine lymphoma resembling Burkitt's tumor, *Am. J. Pathol.* 51:629, 1967.

41. Canellos, G. P., Young, R. C., Berard, C. W., and DeVita, V. T. Combination chemotherapy and survival in advanced Hodgkin's disease, *Arch. Intern. Med.* 131:388, 1973.

42. Canellos, G. P., Young, R. C., and DeVita, V. T. Combination chemotherapy for advanced Hodgkin's disease in relapse following extensive radiotherapy, *Clin. Pharmacol. Ther.* 13:750, 1972.

43. Carbone, P. P. Management with combination therapy, *J.A.M.A.* 223:165, 1973.

44. Carbone, P. P., Berard, C. W., Bennett, J. M., Ziegler, J. L., Cohen, M. H., and Gerber, P. NIH clinical staff conference: Burkitt's tumor, *Ann. Intern. Med.* 70:817, 1969.

45. Carbone, P. P., Kaplan, H. S., Musshoff, K., Smithers, D. W., and Tubiana, M. Report of the committee on Hodgkin's disease staging classification, *Cancer Res.* 31:1860, 1971.

46. Carney, E. K., Oppelt, W. W., Gleason, W. L., and Brindley, C. O. Cardiac Hodgkin's disease. A clinical, hemodynamic, and angiocardiographic evaluation of a case, *Am. Heart J.* 64:106, 1962.

47. Casazza, A. R., Duvall, C. P., and Carbone, P. P. Summary of infectious complications occurring in patients with Hodgkin's disease, *Cancer Res.* 26:1290, 1966.

48. Casazza, A. R., Duvall, C. P., and Carbone, P. P. Infection in lymphoma. Histology, treatment, and duration in relation to incidence and survival, *J.A.M.A.* 197:710, 1966.

49. Case Records of the Massachusetts General Hospital: Case 27-1968. Presentation of a case, *N. Engl. J. Med.* 279:33, 1968.

50. Chabner, B. A., DeVita, V. T., Livingston, D. M., and Oliverio, V. T. Abnormalities of tryptophan metabolism and plasma pyridoxal phosphate in Hodgkin's disease, *N. Engl. J. Med.* 282:838, 1970.

51. Chase, M. W. Delayed-type hypersensitivity and the immunology of Hodgkin's disease, with a parallel examination of sarcoidosis, *Cancer Res.* 26:1097, 1966.

52. Chawla, P. L., Stutzman, L., Dubois, R. E., Kim, U., and Sokal, J. E. Long survival in Hodgkin's disease, *Am. J. Med.* 48:85, 1970.

53. Churg, J., and Strauss, L. Allergic granulomatosis, allergic angiitis, and periarteritis nodosa, *Am. J. Pathol.* 27:277, 1951.

54. Clarkson, B. Formal discussion: on the cellular origins and distinctive features of cultured cell lines derived from patients with leukemias and lymphomas, *Cancer Res.* 27:2483, 1967.

55. Clemmesen, J. Statistical Studies in the Aetiology of Malignant Neoplasms, Munksgaard, Copenhagen, 1965.

56. Clendenning, W. E., Brecher, G., and Van Scott, E. J. Mycosis fungoides. Relationship to malignant cutaneous reticulosis and the Sézary syndrome, *Arch. Dermatol.* 89:785, 1964.

57. Clendenning, W. E., and Van Scott, E. J. Skin autografts and homografts in patients with the lymphoma mycosis fungoides, *Cancer Res.* 25:1844, 1965.

58. Clifford, P. Malignant disease of the nose, paranasal sinuses and postnasal space in East Africa, *J. Laryngol.* 75:707, 1961.

59. Clifford, P. Further studies in the treatment of Burkitt's lymphoma, *East Afr. Med. J.* 43:179, 1966.

60. Clift, R. A., Wright, D. H., and Clifford, P. Leukemia in Burkitt's lymphoma, *Blood* 22:243, 1963.

61. Cline, M. J., and Haskell, C. M. Cancer Chemotherapy, 2nd ed., W. B. Saunders, Philadelphia, 1975.

62. Cline, M. J., and Berlin, N. I. Anemia in Hodgkin's disease, *Cancer* 16:526, 1963.

63. Clinicopathologic conference. Mycosis fungoides with pulmonary and neurologic complications, *Am. J. Med.* 42:129, 1967.

64. Cole, P., MacMahon, B., and Aisen-

berg, A. Mortality from Hodgkin's disease in the United States. Evidence for the multiple-aetiology hypothesis, *Lancet* ii:1371, 1968.

65. Conklin, S. D., and Gent, D. H. Lymphosarcoma of the thyroid: report of a case, *Ann. Intern. Med.* 46:784, 1957.

66. Cooley, J. C., McDonald, J. R., and Clagett, O. T. Primary lymphoma of the lung, *Ann. Surg.* 143:18, 1956.

67. Cooper, M., Peterson, R. D. A., Gabrielsen, A. E., and Good, R. A. Lymphoid malignancy and development, differentiation, and function of the lymphoreticular system, *Cancer Res.* 26:1165, 1966.

68. Cornog, J. L., Jr., and Enterline, H. T. Lymphangiomyoma, a benign lesion of chyliferous lymphatics synonymous with lymphangiopericytoma, *Cancer* 19:1909, 1966.

69. Cottier, H., Turk, J., and Sobin, L. A proposal for a standardized system of reporting human lymph node morphology in relation to immunologic function, *Bull. W.H.O.* 47:375, 1972.

70. Dalldorf, G., Linsell, C. A., Barnhart, F. E., and Martyn, R. An epidemiologic approach to the lymphomas of African children and Burkitt's sarcoma of the jaws, *Perspect. Biol. Med.* 7:435, 1964.

71. Dameshek, W. Immunocytes and immunoproliferative disorders, *in* G. E. W. Wolstenholme and R. Porter (eds.), Ciba Foundation Symposium, The Thymus, p. 399, Little, Brown and Co., Boston, 1966.

72. Dameshek, W., and Schwartz, R. A. Leukemia and auto-immunization — some possible relationships, *Blood* 14:1151, 1959.

73. Davis, F. M., and Olivetti, R. G. Primary lymphosarcomatosis of kidneys, adrenal glands and perirenal adipose tissue, *J. Urol.* 66:106, 1951.

74. DeBast, C., Moriame, N., Wanet, J., Ledoux, M., Achten, G., and Kenis, Y. Bleomycin in mycosis fungoides and reticulum cell lymphoma, *Arch. Dermatol.* 104:508, 1971.

75. DeConti, R. C. Procarbazine in the management of late Hodgkin's disease, *J.A.M.A.* 215:927, 1971.

76. Deeb, P. H., and Stilson, W. L. Roentgenologic manifestations of

lymphosarcoma of the small bowel, *Radiology* 63:235, 1954.

77. Denham, S., Hall, J. G., Wolf, A., and Alexander, P. The nature of the cytotoxic cells in lymph following primary antigenic challenge, *Transplantation* 7:194, 1969.

78. Deodhard, S. D., Kuklinca, A. G., Vidt, D. G., Robertson, A. L., and Hazard, J. B. Development of reticulum cell sarcoma at the site of antilymphocyte globulin injection in a patient with renal transplant, *N. Engl. J. Med.* 280:1104, 1969.

79. DeSchryver, A., Friberg, S., Jr., Klein, G., Henle, W., Henle, G., de-Thé, G., Clifford, P., and Ho, H. C. Epstein-Barr virus-associated antibody patterns in carcinoma of the post-nasal space, *Clin. Exp. Immunol.* 5:443, 1969.

80. DeVita, V. T., Jr., Bagley, C. M., Jr., Goodell, B., O'Kieffe, D. A., and Trujillo, N. P. Peritoneoscopy in the staging of Hodgkin's disease, *Cancer Res.* 31:1746, 1971.

81. DeVita, V. T., Jr., and Canellos, G. P. Treatment of the lymphomas, *Semin. Hematol.* 9:193, 1972.

82. DeVita, V. T., Jr., and Carbone, P. P. Chemotherapeutic implications of staging in Hodgkin's disease, *Cancer Res.* 31:1838, 1971.

83. DeVita, V. T., Jr., Serpick, A. A., and Carbone, P. P. Combination chemotherapy in the treatment of advanced Hodgkin's disease, *Ann. Intern. Med.* 73:881, 1970.

84. Diamandopoulos, G. T., and Smith, E. B. Phagocytosis in reticulum cell sarcoma, *Cancer* 17:329, 1964.

85. Diamond, H. D., Williams, H. M., and Craver, L. F. The pathogenesis and management of neurological complications of malignant lymphomas and leukemia, *Acta Un. Int. contra Cancr.* 16:831, 1960.

86. Donaldson, S. S., Moore, M. R., Rosenberg, S. A., and Vosti, K. L. Characterization of postsplenectomy bacteremia among patients with and without lymphoma, *N. Engl. J. Med.* 287:69, 1972.

87. Dorfman, R. F. Childhood lymphosarcoma in St. Louis, Missouri, clinically and histologically resembling Burkitt's tumor, *Cancer* 18:418, 1965.

88. Dorfman, R. F. Ultrastructural studies of Hodgkin's disease, *Natl. Cancer Inst. Monogr.* 36:221, 1973.

89. Dorfman, R., and Reinhard, E. Hodgkin's disease, *J.A.M.A.* 208:326, 1969.

90. Dörken, H. Über die Altersverteilung der Lymphogranulomatose, *Klin. Wochenschr.* 38:944, 1960.

91. Duke-Elder, S. W. Textbook of Ophthalmology, vol. 5, C. V. Mosby Co., St. Louis, 1952.

92. Easson, E. C., and Russell, M. H. The cure of Hodgkin's disease, *Br. Med. J.* 2:1704, 1963.

93. Ebstein, W. Das chronische Rückfallsfieber, eine neue Infektionskrankheit, *Berl. Klin. Wochenschr.* 24:565, 837; 1887.

94. Edelson, R. L., Kirkpatrick, C. H., Shevach, E. M., et al. Preferential cutaneous infiltration by neoplastic thymus-derived lymphocytes, *Ann. Intern. Med.* 80:685, 1974.

95. Eidelman, S., Parkins, R. A., and Rubin, C. E. Abdominal lymphoma presenting as malabsorption: a clinico-pathologic study of nine cases in Israel and a review of the literature, *Medicine* 45:111, 1966.

96. Elmer, R. F., and Boylan, C. E. Reticulum cell sarcoma of kidney. With a case report, *Ill. Med. J.* 66:83, 1934.

97. Enterline, H. T., and Roberts, B. Lymphangiopericytoma. Case report of a previously undescribed tumor type, *Cancer* 8:582, 1955.

98. Epstein, E., and MacEachern, K. Dermatologic manifestations of the lymphoblastoma-leukemia group, *Arch. Intern. Med.* 60:867, 1937.

99. Epstein, E. H., Levin, D. L., Croft, J. D., and Lutzner, M. A. Mycosis fungoides: survival, prognostic features, response to therapy and autopsy findings, *Medicine* 15:61, 1972.

100. Epstein, M. A., Achong, B. G., and Barr, Y. M. Virus particles in cultured lymphoblasts from Burkitt's lymphoma, *Lancet* 1:702, 1964.

101. Epstein, M. A., Barr, Y. M., and Achong, B. G. Studies with Burkitt's lymphoma, *in* V. Defendi (ed.), Methodological Approaches to the Study of Leukemias, Wistar Inst. Symp. Monogr. 4:69, 1965.

102. Evans, N. Lymphadenitis of secondary syphilis; its resemblance to giant follicular lymphadenopathy, *Arch. Pathol.* 37:175, 1944.

103. Falconer, E. H., and Leonard, M. E. Skeletal lesions in Hodgkin's disease, *Ann. Intern. Med.* 29:1115, 1948.

104. Farago, C. Report of 1160 registered tumor cases in Papua and New Guinea, *Cancer* 16:670, 1963.

105. Fass, L., and Herberman, R. B. Evaluation of a complement-dependent human cytotoxic antibody reactive with Burkitt's lymphoma biopsy cells, *Proc. Soc. Exp. Biol. Med.* 133:286, 1970.

106. Fechner, R. E. Hodgkin's disease of the thymus, *Cancer* 23:16, 1969.

107. Federman, J., Goldstein, M. E., and Weingarten, B. Malignant lymphoma of over fifteen years' duration masquerading as ulcerative colitis, *Am. J. Roentgenol.* 89:771, 1963.

108. Feldaker, M., Kierland, R. R., and Montgomery, H. Cutaneous lymphoblastoma. Report of two unusual cases of reticulum cell sarcoma with emphasis on cutaneous touch smears, *Arch. Dermatol.* 70:583, 1954.

109. Felson, B. The roentgen diagnosis of disseminated pulmonary alveolar diseases, *Semin. Roentgenol.* 2:3, 1967.

110. Fialkow, P. J. "Immunologic" oncogenesis, *Blood* 30:388, 1967.

111. Fisher, E. R., Horvat, B. L., and Wechsler, H. L. Ultrastructural features of mycosis fungoides, *Am. J. Clin. Pathol.* 58:99, 1972.

112. Flatow, F. A., Ultmann, J. E., Hyman, G. A., and Muggia, F. M. Treatment of advanced Hodgkin's disease with vinblastine (NSC-49842) or procarbazine (NSC-77213), *Cancer Chemother. Rep.* 53:39, 1969.

113. Flaxman, B. A., Zelazny, G., and Van Scott, E. J. Nonspecificity of characteristic cells in mycosis fungoides, *Arch. Dermatol.* 104:141, 1971.

114. Frack, M. D., Simon, L., and Dawson, B. H. The lymphangiomyomatosis syndrome, *Cancer* 22:428, 1968.

115. Franssila, K. O., Kalima, T. V., and Voutilainen, A. Histologic classification of Hodgkin's disease, *Cancer* 20:1594, 1967.

116. Fraumeni, J. F., Jr., Herweg, J. C., and Kissane, J. M. Panaortitis complicating Hodgkin's disease, *Ann. Intern. Med.* 67:1242, 1967.

117. Frei, E. III, and Gamble, J. F.

Progress in the chemotherapy of Hodgkin's disease, *Cancer* 19:378, 1966.

118. Frei, E. III, and Gehan, E. A. Definition of cure for Hodgkin's disease, *Cancer Res.* 31:1828, 1971.

119. Frenkel, J. K. Role of corticosteroids as predisposing factors in fungal diseases, *Lab. Invest.* 11:1192, 1962.

120. Friedman, A. I. Primary lymphosarcoma of the stomach. A clinical study of seventy-five cases, *Am. J. Med.* 26:783, 1959.

121. Fuks, Z. Y., Bagshaw, M., and Farber, E. M. Prognostic signs and management of mycosis fungoides, *Cancer* 32:1385, 1973.

122. Gaelen, L. H., and Levitan, S. Solitary intracranial metastasis by Hodgkin's disease, *Arch. Intern. Med.* 120:740, 1967.

123. Gall, E. A. The enlarged lymph node: differential diagnosis, *in* G. T. Pack and I. M. Ariel (eds.), Treatment of Cancer and Allied Diseases, vol. 9, Lymphomas and Related Diseases, p. 28, Harper & Row, New York, 1964.

124. Gall, E. A., and Mallory, T. B. Malignant lymphoma. A clinicopathologic survey of 618 cases, *Am. J. Pathol.* 18:381, 1942.

125. Gall, E. A., and Stout, H. A. The histological lesion in lymph nodes in infectious mononucleosis, *Am. J. Pathol.* 16:433, 1940.

126. Garrison, C. O., Dines, D. E., Harrison, E. G., Jr., et al. The alveolar pattern of pulmonary lymphoma, *Mayo Clin. Proc.* 44:260, 1969.

127. Garvin, A. J., Spicer, S. S., Parmley, R. T., and Munster, A. M. Immunohistochemical demonstration of IgG in Reed-Sternberg and other cells in Hodgkin's disease, *J. Exp. Med.* 139:1077, 1974.

128. Geller, S. A., and Stimmel, B. Diagnostic confusion from lymphatic lesions in heroin addicts, *Ann. Intern. Med.* 78:703, 1973.

129. Gerber, P., and Birch, S. M. Complement-fixing antibodies in sera of human and nonhuman primates to viral antigens derived from Burkitt's lymphoma cells, *Proc. Natl. Acad. Sci. U.S.A.* 58:478, 1967.

130. Gibson, T. E. Lymphosarcoma of kidney, *J. Urol.* 60:838, 1948.

131. Gilbert, R. Radiotherapy in Hodgkin's disease (malignant granulomatosis). Anatomic and clinical foundations governing principles, results, *Am. J. Roentgenol.* 41:198, 1939.

132. Gilbert, T. T., Evjy, J. T., and Edelstein, L. Hodgkin's disease associated with Kaposi's sarcoma and malignant melanoma, *Cancer* 28:293, 1971.

133. Gilliam, A. G. Age, sex, and race selection at death from leukemia and the lymphomas, *Blood* 8:693, 1953.

134. Givler, R. L., Brunk, S. F., Hass, C. A., and Gulesserian, H. P. Problems of interpretation of liver biopsy in Hodgkin's disease, *Cancer* 28:1335, 1971.

135. Glaser, R., and Nonoyama, M. Epstein-Barr virus: detection of genome in somatic cell hybrids of Burkitt's lymphoblastoid cells, *Science* 179:492, 1973.

136. Glatstein, E., Guernsey, J. M., Rosenberg, S. H., and Kaplan, H. S. The value of laparotomy and splenectomy in the staging of Hodgkin's disease, *Cancer* 24:709, 1969.

137. Goldman, L. B. Hodgkin's disease: an analysis of 212 cases, *J.A.M.A.* 114:1611, 1940.

138. Gough, J. Significance of a "starry sky" in lymphosarcomata in Britain, *J. Clin. Pathol.* 20:578, 1967.

139. Green, H. N. An immunological concept of cancer: a preliminary report, *Br. Med. J.* 2:1374, 1954.

140. Greenberg, S. D., Heisler, J. G., Gyorkey, F., and Jenkins, D. E. Pulmonary lymphoma versus pseudolymphoma: a perplexing problem, *South. Med. J.* 65:775, 1972.

141. Greenspan, R. H. Chronic disseminated alveolar diseases of the lung, *Semin. Roentgenol.* 2:77, 1967.

142. Griffin, J. W., Thompson, R. W., Mitchinson, M. J., de Kiewet, J. C., and Welland, F. H. Lymphomatous leptomeningitis, *Am. J. Med.* 51:200, 1971.

143. Groch, G. S., Perillie, P. E., and Finch, S. C. Reticuloenthelial phagocytic function in patients with leukemia, lymphoma and multiple myeloma, *Blood* 26:489, 1965.

144. Haddow, A. J. Age incidence in Burkitt's lymphoma syndrome, *East Afr. Med. J.* 41:1, 1964.

145. Hall, T. C., Choi, O. S., Abadi, A., and Krant, M. J. High-dose corticoid therapy in Hodgkin's disease and other lymphomas, *Ann. Intern. Med.* 66:1144, 1967.

146. Han, T. Chronic lymphocytic leukemia in Hodgkin's disease, *Cancer* 28:300, 1971.

147. Han, T., and Sokal, J. E. Lymphocyte response to phytohemagglutinin in Hodgkin's disease, *Am. J. Med.* 48:728, 1970.

148. Han, T., and Stutzman, L. Mode of spread in patients with localized malignant lymphoma, *Arch. Intern. Med.* 120:1, 1967.

149. Han, T., Stutzman, L., and Rogue, A. L. Bone marrow biopsy in Hodgkin's disease and other neoplastic diseases, *J.A.M.A.* 217:1239, 1971.

150. Hanks, G. E., Terry, L. N., Jr., Bryan, J. A., and Newsome, J. F. Contribution of diagnostic laparotomy to staging non-Hodgkin's lymphoma, *Cancer* 29:41, 1972.

151. Hanson, T. A. S. Histological classification and survival in Hodgkin's disease. A study of 251 cases with special reference to nodular sclerosing Hodgkin's disease, *Cancer* 17:1595, 1964.

152. Harbert, J. C., and Ashburn, W. L. Radiostrontium bone scanning in Hodgkin's disease, *Cancer* 22:58, 1968.

153. Hartsock, R. J. Postvaccinial lymphadenitis-hyperplasia of lymphoid tissue that simulates malignant lymphomas, *Cancer* 21:632, 1968.

154. Hartsock, R. J., Halling, L. W., and King, F. M. Luetic lymphadenitis: an analysis of 18 cases, *Am. J. Clin. Pathol.* 49:260, 1968.

155. Hehlmann, R., Kufe, D., and Spiegelman, S. Viral-related RNA in Hodgkin's disease and other human lymphomas, *Proc. Natl. Acad. Sci. U.S.A.* 69:1727, 1972.

156. Henle, G., and Henle, W. Immunofluorescence in cells derived from Burkitt's lymphoma, *J. Bacteriol.* 91:1248, 1966.

157. Henle, G., and Henle, W. Immunofluorescence, interference and complement fixation technics in the detection of the Herpes-type virus in Burkitt tumor cell lines, *Cancer Res.* 27:2442, 1967.

158. Henle, G., Henle, W., and Diehl, V. Relation of Burkitt's tumor-associated Herpes-type virus to infec-

tious mononucleosis, *Proc. Natl. Acad. Sci. U.S.A.* 59:94, 1968.

159. Hersh, E. M., Bodey, G. P., Nies, B. A., and Freireich, E. J. Causes of death in acute leukemia. A ten-year study of 414 patients from 1954–1963. *J.A.M.A.* 193:105, 1965.

160. Hersh, E. M., and Oppenheim, J. J. Impaired in vitro lymphocyte transformation in Hodgkin's disease, *N. Engl. J. Med.* 273:1006, 1965.

161. Hickling, R. A. "Giant follicle lymphoma of the spleen." A condition closely related to lymphatic leukaemia but apparently curable by splenectomy, *Br. Med. J.* 2:787, 1964.

162. Hilbun, B. M., and Chavez, C. M. Lymphoma of the lung, *J. Thorac. Cardiovasc. Surg.* 53:721, 1967.

163. Hirsch, E. F. Primary lymphosarcoma of the liver with metastases to the marrow and secondary anemia, *Arch. Pathol.* 23:674, 1937.

164. Hoster, H. A., and Dratman, M. B. Hodgkin's disease (Part I and Part II) 1832–1947, *Cancer Res.* 8:1, 1948.

165. Hurst, D. W., and Meyer, O. O. Giant follicular lymphoblastoma, *Cancer* 14:753, 1961.

166. Hurwitt, E. Dermatopathic lymphadenitis: focal granulomatous lymphadenitis associated with chronic generalized skin disorders, *J. Invest. Dermatol.* 5:197, 1942.

167. Hyman, G. A., and Sommers, S. C. The development of Hodgkin's disease and lymphoma during anticonvulsant therapy, *Blood* 28:416, 1966.

168. Isaacs, R. Lymphosarcoma cell leukemia, *Ann. Intern. Med.* 11:657, 1937.

169. Jackson, H., Jr., and Parker, F., Jr. Hodgkin's Disease and Allied Disorders, p. 117, Oxford University Press, New York, 1947.

170. Jackson, H., Jr., Parker, F., Jr., and Brues, A. M. Malignant lymphoma of the tonsil, *Am. J. Med. Sci.* 191:1, 1936.

171. Jackson, S. M., Garrett, J. V., and Craig, A. W. Lymphocyte transformation changes during the clinical course of Hodgkin's disease, *Cancer* 25:843, 1970.

172. Janota, I. Involvement of the nervous system in malignant lymphoma in Nigeria, *Br. J. Cancer* 20:47, 1966.

173. Javier, B. V., Yount, W. J., Crosby, D. J., and Hall, T. C. Cardiac metastases in lymphoma and leukemia, *Dis. Chest* 52:481, 1967.

174. John, H. T., and Nabarro, J. D. N. Intracranial manifestations of malignant lymphoma, *Br. J. Cancer* 9:386, 1955.

175. Johnson, R. E. Modern approaches to the radiotherapy of lymphoma, *Semin. Hematol.* 6:133, 1969.

176. Johnson, R. E., Glover, M. K., and Marshall, S. K. Results of radiation therapy and implications for the clinical staging of Hodgkin's disease, *Cancer Res.* 31:1834, 1971.

177. Jones, B., and Klingberg, W. G. Lymphosarcoma in children. A report of 43 cases and review of the recent literature, *J. Pediatr.* 63:11, 1963.

178. Jones, S. E., Fuks, Z., Bull, M., Kadin, M. E., Dorfman, R. F., Kaplan, H. S., Rosenberg, S. A., and Kim, H. Non-Hodgkin's lymphomas. IV. Clinicopathologic correlation in 405 cases, *Cancer* 31:806, 1973.

179. Kaplan, H. S. Prognostic significance of the relapse-free interval after radiotherapy in Hodgkin's disease, *Cancer* 22:1131, 1968.

180. Kaplan, H. S. Clinical evaluation and radiotherapeutic management of Hodgkin's disease and the malignant lymphomas, *N. Engl. J. Med.* 278:892, 1968.

181. Kaplan, H. S. On the natural history, treatment and prognosis of Hodgkin's disease. Harvey Lect. 1968-1969, p. 215, Academic Press, New York, 1970.

182. Kaplan, H. S. Contiguity and progression in Hodgkin's disease, *Cancer Res.* 31:1811, 1971.

183. Kaplan, H. S., and Smithers, D. W. Auto-immunity in man and homologous disease in mice in relation to the malignant lymphomas, *Lancet* ii:1, 1959.

184. Katz, A., and Lattes, R. Granulomatous thymoma or Hodgkin's disease of thymus, *Cancer* 23:1, 1969.

185. Kawakami, T. G., Huff, S. D., Buckley, P. M., et al. C-type virus associated with Gibbon lymphosarcoma, *Nature (New Biol.)* 235:170, 1972.

186. Keller, A. R., Kaplan, H. S., Lukes, R. J., and Rappaport, H. Correlation of histopathology with other prog-

nostic indicators in Hodgkin's disease, *Cancer* 22:487, 1968.

187. Kellet, H. S., and Sutherland, T. W. Reticulosarcoma of the thyroid gland, *J. Pathol. Bacteriol.* 61:233, 1949.

188. Kelly, W. D., Lamb, D. L., Varco, R. L., and Good, R. A. An investigation of Hodgkin's disease with respect to the problem of homotransplantation, *Ann. N.Y. Acad. Sci.* 87:187, 1960.

189. Kenyon, R., and Ackerman, L. V. Malignant lymphoma of the thyroid apparently arising in struma lymphomatosa, *Cancer* 8:964, 1955.

190. Kiely, J. M. Symptomatic control of fever in lymphoma and leukemia, *Mayo Clin. Proc.* 44:272, 1969.

191. Kimura, I., Onoshi, T., Kumimasa, I., and Takano, J. Treatment of malignant lymphomas with bleomycin, *Cancer* 29:58, 1972.

192. Klein, G. Experimental studies in tumor immunology, *Fed. Proc.* 28:1739, 1969

193. Klein, G., Clifford, P., Klein, E., and Stjernswärd, J. Search for tumor-specific immune reactions in Burkitt lymphoma patients by the membrane immunofluorescence reaction, *Proc. Natl. Acad. Sci. U.S.A.* 55:1628, 1966.

194. Klein, G., Clifford, P., Klein, E., Smith, R. T., Minowada, J., Kourilsky, F. M., and Burchenal, J. H. Membrane immunofluorescence reactions of Burkitt lymphoma cells from biopsy specimens and tissue cultures, *J. Natl. Cancer Inst.* 39:1027, 1967.

195. Klein, G., Klein, E., and Clifford, P. Search for host defenses in Burkitt lymphoma: membrane immunofluorescence tests on biopsies and tissue culture lines, *Cancer Res.* 27:2510, 1967.

196. Klein, G., Pearson, G., Henle, G., Henle, W., Diehl, V., and Niederman, J. C. Relation between Epstein-Barr viral and cell membrane immunofluorescence in Burkitt tumor cells. II. Comparison of cells and sera from patients with Burkitt's lymphoma and infectious mononucleosis, *J. Exp. Med.* 128:1021, 1968.

197. Knoepp, L. F. Lymphosarcoma of the kidney, *Surgery* 39:510, 1956.

198. Krauss, S., and Sokal, J. E. Parapro-

teinemia in the lymphomas, *Am. J. Med.* 40:400, 1966.

199. Lacher, M. J. Long survival in Hodgkin's disease, *Ann. Intern. Med.* 70:7, 1969.

200. Lamb, D., Pilney, F., Kelly, W. D., and Good, R. A. A comparative study of the incidence of anergy in patients with carcinoma, leukemia, Hodgkin's disease and other lymphomas, *J. Immunol.* 89:555, 1962.

201. Lanaro, A. E., Bosch, A., and Frías, Z. Red blood cell survival in patients with Hodgkin's disease, *Cancer* 28:658, 1971.

202. Lee, B. J., Nelson, J. H., and Schwarz, G. Evaluation of lymphangiography, inferior venacavography and intravenous pyelography in the clinical staging and management of Hodgkin's disease and lymphosarcoma, *N. Engl. J. Med.* 271:327, 1964.

203. Levine, P. H., Sandler, S. G., Komp, D. M., O'Conor, G. T., and O'Connor, D. M. Simultaneous occurrence of "American Burkitt's lymphoma" in neighbors, *N. Engl. J. Med.* 288:562, 1973.

204. Levinson, B., Walter, B. A., Wintrobe, M. M., and Cartwright, G. E. A clinical study in Hodgkin's disease, *Arch. Intern. Med.* 99:519, 1957.

205. Levitan, R., Diamond, H. D., and Craver, L. F. Esophageal varices in Hodgkin's disease involving the liver, *Am. J. Med.* 27:137, 1959.

206. Levitan, R., Diamond, H. D., and Craver, L. F. Jaundice in Hodgkin's disease, *Am. J. Med.* 30:99, 1961.

207. Lindström, F. D., Williams, R. C., Jr., and Theologides, A. Urinary light chain excretion in leukaemia and lymphoma, *Clin. Exp. Immunol.* 5:83, 1969.

208. Lobell, M., Boggs, D. R., and Wintrobe, M. M. The clinical significance of fever in Hodgkin's disease, *Arch. Intern. Med.* 117:335, 1966.

209. Lowenbraun, S., DeVita, V. T., and Serpick, A. A. Combination chemotherapy with nitrogen mustard, vincristine, procarbazine, and prednisone in previously treated patients with Hodgkin's disease, *Blood* 36:704, 1970.

210. Lucas, P. F. Lymph node smears in the diagnosis of lymphadenopathy: a review, *Blood* 10:1030, 1955.

211. Luce, J. K., Gamble, J. F., Wilson, H. E., Monto, R. W., Isaacs, B. L., Palmer, R. L., Coltman, C. A., Jr., Hewlett, J. S., Gehan, E. A., and Frei, E. III. Combined cyclophosphamide, vincristine, and prednisone therapy of malignant lymphoma, *Cancer* 28:306, 1971.

212. Lukes, R. J., Butler, J. J., and Hicks, E. B. Natural history of Hodgkin's disease as related to its pathologic picture, *Cancer* 19:317, 1966.

213. Lukes, R. J., Craver, L. F., Hall, T. C., Rappaport, H., and Ruben, P. Report of the nomenclature committee, *in* Symposium: obstacles to the control of Hodgkin's disease, *Cancer Res.* 26:1311, 1966.

214. Lutzner, M. A., and Jordan, H. W. The ultrastructure of an abnormal cell in Sézary's syndrome, *Blood* 31:719, 1968.

215. McFarlane, H., Ngu, V. A., Udeozo, O. K., Osunkoya, B. O., Luzzatto, L., and Mottram, F. C. Some acute phase proteins in Burkitt lymphoma in Nigerians, *Clin. Chim. Acta* 17:325, 1967.

216. MacMahon, B. Epidemiology of Hodgkin's disease, *Cancer Res.* 26:1189, 1966.

217. MacMahon, B. Epidemiological considerations in staging Hodgkin's disease, *Cancer Res.* 31:1854, 1971.

218. McNeer, G., and Berg, J. W. The clinical behavior and management of primary malignant lymphoma of the stomach, *Surgery* 46:829, 1959.

219. Madianos, M., and Sokal, J. E. Cardiac involvement in lymphosarcoma and reticulum cell sarcoma, *Am. Heart J.* 65:322, 1963.

220. Major, R. H., and Leger, L. H. Marked eosinophilia in Hodgkin's disease, *J.A.M.A.* 112:2601, 1939.

221. Manolov, G., and Manolova, Y. Marker band in one chromosome 14 from Burkitt lymphomas, *Nature* 237:33, 1972.

222. Marshall, A. H. E. An Outline of the Cytology and Pathology of the Reticular Tissue, Oliver and Boyd, Edinburgh, 1956.

223. Marshall, G., Roessmann, U., and van den Noort, S. Invasive Hodgkin's disease of the brain. Report of two new cases and review of American and European literature with clinical-pathologic correlations, *Cancer* 22:621, 1968.

224. Mathé, C. P. Retroperitoneal lymphoblastoma simulating kidney neoplasm, *J. Urol.* 17:357, 1927.

225. Melamed, M. R. The cytological presentation of malignant lymphomas and related disease in effusions, *Cancer* 16:413, 1963.

226. Mestel, A. L. Lymphosarcoma of the small intestine in infancy and childhood, *Ann. Surg.* 149:87, 1959.

227. Millburn, L., Hibbs, G. G., and Hendrickson, F. R. Treatment of spinal cord compression from metastatic carcinoma. Review of the literature and presentation of a new method of treatment. *Cancer* 21:447, 1968.

228. Miller, G., Niederman, J. C., and Andrews, L-L. Infectious mononucleosis: prolonged pharyngeal excretion of E-B virus, *N. Engl. J. Med.* 288:229, 1973.

229. Miller, S. P., and Shanbrom, E. Infectious syndromes of leukemias and lymphomas, *Am. J. Med. Sci.* 246:420, 1963.

230. Minot, G. R., and Isaacs, R. Lymphoblastoma (malignant lymphoma), *J.A.M.A.* 86:1185, 1926.

231. Minowada, J., Klein, G., Clifford, P., Klein, E., and Moore, G. E. Studies of Burkitt lymphoma cells. I. Establishment of a cell line (B35M) and its characteristics, *Cancer* 20:1430, 1967.

232. Mones, R. J., Dozier, D., and Berrett, A. Analysis of medical treatment of malignant extradural spinal cord tumors, *Cancer* 19:1842, 1966.

233. Morrow, R. H., Pike, M. C., and Kisuule, A. Survival of Burkitt's lymphoma patients in Mulago hospital, Uganda, *Br. Med. J.* 4:323, 1967.

234. Motulsky, A. G., Weinberg, S., Saphir, O., and Rosenberg, E. Lymph nodes in rheumatoid arthritis, *Arch. Intern. Med.* 90:660, 1952.

235. Mukherji, B., Yagoda, A., Oettgen, H. F., and Krakoff, I. H. Cyclic chemotherapy in lymphoma, *Cancer* 28:886, 1971.

236. Musshoff, K. Prognostic and therapeutic implications of staging in extranodal Hodgkin's disease, *Cancer Res.* 31:1814, 1971.

237. Musshoff, K., and Boutis, L. Therapy results in Hodgkin's disease. Freiburg i.Br., 1948–1966, *Cancer* 21:1100, 1968.

238. Neiman, R. S., Rosen, P. J., and

Lukes, R. J. Lymphocyte-depletion Hodgkin's disease, *N. Engl. J. Med.* 288:751, 1973.

239. Nosanchuck, J. S., and Schnitzer, B. Follicular hyperplasia in lymph nodes from patients with rheumatoid arthritis, *Cancer* 24:343, 1969.

240. Novis, B. H., Bank, S., Marks, I. N., Selzer, G., Kahn, L., and Sealy, R. Abdominal lymphoma presenting with malabsorption, *Q. J. Med.* 40:521, 1971.

241. O'Conor, G. T. Malignant lymphoma in African children—II. A pathological entity, *Cancer* 14:270, 1961.

242. O'Conor, G. T., and Davies, J. N. P. Malignant tumors in African children. With special reference to malignant lymphoma, *J. Pediatr.* 56:526, 1960.

243. O'Conor, G. T., Rappaport, H., and Smith, E. B. Childhood lymphoma resembling "Burkitt tumor" in the United States, *Cancer* 18:411, 1965.

244. Oels, H. C., Harrison, E. G., Jr., and Kiely, J. M. Lymphoblastic lymphoma with histiocytic phagocytosis ("starry sky" appearance) in adults. Guide to prognosis, *Cancer* 21:368, 1968.

245. Oettgen, H. F., Aoki, T., Geering, G., Boyse, E. A., and Old, L. J. Definition of an antigenic system associated with Burkitt's lymphoma, *Cancer Res.* 27:2532, 1967.

246. Old, L. J., Boyse, E. A., Oettgen, H. F., DeHarven, E., Geering, G., Williamson, B., and Clifford, P. Precipitating antibody in human serum to an antigen present in cultured Burkitt's lymphoma cells, *Proc. Natl. Acad. Sci. U.S.A.* 56:1699, 1966.

247. Order, S. E., Chism, S. E., and Hellman, S. Studies of antigens associated with Hodgkin's disease, *Blood* 40:621, 1972.

248. Order, S. E., and Hellman, S. Tumor associated antigens. A new perspective of Hodgkin's disease, *J.A.M.A.* 223:174, 1973.

249. Pagano, J. S., Huang, C. H., and Levine, P. Absence of Epstein-Barr viral DNA in American Burkitt's lymphoma, *N. Engl. J. Med.* 289:1395, 1973.

250. Panciera, R. J., Johnson, L., and Osburn, B. I. A disease of cattle grazing hairy vetch pasture, *J. Am. Vet. Med. Assoc.* 148:804, 1966.

251. Papac, R. J. Lymphocyte transformation in malignant lymphomas, *Cancer* 26:279, 1970.

252. Papaioannou, A. N., and Watson, W. L. Primary lymphoma of the lung: an appraisal of its natural history and a comparison with other localized lymphomas, *J. Thorac. Cardiovasc. Surg.* 49:373, 1965.

253. Pearson, G., Klein, G., Henle, G., Henle, W., and Clifford, P. Relation between Epstein-Barr viral and cell membrane immunofluorescence in Burkitt tumor cells. IV. Differentiation between antibodies responsible for membrane and viral immunofluorescence, *J. Exp. Med.* 129:707, 1969.

254. Pen, I., Hammond, W., Brettschneider, L., and Starzl, E. Malignant lymphomas in transplantation patients, *Transplant. Proc.* 1:106, 1969.

255. Perry, S., Thomas, L. B., Johnson, R. E., Carbone, P. P., and Haynes, H. A. Hodgkin's disease. Combined clinical staff conference at the National Institutes of Health, *Ann. Intern. Med.* 67:424, 1967.

256. Peters, M. V. A study of survivals in Hodgkin's disease treated radiologically, *Am. J. Roentgenol.* 63:299, 1950.

257. Peters, M. V. The contribution of radiation therapy in the control of early lymphomas, *Am. J. Roentgenol.* 90:956, 1963.

258. Peters, M. V. Prophylactic treatment of adjacent areas in Hodgkin's disease, *Cancer Res.* 26:1232, 1966.

259. Pierce, J. C., Madge, G. E., Lee, H. M., and Hume, D. M. Lymphoma, a complication of renal allotransplantation in man, *J.A.M.A.* 219:1593, 1972.

260. Piessens, W. F., Schur, P. H., Moloney, W. C., and Churchill, W. H. Lymphocyte surface immunoglobulins, *N. Engl. J. Med.* 288:176, 1973.

261. Pinsky, S. M., Hoffer, P. B., Turner, D. A., Harper, P. V., and Gottschalk, A. Place of the ^{67}Ga in the staging of Hodgkin's disease, *J. Nucl. Med.* 12:385, 1971.

262. Prosnitz, L. R., Hellman, S., Von Essen, C. F., and Kligerman, M. M. The clinical course of Hodgkin's disease and other malignant lymphomas treated with radical radiation therapy, *Am. J. Roentgenol.* 105:618, 1969.

263. Prosnitz, L. R., Nuland, S. B., and Kligerman, M. M. Role of laparatomy and splenectomy in the management of Hodgkin's disease, *Cancer* 29:44, 1972.

264. Rappaport, H. Tumors of the hematopoietic system. Atlas of Tumor Pathology, sect. 3, fasc. 8, p. 1, Armed Forces Institute of Pathology, Washington, D. C., 1966.

265. Rappaport, H., and Strum, S. B. Vascular invasion in Hodgkin's disease: its incidence and relationship to the spread of the disease, *Cancer* 25:1302, 1970.

266. Rappaport, H., Winter, W. J., and Hicks, E. B. Follicular lymphoma. A re-evaluation of its position in the scheme of malignant lymphoma, based on a survey of 253 cases, *Cancer* 9:792, 1956.

267. Ratner, A. C., Waldorf, D. S., and Van Scott, E. J. Alterations of lesions of mycosis fungoides by direct imposition of delayed hypersensitivity reactions, *Cancer* 21:83, 1968.

268. Razis, D. V., Diamond, H. D., and Craver, L. F. Familial Hodgkin's disease: its significance and implications, *Ann. Intern. Med.* 51:933, 1959.

269. Redd, B. L., Jr. Lymphosarcoma of the stomach, *Am. J. Roentgenol.* 82:634, 1959.

270. Remington, J. S., Dalrymple, W., Jacobs, L., and Finland, M. Toxoplasma antibodies among college students, *N. Engl. J. Med.* 269:1394, 1963.

271. Rewcastle, N. B. Subacute cerebellar degeneration with Hodgkin's disease, *Arch. Neurol.* 9:407, 1963.

272. Rhoads, C. P. Nitrogen mustards in the treatment of neoplastic disease. Official statement, *J.A.M.A.* 131:656, 1946.

273. Richardson, E. P., Jr. Progressive multifocal leukoencephalopathy, *N. Engl. J. Med.* 265:815, 1961.

274. Richmond, J., Sherman, R. S., Diamond, H. D., and Craver, L. F. Renal lesions associated with malignant lymphomas, *Am. J. Med.* 32:184, 1962.

275. Richter, R. B., and Moore, R. Y. Non-invasive central nervous system disease associated with

lymphoid tumors, *Johns Hopkins Med. J.* 122:271, 1968.

276. Robb-Smith, A. H. T. The lymph node biopsy, in S. C. Dyke (ed.), Recent Advances in Clinical Pathology, p. 350, Blakiston, Philadelphia, 1947.

277. Roberts, W. C., Bodey, G. P., and Wertlake, P. T. The heart in acute leukemia: a study of 420 autopsy cases, *Am. J. Cardiol.* 21:388, 1968.

278. Roberts, W. C., Glancy, D. L., and DeVita, V. T. Heart in malignant lymphoma (Hodgkin's disease, lymphosarcoma, reticulum cell sarcoma and mycosis fungoides). A study of 196 autopsy cases, *Am. J. Cardiol.* 22:85, 1968.

279. Rosenberg, S. A. Hodgkin's disease of the bone marrow, *Cancer Res.* 31:1773, 1971.

280. Rosenberg, S. A., Boiron, M., De-Vita, V. T., Jr., Johnson, R. E., Lee, B. J., Ultmann, J. E., and Viamonte, M., Jr. Report of the committee on Hodgkin's disease staging procedures, *Cancer Res.* 31:1862, 1971.

281. Rosenberg, S. A., Diamond, H. D., and Craver, L. F. Lymphosarcoma: survival and the effects of therapy, *Am. J. Roentgenol.* 85:521, 1961.

282. Rosenberg, S. A., Diamond, H. D., Dargeon, H. W., and Craver, L. F. Lymphosarcoma in childhood, *N. Engl. J. Med.* 259:505, 1958.

283. Rosenberg, S. A., Diamond, H. D., Jaslowitz, B., and Craver, L. F. Lymphosarcoma: a review of 1269 cases, *Medicine* 40:31, 1961.

284. Rosenberg, S. A., and Kaplan, H. S. Evidence for an orderly progression in the spread of Hodgkin's disease, *Cancer Res.* 26:1225, 1966.

285. Rosenberg, S. A., and Kaplan, H. S. Hodgkin's disease and other malignant lymphomas, *Calif. Med.* 113:23, 1970.

286. Rowland, L. P., and Schneck, S. A. Neuromuscular disorders associated with malignant neoplastic disease, *J. Chron. Dis.* 16:777, 1963.

287. Saltzstein, S. L. Pulmonary malignant lymphomas and pseudolymphomas: classification, therapy and prognosis, *Cancer* 16:928, 1963.

288. Saltzstein, S. L., and Ackerman, L. V. Lymphadenopathy induced by anticonvulsant drugs and mimicking clinically and pathologically malignant lymphomas, *Cancer* 12:164, 1959.

289. Scheer, A. C. The course of stage I malignant lymphomas following local treatment, *Am. J. Roentgenol.* 90:939, 1963.

290. Scheerer, P. P., Pierre, R. V., Schwartz, D. L., and Linman, J. W. Reed-Sternberg-cell leukemia and lactic acidosis. Unusual manifestations of Hodgkin's disease, *N. Engl. J. Med.* 270:274, 1964.

291. Schier, W. W. Cutaneous anergy and Hodgkin's disease, *N. Engl. J. Med.* 250:353, 1954.

292. Schier, W. W., Roth, A., Ostroff, G., and Schrift, M. H. Hodgkin's disease and immunity, *Am. J. Med.* 20:94, 1956.

293. Schnitzer, B., Nishiyama, R. H., Heidelberger, K. P., and Weaver, D. K. Hodgkin's disease in children, *Cancer* 31:560, 1973.

294. Schrek, R., Rappaport, H., Rubnitz, M. E., and Kwann, H. C. Cytology and reactions of viable cells from malignant lymphoma, *Cancer* 23:1061, 1969.

295. Schricker, J. L., Jr., and Smith, D. E. Primary intracerebral Hodgkin's disease, *Cancer* 8:629, 1955.

296. Schwartz, R., André-Schwartz, J., Armstrong, M. Y. K., and Beldotti, L. Neoplastic sequelae of allogenic disease. I. Theoretical considerations and experimental design, *Ann. N.Y. Acad. Sci.* 129:804, 1966.

297. Schwartz, R. S., and Beldotti, L. Malignant lymphomas following allogenic disease: transition from an immunological to a neoplastic disorder, *Science* 149:1511, 1965.

298. Sears, W. G. The blood in Hodgkin's disease with special reference to eosinophilia, *Guys Hosp. Rep.* 82:40, 1932.

299. Seed, P. G. Burkitt's tumour in Britain, *J. Obstet. Gynaecol. Br. Commonw.* 73:808, 1966.

300. Seltzer, R. A., and Wenlund, D. E. Renal lymphoma. Arteriographic studies, *Am. J. Roentgenol. Radium Ther. Nucl. Med.* 51:692, 1967.

301. Serpick, A. A., Lowenbraun, S., and DeVita, V. T. Combination chemotherapy of lymphosarcoma (LSA) and reticulum cell sarcoma (RCS), *Proc. Am. Assoc. Cancer Res.* 10:78, 1969.

302. Sézary, A. Une nouvelle réticulose cutanée. La réticulose maligne leucémique à histio-monocytes monstrueux et à forme d'érythrodermie

oedémateuse et pigmentée, *Ann. Dermatol. Syphiligr.* (Paris) 9:5, 1949.

303. Sézary, A., and Bouvrain, Y. Erythrodermie avec présence de cellules monstrueuses dans le derme et le sang circulant, *Bull. Soc. Fr. Dermatol. Syphiligr.* 45:254, 1938.

304. Shapiro, J. H., Ramsay, C. G., Jacobson, H. G., Botstein, C. C., and Allen, L. B. Renal involvement in lymphomas and leukemias in adults, *Am. J. Roentgenol.* 88:928, 1962.

305. Shimkin, M. B. Hodgkin's disease. Mortality in the United States, 1921–1951; race, sex and age distribution; comparison with leukemia, *Blood* 10:1214, 1955.

306. Shimkin, M. B., Oppermann, K. C., Bostick, W. L., and Low-Beer, B. V. A. Hodgkin's disease: an analysis of frequency, distribution, and mortality at the University of California Hospital, 1914-1951, *Ann. Intern. Med.* 42:136, 1955.

307. Shimkin, M. B., Oppermann, K. C., Low-Beer, B. V. A., and Mettier, S. R. Lymphosarcoma: an analysis of frequency, distribution and mortality at the University of California Hospital, 1913–1948, *Ann. Intern. Med.* 40:1095, 1954.

308. Shoji, H., and Miller, T. R. Primary reticulum cell sarcoma of bone, *Cancer* 28:1234, 1971.

309. Siim, J. Chr. Toxoplasmosis aquisita lymphonodosa: clinical and pathological aspects, *Ann. N.Y. Acad. Sci.* 64:185, 1956.

310. Smetana, H. F. Hodgkin's disease: a follow-up study of patients surviving more than twenty years after the original diagnosis, *J. Pathol.* 98:231, 1969.

311. Sokal, J. E., and Firat, D. Varicella-zoster infection in Hodgkin's disease, *Am. J. Med.* 39:452, 1965.

312. Sparling, H. J., Adams, R. D., and Parker, F., Jr. Involvement of the nervous system by malignant lymphoma, *Medicine* 26:285, 1947.

313. Spellberg, M. A., and Zivin, S. Lymphosarcoma of the gastrointestinal tract, *Arch. Intern. Med.* 83:135, 1949.

314. Squire, R. A. Feline lymphoma. A comparison with the Burkitt tumor of children, *Cancer* 19:447, 1966.

315. Squire, R. A. Equine infectious ane-

mia: a model of immunoproliferative disease, *Blood* 32:157, 1968.

316. Squire, R. A. Non-neoplastic hyper-
plasias of lymph nodes of animals,
Natl. Cancer Inst. Monogr. 23:257,
1969.

317. Squire, R. A. Burkitt's lymphoma—a comparative study, *Natl.
Cancer Inst. Monogr.* 32:297,
1969.

318. Stanley, N. F. The aetiology and
pathogenesis of Burkitt's African
lymphoma, *Lancet* i:961, 1966.

319. Stanton, M. F., and Pinkerton, H.
Benign acquired toxoplasmosis
with subsequent pregnancy, *Am. J.
Clin. Pathol.* 23:1199, 1953.

320. Stevens, D. A., O'Conor, G. T., Levine, P. H., and Rosen, R. B. Acute
leukemia with "Burkitt's lymphoma cells" and Burkitt's lymphoma. Simultaneous onset in
American siblings; description of a
new entity, *Ann. Intern. Med.*
76:967, 1972.

321. Stolberg, H. O., Patt, N. L., Mac-
Ewen, K. F., Warwick, O. H., and
Brown, T. C. Hodgkin's disease of
the lung. Roentgenologic-pathologic
correlation, *Am. J. Roentgenol.*
92:96, 1964.

322. Strickland, B. The value of arteriography in the diagnosis of bone
tumours, *Br. J. Radiol.* 32:705,
1959.

323. Sugarbaker, E. D., and Craver, L. F.
Lymphosarcoma, *J.A.M.A.* 115:17,
112; 1940.

324. Sullivan, M. P. Leukemic transformation in lymphosarcoma of childhood, *Pediatrics* 29:589, 1962.

325. Suprun, H., and Koss, L. G. The
cytological study of sputum and
bronichial washings in Hodgkin's
disease with pulmonary involvement, *Cancer* 17:674, 1964.

326. Swan, H. T., and Knowelden, J.
Prognosis in Hodgkin's disease re-
lated to the lymphocyte count, *Br.
J. Haematol.* 21:343, 1971.

327. Sweet, E. I., Scalon, G. T., and
Kaplan, S. R. Residual Ethiodol®
after lymphography in diagnosis of
lymphoma, *Ann. Intern. Med.*
69:53, 1968.

328. Sweitzer, S. E., and Winer, L. H.
Ulcerative Hodgkin's disease and
lymph node imprints, *Arch. Dermatol.* 51:229, 1945.

329. Symmers, D. Clinical significance
of the deeper anatomic changes in
lymphoid diseases, *Arch. Intern.
Med.* 74:163, 1944.

330. Symposium. Obstacles to the control of Hodgkin's disease, *Cancer
Res.* 26:1045, 1966.

331. Taswell, H. F., and Winkelmann,
M. D. Sézary syndrome—a malig-
nant reticulemic erythroderma,
J.A.M.A. 177:465, 1961.

332. Ten Seldam, R. E. J., Cooke, R., and
Atkinson, L. Childhood lymphoma
in the territories of Papua and New
Guinea, *Cancer* 19:437, 1966.

333. Terry, L. N., Jr., and Kligerman, M.
M. Pericardial and myocardial
involvement by lymphomas and
leukemias. The role of radiotherapy, *Cancer* 25:1003, 1970.

334. Tindle, B. H., Parker, J. W., and
Lukes, R. J. "Reed-Sternberg cells"
in infectious mononucleosis? *Am.
J. Clin. Pathol.* 58:607, 1972.

335. Tubiana, M., Attié, E., Flamant, R.,
Gérard-Marchant, R., and Hayat,
M. Prognostic factors in 454 cases
of Hodgkin's disease, *Cancer Res.*
31:1801, 1971.

336. Tyler, A. Clues to the etiology,
pathology and therapy of cancer
provided by analogies with transplantation disease, *J. Natl. Cancer
Inst.* 25:1197, 1960.

337. Ultmann, J. E. Current status: the
management of lymphoma, *Semin.
Hematol.* 7:441, 1970.

338. Ultmann, J. E., Fish, W., Osserman,
E., and Gellhorn, A. The clinical
implications of hypogam-
maglobulinemia in patients with
chronic lymphocytic leukemia and
lymphocytic lymphosarcoma, *Ann.
Intern. Med.* 51:501, 1959.

339. Ultmann, J. E., and Nixon, D. D.
The therapy of lymphomas, *Semin.
Hematol.* 6:152, 1969.

340. Van Slyck, E. J., and Schuman, B.
M. Lymphocytic lymphosarcoma of
the gallbladder, *Cancer* 30:810,
1972.

341. Variakojis, D., Rosas-Uribe, A., and
Rappaport, H. Mycosis fungoides:
pathological findings in staging lap-
arotomies, *Cancer* 33:1589, 1974.

342. Viamonte, M., Jr. Current status
of lymphography, *Cancer Res.*
31:1731, 1971.

343. Vianna, N. J., Greenwald, P., Brady,
J., et al. Hodgkin's disease: cases
with features of a community outbreak, *Ann. Intern. Med.* 77:169,
1972.

344. Vieta, J. O., Friedell, H. L., and
Craver, L. F. A survey of Hodgkin's
disease and lymphosarcoma in
bone, *Radiology* 39:1, 1942.

345. Waldorf, D. S., Ratner, A. C., and
Van Scott, E. J. Cells in lesions of
mycosis fungoides lymphoma following therapy. Changes in number
and type, *Cancer* 21:264, 1968.

346. Walford, R. L. Increased incidence
of lymphoma after injections of
mice with cells differing at weak
histocompatibility loci, *Science*
152:78, 1966.

347. Walford, R. L., and Hildemann, W.
H. Life span and lymphoma—incidence of mice injected at birth
with spleen cells across a weak histocompatibility locus, *Am. J.
Pathol.* 47:713, 1965.

348. Welch, J. W., Chesky, V. E., and
Hellwig, C. A. Malignant lymphoma of the thyroid, *Surg. Gynecol. Obstet.* 106:70, 1958.

349. Whisnant, J. P., Siekert, R. G., and
Sayre, G. P. Neurologic manifesta-
tions of the lymphomas, *Med. Clin.
North Am.* 40:1151, 1956.

350. Williams, H. M. Neurological Complications of Lymphomas and Leukemias, Charles C Thomas, Springfield, Ill., 1959.

351. Williams, H. M., Diamond, H. D.,
and Craver, L. F. The pathogenesis
and management of neurological
complications in patients with malignant lymphomas and leukemia,
Cancer 11:76, 1958.

352. Willis, R. A. Pathology of Tumours,
2nd ed., Butterworth, London,
1953.

353. Winkelman, R. K. Symposium on
the Sézary cell, *Mayo Clin. Proc.*
49:513, 1974.

354. Wintrobe, M. M. Clinical Hematology, 6th ed., p. 1108, Lea &
Febiger, Philadelphia, 1967.

355. Wiseman, B. K. The blood pictures
in the primary diseases of the lymphatic system, *J.A.M.A.* 107:2016,
1936.

356. Wolpaw, S. E., Higley, C. S., and
Hauser, H. Intrathoracic Hodgkin's
disease, *Am. J. Roentgenol.* 52:374,
1944.

357. Woodard, H. Q., and Craver, L. F.
Serum phosphatase in the lympho-
matoid diseases, *J. Clin. Invest.*
19:1, 1940.

358. Wright, D. H. Cytology and histochemistry of the Burkitt lym-

phoma, *Br. J. Cancer* 17:50, 1963.

359. Wright, D. H., and Pike, P. A. Bone marrow involvement in Burkitt's tumour, *Br. J. Haematol.* 15:409, 1968.

360. Wychulis, A. R., Beahrs, O. H., and Woolner, L. B. Malignant lymphoma of the colon. A study of 69 cases, *Arch. Surg.* 93:215, 1966.

361. Yardumian, K., and Myers, L. Primary Hodgkin's disease of the lung, *Arch. Intern. Med.* 86:233, 1950.

362. Young, R. C., Corder, M. P., Haynes, H. A., and DeVita, V. T., Jr. Delayed hypersensitivity in Hodgkin's disease. A study of 103 untreated patients, *Am. J. Med.* 52:63, 1972.

363. Young, R. C., DeVita, V. T., and Johnson, R. E. Hodgkin's disease in childhood, *Blood* 42:163, 1973.

364. Ziegler, J. L., and Miller, D. G. Lymphosarcoma resembling the Burkitt tumor in a Connecticut girl, *J.A.M.A.* 198:1071, 1966.

PART III Monocytes and Macrophages

A The Normal Macrophage

Chapter 23   Morphogenesis and Production
of Monocytes and Macrophages

In this and the two following chapters we shall consider the morphogenesis, production, metabolism, and function of mononuclear phagocytes. The concluding chapters are concerned with abnormalities of monocytes and macrophages in disease states.

Morphogenesis of the Monocyte-Macrophage Cell Line

The blood monocyte is an intermediate in a cell line of which the youngest identifiable forms in the bone marrow are the monoblast and the promonocyte and of which the most mature form in the tissue is the macrophage (107). The concept of a continuum of cells from the bone marrow monoblast and promonocyte through the monocyte to the larger tissue macrophage and multinucleate giant cell is critical to an understanding of the metabolism and function of these cells. Figure 23.1 presents in schematic fashion morphologically identifiable cells along the continuum from monoblast to mature macrophage. Figures 23.2 through 23.7 are photomicrographs of the cells shown diagrammatically in Fig. 23.1. Mononuclear phagocytes at different levels of maturation have different metabolic and functional characteristics, as well as distinctive morphologic features.

Cells of the mononuclear phagocyte series are related in their development to other hematopoietic cell lines, most closely to cells of the granulocytic series. These relationships are illustrated in Fig. I.1 in the Introduction.

The Monocyte-Macrophage Continuum

The early histologic observations of Metchnikoff and Aschoff provided the basis for the concept of transitional forms between the blood monocyte and the tissue macrophage (2, 72, 73). It was in 1925 that Lewis (59) first demonstrated clearly that in tissue culture monocytes (Fig. 23.4) transform into macrophages (Figs. 23.5 and 23.6), multinucleate giant cells (Fig. 23.7), and epithelioid cells. Earlier studies had described a similar phenomenon in cultured leukemic blood (4). The Lewises (60) in 1926 showed that circulating large mononuclear phagocytes in all classes of vertebrates were capable of differentiating into "macrophages similar to those found in connective tissues, liver, spleen and lymph nodes, and epithelioid cells and giant cells precisely like those found in tuberculous lesions."

The subsequent observations of Maximow (68) and modern cell biologists (6, 23–26, 102) confirmed and extended these observations. The most convincing evidence for the differentiation of the blood monocytes in the living animal came from the 1939 work of Ebert and Florey (30). Using rabbit ear chambers, these investigators observed that monocytes containing phagocytized carbon particles or stained with supravital dyes migrate from the blood vessels into the connective tissue and there transform into cells indistinguishable from tissue macrophages (histiocytes). With time, some of these monocytes give rise to giant cells.

The transformation from monocyte to macrophage is accompanied by changes in cell composition and metabolism, as well as by changes in cell architecture. After the monocyte enters the tissue or is maintained in tissue culture for days or weeks, it increases in size and may eventually reach five to ten times its original cell diameter. As

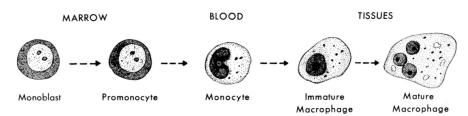

MARROW   BLOOD   TISSUES

Monoblast   Promonocyte   Monocyte   Immature   Mature
Macrophage   Macrophage

Figure 23.1 Sequence of development of cells of the mononuclear phagocyte series. Monoblasts and promonocytes are the least mature cells of the series. Cells through the immature macrophage stage are capable of division.

the size increases, certain cytoplasmic structures, including granules, become more abundant and appear to pack the cytoplasm when the cell is viewed by phase or electron microscopy (24, 102) (Fig. 23.8). Accompanying these morphologic changes are the expected increases in lysosomal enzymes, including acid phosphatase, beta-glucuronidase, cathepsin, lysozyme, and aryl sulfatase (6, 17, 24–26). Thus, as the monocyte differentiates into a macrophage, it increases its arsenal of hydrolytic enzymes.

The transition from monocyte to macrophage is also characterized by increases in the number of mitochondria (Figs. 23.8A and C), in the activity of mitochondrial enzymes such as cytochrome oxidase, and in the rate of cell respiration (23). The rate of glucose oxidation and lactate production also increases with transformation. To sum-

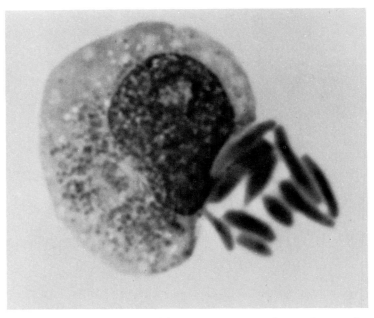

Figure 23.3 A promonocyte from an in vitro culture of normal human bone marrow. The nucleoli and the granules in the Golgi area are prominent features. Note that the cell has not ingested the yeast surrounding it.

marize, the activated macrophage is metabolically more active and has a greater store of acid hydrolases than does the cell of origin. In addition, certain classes of macrophages developing in particular anatomic sites may acquire distinctive characteristics. The predominantly

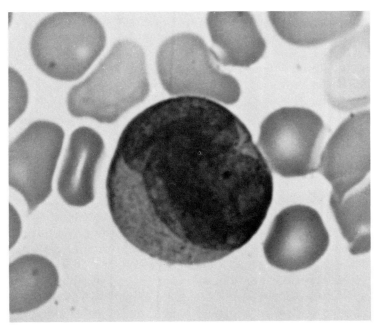

Figure 23.2 A monoblast from the peripheral blood of a patient with acute monocytic leukemia.

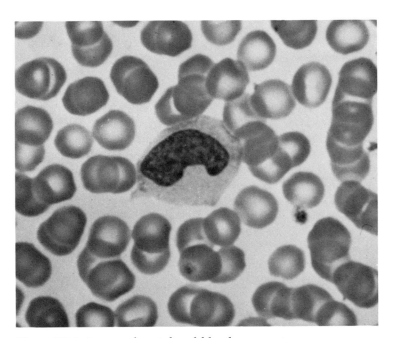

Figure 23.4 A normal peripheral blood monocyte.

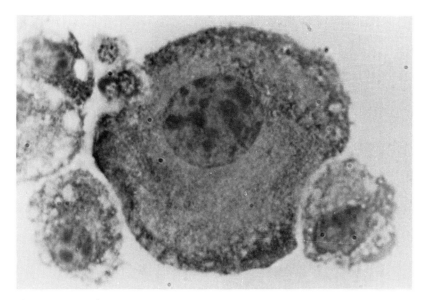

Figure 23.5 A large immature macrophage grown in an in vitro culture system. The large cell is surrounded by smaller macrophages. In the original preparation the cytoplasm was stained blue by Giemsa. The nuclear chromatin is condensed in a patchy manner but is not so dense as that of the fully mature macrophage.

aerobic metabolism of the alveolar macrophage (Fig. 23.6) is an example of such a distinctive characteristic.

Cytoplasmic organelles, thought to be involved in protein synthesis, are abundant in all phases of monocyte differentiation but are particularly numerous in mature epithelioid cells (102). The Golgi apparatus, which is

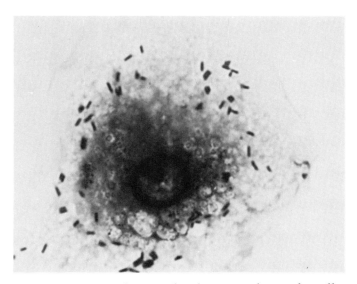

Figure 23.6 A mature human alveolar macrophage. The cell has ingested numerous bacteria.

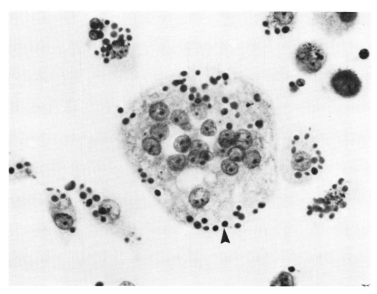

Figure 23.7 A mature multinucleate human macrophage. The *Candida albicans* (arrow) that have been phagocytized by the cell are 1 to 2 microns in diameter.

small in monocytes, increases in size and complexity with cell differentiation.

The multinucleate giant cell is an end stage of monocyte differentiation. It contains massive quantities of lysosomes, mitochondria, and pinocytic vesicles. The origin of such multinucleate giant cells is not certain, but it has frequently been suggested that they arise by fusion of macrophages.

The Monoblast

With currently available techniques, monoblasts are not identifiable in normal bone marrow. They are extremely rare and have no unique ultrastructural features that allow unequivocal identification. Indeed, it is not certain that normal monoblasts are morphologically distinct from myeloblasts. Evidence obtained from in vitro culture of mouse bone marrow suggests that the granulocytic series and the mononuclear series share a common stem cell (see Chapters 1 and 2).

Blast cells (monoblasts), presumed to be the progenitors of differentiated mononuclear cells, are seen with frequency only in monocytic leukemia. These cells are 15 to 25 microns in diameter and have a round or oval nucleus with fine chromatin structure and prominent nucleoli (Figs. 23.2 and 23.9). They show little motility or adhesiveness to a glass surface and are rarely phagocytic. Numerous rod-like mitochondria are demonstrable in the electron microscope.

When these undifferentiated blast cells develop a com-

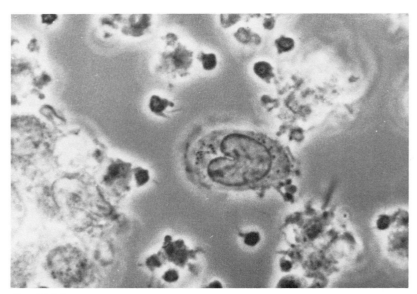

Fig. 23.8A

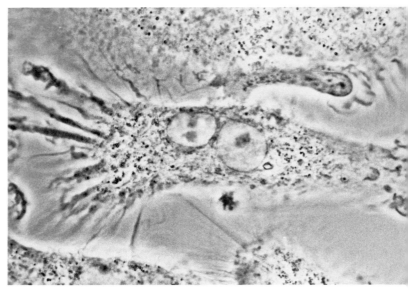

Fig. 23.8C

Figure 23.8 Phase contrast photomicrographs showing the transition from monocyte to macrophage. In the living monocyte (Fig. 23.8A) the nucleus is kidney shaped and a few granules are scattered in the cytoplasm. Figure 23.8B shows a human monocyte that has been cultured in vitro for five days. The cell is larger than in A and has begun to spread out on the surface of the glass cover slip. Cytoplasmic granulation has become prominent. After in vitro culture for ten days (Fig. 23.8C), the cell is much larger than before.

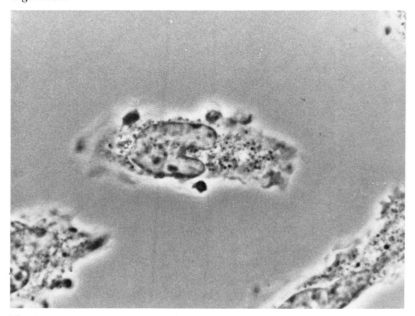

Fig. 23.8B

plex Golgi apparatus and a definite granule population, they can be identified with certainty and are designated *promonocytes*.

The Bone Marrow Promonocyte

Glass-adherent mononuclear phagocytes capable of DNA synthesis have been isolated from mouse bone marrow and called promonocytes by van Furth and Cohn and their collaborators (106, 108). These investigators have constructed a model in which the promonocytes are self-

replicating cells half of whose daughter cells remain promonocytes, the other half giving rise to monocytes.

The promonocyte (Figs. 23.3, 23.10, and 23.11) is characterized by relatively large diameter (10 to 20 microns in man), a high nuclear/cytoplasmic ratio, a basophilic cytoplasm, some peroxidase activity, glass adherence, and the ability to incorporate ^{3}H-thymidine. Details of its fine structure are known (84), including the mechanism of granulogenesis (Fig. 23.12). The cell has a conspicuous Golgi complex, relatively few cisternae of endoplasmic reticulum, numerous free polysomes, and many immature and mature azurophil granules. These granules are usually round or oval, but may be pleomorphic; as a rule, they are homogeneously dense.

Promonocytes are capable of endocytosis, but generally show little phagocytosis (19). With cellular maturation the activity of certain hydrolases increases, but peroxidase activity diminishes.

The Blood Monocyte

In conventional Wright-stained preparations, human monocytes appear as large cells (10 to 18 microns in diameter)

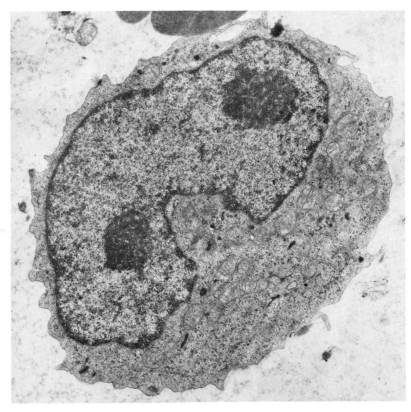

Figure 23.9 An immature cell from a patient with monocytic leukemia. (From Y. Tanaka and J. R. Goodman, Electron Microscopy of Human Blood Cells, Harper & Row, New York, 1972. Reprinted by permission of authors and publisher.)

with grayish-blue cytoplasm that frequently contains small numbers of faint, azurophilic granules (Fig. 23.4). Although large by comparison with other cell types, monocytes are generally smaller than the antecedent promonocytes (84). The centrally located nucleus is indented or horseshoe shaped and has a fine, lacy chromatin structure.

In supravital preparations observed by phase microscopy, granules are often noted in the perinuclear area (Fig. 23.8). These granules stain with neutral red, and the distinct cytoplasmic mitochondria stain with Janus green. In living cell preparations studied by phase microscopy and time-lapse cinematography, the monocyte is seen to be slowly motile by means of blunt pseudopodia. The monocyte has small, lens-shaped surface organelles ("micropapillae"), which are dependent for their preservation on physiological levels of Ca^{++} and Mg^{++} (16).

In thin sections studied under the electron microscope, the monocyte has a characteristic fine structure (8, 62, 84) (Fig. 23.13). The Golgi apparatus is well developed, probably indicating continued granulogenesis. At this stage of

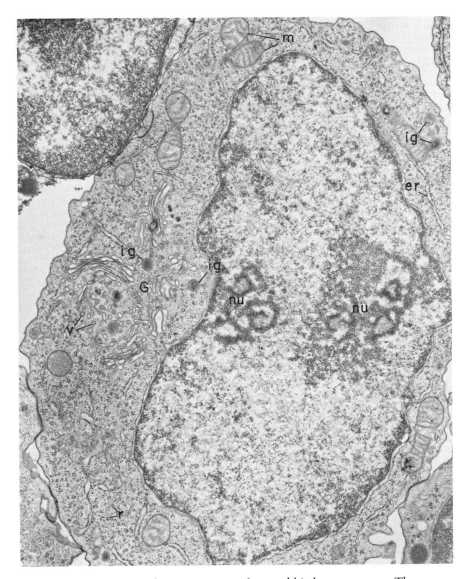

Figure 23.10 Early promonocyte from rabbit bone marrow. The large oval nucleus, which contains two large nucleoli (*nu*) and sparse heterochromatin, almost fills the cell. In the cytoplasm there are numerous free polysomes (*r*), a few flattened cisternae of rough-surfaced endoplasmic reticulum (*er*), mitochondria (*m*), and a conspicuous Golgi complex (*G*). The latter consists of several stacks of four to six cisternae and small vesicles (*v*) with a content of low density. In the Golgi region there are several immature granules (*ig*), ~150 mμ in diameter, characterized by their slightly irregular outline and a content that is typically denser in the center than at the periphery. No fully condensed or mature granules are present in this very young cell. Magnification × 19,000. (From B. A. Nichols, D. F. Bainton, and M. G. Farquhar, *J. Cell Biol.* 50:498, 1971. Reprinted by permission of authors and publisher.)

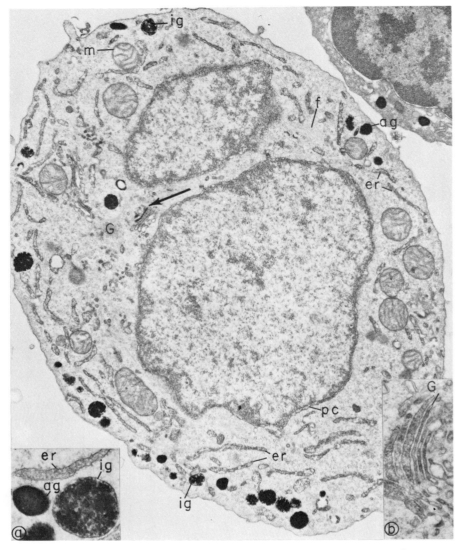

cellular development, the lysosomal granules are more numerous; there are fewer free polysomes, and the mitochondria are evenly distributed. Nuclear density is characteristically increased at the nuclear membrane. Nucleoli are present in about half the cells.

The monocyte, for the most part, is easily distinguished from other types of circulating leukocytes. However, there are some cells, identifiable by both light and electron microscopy, that appear to be intermediate in structure between monocytes and large lymphocytes (42). To distinguish monocytes from such cells, one must apply functional criteria such as phagocytic ability, the presence of specific immunoglobulin receptors, and the presence of certain enzymatic activities (57, 58) (see Chapter 24).

The Tissue Macrophage

Tissue macrophages (also called histiocytes, or tissue histiocytes) are a later stage of development and maturation of monocytes. They are found in the pleural and peritoneal spaces, in the alveolar spaces (alveolar macrophages), and in the tissues. They are particularly abundant in lymph nodes and in the sinusoids of the spleen. In Romanovsky-stained preparations human macrophages are large cells, measuring 20 to 80 microns in diameter. They contain one or more large vesicular nuclei, often with prominent nucleoli (17) (Fig. 23.5). Cytoplasmic granules and inclusions are numerous.

Living cells or surface-adherent cells fixed in glutaraldehyde and viewed by phase microscopy contain numerous dense granules in the perinuclear cytoplasm, and abundant ribbon-like mitochondria in the clear cytoplasmic mantle (17, 23–25, 102) (Fig. 23.8). The living cells are slowly motile and are constantly pushing out giant pseudopods many cell diameters in length. This cell movement appears to depend on the complex of microfilaments found in the cell cytoplasm (1). The pseudopods draw into the main cell body when they encounter and entrap particulate matter such as a yeast or bacterium (Fig. 23.14).

Thin sections of cells studied in the electron microscope have large vesicular nuclei containing multiple nucleoli. The abundant cytoplasm is filled with granules, large mitochondria, microfilaments, microtubules, and digestive vacuoles containing heterogeneous material.

Figure 23.11 Promonocytes from human bone marrow reacted for peroxidase. Reaction product is distributed throughout the entire rough endoplasmic reticulum (*er*), including the perinuclear cisterna (*pc*), all Golgi cisternae (*G* and *arrow*), and all immature granules (*ig*) and mature granules (*ag*). It is not found in the mitochondria (*m*). Note that the reaction is more intense in the granules than in the endoplasmic reticulum and that one Golgi cisterna (*arrow*) is more intensely reactive than the others, suggesting that a concentration gradient exists across the Golgi complex. In the human monocyte clusters of fine filaments (*f*) are common.

Inset *a* is a higher-magnification view showing the dense globular reaction product at low concentration within the rough endoplasmic reticulum and at higher concentration in the immature and mature azurophil granules. In the immature granules, whose content is presumably still undergoing concentration, the aggregates of reaction product are less compact than in the mature granules. Inset *b* shows reaction product

filling six or seven successive cisternae of the Golgi complex of another cell.

Magnification × 12,500; inset *a*, × 39,500; inset *b*, × 34,500. (From B. A. Nichols, D. F. Bainton, and M. G. Farquhar, *J. Cell Biol.* 50:498, 1971. Reprinted by permission of authors and publisher.)

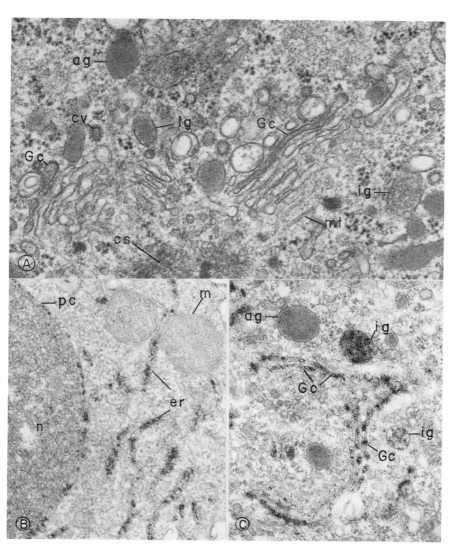

The Golgi apparatus is large and well developed; the rough endoplasmic reticulum is varied in amount (13, 23, 24, 84, 89, 102) (Figs. 23.15 and 23.16).

It is likely that lysosomal enzymes are made in the endoplasmic reticulum and packaged by the Golgi apparatus into structures called primary lysosomes. These primary lysosomes may then fuse with phagocytic or pinocytic vacuoles containing ingested material. The combined structures—called secondary lysosomes—are rich in hydrolytic enzymes and may be more effective than primary lysosomes for the digestion of microorganisms and other ingested particulate matter. Nichols and her colleagues (84) have suggested that the monocyte produces two types of granules during different phases of its life cycle: azurophil granules that are made by developing monocytes in bone marrow and blood, and coated vesicles that are made by macrophages in the tissues.

Pinocytosis and phagocytosis appear to stimulate hydrolytic enzyme production in vitro (23, 26, 120). It seems clear that cellular maturation toward the macrophage, and the accompanying increase in specific activity of certain lysosomal enzymes, are dependent upon intact protein synthesis (23, 25). When macrophages are cultivated in vitro under circumstances in which pinocytic activity is reduced, the numerous secondary lysosomes formed by fusion of pinocytic vesicles and primary lysosomes gradually disappear from the cytoplasm. This influence of environmental factors on the cellular level of lysosomal enzymes may reflect the situation in the intact animal, where the metabolic and functional status of the macrophage adapts to external factors.

By a process of cell fusion, human and other mammalian macrophages may form multinucleate giant cells (Fig. 23.7). The continued maturation of these cells results in the typical epithelioid cells seen in chronic granulomatous reactions (31). These giant cells are extremely rich in granules, hydrolytic enzymes, and mitochondria.

The macrophage must not be viewed simply as an end cell arising from promonocyte and monocyte proliferation. Immature macrophages are capable of DNA synthesis and cell division. Ultimately, this immature (A) macrophage gives rise to the nonreplicating mature (B) macrophage. The immature cell has loose nuclear chromatin and basophilic cytoplasm; the mature macrophage

Figure 23.12 Fields from developing promonocytes in the bone marrow, illustrating immature or forming azurophil granules. *A* shows that in the rabbit an occasional Golgi cisterna (*Gc*) contains homogeneous material of moderate density similar to the content of immature granules (*ig*). It is believed that as granule formation proceeds, small vesicles pinch off the Golgi cisternae; subsequently, several coalesce and the content condenses to form the mature azurophil granule (*ag*). Note that several coated vesicles (*cv*) are also present in the Golgi region, and that microtubules (*mt*) are converging on centriolar satellites (*cs*).

B and *C* are preparations of developing promonocytes collected from the guinea pig and rabbit, respectively, and reacted for acid phosphatase. Reaction product is seen in the rough endoplasmic reticulum (*er*) and perinuclear cisterna (*pc*), and within the Golgi cisternae and immature granules. All the endoplasmic reticulum cisternae and all the cisternae in the Golgi stack (three to four) contain reaction product, but none

is present in the mature granule. Mitochondria (*m*) and part of the nucleus (*n*) are shown.

Magnifications: *A*, × 45,000; *B*, × 38,000; *C*, × 39,000. (From B. A. Nichols, D. F. Bainton, and M. G. Farquhar, *J. Cell Biol.* 50:498, 1971. Reprinted by permission of authors and publisher.)

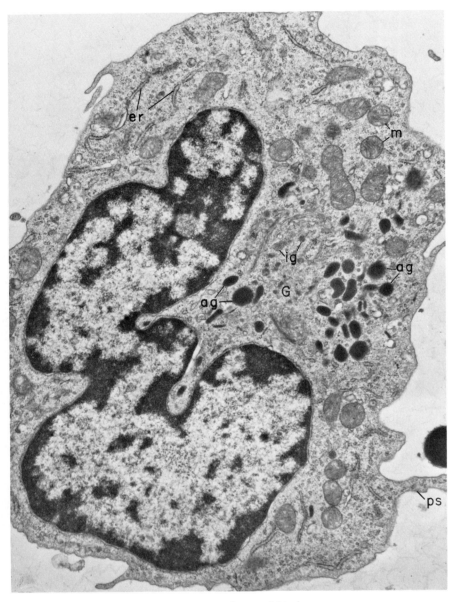

Figure 23.13 Mature monocyte from rabbit bone marrow, showing its characteristic features: the eccentric, kidney-shaped nucleus with moderately condensed chromatin, and the "rosette" of azurophil granules (*ag*) clustered near the Golgi complex (*G*) at the "hof" of the nucleus. About 30 mature, homogeneously dense azurophil granules (variable in shape) can be counted. In addition, numerous small, immature granules (*ig*) are seen in the center of the Golgi region. A few endoplasmic reticulum cisternae (*er*) are present near the cell periphery, and scattered mitochondria (*m*) are seen. Note that a few pseudopodia (*ps*) extend from the surface. Magnification × 16,000. (From B. A. Nichols, D. F. Bainton, and M. G. Far-quhar, *J. Cell Biol.* 50:498, 1971. Reprinted by permission of authors and publisher.)

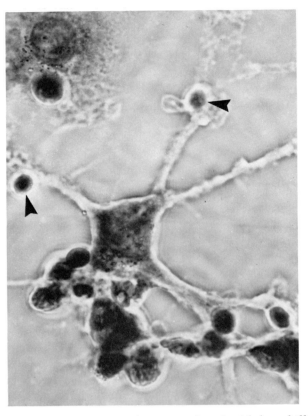

Figure 23.14 Human macrophages incubated with heat-killed *Candida albicans* (*arrows*), showing how the cells have trapped the yeast with their long pseudopods. Cells and yeast were fixed with glutaraldehyde and photographed with phase contrast illumination.

has condensed nuclear chromatin and cytoplasm that stains pink or light red with Romanovsky stains (19).

Table 23.1 provides a partial summary of enzymes that have been identified in macrophages by histochemical techniques. Like the monocyte, the macrophage appears to have a rough surface membrane with microprojections (119) (Fig. 23.17). Macrophage surface membranes may have distinctive antigenic features not found on lymphoid cells (32).

The Alveolar Macrophage

The alveolar macrophage is an example of a tissue macrophage maturing in a unique environment—the alveolar space. Like other tissue macrophages, it probably originates (at least in part) from precursors in the bone marrow that are distributed via the blood.

Three types of large mononuclear cells can be distinguished morphologically in lavages of human lung (21) (Fig. 23.18); for convenience, these cells are termed types

Table 23.1 Enzymes identified in macrophages by histochemical techniques (3, 7, 27, 29, 84, 90, 109, 130).

Nonlysosomal enzymes
    Succinic dehydrogenase
    Cytochrome oxidase
    Aminopeptidase
Lysosomal enzymes (probable)
    Beta-glucuronidase
    Beta-galactosidase
    Esterases
    Acid phosphatase
    Aryl sulfatase
    Peroxidase (young cells)

A, B, and C. Type A cells (Fig. 23.18A) account for 94 to 98 percent of the mononuclear cells in the lavage fluid from normal lung tissue. The cells have a mean diameter of 25 microns, with a range of 10 to 45 microns. The cytoplasm is stained dark and muddy gray and contains many small, dark blue granules with Giemsa stain, but shows no staining with peroxidase. The nucleus is oval or irregular and stains dark blue to aqua. Vacuoles are often present, especially at the outer border of the cell. Spontaneous ingestion of autologous red blood cells by viable macrophages is occasionally observed by phase microscopy. Electron micrographs of these cells show numerous mitochondria and lysosomes and abundant quantities of granular endoplasmic reticulum. Large inclusions are seen, especially in cells from smokers (Fig. 23.19).

About 5 percent of the mononuclear cells in the lavage fluid are type B, shown in Figure 23.18B. The cells have a mean diameter of 30 microns, with a range of 25 to 40 microns. The most easily identifiable difference between type A and type B cells is in the nucleus. The nucleolus of the type B cell is red to pink with Giemsa stain and the nuclear/cytoplasmic ratio is about 1:6 or 1:7, whereas in the type A cell the ratio is closer to 1:3. The cytoplasm of the type B cell contains fewer granules than the type A cell and has large, green-staining inclusion bodies.

Type C cells account for less than 1 percent of the mononuclear cells washed from normal lungs, but contribute up to 95 percent of the macrophages washed from the lungs of patients with postobstructive endogenous lipoid pneumonia (Fig. 23.18C). They are the only variety of alveolar macrophage in which phagocytized intact nucleated cells are observed. Their mean diameter is 40 microns, and the cytoplasm is packed with vacuoles. When attached to glass, the vacuoles become less prominent or disappear completely; the cells then look like macrophages washed from normal lungs.

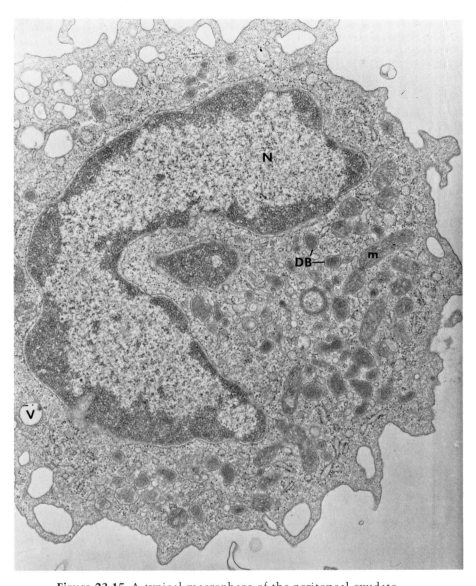

Figure 23.15 A typical macrophage of the peritoneal exudate with a large eccentric kidney-shaped nucleus (*N*). The centrosomal region contains many dense bodies (*DB*) varying from 50 to 400 mμ in diameter and a moderately large Golgi complex (not shown here). Invaginations and clear vacuoles (*V*) are found throughout the cell periphery. Moderate numbers of mitochondria (*m*) with lamellar cristae and cisternae of the rough-surfaced endoplasmic reticulum are evenly distributed in the cytoplasm. The nuclei of both control macrophages and those incubated with bacteriophage frequently contain one to four dense perichromatin granules 75 to 100 mμ in diameter. Magnification × 9,000. (From D. S. Friend, W. Rosenau, J. S. Winfield, and H. D. Moon, *Lab. Invest.* 20:275, 1969. Reprinted by permission of authors and publisher.)

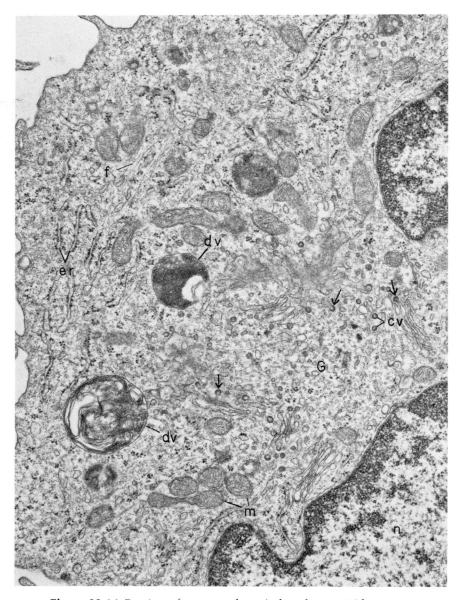

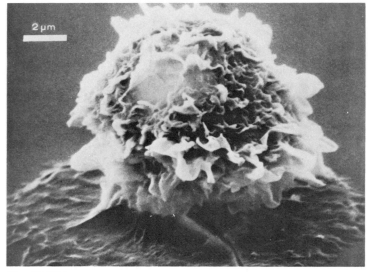

Fig. 23.17A

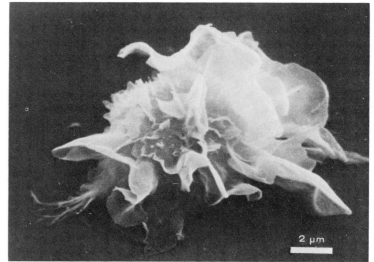

Fig. 23.17B

Figure 23.16 Portion of a macrophage (taken from a 96-hour peritoneal exudate produced in a rabbit) showing the Golgi region and surrounding cytoplasm. Numerous digestive vacuoles (*dv*) that vary in size and content are present, but no azurophil granules are seen. The Golgi complex (*G*) is large and contains many vesicles, most of which are coated (*cv*). Some of the coated vesicles (*arrows*) appear to be in direct continuity with Golgi cisternae. Rough endoplasmic reticulum (*er*) is moderately abundant, and mitochondria (*m*) are numerous. The cytoplasm is interlaced with fine (~100 Å) filaments (*f*), which are sometimes oriented in bundles and sometimes scattered randomly. Part of the nucleus (*n*) is shown. Magnification × 19,000. (From B. A. Nichols, D. F. Bainton, and M. G. Farquhar, *J. Cell Biol.* 50:498, 1971. Reprinted by permission of authors and publisher.)

Figure 23.17 Two views of macrophage membranes through a scanning electron microscope. (From A. H. Warfel and S. S. Elberg, *Science* 170:446, 1970. Reprinted by permission of authors and publisher.)

The population of macrophages that adhere to glass appears to be homogeneous and resembles type A cells. Type B cells either do not adhere to glass and phagocytize, or they do adhere but change their morphologic characteristics after adherence. Type C macrophages adhere to glass and phagocytize, and probably represent type A cells that have been modified by the environment distal to the obstructed bronchus. Adherent cells transform into multinucleated, large, vacuolated cells after three to four weeks in vitro (Fig. 23.18D).

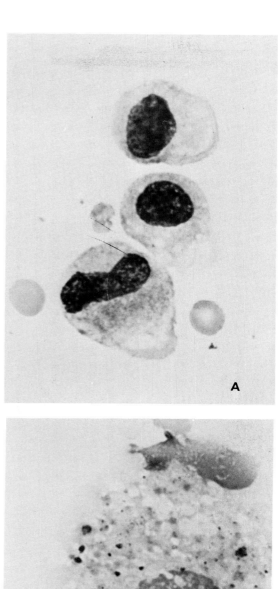

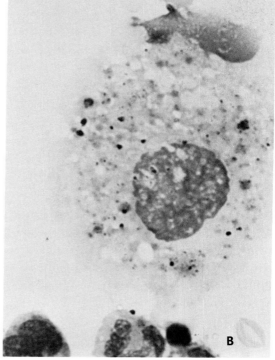

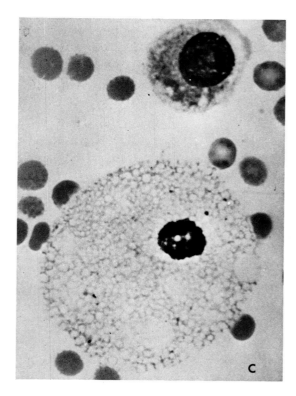

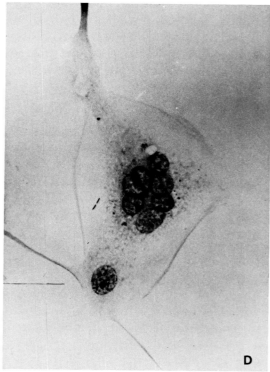

Figure 23.18 Various forms of human alveolar macrophages stained with Giemsa and photographed with bright-field illumination. Type A cells (shown in *A*) constitute between 94 and 98 percent of the normal population. About 5 percent of the population is type B (seen in *B*), and less than 1 percent is type C cells (*C*) with foamy-appearing cytoplasm. Multinucleate, glass-adherent cells (*D*) develop after three to four weeks of in vitro culture. (From A. B. Cohen and M. J. Cline, *J. Clin. Invest.* 50:1390, 1971. Reprinted by permission of authors and publisher.)

The numerous mitochondria of the alveolar macrophage are reflected in a rich oxidative metabolism.

The fine structure of the human alveolar macrophage is described in a number of recent publications (21, 22, 39, 66, 87). Alveolar macrophages from smokers' lungs often contain numerous dense inclusions, or residual bodies (39, 66) (Fig. 23.19).

Fetal Origin of the Macrophage

In the chick embryo the blood islands of the yolk sac are the first identifiable site of appearance of hematopoietic stem cells (77, 78). The available evidence indicates that stem cells migrate from the yolk sac to colonize and proliferate within the other sites of hematopoiesis of the older embryo and ultimately of the postnatal animal (79). Cells of avian yolk sac origin can repopulate the granulopoietic and lymphopoietic systems of irradiated host animals. A similar yolk sac origin of mammalian hematopoietic progenitor cells is suggested by the observation that in the mouse this embryonic organ is the first identifiable site containing cells capable of forming mixed hemic colonies in vitro and in the spleens of irradiated hosts in vivo (80).

On the seventh day of gestation the mouse yolk sac appears as the central part of the egg cylinder wall and then grows rapidly, forming an extensive membrane that envelops the amnion and exocoelomic cavity. During this period blood islands appear in the mesodermal layer of the yolk sac (80). In these islands the hemangioblasts develop either as undifferentiated blast cells or as progressively more mature erythroid precursors. In the yolk sac of seven to nine days' gestational age, differentiated cells of the monocytic or granulocytic series are never observed. Furthermore, no cells can be identified in the early yolk sac that are similar to immature bone marrow promonocytes of the adult animal—the cells characterized by glass adherence, limited phagocytic ability, and some surface IgG receptor activity (see Chapter 24). Despite the absence of identifiable monocyte-macrophage precursors, early yolk sac cells are capable of giving rise in culture to typical mature macrophages characterized by abundant lysosomes, avid phagocytosis, and surface receptor activity for IgG immunoglobulin (18).

In the late yolk sac (11 to 14 days), monocytes, macrophages, and cells with the characteristics of promonocytes are readily identifiable. At this time the yolk sac is open to the fetal circulation; consequently, it is not known whether these macrophages originate in situ or outside the yolk sac.

From these observations it appears that the fetal yolk sac is the site of origin of the macrophage precursor in the

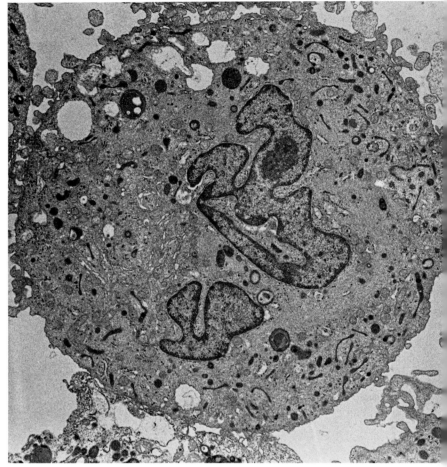

Fig. 23.19A

mouse embryo. The yolk sac appears to serve a similar function in the production of immunoglobulin-producing cells (105). The macrophage progenitor in the yolk sac is "proximal" to the bone marrow promonocyte in the pathway of sequential development that culminates in the monocyte and the mature macrophage; that is, it is a less differentiated cell than the promonocyte. The early yolk sac does not itself support differentiation of the progenitor to the promonocyte stage or beyond until after the ninth or tenth day of gestation in the mouse. Thereafter, the opening of the yolk sac to the fetal circulation obscures the origin of the macrophages observed in this organ. Thus, the situation described for the macrophage progenitor appears to be similar to that of the progenitor of granulopoiesis. Precursors of the granulocyte exist in the early yolk sac, but granulopoiesis does not occur there (80).

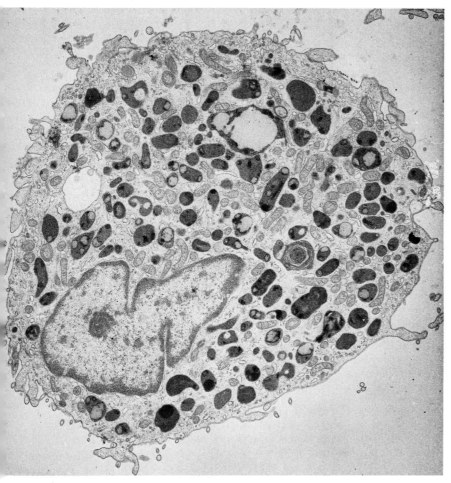

Fig. 23.19B

Figure 23.19 Electron micrographs of alveolar macrophages washed from the lungs of a normal, nonsmoking subject (Fig. 23.19A) and a normal, tobacco-smoking subject (Fig. 23.19B). Note the "smoker inclusions" in the latter. (Photographs courtesy of Dr. P. E. G. Mann.)

Production of Macrophages and Monocytes

Relation to Other Cell Lines

Evidence that monocytes share a common progenitor cell with the granulocytic series is suggested by the frequently observed mixed cellular proliferation in certain varieties of acute leukemia and chronic myelocytic leukemia. Further evidence for a common progenitor cell has come from observations of proliferation of bone marrow cells in soft nutrient agar medium. Under appropriate stimuli the bone marrow cells give rise to colonies comprised of granulocytic and macrophage elements (11, 46). The granulocytes are identified largely on morphologic criteria, and

the macrophages on morphologic and functional criteria (20). The colonies appear to be predominantly granulocytic at the early stages of their growth (70). Transfer of single cells at this time results in colonies that are predominantly granulocytic, predominantly macrophage, or mixed—the final cell pattern depending on the time after transfer at which the daughter colony is examined (71).

A similar relation between monocyte precursors and early granulocytes has been deduced from cytochemical studies of human bone marrow (58) and by examination of spleen colonies developing in irradiated mice after the administration of cell populations containing pluripotent stem cells (112). Other studies, both in vivo and in vitro, have provided generally similar conclusions (14, 15, 126, 127).

These observations suggest that the granulocyte and the macrophage share a common progenitor cell and that under certain experimental conditions early myeloid precursors may give rise to monocytic cells. This concept is illustrated in Fig. I.1 of the Introduction. It is not known at what level of maturation a cell is irrevocably committed to granulocyte development as opposed to monocyte differentiation; presumably it is at a stage preceding the promyelocyte. Nor is it known whether the process can go in the reverse direction—from the monocytic to the granulocytic series. The data available from in vitro leukocyte culture work suggest that the monocyte-to-granulocyte sequence is unlikely (see Chapter 2).

Certain subpopulations of lymphocytes are difficult to distinguish from monocytes on morphologic grounds, either by light or by electron microscopy. There is no evidence that such cells are related to monocytes either functionally or as precursors. These morphologically nonspecific lymphocytes must of necessity be defined on the grounds of function: the capacity to initiate immunologic responses or to undergo blastogenic transformation in response to appropriate stimuli (36, 83, 115). Those cells that meet the morphologic criteria for lymphocytes but (for the present) lack definable functions should be referred to as lymphocyte-like cells. It is possible that the early bone marrow precursor of the monocyte is such a lymphocyte-like cell, but the existing evidence is not definitive (115).

Origin of the Tissue Macrophage in Inflammation

By the use of tritiated thymidine it is possible to label cells in the DNA synthetic (S) phase of the cell cycle preceding mitosis. When such a label is given as a pulse before the initiation of an inflammatory lesion, it is possible to show that the mononuclear leukocytes accumulating in the focus of inflammation originate almost entirely in the circulation (28, 54). If colloidal carbon is given at the same time to identify phagocytic leukocytes, it can be shown that the mononuclear phagocytes originate from blood monocytes (99). Similar conclusions about the blood monocyte origin of the inflammatory mononuclear cell have been reached on the basis of other experimental models such as parabiotic animals, one of which is labeled with tritiated thymidine (117) or with chromosome markers (110).

Volkman and Gowans (118) transfused tritium-thymidine-labeled bone marrow and lymph node cells into rats and found that only the bone marrow cells have the capacity to become macrophages. Similar conclusions have been reached by other investigators using other experimental systems (12, 41, 42, 95, 97, 100, 104, 128, 129). Under certain experimental inflammatory conditions, the liver macrophage appears to have its origin in the bone marrow via the blood monocyte (9, 43).

To summarize: As determined from a wealth of data, the major source of monocytes and macrophages at inflammatory sites is the bone marrow. Labeling patterns indicate that these inflammatory mononuclear cells arise from continuously and rapidly proliferating bone marrow cells. They reach the inflammatory site via the bloodstream.

In the tissues, under normal circumstances, macrophages show little evidence of mitotic activity; they are in a dormant, or G_0, state (55, 110). The same pattern is true for macrophages cultivated in vitro; they show little proliferative activity unless a stimulus is applied (38, 47, 110, 111).

Inflammatory lesions induced by antigen-antibody interactions generally contain abundant macrophages. These cells, like those of other inflammatory lesions, almost certainly arise from bone marrow progenitors (61, 63, 64).

Kinetic Behavior of the Monocyte and its Precursors

From a variety of rodent studies using tritiated thymidine and radioautographic techniques, we may draw the following conclusions (99, 106, 113, 117, 118, 122–124):

(a) The blood monocyte is derived from a rapidly proliferating cell in the bone marrow.
(b) Within 24 hours of a pulse of tritiated thymidine, labeled monocytes appear in the peripheral blood.
(c) The immediate progenitor of the monocytes remains in the bone marrow about 18 hours after the last DNA synthesis.
(d) The number of divisions between stem cell and monocyte is three, or possibly four (19).

(e) Monocytes seem to leave the circulation in random fashion; that is, independent of age. The half-survival time in the rat is between 13 and 74 hours.
(f) Once the monocyte leaves the circulation, it does not return.
(g) In the tissues the monocyte undergoes transformation to a macrophage.
(h) The macrophage may live many months, perhaps even years (98).

In studies of patients with monocytic leukemia, the life-span of the blood monocyte has been estimated to be about 3 days (85). In another study, the mean circulation time of leukemic monocytes in man was calculated to be about 6 days (51). In the rat, labeled monocytes appear in the blood as early as 6 hours after injection of tritiated thymidine. By 18 hours 18 percent of the cells are labeled. This proportion remains stable for approximately 72 hours, after which it declines (117). A roughly similar pattern of monocyte labeling has been described in the mouse (67). Thus, in three species—man, the rat, and the mouse—the pattern emerges of a rapid turnover of monocytes in the blood. The data of Whitelaw (122) and Volkman (114, 115), obtained from rodent studies, indicate a maximal intramarrow transit time of 6 to 8 days, an exponential clearance of monocytes from the blood of 2.6 to 3.1 days, and a mean generation time for monocyte precursors of approximately 21 to 24 hours.

The recent studies of Meuret and Hoffman (74) provide the following information on monocyte kinetics in man: (a) the total blood monocyte pool is comprised of a circulating pool (CMP) and a marginated pool (MMP), with the latter about three times the size of the former; (b) monocytes leave the vascular space in an exponential fashion with a $T_{1/2}$ of 8.4 hours; (c) the $T_{1/2}$ may be prolonged in some patients with monocytosis and shortened in others with acute infection or splenomegaly; and (d) the normal monocyte turnover rate averages 7×10^6 cells/hour/kg of body weight.

In the mouse the disappearance of monocytes from the blood is also exponential, with a half-time of about 22 hours (106).

Factors Influencing Monocyte Numbers,
Development, and Turnover

A variety of factors influences the numbers of circulating monocytes. In the normal adult the relative monocyte count is between 1 and 6 percent of the total leukocyte count, rarely exceeding 10 percent (56, 75, 101, 125). The absolute monocyte count in the adult ranges between 285 and 500 cells/mm³ of blood (75, 125). In children the average count is about 9 percent (121), and the absolute number ranges up to 750 or 800 cells/mm³ (8, 75). Monocytosis is normal in the first two weeks of life (49).

Some of the disease states in which there is characteristically a blood monocytosis are the following (65):

Infections
    Tuberculosis
    Brucellosis
    Subacute bacterial endocarditis
Malignancies
    Hodgkin's disease
Miscellaneous
    Hepatic cirrhosis
    Systemic lupus erythematosus
    Polycythemia vera
    Myeloid metaplasia
    Rheumatoid arthritis

Diseases associated with monocytosis are discussed more fully in Chapter 26.

Administration of endotoxin results in a monocytopenia followed by a recovery phase that is slow and incomplete relative to the granulocyte response (96). Injection in man of antibody-coated erythrocytes results in a prompt fall in circulating monocytes, persisting for at least three to six hours (48).

Glucocorticoid administration may induce a monocytopenia, probably by interfering with the release of monocytes from the bone marrow (103). *Listeria monocytogenes* and some of its components are capable of inducing a striking blood monocytosis in some experimental animals (40). Infection with a variety of parasitic intracellular microorganisms produces notable changes in the kinetics, metabolism, and function of mononuclear phagocytes. These changes are discussed in the next three chapters.

Monocytes and their progeny appear to be relatively insensitive to irradiation (53, 118). However, whole-body irradiation produces a sharp fall in the number of circulating monocytes (45, 106, 116) and of newly formed macrophages (118). It appears, therefore, that the dividing progenitors of the monocyte are radio-sensitive. Presumably these include the promonocyte and its antecedents in the bone marrow.

Origin of Other Tissue Macrophages

Earlier in this chapter data were summarized which indicated that macrophages in foci of inflammation arise from progenitor cells in the bone marrow. At some stage, these macrophages pass through the circulation as monocytes. Let us examine whether the population of normal macrophages that inhabits noninflamed tissues has a similar origin.

Liver Macrophages   Some quite recent observations in parabiotic, chromosomally marked mice suggest that normal Kupffer cells of the liver may be partially of hemic origin (52, 92). The morphology of peripheral blood monocytes and Kupffer cells may be very similar (76). However, some—perhaps most—of these hepatic macrophages probably arise from local cellular proliferation (50).

Peritoneal Macrophages   A number of observations indicate that the source of peritoneal macrophages is the bone marrow (5, 35, 106, 110); many of these studies utilize irradiated chimeric mice that have received various cell populations from intact animals. The donor cells have been labeled either with a chromosome marker or with tritiated thymidine.

Peritoneal macrophages may also be derived from cells present in thoracic duct lymph draining the site of a graft-vs-host reaction (44).

Tissue Histiocytes   Although blood monocytes clearly can give rise to tissue histiocytes (30), it is not known whether this is the major mechanism of histiocyte renewal in the intact animal. Recent evidence suggests that tissue macrophages may be capable of migration or localization within specific organs (33, 91, 94).

Alveolar Macrophages   Several investigators have reported that a portion of alveolar macrophages is derived from circulating monocytes and a bone marrow precursor. For example, when X-irradiated CBA mice are given bone marrow cells from CBA/T6T6 animals, between 60 and 80 percent of the alveolar macrophages in mitosis carry the T6 markers; that is, they are of donor bone marrow origin (86). Similar conclusions have been reached by other investigators (10, 34, 82, 106). One must express the reservation, however, that irradiated animals may not be a perfect model for the study of normal cell kinetics.

Moore and Schoenberg (81) have published electron micrographs of rabbit cells identified as "histiocytes" in transit through the alveolar lining cells.

Fibroblasts   The occasional reports that blood mononuclear cells can give rise to fibroblasts are probably unfounded. Many sound data refute such a possibility (37, 69, 88, 93).

Summary

The mononuclear leukocyte series has its origin in the bone marrow monoblast and promonocyte. Only the intermediate-stage cell (the monocyte) is normally encountered in the circulation. In the tissues the monocytes differentiate into large, phagocytic, mononuclear cells called macrophages or histiocytes. These may have a variety of forms: the alveolar macrophage, the Kupffer cell, the peritoneal macrophage. The mononuclear phagocyte series may be regarded as a morphologically heterogeneous, geographically dispersed tissue.

Maturation is accompanied by increase in cell size and in numbers of cytoplasmic organelles, including mi-tochondria and lysosomes. The precise pattern of development is influenced by the tissue in which the macrophage matures. For example, the alveolar macrophage developing within the alveolar space has certain unique biochemical properties.

In its development the mononuclear phagocyte system is related closely to the granulocyte series, and more distantly to other hematopoietic cells. Like other hematopoietic cells, the mononuclear phagocyte is originally derived from the fetal yolk sac.

Chapter 23 References

1. Allison, A. C., Davies, P., and De Petris, S. Role of contractile microfilaments in macrophage movement and endocytosis, *Nature (New Biol.)* 232:153, 1971.
2. Aschoff, L. Lectures on Pathology, Paul B. Hoeber, New York, 1924.
3. Atwal, O. S. Cytoenzymological behavior of peritoneal exudate cells of rat in vivo, *J. Reticuloendothel. Soc.* 10:163, 1971.
4. Awrorow, P. P., and Timofejewskij, A. D. Kultivierungsversuche von leukämischem Blute, *Virchows Arch. (Pathol. Anat. Physiol.)* 216:184, 1914.
5. Balner, H. Identification of peritoneal macrophages in mouse radiation chimeras, *Transplantation* 1:217, 1963.
6. Bennett, W. E., and Cohn, Z. A. The isolation and selected properties of blood monocytes, *J. Exp. Med.* 123:145, 1966.
7. Bennett, W. E., and Pearson, B. A study of the indigogenic principle and in vitro macrophage differentiation, *J. Reticuloendothel. Soc.* 6:158, 1969.
8. Bessis, M. Cytology of the Blood and Blood Forming Organs, p. 629, Grune & Stratton, New York, 1956.
9. Boak, J. L., Christie, G. H., Ford, W. L., and Howard, J. G. Pathways in the development of liver macrophages: alternative precursors contained in populations of lymphocytes and bone marrow cells, *Proc. R. Soc. Lond. (Biol.)* 169:307, 1968.
10. Bowden, D. H., Adamson, I. Y. R., Grantham, W. G., and Wyatt, J. P. Origin of the lung macrophage, *Arch. Pathol.* 88:540, 1969.
11. Bradley, T. R., and Metcalf, D. The growth of mouse bone marrow cells *in vitro, Aust. J. Exp. Biol. Med.* 44:287, 1966.
12. Braunsteiner, H. Expériences de marquage des lymphocytes par la thymidine tritiée, *Nouv. Rev. Fr. Hematol.* 1:733, 1961.
13. Chapman, J. A., Gough, J., and Elves, M. W. An electron-microscope study of the *in vitro* transformation of human leucocytes. II. Transformation to macrophages, *J. Cell Sci.* 2:371, 1967.
14. Chen. M. G., and Schooley, J. C. Recovery of proliferative capacity of agar colony-forming cells and spleen colony-forming cells following ionizing radiation or vinblastine, *J. Cell. Physiol.* 75:89, 1970.
15. Chen, M. G., and Schooley, J. C. Effects of ionizing radiation and vinblastine on the proliferation of peritoneal macrophage precursors in the mouse, *Radiat. Res.* 41:623, 1970.
16. Clawson, C. C., and Good, R. A. Micropapillae. A surface specialization of human leukocytes, *J. Cell Biol.* 48:207, 1971.
17. Cline, M. J. Monocytes and macrophages: differentiation and function, *in* T. J. Greenwalt and G. A. Jamieson (eds.), Third Annual Red Cross Symposium on Formation and Destruction of Blood Cells, p. 222, J. B. Lippincott, Philadelphia, 1970.
18. Cline, M. J., and Moore, M. A. S. Embryonic origin of the mouse macrophage, *Blood* 39:842, 1971.
19. Cline, M. J., and Sumner, M. A. Bone marrow macrophage precursors. I. Some functional characteristics of the early cells of the mouse macrophage series, *Blood* 40:62, 1972.
20. Cline, M. J., Warner, N. L., and Metcalf, D. Identification of the bone marrow colony mononuclear phagocytes as a macrophage, *Blood* 39:326, 1971.
21. Cohen, A. B., and Cline, M. J. The human alveolar macrophage. Isolation, cultivation in vitro and studies of morphologic and functional characteristics, *J. Clin. Invest.* 50:1390, 1971.
22. Cohen, A. B., and Cline, M. J. In vitro studies of the foamy macrophage of postobstructive endogenous lipoid pneumonia in man, *Am. Rev. Respir. Dis.* 106:69, 1972.
23. Cohn, Z. A. The structure and function of monocytes and macrophages, *Adv. Immunol.* 9:163, 1968.
24. Cohn, Z. A., and Benson, B. The differentiation of mononuclear phagocytes. Morphology, cytochemistry and biochemistry, *J. Exp. Med.* 121:153, 1965.
25. Cohn, Z. A., and Benson, B. The in vitro differentiation of mononuclear phagocytes. I. The influence of inhibitors and the results of autoradiography, *J. Exp. Med.* 121:279, 1965.
26. Cohn, Z. A., and Benson, B. The in vitro differentiation of mononuclear phagocytes. II. The influence of serum on granule formation, hydrolase production and pinocytosis, *J. Exp. Med.* 121:835, 1965.
27. Cotran, R. S., and Litt, M. Ultrastructural localization of horseradish peroxidase and endogenous peroxidase activity in guinea pig peritoneal macrophages, *J. Immunol.* 105:1536, 1970.
28. Cronkite, E. P., Bond, V. P., Fliedner, T. M., and Killman, S-A. The use of tritiated thymidine in the study of haemopoietic cell proliferation, *in* G. E. W. Wolstenholme and H. O'Connor (eds.), Haemopoiesis (Ciba Found. Symp.), p. 70, Little, Brown, and Co., Boston, 1960.
29. Dannenberg, A. M., Jr., Burstone, M. S., Walter, P. C., and Kinsley, J. W. A histochemical study of phagocytic and enzymatic functions of rabbit mononuclear and polymorphonuclear exudate cells and alveolar macrophages. I. Survey and quantitation of enzymes, and states of cellular activation, *J. Cell Biol.* 17:465, 1963.
30. Ebert, R. H., and Florey, H. W. The extravascular development of the monocyte observed in vitro, *Br. J. Exp. Pathol.* 20:342, 1939.
31. Epstein, W. L. Granulomatous hypersensitivity, *Prog. Allergy* 11:36, 1967.
32. Gallily, R., and Bornostansky, M. Specificity and nature of binding of antimacrophage serum, *Immunology* 22:431, 1972.
33. Gillette, R. W., and Lance, E. M. Kinetic studies of macrophages. I. Distributional characteristics of radiolabeled peritoneal cells, *J. Reticuloendothel. Soc.* 10:223, 1971.
34. Godleski, J. J., and Brain, J. D. The origin of alveolar macrophages in mouse radiation chimeras, *J. Exp. Med.* 136:630, 1972.
35. Goodman, J. W. On the origin of peritoneal fluid cells, *Blood* 23:18, 1964.
36. Gowans, J. L., and McGregor, D. D. The immunological activities of lymphocytes, *Prog. Allergy* 9:1, 1965.
37. Hall, J. W., and Furth, J. Cultural studies on the relationship of lymphocytes to monocytes and fibroblasts, *Arch. Pathol.* 25:46, 1938.
38. Hanifin, J., and Cline, M. J. Human

monocytes and macrophages: interaction with antigen and lymphocytes, *J. Cell Biol.* 46:97, 1970.

39. Harris, J. O., Swenson, E. W., and Johnson, J. E. III. Human alveolar macrophages: comparison of phagocytic ability, glucose utilization and ultrastructure in smokers and nonsmokers, *J. Clin. Invest.* 49:2086, 1970.

40. Holder, I. A., and Sword, C. P. Characterization and biological activity of the monocytosis-producing agent of *Listeria monocytogenes*, *J. Bacteriol.* 97:603, 1969.

41. Horwitz, D. A. The development of macrophages from large mononuclear cells in the blood of patients with inflammatory disease, *J. Clin. Invest.* 51:760, 1972.

42. Horwitz, D. A., Stastny, P., and Ziff, M. Circulating deoxyribonucleic acid-synthesizing mononuclear leukocytes. I. Increased numbers of proliferating mononuclear leukocytes in inflammatory diseases. *J. Lab. Clin. Med.* 76:391, 1970.

43. Howard, J. G., Boak, J. L., and Christie, G. H. Further studies on the transformation of thoracic duct cells into liver macrophages, *Ann. N.Y. Acad. Sci.* 129:327, 1966.

44. Howard, J. G., Christie, G. H., Boak, J. L., and Kinsky, R. G. Peritoneal and alveolar macrophages derived from lymphocyte populations during graft-*versus*-host reaction, *Br. J. Exp. Pathol.* 50:448, 1969.

45. Hulse, E. V. The total white cell count of the blood as an indicator of acute radiation damage and its value during the first few hours after exposure, *J. Clin. Pathol.* 13:37, 1959.

46. Ichikawa, Y., Pluznik, D. H., and Sachs, L. In vitro control of the development of macrophage and granulocyte colonies, *Proc. Natl. Acad. Sci. U.S.A.* 56:488, 1966.

47. Jacoby, F. Macrophages, *in* E. N. Willmer (ed.), Cells and Tissues in Culture: Methods, Biology and Physiology, vol. 2, p. 1, Academic Press, New York, 1965.

48. Jandl, J. H., and Tomlinson, A. S. The destruction of red cells by antibodies in man. II. Pyrogenic, leukocytic and dermal responses to

immune hemolysis, *J. Clin. Invest.* 37:1202, 1958.

49. Kato, K. Leucocytes in infancy and childhood: a statistical analysis of 1,081 total and differential counts from birth to fifteen years, *J. Pediatr.* 7:7, 1935.

50. Kelly, L. S., and Dobson, E. L. Evidence concerning the origin of liver macrophages, *Br. J. Exp. Pathol.* 52:88, 1971.

51. Killmann, S-A., Cronkite, E. P., Bond, V. P., and Fliedner, T. M. Proliferation of human leukemic cells studied with tritiated thymidine in vivo, *in* Proc. VIII Congress of the European Society of Hematology, Vienna, p. 63, S. Karger, Basel, 1962.

52. Kinsky, R. G., Christie,G. H., Elson, J., and Howard, J. G. Extrahepatic derivation of Kupffer cells during oestrogenic stimulation of parabiosed mice, *Br. J. Exp. Pathol.* 50:438, 1969.

53. Kornfeld, L., and Greenman, V. Effects of total-body X-irradiation on peritoneal cells of mice, *Radiat. Res.* 29:433, 1966.

54. Kosunen, T. V., Waksman, B. H., Flax, M. H., and Tihen, W. S. Radioautographic study of cellular mechanisms in delayed hypersensitivity. I. Delayed reactions to tuberculin and purified proteins in the rat and guinea-pig, *Immunology* 6:276, 1963.

55. Lajtha, L. G., Gilbert, C. W., Porteous, D. D., and Alexanian, R. Kinetics of a bone-marrow stem-cell population, *Ann. N.Y. Acad. Sci.* 113:742, 1964.

56. Leavell, B. S., and Thorup, O. A., Jr. Fundamentals of Clinical Hematology, p. 314, W. B. Saunders Co., Philadelphia, 1960.

57. Leder, L-D. Fermentcytochemische Untersuchungen zur Herkunft des Blutmonocyten, *Klin. Wochenschr.* 44:25, 1966.

58. Leder, L-D. The origin of blood monocytes and macrophages, *Blut* 16:86, 1967.

59. Lewis M. R. The formation of macrophages, epithelioid cells and giant cells from leucocytes in incubated blood, *Am. J. Pathol.* 1:91, 1925.

60. Lewis, M. R., and Lewis, W. H. Transformation of mononuclear blood cells into macrophages,

epithelioid cells and giant cells in hanging drop cultures of lower vertebrates, Carnegie Inst. Wash. Publ. 96, *Contrib. Embryol.* 18:95, 1926.

61. Liden, S. The mononuclear-cell infiltrate in allergic contact dermatitis, *Acta Pathol. Microbiol. Scand.* 70:58, 1967.

62. Low, F. N., and Freeman, J. A. Electron Microscopic Atlas of Normal and Leukemic Human Blood, McGraw-Hill, New York, 1958.

63. Lubaroff, D. M., and Waksman, B. H. Bone marrow as source of cells in reactions of cellular hypersensitivity. II. Identification of allogenic or hybrid cells by immunofluorescence in passively transferred tuberculin reactions, *J. Exp. Med.* 128:1437, 1968.

64. McCluskey, R. T., Benacerraf, B., and McCluskey, J. W. Studies on the specificity of the cellular infiltrate in delayed hypersensitivity reactions, *J. Immunol.* 90:466, 1963.

65. Maldonado, J. E., and Hanlon, D. G. Monocytosis: a current appraisal, *Mayo Clin. Proc.* 40:248, 1965.

66. Mann, P. E. G., Cohen, A. B., Finley, T. N., and Ladman, A. J. Alveolar macrophages. Structural and functional differences between nonsmokers and smokers of marijuana and tobacco, *Lab. Invest.* 25:111, 1971.

67. Matsuyama, M., Wiadrowski, M. N., and Metcalf, D. Autoradiographic analysis of lymphopoiesis and lymphocyte migration in mice bearing multiple thymus grafts, *J. Exp. Med.* 123:559, 1965.

68. Maximow, A. A. The macrophages or histiocytes, *in* E. V. Cowdrey (ed.), Special Cytology. The Form and Functions of the Cell in Health and Disease, 2nd ed., vol. 2, sec. 19, pp. 709–770, Paul B. Hoeber, New York, 1932.

69. Medawar, J. Observations on lymphocytes in tissue culture, *Br. J. Exp. Pathol.* 21:205, 1940.

70. Metcalf, D. Studies on colony formation *in vitro* by mouse bone marrow cells. I. Continuous cluster formation and relation of clusters to colonies, *J. Cell. Physiol.* 74:323, 1969.

71. Metcalf, D. Transformation of granulocytes to macrophages in bone

marrow colonies in vitro, *J. Cell. Physiol.* 77:277, 1971.

72. Metchnikoff, E. Ueber die phagocytäre Rolle der Tuberkelriesenzellen, *Arch. Pathol. Anat. Physiol. Klin. Med.* 113:63, 1888.
73. Metchnikoff, E. Immunity in Infective Diseases (F. G. Binnie, trans.), Cambridge University Press, Cambridge, England, 1905.
74. Meuret, G., and Hoffman, G. Monocyte kinetic studies in normal and disease states, *Br. J. Haematol.* 24:275, 1973.
75. Miale, J. B. Laboratory Medicine—Hematology, 2nd ed., p. 600, C. V. Mosby Co., St. Louis, 1962.
76. Mills, D. M., and Zucker-Franklin, D. Electron microscopic study of isolated Kupffer cells, *Am. J. Pathol.* 54:147, 1969.
77. Moore, M. A. S., and Owen, J. J. T. Chromosome marker studies on the development of the haemopoietic system in the chick embryo, *Nature* 208:956, 1965.
78. Moore, M. A. S., and Owen, J. J. T. Stem-cell migration in developing myeloid and lymphoid systems, *Lancet* ii:658, 1967.
79. Moore, M. A. S., and Owen, J. J. T. Chromosome studies in the irradiated chick embryo, *Nature* 215:1081, 1967.
80. Moore, M. A. S., and Metcalf, D. Ontogeny of the haemopoietic system: yolk sac origin of *in vivo* and *in vitro* colony forming cells in the developing embryo, *Br. J. Haematol.* 18:279, 1970.
81. Moore, R. D., and Schoenberg, M. D. Alveolar lining cells and pulmonary reticuloendothelial system of the rabbit, *Am. J. Pathol.* 45:991, 1964.
82. Myrvik, Q. N., Leake, E. S., and Oshima, S. A study of macrophages and epithelioid-like cells from granulomatous (BCG-induced) lungs of rabbits, *J. Immunol.* 89:745, 1963.
83. Nelson, D. S. Macrophages and Immunity, North-Holland Publishing Co., Amsterdam, 1969.
84. Nichols, B. A., Bainton, D. F., and Farquhar, M. G. Differentiation of monocytes. Origin, nature and fate of their azurophil granules, *J. Cell Biol.* 50:498, 1971.
85. Osgood, E. E., Tivey, H., Davison, K. B., Seaman, A. J., and Li, J. G. The relative rates of formation of new leukocytes in patients with acute and chronic leukemias. Measured by the uptake of radioactive phosphorous in the isolated desoxyribosenucleic acid, *Cancer* 5:331, 1952.
86. Pinkett, M. O., Cowdrey, C. R., and Nowell, P. C. Mixed hematopoietic and pulmonary origin of "alveolar macrophages" as demonstrated by chromosome markers, *Am. J. Pathol.* 48:859, 1966.
87. Pratt, S. A., Finley, T. N., Smith, M. H., and Ladman, A. J. A comparison of alveolar macrophages and pulmonary surfactant (?) obtained from the lungs of human smokers and nonsmokers by endobronchial lavage, *Anat. Rec.* 163:497, 1969.
88. Rangan, S. R. S. Origin of the fibroblastic growths in chicken buffy coat macrophage cultures, *Exp. Cell Res.* 46:477, 1967.
89. Robineaux, R., Anteunis, A., and Bona, C. Ultrastructure des macrophages de cobaye, *Ann. Inst. Pasteur* 120:329, 1971.
90. Rosenszajn, L., Leibovich, M., Shoham, D., and Epstein, J. The esterase activity in megaloblasts, leukaemic and normal haemopoietic cells, *Br. J. Haematol.* 14:605, 1968.
91. Roser, B. The distribution of intravenously injected peritoneal macrophages in the mouse, *Aust. J. Exp. Biol. Med. Sci.* 43:553, 1965.
92. Roser, B. The distribution of intravenously injected Kupffer cells in the mouse, *J. Reticuloendothel. Soc.* 5:455, 1968.
93. Ross, R., and Lillywhite, J. W. The fate of buffy coat cells grown in subcutaneously implanted diffusion chambers. A light and electron microscopic study, *Lab. Invest.* 14:1568, 1966.
94. Russell, P., and Roser, B. The distribution and behaviour of intravenously injected pulmonary alveolar macrophages in the mouse, *Aust. J. Exp. Biol. Med. Sci.* 44:629, 1966.
95. Schmalzl, F., Huber, H., Asamer, H., Abbrederis, K., and Braunsteiner, H. Cytochemical and immunohistologic investigations on the source and the functional changes of mononuclear cells in skin window exudates, *Blood* 34:129, 1969.
96. Scully, F. J. The reaction after intravenous injections of foreign protein, *J.A.M.A.* 69:20, 1917.
97. Spector, W. G., Lykke, A. W. J., and Willoughby, D. A. A quantitative study of leucocyte emigration in chronic inflammatory granulomata, *J. Pathol. Bacteriol.* 93:101, 1967.
98. Spector, W. G., and Ryan, G. B. New evidence for the existence of long lived macrophages, *Nature* 221:860, 1969.
99. Spector, W. G., Walters, M. N-I., and Willoughby, D. A. The origin of the mononuclear cells in inflammatory exudates induced by fibrinogen, *J. Pathol. Bacteriol.* 90:181, 1965.
100. Spector, W. G., and Willoughby, D. A. The origin of mononuclear cells in chronic inflammation and tuberculin reactions in the rat, *J. Pathol. Bacteriol.* 96:389, 1968.
101. Sturgis, C. C. Hematology, 2nd ed., p. 708, Charles C Thomas, Springfield, Ill., 1955.
102. Sutton, J. S. Ultrastructural aspects of in vitro development of monocytes into macrophages, epithelioid cells, and multinucleated giant cells, *Natl. Cancer Inst. Monogr.* 26:71, 1967.
103. Thompson, J., and van Furth, R. The effect of glucocorticosteroids on the proliferation and kinetics of promonocytes and monocytes of the bone marrow, *J. Exp. Med.* 137:10, 1973.
104. Trepel, F., and Begemann, H. On the origin of the skin window macrophages, *Acta Haematol.* 36:386, 1966.
105. Tyan, M. L., and Herzenberg, L. A. Studies on the ontogeny of the immune response. II. Immunoglobulin-producing cells, *J. Immunol.* 101:446, 1968.
106. van Furth, R., and Cohn, Z. A. The origin and kinetics of mononuclear phagocytes, *J. Exp. Med.* 128:415, 1968.
107. van Furth, R., Cohn, Z. A., Hirsch, J. G., Humphrey, J. H., Spector, W. G., and Langevoort, H. L. The mononuclear phagocyte system: a new classification of macrophages, monocytes, and their precursor cells, *Bull. W.H.O.* 46:845, 1972.
108. van Furth, R., and Diesselhoff-Den-

Dulk, M. M. C. The kinetics of promonocytes and monocytes in the bone marrow, *J. Exp. Med.* 132:813, 1970.

109. van Furth, R., Hirsch, J. G., and Fedorko, M. E. Morphology and peroxidase cytochemistry of mouse promonocytes, monocytes and macrophages, *J. Exp. Med.* 132:794, 1970.

110. Virolainen, M. Hematopoietic origin of macrophages as studied by chromosome markers in mice, *J. Exp. Med.* 127:943, 1968.

111. Virolainen, M., and Defendi, V. Dependence of macrophage growth in vitro upon interaction with other cell types, *in* V. Defendi and M. Stoker (eds.), Growth Regulating Substances for Animal Cells in Culture, p. 67, Wistar Inst. Symp. Monogr. No. 7, Philadelphia, 1967.

112. Virolainen, M., and Defendi, V. Ability of haematopoietic spleen colonies to form macrophages *in vitro*, *Nature* 217:1069, 1968.

113. Volkman, A. The origin and turnover of mononuclear cells in peritoneal exudates in rats, *J. Exp. Med.* 124:241, 1966.

114. Volkman, A. The production of monocytes and related cells, *Haematol. Lat. (Milan)* 10:61, 1967.

115. Volkman, A. The origin and fate of the monocyte, *Ser. Haematol.* 3:62, 1970.

116. Volkman, A., and Collins, F. M. Recovery of delayed-type hypersensitivity in mice following suppressive doses of X-radiation, *J. Immunol.* 101:846, 1968.

117. Volkman, A., and Gowans, J. L. The production of macrophages in the rat, *Br. J. Exp. Pathol.* 46:50, 1965.

118. Volkman, A., and Gowans, J. L. The origin of macrophages from bone marrow in the rat, *Br. J. Exp. Pathol.* 46:62, 1965.

119. Warfel, A. H., and Elberg, S. S. Macrophage membranes viewed through a scanning electron microscope, *Science* 170:446, 1970.

120. Weiss, L. P., and Fawcett, D. W. Cytochemical observations on chicken monocytes, macrophages, and giant cells in tissue culture, *J. Histochem. Cytochem.* 1:47, 1953.

121. Whitby, L. E. H., and Britton, C. J. C. Disorders of the Blood: Diagnosis; Pathology; Treatment; Technique, 7th ed., p. 421, Grune & Stratton, New York, 1953.

122. Whitelaw, D. M. The intravascular life span of monocytes, *Blood* 28:455, 1966.

123. Whitelaw, D. M., and Batho, H. F. The distribution of monocytes in the rat, *Cell Tissue Kinet.* 5:215, 1972.

124. Whitelaw, D. M., Bell, M. F., and Batho, H. F. Monocyte kinetics: observations after pulse labeling, *J. Cell. Physiol.* 72:65, 1968.

125. Wintrobe, M. M. Clinical Hematology, 6th ed. p. 241, Lea & Febiger, Philadelphia, 1967.

126. Worton, R. G., McCulloch, E. A., and Till, J. E. Physical separation of haemopoietic stem cells from cells forming colonies in culture, *J. Cell. Physiol.* 74:171, 1969.

127. Wu, A. M., Siminovitch, L., Till, J. E., and McCulloch, E. A. Evidence for a relationship between mouse haemopoietic cells and cells forming colonies in culture, *Proc. Natl. Acad. Sci. U.S.A.* 59:1209, 1968.

128. Wulff, H. R. Histochemical studies of leukocytes from an inflammatory exudate. V. Alkaline and acid phosphatases and esterases, *Acta Haematol. (Basel)* 30:159, 1963.

129. Wulff, H. R., and Sparrevohn, S. The origin of mononuclear cells in human skin windows, *Acta Pathol. Microbiol. Scand.* 68:401, 1966.

130. Yarborough, D. J., Meyer, O. T., Dannenberg, A. M., Jr., and Pearson, B. Histochemistry of macrophage hydrolases. III. Studies on beta-galactosidase, beta-glucuronidase and aminopeptidase with indolyl and naphthyl substrates, *J. Reticuloendothel. Soc.* 4:390, 1967.

Chapter 24   Metabolism of Monocytes and Macrophages

Any description of the enzymatic activity and metabolism of monocytes and macrophages must take into account the profound changes that occur in these cells with maturation, with changes in cellular environment, and with activities such as pinocytosis and phagocytosis (13, 22, 32). It is clear that the mononuclear phagocytes of the reticuloendothelial system represent a spectrum of cells that are at various levels of differentiation and that originate from a common progenitor. Within the bone marrow the earliest identifiable cells of the series—blast cells and promonocytes—are characterized by a high rate of nucleic acid synthesis. The mature macrophages of the tissues (histiocytes) are characterized by high rates of protein synthesis and a high content of lysosomal enzymes. Mature macrophages in unique environments may develop a unique cellular physiology; for example, the highly developed aerobic metabolism of the alveolar macrophage. Furthermore, macrophages may alter their metabolism in response to environmental stress. For instance, "activated" macrophages from an animal infected by an intracellular parasite may have higher levels of lysosomal enzyme activity than do nonactivated macrophages. Activation and changes in metabolism may be mediated by interaction with other cell types, particularly the lymphocyte.

Carbohydrate and Energy Production

The relative contribution to energy production of oxidative respiration and of glycolysis varies with the level of mononuclear cell differentiation and with the type of macrophage. The principal energy source for the mono-cyte and tissue macrophage (such as the peritoneal macrophage) appears to be glycolysis, even under aerobic conditions (77, 138, 157, 182). In contrast, the metabolism of the alveolar macrophage appears to be primarily aerobic (21, 28).

Frei and his colleagues (77) and Vanotti (173) were among the first to observe aerobic glycolysis in blood monocytes and to document aerobic production of lactic acid. Later studies indicated that with progressive maturation from monocyte to macrophage in vitro, the rate of glucose utilization increases and the rate of lactate production per cell may double (17). Glycolysis accounts for most of the glucose utilization of these cells. A relatively small amount (1 to 2 percent) of the total glucose is metabolized via the hexose monophosphate shunt (182).

A "Pasteur effect" (depression of glycolysis under aerobic conditions) is demonstrable in mammalian peritoneal macrophages, indicating at least a partial utilization of oxidative energy sources (89, 139). The human monocyte, which has a less well-developed mitochondrial system, does not demonstrate this phenomenon (77). A "Crabtree effect" (depression of respiration by glucose) is found in guinea pig peritoneal macrophages (139).

The alveolar macrophage differs from the monocyte and the peritoneal macrophage in several respects: its rate of glucose utilization and lactic acid production is higher, and a Crabtree effect is not demonstrable. Moreover, the rate of oxygen consumption is many times higher in the alveolar macrophage—an observation consistent with its large number of mitochondria and its content of mitochondrial enzymes (103).

When the environmental oxygen tension falls below 20 mm of mercury, critical cellular energy-dependent processes such as phagocytosis fail in the alveolar macrophage (28). In contrast, the phagocytic function of monocytes and other tissue macrophages is not so critically dependent on available oxygen. Phagocytosis by these cells occurs in the presence of inhibitors of oxidative metabolism, but it is depressed by inhibitors of glycolysis (23, 25, 32).

To generate hydrogen peroxide during the phagocytic process, monocytes may utilize molecular oxygen much as neutrophils do (23). Similarly, in a manner analogous to that of the granulocyte, monocytes increase the fraction of glucose metabolized via the hexose monophosphate shunt with phagocytosis (25).

Lipid Metabolism

Fatty Acids

The principal fatty acids synthesized from acetate by peritoneal macrophages are palmitic, oleic, and linoleic acid (50). Elsbach (64) studied the uptake of ^{14}C-labeled fatty acids by rabbit alveolar macrophages. Linoleic acid is esterified and incorporated into triglyceride phospholipids in a process that does not depend on oxidative phosphorylation, but that is inhibited by substances interfering with glycolytic enzymes. Palmitic acid from triglyceride or chylomicrons is similarly incorporated. Homogenates of peritoneal macrophages also incorporate labeled fatty acids into triglyceride, provided a source of adenosine triphosphate is present (55). These observations indicate that macrophages are capable of utilizing either free or bound fatty acids for intracellular esterification reactions. They also oxidize free fatty acid and triglycerides (47, 48).

Cholesterol Metabolism

Rabbit peritoneal macrophages can synthesize cholesterol from small precursors such as acetate (50). They can also esterify cholesterol (53, 55). Radioactive cholesterol, either as an aqueous suspension or as a component of chylomicrons, is incorporated rapidly by macrophages (48). Exogenous cholesterol esters are similarly incorporated and rapidly hydrolyzed (49, 51, 54).

Macrophages are rich in cholesterol and maintain a constant ratio of cholesterol to protein (181). More than 95 percent of the cholesterol is associated with membranes, most in association with lysosomes and plasma membranes. A rapid exchange occurs between serum and membrane cholesterol. Alveolar macrophages also have the enzymatic machinery for cholesterol esterification (167).

Phospholipids

Phosphatidyl choline, phosphatidyl ethanolamine, and sphingomyelin together constitute about 80 percent of total macrophage phospholipid. Of these, phosphatidyl choline accounts for about 40 percent of the total.

Lecithin is a constituent of cell membrane phospholipid. Homogenates of alveolar macrophages in the presence of adenosine triphosphate and coenzyme A-SH convert lysolecithin to lecithin. Intact cells incorporate radioactive lysolecithin; the label is then found in the lecithin fraction (65–68). The reaction is assumed to proceed via the direct acylation of lysolecithin (106).

A number of interconversions of phospholipids within the cell have been described (65, 67). During phagocytosis, phospholipid synthesis is increased (66, 68)—presumably as a consequence of new membrane synthesis. The uptake of cholesterol by peritoneal macrophages facilitates the incorporation of inorganic ^{32}P into phospholipid (52).

Nucleic Acid Synthesis

DNA Synthesis

Most studies have shown that the early precursors of monocytes within the bone marrow are capable of DNA synthesis as measured by incorporation of tritiated thymidine (26, 161, 170, 171, 175, 176). Under ordinary conditions of culture, monocytes and more mature cells do not synthesize DNA (22, 97, 170, 178), although they can incorporate tritiated thymidine to repair ultraviolet-damaged DNA (22). Following intense antigen stimulation or exposure to stimulating substances produced by other cells, bone marrow and peritoneal macrophages are capable of DNA synthesis and proliferation (6, 26, 75, 104, 132, 133, 174, 183). Proliferation may continue up to the stage of morphologically mature cells, which have condensed nuclear chromatin and acidophilic cytoplasm (26). Macrophage nuclei are also able to synthesize DNA when they are part of a heterokaryon produced by the fusion of macrophages with replicating cells by means of Sendai virus (83, 90), or when they are infected by oncogenic virus (116).

RNA Metabolism

Monocytes, macrophages, and their early precursors are capable of active RNA synthesis (32, 178). A special role in the induction of antibody synthesis has been ascribed to "immunogenic" RNA synthesized by macrophages after exposure to specific antigen (3, 8, 72, 73, 78, 79, 84, 105, 151, 168). The validity of this hypothesis is reviewed in more detail in the next chapter.

Using agarose-acrylamide electrophoresis, Soderberg

and his colleagues (156) have recently separated newly synthesized macrophage RNA into multiple components. Macrophage RNA labeling reaches equilibrium only slowly when the cells are exposed to ^{3}H-uridine.

Pinocytic activity of macrophages is reduced by inhibition of RNA synthesis, whereas phagocytosis of large particles by monocytes is unimpaired (25, 32).

Protein Synthesis

Consistent with their abundant, rough-surfaced, endoplasmic reticulum, macrophages are active in protein synthesis (32, 33, 37, 38, 135, 164, 165). Much of this activity is directed toward synthesis of lysosomal enzymes (see Chapter 23 and the next section of this chapter). Blocking of protein synthesis inhibits the normal increment in lysosomal enzyme activity that occurs with maturation from the monocyte to the macrophage or that occurs with pinocytic activity (14). Inhibition of cellular protein synthesis has no effect on the ability of monocytes to phagocytize a variety of particles and has little effect on the ability of macrophages to kill certain species of bacteria (25, 123). It is likely that these functions simply require preformed protein rather than new protein synthesis.

Macrophages may make other biologically active proteins in addition to lysosomal enzymes, including endogenous pyrogen (9) and perhaps complement components (158). The characteristics of the amino acid transport systems of the macrophage are poorly understood (166).

Lysosomes and Lysosomal Enzymes

Functions of Lysosomes

A prominent feature of the mature macrophage is the large number of phase-dense cytoplasmic inclusions (Fig. 24.1). In the 1930s, these inclusions were shown to accumulate the vital stain, neutral red; and in the 1950s, histochemical studies demonstrated acid phosphatase activity in the perinuclear region, where the cytoplasmic inclusions are most prominent (179). These organelles were subsequently identified as lysosomes on the basis of cell fractionation techniques and enzymatic studies (42, 43). They have the characteristics of lysosomes isolated from other tissue, such as liver (56–58, 180).

The role of lysosomal enzymes from macrophages and other tissues in intracellular digestive processes was predicated on the basis of their hydrolytic nature and was subsequently substantiated by electron microscopy (57, 135, 136). With phagocytosis the enzymes of the lysosome are discharged into the phagocytic vacuole, where they ef-

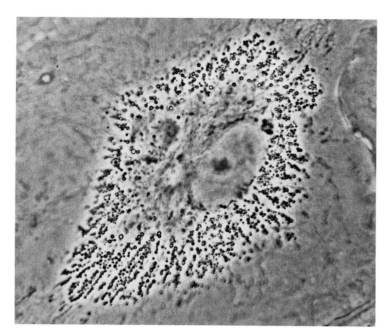

Figure 24.1 A mature human macrophage cultured in vitro for two weeks and photographed under phase contrast illumination. Note the prominent nucleolus, the dense cytoplasmic granules clustered about the nucleus, and the ribbon-like mitochondria in the periphery of the cytoplasm.

fect digestion of degradable materials (70, 108, 128) (Figs. 4.2 and 24.2). Phagocytized bacteria are degraded in this manner (29, 30). The process of fusion of the phagocytic vacuole with the primary lysosome may be inhibited by high concentrations of corticosteroids (118).

Soluble protein taken up by macrophages into small pinocytic vesicles is eventually exposed to the hydrolytic action of lysosomal enzymes within the cell, by the process of fusion of primary lysosomes with the pinocytic vesicles. Within hours or days, proteins such as albumin and hemoglobin are broken down to amino acids or dipeptides (60–63). Small peptides released within the lysosome may then leak out into the cell and into the surrounding fluid. Carbohydrates may be handled in similar fashion (36).

In addition to digestion of bacteria (15, 81), other microorganisms, and soluble proteins, macrophage lysosomes may be involved in collagen resorption (185). This thesis is supported by the observation of collagen fibers within lysosomes of macrophages from involuting mouse uterus (141).

Formation of Lysosomes

From available evidence one can reasonably conclude that lysosomal enzymes of the macrophages are made in the

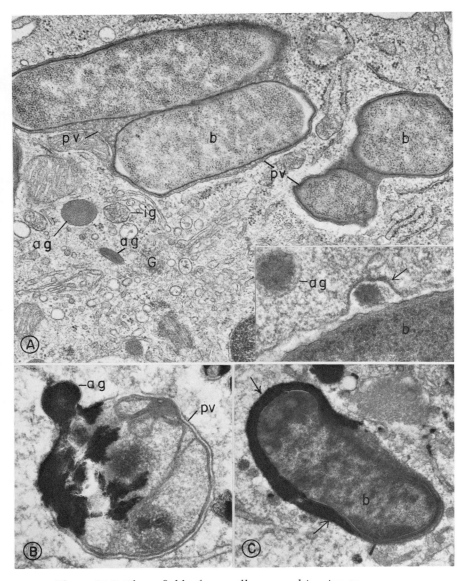

endoplasmic reticulum and then packaged inside lysosomes in the Golgi apparatus (32, 126) (Chapter 23). These primary lysosomes may then fuse with phagocytic vacuoles or pinocytic vesicles; as a result, combined structures called secondary lysosomes are produced.

The formation of lysosomes and lysosomal enzymes is influenced by the extracellular environment. At low concentrations of serum, macrophages develop only a few small lysosomes and show little increase in lysosomal enzyme activity during cultivation in vitro. As serum concentration increases, granule formation and enzyme activity increase (33). The rate of pinocytic activity is also directly related to serum concentration. In addition to some serum components (including fetoin, albumin, and a macroglobulin), a number of other substances (including nucleosides and nucleotides) stimulate pinocytosis and the formation of pinocytic vesicles (40, 41). These pinocytic vesicles contribute directly to lysosome formation by fusing with preexisting secondary lysosomes and primary lysosomes derived from the Golgi apparatus (37,38). Thus, *there is a relation between endocytic activity and the formation of lysosomes.*

The mechanism of lysosome formation has been investigated by Axline and Cohn (14), who used a phagocytic system to place defined substances within the interior of the macrophage. Phagocytosis of digestible erythrocytes produces a greater synthesis of several lysosomal enzymes than does phagocytosis of nondigestible particles such as polystyrene or insoluble starch. The endocytic stimulus to lysosomal enzyme production is therefore presumed to be related to the digestive process or to the products of digestion. Using homopolymers of L- and D-amino acids, these investigators demonstrated that both the quantity of phagocytized material and its rate of enzymatic hydrolysis control the level and persistence of lysosomal hydrolytic enzymes.

Figure 24.2 These fields, from cells exposed in vivo to *Escherichia coli,* illustrate the events that occur during phagocytosis of microorganisms by macrophages. Fig. *A* (and *inset*) is from a 4-hour exudate produced in the guinea pig and fixed 15 minutes after intraperitoneal injection of *E. coli.* A number of bacteria (*b*) have been taken up and segregated into phagocytic vacuoles (*pv*). Two mature azurophil granules (*ag*), as well as several immature granules (*ig*), are present in the Golgi region (*G*). The inset depicts a field in which fusion has occurred between an azurophil granule and a phagosome containing a bacterium. The content of the azurophil granule is visible in the membrane pocket (*arrow*). Note the high density of the content of the phagocytic vacuole. Another azurophil granule with a content of comparable texture and density is present in the same field.

Figs. *B* and *C* are from a 20-hour rabbit exudate fixed 30 minutes after exposure to *E. coli* and reacted for aryl sulfatase.

They illustrate stages that presumably occur shortly after fusion of a phagocytic vacuole with an azurophil granule. In *B* an azurophil granule containing dense reaction product is observed in continuity with a phagocytic vacuole (*pv*); *C* shows reaction product (*arrows*) around a bacterium in a phagocytic vacuole.

Specimens were fixed for 4 hours at 23° C (Fig. *A*) or 10 minutes at 4° C (Figs. *B* and *C*) in formaldehyde-glutaraldehyde. The cells in *B* and *C* were then incubated in Goldfischer's aryl sulfatase medium (pH 5.5) at 23° C for 3 hours and treated with $(NH_4)_2S$. Figure *A*, magnification × 25,000; inset, × 60,000; Fig. *B*, × 33,000; Fig. *C*, × 27,000. (From B. A. Nichols, D. F. Bainton, and M. G. Farquhar, *J. Cell Biol.* 50:498, 1971. Reprinted by permission of authors and publisher.)

The number of lysosomes in the cytoplasm of the macrophage and the activity of cellular lysosomal hydrolases are also related to the degree of cellular maturation. As a generalization, *with cellular maturation there is a progressive increase in the numbers of these structures and in hydrolytic enzyme activity* (22, 32, 33, 126, 187) (Chapter 23).

The level of activity of several of the acid hydrolases is higher in alveolar macrophages than in peritoneal exudate macrophages (108). A correlation is said to exist between resistance to tuberculosis and the activity of lysosomal acid phosphatases (5,45). Thyroid hormones also may influence enzyme activity levels (99).

Lysosomal Enzymes

A large number of hydrolytic enzymes have been localized within the lysosome fraction. In general, their activity has been associated with digestive processes rather than with bactericidal activity. These enzymes probably have a major role in digestion of phagocytized microorganisms and other organic particles (29, 30). Beta-hyaluronidase is also probably lysosomal (82).

Acid Phosphatase Five electrophoretically distinct forms of acid phosphatase have been found in the lysosomal fraction of rabbit alveloar macrophages (12). Isozymes have been identified in the mouse (11). Macrophage acid phosphatase works on a wide variety of artificial substrates (13); the natural substrates are unknown.

Lysozyme Alveolar macrophages from rabbits are said to contain high levels of lysozyme, whereas peritoneal macrophages contain little, if any (42, 93, 121). However, we have observed significant levels of lysozyme activity in normal human macrophages grown in tissue cultures, and there are apparently high levels associated with malignant human monocytes (140).

Beta-glucuronidase Beta-glucuronidase is predominantly lysosomal in distribution, although small amounts have been found in the endoplasmic reticulum by electron microscopy and in the microsomal fraction of the cell (42, 74).

Lipase A variety of lipase activities has been identified in the peritoneal and alveolar macrophage (42, 45, 64, 76, 100). Although some of these enzymes are clearly localized in the lysosomal fraction (42), others may be present in the soluble fraction of the cell.

BPN-hydrolase A chymotrypsin-like enzyme activity that hydrolyzes a number of amino acid and oligopeptide esters and N-benzoyl-DL-phenylalanine-β-naphthol esters (hence BPN-hydrolase) has been found in rabbit peritoneal macrophages (45). This activity can clearly be distinguished from cathepsin-D in its substrate specificity, response to inhibitors, and pH optimum. It may be the same as cathepsin-C.

Hyaluronidase This activity, with pH optimum near 3.9, has been described in rabbit alveolar macrophages (82). It is probably an endohexosaminidase. Evidence from other cell types suggests that it may well be a lysosomal enzyme (7).

Myeloperoxidase Although myeloperoxidase has not definitely been localized within the lysosomal fraction of mononuclear phagocytes, evidence from other types of leukocytes strongly suggests such a localization. Myeloperoxidase is found in the monocyte precursors within the bone marrow (the promonocyte) and in monocytes, but not in more mature macrophages (26, 171, 172).

Immunologic studies suggest a close relation, and probably identity, between granulocyte and monocyte peroxidase (154). In genetic absence of neutrophil myeloperoxidase, the enzyme is absent from monocytes also (110).

Metabolic Changes with Cell Maturation and Activation

The cytologic aspects of the maturation of monocytes to macrophages was discussed in Chapter 23. The principal features are increases in size, in complexity of the Golgi apparatus, and in number and size of the cytoplasmic lysosomes, mitochondria, and lipid droplets (33, 38, 59, 125, 164). This transformation from monocyte to macrophage is associated with changes in cell composition and metabolism, as well as with changes in cell structure and function. These changes are summarized in Fig. 24.3.

As the number of cytoplasmic lysosomes increases, the activity level from associated enzymes increases dramatically. These enzymes include acid phosphatase, beta-glucuronidase, cathepsin, and lysozyme (17, 22, 34, 35). Studies with inhibitors of protein synthesis demonstrate that the increase in enzyme activity results from the increased enzyme synthesis accompanying cellular differentiation (34, 37). Some of these increases in enzyme activity may be inhibited by high concentrations of adrenocorticosteroids (184).

The transition from monocyte to macrophage is also characterized by increases in the number of mitochondria, in the activity of mitochondrial enzymes such as cyto-

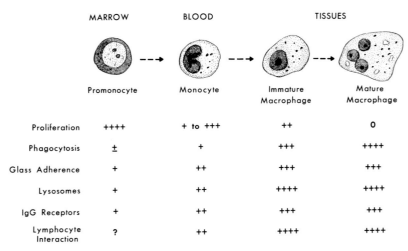

	MARROW	BLOOD	TISSUES	
	Promonocyte	Monocyte	Immature Macrophage	Mature Macrophage
Proliferation	++++	+ to +++	++	0
Phagocytosis	±	+	+++	++++
Glass Adherence	+	++	+++	+++
Lysosomes	+	++	++++	++++
IgG Receptors	+	++	+++	+++
Lymphocyte Interaction	?	++	++++	++++

Figure 24.3 Development of certain functional characteristics with maturation of mononuclear leukocytes. (From M. J. Cline and D. W. Golde, *Am. J. Med.* 55:49, 1973. Reprinted by permission of authors and publisher.)

chrome oxidase, and in the rate of cellular respiration (17, 32).

The differentiation from monocytes to macrophages in vivo is almost certainly influenced by environmental factors such as the presence of infection and inflammatory agents. In animals infected by intracellular parasites, macrophages may be "activated" in the sense that they are more active as phagocytes, have a greater digestive capacity, contain higher levels of most hydrolytic enzymes, and have a more active glucose oxidative metabolism (5, 10, 18, 44-46, 59, 76, 86, 88, 112-115, 119, 129, 149, 153, 160, 162, 163). Such activated macrophages may also have a higher rate of DNA synthesis and cell division (104, 131, 132).

Nathan and his colleagues found that a "factor" produced by antigen-stimulated lymphocytes converted normal macrophages to an activated state (124). The mechanism of macrophage activation and its relation to cellular immunity is considered in more detail in the next chapter. It should be noted, however, that the mechanism of activation is largely unknown.

Metabolic Changes with Endocytosis

Endocytosis is a term that embraces the terms *phagocytosis* and *pinocytosis*, signifying the cellular ingestion of solids and fluid droplets respectively. Endocytosis therefore is the process by which a cell internalizes part of its external environment, enclosing it in an invagination of its plasma membrane (98).

Phagocytosis

The morphologic events that accompany phagocytosis by alveolar and peritoneal macrophages and Kupffer cells have been well described, including the process of surface membrane invagination, phagocytic vacuole formation, and union of lysosomes with the phagocytic vacuole (32, 43, 128, 137) (Fig. 4.2). The phagocytic process is often considered to comprise two phases: an attachment phase in which the particle is bound to the cell, and an ingestion phase in which the particle is internalized within the cell (120, 146-148). It has been suggested that the spreading of macrophages on a glass surface has many of the features of the ingestion phase of phagocytosis (129, 130, 134).

The attachment phase of the phagocytic process has complex and poorly understood requirements that are in part dependent upon the nature of the particle (109, 147, 148). For some particles, cation is required. Others may require opsonization with immunoglobulin, complement, or other thermolabile serum factors (16, 107, 148, 152, 159). Such opsonins may interact with receptors on the surface of the macrophage (1, 2, 25, 27, 95, 96, 111, 125, 144). The receptors appear to be phospholipid proteins, on the basis of enzyme degradation studies (95). Opsonization may be necessary to overcome the repellent effects of negative charges on the surface of the macrophage and the bacteria (138, 143).

Energy Source   The human monocyte, like the neutrophil, appears to derive its energy for particle ingestion from glycolytic mechanisms rather than from aerobic metabolism. Phagocytosis proceeds under anaerobic conditions and in the presence of cyanide, whereas inhibitors of glycolysis, such as fluoride and iodoacetate, impair particle ingestion (25) (Table 24.1). The same dependence on glycolytic mechanisms is demonstrable in macro-

Table 24.1 Effect of metabolic inhibitors on phagocytosis.

Metabolic inhibitor of—	Inhibitor	Mean inhibition of phagocytosis (percent)
Glycolysis	Iodoacetate 1×10^{-4} M	51
Glycolysis	Fluoride 2×10^{-3} M	26
Cytochrome electron transport	Cyanide 1×10^{-3} M	20
Oxidative phosphorylation	Dinitrophenol 2×10^{-4} M	9
Oxidative metabolism	Nitrogen (100%)	40

phages derived from monocytes in vitro (23). In contrast, phagocytosis by human alveolar macrophages is largely dependent upon the availability of oxygen and is reduced below an oxygen tension of 25 mm of mercury (28). The same general pattern holds for animal macrophages. Thus, animal peritoneal macrophages derive their energy for phagocytosis from glycolysis (101, 102), whereas alveolar macrophages are dependent on oxidative metabolism (139).

Phagocytosis by animal macrophages is resistant to kiloroentgen doses of X ray (142).

Metabolic Changes   Human monocytes resemble neutrophils in demonstrating a postphagocytic burst in oxygen consumption (Fig. 24.4), hydrogen peroxide generation, and hexose monophosphate shunt stimulation (24, 25). Neither monocytes nor neutrophils increase their rate of protein synthesis, and monocytes do not increase their rate of RNA synthesis with phagocytosis. Particle ingestion by human monocytes is not dependent on new protein or RNA synthesis.

In animal peritoneal macrophages glycolysis, oxygen consumption, and the hexose monophosphate shunt also are transiently stimulated by phagocytosis (101, 102, 139,

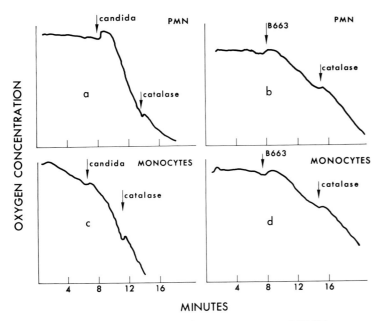

Figure 24.4 Oxygen utilization by monocytes and PMN neutrophils. The steepness of the curve is a function of the rate of oxygen utilization, which is enhanced by phagocytosis (addition of *Candida* particles) and by a phenazine drug (B663). Oxygen consumption, on the other hand, is reduced by the addition of catalase, which releases O_2 from the H_2O_2 generated during the phagocytic process.

Table 24.2 Changes in mononuclear phagocyte metabolism with phagocytosis. Alveolar macrophages are not included.

Increased glycolysis (supplying energy for phagocytosis).
Increased oxygen consumption (cyanide insensitive).
Increased hydrogen peroxide generation.
Increased hexose monophosphate shunt activity.
Increased turnover of phospholipids.

182). As in the neutrophil, the oxygen burst of the human monocytes (24) and the animal macrophages (102) is cyanide-insensitive. In contrast, with particle ingestion human alveolar macrophages show little increment in oxygen consumption (28). With phagocytosis rabbit alveolar macrophages display some increase in shunt activity (71). In both tissue and alveolar macrophages there is an increased turnover of phospholipid as new membrane is synthesized (66, 67, 102, 139).

From the foregoing it is reasonable to conclude that the monocyte and tissue macrophages resemble the neutrophil in metabolic changes associated with phagocytosis, whereas the alveolar macrophage appears to be distinctive. The reactions linking particle uptake and the dramatic metabolic changes associated with this event are almost entirely unknown at the present time. Surface-active compounds such as deoxycholate and digitonin may stimulate respiration, glucose oxidation, and phospholipid turnover in a manner analogous to that of phagocytosis (85). These observations suggest that there is a link between membrane phenomena and postphagocytic metabolic events. For mononuclear phagocyte metabolism the postphagocytic changes are listed in Table 24.2.

Metabolic Requirements for Pinocytosis
The pinocytic vesicle is formed by the invagination and pinching off of the external cell membrane in a process analogous to the formation of the phagocytic vacuole. Like the phagocytic vacuole, the pinocytic vesicle moves from the peripheral to the central cytoplasm and perinuclear area, fusing with primary lysosomes and acquiring acid hydrolases. In this combined structure the pinocytosed material is degraded (94). Surprisingly, pinocytosis and phagocytosis appear to have different metabolic requirements. In mouse peritoneal macrophages, pinocytosis is inhibited by interference with oxidative metabolism (for example, anaerobiasis, cyanide, antimycin-A, 2,4-dinitrophenol), whereas phagocytosis depends primarily upon glycolytic metabolism.

Another point of diversion in these two processes is that RNA synthesis and protein synthesis are required for pinocytosis (32). Inhibition of anaerobic glycolysis will also block pinocytosis (31). Presumably, inhibition of glycolytic or aerobic energy production exerts its effect by reducing available adenosine triphosphate. Exogenous adenosine triphosphate can counteract these effects of endogenous adenosine triphosphate deprivation in macrophages (40) and other cells (87).

The level of pinocytic activity of macrophages in vitro is influenced by the presence in the culture medium of certain types of molecules. Anionic proteins, carbohydrates, and amino acids may increase the rate of pinocytosis (39); neutral and cationic proteins have little effect. A similar phenomenon occurs in amoebae (122). Additionally, in newborn calf serum there is a protein that can interact with the macrophage membrane to increase pinocytic activity (41).

Another difference between phagocytosis and pinocytosis is that the latter process does not stimulate the dramatic changes in cell metabolism that accompany solid particle ingestion. The size of the particle is the critical factor that determines whether phagocytosis or pinocytosis is stimulated. The cutoff point is probably in the range of 0.1 micron or less (94, 133). Thus, protein antigens could accumulate on a macrophage surface without stimulating phagocytosis until a critical mass is reached (169).

Mechanism of Endocytosis

The mechanism of endocytosis is almost completely unknown. Because of the requirement for adenosine triphosphate and the obvious analogy with other biologic systems involving cell movement, it has been suggested that an adenosine triphosphatase system may be involved (134, cf. 177). Such systems are found in muscle myosin (69), in the mitotic apparatus (92), and in flagellae (20). In the macrophage and the neutrophil, adenosine triphosphatase appears in the plasma membrane (127, 186). This observation suggests a key role in endocytic events for the membrane itself and for associated microfilaments (4). Evidence to support such a suggestion has been obtained in pinocytosing amoebae (19).

The Alveolar Macrophage

The distinctive features of the metabolism of alveolar macrophages have already been alluded to in preceding sections of this chapter. They are summarized in Table 24.3 and relate primarily to differences in oxidative metabolism and energy production. The critical point is that human alveolar macrophages fail to carry out some

Table 24.3 Distinctive features of the alveolar macrophage.

High basal level of oxygen consumption.
Primarily oxidative metabolism; no Crabtree effect.
Dependence on oxidative metabolism to provide energy
  for phagocytosis.
Small respiratory burst with phagocytosis.

key cellular functions below a partial pressure of oxygen of 25 mm of mercury, whereas monocytes and tissue macrophages function effectively under anaerobic conditions (28). Human alveolar macrophages also lack the typical respiratory burst seen in the monocyte with phagocytosis. The energy for phagocytosis (28, 102) and for sodium ion transport (150) by alveolar macrophages is derived from oxidative phosphorylation, whereas in monocytes and other tissue macrophages this energy is derived primarily from glycolysis. With phagocytosis by alveolar macrophages, catalase-dependent peroxidative metabolism may be stimulated (80) and cyclic-AMP concentration increases (155).

The reasons for the differences in metabolism between alveolar and tissue macrophages are not known. It is presumed that at least some of the alveolar macrophages arise from the same pool of bone marrow precursors that gives rise to tissue macrophages (145).

Many of the distinctive features of the alveolar macrophage are especially prominent in cells derived from smokers' lungs (91, 117).

Summary

The metabolism of mononuclear phagocytes is determined by a number of factors, of which the most important are the degree of cellular maturity and the level of endocytic activity. Environmental factors influence the rate of both mononuclear cell maturation and endocytic activity. Consequently, the metabolism of the mononuclear leukocyte is strikingly influenced by its microenvironment. These external factors induce major metabolic differences between cells such as the peritoneal and alveolar macrophages, which arise from a common progenitor. Similarly, the "activated" macrophage is metabolically and functionally more active than its unstimulated counterpart. It is only within the last few years that we have begun to understand the mechanisms by which certain external stimuli and the ingestion of degradable materials influence macrophage metabolism and composition.

Chapter 24 References

1. Abramson, N., Gelfand, E. W., Jandl, J. H., and Rosen, F. S. The interaction between human monocytes and red cells. Specificity for IgG subclasses and IgG fragments, *J. Exp. Med.* 132:1207, 1970.
2. Abramson, N., Lo Buglio, A. F., Jandl, J. H., and Cotran, R. S. The interaction between human monocytes and red cells. Binding characteristics, *J. Exp. Med.* 132:1191, 1970.
3. Adler, F. L., Fishman, M., and Dray, S. Antibody formation initiated in vitro. III. Antibody formation and allotypic specificity directed by ribonucleic acid from peritoneal exudate cells, *J. Immunol.* 97:554, 1966.
4. Allison, A. C., Davies, P., and De Petris, S. Role of contractile microfilaments in macrophage movement and endocytosis, *Nature (New Biol.)* 232:153, 1971.
5. Allison, M. J., Zappasodi, P., and Lurie, M. D. Metabolic studies on mononuclear cells from rabbits of varying genetic resistance to tuberculosis. I. Studies on cells of normal noninfected animals. *Am. Rev. Respir. Dis.* 84:364, 1961.
6. Aronson, M., and Elberg, S. Proliferation of rabbit peritoneal histiocytes as revealed by autoradiography with tritiated thymidine, *Proc. Natl. Acad. Sci. U.S.A.* 48:208, 1962.
7. Aronson, N. N., Jr., and Davidson, E. A. Lysosomal hyaluronidase, *J. Biol. Chem.* 240:3222, 1965.
8. Askonas, B. A., and Rhodes, J. M. Immunogenicity of antigen-containing ribonucleic acid preparations from macrophages, *Nature* 205:470, 1965.
9. Atkins, E., Bodel, P., and Francis, L. Release of an endogenous pyrogen in vitro from rabbit mononuclear cells, *J. Exp. Med.* 126:357, 1967.
10. Auzins, I., and Rowley, D. On the question of the specificity of cellular immunity, *Aust. J. Exp. Biol. Med. Sci.* 40:283, 1962.
11. Axline, S. G. Acid phosphatase isozymes in cultivated mouse peritoneal macrophages, *Fed. Proc.* 27:480, 1968.
12. Axline, S. G. Isozymes of acid phosphatase in normal and Calmette-Guérin bacillus-induced rabbit alveolar macrophages, *J. Exp. Med.* 128:1031, 1968.
13. Axline, S. G. Functional biochemistry of the macrophage, *Semin. Hematol.* 7:142, 1970.
14. Axline, S. G., and Cohn, Z. A. The in vitro induction of lysosomal enzymes by phagocytosis, *J. Clin. Invest.* 48:4a, 1969.
15. Ayoub, E. M., and McCarty, M. Intraphagocytic β-N-acetylglucosaminidase. Properties of the enzyme and its activity on group A streptococcal carbohydrate in comparison with a soil bacillus enzyme, *J. Exp. Med.* 127:833, 1968.
16. Benacerraf, B., and Miescher, P. Bacterial phagocytosis by the reticuloendothelial system *in vivo* under different immune conditions, *Ann. N.Y. Acad. Sci.* 88:184, 1960.
17. Bennett, W. E., and Cohn, Z. A. The isolation and selected properties of blood monocytes, *J. Exp. Med.* 123:145, 1966.
18. Blanden, R. V. Modification of macrophage function, *J. Recticuloendothel. Soc.* 5:179, 1968.
19. Brandt, P. W., and Freeman, A. R. Plasma membrane: substructural changes correlated with electrical resistance and pinocytosis, *Science* 155:582, 1967.
20. Claybrook, J. R., and Nelson, L. Flagellar adenosine triphosphatase from sea urchin sperm. Properties and relation to motility, *Science* 162:1134, 1968.
21. Cline, M. J. Metabolism of the circulating leukocyte, *Physiol. Rev.* 45:674, 1965.
22. Cline, M. J. Monocytes and macrophages: differentiation and function, *in* T. J. Greenwalt and G. A. Jamieson (eds.), Third Annual Red Cross Symposium on Formation and Destruction of Blood Cells, p. 222, J. B. Lippincott, Philadelphia, 1970.
23. Cline, M. J. Bactericidal activity of human macrophages: analysis of factors influencing the killing of *Listeria monocytogenes, Infect. Immun.* 2:156, 1970.
24. Cline, M. J. Drug potentiation of macrophage function, *Infect. Immun.* 2:601, 1970.
25. Cline, M. J., and Lehrer, R. I. Phagocytosis by human monocytes, *Blood* 32:423, 1968.
26. Cline, M. J., and Sumner, M. A. Bone marrow macrophage precursors. I. Some functional characteristics of the early cells of the mouse macrophage series, *Blood* 40:62, 1972.
27. Cline, M. J., Warner, N. L., and Metcalf, D. Identification of the bone marrow colony mononuclear phagocyte as a macrophage, *Blood* 39:326, 1972.
28. Cohen, A. B., and Cline, M. J. The human alveolar macrophage: isolation, cultivation in vitro, and studies of morphologic and functional characteristics, *J. Clin. Invest.* 50:1390, 1971.
29. Cohn, Z. A. The fate of bacteria within phagocytic cells. I. The degradation of isotopically labeled bacteria by polymorphonuclear leucocytes and macrophages, *J. Exp. Med.* 117:27, 1963.
30. Cohn, Z. A. The fate of bacteria within phagocytic cells. II. The modification of intracellular degradation, *J. Exp. Med.* 117:43, 1963.
31. Cohn, Z. A. The regulation of pinocytosis in mouse macrophages. I. Metabolic requirements as defined by the use of inhibitors, *J. Exp. Med.* 124:557, 1966.
32. Cohn, Z. A. The structure and function of monocytes and macrophages, *Adv. Immunol.* 9:163, 1968.
33. Cohn, Z. A., and Benson, B. The differentiation of mononuclear phagocytes: morphology, cytochemistry, and biochemistry, *J. Exp. Med.* 121:153, 1965.
34. Cohn, Z. A., and Benson, B. The in vitro differentiation of mononuclear phagocytes. I. The influence of inhibitors and the results of autoradiography, *J. Exp. Med.* 121:279, 1965.
35. Cohn, Z. A., and Benson, B. The in vitro differentiation of mononuclear phagocytes. II. The influence of serum on granule formation, hydrolase production, and pinocytosis, *J. Exp. Med.* 121:835, 1965.
36. Cohn, Z. A., and Ehrenreich, B. A. The uptake, storage, and intracellular hydrolysis of carbohydrates by macrophages, *J. Exp. Med.* 129:201, 1969.

37. Cohn, Z. A., Fedorko, M. E., and Hirsch, J. G. The in vitro differentiation of mononuclear phagocytes. V. The formation of macrophage lysosomes, *J. Exp. Med.* 123:757, 1966.

38. Cohn, Z. A., Hirsch, J. G., and Fedorko, M. E. The in vitro differentiation of mononuclear phagocytes. IV. The ultrastructure of macrophage differentiation in the peritoneal cavity and in culture, *J. Exp. Med.* 123:747, 1966.

39. Cohn, Z. A., and Parks, E. The regulation of pinocytosis in mouse macrophages. II. Factors inducing vesicle formation, *J. Exp. Med.* 125:213, 1967.

40. Cohn, Z. A., and Parks, E. The regulation of pinocytosis in mouse macrophages. III. Induction of vesicle formation by nucleosides and nucleotides, *J. Exp. Med.* 125:457, 1967.

41. Cohn, Z. A., and Parks, E. The regulation of pinocytosis in mouse macrophages. IV. The immunological induction of pinocytic vesicles, secondary lysosomes, and hydrolytic enzymes, *J. Exp. Med.* 125:1091, 1967.

42. Cohn, Z. A., and Wiener, E. The particulate hydrolases of macrophages. I. Comparative enzymology, isolation, and properties, *J. Exp. Med.* 118:991, 1963.

43. Cohn, Z. A., and Wiener, E. The particulate hydrolases of macrophages. II. Biochemical and morphological response to particle ingestion, *J. Exp. Med.* 118:1009, 1963.

44. Dannenberg, A. M., Jr. Cellular hypersensitivity and cellular immunity in the pathogenesis of tuberculosis: specificity, systemic and local nature, and associated macrophage enzymes, *Bacteriol. Rev.* 32:85, 1968.

45. Dannenberg, A. M., Jr., and Bennett, W. E. Hydrolytic enzymes of rabbit mononuclear exudate cells. I. Quantitative assay and properties of certain proteases, nonspecific esterases, and lipases of mononuclear and polymorphonuclear cells and erythrocytes, *J. Cell Biol.* 21:1, 1964.

46. Dannenberg, A. M., Jr., Walter, P. C., and Kapral, F. A. A histochemical study of phagocytic and enzymatic functions of rabbit mononuclear and polymorphonuclear exudate cells and alveolar macrophages. II. The effect of particle ingestion on enzyme activity; two phases of *in vitro* activation, *J. Immunol.* 90:448, 1963.

47. Day, A. J. Oxidation of ^{14}C-labelled chylomicron fat and ^{14}C-labelled unesterified fatty acids by macrophages *in vitro* and the effect of clearing factor, *Q. J. Exp. Physiol.* 45:220, 1960.

48. Day, A. J. A comparison of the oxidation of cholesterol-26-^{14}C, palmitate-1-^{14}C and tripalmitin-1-^{14}C by macrophages *in vitro*, *Q. J. Exp. Physiol.* 46:383, 1961.

49. Day, A. J. Lipid metabolism by macrophages and its relationship to atherosclerosis, *Adv. Lipid Res.* 5:185, 1967.

50. Day, A. J., and Fidge, N. H. Incorporation of C^{14}-labelled acetate into lipids by macrophages in vitro, *J. Lipid Res.* 5:163, 1964.

51. Day, A. J., Fidge, N. H., and Wilkinson, G. K. The incorporation of ^{14}C-labelled acetate into long chain fatty acids by macrophages *in vitro*, *Biochim. Biophys. Acta* 84:149, 1964.

52. Day, A. J., Fidge, N. H., and Wilkinson, G. K. Effect of cholesterol in suspension on the incorporation of phosphate into phospholipid by macrophages in vitro, *J. Lipid Res.* 7:132, 1966.

53. Day, A. J., and Gould-Hurst, P. R. S. Esterification of ^{14}C-labelled cholesterol by reticulo-endothelial cells, *Q. J. Exp. Physiol.* 46:376, 1961.

54. Day, A. J., Gould-Hurst, P. R. S., and Wahlquist, M. L. The uptake and metabolism of cholesterol-H^3 labeled lipoprotein by macrophages *in vitro*, *J. Reticuloendothel. Soc.* 1:40, 1964.

55. Day, A. J., and Tume, R. K. Cholesterol-esterifying activity of cell-free preparations of rabbit peritoneal macrophages, *Biochim. Biophys. Acta* 176:367, 1969.

56. de Duve, C. *In* T. Hayashi (ed.), Subcellular Particles, p. 128, Ronald Press, New York, 1959.

57. de Duve, C., Pressman, B. C., Gianetto, R., Wattiaux, R., and Applemans, F. Tissue fractionation studies. 6. Intracellular distribution patterns of enzymes in rat-liver tissue, *Biochem. J.* 60:604, 1955.

58. de Duve, C., and Wattiaux, R. Functions of lysosomes, *Ann. Rev. Physiol.* 28:435, 1966.

59. Ebert, R. H., and Florey, H. W. The extravascular development of the monocyte observed *in vivo*, *Br. J. Exp. Pathol.* 20:342, 1939.

60. Ehrenreich, B. A., and Cohn, Z. A. The uptake and digestion of iodinated human serum albumin by macrophages in vitro, *J. Exp. Med.* 126:941, 1967.

61. Ehrenreich, B. A., and Cohn, Z. A. Fate of hemoglobin pinocytosed by macrophages in vitro, *J. Cell Biol.* 38:244, 1968.

62. Ehrenreich, B. A., and Cohn, Z. A. Pinocytosis by macrophages, *J. Reticuloendothel. Soc.* 5:230, 1968.

63. Ehrenreich, B. A., and Cohn, Z. A. The fate of peptides pinocytosed by macrophages in vitro, *J. Exp. Med.* 129:227, 1969.

64. Elsbach, P. Uptake of fat by phagocytic cells. An examination of the role of phagocytosis. II. Rabbit alveolar macrophages, *Biochim. Biophys. Acta* 98:420, 1965.

65. Elsbach, P. Phospholipid metabolism by phagocytic cells. I. A comparison of conversion of ^{32}P-lysolecithin to lecithin and glycerlyphosphorylcholine by homogenates of rabbit polymorphonuclear leukocytes and alveolar macrophages, *Biochim. Biophys. Acta* 125:510, 1966.

66. Elsbach, P. Stimulation of lecithin synthesis from medium lysolecithin during phagocytosis, *J. Clin. Invest.* 46:1052, 1967.

67. Elsbach, P. Metabolism of lysophosphatidyl ethanolamine and lysophosphatidyl choline by homogenates of rabbit polymorphonuclear leukocytes and alveolar macrophages, *J. Lipid Res.* 8:359, 1967.

68. Elsbach, P. Increased synthesis of phospholipid during phagocytosis, *J. Clin. Invest.* 47:2217, 1968.

69. Engelhardt, W. H., and Ljubimowa, M. N. Myosine and adenosine-triphosphatase, *Nature* 144:668, 1939.

70. Essner, E. An electron microscope study of erythrophagocytosis,

J. Biophys. Biochem. Cytol. 7:329, 1960.

71. Evans, D. G., and Myrvik, Q. N. Increased phagocytic and bactericidal activities of alveolar macrophages after vaccination with killed BCG, *J. Reticuloendothel. Soc.* 4:428, 1967.

72. Fishman, M. Antibody formation in vitro, *J. Exp. Med.* 114:837, 1961.

73. Fishman, M., and Adler, F. L. Antibody formation initiated in vitro. II. Antibody synthesis in x-irradiated recipients of diffusion chambers containing nucleic acid derived from macrophages incubated with antigen, *J. Exp. Med.* 117:595, 1963.

74. Fishman, W. H., Goldman, S. S., and DeLellis, R. Dual localization of β-glucuronidase in endoplasmic reticulum and in lysosomes, *Nature* 213:457, 1967.

75. Forbes, I. J., and Mackaness, G. B. Mitosis in macrophages, *Lancet* ii:1203, 1963.

76. Franson, R. C., and Waite, M. Lysosomal phospholipases A_1 and A_2 of normal and bacillus Calmette Guerin-induced alveolar macrophages, *J. Cell Biol.* 56:621, 1973.

77. Frei, J., Borel, C., Horvath, G., Cullity, B., and Vannotti, A. Enzymatic studies in the different types of normal and leukemic human white cells, *Blood* 18:317, 1961.

78. Friedman, H. Antibody plaque formation by normal mouse spleen cell cultures exposed in vitro to RNA from immune mice, *Science* 146:934, 1964.

79. Friedman, H. P., Stravitsky, A. B., and Solomon, J. M. Induction in vitro of antibodies to phage T2: antigens in the RNA extract employed, *Science* 149:1106, 1965.

80. Gee, J. B. L., Vassallo, C. L., Bell, P., Kaskin, J., Basford, R. E., and Field, J. B. Catalase-dependent peroxidative metabolism in the alveolar macrophage during phagocytosis, *J. Clin. Invest.* 49:1280, 1970.

81. Gladstone, G. P., and Johnston, H. H. The effect of cultural conditions on the susceptibility of *Bacillus anthracis* to lysozyme, *Br. J. Exp. Pathol.* 36:363, 1955.

82. Goggins, J. F., Lazarus, G. S., and Fullmer, H. M. Hyaluronidase activity of alveolar macrophages,

J. Histochem. Cytochem. 16:688, 1968.

83. Gordon, S., and Cohn, Z. Macrophage-melanocyte heterokaryons. II. The activation of macrophage DNA synthesis. Studies with inhibitors of RNA synthesis, *J. Exp. Med.* 133:321, 1971.

84. Gottlieb, A. A., Glisin, V. R., and Doty, P. Studies on macrophage RNA involved in antibody production, *Proc. Natl. Acad. Sci. U.S.A.* 57:1849, 1967.

85. Graham, R. C., Jr., Karnovsky, M. J., Shafer, A. W., Glass, E. A., and Karnovsky, M. L. Metabolic and morphological observations on the effect of surface-active agents on leukocytes, *J. Cell Biol.* 32:629, 1967.

86. Grogg, E., and Pearse, A. G. E. The enzymic and lipid histochemistry of experimental tuberculosis, *Br. J. Exp. Pathol.* 33:567, 1952.

87. Gropp, A. Phagocytosis and pinocytosis, *in* G. D. Rose (ed.), Cinemicrography in Cell Biology, p. 279, Academic Press, New York, 1963.

88. Hard, G. C. Some biochemical aspects of the immune macrophage, *Br. J. Exp. Pathol* 51:97, 1970.

89. Harris, H., and Barclay, W. R. A method for measuring the respiration of animal cells *in vitro* with some observations on the macrophages of the rabbit, *Br. J. Exp. Pathol.* 36:592, 1955.

90. Harris, H., Watkins, J. F., Ford, C. E., and Schoefl, G. I. Artificial heterokaryons of animal cells from different species, *J. Cell Sci.* 1:1, 1966.

91. Harris, J. O., Swenson, E. W., and Johnson, J. E. III. Human alveolar macrophages: comparison of phagocytic ability, glucose utilization, and ultrastructure in smokers and nonsmokers, *J. Clin. Invest.* 49:2086, 1970.

92. Hartmann, J. F. Cytochemical localization of adenosine triphosphatase in the mitotic apparatus of HeLa and sarcoma 180 tissue culture cells, *J. Cell Biol.* 23:363, 1964.

93. Heise, E. R., and Myrvik, Q. N. Secretion of lysozyme by rabbit alveolar macrophages *in vitro*, *J. Reticuloendothel. Soc.* 4:510, 1967.

94. Hirsch, J. G., Fedorko, M. E., and Cohn, Z. A. Vesicle fusion and formation at the surface of pinocytotic

vacuoles in macrophages, *J. Cell Biol.* 38:629, 1968.

95. Howard, J. G., and Benacerraf, B. Properties of macrophage receptors for cytophilic antibodies, *Br. J. Exp. Pathol.* 47:193, 1966.

96. Huber, H., Polley, M. J., Linscott, W. D., Fudenberg, H. H., and Müller-Eberhard, H. J. Human monocytes: distinct receptor sites for the third component of complement and for immunoglobulin G, *Science* 162:1281, 1968.

97. Jacoby, F. Macrophages, *in* E. N. Willmer (ed.), Cells and Tissues in Culture: Methods, Biology, and Physiology, vol. 2, p. 1, Academic Press, New York, 1965.

98. Jacques, P. J. Endocytosis, *in* J. T. Dingle and H. B. Fell (eds.), Lysosomes in Biology and Pathology, vol. 2, p. 395, North-Holland Publishing Co., Amsterdam, 1969.

99. Janoff, A. Total acid phosphatase content of peritoneal leucocytes obtained from 1-triiodothyronine treated guinea pigs, *Proc. Soc. Exp. Biol. Med.* 110:372, 1962.

100. Johnson, L. D., and Moskowitz, M. The presence of two distinct and separable lipases in peritoneal exudate cells, *Fed. Proc.* 24:553, 1965.

101. Karnovsky, M. L. Metabolic shifts in leucocytes during the phagocytic event, *Ciba Found. Study Group* 10:60, 1961.

102. Karnovsky, M. L. Metabolic basis of phagocytic activity, *Physiol. Rev.* 42:143, 1962.

103. Karrer, H. E. The ultrastructure of mouse lung: the alveolar macrophage, *J. Biophys. Biochem. Cytol.* 4:693, 1958.

104. Khoo, K. K., and Mackaness, G. B. Macrophage proliferation in relation to acquired cellular resistance, *Aust. J. Exp. Biol. Med. Sci.* 42:707, 1964.

105. Kolsch, E., and Mitchison, N. A. The subcellular distribution of antigen in macrophages, *J. Exp. Med.* 128:1059, 1968.

106. Lands, W. E. M. Metabolism of glycerolipids. II. The enzymatic acylation of lysolecithin, *J. Biol. Chem.* 235:2233, 1960.

107. Lay, W. H., and Nussenzweig, V. Receptors for complement on leukocytes, *J. Exp. Med.* 128:991, 1968.

108. Leake, E. S., and Myrvik, Q. N. Digestive vacuole formation in alveolar macrophages after phagocytosis of Mycobacterium smegmatis in vivo, *J. Reticuloendothel. Soc.* 3:83, 1966.

109. Lee, A., and Cooper, G. N. Adhesion of homologous and heterologous red cells to peritoneal macrophages, *Aust. J. Exp. Biol. Med. Sci.* 44:527, 1966.

110. Lehrer, R. I., and Cline, M. J. Leukocyte myeloperoxidase deficiency and disseminated candidiasis: the role of myeloperoxidase in resistance to Candida infection, *J. Clin. Invest.* 48:1478, 1969.

111. Lo Buglio, A. F., Cotran, R. S., and Jandl, J. H. Red cells coated with immunoglobulin G: binding and sphering by mononuclear cells in man, *Science* 158:1582, 1967.

112. Lurie, M. B. Studies on the mechanism of immunity in tuberculosis. The mobilization of mononuclear phagocytes in normal and immunized animals and their relative capacities for division and phagocytosis, *J. Exp. Med.* 69:579, 1939.

113. Lurie, M. B. Experimental studies in native and acquired defense mechanisms, *in* Resistance to Tuberculosis, Harvard University Press, Cambridge, Mass., 1964.

114. Mackaness, G. B. Cellular resistance to infection, *J. Exp. Med.* 116:381, 1962.

115. Mackaness, G. B., and Blanden, R. V. Cellular immunity, *Prog. Allergy* 11:89, 1967.

116. Malluci, L. T-antigen and DNA synthesis in macrophages infected with polyoma virus, *Nature* 223:630, 1969.

117. Mann, P. E. G., Cohen, A. B., Finley, T. N., and Ladman, A. J. Alveolar macrophages. Structural and functional differences between nonsmokers and smokers of marijuana and tobacco. *Lab. Invest.* 25:111, 1971.

118. Merkow, L., Pardo, M., Epstein, S. M., Verney, E., and Sidransky, H. Lysosomal stability during phagocytosis of Aspergillus flavus spores by alveolar macrophages of cortisone-treated mice, *Science* 160:79, 1968.

119. Mizunoe, K., and Dannenberg, A. M. Hydrolases of rabbit macrophages. III. Effect of BCG vaccination, tissue culture, and ingested tubercle bacilli, *Proc. Soc. Exp. Biol. Med.* 120:284, 1965.

120. Mudd, E. B. H., and Mudd, S. The process of phagocytosis. The agreement between direct observation and deductions from theory, *J. Gen. Physiol.* 16:625, 1933.

121. Myrvik, Q. N., Leake, E. S., and Fariss, B. Lysozyme content of alveolar and peritoneal macrophages from the rabbit, *J. Immunol.* 86:133, 1961.

122. Nachmias, V. T., and Marshall, J. M., Jr. Protein uptake by pinocytosis in amoebae: studies on ferritin and methylated ferritin, *in* T. W. Goodwin and O. Lindberg (eds.), Biological Structure and Function, vol. 11, p. 605, Academic Press, New York, 1961.

123. Nakae, T., Nakano, M., and Saito, K. Metabolic study of intracellular killing of bacteria by mouse macrophages, *Jap. J. Microbiol.* 11:189, 1967.

124. Nathan, C. F., Karnovsky, M. L., and David, J. R. Alterations of macrophage functions by mediators from lymphocytes, *J. Exp. Med.* 133:1356, 1971.

125. Nelson, D. S. Macrophages and Immunity, North-Holland Publishing Co., Amsterdam, 1969.

126. Nichols, B. A., Bainton, D. F., and Farquhar, M. G. Differentiation of monocytes. Origin, nature and fate of their azurophil granules, *J. Cell Biol.* 50:498, 1971.

127. North, R. J. The localization by electron microscopy of nucleoside phosphatase activity in guinea pig phagocytic cells, *J. Ultrastruct. Res.* 16:83, 1966.

128. North, R. J. The localization by electron microscopy of acid phosphatase activity in guinea pig macrophages, *J. Ultrastruct. Res.* 16:96, 1966.

129. North, R. J. The uptake of particulate antigens, *J. Reticuloendothel. Soc.* 5:203, 1968.

130. North, R. J. The additive effects on the spreading of guinea pig macrophages of exogenous ATP and a surface coated with antigen-antibody, *Exp. Cell Res.* 54:267, 1969.

131. North, R. J. Cellular kinetics associated with the development of acquired cellular resistance, *J. Exp. Med.* 130:299, 1969.

132. North, R. J. The mitotic potential of fixed phagocytes in the liver as revealed during the development of cellular immunity, *J. Exp. Med.* 130:315, 1969.

133. North, R. J. The relative importance of blood monocytes and fixed macrophages to the expression of cell-mediated immunity to infection, *J. Exp. Med.* 132:521, 1970.

134. North, R. J. Endocytosis, *Semin. Hematol.* 7:161, 1970.

135. North, R. J., and Mackaness, G. B. Electronmicroscopical observations on the peritoneal macrophages of normal mice and mice immunised with *Listeria monocytogenes*. I. Structure of normal macrophages and the early cytoplasmic response to the presence of ingested bacteria, *Br. J. Exp. Pathol.* 44:601, 1963.

136. North, R. J., and Mackaness, G. B. Electronmicroscopical observations on the peritoneal macrophages of normal mice and mice immunised with *Listeria monocytogenes*. II. Structure of macrophages from immune mice and early cytoplasmic response to the presence of ingested bacteria, *Br. J. Exp. Pathol.* 44:608, 1963.

137. Novikoff, A. B., and Essner, E. The liver cell. Some new approaches to its study, *Am. J. Med.* 29:102, 1960.

138. Nungester, W. J., Ames, A. M., and Lanning, W. Electrophoresis studies of leucocytes and bacteria in relation to mechanisms of phagocytosis, *J. Infect. Dis.* 90:61, 1952.

139. Oren, R., Farnham, A. E., Saito, K., Milosky, E., and Karnovsky, M. L. Metabolic patterns in three types of phagocytizing cells, *J. Cell Biol.* 17:487, 1963.

140. Osserman, E. F., and Lawlor, D. P. Serum and urinary lysozyme (muramidase) in monocytic and monomyelocytic leukemia, *J. Exp. Med.* 124:921, 1966.

141. Parakkal, P. F. Involvement of macrophages in collagen resorption, *J. Cell Biol.* 41:345, 1969.

142. Perkins, E. H., Nettesheim, P., and Morita, T. Radioresistance of the engulfing and degradative capacities of peritoneal phagocytes to ki-

loroentgen x-ray doses, *J. Reticuloendothel. Soc.* 3:71, 1966.

143. Pethica, B. A. The physical chemistry of cell adhesion, *Exp. Cell Res.* 8:123, 1961 (suppl.).

144. Phillips-Quagliata, J. M., Levine, B. B., Quagliata, F., and Uhr, J. W. Mechanisms underlying binding of immune complexes to macrophages, *J. Exp. Med.* 133:589, 1971.

145. Pinkett, M. O., Cowdrey, C. R., and Nowell, P. C. Mixed hematopoietic and pulmonary origin of alveolar macrophages as demonstrated by chromosome markers, *Am. J. Pathol.* 48:859, 1966.

146. Rabinovitch, M. The dissociation of the attachment and ingestion phases of phagocytosis by macrophages, *Exp. Cell Res.* 46:19, 1967.

147. Rabinovitch, M. Attachment of modified erythrocytes to phagocytic cells in absence of serum, *Proc. Soc. Exp. Biol. Med.* 124:396, 1967.

148. Rabinovitch, M. Phagocytosis: the engulfment stage, *Semin. Hematol.* 5:134, 1968.

149. Ratzan, K. R., Musher, D. M., Keusch, G. T., and Weinstein, L. Correlation of increased metabolic activity, resistance to infection, enhanced phagocytosis, and inhibition of bacterial growth by macrophages from Listeria- and BCG-infected mice, *Infect. Immun.* 5:499, 1972.

150. Robin, E. D., Smith, J. D., Tanser, A. R., Adamson, J. S., Millen, J. E., and Packer, B. Ion and macromolecular transport in the alveolar macrophage, *Biochim. Biophys. Acta* 241:117, 1971.

151. Roelants, G. E., and Goodman, J. W. The chemical nature of macrophage RNA-antigen complexes and their relevance to immune induction, *J. Exp. Med.* 130:557, 1969.

152. Rowley, D. Antibacterial systems of serum in relation to nonspecific immunity to infection, *Bacteriol. Rev.* 24:106, 1960.

153. Saito, K., and Suter, E. Lysosomal acid hydrolases in mice infected with BCG, *J. Exp. Med.* 121:727, 1965.

154. Salmon, S. E., Cline, M. J., Schultz, J., and Lehrer, R. I. Myeloperoxidase deficiency: immunologic study of a genetic leukocyte defect, *N. Engl. J. Med.* 282:250, 1970.

155. Seyberth, H. W., Schmidt-Gayk, H.,

Jakobs, K. H., and Hackenthal, E. Cyclic adenosine monophosphate in phagocytizing granulocytes and alveolar macrophages, *J. Cell Biol.* 57:567, 1973.

156. Soderberg, L. S. F., Rubin, A., Kuchler, R. J., and Solotorovsky, M. Ribonucleic acid synthesis in mouse peritoneal macrophages *in vitro, Cell. Immunol.* 3:672, 1972.

157. Stähelin, H., Suter, E., and Karnovsky, M. L. Studies on the interaction between phagocytes and tubercle bacilli. I. Observations on the metabolism of guinea pig leucocytes and the influence of phagocytosis, *J. Exp. Med.* 104:121, 1956.

158. Stecher, V. J., and Thorbecke, G. J. Sites of synthesis of serum proteins: I. Serum proteins produced by macrophages in vitro, *J. Immunol.* 99:643, 1967.

159. Stollerman, G. H., Rytel, M., and Ortiz, J. Accessory plasma factors involved in the bactericidal test for type-specific antibody to group A streptococci, *J. Exp. Med.* 117:1, 1963.

160. Stubbs, M., Kühner, A. V., Glass, E. A., David, J. R., and Karnovsky, M. L. Metabolic and functional studies on activated mouse macrophages, *J. Exp. Med.* 137:537, 1973.

161. Sumner, M. A., Bradley, T. R., Hodgson, G. S., Cline, M. J., Fry, P. A., and Sutherland, L. The growth of bone marrow cells in liquid culture, *Br. J. Haematol.* 23:221, 1972.

162. Suter, E., and Hulliger, L. Nonspecific and specific cellular reactions to infections, *Ann. N.Y. Acad. Sci.* 88:1237, 1960.

163. Suter, E., and Ramseier, H. Cellular reactions in infection, *Adv. Immunol.* 4:117, 1964.

164. Sutton, J. S. Ultrastructural aspects of *in vitro* development of monocytes into macrophages, epithelioid cells, and multinucleated giant cells, *in* Conference on Cell Tissue and Organ Culture, Natl. Cancer Inst. Monogr. 26:71, National Cancer Institute, Bethesda, 1967.

165. Sutton, J. S., and Weiss, L. Transformation of monocytes in tissue culture into macrophages, epithelioid cells, and multinucleated giant cells. An electron microscope study, *J. Cell Biol.* 28:303, 1966.

166. Tsan, M-F., and Berlin, R. D.

Membrane transport in the rabbit alveolar macrophage. The specificity and characteristics of amino acid transport systems, *Biochim. Biophys. Acta* 241:155, 1971.

167. Tume, R. K., and Day, A. J. Cholesterol esterifying activity of rabbit alveolar macrophages, *J. Reticuloendothel. Soc.* 7:338, 1970.

168. Unanue, E. R., and Askonas, B. A. Persistence of immunogenicity of antigen after uptake by macrophages, *J. Exp. Med.* 127:915, 1968.

169. Unanue, E. R., and Cerottini, J-C. Persistence of antigen on the surface of macrophages, *Nature* 222:1193, 1969.

170. van Furth, R., and Cohn, Z. A. The origin and kinetics of mononuclear phagocytes, *J. Exp. Med.* 128:415, 1968.

171. van Furth, R., and Diesselhoff-Den Dulk, M. M. C. The kinetics of promonocytes and monocytes in the bone marrow, *J. Exp. Med.* 132:813, 1970.

172. van Furth, R., Hirsch, J. G., and Fedorko, M. E. Morphology and peroxidase cytochemistry of mouse promonocytes, monocytes, and macrophages, *J. Exp. Med.* 132:794, 1970.

173. Vannotti, A. Metabolic pattern of leucocytes within the circulation and outside it, *Ciba Found. Study Group* 10:79, 1961.

174. Virolainen, M., and Defendi, V. Dependence of macrophage growth *in vitro* upon interaction with other cell types, *Wistar Inst. Symp. Monogr.* 7:67, 1967.

175. Volkman, A., and Gowans, J. L. The production of macrophages in the rat, *Br. J. Exp. Pathol.* 46:50, 1965.

176. Volkman, A., and Gowans, J. L. The origin of macrophages from bone marrow in the rat, *Br. J. Exp. Pathol.* 46:62, 1965.

177. Ward, P. A. Chemotaxis of mononuclear cells, *J. Exp. Med.* 128:1201, 1968.

178. Watts, J. W., and Harris, H. Turnover of nucleic acids in a non-multiplying animal cell, *Biochem. J.* 72:147, 1959.

179. Weiss, L. P., and Fawcett, D. W. Cytochemical observations on chicken monocytes, macrophages

and giant cells in tissue culture, *J. Histochem. Cytochem.* 1:47, 1953.

180. Weissmann, G. The role of lysosomes in inflammation and disease, *Ann. Rev. Med.* 18:97, 1967.

181. Werb, Z., and Cohn, Z. A. Cholesterol metabolism in the macrophage. I. The regulation of cholesterol exchange, *J. Exp. Med.* 134:1545, 1971.

182. West, J., Morton, D. J., Esmann, V., and Stjernholm, R. L. Carbohydrate metabolism in leukocytes. VIII. Metabolic activities of the macro-

phage, *Arch. Biochem. Biophys.* 124:85, 1968.

183. Wiener, E. DNA-synthesis in peritoneal mononuclear leucocytes, *Exp. Cell Res.* 45:450, 1967.

184. Wiener, E., and Marmary, Y. The in vitro effect of hydrocortisone on cultures of peritoneal monocytes, *Lab. Invest.* 21:505, 1969.

185. Woessner, J. F. Biological mechanisms of collagen resorption, *in* B. S. Gould (ed.), Treatise on Collagen, pt. B, p. 253, Academic Press, New York, 1968.

186. Woodin, A. M., and Wieneke, A. A. Composition and properties of a cell-membrane fraction from the polymorphonuclear leucocyte, *Biochem. J.* 99:493, 1966.

187. Yarborough, D. J., Meyer, O. T., Dannenberg, A. M., and Pearson, B. Histochemistry of macrophage hydrolases. III. Studies on β-galactosidase, and aminopeptidase with indolyl and naphthyl substrates, *J. Reticuloendothel. Soc.* 4:390, 1967.

Chapter 25   Function of Monocytes and Macrophages

The monocyte-macrophage group of cells—whether free in the blood, migrating in the tissues, or fixed in the tissues—appears to have three well-defined functions: (a) removal of damaged or dying cells and cell debris (for example, the phagocytosis of damaged or effete red cells); (b) interaction with lymphoid cells in certain phases of immunologic reactions; and (c) defense reactions against certain classes of microorganisms. In addition, it has been suggested that mononuclear leukocytes may function in control of granulopoiesis, in the defense against spontaneously arising tumors, in wound repair, and in remodeling of embryonic tissues and bone (73). "Reticulum cells," perhaps related to macrophages in function and ontogeny, may be important in erythropoiesis. Reticulum cells may possibly provide utilizable iron to developing erythroblasts by forming an "erythroblastic island" (20, 21, 228).

In the succeeding sections of this chapter we shall consider first the three well-defined macrophage functions set forth above. Subsequently, materials related to other possible physiologic roles of the macrophage will be considered.

Erythrophagocytosis

The appearance of hemosiderin-laden macrophages in diseases characterized by excessive erythrocyte destruction (such as hereditary spherocytosis) or by extravasation of red cells into tissues (for example, tight mitral stenosis with pulmonary hypertension) has been recognized by morphologists and pathologists for many years (see Fig. 26.6). Erythrophagocytosis is also a feature of many of the diseases of proliferation of malignant macrophages; for example, monocytic leukemia and histiocytic medullary reticulosis (81) (Chapter 27).

The phagocytosis of erythrocytes by macrophages has been studied under a variety of conditions in vitro (39, 61, 150, 194-196, 247, 248). It is convenient to think of erythrophagocytosis as occurring in three phases: attachment, ingestion, and digestion. During the attachment phase (194, 195) the macrophage fixes the red cell to its surface. The phagocyte appears to recognize changes in the erythrocyte surface membrane induced by immunoglobulin coating, chemical injury, or by the aging process. These recognition processes for immunoglobulins are known in considerable detail.

The ingestion phase of erythrophagocytosis is similar to the ingestion process for other particles of organic matter. Ingestion was considered briefly in Chapter 24 and will be discussed again later in this chapter.

Immunoglobulin Receptors and the Attachment Phase

The study of Lo Buglio and his colleagues in 1967 placed in sharp focus the mechanism of monocyte attachment to, and subsequent phagocytosis of, antibody-coated erythrocytes (133). These investigators demonstrated that human monocytes have receptors for IgG at their surface that bind to IgG-coated red cells (Fig. 25.1). These receptors do not recognize IgM or IgA immunoglobulin. Lo Buglio's observations have been confirmed and extended by many other investigators (1-3, 39, 41, 61, 112, 166, 178,

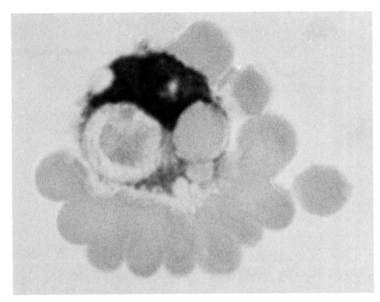

Figure 25.1 Erythrocytes coated with IgG anti-D antibody surround a monocyte. Several of the red cells have been phagocytized. The erythrocytes attach to monocyte membrane receptors.

185, 186). The salient features of the receptors for immunoglobulins are summarized in Table 25.1.

The monocyte-macrophage surface receptor is limited in its specificity. In man this specificity is directed toward IgG$_1$ and IgG$_3$ immunoglobulin. Most naturally occurring IgG antibodies are a mixture of IgG$_1$, IgG$_2$, IgG$_3$, and IgG$_4$. Anti-Rh antibodies are primarily IgG$_1$ and IgG$_3$ (165), and some other antibodies may be composed primarily of a single class of immunoglobulin (132, 261).

Because the surface receptor binds complexes of IgG and antigen more avidly than IgG alone, the macrophage can selectively identify such immune complexes in plasma or extracellular fluid containing many immunoglobulins. Perhaps this difference in binding avidity reflects conformational changes in the IgG molecule once it unites with its specific antigen.

Although the IgG molecule reacts with antigen through its Fab piece, it interacts with the macrophage receptor through its Fc fragment (see Fig. 8.1 and Chapter 16). The

Table 25.1 Characteristics of macrophage surface receptors for IgG immunoglobulins.

Specificity for certain IgG subclasses; for example, IgG$_1$ and IgG$_3$ in man, IgG$_{2a}$ in the mouse.
Requirement for an intact IgG Fc fragment.
More avid binding of IgG-antigen complex than of IgG alone.
Protease-resistant receptor; destruction by phospholipase C.

receptor is probably a phospholipid or a phospholipoprotein, although recent observations suggest the possibility of glycoprotein structure (6). It is almost certainly similar or identical to the macrophage surface receptor that binds cytophilic antibody (18, 19, 56, 109, 166). The macrophage surface receptor disappears with phagocytosis (probably because it enters the cell's interior) and is then slowly reconstituted (214). Similar IgG receptors have been identified on normal and malignant mast cells (44, 234), on B lymphocytes (41), and on neutrophils (see Chapter 4).

The surface receptors of monocytes and macrophages provide a mechanism for these cells to identify and bind red cells coated with IgG antibody—as, for example, in erythroblastosis fetalis. They also constitute a mechanism for the mononuclear phagocyte to attach to microorganisms coated with IgG antibody. The presence of such surface receptors may be used in identifying cells of the mononuclear leukocyte series (45, 111).

Human monocytes do not bind red cells coated with IgM antibody. Some investigators have suggested that the macrophage has surface receptors for some complement components bound to IgM or IgA (112, 119). Similarly, the possibility exists that some animal macrophages have receptors for IgM-antigen complexes (130).

Phagocytic and Digestion Phases

Once the monocyte or macrophage binds an antibody-coated red cell, it then proceeds to ingest it, provided energy is available from glycolytic processes (see Fig. 4.2 and Chapter 24). The red cell is internalized within the monuclear phagocyte in a phagocytic vacuole. As the lysosomes fuse with the vacuole and discharge their contents into it, the erythrocyte is exposed to the action of hydrolytic enzymes. The subsequent digestion occurs without expenditure of metabolic energy. The globin moiety of the red cell is digested to amino acids and peptides (67). The heme moiety is catabolized by a macrophage enzyme—heme oxygenase (192, 229–231; cf. 168). This cellular enzyme activity, normally present at low levels, increases greatly after exposure of the cells to hemoglobin (190, 191). Heme oxygenase in the macrophage appears to be an inducible enzyme. It is likely that the mononuclear phagocytes equipped with this enzyme are critically important in clearing extravasated hemoglobin from tissues and in converting it to amino acid and bilirubin.

Under some circumstances red cells coated with IgG antibodies may be bound to a monocyte, but are not phagocytized. These attached erythrocytes become deformed and are abnormally sensitive to osmotic lysis (9, 99, 117, 133). Antibody-injured red cells thus may be removed by two macrophage-dependent processes: phagocytosis and osmotic lysis.

Circumstantial evidence suggests that the specificity of the bound antibody may determine which red cells are destroyed in vivo and which survive (85). It is likely that in vivo the splenic macrophage plays a key role in sequestration of antibody-coated red cells (114).

Disposal of Senescent and Chemically Injured Red Cells
Senescent red blood cells disappear from the circulation of man at a rate of about 0.9 percent per day (99). Sequestration and destruction are thought to occur in organs with large numbers of phagocytic reticuloendothelial cells—the spleen, liver, and bone marrow (115, 116, 121). In these organs red cell destruction proceeds by osmotic lysis, fragmentation, and erythrophagocytosis (99, 163).

Descriptions of the microanatomy of the spleen (32, 254-256) and of the liver (14, 206, 258, 260) have led to a better understanding of the role of these organs in sequestration and destruction of blood cells. The red pulp of the spleen is formed by cords and sinuses lined with phagocytic macrophages. Blood cells enter the splenic cords through terminal arterioles. They pass through fenestrations in the basement membranes between cords and sinuses and traverse the narrow spaces between sinus endothelial cells before collecting in the splenic sinuses. These fenestrations and spaces comprise an effective biological filtration system, which places the percolating blood cells in intimate contact with the lining cells. Successful passage through this filtration device requires a normally deformable erythrocyte. Red cells with abnormal deformability, such as those that are senescent or from patients with diseases such as hereditary spherocytosis, have difficulty navigating the small passages of the spleen and are sequestered and then lysed or phagocytized (255). A similar phenomenon probably occurs in the liver (23).

Red cells with inclusions from oxidant drugs (Heinz bodies) or parasites may also have difficulty getting the nondeformable inclusions through the narrow spaces of these reticuloendothelial organs. Such erythrocytes are at high risk of sequestration and subsequent destruction. Several lines of evidence suggest that the phagocytic cells of the spleen may "pit" or "cull" these and other inclusions from red cells, ultimately destroying the red cell or returning the inclusion-free ("pitted") erythrocyte to the circulation (51, 52, 129, 198, 216).

Macrophage Function in the Immune Response
The interaction of mononuclear phagocytes with lymphoid cells in certain phases of the immune response is supported by several observations:

(a) Pure populations of lymphocytes containing no phagocytes show a reduced blastogenic and antibody response to specific antigens in vitro; addition of macrophages restores this response to normal levels (104, 161, 162, 187, 188).
(b) RNA containing trace amounts of antigen prepared from animal macrophages can induce lymphocytes to produce the corresponding antibody (5, 13, 75, 79, 80, 89-91).
(c) Human monocytes and macrophages exposed to antigen in vitro and then washed free of extracellular antigen can induce transformation of autologous lymphocytes (43, 94).
(d) Normal, nonimmune lymphoid cells can induce antibody synthesis in X-irradiated recipient animals when living macrophages containing antigen are also transferred (128, 241, 242).
(e) Close cellular contact and cytoplasmic connections have been demonstrated between lymphocytes and macrophages (217, 220).
(f) Addition of macrophages to lymphocytes augments the production of certain effector substances, such as interferon, in response to specific antigen and nonspecific mitogen (68, 69).
(g) After administration of radioactive antigen to an experimental animal, the label is found associated with medullary macrophages, as well as surface processes, of dendritic reticular cells within the cortical areas of lymph nodes. The reticular cells are in intimate contact with the surfaces of surrounding lymphocytes (173, 174, 176).

This series of observations has led to the concept that macrophages function during two phases of the immune response: in the "afferent" limb during the induction of immunity by antigen, and in the "efferent" limb during the expression of cellular immunity.

Macrophages and Antigen Processing
The role of the macrophage in the handling of antigen during the inductive phase (afferent limb) of the immune response appears to be quite separate from its role in cell-mediated immune reactions (efferent limb) (see Fig. 15.3).

The first evidence of a role for macrophages in antigen processing came from observations that better immune responses were obtained when animals were immunized with particulate, readily phagocytized antigen rather than with soluble, poorly phagocytized antigen (22, 34, 62, 78, 88, 225). In general, aggregation of antigen enhanced the immune response. However, attempts to exploit this observation by manipulations such as reticuloendothelial blockade or by injury of macrophages with specific antiserum were, in general, inconclusive (59, 63, 84, 180, 208, 239, 244).

The second line of evidence for macrophage involvement in the afferent limb of the immune response came from studies of the distribution of labeled antigen within the reticuloendothelial system after administration to an intact animal. A variety of antigens and labels was used (4, 31, 83, 96, 113, 139, 173-176, 257). The broad conclusion of these studies was that antigen may be found in association with macrophages and the dendritic processes of reticular cells for long periods of time. However, these studies suffer from the deficiency that they localized but did not define the function of retained antigen.

The next phase of the study of antigen processing came with the use of isolated cell populations. Two types of experiments were performed. First, antigen was administered to macrophages, and the living cells were transferred to histocompatible recipients. The immune response to the macrophage-bound antigen was then observed. Second, macrophages plus free or bound antigen were added to lymphocytes in vitro and the proliferative and/or antibody response of the lymphocytes was measured.

Such experiments demonstrated that with administration of antigen bound to macrophages, one can indeed initiate an immune response in intact animals (10, 47, 157, 193, 240, 241, 244, 245). By labeling techniques the macrophages can be shown to migrate to spleen and lymph nodes (205, 207). The immunologic response may be 19 S or 7 S antibody immunoglobulin, depending on the character of the inducing antigen (240, 241). In such transfer experiments one requires a lymphocyte capable of antigen recognition and of antibody response.

In in vitro studies, antigen bound to macrophages can direct specific blastogenic transformation of lymphocytes and production of antibody, as illustrated in Fig. 25.2 (43, 94, 97, 104, 179).

It has been speculated that the immunologic unresponsiveness of some newborn animals to antigen may be the result of immaturity of the reticuloendothelial system. Consistent with this thesis is the observation that injection of adult macrophages into newborn mice may enhance their response to sheep red cells (11, 28).

Persistence of Antigen Many factors influence the uptake of antigen by macrophages, including the state of aggregation of the antigen and its binding to serum proteins (210). Once protein antigens are taken up by macrophages, the majority are rapidly degraded to amino acids and oligopeptides (66, 240). Some antigen escapes degrada-

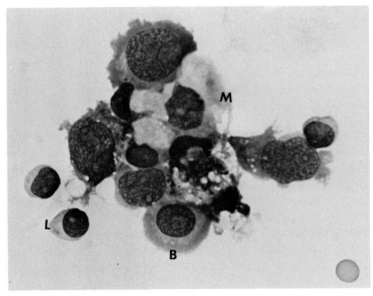

Figure 25.2 An "immunologic island" composed of central macrophage (*M*) surrounded by untransformed lymphocytes (*L*) and lymphocytes undergoing blastogenic transformation (*B*). (From M. J. Cline and V. C. Swett, *J. Exp. Med.* 128:1309, 1968. Reprinted by permission of authors and publisher.)

tion and may persist for long periods of time (77, 244). Concomitantly, immunogenicity may persist. It appears that most of the antigen is degraded within phagolysosomes, but that a small fraction—probably less than 10 percent of the total—finds its way into other cell fractions, thereby escaping degradation (126, 238, 242). Antigen may also persist in association with the membrane of the macrophage.

Handling of Antigen The key questions that arise from the foregoing observation are, How does the macrophage handle antigen in order to stimulate a lymphocyte response? Does the cell metabolize antigen in some way to enhance its immunogenicity? Does it synthesize an informational molecule in response to antigen? Or does the cell merely retain antigen for long periods of time in a form that is accessible to lymphocytes?

The answers to these questions are not known with certainty. It is probable that macrophages function primarily to accumulate antigen and to maintain it in the form to which lymphocytes have access. It is possible that the small amount of antigen that escapes degradation has enhanced immunogenicity.

Early in the studies of the interaction of monocytes with lymphocytes it was suggested that the mononuclear phagocytes synthesized an informational RNA that instructed the lymphocyte (5, 74-76). Further studies demonstrated that RNA preparations from antigen-primed macrophages contain antigen fragments and that these probably account for lymphocyte antibody response when lymphocytes are interacted with the macrophages (13, 30, 80, 89-91). When combined with RNA, certain antigens appear to be more effective as immunologic stimulants. Such enhancement may be akin to that achieved by aggregating antigens or binding them to insoluble particles. Nonantigenic molecules are not rendered immunogenic by binding them to RNA (202, 203). It is quite possible, however, that the association between RNA and antigen does not occur in the intact cell and is merely an artifact of laboratory handling.

Contact between cells occurs at their surfaces. It is probable that at least some antigen is retained for long periods of time on the surface of the macrophage (243, 245).

Unanue and Cerottini (244) have summarized the handling of the soluble antigen hemocyanin; of 100 molecules taken up by the macrophage, 97 are immediately endocytosed and 2 or 3 are retained at the plasma membrane. Some of the membrane-bound molecules are immunogenic. Of the endocytosed molecules, 90 are ultimately expelled from the cell, usually in a catabolized form. The remaining 7 are retained in the cell, probably in lysosomes.

Interaction with Lymphocytes Antigen-primed macrophages can induce specific antibody synthesis or blas-

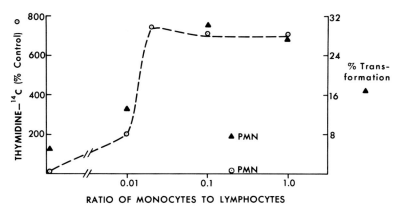

Figure 25.4 Degree of stimulation of blastogenic transformation when monocytes and PPD are added to sensitized lymphocytes. Ratios of monocytes to lymphocytes as low as 1:100 are stimulatory. Neutrophils (PMN) are nonstimulatory. (From M. J. Cline and V. C. Swett, *J. Exp. Med.* 128:1309, 1968. Reprinted by permission of authors and publisher.)

togenic transformation in responsive lymphocytes (43, 160). The response has certain requirements: a metabolically intact macrophage, a metabolically intact lymphocyte, and physical contact between the cells. As shown in Fig. 25.3, macrophages are superior to monocytes at inducing lymphocyte blastogenic transformation (35, 94). However, even one monocyte per 100 lymphocytes suffices to initiate transformation (43) (Fig. 25.4).

When the antigen-primed macrophage is poisoned by an inhibitor of glycolysis, it no longer induces blastogenic transformation of lymphocytes (43). The mononuclear cells are relatively resistant to irradiation, whereas the antibody-synthesizing lymphocytes are radiosensitive (204, 215). The suggestion that the immunogenicity of antigen in macrophages is dependent on a radiosensitive process needs corroboration (17, 60, 82, 193).

In addition to their involvement in the blastogenic transformation of lymphocytes, macrophages also enhance the production of certain lymphocyte mediators, such as interferon (68, 69) (see Chapter 17).

The necessity for intimate contact between an antigen-binding macrophage and the potential antibody-forming cell was suggested by the observation of islands of antibody-forming cells around macrophages in antibody-forming organs of the whole animal. It was further supported by the observation of cell fusion between lymphocytes and macrophages (217). In vitro, "immune clusters" with the central mononuclear cell and a halo of adherent lymphocytes are readily demonstrable (43, 94, 232) (Figs. 25.2 and 25.5).

In such clusters there is a close anatomic association

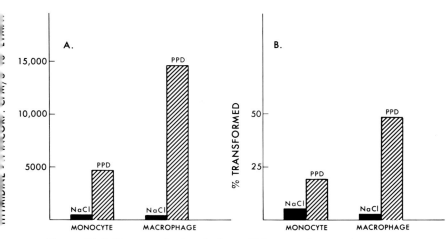

Figure 25.3 Degree of stimulation of blastogenic transformation when monocytes, macrophages, and specific antigen (PPD) are added to purified populations of lymphocytes from tuberculin-positive subjects. Measurement is by ³H-thymidine incorporation (part *A*) and by morphology (part *B*). (From J. Hanifin and M. J. Cline, *J. Cell Biol.* 46:97, 1970. Reprinted by permission of authors and publisher.)

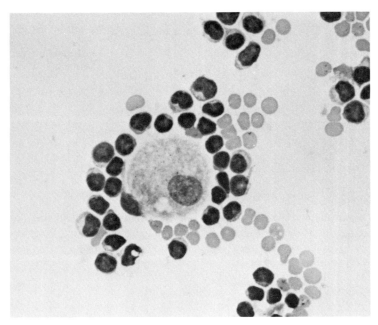

Figure 25.5 A cluster of lymphocytes around a large macrophage previously exposed to antigen.

between the lymphocyte and the mononuclear cell (140-142). The attachment between cells is by means of the microspikes of the lymphocyte uropod (see Chapter 12 and Figs. 12.8 and 12.9). Separation of lymphocytes from macrophages by a cell-impermeable membrane or by repeated agitation of the culture inhibits lymphocyte response to antigen (43, 97, 104, 160, 161).

Effect of Adjuvants Many of the well-known immunologic adjuvants are readily phagocytized by cells of the reticuloendothelial system (84, 233). Some of these adjuvants also exert toxic effects on macrophages, including silica (7, 124), endotoxin (101, 123), and beryllium (243, 245). Viruses that are phagocytized by macrophages may also exert an adjuvant effect (151, 177). The relation between the phagocytosis of these particles and the enhancement of immunogenicity is uncertain.

Macrophages and Cellular Immunity
Cellular immunity is a form of immune response that is expressed by cells rather than humoral antibodies. Cellular immune responses impart resistance to certain classes of microbial and multicellular parasites and are involved in antitumor immunity and allograft rejection. At the turn of the century, Metchnikoff (155) thought that an animal recovered from an infection through the "perfection of the phagocytic and digestive processes of the leukocytes." From a lifetime of studying host-defense mecha-

nisms, Lurie (137) concluded that acquired resistance to *Mycobacterium tuberculosis* was mediated through the epithelioid cells of the granulomata and that the maturation of monocytes to epithelioid cells was accompanied by changes that increased the antimicrobial capabilities of the cell. As we shall see, both of these biologists were fundamentally correct in their views.

The Activated Macrophage When an animal is sublethally infected by a facultative intracellular parasite such as *M. tuberculosis*, its tissue macrophages differ in certain respects from cells obtained from normal, uninfected animals (143-147, 237). The activated macrophage of the infected host has a more highly developed antimicrobial system; it has enhanced phagocytic activity and ability to spread on a glass surface; it is larger, has a greater acid hydrolase content and digestive capacity, a higher rate of glucose oxidation, and a higher mitotic rate than the unactivated cell (see Chapter 24). These characteristics of activation are summarized in Table 25.2 and Fig. 25.6.

Activation of macrophages varies with the time and extent of infection. For example, a small intravenous dose of *Mycobacterium bovis* in mice produces only minor activation, whereas a large dose produces a rapid effect (25). Similarly, in mild infection free peritoneal macrophages may be essentially unchanged, while fixed tissue macrophages may be activated. With an intracellular parasite such as *Listeria monocytogenes*, peak resistance may not develop for 12 to 14 days. With other parasites, such as *Mycobacterium tuberculosis* and *Brucella*, resistance grows more slowly (25, 144); with *Salmonella* it may develop more rapidly (26).

A critical observation is that activation is nonspecific in the following sense: induction under appropriate conditions by any intracellular parasite produces an activated state that is reflected in the enhanced ability of the cells to deal with a variety of intracellular parasites. Adrenocorticosteroids in high concentrations may inhibit macro-

Table 25.2 Characteristics of activated macrophages.

Characteristic	References
Larger than normal	147
Increased activity of acid hydrolases	54, 209, 227
Increased digestive capacity	24
Increased phagocytic capacity and glass spreading	169, 226
Increased microbicidal activity	147
Increased glucose oxidation	164, 226

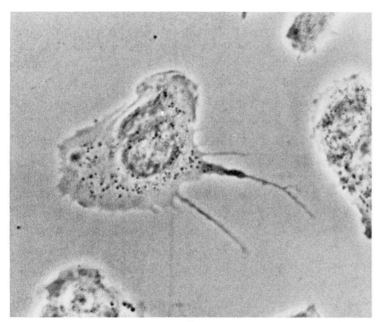

Fig. 25.6A

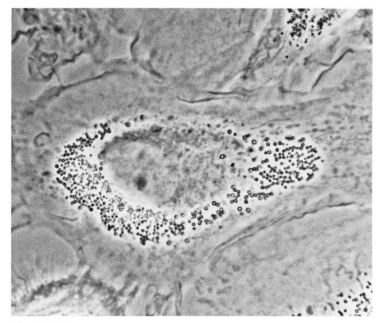

Fig. 25.6B

Figure 25.6 Living monocytes, cultivated in vitro for four days, from a normal subject (Fig. 25.6A) and from a subject with hypersensitivity to beryllium (Fig. 25.6B). The first cell has just begun to spread on the glass cover slip and to develop cytoplasmic granulation. The second cell has enlarged greatly, spread out much more, and developed more prominent cytoplasmic granules. Both cells were photographed under phase contrast illumination.

phage activation and accumulation in infective foci in the tissues (172).

Immunologic Mediation of Macrophage Activation and Cellular Immunity From a variety of observations it is clear that four phenomena go hand in hand after a sublethal intracellular infection: (a) development of enhanced microbial resistance, (b) macrophage activation, (c) increased macrophage proliferation (125, 144, 147, 170, 171), and (d) development of delayed hypersensitivity (147, 212).

Resistance to an intracellular parasite such as *Listeria* may be accomplished by the transfer of immune lymphoid cells to syngeneic recipient animals, but not by the administration of humoral antibody (143, 146). Similarly, antilymphocyte serum blocks the adoptive transfer of immunity (148). These observations suggest that lymphoid cells are involved in mediating the enhanced resistance to the parasite. The macrophage is the "effector" cell in this response.

In such adoptive immune responses, delayed hypersensitivity and resistance develop in parallel in the recipient animal. It seems clear from experiments using irradiated recipient animals that it is the monocyte and macrophage derived from bone marrow precursors (250, 251) that are necessary both for the expression of resistance to microorganisms and for development of delayed hypersensitivity (135, 136, 236, 249).

The mechanisms of macrophage activation and of the stimulation of macrophage proliferation are largely unknown. Presumably the process is mediated by immunologically competent lymphocytes and their products. Replication of the lymphoid cells is probably necessary for activation of macrophages, as indicated by experiments with mitomycin-C (147). The lymphocyte stimulated by antigen makes a great many effector substances (Chapter 17). Some of these have an effect on macrophage function—as, for example, migration inhibitory factor (MIF) (57). Several investigators recently have demonstrated that antigen-stimulated lymphocytes produce a substance(s) capable of activating normal macrophages (158, 164, 222). However, no one lymphocyte factor has been clearly identified as a critical mediator of macrophage activation (cf. 223).

As an alternative to lymphocyte mediators, cytophilic antibody has been suggested as a possible mechanism of macrophage activation: lymphocytes and plasma cells are postulated to secrete a high-affinity antibody that binds to the macrophages and captures circulating antigens (166, 235). Cytophilic antibody is found in animals with delayed hypersensitivity (167, cf. 65) and may be important in the recognition by macrophages of foreign antigens on the surface of tumor cells (156). Despite these observations, the weight of evidence does not suggest a critical role for cytophilic antibody in macrophage activation (143). It must be admitted that the present state of our knowledge is inadequate to define the precise mechanism of macrophage activation. For further discussion on macrophages in delayed hypersensitivity and cellular immunity, several excellent reviews are available (27, 48, 147).

Antimicrobial Defense Function

Mononuclear phagocytes are involved in the defense against a variety of infectious agents. They form the principal cellular defense system against intracellular pathogenic bacteria and fungi, and a variety of other intracellular parasites. For example, macrophages kill or limit the growth of *Mycobacteria* (8, 12, 54, 64, 181), *Salmonella* (49, 110), *Listeria* (29, 36, 37), *Cryptococcus* (219), *Toxoplasma* (197), malaria organisms (138), and probably *Brucella* (107).

In their reaction to invading microorganisms, macrophages must accumulate at an infective focus; they must ingest and ultimately kill or limit the intracellular replication of the organism. In carrying out these functions, the immunologically activated macrophage is more effective than is the unstimulated macrophage (see Chapter 24, the section on macrophages and cellular immunity above, and references 25, 49, 146, 147, 181, 197). Activation of macrophages requires cooperation between these cells and lymphocytes.

Phagocytosis

In 1960 Harris used the dark-ground trace technique to demonstrate the chemotactic response of monocytes to bacteria (98). More recent investigators have adapted the Boyden double chamber to the study of mononuclear cell chemotaxis (122, 224, 252, 259) (see Chapter 4). However, considerably less is known about oriented movement in these cells than in neutrophils. One serum factor that is chemotactic for mononuclear leukocytes is the activated fifth component of complement (C'5) (224). In addition, guinea pig serum contains a chemotactically active factor of molecular weight 90,000 that is heat-labile (100).

Little is known about factors that may influence mononuclear leukocyte mobilization into areas of inflammation. Both ethanol (93, 134) and high concentrations of adrenocorticosteroids (172) can inhibit this directed cell movement. A comprehensive discussion of humoral mediators of chemotaxis is available in the recent report of Hausman and his colleagues (100).

The major features of phagocytosis, including the morphologic events, metabolic considerations, biochemical changes, and requirements for opsonins and cations, have been discussed in Chapter 24 and will not be reviewed here. It is sufficient to note that with progressive maturation from the bone marrow promonocyte to the tissue macrophage there is progressive increase in phagocytic capacity (35, 42).

Macrophages and monocytes are capable of ingesting a wide variety of particles, including red cells (Fig. 25.1), damaged leukocytes and other nucleated cells (Fig. 25.7), microorganisms (Fig. 25.8), and crystals (Fig. 25.9). Within the tissues macrophages localize certain metals, metal salts, and other particles, including plutonium oxide (213), silica (182), beryllium (95), coal dust, carbon, iron oxide, and barium salts. All the cells of this series, with the exception of the alveolar macrophage, are largely dependent upon glycolytic energy production for particle ingestion (120). The alveolar macrophage is dependent upon available oxygen for phagocytosis (46, 120).

As noted earlier, phagocytosis of any particle may be subdivided into the attachment and ingestion phases (see Fig. 4.2). The attachment phase involves the establishment of a firm contact between the particle and the macrophage plasma membrane. For most bacteria this requires cation and surface coating with IgG. The Fc fragment of the IgG antibody molecule binds to receptors on the macrophage surface. Organisms coated with IgM and activated com-

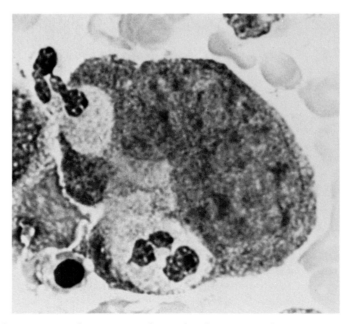

Figure 25.7 A large macrophage that has ingested one neutrophil and is in the process of ingesting another.

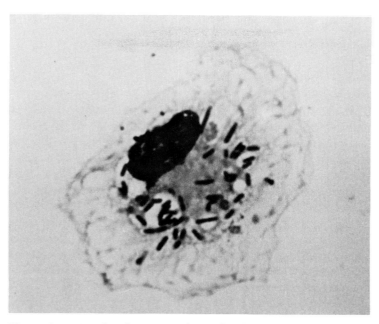

Figure 25.8 An alveolar macrophage that has ingested numerous bacilli.

plement components may bind to other surface receptors. Both IgG and complement receptors may be blocked by antibody to the plasma membrane of the macrophage (108). For some microorganisms such as *Mycoplasma* immunoglobulins, complement and cations are not required for the attachment phase (118).

Subsequent to attachment of the particle, the cell's plasma membrane invaginates to form a vacuole enclosing the particle. This process is probably mediated by the subplasmalemmal network of microfilaments and microtubules. As the phagocytic vacuole moves into the cell cytoplasm, the surface membranes of neighboring lysosomes fuse with the membrane of the vacuole. Particle ingestion is then accompanied by discharge of lysosomes into the phagocytic vacuole. This process of degranulation may be inhibited by high concentrations of corticosteroids (152) and perhaps by the products of certain virulent bacteria (12).

Killing

The mononuclear cell complex provides a critical tissue defense system against a variety of microorganisms. We tend to think of the neutrophil as the primary defense unit against pyogenic organisms such as *Staphylococcus* and *Pneumococcus* and regard the macrophage as a cellular defense unit against intracellular organisms such as *Mycobacterium tuberculosis* and *M. leprae.*

The mechanisms by which monocytes and macro-

phages kill bacteria is largely unknown. The available evidence is derived from two sources: studies of genetic defects of host functions, and in vitro manipulation of the environment of the mononuclear phagocyte to alter its bactericidal capabilities.

Oxygen Requirement and H_2O_2 Generation In the absence of oxygen, the ability of human macrophages to kill certain bacteria is impaired (36). In the presence of oxygen and an agent that stimulates H_2O_2 generation, killing is enhanced (37, 50). Furthermore, monocyte bactericidal capacity is reduced in chronic granulomatous disease, a condition in which leukocyte hydrogen peroxide generation is impaired (58, 201) (see Chapter 8 for details). These observations strongly suggest that the monocyte-macrophage utilizes a hydrogen-peroxide–generating system as an important bactericidal mechanism. Similar systems comprise the major antibacterial armament of the neurophil.

Myeloperoxidase The enzyme myeloperoxidase is present in macrophage precursors up to the stage of the monocyte. It is not present in more mature cells of this series (42, 246). In the genetic absence of this enzyme impaired monocyte microbicidal activity is demonstrable, but macrophage killing is normal (131, 210). It appears,

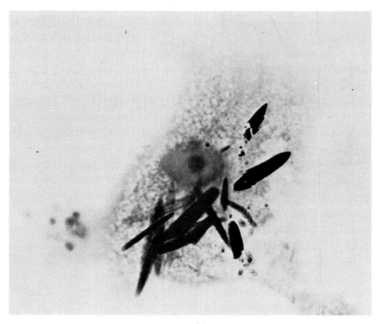

Figure 25.9 A macrophage that has been incubated in vitro with a poorly soluble crystalline compound and has phagocytized several of the crystals.

therefore, that in the monocyte—as in the neu-trophil—myeloperoxidase provides an ancillary killing mechanism in conjunction with hydrogen peroxide. In the macrophage, microbicidal mechanisms are independent of myeloperoxidase; perhaps the abundant catalase of the mature cell serves the same function.

Other Factors

A variety of mechanisms, unidentified as yet, may exist in the macrophage for microbial killing. Macrophages activated by immune lymphocytes are better killers than nonactivated cells. Whether the enhanced killing capacity of the activated leukocyte is based on oxygen-dependent or other mechanisms is not known. It has been suggested that surfactants and other membrane-active substances may be important in the control of *Mycobacterium tuberculosis* by macrophages (55).

Defective mononuclear leukocyte microbicidal function has been observed in chronic granulomatous disease (a genetic disorder of childhood), and in some patients with lymphoma and myelomonocytic leukemia (38). In the latter conditions the mononuclear cells can ingest microorganisms, but fail to inhibit their intracellular replication.

Other Macrophage Functions

Antitumor Activity

The role of cellular immunity in host defense against autochthonous neoplasms has been discussed in detail in Chapter 17. Such defense involves the interplay of humoral factors (antibody and complement) and diverse types of blood cells, particularly lymphocytes and macrophages (16, 72, 103, 183, 184, 221). Some evidence indicates that part of the antitumor activity of macrophages from immunized animals is immunologically specific (70, 92). This specificity probably applies to the first phase of tumor antigen recognition; the second phase of the killing reaction appears to be nonspecific (71). In another mechanism, macrophage killing of tumor cells may be wholly nonspecific. For example, following infection of mice with *Toxoplasma*, the activated macrophages kill L cells more readily than cells from uninfected animals (105, 106).

The macrophage attack on the target tumor cell may involve the participation of cytophilic antibody (72, 156), which may thus explain immunologically specific antitumor activity. Furthermore, recent observations suggest that macrophages may recognize and subsequently destroy malignantly transformed cells by mechanisms that are nonimmunologic (105, 106). The macrophage attack on target cells may be mediated by hydrolytic ly-

sosmal enzymes and perhaps other soluble factors (102, 127).

Control of Granulopoiesis and Involvement in Erythropoiesis

The growth of human and mouse bone marrow in vitro in semisolid supporting medium requires a factor or factors usually designated colony-stimulating factor (CSF) (see Chapter 2). In the mouse, diverse embryonic and adult tissues serve as a source of CSF (153).At the present time, the only known effective source of CSF stimulating the growth of human bone marrow in vitro is the peripheral blood leukocyte (189, 200). The observation that these white cells may be used as a "feeder layer," or as a source of conditioned medium containing CSF, led to a concept of feedback regulation of granulopoiesis by peripheral blood granulocytes or their breakdown products (200). Recently, however, three groups of investigators independently demonstrated that it is the monocyte and the macrophage, rather than the granulocyte, that normally produce CSF (33, 86, 87, 159). This assertion does not exclude the possibility that under some circumstances granulocytes also may produce CSF.

It is not certain that CSF, which stimulates the growth of granulocytic and mononuclear colonies in vitro, is a physiologic regulator of leukopoiesis in vivo. But several lines of evidence suggest that CSF may indeed play a role in the control of granulopoiesis in the intact animal and in man. For example, urinary CSF levels rise as the peripheral granulocyte count falls in patients undergoing surgery (253). Urinary CSF levels are low in patients with aplastic anemia and rise after administration of large numbers of leukocytes (200). Acute granulocyte destruction is associated with increased levels of CSF activity (218). Partially purified CSF injected into mice causes an elevation of the granulocyte count (154), and CSF activity correlates with granulocyte levels in cyclic neutropenia in dogs and man (53, 149). If CSF proves to be the physiologic regulator of leukopoiesis (that is, a "leukopoietin"), then the scheme presented in Fig. 2.6 is a reasonable hypothesis at the present state of our knowledge: monocytes and macrophages produce CSF, which can stimulate the proliferation of cells of the granulocyte series and the mononuclear leukocyte series. These cell lines originate from a common committed progenitor cell. Malignant monocytes may retain the capacity to produce CSF, provided they demonstrate some degree of morphologic and functional differentiation (40). Whether granulocytes also operate a positive feedback loop to the committed stem cell is presently uncertain.

There are occasional reports in the literature suggesting that macrophages and reticulum cells may also be involved in cell interactions leading to erythropoiesis. These suggestions that macrophages or reticulum cells may serve as central "nurse" cells in an island of developing normoblasts are based mainly on morphologic, rather than physiologic, observations (20, 21). Interestingly, macrophages do have an active transport system for ferritin (199)—an observation consistent with the hypothesis that the macrophage may be a source of iron for the developing erythrocyte.

Summary

The primary roles of monoculear phagocytes are in the complex defenses against invading microorganisms and in the removal of damaged or altered host cells. The macrophage functions indirectly in the defense system by interacting with lymphoid cells in both the afferent (recognition) and efferent (effector) limbs of the immune response. In afferent limb reactions, the mononuclear cell accumulates and retains antigen in immunogenic form. The macrophage functions directly in defense reactions by its phagocytic and microbicidal activities. Again, in these defense reactions the macrophage interacts with lymphoid cells.

Cells of the mononuclear leukocyte system phagocytize senescent or damaged cells. The mechanisms of this microscopic debridement are best understood in the interaction between mononuclear phagocytes and erythrocytes.

Less well understood functions of monocytes and macrophages are those of surveillance against neoplastic cells and interaction with other hematopoietic cells in the control of granulopoiesis.

Chapter 25 References

1. Abramson, N., Gelfand, E. W., Jandl, J. H., and Rosen, F. S. The interaction between human monocytes and red cells. Specificity for IgG subclasses and IgG fragments, *J. Exp. Med.* 132:1207, 1970.

2. Abramson, N., Lo Buglio, A. F., Jandl, J. H., and Cotran, R. S. The interaction between human monocytes and red cells. Binding characteristics, *J. Exp. Med.* 132:1191, 1970.

3. Abramson, N., and Schur, P. H. The IgG subclasses of red cell antibodies and relationship to monocyte binding, *Blood* 40:500, 1972.

4. Ada, G. L., Nossal, G. J. V., and Austin, C. M. Antigens in immunity. V. The ability of cells in lymphoid follicles to recognize foreignness, *Aust. J. Exp. Biol. Med. Sci.* 42:331, 1964.

5. Adler, F. L., Fishman, M., and Dray, S. Antibody formation initiated *in vitro*. III. Antibody formation and allotypic specificity directed by ribonucleic acid from peritoneal exudate cells, *J. Immunol.* 97:554, 1966.

6. Allen, J. M., and Cook, G. M. W. A study of the attachment phase of phagocytosis by murine macrophages, *Exp. Cell Res.* 59:105, 1970.

7. Allison, A. C., Harrington, J. S., and Birbeck, M. An examination of the cytotoxic effects of silica on macrophages, *J. Exp. Med.* 124:141, 1966.

8. Ando, M., and Dannenberg, A. M., Jr. Macrophage accumulation, division, maturation, and digestive and microbicidal capacities in tuberculous lesions. IV. Macrophage turnover, lysosomal enzymes, and division in healing lesions, *Lab. Invest.* 27:466, 1972.

9. Archer, G. T. Phagocytosis by human monocytes of red cells coated by Rh antibodies, *Vox Surg.* 10:590, 1965.

10. Argyris, B. F. Role of macrophages in antibody production. Immune response to sheep red blood cells, *J. Immunol.* 99:744, 1967.

11. Argyris, B. F. Role of macrophages in immunological maturation, *J. Exp. Med.* 128:459, 1968.

12. Armstrong, J. A., and D'Arcy Hart, P. Response of cultured macrophages to Mycobacterium tuberculosis with observations on fusion of lysosomes with phagosomes, *J. Exp. Med.* 134:713, 1971.

13. Askonas, B. A., and Rhodes, J. M. Immunogenicity of antigen-containing ribonucleic acid preparations from macrophages, *Nature* 205:470, 1965.

14. Aterman, K. The structure of the liver sinusoids and the sinusoidal cells, *in* Ch. Rouiller (ed.), The Liver, vol. 1, p. 61, Academic Press, New York, 1963.

15. Baehner, R. L., and Johnston, R. B., Jr. Monocyte function in children with neutropenia and chronic infections, *Blood* 40:31, 1972.

16. Bennett, B. Specific suppression of tumor growth by isolated peritoneal macrophages from immunized mice, *J. Immunol.* 95:656, 1965.

17. Bercovici, B. The effect of local radiation on the phagocytic activity of macrophages, *Isr. J. Med. Sci.* 2:564, 1966.

18. Berken, A., and Benacerraf, B. Properties of antibodies cytophilic for macrophages, *J. Exp. Med.* 123:119, 1966.

19. Berken, A., and Benacerraf, B. Sedimentation properties of antibody cytophilic for macrophages, *J. Immunol.* 100:1219, 1968.

20. Bessis, M. C., and Breton-Gorius, J. Iron particles in normal erythroblasts and normal pathological erythrocytes, *J. Biophys. Biochem. Cytol.* 3:503, 1957.

21. Bessis, M. C., and Breton-Gorius, J. Iron metabolism in the bone marrow as seen by electron microscopy: a critical review, *Blood* 19:635, 1962.

22. Biro, C. E., and García, G. The antigenicity of aggregated and aggregate-free human gamma-globulin for rabbits, *Immunology* 8:411, 1965.

23. Bissell, D. M., Hammaker, L., and Schmid, R. Liver sinusoidal cells. Identification of a subpopulation for erythrocyte catabolism, *J. Cell Biol.* 54:107, 1972.

24. Blanden, R. V. Modification of macrophage function, *J. Reticuloendothel. Soc.* 5:179, 1968.

25. Blanden, R. V., Lefford, M. J., and Mackaness, G. B. The host response to Calmette-Guerin bacillus infection in mice, *J. Exp. Med.* 129:1079, 1969.

26. Blanden, R. V., Mackaness, G. B., and Collins, F. M. Mechanisms of acquired resistance in mouse typhoid, *J. Exp. Med.* 124:585, 1966.

27. Bloom, B. R., and Bennett, B. Macrophages and delayed-type hypersensitivity, *Semin. Hematol.* 7:215, 1970.

28. Braun, W., and Lasky, L. J. Antibody formation in newborn mice initiated through adult macrophages, *Fed. Proc.* 26:642, 1967.

29. Buchner, L. H., and Schneierson, S. S. Clinical and laboratory aspects of Listeria monocytogenes infections, *Am. J. Med.* 45:904, 1968.

30. Campbell, D. H., and Garvey, J. S. The fate of foreign antigen and speculations as to its role in immune mechanisms, *Lab. Invest.* 10:1126, 1961.

31. Campbell, D. H., and Garvey, J. S. Nature of retained antigen and its role in immune mechanisms, *Adv. Immunol.* 3:261, 1963.

32. Chen, L., and Weiss, L. Electron microscopy of the red pulp of human spleen, *Am. J. Anat.* 134:425, 1972.

33. Chervenick, P. A., and Lo Buglio, A. F. Human blood monocytes: stimulators of granulocyte and mononuclear colony formation in vitro, *Science* 178:164, 1972.

34. Claman, H. N. Tolerance to a protein antigen in adult mice and the effect of nonspecific factors, *J. Immunol.* 91:833, 1963.

35. Cline, M. J. Monocytes and macrophages: differentiation and function, *in* T. J. Greenwalt and G. A. Jamieson (eds.), Third Annual Red Cross Symposium on Formation and Destruction of Blood Cells, p. 22, J. B. Lippincott, Philadelphia, 1970.

36. Cline, M. J. Bactericidal activity of human macrophages: analysis of factors influencing the killing of *Listeria monocytogenes, Infect. Immun.* 2:156, 1970.

37. Cline, M. J. Drug potentiation of macrophage function, *Infect. Immun.* 2:601, 1970.

38. Cline, M. J. Defective mononuclear phagocyte function in patients with myelomonocytic leukemia and in

some patients with lymphoma, *J. Clin. Invest.* 52:2185, 1973.

39. Cline, M. J., and Lehrer, R. I. Phagocytosis by human monocytes, *Blood* 32:423, 1968.

40. Cline, M. J., and Golde, D. W. Hematopoiesis in liquid culture, *in* W. A. Robinson (ed.), Proc. Second Int. Conf. on Bone Marrow Culture, p. 200, DHEW publ. (NIH) 74-205, 1974.

41. Cline, M. J., Sprent, J., Warner, N. L., and Harris, A. W. Receptors for immunoglobulin on B lymphocytes and cells of a cultured plasma cell tumor, *J. Immunol.* 108:1126, 1972.

42. Cline, M. J., and Sumner, M. A. Bone marrow macrophage precursors. I. Some functional characteristics of the early cells of the mouse macrophage series, *Blood* 40:62, 1972.

43. Cline, M. J., and Swett, V. C. The interaction of human monocytes and lymphocytes, *J. Exp. Med.* 128:1309, 1968.

44. Cline, M. J., and Warner, N. L. Immunoglobulin receptors on a mouse mast cell tumor, *J. Immunol.* 108:339, 1972.

45. Cline, M. J., Warner, N. L., and Metcalf, D. Identification of the bone marrow colony mononuclear phagocyte as a macrophage, *Blood* 39:326, 1972.

46. Cohen, A. B., and Cline, M. J. The human alveolar macrophage: isolation, cultivation in vitro, and studies of morphologic and functional characteristics, *J. Clin. Invest.* 50:1390, 1971.

47. Cohn, Z. A. Influence of rabbit polymorphonuclear leucocytes and macrophages on the immunogenicity of *Escherichia coli, Nature* 196:1066, 1962.

48. Collins, F. M. Mechanisms in antimicrobial immunity, *J. Reticuloendothel. Soc.* 10:58, 1971.

49. Collins, F. M., and Mackaness, G. B. Delayed hypersensitivity and Arthus reactivity in relation to host resistance in Salmonella-infected mice, *J. Immunol.* 101:830, 1968.

50. Conalty, M. L., Barry, V. C., and Jina, A. The antileprosy agent B. 663 (Clofazimine) and the reticuloendothelial system, *Int. J. Lepr.* 39:479, 1971.

51. Conrad, M. E., and Dennis, L. H. Splenic function in experimental malaria, *Am. J. Trop. Med. Hyg.* 17:170, 1968.

52. Crosby, W. H. Siderocytes and the spleen, *Blood* 12:165, 1957.

53. Dale, D. C., Brown, C. H., Carbone, P., and Wolff, S. M. Cyclic urinary leukopoietic activity in grey collie dogs, *Science* 173:152, 1971.

54. Dannenberg, A. M., Jr. Cellular hypersensitivity and cellular immunity in the pathogenesis of tuberculosis: specificity, systemic and local nature and associated macrophage enzymes, *Bacteriol. Rev.* 32:85, 1968.

55. D'Arcy Hart, P. Mycobacterium tuberculosis in macrophages: effect of certain surfactants and other membrane-active compounds, *Science* 162:686, 1968.

56. Davey, M. J., and Asherson, G. L. Cytophilic antibody. I. Nature of the macrophage receptor, *Immunology* 12:13, 1967.

57. David, J. R. Delayed hypersensitivity in vitro: its mediation by cell-free substances formed by lymphoid cell-antigen interaction, *Proc. Natl. Acad. Sci. U.S.A.* 56:72, 1966.

58. Davis, W. C., Huber, H., Douglas, S. D., and Fudenberg, H. H. A defect in circulating mononuclear phagocytes in chronic granulomatous disease of childhood, *J. Immunol.* 101:1093, 1968.

59. Despont, J. P., and Cruchaud, A. *In vivo* and *in vitro* effects of antimacrophage serum, *Nature* 223:838, 1969.

60. Donaldson, D. M., Marcus, S., Gyi, K. K., and Perkins, E. H. The influence of immunization and total body x-irradiation on intracellular digestion by peritoneal phagocytes, *J. Immunol.* 76:192, 1956.

61. Douglas, S. D., and Huber, H. Electron microscopic studies of human monocyte and lymphocyte interaction with immunoglobulin and complement-coated erythrocytes, *Exp. Cell Res.* 70:161, 1972.

62. Dresser, D. W. Specific inhibition of antibody production. II. Paralysis induced in adult mice by small quantities of protein antigen, *Immunology* 5:378, 1962.

63. Dresser, D. W., and Mitchison, N. A. The mechanism of immunological paralysis, *Adv. Immunol.* 8:129, 1968.

64. Drutz, D. J., and Cline, M. J. Incorporation of tritiated thymidine by leprosy bacilli in cultures of human lepromatous macrophages, *J. Infect. Dis.* 125:416, 1972.

65. Dumonde, D. C. The role of the macrophage in delayed hypersensitivity, *Br. Med. Bull.* 23:9, 1967.

66. Ehrenreich, B. A., and Cohn, Z. A. The uptake and digestion of iodinated human serum albumin by macrophages in vitro, *J. Exp. Med.* 126:941, 1967.

67. Ehrenreich, B. A., and Cohn, Z. A. Pinocytosis by macrophages, *J. Reticuloendothel. Soc.* 5:230, 1968.

68. Epstein, L. B., Cline, M. J., and Merigan, T. C. The interaction of human macrophages and lymphocytes in the PHA-stimulated production of interferon, *J. Clin. Invest.* 50:744, 1971.

69. Epstein, L. B., Cline, M. J., and Merigan, T. C. Macrophage-lymphocyte interaction in the PHA-stimulated production of interferon in vitro, Proc. Fifth Annual Leukocyte Culture Conf., p. 501, Academic Press, New York, 1971.

70. Evans, R., and Alexander, P. Cooperation of immune lymphoid cells with macrophages in tumor immunity, *Nature* 228:620, 1970.

71. Evans, R., and Alexander, P. Mechanism of immunologically specific killing of tumor cells by macrophages, *Nature* 236:168, 1972.

72. Fakhri, O., McLaughlin, H., and Hobbs, J. R. 7S anti-tumor antibodies and activated Fc in macrophage tumor cell interaction, *Eur. J. Cancer* 9:19, 1973.

73. Fischman, D. A., and Hay, E. D. Origin of osteoclasts from mononuclear leucocytes in regenerating newt limbs, *Anat. Rec.* 143:329, 1962.

74. Fishman, M. Antibody formation in vitro, *J. Exp. Med.* 114:837, 1961.

75. Fishman, M., and Adler, F. L. Antibody formation initiated in vitro. II. Antibody synthesis in X-irradiated recipients of diffusion chambers containing nucleic acid derived from macrophages incubated with antigen, *J. Exp. Med.* 117:595, 1963.

76. Fishman, M., and Adler, F. L. An-

tibody formation in vitro, *in* P. Grabar and P. A. Miescher (eds.), Third International Symposium on Immunopathology, p. 79, Grune & Stratton, New York, 1963.

77. Franzl, R. E. Immunogenic subcellular particles obtained from spleens and antigen-injected mice, *Nature* 195:457, 1962.

78. Frei, P. C., Benacerraf, B., and Thorbecke, G. J. Phagocytosis of the antigen, a crucial step in the induction of the primary response, *Proc. Natl. Acad. Sci. U.S.A.* 53:20, 1965.

79. Friedman, H. Antibody plaque formation by normal mouse spleen cell cultures exposed in vitro to RNA from immune mice, *Science* 146:934, 1964.

80. Friedman, H. P., Stavitsky, A. B., and Solomon, J. M. Induction in vitro of antibodies to Phage T2:antigens in the RNA extract employed, *Science* 149:1106, 1965.

81. Friedman, R. M., and Steigbigel, N. H. Histiocytic medullary reticulosis, *Am. J. Med.* 38:130, 1965.

82. Gallily, R., and Feldman, M. The role of macrophages in the induction of antibody in x-irradiated animals, *Immunology* 12:197, 1967.

83. Garvey, J. S., Campbell, D. H., and Das, M. L. Urinary excretion of foreign antigens and RNA following primary and secondary injections of antigens, *J. Exp. Med.* 125:111, 1967.

84. Gay, F. P., and Clark, A. R. The reticulo-endothelial system in relation to antibody formation, *J.A.M.A.* 83:1296, 1924.

85. Gelfand, E. W., Abramson, N., Segel, G. S., and Nathan, D. G. Buffy coat observations and red cell antibodies in acquired hemolytic anemia, *N. Engl. J. Med.* 284:1250, 1971.

86. Golde, D. W., and Cline, M. J. Identification of the colony-stimulating cell in human peripheral blood, *J. Clin. Invest.* 51:2981, 1972.

87. Golde, D. W., Finley, T. N., and Cline, M. J. Production of colony stimulating factor by human macrophages, *Lancet* ii:1397, 1972.

88. Golub, E. S., and Weigle, W. O. Studies on the induction of immunologic unresponsiveness. III. Antigen form and mouse strain variation, *J. Immunol.* 102:389, 1969.

89. Gottlieb, A. A. Studies on the binding of soluble antigens to a unique ribonucleoprotein fraction of macrophage cells, *Biochemistry* 8:2111, 1969.

90. Gottlieb, A. A., Glišin, V. R., and Doty, P. Studies on macrophage RNA involved in antibody production, *Proc. Natl. Acad. Sci. U.S.A.* 57:1849, 1967.

91. Gottlieb, A. A., and Straus, D. S. Physical studies on the light density ribonucleoprotein complex of macrophage cells, *J. Biol. Chem.* 244:3324, 1969.

92. Granger, G. A., and Weiser, R. S. Homograft target cells: specific destruction in vitro by contact interaction with immune macrophages, *Science* 145:1427, 1964.

93. Guarneri, J. J., and Laurenzi, G. A. Effect of alcohol on the mobilization of alveolar macrophages, *J. Lab. Clin. Med.* 72:40, 1968.

94. Hanifin, J. M., and Cline, M. J. Human monocytes and macrophages: interaction with antigen and lymphocytes, *J. Cell Biol.* 46:97, 1970.

95. Hanifin, J. M., Epstein, W. L., and Cline, M. J. In vitro studies of granulomatous hypersensitivity to beryllium, *J. Invest. Dermatol.* 55:238, 1970.

96. Hanna, M. G., Jr., Francis, M. W., and Peters, L. C. Localization of ^{125}I-labelled antigen in germinal centres of mouse spleen: effects of competitive injection of specific or non-cross-reacting antigen, *Immunology* 15:75, 1968.

97. Harris, G. Studies of the mechanism of antigen stimulation of DNA synthesis in rabbit spleen cultures, *Immunology* 9:529, 1965.

98. Harris, H. Mobilization of defensive cells in inflammatory tissue, *Bacteriol. Rev.* 24:3, 1960.

99. Harris, J. W., and Kellermeyer, R. W. The Red Cell, rev. ed., p. 526, Harvard University Press, Cambridge, Mass., 1970.

100. Hausman, M. S., Snyderman, R., and Mergenhagen, S. E. Humoral mediators of chemotaxis of mononuclear leukocytes, *J. Infect. Dis.* 125:595, 1972.

101. Heilman, D. H. The selective toxicity of endotoxin for phagocytic cells of the reticuloendothelial

system, *Int. Arch. Allergy* 26:63, 1965.

102. Heise, E. R., and Weiser, R. S. Factors in delayed sensitivity: lymphocyte and macrophage cytotoxins in the tuberculin reaction, *J. Immunol.* 103:570, 1969.

103. Hellström, K. E., and Hellström, I. Cellular immunity against tumor antigens, *Adv. Cancer Res.* 12:167, 1969.

104. Hersh, E. M., and Harris, J. E. Macrophage-lymphocyte interaction in the antigen-induced blastogenic response of human peripheral blood leukocytes, *J. Immunol.* 100:1184, 1968.

105. Hibbs, J. B., Jr., Lambert, L. H., Jr., and Remington, J. S. Possible role of macrophage mediated non-specific cytotoxicity in tumour resistance, *Nature (New Biol.)* 235:48, 1972.

106. Hibbs, J. B., Jr., Lambert, L. H., Jr., and Remington, J. S. Control of carcinogenesis: a possible role for the activated macrophage, *Science* 177:998, 1972.

107. Hinsdill, R. D., and Berman, D. T. Antigens of Brucella abortus. II. Toxicity for macrophages in culture, *J. Infect. Dis.* 118:307, 1968.

108. Holland, P., Holland, N. H., and Cohn, Z. A. The selective inhibition of macrophage phagocytic receptors by anti-membrane antibodies, *J. Exp. Med.* 135:458, 1972.

109. Howard, J. G., and Benacerraf, B. Properties of macrophage receptors for cytophilic antibodies, *Br. J. Exp. Pathol.* 47:193, 1966.

110. Hsu, H. S., and Radcliffe, A. S. Interactions between macrophages of guinea pigs and Salmonellae, *J. Bacteriol.* 96:191, 1968.

111. Huber, H., Douglas, S. D., and Fudenberg, H. H. The IgG receptor: an immunological marker for the characterization of mononuclear cells, *Immunology* 17:7, 1969.

112. Huber, H., and Fudenberg, H. H. Receptor sites of human monocytes for IgG, *Int. Arch. Allergy* 34:18, 1968.

113. Humphrey, J. H., and Frank, M. M. The localization of non-microbial antigens in the draining lymph nodes of tolerant, normal, and primed rabbits, *Immunology* 13:87, 1967.

114. Jandl, J. H. Sequestration by the spleen of red cells sensitized with incomplete antibody and with metallo-protein complexes, *J. Clin. Invest.* 32:912, 1955.

115. Jandl, J. H. The spleen and reticuloendothelial system, *in* W. A. Sodeman and W. A. Sodeman, Jr. (eds.), Pathologic Physiology: Mechanisms of Disease, 4th ed., p. 897, W. B. Saunders Co., Philadelphia, 1967.

116. Jandl, J. H., Jones, A. R., and Castle, W. B. The destruction of red cells by antibodies in man. I. Observations on the sequestration and lysis of red cells altered by immune mechanisms, *J. Clin. Invest.* 36:1428, 1957.

117. Jandl, J. H., and Tomlinson, A. S. The destruction of red cells by antibodies in man. II. Pyrogenic, leukocytic and dermal responses to immune hemolysis, *J. Clin. Invest.* 37:1202, 1958.

118. Jones, T. C., Yeh, S., and Hirsch, J. G. Studies on attachment and ingestion phases of phagocytosis of *Mycoplasma pulmonis* by mouse peritoneal macrophages, *Proc. Soc. Exp. Biol. Med.* 139:464, 1972.

119. Kaplan, M. E., Dalmasso, A. P., and Woodson, M. Complement-dependent opsonization of incompatible erythrocytes by human secretory IgA, *J. Immunol.* 108:275, 1972.

120. Karnovsky, M. L. The physiological basis of phagocytosis, *Physiol. Rev.* 42:1143, 1962.

121. Keene, W. R., and Jandl, J. H. Studies of the reticuloendothelial mass and sequestering function of rat bone marrow, *Blood* 26:157, 1965.

122. Keller, H. U., and Sorkin, E. Studies on chemotaxis. VI. Specific chemotaxis in rabbit polymorphonuclear leucocytes and mononuclear cells, *Int. Arch. Allergy Appl. Immunol.* 31:575, 1967.

123. Kessel, R. W. I., and Braun, W. Cytotoxicity of endotoxin *in vitro*. Effects on macrophages from normal guinea pigs, *Aust. J. Exp. Biol. Med. Sci.* 43:511, 1965.

124. Kessel, R. W. I., Monaco, L., and Marchisio, M. A. The specificity of the cytotoxic action of silica—a study *in vitro*, *Br. J. Exp. Pathol.* 44:351, 1963.

125. Khoo, K. K., and Mackaness, G. B. Macrophage proliferation in relation to acquired cellular resistance, *Aust. J. Exp. Biol. Med. Sci.* 42:707, 1964.

126. Kölsch, E., and Mitchison, N. A. The subcellular distribution of antigen in macrophages, *J. Exp. Med.* 128:1059, 1968.

127. Kramer, J. J., and Granger, G. A. The *in vitro* induction and release of a cell toxin by immune C57B1/6 mouse peritoneal macrophages, *Cell. Immunol.* 3:88, 1972.

128. Kunin, S., Shearer, G. M., Globerson, A., and Feldman, M. Immunogenic function of macrophages: in vitro production of antibodies to a hapten-carrier conjugate, *Cell. Immunol.* 5:288, 1972.

129. Lawson, N. S., Schnitzer, B., and Smith, E. B. Splenic ultrastructure in drug-induced Heinz body hemolysis, *Arch. Pathol.* 87:491, 1969.

130. Lay, W. H., and Nussenzweig, V. Ca^{++}-dependent binding of antigen-19S antibody complexes to macrophages, *J. Immunol.* 102:1172, 1969.

131. Lehrer, R. I., and Cline, M. J. Leukocyte myeloperoxidase deficiency and disseminated candidiasis: the role of myeloperoxidase in resistance to *Candida* infection, *J. Clin. Invest.* 48:1478, 1969.

132. Lewis, E. J., Busch, G. J., and Schur, P. H. Gamma G globulin subgroup composition of the glomerular deposits in human renal diseases, *J. Clin. Invest.* 49:1103, 1970.

133. Lo Buglio, A. F., Cotran, R. S., and Jandl, J. H. Red cells coated with immunoglobulin G. Binding and sphering by mononuclear cells in man, *Science* 158:1582, 1967.

134. Louria, D. B. Susceptibility to infection during experimental alcohol intoxication, *Trans. Assoc. Am. Physicians* 76:102, 1963.

135. Lubaroff, D. M., and Waksman, B. H. Delayed hypersensitivity: bone marrow as the source of cells in delayed skin reactions, *Science* 157:322, 1967.

136. Lubaroff, D. M., and Waksman, B. H. Bone marrow as source of cells in reactions of cellular hypersensitivity. I. Passive transfer of tuberculin sensitivity in syngeneic systems, *J. Exp. Med.* 128:1425, 1968.

137. Lurie, M. B. Resistance to Tuberculosis: Experimental Studies in Native and Acquired Defensive Mechanisms, Harvard University Press, Cambridge, Mass., 1964.

138. MacCallum, D. K. Time sequence study on the hepatic system of macrophages in malaria-infected hamsters, *J. Reticuloendothel. Soc.* 6:232, 1969.

139. McDevitt, H. O., Askonas, B. A., Humphrey, J. H., Schechter, I., and Sela, M. The localization of antigen in relation to specific antibody-producing cells. I. Use of a synthetic polypeptide [(T,G)-A−L] labelled with iodine-125, *Immunology* 11:337, 1966.

140. McFarland, W. Microspikes on the lymphocyte uropod, *Science* 163:818, 1969.

141. McFarland, W., and Heilman, D. H. Lymphocyte foot appendage: its role in lymphocyte function and in immunological reactions, *Nature* 205:887, 1965.

142. McFarland, W., Heilman, D. H., and Moorhead, J. F. Functional anatomy of the lymphocyte in immunological reactions in vitro, *J. Exp. Med.* 124:851, 1966.

143. Mackaness, G. B. Cellular resistance to infection, *J. Exp. Med.* 116:381, 1962.

144. Mackaness, G. B. The immunological basis of acquired cellular resistance, *J. Exp. Med.* 120:105, 1964.

145. Mackaness, G. B. The behavior of microbial parasites in relation to phagocytic cells in vitro and in vivo, *in* 14th Sympos. Soc. Gen. Microbiol., p. 213, University Press, Cambridge, England, 1964.

146. Mackaness, G. B. The influence of immunologically committed lymphoid cells on macrophage activity in vivo, *J. Exp. Med.* 129:973, 1969.

147. Mackaness, G. B. The monocyte in cellular immunity, *Semin. Hematol.* 7:172, 1970.

148. Mackaness, G. B., and Hill, W. C. The effect of anti-lymphocyte globulin on cell-mediated resistance to infection, *J. Exp. Med.* 129:993, 1969.

149. Mangalik, A., and Robinson, W. A. Cyclic neutropenia: the relationship between urine granulocyte colony stimulating activity and neutrophil count, *Blood* 41:79, 1973.

150. Maruta, H., and Mizuno, D. Selective recognition of various erythrocytes in endocytosis by mouse peritoneal macrophages, *Nature (New Biol.)* 234:246, 1971.

151. Mergenhagen, S. E., Notkins, A. L., and Dougherty, S. F. Adjuvanticity of lactic dehydrogenase virus: influence of virus infection on the establishment of immunologic tolerance to a protein antigen in adult mice, *J. Immunol.* 99:576, 1967.

152. Merkow, L., Pardo, M., Epstein, S. M., Verney, E., and Sidransky, H. Lysosomal stability during phagocytosis of Aspergillus flavus spores by alveolar macrophages of cortisone-treated mice, *Science* 160:79, 1968.

153. Metcalf, D., and Moore, M. A. S. Haematopoietic Cells: Frontiers of Biology, North-Holland Publishing Co., Amsterdam, 1971.

154. Metcalf, D., and Stanley, E. R. Haematological effects in mice of partially purified colony stimulating factor (CSF) prepared from human urine, *Br. J. Haematol.* 21:481, 1971.

155. Metchnikoff, E. Immunity in Infective Diseases, University Press, Cambridge, England, 1905.

156. Mitchell, M. S., and Mokyr, M. B. Specific inhibition of receptors for cytophilic antibody on macrophages by isoantibody, *Cancer Res.* 32:832, 1972.

157. Mitchison, N. A. The immunogenic capacity of antigen taken up by peritoneal exudate cells, *Immunology* 16:1, 1969.

158. Mooney, J. J., and Waksman, B. H. Activation of normal rabbit macrophage monolayers by supernatants of antigen-stimulated lymphocytes, *J. Immunol.* 105:1138, 1970.

159. Moore, M. A. S., Williams, N., and Metcalf, D. In vitro colony formation by normal and leukemic human hematopoietic cells: interaction between colony-forming and colony-stimulating cells, *J. Natl. Cancer Inst.* 50:591, 1973.

160. Mosier, D. E. A requirement for two cell types for antibody formation in vitro, *Science* 158:1573, 1967.

161. Mosier, D. E. Cell interactions in the primary immune response in vitro: a requirement for specific cell clusters, *J. Exp. Med.* 129:351, 1969.

162. Mosier, D. E., and Coppleson, L. W. A three-cell interaction required for the induction of the primary immune response in vitro, *Proc. Natl. Acad. Sci. U.S.A.* 61:542, 1968.

163. Motulsky, A. G., Casserd, F., Giblett, E. R., Brown, G. O., and Finch, C. A. Anemia and the spleen, *N. Engl. J. Med.* 259:1164, 1215; 1958.

164. Nathan, C. F., Karnovsky, M. L., and David, J. R. Alterations of macrophage functions by mediators from lymphocytes, *J. Exp. Med.* 133:1356, 1971.

165. Natvig, J. B., Kunkel, H. G., and Gedde-Dahl, T., Jr. Genetic studies of the heavy chain sub-groups G globulin, in J. Killander (ed.), Gamma Globulins: Proceedings of the Third Nobel Symposium, J. Wiley and Sons, Interscience Publishers, New York, 1967.

166. Nelson, D. S. Macrophages and Immunity, North-Holland Publishing Co., Amsterdam, 1969.

167. Nelson, D. S., and Boyden, S. V. Macrophage cytophilic antibodies and delayed hypersensitivity, *Br. Med. Bull.* 23:15, 1967.

168. Nichol, A. W. The formation of biliverdin from haemin suspensions by chicken macrophages in culture, *Biochim. Biophys. Acta* 244:595, 1971.

169. North, R. J. The uptake of particulate antigens, *J. Reticuloendothel. Soc.* 5:203, 1968.

170. North, R. J. Cellular kinetics associated with the development of acquired cellular resistance, *J. Exp. Med.* 130:299, 1969.

171. North, R. J. The mitotic potential of fixed phagocytes in the liver as revealed during the development of cellular immunity, *J. Exp. Med.* 130:315, 1969.

172. North, R. J. The action of cortisone acetate on cell-mediated immunity to infection, *J. Exp. Med.* 134:1485, 1971.

173. Nossal, G. J. V., Abbot, A., and Mitchell, J. Antigens in immunity. XIV. Electron microscopic-radioautographic studies of antigen capture, *J. Exp. Med.* 127:263, 1968.

174. Nossal, G. J. V., Abbot, A., Mitchell, J., and Lummus, A. Antigens in immunity. XV. Ultrastructural features of antigen capture in pri-

mary and secondary lymphoid follicles, *J. Exp. Med.* 127:277, 1968.

175. Nossal, G. J. V., Ada, G. L., and Austin, C. M. Antigens in immunity. IV. Cellular localization of ^{125}I- and ^{131}I-labelled flagella in lymph nodes, *Aust. J. Exp. Biol. Med. Sci.* 42:311, 1964.

176. Nossal, G. J. V., Ada, G. L., Austin, C. M., and Pye, J. Antigens in immunity. VIII. Localization of ^{125}I-labelled antigens in the secondary response, *Immunology* 9:349, 1965.

177. Notkins, A. L., Mergenhagen, S. E., Rizzo, A. A., Shelle, C., and Waldmann, T. A. Elevated γ-globulin and increased antibody production in mice infected with lactic dehydrogenase virus, *J. Exp. Med.* 123:347, 1966.

178. Okafor, G. O., Turner, M. W., and Hay, F. C. Localization of monocyte binding site of human immunoglobulin G, *Nature* 248:228, 1974.

179. Oppenheim, J. J., Leventhal, B. G., and Hersh, E. M. The transformation of column-purified lymphocytes with nonspecific and specific antigenic stimuli, *J. Immunol.* 101:262, 1968.

180. Panijel, J., and Cayeux, P. Immunosuppressive effects of macrophage antiserum, *Immunology* 14:769, 1968.

181. Patterson, R. J., and Youmans, G. P. Multiplication of *Mycobacterium tuberculosis* within normal and "immune" mouse macrophages cultivated with and without streptomycin, *Infect. Immun.* 1:30, 1970.

182. Pearsall, N. N., and Weiser, R. S. The macrophage in allograft immunity. I. Effects of silica as a specific macrophage toxin, *J. Reticuloendothel. Soc.* 5:107, 1968.

183. Penn, I., and Starzl, T. E. Malignant tumors arising de novo in immunosupressed organ transplant recipients, *Transplantation* 14:407, 1972.

184. Perlmann, P., and Holm, G. Cytotoxic effects of lymphoid cells *in vitro*, *Adv. Immunol.* 11:117, 1969.

185. Phillips-Quagliata, J. M., Levine, B. B., Quagliata, F., and Uhr, J. W. Mechanisms underlying binding of immune complexes to macrophages, *J. Exp. Med.* 133:589, 1971.

186. Phillips-Quagliata, J. M., Levine, B.

B., and Uhr, J. W. Studies on the mechanism of binding of immune complexes to phagocytes, *Nature* 222:1290, 1969.

187. Pierce, C. W. Immune responses in vitro. I. Cellular requirements for the immune response by non-primed and primed spleen cells in vitro, *J. Exp. Med.* 130:345, 1969.

188. Pierce, C. W. Immune responses in vitro. II. Suppression of the immune response in vitro by specific antibody, *J. Exp. Med.* 130:365, 1969.

189. Pike, B. L., and Robinson, W. A. Human bone marrow colony growth in agar-gel, *J. Cell. Physiol.* 76:77, 1970.

190. Pimstone, N. R., Engel, P., Tenhunen, R., Seitz, P. T., Marver, H. S., and Schmid, R. Inducible heme oxygenase in the kidney: a model for the homeostatic control of hemoglobin catabolism, *J. Clin. Invest.* 50:2042, 1971.

191. Pimstone, N. R., Tenhunen, R., Seitz, P. T., Marver, H. S., and Schmid, R. The enzymatic degradation of hemoglobin to bile pigments by macrophages, *J. Exp. Med.* 133:1264, 1971.

192. Pimstone, N. R., Tenhunen, R., Seitz, P. T., Schmid, R., and Marver, H. S. The enzymatic degradation of hemoglobin to bile pigment by macrophages, *Gastroenterology* 58:304, 1970.

193. Pribnow, J. F., and Silverman, M. S. Studies on the radiosensitive phase of the primary antibody response in rabbits. I. The role of the macrophage, *J. Immunol.* 98:225, 1967.

194. Rabinovitch, M. The dissociation of the attachment and ingestion phases of phagocytosis by macrophages, *Exp. Cell Res.* 46:19, 1967.

195. Rabinovitch, M. Attachment of modified erythrocytes to phagocytic cells in absence of serum, *Proc. Soc. Exp. Biol. Med.* 124:396, 1967.

196. Rabinovitch, M. Phagocytosis: the engulfment stage, *Semin. Hematol.* 5:134, 1968.

197. Remington, J. S., Krahenbuhl, J. L., and Mendenhall, J. W. A role for activated macrophages in resistance to infection with *Toxoplasma, Infect. Immun.* 6:829, 1972.

198. Rifkind, R. A. Heinz body anemia: an ultrastructural study. II. Red cell sequestration and destruction, *Blood* 26:433, 1965.

199. Robin, E. D., Smith, J. D., Tanser, A. R., Adamson, J. S., Millen, J. E., and Packer, B. Ion and macromolecular transport in the alveolar macrophage, *Biochim. Biophys. Acta* 241:117, 1971.

200. Robinson, W. A., and Mangalik, A. Regulation of granulopoiesis: a positive feedback, *Lancet* ii:742, 1972.

201. Rodey, G. E., Park, B. H., Windhorst, D. B., Holmes, B., and Good, R. A. Defective bactericidal activity of monocytes in fatal granulomatous disease, *Blood* 33:813, 1969.

202. Roelants, G. E., and Goodman, J. W. Immunochemical studies on the poly-γ-D-glutamyl capsule of *Bacillus anthracis.* IV. The association with peritoneal exudate cells ribonucleic acid of the polypeptide in immunogenic and nonimmunogenic forms, *Biochemistry* 7:1432, 1968.

203. Roelants, G. E., and Goodman, J. W. The nature of macrophage RNA-antigen complexes, *Fed. Proc.* 28:427, 1969.

204. Roseman, J. M., Fitch, F. W., and Rowley, D. A. Cell populations required for the primary immune response in vitro. I. A radiosensitive population, *Fed. Proc.* 28:814, 1969.

205. Roser, B. The distribution of intravenously injected peritoneal macrophages in the mouse, *Aust. J. Biol. Med. Sci.* 43:553, 1965.

206. Roser, B. The distribution of intravenously injected Kupffer cells in the mouse, *J. Reticuloendothel. Soc.*, 5:455, 1968.

207. Russell, P., and Roser, B. The distribution and behavior of intravenously injected pulmonary alveolar macrophages in the mouse, *Aust. J. Biol. Med. Sci.* 44:629, 1966.

208. Sabet, T., Newlin, C., and Friedman, H. Effects of RES "blockade" on antibody-formation. I. Suppressed cellular and humoral haemolysin responses in mice injected with carbon particles, *Immunology* 16:433, 1969.

209. Saito, K., and Suter, E. Lysosomal acid hydrolases in mice infected with BCG, *J. Exp. Med.* 121:727, 1965.

210. Salmon, S. E., Cline, M. J., Schultz, J., and Lehrer, R. I. Myeloperoxidase deficiency: immunologic study of a genetic leukocyte defect, *N. Engl. J. Med.* 282:250, 1970.

211. Salmon, S. E., Morhenn, V. B., and Cline, M. J. Uptake of radioiodinated antigens by human monocytes, *J. Clin. Exp. Immunol.* 8:409, 1971.

212. Salvin, S. B., Sell, S., and Nishio, J. Activity in vitro of lymphocytes and macrophages in delayed hypersensitivity, *J. Immunol.* 107:655, 1971.

213. Sanders, C. L., and Adee, R. R. Phagocytosis of inhaled plutonium oxide—^{239}Pu particles by pulmonary macrophages, *Science* 162:918, 1968.

214. Schmidt, M. E., and Douglas, S. D. Disappearance and recovery of human monocyte IgG receptor activity after phagocytosis, *J. Immunol.* 109:914, 1972.

215. Schmidtke, J. R., and Dixon, F. J. The functional capacity of x-irradiated macrophages, *J. Immunol.* 108:1624, 1972.

216. Schnitzer, B., Sodeman, T., Mead, M. L., and Contacos, P. G. Pitting function of the spleen in malaria: ultrastructural observations, *Science* 177:175, 1972.

217. Schoenberg, M. D., Mumaw, V. R., Moore, R. D., and Weisberger, A. S. Cytoplasmic interaction between macrophages and lymphocytic cells in antibody synthesis, *Science* 143:964, 1964.

218. Shadduck, R. K., and Nagabhushanam, N. G. Granulocyte colony stimulating factor. I. Response to acute granulocytopenia, *Blood* 38:559, 1971.

219. Shahar, A., Kletter, Y., and Aronson, M. Granuloma formation in cryptococcosis, *Isr. J. Med. Sci.* 5:1164, 1969.

220. Sharp, J. A., and Burwell, R. G. Interaction ("peripolesis") of macrophages and lymphocytes after skin homografting or challenge with soluble antigens, *Nature* 188:474, 1960.

221. Shin, H. S., Kaliss, N., Borenstein, D., and Gately, M. K. Antibody-mediated suppression of grafted lymphoma cells, *J. Exp. Med.* 136:375, 1972.

222. Simon, H. B., and Sheagren, J. N.

Enhancement of macrophage bactericidal capacity by antigenically stimulated immune lymphocytes, *Cell. Immunol.* 4:163, 1972.

223. Simon, H. B., and Sheagren, J. N. Migration inhibitory factor and macrophage bactercidal function, *Infect. Immun.* 6:101, 1972.

224. Snyderman, R., Shin, H. S., and Hausman, M. S. Chemotactic factor for mononuclear leucocytes, *Proc. Soc. Exp. Biol. Med.* 138:387, 1971.

225. Spiegelberg, H. L., and Weigle, W. O. The immune response to human γ G-immunoglobulin in rabbits unresponsive to Fc fragment and H chain protein, *J. Immunol.* 98:1020, 1967.

226. Stubbs, M., Kühner, A. V., Glass, E. A., David, J. R., and Karnovsky, M. L. Metabolic and functional studies on activated mouse macrophages, *J. Exp. Med.* 137:537, 1973.

227. Suter, E., and Ramseier, H. Cellular reactions in infection, *Adv. Immunol.* 4:117, 1964.

228. Tanaka, Y., Brecher, G., and Bull, B. Ferritin localization on the erythroblast cell membrane and ropheocytosis in hypersiderotic human bone marrow, *Blood* 28:758, 1966.

229. Tenhunen, R., Marver, H. S., and Schmid, R. The enzymatic conversion of heme to bilirubin by microsomal heme oxygenase, *Proc. Natl. Acad. Sci. U.S.A.* 61:748, 1968.

230. Tenhunen, R., Marver, H. S., and Schmid, R. Microsomal heme oxygenase. Characterization of the enzyme, *J. Biol. Chem.* 244:6388, 1969.

231. Tenhunen, R., Marver, H. S., and Schmid, R. The enzymatic catabolism of hemoglobin: stimulation of microsomal heme oxygenase by hemin, *J. Lab. Clin. Med.* 75:410, 1970.

232. Thiéry, J. P. Microcinematographic contribution to the study of plasma cells, *in* G. E. W. Wolstenholme and M. O'Connor (eds.), Ciba Found. Symp., Cellular Aspects of Immunity, vol. 59, p. 59, Little, Brown and Co., Boston, 1960

233. Thorbecke, G. J., and Benacerraf, B. The reticulo-endothelial system and immunological phenomena, *Prog. Allergy* 6:559, 1962.

234. Tigelaar, R. E., Vaz, N. M., and Ovary, Z. Immunoglobulin receptors on mouse mast cells, *J. Immunol.* 106:661, 1971.

235. Tizard, I. R. Macrophage cytophilic antibodies in mice: the adsorption of cytophilic antibodies from solution by mouse peritoneal cells and cooperative interaction between receptors for immunoglobulin, *J. Reticuloendothel. Soc.* 10:449, 1971.

236. Tripathy, S. P., and Mackaness, G. B. The effect of cytotoxic agents on the primary immune response to *Listeria monocytogenes, J. Exp. Med.* 130:1, 1969.

237. Tripathy, S. P., and Mackaness, G. B. The effect of cytotoxic agents on the passive transfer of cell-mediated immunity, *J. Exp. Med.* 130:17, 1969.

238. Uhr, J. W., and Weissman, G. Intracellular distribution and degradation of bacteriophage in mammalian tissues, *J. Immunol.* 94:544, 1965.

239. Unanue, E. R. Properties and some uses of anti-macrophage antibodies, *Nature* 218:36, 1968.

240. Unanue, E. R. The immune response of mice to keyhole limpet hemocyanin bound to macrophages, *J. Immunol.* 102:893, 1969.

241. Unanue, E. R., and Askonas, B. A. The immune response of mice to antigen in macrophages, *Immunology* 15:287, 1968.

242. Unanue, E. R., and Askonas, B. A. Persistence of immunogenicity of antigen after uptake by macrophages, *J. Exp. Med.* 127:915, 1968.

243. Unanue, E. R., Askonas, B. A., and Allison, A. C. A role of macrophages in the stimulation of immune responses by adjuvants, *J. Immunol.* 103:71, 1969.

244. Unanue, E. R., and Cerottini, J. C. The function of macrophages in the immune response, *Semin. Hematol.* 7:225, 1970.

245. Unanue, E. R., Cerottini, J. C., and Bedford, M. Persistence of antigen on the surface of macrophages, *Nature* 222:1193, 1969.

246. van Furth, R., Hirsch, J. G., and Fedorko, M. E. Morphology and peroxidase cytochemistry of mouse promonocytes, monocytes, and macrophages, *J. Exp. Med.* 132:794, 1970.

247. Vaughan, R. B. Interactions of macrophages and erythrocytes: some further experiments, *Immunology* 8:245, 1965.

248. Vaughan, R. B., and Boyden, S. V. Interactions of macrophages and erythrocytes, *Immunology* 7:118, 1964.

249. Volkman, A., and Collins, F. M. Recovery of delayed-type hypersensitivity in mice following suppressive doses of X-radiation, *J. Immunol.* 101:846, 1968.

250. Volkman, A., and Gowans, J. L. The production of macrophages in the rat, *Br. J. Exp. Pathol.* 46:50, 1965.

251. Volkman, A., and Gowans, J. L. The origin of macrophages from bone marrow in the rat, *Br. J. Exp. Pathol.* 46:62, 1965.

252. Ward, P. A. Chemotaxis of mononuclear cells, *J. Exp. Med.* 128:1201, 1968.

253. Weiner, H. L., and Robinson, W. A. Leukopoietic activity in human urine following operative procedures, *Proc. Soc. Exp. Biol. Med.* 136:29, 1971.

254. Weiss, L. A note on the functional anatomy of the spleen, *in* A. S. Gordon (ed.), Regulation of Hematopoiesis, p. 93, Appleton-Century-Crofts, New York, 1970.

255. Weiss, L., and Tavassoli, M. Anatomical hazards to the passage of erythrocytes through the spleen, *Semin. Hematol.* 7:372, 1970.

256. Weiss, L., and Tavassoli, M. The spleen, *in* R. O. Greep and L. Weiss (eds.), Histology, McGraw-Hill, New York, 1972.

257. White, R. G., French, V. I., and Stark, J. M. Germinal center formation and antigen localization in Malpighian bodies of the chicken spleen, *in* H. Cottier, N. Odartchenko, R. Schindler, and C. C. Congdon (eds.), Germinal Centers in Immune Responses, p. 131, Springer-Verlag, New York, 1967.

258. Widmann, J-J., Cotran, R. S., and Fahimi, H. D. Mononuclear phagocytes (Kupffer cells) and endothelial cells. Identification of two functional cell types in rat liver sinusoids by endogenous peroxidase

activity, *J. Cell Biol.* 52:159, 1972.

259. Wilkinson, P. C., Borel, J. F., Stecher-Levin, V. J., and Sorkin, E. Macrophage and neutrophil specific chemotactic factors in serum, *Nature* 222:244, 1969.

260. Wisse, E., and Daems, W. T. Fine structural study on the sinusoidal lining cells of rat liver, *in* R. van Furth (ed.), Mononuclear Phagocytes, p. 200, F. A. Davis Co., Philadelphia, 1970.

261. Yount, W. J., Dorner, M. M., Kunkel, H. G., and Kabat, E. A. Studies on human antibodies. VI. Selective variations in subgroup composition and genetic markers, *J. Exp. Med.* 127:633, 1968.

B The Abnormal Macrophage

Chapter 26 The Macrophage and Nonmalignant Diseases of the Reticuloendothelial System

Largely from the studies and writings of Aschoff (8), and later of Maximow (143), a concept has arisen of the reticuloendothelial system as a collection of widely dispersed mesenchymal cells capable of phagocytosis. The cellular elements of this system include monocytes in the blood, macrophages in the tissues, Kupffer cells in the liver, and the reticular and endothelial cells of the lymph nodes, bone marrow, and spleen.

Origin of Cells of the Reticuloendothelial System

The origin of tissue macrophages (histiocytes) from precursor cells in the bone marrow was discussed in Chapter 23. Histiocytes, including inflammatory macrophages, peritoneal macrophages, hepatic Kupffer cells, alveolar macrophages, and splenic sinusoidal lining cells, arise wholly or in part from bone marrow precursors.

Although it is comparatively simple to summarize the existing information about the monocyte-macrophage complex (Chapters 23 to 25), it is extremely difficult to characterize the reticulum cell in a similiar manner. This difficulty stems from the fact that at present reticulum cells cannot always be unequivocally identified in tissues, nor can they be isolated or cultivated free of other tissue elements; consequently, one must rely on qualitative, or at best semiquantitative, histochemical techniques to identify and characterize them (140).

The existence of a framework of stellate cells in the pulp of the spleen was recognized in the mid-nineteenth century. By the early years of the twentieth century, the use of vital staining techniques permitted the recognition in lymph nodes, spleen, bone marrow, and other tissues of stellate cells capable of removal and storage of foreign particulate matter. The capacity to take up certain metal stains is a property of these cells. Such cells were considered to be involved in the formation of a syncytium of fibrils (reticulin) and consequently were called reticulum cells. The relation between cells and fibrils is, however, not wholly defined, nor is the relation between these cells and other elements of the reticuloendothelial system (140).

Aschoff conceived an association of the reticulum cells and the endothelial cells based on the common property of phagocytosis of colloidal dyes (8). He did not conclude that this common feature implied anatomic or embryologic identity. Later authors have had little success in unraveling the interrelations between these complex classes of cells. At the present time the best operational definition of reticulum cells takes cognizance of the following characteristics: (a) they are widely disseminated in a number of tissues and lie in close apposition to blood vessels; (b) they are distributed in association with a syncytium of reticulin fibers; (c) they have ill-defined, pale-staining, and often stellate cytoplasm and large, ovoid nuclei often with prominent nucleoli; (d) they are metalophilic; and (e) they demonstrate endocytic activity.

The composition and metabolism of reticulum cells are largely unknown. They stain intensely for alkaline phosphatase and adenosine tri-, di-, and monophosphatase;

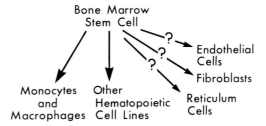

Figure 26.1 Aschoff's concept of the origin of the cells of the reticuloendothelial system. The derivation of mononuclear leukocytes and other hematopoietic cell lines from a common stem cell is well established. Although all reticuloendothelial cells were originally thought to be derived from a common progenitor, the relation of reticulum cells, fibroblasts, and endothelial cells to the hematopoietic progenitor cells is uncertain.

they may contain large granules of hemosiderin and may have acid phosphatase activity (206). They do not stain with periodic acid Schiff.

Aschoff's concept of the origin of the cells of the reticuloendothelial system, with certain modern adaptations, is seen in Fig. 26.1. The evidence that there exists a pluripotent bone marrow stem cell capable of giving rise to monocytes and macrophages, as well as to granulocytes and erythroid and megkaryocytic precursors, is summarized in Chapters 2 and 10. Evidence for the origin of reticulum cells, endothelial cells, and fibroblasts from a similiar precursor is poor or inconclusive.

Hyperplasia — Reactive and Autonomous

In Chapters 10 and 22 it was pointed out that myeloid, erythroid, and lymphoid cells can proliferate in response to appropriate stimuli; for example, granulocytosis occurs in response to infection, and erythrocytic hyperplasia in response to chronic bleeding. Lymphocytosis may be an appropriate response to certain viral and bacterial infections. These cell lines may also proliferate autonomously or in response to unidentified stimuli. In such circumstances we speak of lymphoproliferative disorders (Chapters 19 to 22) or myeloproliferative disorders (Chapters 10 and 11). These may be either relatively benign (as, for example, polycythemia vera), or malignant (acute myelocytic leukemia). In an analogous manner, cells of the monocyte-macrophage series may proliferate appropriately in response to a stimulus such as *Mycobacterium tuberculosis*. In such a circumstance the mononuclear leukocyte response is often termed "reactive" hyperplasia. Clinically reactive hyperplasia is manifested by enlargement of reticuloendothelial organs such as the spleen and lymph nodes.

On the other hand, these cells may proliferate "inappro-

Table 26.1 Summary of histiocytic proliferative disorders and the stimuli to which they respond.

Category	Examples	Inciting agent
Reactive	Tuberculosis	*M. tuberculosis*
	Toxoplasmosis	Toxoplasma
	Silicosis	Silica
	Hemolytic anemia	Antibody-coated erythrocytes
Neoplastic (malignant histiocytic proliferative disorders)	Monocytic leukemia	?
	Malignant histiocytosis	?
Storage diseases	Gaucher's disease	Glucocerebroside
	Hemochromatosis	? Iron
Of unknown origin	Sarcoidosis	?
	Felty's syndrome	?
	Rheumatoid arthritis	?

priately" (autonomously and to an extent exceeding normal levels) as, for example, in monocytic leukemia. A variety of terms has been used to describe neoplastic histiocytic proliferation: reticuloendotheliosis, histiocytic malignancy, reticuloendothelial malignancy. Some of these terms are probably misnomers, since we do not have firm evidence that endothelial elements participate in the proliferative process. Perhaps *malignant histiocytic proliferative disorders* would be a more appropriate term to cover this spectrum of diseases.

A third category of disorders in which one observes hyperplasia of tissue macrophages is that in which a phagocytizable material accumulates more rapidly than it can be disposed of by metabolic processes. An example would be glucocerebroside in Gaucher's disease. For convenience we identify these as *storage diseases.*

Finally, histiocytes may proliferate in a variety of disorders in which the inciting agent has not yet been identified — for instance, in sarcoidosis and in rheumatoid arthritis.

The categories of histiocytic proliferative disorders are summarized in Table 26.1. In this chapter we shall consider reactive hyperplasia of the monocyte-macrophage cell line and storage diseases. In the next chapter the malignant histiocytic proliferative syndromes will be discussed.

Reactive Hyperplasia

Response to Intracellular Parasites

A variety of intracellular parasites is associated with clinical enlargement of the liver, spleen, and sometimes

Table 26.2 Categories of agents that stimulate reactive histiocytic proliferation.

Intracellular parasites

　Bacterial agents
　　Subacute bacterial endocarditis
　　Tuberculosis
　　Brucellosis
　　Typhoid fever
　　Syphilis
　Fungal agents
　　Histoplasmosis
　　Cryptococcosis
　Parasitic agents
　　Malaria
　　Leishmaniasis
　　Trypanosomiasis
　　Toxoplasmosis

Diseases with excessive erythrocyte destruction

　Acquired hemolytic anemia
　Congenital hemolytic syndromes (for example, hemolytic
　　disease of the newborn)
　Pulmonary hemosiderosis

Heavy metal compounds

　Silicosis
　Berylliosis

Organic compounds

　Molds

lymph nodes, and with microscopic evidence of histiocytic hyperplasia throughout the reticuloendothelial system. A partial listing of diseases with such an association is given in Table 26.2.

Tuberculosis as a Prototype　Tuberculosis is still one of the more common chronic infectious diseases in this country and may be taken as the prototype of histiocytic proliferation in response to an intracellular parasite. Splenomegaly as a feature of reticuloendothelial hyperplasia in generalized tuberculosis is well recognized in the literature (32, 37, 64, 66, 78). In the early days of human and animal macrophage cultivation, the multinucleate giant cell (macrophage) of the tuberculoid lesion was taken as the prototype of histiocytic response to a facultative intracellular parasite (119, 120).

The macrophage appears to be the primary cell in defense against this organism. Differences in enzyme content and activity of macrophages from nonresistant and tuberculosis-resistant animals have been described (5, 11, 53). Macrophages from animals that are infected but able to control the infection are said to be activated. As dis-

cussed in Chapters 24 and 25, the activated macrophage has many distinctive features, including greater content of hydrolytic enzymes, greater adhesiveness and spreading on a glass surface, and greater microbicidal activity than its nonactivated counterpart. The mechanism of this activation appears to be dependent upon antigen-responsive lymphoid cells and requires a living proliferating microorganism and not just a killed vaccine (53, 90, 133–135, 150). Activation appears to be nonspecific in the sense that once it is initiated it is directed against several intracellular parasites and not just the inciting organism (44, 81); for example, tuberculosis infection may increase host resistance to *Listeria* and other intracellular organisms.

The mechanism of macrophage activation by lymphoid cells is obscure. It may involve soluble lymphocyte mediator substances (Chapter 17), but the precise one has yet to be identified.

In a tuberculous lesion one sees macrophages at all stages of development, from the newly arrived monocyte to the mature multinucleated giant cell (53) (Fig. 26.2; see also Figs. 23.7 and 23.18). Many of the phagocytes contain ingested organisms. One of the interesting features of this infection, as well as other infections with facultative and obligate intracellular parasites, is that many organisms survive and even proliferate within the macrophage (202) (Fig. 26.3). The reason some organisms survive while others are killed is unclear. Armstrong and D'Arcy Hart (7) recently have suggested that surviving organisms are sequestered in phagosomes that do not receive a complement of hydrolytic enzymes from the discharge of primary

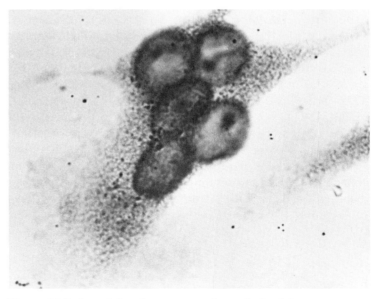

Figure 26.2 A multinucleate macrophage derived from a monocyte cultured in vitro.

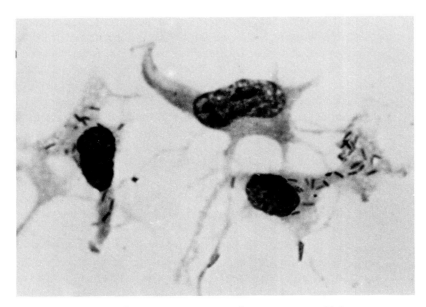

Figure 26.3 Macrophages containing replicating intracellular *Listeria monocytogenes.*

and secondary lysosomes (147) (cf. Chapters 4 and 25).

The course of tuberculosis is governed by the overall function of the macrophage system: effectiveness of individual cells and total number of responding cells. Although the organisms initially may multiply within the cell, with the development of cellular immunity they are destroyed (53, 129). Thus the development of delayed hypersensitivity and full expression of macrophage microbicidal function are concomitant phenomena (Chapter 25).

Other Intracellular Infections Histiocytic proliferation, evident clinically as splenomegaly and lymphadenopathy and histologically as reticuloendothelial hyperplasia, has been documented in association with a variety of intracellular infections and parasitic diseases: syphilis (226, 227), brucellosis (200), listeriosis (110), leprosy (163), malaria (57, 131, 139), schistosomiasis (172), leishmaniasis (6, 30), cryptococcosis (184, 185), histoplasmosis (50, 194), and toxoplasmosis (102, 168).

There have been detailed studies of the mechanisms or consequences of histiocytic proliferation in some of these disorders; for example, *Listeria* infection (134, 135), histoplasmosis (16), and toxoplasmosis (72, 113, 176, 177).

Response to Chemicals

Beryllium Chronic pulmonary disease caused by exposure to beryllium was first reported in 1933 (219). Thereafter, as the increased use of this metal in industry led to an increased incidence of disease (91), the number

of case reports and descriptions increased. The lesions of berylliosis may be widespread in reticuloendothelial tissues and may mimic those of sarcoidosis; they are characterized by large macrophages, giant cells, and organized epithelioid cells (225).

In 1951 Sterner and Eisenbud suggested that the lesions of chronic beryllium disease were caused by a delayed hypersensitivity reaction (197), a suggestion supported by subsequent studies of cutaneous delayed hypersensitivity reactions to beryllium salts (3, 67, 157). Injection of twenty normal volunteers with insoluble beryllium salts produced foreign-body granulomatous reactions without concomitant delayed hypersensitivity in nineteen; in one subject, true granulomatous hypersensitivity with reaction to as little as 1 μgm of beryllium oxide resulted (67).

Our own studies demonstrated that lymphocytes from hypersensitive subjects undergo blastogenic transformation when exposed to poorly soluble beryllium salts in vitro. Such lymphocytes interact with macrophages in producing clusters of responding cells (89). The macrophages of these subjects appear to be activated by morphologic criteria in their rate of differentiation from monocytes. However, they do not show the enhanced ability to kill an intracellular parasite that characterizes the macrophages of patients with active tuberculosis or leprosy (39). These observations indicate that intracellular parasitosis, rather than granulomatous hypersensitivity per se, is necessary for functionally activated macrophages (that is, those showing enhanced microbicidal activity).

If we may extrapolate from these studies with beryllium, the histiocytic proliferative reactions to certain heavy metals appear to involve two components: a foreign-body reaction to poorly soluble particulate matter, and a delayed hypersensitivity reaction involving lymphocyte participation.

Zirconium Zirconium salts were widely used in deodorants in the mid-1950s and were associated with a high incidence of granulomatas of the skin (187, 220). Zirconium reacts readily with body proteins (145), and the complexes formed—rather than the metal salts themselves—are probably immunogenic; the same phenomenon is likely to hold true for beryllium compounds.

The histiocytic response to zirconium salts appears to be similar, in general, in histologic appearance and pathogenesis to the response to beryllium compounds (67). The lesions are characterized by histiocytic proliferation and accumulations of lymphocytes.

Silica Compounds Injection of colloidal silica into the skin of man produces a foreign-body macrophage/giant-cell response in all individuals (68, 189). A similar response to micron- and millimicron-sized silica particles is seen in the lung (182). Superficially, silicosis has a number of features in common with diseases such as berylliosis, tuberculosis, and sarcoidosis. Histologically, the lesions produced by these diseases have many similarities also (76, 85). Although there have been occasional proponents of an immunologic pathogenesis of silicosis (211), the available evidence does not lend strong support to such a concept. The current concept of the pathogenesis of silicosis is that phagocytized silica particles are toxic for cells. The necrotic cells are chemotactic for other phagocytes, which accumulate, proliferate, and form a granulomatous lesion (4, 49, 108, 153).

Organic Compounds

A variety of organic substances stimulate localized histiocytic proliferation. Since the portal of entry of such compounds is often the airway, the lungs are a common site of granulomatous lesions. Examples of such diseases are "farmer's lung" (59, 112), bagassosis (26), maple-bark disease (65), pigeon-breeder's lungs (122, 165), and the pulmonary granulomas produced by hairspray polymers (PAS-positive) (15). In some instances the principal pathogenetic mechanism appears to be a cytolytic foreign-body type reaction (cf. silicosis); in others, delayed hypersensitivity reactions play a role (158).

From the foregoing one can conclude that there are two general categories of histiocytic response to small, phagocytizable, inorganic compounds and certain organic substances:

(a) A "foreign-body/giant-cell reaction" in which the phagocytized substance is nondigestible and is ultimately cytotoxic for the phagocyte; in this circumstance, cell death attracts other phagocytes.

(b) Delayed hypersensitivity reactions to organic substances or inorganic compounds bonded to tissue proteins; in this type of reaction, lymphoid participation is a prominent feature.

Histiocytic Response to Hematopoietic
Cell Destruction

Hemolytic Anemia   In most hemolytic anemias the primary site of destruction of damaged, intrinsically abnormal, or antibody-coated erythrocytes is the reticuloendothelial elements of the spleen and, to a lesser extent, of the liver. Several mechanisms of cell destruction may be operative, including stasis of erythrocytes and subsequent osmotic lysis in the splenic sinusoids, and phagocytosis by the reticuloendothelial cells of the spleen, liver, and blood (88, 97, 232) (see Chapter 25). Splenomegaly is clini-

cally apparent in most long-standing hemolytic anemias (227, 231). It is probable that part of this increase in spleen size is the result of hyperplasia of the phagocytic histiocytes. This hyperplasia may also be seen in the liver and to some extent in the lymph nodes. Erythrophagocytosis and its consequence (hemosiderin pigments) may be more or less prominent in histiocytes (see Fig. 25.1).

Hemolysis induced in the experimental animal produces an increase in spleen size and hyperplasia of the phagocytic histiocytes (96, 98). The mechanism by which this "work hypertrophy" occurs is not known. Clearly there must be some signal by which tissue macrophages are induced to proliferate and expand the size of the tissue available for handling the defective red cells.

There is reason to believe that once histiocytic hyperplasia is established in the spleen, a vicious cycle may be instituted in which even normal red cells are destroyed prematurely in this organ. Again, the mechanism of erythrocyte destruction may involve stasis and phagocytosis. For example, in a model system in which splenomegaly and macrophage hyperplasia is induced in animals by methyl cellulose, hemolytic anemia is produced (221).

It is probable that the induction of histiocytic proliferation by red cells undergoing lysis can take place locally in many areas of the body. Perhaps the best example is the occurrence of large numbers of hemoglobin- and hemosiderin-laden alveolar macrophages in a variety of diseases where red cell extravasation into the alveoli occurs; for example, pulmonary hemosiderosis, Goodpasture's syndrome, and severe mitral valve stenosis. There is some evidence that erythrophagocytosis interferes with the ability of macrophages to simultaneously phagocytize and destroy certain intracellular bacteria (79). The fate of hemoglobin pinocytosed by macrophages was discussed more fully in Chapter 25.

Destruction of Other Hematopoietic Cells   It is possible that hyperplasia of histiocytes may occur in disorders in which there is a high turnover and excessive destruction of granulocytes. This is difficult to document, however. Inferential evidence is provided by the observation of large, lipid-laden phagocytes in patients with chronic myelocytic leukemia (107). These cells resemble Gaucher's cells (62) (see Fig. 10.6).

Storage Diseases

As a generalization, one can say that when a phagocytizable organic material accumulates more rapidly than it can be disposed of by normal catabolic or excretory processes, it will accumulate in cells of the reticuloendothelial system and, in particular, in macrophages. Such accumulation may occur in genetic defects of enzyme function in which a poorly catabolized product accumulates. It may also occur in diseases characterized by excessive cell death or turnover and in diseases in which the normal excretory pathways are blocked. Examples of diseases associated with each of these mechanisms are listed in Table 26.3. Clearly in some of the diseases, such as localized bronchial obstruction with foamy alveolar macrophages, more than one mechanism may be operative in inducing reticuloendothelial hyperplasia.

A common feature of all these storage diseases is the accumulation of tissue macrophages that appear prominent because of their ingested products; for example, lipid-laden macrophages in the lipidoses. Whether there is in addition a true hyperplasia of the histiocyte is not certain.

The Lipidoses

Gaucher's disease and Niemann-Pick disease are classic examples of the lipidoses, in which lipid-laden macrophages accumulate. The characteristic cells in the bone marrow, of which an example is shown in Fig. 26.4, are well known to students of hematology. The pathology, histochemistry, and biochemical abnormalities of these two most common lipidoses are fully documented (46, 47, 132, 201, 203). Enzymes that catalyze the hydrolysis of glucose cerebroside and sphingomyelin are reduced in the leukocytes and other tissues of patients with Gaucher's disease and Niemann-Pick disease respectively (23, 161). Gaucher cells are found in the bone marrow (58, 101), spleen (74), and liver (214). Cerebroside is aggregated into tubular elements within the histiocytic cells. A variable amount of tubular material together with matrix is con-

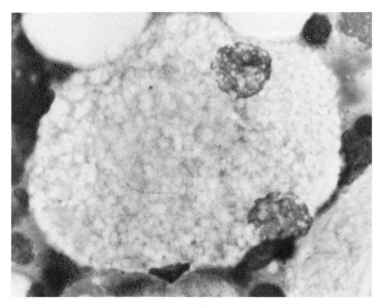

Figure 26.4 A Gaucher cell from the bone marrow.

tained within cytoplasmic vacuoles called Gaucher bodies. These structures have high acid phosphatase activity and are probably secondary lysosomes. Whether the cerebroside comes from metabolism of the macrophage itself or from sources outside the cell is not clear. There is reasonable evidence favoring the thesis that the material enters the cell by phagocytosis (75, 115, 160) and that erythrocyte membranes are the principal source of cerebroside. Considerable amounts of intracellular iron may occur in Gaucher cells (125, 126).

The morphologic and histochemical features of Gaucher's cells and Niemann-Pick cells are listed in Table 26.4.

A variety of other diseases are grouped together under the category of lipidoses, although they encompass a variety of enzyme defects: (a) Tay-Sachs disease (104, 117); (b) Farber's disease (1, 71); (c) xanthomas associated with hyperlipemia and hypercholesterolemia (164, 203); and (d) a benign, chronic, reticuloendothelial lipid storage disease or diseases occurring in infancy, childhood, and adult life and histochemically distinct from other lipidoses (94, 137, 179–181, 191–193). This last disease has recently been called the "sea-blue histiocyte" syndrome (see Fig. 26.5). Sea-blue histiocytes are, however, not unique to familial lipidoses (62, 138). Excellent reviews of the sphingolipidoses have recently appeared (22, 181, 213).

Hemochromatosis

In hemochromatosis, hemosiderin-laden macrophages are found throughout reticuloendothelial tissues and particularly in the liver and spleen. In addition, iron-containing

Table 26.3 Storage diseases in which cellular products accumulate in tissue histiocytes.

Characteristics of disease	Examples of disease	Product	Tissue distribution of product
Enzyme defects with metabolic overproduction or diminished catabolism	Gaucher's	Glucocerebroside	General
	Niemann-Pick	Sphingomyelin	General
	Gout	Microcrystalline uric acid	Local or general
	Hemochromatosis	Iron-hemosiderin	General
Excessive production from cell death or turnover	Secondary gout	Uric acid	Local or general
	Chronic myelocytic leukemia	? Phospholipid	Bone marrow
Impaired clearance	Bronchial obstruction with foamy alveolar macrophages	? Phospholipid	Alveolar macrophages

Table 26.4 Morphologic and cytochemical features of storage cells in lipidoses.

Characteristic	Manifestation in Gaucher's disease	Manifestation in Niemann-Pick disease
Size	20–60 microns	20–40 microns
Wright's stain	Usually non-vacuolated, faint fibrils	Often vacuolated = "foam cell," no fibrils
PAS	++	+
Sudan black B	Gray	Gray-black
Sudan IV	– – –	Faint orange
Toluidine blue (metachromasia)	– – –	+
Acid phosphatase	++	+
Prussian blue (iron)	+ or −	– – –

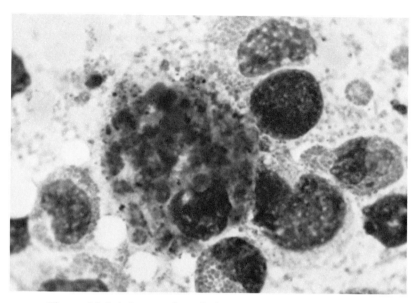

Figure 26.6 A hemosiderin-laden macrophage from the bone marrow of a patient with hemochromatosis.

macrophages occur at various levels of the intestinal villi (48) and have been demonstrated to pass from the villus into the intestinal lumen (9). Certain investigators have suggested that the macrophages may be performing an iron-excretory function in this iron storage disease (204, 230).

Iron-containing macrophages are occasionally found also in the circulating blood and bone marrow (Fig. 26.6) of patients with hemochromatosis and hemosiderosis (175, 188, 230). In transfusion hemosiderosis, the hemosiderin granules in the blood and tissue macrophages are larger than those in hemochromatosis (19).

The Foamy Alveolar Macrophage

The occurrence of lipid-laden macrophages (see Fig. 23.18) in areas of pneumonitis behind an obstructed or partially obstructed bronchus has long been recognized in the pathology literature. Recently it has been shown that such foamy alveolar macrophages may release their lipid upon isolation and cultivation in vitro and that such lipid has the properties of pulmonary surfactant (43). A major constituent of this lipid is dipalmatyllecithin, which is also a major component of surfactant. These observations suggest that surfactant normally may be cleared upward through the bronchial tree, and that in circumstances in which clearance is obstructed the material may be endocytosed by alveolar macrophages. Cell death and subsequent phagocytosis in the area behind the obstruction may be a contributing factor in the production of foamy alveolar macrophages.

Histiocytic Proliferative Disorders of Uncertain Origin

Histiocytic proliferation, either localized or generalized, occurs in a variety of disease states of unknown etiology. Consequently, the pathogenetic mechanisms leading to cellular proliferation are obscure. Sarcoidosis and rheumatoid arthritis are examples of such diseases.

Sarcoidosis

There is a rich and complex literature on sarcoidosis that unfortunately provides little insight into the pathogenesis of the disease. The important features relevant to the present discussion are that splenomegaly and lymphaden-

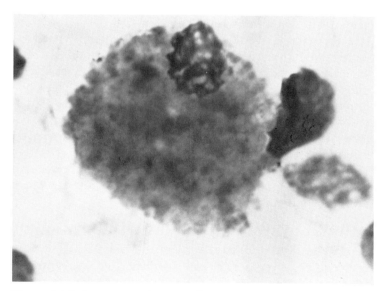

Figure 26.5 A pigmented macrophage from the bone marrow of a patient with the sea-blue histiocyte syndrome.

opathy are frequent features of this disease and monocytosis an occasional feature. Lymph nodes likely to be involved include the pre- and postauriculars, the submaxillary and submental nodes, and particularly the mediastinal nodes, which are often symmetrically enlarged and without calcification. The histologic features of the affected nodes and spleen resemble those of miliary epithelioid tubercles without necrosis and generally without a surrounding inflammatory zone. The spleen may be slightly or greatly enlarged. Secondary thrombocytopenia, neutropenia, or hemolytic anemia may occur (17, 124).

Felty's Syndrome

Splenomegaly and hyperplasia of the histiocytic elements of the spleen and lymph nodes occur in Felty's syndrome, in Still's disease, and in the more common varieties of rheumatoid arthritis.

Felty's syndrome is thought to be a variant of rheumatoid arthritis (see Chapter 9). The marrow usually contains granulocyte precursors and is hyperplastic—rarely hypoplastic. The degree of splenomegaly, which may vary from slight to marked, is not generally correlated with the activity of the arthritis or the magnitude of the hematologic changes (141). Splenectomy often produces a transient improvement in the white blood cell count (84).

Other Localized Histiocytic Proliferative Disorders

There are a number of rare diseases in which histiocytic proliferation and granulomatous infiltration occur in the tissues, particularly around damaged blood vessels. These include "allergic" granulomatosis (35), Wegener's granulomatosis (28, 70, 80, 95, 111), midline granuloma (224), giant cell arteritis (159, 178), Cogan's syndrome (42, 45), and multicentric reticulohistiocytosis (82). Attempts have been made to analyze and classify these diseases (2, 34, 196); however, no clear, completely acceptable explanation of the clinical and histologic features of these disorders has yet emerged.

Macrophage Dysfunction Syndromes

Several macrophage dysfunction syndromes in man have recently been described. These include genetic abnormalities such as chronic granulomatous disease (24, 29, 56, 69, 171) and acquired disorders such as lymphoma and myelomonocytic leukemia (40) but not chronic neutropenia of childhood (12). These disorders are all associated with an increased incidence of opportunistic infection. The mononuclear defect in chronic granulomatous disease is probably related to deficient postphagocytic H_2O_2 generation. In acute myelomonocytic leukemia the defective leuko-

Table 26.5 Summary of proven and possible macrophage dysfunction syndromes.

Macrophage dysfunction syndromes supported by experimental evidence
    Chronic granulomatous disease
    Myelomonocytic leukemia
    Lymphoma (some patients)
    Adrenocorticosteroid therapy

Putative macrophage dysfunction syndromes
    Lepromatous leprosy
    Disseminated tuberculosis
    Disseminated fungal disease
    Hodgkin's disease

cytes phagocytize organisms, but fail to inhibit their intracellular replication.

High concentrations of adrenocorticosteroids and ionizing irradiation also may interfere with the macrophage defense system (25, 130, 147). With high doses of ionizing irradiation the proliferation of macrophage precursors is impaired, but the metabolic development of the cells appears to be intact (54, 103). Thus the main effect on macrophage defense function of high doses of X ray is against the proliferating cell in the bone marrow rather than the functional cell in the periphery (128, 209, 212, 215–217).

In addition to these documented macrophage dysfunction syndromes, defective mononuclear cell function has been thought to occur in several other disorders. For obvious reasons the patient who fails to control intracellular parasitosis adequately must be suspected of having a defective macrophage defense system. Therefore patients with lepromatous leprosy (218), miliary tuberculosis, disseminated fungal infections, and Hodgkin's disease (25) may be considered as possibly having macrophage dysfunction syndromes (Table 26.5). However, in these disorders intrinsic or acquired defects of macrophage function or of macrophage-lymphoid interaction have been inferred, not proven.

In many of the putative macrophage dysfunction syndromes, abnormalities of delayed hypersensitivity are a prominent feature of the disease.

Lepromatous Leprosy

Leprosy may be divided clinically and histopathologically into two polar types of disease—tuberculoid and lepromatous—with intermediate stages linking these extremes (41) (see also Chapter 18). Although intermediate forms of the disease may evolve toward either pole, it is rare for lepromatous leprosy to develop into tuberculoid leprosy, and vice versa. The characteristic histologic feature of tuberculoid leprosy is an organized granuloma composed of macrophages and epithelioid cells. In lepromatous leprosy such granulomas fail to evolve and the characteristic feature is the large, foamy "lepra" cell filled with acid-fast bacilli. Tuberculoid leprosy tends to be relatively benign and circumscribed; lepromatous leprosy is widely disseminated (109). The administration of a mycobacterial antigen—lepromin—elicits a delayed hypersensitivity reaction and granuloma formation in tuberculoid, but not lepromatous, leprosy (41, 166). As a generalization, a positive delayed response (Mitsuda reaction) correlates with intact defenses against the severe form of the disease.

Macrophages from patients with tuberculoid leprosy phagocytize and then lyse ingested *Mycobacterium leprae*. Some investigators have reported that macrophages from patients with lepromatous leprosy phagocytize but do not lyse the organisms (10, 13, 14). Our own experiments do not confirm these reports. Rather, we find macrophages from both tuberculoid and lepromatous leprosy to be functionally equivalent to normal cells (63). Macrophages from both types of disease appear to have the same content of lysosomal enzymes (10).

The cellular immune defect in patients with lepromatous leprosy is not restricted to lepromin; it may be deficient in response to tuberculin (86) and to skin sensitization to picryl chloride (27) and dinitrochlorobenzene (218). Lymphocytes from such patients may show impaired blastogenic response to phytohemagglutinin (60) and to streptolysin-O (186). Rejection of allogeneic skin grafts may also be delayed (55). On the other hand, humoral immune responses appear to be intact in such patients (167). Turk and Waters (207) have suggested that in lepromatous leprosy there is a correlation between depression of cellular immunity and replacement of the normal lymphoid population of the paracortical areas of lymph nodes by histiocytes.

The basic question arising from these observations is this: Is the abnormality of cellular immunity the primary genetically determined event (21, 154) that leads to impaired defense against *M. leprae,* or does overwhelming infection based on environmental factors lead to a secondary immunosuppression? Recent studies in an animal model of murine leprosy suggest that overwhelming infection leads to impaired cellular immune responses (163).

Lymphoreticular Malignancies

Malignant diseases of the lymphoid and reticuloendothelial systems are associated with an unusually high incidence of infection with intracellular organisms. Many of these organisms are nonpathogenic or are of low-grade pathogenicity for normal individuals; consequently, the infections they cause in the impaired host are called *opportunistic infections.* For example, infection with *Listeria monocytogenes* occurs with unusually high frequency in patients with reticulum cell sarcoma, Hodgkin's disease, and chronic lymphocytic leukemia (25). Toxoplasmosis (210), as well as *Candida albicans* infection (116), also occurs with unusual frequency in this group of patients. Abnormalities of cellular or humoral immune responses are well documented in such disorders (see Chapters 18 to 22); still, it is difficult to know whether these are critical factors in the association with opportunistic infection or whether related phenomena are more important—for instance, the frequent occurrence of neutropenia, of indwelling venous catheters, of immunosuppressant therapy, and of high doses of adrenocorticosteroids (127).

It has been demonstrated recently that mononuclear phagocytes from patients with myelomonocytic leukemia and some patients with lymphoma phagocytize certain organisms, but fail to kill them (40, 99).

Adrenocorticosteroids

In patients receiving adrenocorticosteroids, opportunistic infections are frequent (25, 83, 100, 116, 190) and may carry a grave prognosis—diseases in which such infections occur and in which corticosteroids are used include malignancy (127), collagen vascular disease (173, 183), and vasculitis (25, 100).

While the mechanism is not known with certainty, it has been shown that in animals treated with high doses of corticosteroids the lysosomes of alveolar macrophages fail to fuse properly with phagosomes containing ingested microorganisms (147). This enhanced lysosomal stability may be one mechanism by which corticosteroids promote enhanced susceptibility to opportunistic pathogens (149).

Monocytosis

The normal relative monocyte count in the adult varies between 1 and 6 percent of the circulating leukocyte population (114, 148, 199, 226). The relative monocyte count is significantly elevated when it exceeds 10 percent. In children the average relative count is 9 percent (222). It is clear that a relative count is not so meaningful or useful as an absolute count. The latter varies between 285 and 500 cells/mm^3 in adults (148, 226) and between 750 and 800 in children (18, 148).

Relative monocytosis is normal in the neonate and may persist for several weeks (106). The variety of infectious

Table 26.6 Causes of monocytosis as found in the literature.

Cause	References
Infectious and parasitic diseases	
Subacute bacterial endocarditis	51, 52, 93
Tuberculosis	61, 136, 222
Rickettsial diseases	208
Syphilis	146, 223
Brucellosis	151
Malaria	170
Trypanosomiasis	148, 226
Leishmaniasis	148, 226
Typhoid fever	222
Following acute infection	92, 148
Neoplastic diseases	
Myelomonocytic leukemia	136, 195
Hodgkin's disease and lymphomas	106, 118, 136, 228
"Preleukemia"	20, 136, 144, 195
Multiple myeloma	136
Nonhematologic malignant disease	136
Miscellaneous hematologic diseases	
Polycythemia vera	114, 136
Recovery phase of agranulocytosis	136, 169, 174, 198
Postsplenectomy	121
Myeloid metaplasia	136
Hemolytic anemia	136
Collagen vascular diseases	
Rheumatic endocarditis	52, 136
Systemic lupus erythematosus	136
Rheumatoid arthritis	136
Chronic inflammatory gastrointestinal diseases	
Ulcerative colitis	77, 136
Regional enteritis	136
Cirrhosis	136
Miscellaneous disorders	
Sarcoidosis	205
Fever of unknown origin	136
Drug reactions	31

diseases that may cause monocytosis are summarized in Table 26.6. These are usually chronic infections with intracellular microorganisms and parasites. For example, the facultative intracellular parasite *Listeria monocytogenes* produces a striking monocytosis in some animal species (153, 229) and in some of the rare human patients infected with this organism.

Monocytosis and abnormal monocytes may be associated with a variety of malignant diseases, but especially the lymphoproliferative and histiocytic proliferative disorders (33, 35, 87, 142, 155, 156). For example, chronic monocytosis may antedate the development of acute leukemia (31, 162). Although monocytosis is not apt to be a prominent feature of the collagen-vascular and inflammatory bowel diseases, the association in some patients is well described. It is quite clear that monocytosis may also be present without definable organic disease (136).

Summary

Proliferation of mononuclear leukocyte precursors in the bone marrow and of immature macrophages in the tissues may occur in response to a variety of stimuli. The proliferation results in cellular hyperplasia in reticuloendothelial organs with resultant organ enlargement. The stimuli may be conveniently divided into several categories: intracellular parasitic microorganisms; damaged cells, especially hematopoietic cells; certain heavy metals and organic compounds; and storage diseases, in which normal metabolites accumulate. Furthermore, histiocytic hyperplasia occurs in a variety of nonneoplastic diseases of uncertain etiology and in malignant diseases of the mononuclear leukocyte system.

Recently, monocyte dysfunction syndromes have been identified in several neoplastic and nonneoplastic disorders.

Chapter 26 References

1. Abul-Haj, S. K., Martz, D. G., Douglas, W. F., and Geppert, L. J. Farber's disease: report of a case with observations on its histogenesis and notes on the nature of stored material, *J. Pediatr.* 61:221, 1962.

2. Alarcón-Segovia, D., and Brown, A. L., Jr. Classification and etiologic aspects of necrotizing angiitides: an analytic approach to a confused subject with a critical review of the evidence for hypersensitivity in polyarteritis nodosa, *Mayo Clin. Proc.* 39:205, 1964.

3. Alekseeva, O. G. Ability of beryllium compounds to cause allergy of the delayed type, *Fed. Proc. Transpl.* 25:T843, 1966 (suppl.).

4. Allison, A. C., Harington, J. S., and Birbeck, M. An examination of the cytotoxic effects of silica on macrophages, *J. Exp. Med.* 124:141, 1966.

5. Allison, M. J., Zappasodi, P., and Lurie, M. B. Metabolic studies on mononuclear cells from rabbits of varying genetic resistance to tuberculosis. I. Studies on cells of normal noninfected animals, *Am. Rev. Respir. Dis.* 84:364, 1961.

6. Angevine, D. M., Hamilton, T. R., Wallace, F. G., and Hazard, J. B. Lymph nodes in leishmaniasis. Report on 2 cases, *Am. J. Med. Sci.* 210:33, 1945.

7. Armstrong, J. A., and D'Arcy Hart, P. Response of cultured macrophages to *Mycobacterium tuberculosis*, with observations on fusion of lysosomes with phagosomes, *J. Exp. Med.* 134:713, 1971.

8. Aschoff, L. Das reticulo-endotheliale System, *Ergeb. Inn. Med. Kinderheilkd.* 26:1, 1924.

9. Astaldi, G., Meardi, G., and Lisino, T. The iron content of jejunal mucosa obtained by Crosby's biopsy in hemochromatosis and hemosiderosis, *Blood* 28:70, 1966.

10. Avila, J. L., and Convit, J. Studies on cellular immunity in leprosy. I. Lysosomal enzymes, *Int. J. Lepr.* 38:359, 1970.

11. Axline, S. G. Isozymes of acid phosphatase in normal and Calmette-Guérin bacillus-induced rabbit alveolar macrophages, *J. Exp. Med.* 128:1031, 1968.

12. Baehner, R. L., and Johnston, R. B., Jr. Monocyte function in children with neutropenia and chronic infections, *Blood* 40:31, 1972.

13. Barbieri, T. A., and Correa, W. M. Human macrophage culture. The leprosy prognostic test (LPT), *Int. J. Lepr.* 35:377, 1967.

14. Beiguelman, B. Leprosy and genetics. A review of past research with remarks concerning future investigations, *Bull. W.H.O.* 37:461, 1967.

15. Bergmann, M., Flance, I. J., and Blumenthal, H. T. Thesaurosis following inhalation of hair spray. A clinical and experimental study, *N. Engl. J. Med.* 258:471, 1958.

16. Berry, C. L. The production of disseminated histoplasmosis in the mouse: the effects of changes in reticulo-endothelial function, *J. Pathol.* 97:441, 1969.

17. Bertino, J., and Myerson, R. M. The role of splenectomy in sarcoidosis, *Arch. Intern. Med.* 106:213, 1960.

18. Bessis, M. Cytology of the Blood and Blood-forming Organs, Grune & Stratton, New York, 1956.

19. Bessis, M., and Caroli, J. A comparative study of hemochromatosis by electron microscopy, *Gastroenterology* 37:538, 1959.

20. Block, M., Jacobson, L. O., and Bethard, W. F. Preleukemic acute human leukemia, *J.A.M.A.* 152:1018, 1953.

21. Blumberg, B. S., and Melartin, L. Conjectures on inherited susceptibility to lepromatous leprosy, *Int. J. Lepr.* 34:60, 1966.

22. Brady, R. O. Biochemical and metabolic basis of familial sphingolipidoses, *Semin. Hematol.* 9:273, 1972.

23. Brady, R. O., Kanfer, J. N., and Shapiro, D. Metabolism of glucocerebrosides. II. Evidence of an enzymatic deficiency in Gaucher's disease, *Biochem. Biophys. Res. Commun.* 18:221, 1965.

24. Bridges, R. A., Berendes, H., and Good, R. A. A fatal granulomatous disease of childhood. The clinical, pathological, and laboratory features of a new syndrome, *Am. J. Dis. Child.* 97:387, 1959.

25. Buchner, L. H., and Schneierson, S. S. Clinical and laboratory aspects of Listeria monocytogenes infections, with a report of ten cases, *Am. J. Med.* 45:904, 1968.

26. Buechner, H. A., Prevatt, A. L., Thompson, J., and Blitz, O. Bagassosis. A review, with further historical data studies of pulmonary function, and results of adrenal steroid therapy, *Am. J. Med.* 25:234, 1958.

27. Bullock, W. E. Depression of the delayed type allergic response by leprosy, *Clin. Res.* 14:337, 1966.

28. Carrington, C. B., and Leibow, A. A. Limited forms of angiitis and granulomatosis of Wegener's type, *Am. J. Med.* 41:497, 1966.

29. Carson, M. J., Chadwick, D. L., Brubaker, C. A., Cleland, R. S., and Landing, B. H. Thirteen boys with progressive septic granulomatosis, *Pediatrics* 35:405, 1965.

30. Cartwright, G. E., Chung, H-L., and Chang, A. Studies on the pancytopenia of Kala-Azar, *Blood* 3:249, 1948.

31. Cassileth, P. A. Monocytosis in chlorpromazine-associated agranulocytosis, *Am. J. Med.* 43:471, 1967.

32. Chapman, A. Z., Reeder, P. S., and Baker, L. A. Neutropenia secondary to tuberculous splenomegaly: report of a case, *Ann. Intern. Med.* 41:1225, 1954.

33. Chomet, B., LaPorte, J., and McGrew, E. A. Atypical monocytes in patients with malignant tumors, *Acta Cytol.* 10:197, 1966.

34. Churg, J. Allergic granulomatosis and granulomatous-vascular syndromes, *Ann. Allergy* 21:619, 1963.

35. Churg, J., and Strauss, L. Allergic granulomatosis, allergic angiitis and periarteritis nodosa, *Am. J. Pathol.* 27:277, 1951.

36. Clausen, K. P., and Von Haam, E. Fine structure of malignancy-associated changes (MAC) in peripheral blood human leukocytes, *Acta Cytol.* 13:435, 1969.

37. Cline, M. J. The hematologic manifestations of tuberculosis, *Calif. Med.* 106:215, 1967.

38. Cline, M. J. Bactericidal activity of human macrophages: analysis of factors influencing the killing of *Listeria monocytogenes*, *Infect. Immun.* 2:156, 1970.

39. Cline, M. J. Drug potentiation of macrophage function, *Infect. Immun.* 2:601, 1970.

40. Cline, M. J. Defective mononuclear phagocyte function in myelomonocytic leukemia and in some patients with lymphoma, *J. Clin. Invest.* 52:2185, 1973.

41. Cochrane, R. G. Leprosy in Theory and Practice, 2nd ed., John Wright and Sons, Bristol, England, 1959.

42. Cody, D. T. R., and Williams, H. L. Cogan's syndrome, *Laryngoscope* 70:447, 1960.

43. Cohen, A. B., and Cline, M. J. In vitro studies of the foamy macrophage of postobstructive endogenous lipoid pneumonia in man, *Ann. Rev. Respir. Dis.* 106:69, 1972.

44. Coppel, S., and Youmans, G. P. Specificity of the anamnestic response produced by *Listeria monocytogenes* or *Mycobacterium tuberculosis* to challenge with *Listeria monocytogenes*, *J. Bacteriol.* 97:127, 1969.

45. Crawford, W. J. Cogan's syndrome associated with polyarteritis nodosa. A report of three cases, *Pa. Med. J.* 60:835, 1957.

46. Crocker, A. C., and Farber, S. Niemann-Pick disease: a review of eighteen patients, *Medicine* 37:1, 1958.

47. Crocker, A. C., and Landing, B. H. Phosphatase studies in Gaucher's disease, *Metabolism* 9:341, 1960.

48. Crosby, W. H. The control of iron balance by the intestinal mucosa, *Blood* 22:441, 1963.

49. Curran, R. C., and Ager, J. A. M. The diffusion chamber in experimental silicosis, *J. Pathol. Bacteriol.* 83:1, 1962.

50. Curtis, A. C., and Grekin, J. N. Histoplasmosis. A review of the cutaneous and adjacent mucous membrane manifestations with a report of three cases, *J.A.M.A.* 134:1217, 1947.

51. Daland, G. A., Gottlieb, L., Wallerstein, R. O., and Castle, W. B. Hematologic observations in bacterial endocarditis. Especially the prevalence of histiocytes and the elevation and variation of the white cell count in blood from the ear lobe, *J. Lab. Clin. Med.* 48:827, 1956.

52. Dameshek, W. The appearance of histiocytes in the peripheral blood, *Arch. Intern. Med.* 47:968, 1931.

53. Dannenberg, A. Cellular hypersensitivity and cellular immunity in the pathogenesis of tuberculosis: specificity, systemic and local nature, and associated macrophage enzymes, *Bacteriol. Rev.* 32:85, 1968.

54. Dannenberg, A. M., Jr., Roessler, W. G., Meyer, O. T., et al. Radiation, infection, and macrophage function. III. Recovery from the effects of radiation illustrated by dermal BCG lesions; resistance of pulmonary alveolar macrophages to radiation illustrated by tuberculosis produced by the airborne route, *J. Reticuloendothel. Soc.* 7:91, 1970.

55. D'Arcy Hart, P., and Rees, R. J. W. Lepromin and Kveim antigen reactivity in man, and their relation to tuberculin reactivity, *Br. Med. Bull.* 23:80, 1967.

56. Davis, W. C., Huber, H., Douglas, S. D., and Fudenberg, H. H. A defect in circulating mononuclear phagocytes in chronic granulomatous disease of childhood, *J. Immunol.* 101:1093, 1968.

57. De, M. N., and Tribedi, B. P. The pathogenesis of the commoner type of splenomegaly met with in India, *Indian Med. Gaz.* 74:9, 1939.

58. DeMarsh, Q. B., and Kautz, J. The submicroscopic morphology of Gaucher cells, *Blood* 12:324, 1957.

59. Dickie, H. A., and Rankin, J. Farmer's lung. An acute granulomatous interstitial pneumonitis occurring in agricultural workers, *J.A.M.A.* 167:1069, 1958.

60. Dierks, R. E., and Shepard, C. C. Effect of phytohemagglutinin and various mycobacterial antigens on lymphocyte cultures from leprosy patients, *Proc. Soc. Exp. Biol. Med.* 127:391, 1968.

61. Doan, C. A., and Wiseman, B. K. The monocyte, monocytosis and monocytic leukosis: a clinical and pathological study, *Ann. Intern. Med.* 8:383, 1934.

62. Dosik, H., Rosner, F., and Sawitsky, A. Acquired lipoidosis: Gaucher-like cells and "blue cells" in chronic granulocytic leukemia, *Semin. Hematol.* 9:309, 1972.

63. Drutz, D., Cline, M. J., and Levy, L. Leukocyte antimicrobial function in patients with leprosy, *J. Clin. Invest.* 53:380, 1974.

64. Dubos, R. J., and Dubos, J. The White Plague, Little, Brown and Co., Boston, 1952.

65. Emmanuel, D. A., Lawton, B. R., and Wenzel, F. J. Maple bark disease. Pneumonitis due to *Coniosporium corticale*, *N. Engl. J. Med.* 266:333, 1962.

66. Engelbreth-Holm, J. A study of tuberculous splenomegaly and splenogenic controlling of the cell emission from the bone marrow, *Am. J. Med. Sci.* 195:32, 1938.

67. Epstein, W. L. Granulomatous hypersensitivity, *Prog. Allergy* 11:36, 1967.

68. Epstein, W. L., Skahen, J. R., and Krasnobrod, H. The organized epithelioid cell granuloma: differentiation of allergic (zirconium) from colloidal (silica) types, *Am. J. Pathol.* 43:391, 1963.

69. Evans, H. E., and Edgecomb, J. H. Unexplained granulomatosis in childhood. A clinicopathological dilemma, *Arch. Pathol.* 74:360, 1962.

70. Fahey, J. L., Leonard, E., Churg, J., and Godman, G. Wegener's granulomatosis, *Am. J. Med.* 17:168, 1954.

71. Farber, S., Cohen, J., and Uzman, L. L. Lipogranulomatosis: a new lipo-glyco-protein "storage" disease, *J. Mount Sinai Hosp.* 24:816, 1957.

72. Feldman, H. A. Toxoplasmosis, *N. Engl. J. Med.* 279:1370, 1431; 1968.

73. Felty, A. R. Chronic arthritis in the adult, associated with splenomegaly and leucopenia. A report of five cases of an unusual clinical syndrome, *Bull. Johns Hopkins Hosp.* 35:16, 1924.

74. Fisher, E. R., and Reidbord, H. Gaucher's disease: pathogenetic considerations based on electron microscopic and histochemical observations, *Am. J. Pathol.* 41:679, 1962.

75. Fraccaro, M., Magrini, U., Scappaticci, S., and Zacchellos, F. *In vitro* culture of spleen cells from a case of Gaucher's disease, *Ann. Hum. Genet.* 32:209, 1968.

76. Gardner, L. U. The similarity of the lesions produced by silica and by the tubercle bacillus, *Am. J. Pathol.* 13:13, 1937.

77. Garvin, R. O., and Bargen, J. A. The hematologic picture of chronic ulcerative colitis: its relation to prog-

nosis and treatment, *Am. J. Med. Sci.* 193:744, 1937.

78. Gelin, G. Les splénomégalies tuberculeuses, *Sang* 25:172, 1954.

79. Gill, F. A., Kaye, D., and Hook, E. W. The influence of erythrophagocytosis on the interaction of macrophages and Salmonella in vitro, *J. Exp. Med.* 124:173, 1966.

80. Godman, G. C., and Churg, J. Wegener's granulomatosis, *Arch. Pathol.* 58:533, 1954.

81. Goihman-Yahr, M., Raffel, S., and Ferraresi, R. W. Delayed hypersensitivity in relation to suppression of growth of *Listeria monocytogenes* by guinea pig macrophages, *J. Bacteriol.* 100:635, 1969.

82. Goltz, R. W., and Laymon, C. W. Multicentric reticulohistiocytosis of the skin and synovia. Reticulohistiocytoma or ganglioneuroma, *Arch. Dermatol. Syph.* 69:717, 1954.

83. Gray, M. L., and Killinger, A. H. Listeria monocytogenes and listeric infections, *Bact. Rev.* 30:309, 1966.

84. Green, R. A., and Fromke, V. L. Splenectomy in Felty's syndrome, *Ann. Intern. Med.* 64:1265, 1966.

85. Gross, P. Pathology of pneumoconioses, *in* A. J. Lanza (ed.), The Pneumoconioses, p. 34, Grune & Stratton, New York, 1963.

86. Guinto, R. S., and Mabalay, M. C. A note on the tuberculin reaction in leprosy, *Int. J. Lepr.* 30:278, 1962.

87. Haas, H. G., and Koller, F. Kernveränderungen der Monocyten bei malignen Tumoren, *Schweiz. Med. Wochenschr.* 92:1354, 1962.

88. Ham, T. H., Weisman, R., Jr., and Hinz, C. F., Jr. Mechanisms of destruction of red cells in certain hemolytic conditions, *Arch. Intern. Med.* 98:574, 1956.

89. Hanifin, J. M., Epstein, W. L., and Cline, M. J. *In vitro* studies of granulomatous hypersentivity to beryllium, *J. Invest. Dermatol.* 55:284, 1970.

90. Hard, G. C. Some biochemical aspects of the immune macrophage, *Br. J. Exp. Pathol.* 51:97, 1970.

91. Hardy, H. L., and Tabershaw, I. R. Delayed chemical pneumonitis occurring in workers exposed to beryllium compounds, *J. Indust. Hyg. Toxicol.* 28:197, 1964.

92. Hickling, R. A. The monocytes in pneumonia: a clinical and hematologic study, *Arch. Intern. Med.* 40:594, 1927.

93. Hill, R. W., and Bayrd, E. D. Phagocytic reticuloendothelial cells in subacute bacterial endocarditis with negative cultures, *Ann. Intern. Med.* 52:310, 1960.

94. Holland, P., Hug, G., and Schubert, W. K. Chronic reticuloendothelial cell storage disease, *Am. J. Dis. Child.* 110:117, 1965.

95. Hollander, D., and Manning, R. T. The use of alkylating agents in the treatment of Wegener's granulomatosis, *Ann. Intern. Med.* 67:393, 1967.

96. Jacobs, H. S., MacDonald, R. A., and Jandl, J. H. Regulation of spleen growth and sequestering function, *J. Clin. Invest.* 42:1476, 1963.

97. Jandl, J. H. (ed.), Symposium on disorders of the red cell: the pathophysiology of hemolytic anemias, *Am. J. Med.* 41:657, 1966.

98. Jandl, J. H., Files, N. M., Barnett, S. B., and MacDonald, R. A. Proliferative response of the spleen and liver to hemolysis, *J. Exp. Med.* 122:299, 1965.

99. Johnson, D. E., Griep, J. A., and Baehner, R. L. Histiocytic leukemia following lifelong infection and thrombocytopenia: histologic, metabolic, and bactericidal studies, *J. Pediatr.* 82:664, 1973.

100. Johnson, M. L., and Colley, E. W. *Listeria monocytogenes* encephalitis associated with corticosteroid therapy, *J. Clin. Pathol.* 22:465, 1969.

101. Jordan, S. W. Electron microscopy of Gaucher cells, *Exp. Mol. Pathol.* 3:76, 1964.

102. Kalderon, A. E., Kikkawa, Y., and Bernstein, J. Chronic toxoplasmosis associated with severe hemolytic anemia. Case report and electron microscopic studies, *Arch. Intern. Med.* 114:95, 1964.

103. Kambara, T., Chandrasekhar, S., Dannenberg, A. M., Jr., et al. Radiation, infection, and macrophage function. I. Effects of whole body radiation on dermal tuberculous lesions in rabbits: development, histology, and histochemistry, *J. Reticuloendothel. Soc.* 7:53, 1970.

104. Kanof, A., Aronson, S. M., and Volk, B. W. Clinical progression of amaurotic familial idiocy. Anthropometric studies, *Am. J. Dis. Child.* 97:656, 1959.

105. Kaplan, H. S. Long-term results of palliative and radical radiotherapy of Hodgkin's disease, *Cancer Res.* 26:1250, 1966.

106. Kato, K. Leucocytes in infancy and childhood. A statistical analysis of 1,081 total and differential counts from birth to 15 years, *J. Pediatr.* 7:7, 1935.

107. Kattlove, H. E., Williams, J. C., Gaynor, E., et al. Gaucher cells in chronic myelocytic leukemia: an acquired abnormality, *Blood* 33:379, 1969.

108. Kessel, R. W. I., Monaco, L., and Marchisio, M. A. The specificity of the cytotoxic action of silica—a study *in vitro*, *Br. J. Exp. Pathol.* 44:351, 1963.

109. Khanolkar, V. R. Pathology of leprosy, *in* R. G. Cochrane (ed.), Leprosy in Theory and Practice, p. 78, John Wright and Sons, Bristol, England, 1959.

110. Khoo, K. K., and Mackaness, G. B. Macrophage proliferation in relation to acquired cellular resistance, *Aust. J. Exp. Biol. Med. Sci.* 42:707, 1964.

111. Kinney, V. R., Olsen, A. M., Hepper, N. G. G., and Harrison, E. G., Jr. Wegener's granulomatosis. Report of two cases and brief review, *Arch. Intern. Med.* 108:269, 1961.

112. Kobayashi, M., Stahmann, M. A., Rankin, J., and Dickie, H. A. Antigens in moldy hay as the cause of farmer's lung, *Proc. Soc. Exp. Biol. Med.* 113:472, 1963.

113. Krahenbuhl, J. L., and Remington, J. S. In vitro induction of nonspecific resistance in macrophages by specifically sensitized lymphocytes, *Infect. Immun.* 4:337, 1971.

114. Leavell, B. S., and Thorup, O. A., Jr. Fundamentals of Clinical Hematology, p. 503, W. B. Saunders Co., Philadelphia, 1960.

115. Lee, R. E., Balcerzak, S. P., and Westerman, M. P. Gaucher's disease. A morphologic study and measurements of iron metabolism, *Am. J. Med.* 42:891, 1967.

116. Lehrer, R. I., and Cline, M. J. Leu-

kocyte candidacidal activity and resistance to systemic candidiasis in patients with cancer, *Cancer* 27:1211, 1971.

117. Lester, R., Hill, M. W., and Bangham, A. D. Molecular mechanism of Tay-Sachs disease, *Nature* 236:32, 1972.

118. Levinson, B., Walter, B. A., Wintrobe, M. M., and Cartwright, G. E. A clinical study in Hodgkin's disease, *Arch. Intern. Med.* 99:519, 1957.

119. Lewis, M. R. The formation of macrophages, epithelioid cells and giant cells from leucocytes in incubated blood, *Am. J. Pathol.* 1:91, 1925.

120. Lewis, M. R., and Lewis, W. H. Transformation of mononuclear blood-cells into macrophages, epithelioid cells, and giant cells in hanging-drop blood-cultures from lower vertebrates, Carnegie Inst. Wash. Publ. 96, *Contrib. Embryol.* 18:95, 1926.

121. Lipson, R. L., Bayrd, E. D., and Watkins, C. H. The postsplenectomy blood picture, *Am. J. Clin. Pathol.* 32:526, 1959.

122. Littman, M. L., and Walter, J. E. Cryptococcosis: current status, *Am. J. Med.* 45:922, 1968.

123. Lockie, L. M., Sanes, S., and Vaughn, S. L. Chronic arthritis; associated with neutrophilic leukopenia, splenomegaly and hepatomegaly, *Am. J. Clin. Pathol.* 12:372, 1942.

124. Longcope, W. T., and Freiman, D. G. A study of sarcoidosis. Based on a combined investigation of 160 cases including 30 autopsies from the Johns Hopkins Hospital and Massachusetts General Hospital, *Medicine* 31:1, 1952.

125. Lorber, M. The occurrence of intracellular iron in Gaucher's disease, *Ann. Intern. Med.* 53:293, 1960.

126. Lorber, M. Adult-type Gaucher's disease: a secondary disorder of iron metabolism, *J. Mount Sinai Hosp.* 37:404, 1970.

127. Louria, D. B., Hensle, T., Armstrong, D., Collins, H. S., Blevins, A., Krugman, D., and Buse, M. Listeriosis complicating malignant disease. A new association, *Ann. Intern. Med.* 67:261, 1967.

128. Lubaroff, D. M., and Waksman, B. H. Bone marrow as source of cells in reactions of cellular hypersensitivity. II. Identification of allogeneic or hybrid cells by immunofluorescence in passively transferred tuberculin reactions, *J. Exp. Med.* 128:1437, 1968.

129. Lurie, M. B. Resistance to Tuberculosis: Experimental Studies in Native and Acquired Defensive Mechanisms, Harvard University Press, Cambridge, Mass., 1964.

130. Lurie, M. B., Zappasodi, P., Dannenberg, A. M., Jr., and Cardona-Lynch, E. The effect of cortisone and ACTH on the pathogenesis of tuberculosis, *Ann. N.Y. Acad. Sci.* 56:779, 1953.

131. MacCallum, D. K. Time sequence study on the hepatic system of macrophages in malaria-infected hamsters, *J. Reticuloendothel. Soc.* 6:232, 1969.

132. McCusker, J. J., and Parsons, D. B. Niemann-Pick disease. Report of two cases in siblings including necropsy and histochemical findings in one, *Arch. Pathol.* 74:127, 1962.

133. Mackaness, G. B. The immunological basis of acquired cellular resistance, *J. Exp. Med.* 120:105, 1964.

134. Mackaness, G. B. The immunology of antituberculous immunity (editorial), *Am. Rev. Respir. Dis.* 97:337, 1968.

135. Mackaness, G. B. Resistance to intracellular infection, *J. Infect. Dis.* 123:439, 1971.

136. Maldonado, J. E., and Hanlon, D. G. Monocytosis: a current appraisal, *Mayo Clin. Proc.* 40:248, 1965.

137. Malinin, T. I. Unidentified reticuloendothelial cell storage disease, *Blood* 17:675, 1961.

138. Maranoff, R., Fite, F. K., and Frumin, A. M. Greenish-blue granular marrow histiocytes associated with low serum cholesterol, *Am. J. Clin. Pathol.* 57:103, 1972.

139. Marsden, P. D., Hutt, M. S. R., Wilks, N. E., Voller, A., Blackman, V., Shah, K. K., Connor, D. H., Hamilton, P. J. S., Banwell, J. G., and Lunn, H. F. An investigation of tropical splenomegaly at Mulago Hospital, Kampala, Uganda, *Br. Med. J.* 1:89, 1965.

140. Marshall, A. H. E. An Outline of the Cytology and Pathology of the Reticular Tissue, Oliver and Boyd, London, 1956.

141. Mason, D. T., and Morris, J. J., Jr. The variable features of Felty's syndrome. Review of the literature, and report of a case with massive splenomegaly, *Am. J. Med.* 36:463, 1964.

142. Mattson, J. C., and Von Haam, E. The presence of "malignancy-associated changes" in the monocytes of the peripheral blood of cancer patients, *Acta Cytol.* 11:308, 1967.

143. Maximow, A. A. The macrophages or histiocytes, *in* E. V. Cowdry (ed.), Special Cytology: The Form and Functions of the Cell in Health and Disease, 2nd ed., vol. 2, p. 711, Paul B. Hoeber, New York, 1932.

144. Meacham, G. C., and Weisberger, A. S. Early atypical manifestations of leukemia, *Ann. Intern. Med.* 41:780, 1954.

145. Mealey, J. Turnover of carrier-free zirconium-89 in man, *Nature* 179:673, 1957.

146. Mercer, S. T. Preliminary observations on human blood in early syphilis by the supravital method, *Proc. Soc. Exp. Biol. Med.* 28:1033, 1931.

147. Merkow, L., Pardo, M., Epstein, S. M., Verney, E., and Sidransky, H. Lysosomal stability during phagocytosis of Aspergillus flavus spores by alveolar macrophages of cortisone-treated mice, *Science* 160:79, 1968.

148. Miale, J. B. Laboratory Medicine—Hematology, 2nd ed., p. 600, C. V. Mosby Co., St. Louis, 1962.

149. Miller, J. K., and Hedberg, M. Effects of cortisone on susceptibility of mice to *Listeria monocytogenes*, *Am. J. Clin. Pathol.* 43:248, 1965.

150. Mooney, J. J., and Waksman, B. H. Activation of normal rabbit macrophage monolayers by supernatants of antigen-stimulated lymphocytes, *J. Immunol.* 105:1138, 1970.

151. Munger, M., and Huddleson, I. F. A preliminary report of the blood picture in brucellosis, *J. Lab. Clin. Med.* 24:617, 1939.

152. Murray, E. G. D., Webb, R. A., and Swann, M. B. R. Disease of rabbits characterized by a large mononu-

clear leucocytosis. Caused by a hitherto undescribed bacillus bacterium monocytogenes, *J. Pathol. Bacteriol.* 29:407, 1926.

153. Nash, T., Allison, A. C., and Harington, J. S. Physico-chemical properties of silica in relation to its toxicity, *Nature* 210:259, 1966.

154. Newell, K. W. An epidemiologist's view of leprosy, *Bull. W.H.O.* 34:827, 1966.

155. Nieburgs, H. E., et al. Systemic cellular changes in material from human and animal tissues in the presence of tumors, Trans. 7th Ann. Mtg., Intersoc. Cytol. Council, p. 137, 1959.

156. Nieburgs, H. E., Herman, B. E., and Reisman, H. Buccal cell changes in patients with malignant tumors, *Lab. Invest.* 11:80, 1962.

157. Norris, G. F., and Peard, M. C. Berylliosis: report of two cases, with special reference to the patch test, *Br. Med. J.* 1:378, 1963.

158. Parish, W. E., and Pepys, J. Allergic reactions in the lung, *in* P. G. H. Gell and R. R. A. Coombs (eds.), Clinical Aspects of Immunology, p. 390, Blackwell Scientific Publications, Oxford, 1963.

159. Paulley, J. W., and Hughes, J. P. Giant-cell arteritis or arteritis of the aged, *Br. Med. J.* 3:1562, 1960.

160. Pennelli, N., Scaravilli, F., and Zacchello, F. The morphogenesis of Gaucher cells investigated by electron microscopy, *Blood* 34:331, 1969.

161. Philippart, M., and Menkes, J. Isolation and characterization of the main splenic glycolipids in Gaucher's disease. Evidence for the site of metabolic block, *Biochem. Biophys. Res. Commun.* 15:551, 1964.

162. Pretlow, T. G. II. Chronic monocytic dyscrasia culminating in acute leukemia, *Am. J. Med.* 46:130, 1969.

163. Ptak, W., Gaugas, J. M., Rees, R. J., et al. Immune responses in mice with murine leprosy, *Clin. Exp. Immunol.* 6:117, 1970.

164. Rausen, A. R., and Adlersberg, D. Idiopathic (hereditary) hyperlipemia and hypercholesteremia in children, *Pediatrics* 28:276, 1961.

165. Reed, C. E., Sosman, A., and Barbee, R. A. Pigeon-breeder's lung.

A newly observed interstitial pulmonary disease, *J.A.M.A.* 193:261, 1965.

166. Rees, R. J. W. The significance of the lepromin reaction in man, *Prog. Allergy* 8:224, 1964.

167. Rees, R. J. W., Chatterjee, K. R., Pepys, J., and Tee, R. D. Antigen studies of other fungi and *Mycobacterium leprae*. Some immunologic aspects of leprosy, *Am. Rev. Respir. Dis.* 92:139, 1965 (suppl.).

168. Remington, J. S., Barnett, C. G., Meikel, M., and Lunde, M. N. Toxoplasmosis and infectious mononucleosis, *Arch. Intern. Med.* 110:744, 1962.

169. Reznikoff, P. The etiologic importance of fatigue and the prognostic significance of monocytosis in neutropenia (agranulocytosis), *Am. J. Med. Sci.* 195:627, 1938.

170. Riley, J. A., and Robins, G. M. Leukemoid reaction due to mixed malaria infection. Report of a case, *Blood* 4:283, 1949.

171. Rodey, G. E., Park, B. H., Windhorst, D. B., and Good, R. A. Defective bactericidal activity of monocytes in fatal granulomatous disease, *Blood* 33:813, 1969.

172. Rodríguez-Molina, F., and Pons, J. A. Hematological studies on Schistosomiasis Mansoni in Puerto Rico, *Puerto Rico J. Public Health Trop. Med.* 11:369, 1936.

173. Rosengarten, R., and Bourn, J. M. Listeria septicemia and meningitis in a case of lupus erythematosus, *Neurology* 9:704, 1959.

174. Rosenthal, N., and Abel, H. A. The significance of the monocytes in agranulocytosis (leukopenic infectious monocytosis), *Am. J. Clin. Pathol.* 6:205, 1936.

175. Rous, P. Urinary siderosis. Hemosiderin granules in urine as aid in the diagnosis of pernicious anemia, hemochromatosis and other diseases causing siderosis of kidney, *J. Exp. Med.* 28:645, 1918.

176. Ruskin, J., McIntosh, J., and Remington, J. S. Studies on the mechanisms of resistance to phylogenetically diverse intracellular organisms, *J. Immunol.* 103:252, 1969.

177. Ruskin, J., and Remington, J. S. Role for the macrophage in acquired immunity to phylogenet-

ically unrelated intracellular organisms, *Antimicrob. Agents Chemother.*, p. 474, 1969.

178. Russell, R. W. R. Muscular involvement in giant-cell arteritis, *Ann. Rheum. Dis.* 21:171, 1962.

179. Rywlin, A. M., Lopez-Gomez, A., Tachmes, P., and Pardo, V. Ceroid histiocytosis of the spleen in hyperlipemia, relationship to the syndrome of the sea-blue histiocyte, *Am. J. Clin. Pathol.* 56:572, 1971.

180. Sawitsky, A., Hyman, G. A., and Hyman, J. B. An unidentified reticuloendothelial cell in bone marrow and spleen. Report of two cases with histochemical studies, *Blood* 9:977, 1954.

181. Sawitsky, A., Rosner, F., and Chodsky, S. The sea-blue histiocyte syndrome, a review: genetic and biochemical studies, *Semin. Hematol.* 9:285, 1972.

182. Schepers, G. W. H. Theories of the causes of silicosis—Parts I, II, and III, *Ind. Med. Surg.* 29:326, 359, 434; 1960.

183. Schulze, M. L., Wahle, G. H., and White, J. B. Meningitis due to Listeria monocytogenes in a case of disseminated lupus erythematosus, *Am. J. Clin. Pathol.* 23:1028, 1953.

184. Sharar, A. Some aspects of the defense mechanism against Cryptococcus neoformans, *G. Accad. Med. Torino* 81:140, 1968.

185. Sharar, A., Kletter, Y., and Aronson, M. Granuloma formation in cryptococcosis, *Isr. J. Med. Sci.* 5:1164, 1969.

186. Sheagren, J. W., Block, J. B., Trautman, J. R., and Wolff, S. M. Immunologic reactivity in leprosy, *Clin. Res.* 15:300, 1967.

187. Sheard, C., Jr., Cormia, F. E., Atkinson, S. C., and Worthington, E. L. Granulomatous reactions to deodorant sticks, *J.A.M.A.* 164:1085, 1957.

188. Sheldon, J. H. Haemochromatosis, Oxford University Press, London, 1935.

189. Shelley, W. B., and Hurley, H. J. The pathogenesis of silica granulomas in man: a non-allergic colloidal phenomenon, *J. Invest. Dermatol.* 34:107, 1960.

190. Sidransky, H., Verney, E., and Beede, H. Experimental pulmonary

aspergillosis, *Arch. Pathol.* 79:299, 1965.

191. Silverstein, M. N., and Ellefson, R. D. The syndrome of the sea-blue histiocyte, *Semin. Hematol.* 9:299, 1972.

192. Silverstein, M. N., Ellefson, R. D., and Ahern, E. J. The syndrome of the sea-blue histiocyte, *N. Engl. J. Med.* 282:1, 1970.

193. Silverstein, M. N., Young, D. G., ReMine, W. H., and Pease, G. L. Splenomegaly with rare morphologically distinct histiocyte. A syndrome, *Arch. Intern. Med.* 114:251, 1964.

194. Simson, F. W., and Barnetson, J. Histoplasmosis: report of a case, *J. Pathol. Bacteriol* 54:299, 1942.

195. Sinn, C. M., and Dick, F. W. Monocytic leukemia, *Am. J. Med.* 20:588, 1956.

196. Sokolov, R. A., Rachmaninoff, N., and Kaine, H. D. Allergic granulomatosis, *Am. J. Med.* 32:131, 1962.

197. Sterner, J. H., and Eisenbud, M. Epidemiology of beryllium intoxication, *Arch. Ind. Hyg.* 4:123, 1951.

198. Stone, G. E., and Redmond, A. J. Leukopenic infectious monocytosis. Report of a case closely simulating acute monocytic leukemia, *Am. J. Med.* 34:541, 1963.

199. Sturgis, C. C. Hematology, 2nd ed., p. 1222, Charles C Thomas, Springfield, Ill., 1955.

200. Sundberg, R. D., and Spink, W. W. The histopathology of lesions in the bone marrow of patients having active brucellosis, *Blood* 1:7, 1947 (suppl.).

201. Suomi, W. D., and Agranoff, B. W. Lipids of the spleen in Gaucher's disease, *J. Lipid Res.* 6:211, 1965.

202. Suter, E. Multiplication of tubercle bacilli within mononuclear phagocytes in tissue cultures derived from normal animals and animals vaccinated with BCG, *J. Exp. Med.* 97:235, 1953.

203. Thannhauser, S. J. Lipidoses: Diseases of the Intracellular Lipid Metabolism, 3rd ed., Grune & Stratton, New York, 1958.

204. Thirayothin, P., and Crosby, W. H. Distribution of iron injected intraperitoneally. Evidence of serosal "absorption" by the small intestine, *J. Clin. Invest.* 41:1206, 1962.

205. Thomas, C. C. Sarcoidosis, *Arch. Dermatol. Syph.* 47:58, 1943.

206. Trubowitz, S., and Masek, B. A histochemical study of the reticuloendothelial system of human marrow—its possible transport role, *Blood* 32:610, 1968.

207. Turk, J. L., and Waters, M. F. R. Immunological basis for depression of cellular immunity and the delayed allergic response in patients with lepromatous leprosy, *Lancet* ii:436, 1968.

208. Van Den Ende, M., Harries, E. H. R., Stuart-Harris, C. H., Steigman, A. J., and Cruickshank, R. Laboratory infection with murine typhus, *Lancet* i:328, 1943.

209. van Furth, R., and Cohn, Z. A. The origin and kinetics of mononuclear phagocytes, *J. Exp. Med.* 128:415, 1968.

210. Vietzke, W. M., Gelderman, A. H., Grimley, P. M., et al. Toxoplasmosis complicating malignancy. Experience at the National Cancer Institute, *Cancer* 21:816, 1968.

211. Vigliani, E. C., and Pernis, B. An immunological approach to silicosis, *J. Occup. Med.* 1:319, 1959.

212. Virolainen, M. Hematopoietic origin of macrophages as studied by chromosome markers in mice, *J. Exp. Med.* 127:943, 1968.

213. Volk, B. W., Adachi, M., and Schneck, L. The pathology of sphingolipidoses, *Semin. Hematol.* 9:317, 1972.

214. Volk, B. W., and Wallace, B. J. The liver and lipoidosis. An electron microscopic and histochemical study, *Am. J. Pathol.* 49:203, 1966.

215. Volkman, A. The origin and turnover of mononuclear cells in peritoneal exudates in rats, *J. Exp. Med.* 124:241, 1966.

216. Volkman, A., and Collins, F. M. Recovery of delayed-type hypersensitivity in mice following suppressive doses of X-radiation, *J. Immunol.* 101:846, 1968.

217. Volkman, A., and Gowans, J. L. The production of macrophages in the rat, *Br. J. Exp. Pathol.* 46:50, 1965.

218. Waldorf, D. S., Sheagren, J. N., Trautman, J. R., and Block, J. B. Impaired delayed hypersensitivity in patients with lepromatous leprosy, *Lancet* ii:773, 1966.

219. Weber, H. H., and Engelhardt, W. E. Untersuchung von Stauben aus der Berylliumgewinnung, *Zentralbl. Geweberhyg. Unfall.* 10:41, 1933.

220. Weber, L., Neuhauser, I., Rubin, L., Slepyan, A. H., and Shellow, H. Granuloma of axillas, *J.A.M.A.* 162:65, 1956.

221. Wennberg, E., and Weiss, L. Splenomegaly and hemolytic anemia induced in rats by methylcellulose—an electron microscopic study, *J. Morphol.* 122:35, 1967.

222. Whitby, L. E. H., and Britton, C. J. C. Disorders of the blood: diagnosis, pathology, treatment, technique, 7th ed., p. 421, Grune & Stratton, New York, 1953.

223. Wile, U. J., Isaacs, R., and Knerler, C. W. The blood cells in early syphilis, *Am. J. Syph. Gonor. Ven. Dis.* 25:133, 1941.

224. Williams, H. L. Lethal granulomatous ulceration involving midline facial tissues, *Ann. Otol. Rhinol. Laryngol.* 58:1013, 1949.

225. Williams, W. J. A histological study of the lungs of 52 cases of chronic beryllium disease, *Br. J. Ind. Med.* 15:84, 1958.

226. Wintrobe, M. M. Clinical Hematology, 5th ed., p. 1186, Lea & Febiger, Philadelphia, 1961.

227. Wintrobe, M. M. Clinical Hematology, 6th ed., p. 1157, Lea & Febiger, Philadelphia, 1967.

228. Wiseman, B. K. The blood pictures in the primary diseases of the lymphatic systems: their character and significance, *J.A.M.A.* 107:2016, 1936.

229. Witts, L. J., and Webb, R. A. The monocytes of the rabbit in B. monocytogenes infection: a study of their staining reactions and histogenesis, *J. Pathol. Bacteriol.* 30:687, 1927.

230. Yam, L. T., Finkel, H. E., Weintraub, L. R., and Crosby, W. H. Circulating iron-containing macrophages in hemochromatosis, *N. Engl. J. Med.* 279:512, 1968.

231. Young, L. E., Izzo, M. J., and Platzer, R. F. Hereditary spherocytosis. I. Clinical, hematologic and genetic features in 28 cases, with particular reference to the somatic and mechanical fragility of incubated erythrocytes, *Blood* 6:1073, 1951.

232. Zinkham, W. H., and Diamond, L. K. In vitro erythrophagocytosis in acquired hemolytic anemia, *Blood* 7:592, 1952.

Chapter 27 Monocytic Leukemia and the Malignant Histiocytic Disorders

Considerable confusion exists in the clinical and pathological literature regarding the nosology of the various histiocytic malignancies. Uncertainties in classification result from the overlapping of clinical syndromes and the inadequacy of histology in defining the proliferative and functional capacity of early cells of the monocyte-macrophage (histiocytic) series. These disorders are most easily distinguished at the extremes of the clinical and cytological spectrum. For example, acute monocytic leukemia with monoblasts and immature mononuclear cells in peripheral blood is readily differentiated from multifocal eosinophilic granuloma of bone with its characteristic clinical and cytological picture. It is in the intermediate, or "mixed," forms of these diseases that diagnostic difficulties arise.

Classification of the Malignant Histiocytic Disorders

The histiocytic disorders have been classified largely on the basis of histopathology and clinical manifestations. It is now possible to construct a classification of the malignant histiocytoses based on current knowledge of cell biology relative to the morphogenesis and functional capacity of cells of the histiocytic series. One such classification is illustrated in Fig. 27.1 and Table 27.1.

The histiocytic cell series may be viewed as a continuum of progressively more mature cells, which begins with progenitors in the bone marrow (monoblasts and promonocytes) and culminates in the mature tissue macrophage. The blood monocyte is an intermediate cell between the bone marrow precursor and the tissue macro-phage (see Chapter 23). Macrophages may be further subdivided into immature A macrophages, which have loose nuclear chromatin and basophilic cytoplasm, and mature B macrophages, with dense chromatin and acidophilic cytoplasm (35). This distinction is important because the A macrophage retains proliferative capacity, whereas the B macrophage is generally a terminal, nonreplicating cell. Both mature and immature macrophages may assume a variety of morphologic forms, including those of the peritoneal macrophage, the alveolar macrophage, the giant cell of granulomata, and probably the Kupffer cell of the liver.

Coincident with morphologic maturation there is a progressive expression of functional characteristics (33-35, 38, 182). Functional attributes that develop with maturation include phagocytic ability, adhesiveness to a charged surface, the presence on the cell surface of receptors for IgG immunoglobulins and immunoglobulin complexes, and interaction with lymphocytes in antigen processing (see Chapters 24 and 25). The cellular content of lysosomal enzymes also changes with maturation.

The reticulum cell is another component of the reticuloendothelial system. We are uncertain about the maturational sequence and morphogenesis of reticulum cells, and we do not know the exact relation between cells of this type and those of the monocyte-macrophage series. Cells identified as mature reticulum cells do, however, resemble the macrophage in having acid phosphatase and esterase activity. They may be phagocytic, but less avidly than macrophages. Normal reticulum cells are rarely ob-

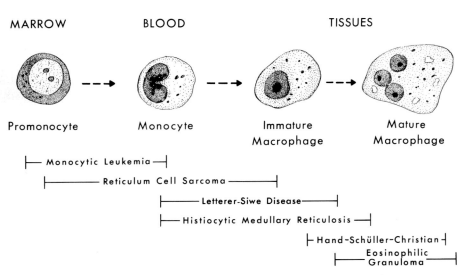

MARROW   BLOOD   TISSUES

Promonocyte   Monocyte   Immature   Mature
                                          Macrophage   Macrophage

├── Monocytic Leukemia ──┤
├──── Reticulum Cell Sarcoma ────────┤
            ├──── Letterer-Siwe Disease────┤
            ├── Histiocytic Medullary Reticulosis ──┤
                              ├─ Hand-Schüller-Christian ┤
                                      Eosinophilic
                              ├───── Granuloma ──────┤

Figure 27.1 A classification of the malignant histiocytic disorders based on mononuclear leukocyte differentiation. The least differentiated cells and the clinically acute diseases are on the left of the figure. (From M. J. Cline and D. W. Golde, *Am. J. Med.* 55:49, 1973. Reprinted by permission of authors and publisher.)

served in mitosis. The origin of the reticulin network, a distinctive feature of some histiocytic malignancies, is unclear. Reticulin is considered to be a collagen precursor and is thought to arise from fibroblasts. Reticulin associated with malignancies may therefore represent a stroma formed by nonneoplastic cell elements or may in-

Table 27.1 Correlation between differentiation of proliferating cells and clinical syndrome in malignant histiocytic disorders.

Predominant cell	Clinical disorder
Diseases with little or variable cellular differentiation	
Monoblast, promonocyte	Acute monocytic leukemia
Promonocyte, immature macrophage	Reticulum cell sarcoma (poorly differentiated)
Diseases with moderate cellular differentiation	
Monocyte, immature macrophage	Letterer-Siwe disease (acute differentiated histiocytosis)
Immature macrophage	Histiocytic medullary reticulosis
Diseases with well-differentiated histiocytes	
Immature and mature macrophage	Hand-Schüller-Christian disease
Immature and mature macrophage	Eosinophilic granuloma
Immature and mature macrophage	Localized histiocytoma

dicate that the tumor cell itself is capable of reticulin synthesis (145).

The relation between the reticulum cell and a recently identified glass-adherent "stellate" cell present in mouse lymphoid tissues is uncertain (176).

The monocyte-macrophage cell line has its origin in the bone marrow. The relation of monocytes and macrophages to other hematopoietic cells is shown in Fig. I.1 of the Introduction. It can be seen that monocytes and granulocytes derive from a common progenitor. Failure of normal differentiation resulting from neoplastic transformation can lead to proliferation of stem cells, which produce a wide range of clinical and cytological manifestations.

From our knowledge of malignant myeloproliferative and lymphoproliferative disorders, we can construct an analogous model for the malignant histiocytoses within the following general framework:

(a) Histiocytic disease with the least cellular differentiation will have the highest degree of cellular proliferative activity and will be clinically the most acute.

(b) Histiocytic disease in which mature macrophages of low proliferative capacity predominate will be clinically more chronic.

(c) Although one cell type will predominate in a given patient, a spectrum of cells at different levels of maturation may be seen.

A certain overlap among disease syndromes can therefore be expected, although clinical and pathological features relate mainly to the accumulation of histiocytes at a given stage of maturation.

Disease manifestations may result from unrestrained proliferation of neoplastically transformed cells within the bone marrow or tissues, from phagocytosis of the formed elements of the blood by mature histiocytes, or from resorption of bone. Monocytes and macrophages may also produce endogenous pyrogen (18). Consequently, the anticipated clinical findings include those related to anemia, leukopenia, thrombocytopenia, fever, osteolysis, and tissue infiltration.

Neoplastic proliferations of histiocytes must be distinguished from the accumulation of histiocytic cells in response to an "appropriate" stimulus. As noted earlier, the macrophage is part of the body's defense against infection and normally is involved in the removal of damaged or senescent cells. Hyperplasia of the histiocytic elements of the spleen and lymph nodes, therefore, may be an appropriate response either to invasion by certain microorganisms or to the presence of abnormal or damaged erythrocytes.

In the response to parasites or tissue destruction, histiocyte proliferation is restrained and self-limited. In malignant proliferation, no such constraints are evident. In the subsequent sections of this chapter we shall proceed from the least differentiated to the most differentiated histiocytic proliferative diseases, realizing that in individual patients with a given disorder the degree of neoplastic differentiation may vary widely from the norm. *The thesis presented here is that these diseases represent clinically identifiable points along a spectrum of histiocytic proliferative disorders with varying degrees of cellular differentiation.*

Malignant Histiocytic Diseases with Little or Variable Cellular Differentiation

Monocytic Leukemia

Cytological Aspects   Monocytic leukemia is recognized morphologically by the presence in blood, bone marrow, and tissues of immature cells of the monocyte-macrophage cell line (Figs. 27.2 and 27.3). These cells vary from primitive blast forms to morphologically and functionally well-differentiated monocytes and macrophages. A similar spectrum may be seen in murine myelomonocytic leukemia (33). In general, the malignant monoblasts, promonocytes, and monocytes are characterized by lacy nuclear chromatin. The later cells have inconspicuous nucleoli and gray-blue cytoplasm with small, reddish

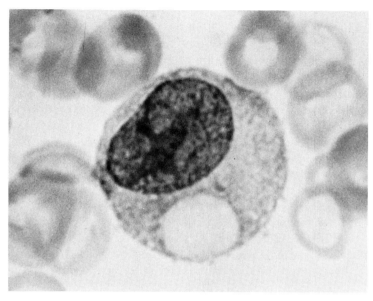

Figure 27.3 An immature mononuclear cell from the peripheral blood of a patient with acute monocytic leukemia. The cell, which corresponds to the promonocyte stage of development, has phagocytized an erythrocyte.

granules. The early cells have round-to-ovoid nuclei, nucleoli, and darker blue cytoplasm. Occasionally, elongate cells with irregular cytoplasm and a high cytoplasmic/nuclear ratio resembling tissue macrophages may be seen in the peripheral blood (15, 36, 48).

In most cases of monocytic leukemia there is a variable admixture of myeloblasts and more differentiated granulocytes. This is not surprising in view of the evidence favoring a common stem cell origin for granulocytes and monocytes (123, 156) (see Chapter 2).

Historically the term *Naegeli type* has been applied to that form of monocytic leukemia in which relatively large numbers of myelocytes and less mature granulocytes are found. The term *Schilling type* (148, 186, 194) has been used where more typical monoblasts and monocytes predominate. These terms are used to define rather arbitrary distinctions. The situation is simply that cellular heterogeneity prevails in monocytic leukemia (46, 56, 60, 63, 134, 171).

The variation in cellular maturation among patients with monocytic leukemia may be great. At one end of the spectrum there is overlap with the so-called stem cell or undifferentiated cell leukemias (hemoblastic or hemocytoblastic leukemia) (91). At the other extreme, mature macrophages are seen in the circulating blood, often with phagocytized red cells or other blood elements. The variation in cytological maturity is reflected in variation of

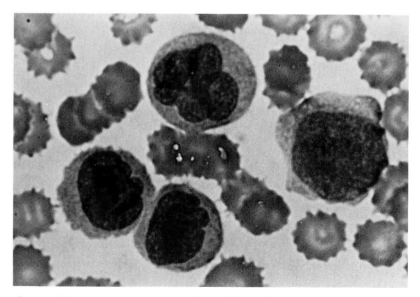

Figure 27.2 Immature mononuclear cells in the peripheral blood of a patient with acute monocytic leukemia. (From M. J. Cline and D. W. Golde, *Am. J. Med.* 55:49, 1973. Reprinted by permission of authors and publisher.)

negative surface charge density, deformability, and surface adhesiveness (110).

Histochemical stains are of some value in the study of monocytic leukemia (Table 27.2). Immature monocytes in both man and the mouse are peroxidase-positive; mature cells are peroxidase-negative (33, 101, 158, 182). In general, more than 5 percent of the cells are positive with Sudan black staining, usually without the heavy localization seen in the myeloblastic leukemias (78). The PAS reaction is variable.

Functionally the very early monocyte precursors of the marrow are characterized by mitotic activity, lack of phagocytic ability, little glass adhesiveness, and lack of surface receptors for IgG. With maturation, functional capabilities increase and peroxidase activity disappears (33, 35) (see Chapter 24, esp. Fig. 24.3). The morphologically differentiated mononuclear cells of monocytic leukemia qualitatively resemble their normal counterpart in these respects. So-called leukemic reticuloendotheliosis (21) or reticulum cell leukemia (196) may be related to hairy cell leukemia (165) and is often classified among the histocytic malignancies. However, the origin of the proliferating neoplastic cell is ill-defined and may well be related to the lymphoid series (70).

Pathology In addition to proliferation within the bone marrow, monocytic cells may be observed throughout the parenchymal and connective tissues of the body, especially in the spleen, lymph nodes, and liver (36, 71, 79, 97). Mitoses are frequent, and the normal architecture of nodes and spleen is destroyed. Myeloid hyperplasia may

be seen (184). In general, the histology of the tissues resembles that described in acute myelocytic leukemia. An occasional additional feature is the presence of erythrophagocytosis.

Clinical Features and Course of the Disease The major clinical manifestations and course of monocytic leukemia resemble those already described for acute myelocytic leukemia. Clinical manifestations include anemia, granulocytopenia with infection, thrombocytopenia with bleeding, and organ infiltration. The course is usually acute, and most patients succumb within a year. It has been pointed out, however, that the course of monocytic leukemia is more likely to be variable than that of acute lymphocytic or myelocytic leukemia (171, 194). Patients with survival of four to eleven years are known (88, 134, 140, 186).

Some authors have divided monocytic leukemia into acute and chronic forms on the basis of survival of less than or greater than one year. This is a rather arbitrary distinction that probably is meaningless in the modern era of effective chemotherapy. It is clear, however, that some patients with this disorder may survive for long periods of time. The group with chronic disease probably comprises less than 5 percent of all patients, although Osgood (134) put the figure at 11 percent. Patients with the chronic form of monocytic leukemia usually have monocytes and macrophages that are moderately or highly differentiated. This variant of the disease probably should be classified among the disorders with moderately differentiated malignant histiocytes.

Monocytic leukemia customarily presents in an acute form. Rarely, presentation is insidious or with a long prodromal "preleukemia phase" (24, 88, 121, 140, 189). A variety of unusual variants in monocytic leukemia has been described, including prominent oroglossopharyngeal involvement (199) and chronic erythromonocytic leukemia (24).

Biochemical Abnormalities In 1966 Osserman and Lawlor reported that untreated patients with acute monocytic or myelomonocytic leukemia have increased concentrations of lysozyme (muramidase) in their serum and urine (135). The enzyme in these patients was antigenically and electrophoretically identical to the normal leukocyte enzyme. Shortly thereafter, other investigators described high levels of serum lysozyme in chronic myelocytic leukemia and low levels in the lymphocytic leukemias (84, 89, 133, 138).

Lysozyme is a cationic lysosomal protein having a molecular weight of about 15,000 (139, 155), whose natu-

Table 27.2 Histiochemical reactions of mononuclear leukocytes. The scale used ranges from 0 (no reaction) to 4+ (strongly positive).

Stain	Normal monocyte	Malignant monocyte	Malignant histiocyte	Granulocyte	Lymphocyte
Peroxidase	2+	0–2+	0	4+	0
Alkaline phosphatase	0	0	0	3+	0
Acid phosphatase	3+	2+	3+	3+	0–1+
PAS	2+ (diffuse)	?	1+ (diffuse)	2+ (diffuse)	3+ (granules)
Sudan black	2+	±	1+	3+	0
Beta-glucuronidase	+	±	±	3+	0
Esterase ASD chloroacetate	0	0	?	4+	0
Esterase alphanaphthyl acetate	4+	2+	±	0	0

ral substrate is a bacterial cell wall polysaccharide (159). Lysozyme occurs in many mammalian tissues but most notably in leukocytes, kidney, and lung. Among leukocytes it is restricted to cells of the monocytic and neutrophilic series (9, 23, 113). From animal studies has come the suggestion that most of the serum lysozyme derives from granulocyte turnover (62). Lysozyme activity has been reported to be increased in the stools and colonic mucus of patients with ulcerative colitis, presumably as a result of the infiltration of leukocytes into the inflammatory tissues (129, 142). Enzyme activity may be increased in the serum and urine of patients with a variety of renal diseases, especially those with abnormalities of tubular function (126, 141).

In acute myelocytic leukemias, serum lysozyme activity may be high, low, or normal (133, 135, 138, 193). Activity levels are generally high in patients with acute myelomonocytic leukemia and acute monocytic leukemia. Even leukopenic patients with these disorders have a high level of serum enzyme activity. The ratio of urine to serum lysozyme activity tends to be elevated much above normal in patients with monocytic leukemia.

It is probable that the origin of the increased activity levels of lysozyme in serum and urine of patients with monocytic leukemia is the rapid turnover rate of malignant mononuclear cells (26, 133). However, a contribution by abnormal renal function in this disorder has not been excluded (135, 193). The elevated lysozyme may itself result in impaired proximal renal tubule function (174).

In a group of 18 patients with mono- or myelomonocytic leukemia, 9 had impaired renal function with azotemia (143). Serum lysozyme levels were higher in the azotemic group. Abnormalities of glomerular filtration and tubular function were noted. All patients had increased levels of serum immunoglobulins, especially IgG, IgA, and IgM. Whether the increased concentrations of immunoglobulins (cf. 127) or the greatly increased filtered levels of lysozyme contribute to renal failure in patients with myelomonocytic leukemia is not known with certainty.

Serum lysozyme activity may be used to follow patients with monocytic leukemia, since the levels generally fall to the normal range with the induction of hematologic remission (193). Enzyme activity levels do not necessarily decline in parallel with the peripheral mononuclear leukocyte count. It is well recognized that extramedullary foci of leukemic cells often exist during a "complete hematologic remission" (120, 131). Quite likely the enzyme activity reflects the total body mass of leukemia cells rather than the number of circulating cells.

Reticulum Cell Sarcoma (Histiocytic Lymphoma)
Traditionally, reticulum cell sarcoma is classified with the lymphomas and lymphoproliferative disorders. The reasons for this are the origin of the malignancy within the lymphoid system and the clinical resemblance to lymphomas such as lymphosarcoma. We should, however, distinguish between the cellular elements of the lymphoid system and those of the mononuclear phagocyte system, even though they are intimately related physically in lymphoid tissues and spleen and function cooperatively in antigen processing and cellular immune responses (41, 65, 69) (Chapters 15 and 25).

Since the cells in the tissues of patients with reticulum cell sarcoma resemble poorly differentiated histiocytes more than they resemble lymphocytes, it is logical to classify reticulum cell sarcoma among the histiocytic proliferative disorders (145). However, future studies may indicate that many of these lymphomas are really of lymphoid origin. Sinus histiocytosis with lymphadenopathy probably belongs in the histiocytic category (51, 150).

Cytological Features and Pathology   In the undifferentiated syncytial form of reticulum cell sarcoma, the predominant cell is relatively large with a diameter of 15 to 35 microns. The nucleus is large, "vesicular," round or oval in shape, with a delicate chromatin structure and prominent nucleolus (Fig. 27.4). The cytoplasm is pale-

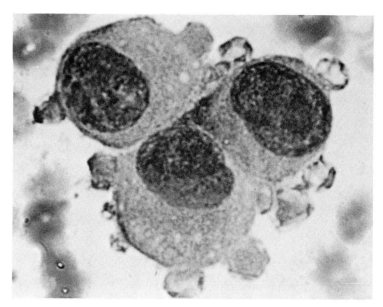

Figure 27.4 Malignant leukocytes from the bone marrow of a patient with poorly differentiated histiocytic lymphoma (reticulum cell sarcoma). (From M. J. Cline and D. W. Golde, *Am. J. Med.* 55:49, 1973. Reprinted by permission of authors and publisher.)

staining, varies in amount, and often appears to form a syncytium (16). Reticulin fibers are scanty and there is little evidence of histiocytic differentiation.

In the differentiated or histiocytic variety of reticulum cell sarcoma, the predominant cell type resembles the tissue histiocyte. It is generally 15 to 25 microns in diameter. The nucleus is oval or reniform, occasionally round. Chromatin is fine. Nucleoli are relatively rare. The cytoplasm is abundant, pale-staining, and usually acidophilic. Phagocytized red cells, nucleated cells, and cell debris sometimes are found within the cytoplasm (45). This type of tumor has been called a "plasmacytic lymphoma," or "monocytoma" (16). The reticulin meshwork may be highly developed as in Fig. 27.5. Undifferentiated reticulum cells have acid phosphatase activity, but lack esterase and beta glucuronidase activity. With maturation, beta glucuronidase appears (132). The proliferating cells of reticulum cell sarcoma therefore encompass a spectrum ranging between the promonocyte and the A macrophage.

Primary reticulum cell sarcoma of the brain probably represents a separate nosologic entity with a histology and a natural history distinct from that of reticulum cell sarcoma occurring in other parts of the body (162).

Incidence Reticulum cell sarcoma has been reported in all parts of the world. In the United States the disease accounts for about 6 percent of all lymphomas; however, the relative incidence varies from institution to institu-

tion depending upon the cytological features used to classify lymphomas. For example, at the Massachusetts General Hospital in Boston, 13 percent of the 618 cases of lymphoma were classified as "plasmacytomas" (68). In a series at Sloan-Kettering Memorial Hospital in New York City, the proportion of reticulum cell sarcoma cases among lymphomas was greater than 20 percent (152).

Unlike Hodgkin's disease, reticulum cell sarcoma occurs relatively rarely in youth (151, 152), although cases in children are well documented (20). In general, it is a disease of middle life.

Clinical Manifestations The general symptomatology associated with reticulum cell sarcomas is similar to that already described for Hodgkin's disease and lymphocytic lymphoma. There are, however, several important differences between histiocytic lymphoma and the other lymphomas. An extranodal primary site is much more common in reticulum cell sarcoma and may occur in up to one-fourth of all patients with this disease (152). Extranodal sites frequently involved include the tonsils and lymphoid tissues of Waldeyer's ring (85) and the gastrointestinal tract, particularly the stomach and jejunum. Rarer sites of involvement include bone, the thyroid, the testes, the genitourinary system, and the lung (175). Symptoms of Waldeyer's ring involvement include sore throat and dysphagia. Ulcerations of the tonsils are frequent.

Reticulum cell sarcoma accounts for about a third of gastric lymphomas (169). Signs and symptoms include weight loss, pain, hematemesis, melena, and a palpable abdominal mass. Roentgenologic manifestations of gastric involvement may vary: a smooth defect in the stomach, a localized mass lesion, a diffuse lesion infiltrating the walls of the stomach, giant rugae, or an annular lesion of the pylorus (190). Gastric emptying may be sluggish.

The small bowel may be involved at any level from the pylorus to the ileocecal valve. Manifestations may include an abdominal mass, pain, diarrhea, intussusception, and malabsorption syndrome (52, 152). Intestinal lymphoma may masquerade as ulcerative colitis (61). Roentgenologic foci may be discrete or diffuse. The walls of the small bowel may appear thickened and the mucosal pattern obliterated (44).

Bony lesions can be identified radiologically in about 20 percent of patients with reticulum cell sarcoma (39, 183). Such lesions are usually a manifestation of disseminated disease; rarely is bone the primary site of involvement (64, 170). Clinical symptomatology includes tenderness and localized pain, occasionally tumors or neurological lesions as a result of nerve or spinal cord compression. In

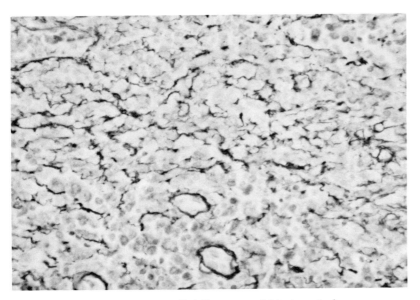

Figure 27.5 A section of a well-differentiated histiocytic lymphoma stained for reticulin.

reticulum cell sarcoma the bony lesions are generally osteolytic, rarely osteoblastic.

Reticulum cell sarcoma infrequently involves the thyroid gland; when it does, the clinical picture consists of goiter, hoarseness, and dysphagia (191). The tumor may stay within the thyroid capsule or invade locally (124, 195).

Histiocytic lymphoma, as well as other lymphomas, may be found anywhere within the genitourinary system (4, 50, 104, 152, 192). Manifestations may include pain, a localized mass, and hematuria. Rarely, uric acid nephropathy may occur from hyperuricemia associated with chemotherapy.

Involvement of the lung and intrathoracic structures occurs in reticulum cell sarcoma as in the other lymphomas (10, 98, 122, 152). Symptoms may include cough, pain, or those of pleural effusions or of superior vena cava obstruction. Hypertrophic pulmonary osteoarthropathy is rare.

Reticulum cell sarcoma tends to be an aggressive tumor, and the median survival time is less than one year. This neoplasm may be quite radiosensitive, however, and frequently responds to chemotherapy. In cases where a remission can be achieved with therapy, survival is significantly prolonged (105, 114). No comprehensive data exist that establish a relation between the degree of histiocytic differentiation and the acuteness of the clinical course. The clinical disease tends to reflect the rapid proliferation of poorly differentiated histiocytic precursors.

In occasional patients the overlap between reticulum cell sarcoma and acute monocytic leukemia is clearly demonstrable. Starting within the lymph nodes, the malignant reticulum cells may subsequently involve the bone marrow and blood, thereby producing a leukemia picture (132, 152, 163).

Principles of Management   At the time the diagnosis is first made, reticulum cell sarcoma usually is already widely disseminated. Consequently, the disease is not curable by radical radiation therapy—unlike Hodgkin's disease, which is often curable at the time of initial diagnosis. Nevertheless, an attempt must be made to identify those rare patients with reticulum cell sarcoma who have limited disease. The principles and techniques of staging are the same as for other lymphomas. For the moment, radical radiation therapy is probably the treatment of choice for stage I and II disease (92). Local disease can also be treated by radiotherapy with the objective of palliation (147). In controlling stage III and IV disease, the quality and duration of remission may be improved with a combination of agents (82, 105, 114, 128).

Histiocytic Disorders with Moderate Cellular Differentiation

Letterer-Siwe Disease (Acute Differentiated Histiocytosis)

Clinical and Pathological Features   In 1924 Letterer described a six-month-old boy with a ten-week history of fever, bilateral purulent otitis media, generalized purpura, lymphadenopathy, hepatosplenomegaly, and purulent material draining from an incision over a postauricular lymph node (102). The white blood count was 26,000/mm³ with 25 percent lymphocytes, 8 percent mononuclear cells, and 2 percent "transitional forms." The child died, and microscopic examination of autopsy material revealed disruption of the architecture of the lymphoid tissues by collections of cells characterized by abundant cytoplasm and large, "endothelial-like" nuclei with granular chromatin and prominent nucleoli. Similar cells were seen in the liver, spleen, bone marrow, large intestine, skin, and adventitia of blood vessels. Letterer was uncertain whether these findings reflected an infectious or a neoplastic process.

In 1933 Siwe described a sixteen-month-old child with a three-month history of fever, hepatosplenomegaly, lymphadenopathy, and destruction of bone (172). At autopsy, proliferation of cells that were interpreted as histiocytes, reticulum cells, and endothelial cells were noted. Siwe then described five cases from the literature, including the original case described by Letterer, and concluded that these comprised a single clinical entity. By this time the terms "reticulosis" and "reticuloendotheliosis" had been coined. By 1936 "Letterer-Siwe disease" was an established entity (1) with the following features: (a) occurrence in infancy, (b) hepatosplenomegaly, (c) lymphadenopathy, (d) bleeding diathesis, (e) tumors of bone (Fig. 27.6), (f) generalized hyperplasia of nonlipid-storing macrophages in many organs but prominently in the skin, and (g) rapidly fatal downhill course.

A number of authors contributed cases (and new nomenclature) which more or less matched the original descriptions (cf. 111). In general, the pathology of these cases resembled the well-differentiated form of reticulum cell sarcoma. In 1940 Wallgren (185) suggested that there were cases intermediate in character between Letterer-Siwe disease and other diseases with more localized, nonlipid, histiocytic proliferation, such as Hand-Schüller-Christian disease. A number of other authors began to classify Letterer-Siwe disease, Hand-Schüller-Christian disease, and eosinophilic granuloma of bone as variants of a single disease entity (53, 59, 74, 86, 107, 108). In 1953 Lichten-

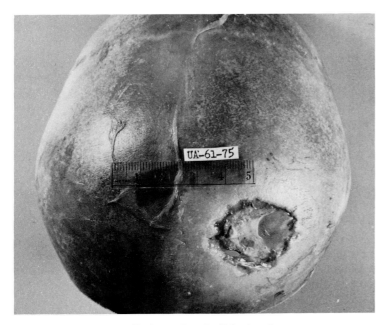

Figure 27.6 Autopsy finding of a skull lesion in a young patient with Letterer-Siwe disease.

stein (107) coined the term *histiocytosis-X* to designate these diseases as a single nosologic category. This concept has not, however, been universally accepted (2, 111, 117, 136, 173), and at the present time opinion favors the view that some of these are independent disease processes.

The clinical syndrome that characterizes Letterer-Siwe disease probably comprises several histiocytic proliferative disorders and some undiagnosed infectious processes (40). For the moment it is best to restrict the term to the malignant and usually rapidly fatal histiocytic proliferative disorder with bone and skin involvement that occurs in infancy and early childhood and has the characteristics cited above.

There are two basic types of skin lesions in Letterer-Siwe disease, as well as a number of "nonspecific dermatoses": (a) granulomata with a varying proportion of histiocytes, eosinophils, and mononuclear cells; and (b) histiocytic infiltration in which a blending of the lower layers of epidermal cells with histiocytes occurs. In ultrastructural examination of the skin lesions "peculiar bodies" have been described (13, 25). Clinically the skin lesions may be papular or resemble seborrheic dermatitis (54, 55).

Most reports of Letterer-Siwe disease have dated the onset from infancy (1). Congenital forms have been described (37, 90, 146). The disease occurs in blacks and Caucasians and with rare exception is not familial (12, 58, 112, 164). Few patients live beyond the first few years of

childhood, generally dying from a complication of disease, such as bleeding or infection. The disease is not, however, uniformly fatal. Lahey (100) reported a mortality rate of 70 percent when the disease occurred up to the age of six months and concluded that the younger the child, the worse the prognosis. However, several patients with onset before four months of age have been reported to be alive and well after several years. Therapy has varied and has included prednisone, vinca alkaloids, and methotrexate (14, 47, 55, 80, 90, 112).

The major cytological feature of Letterer-Siwe disease is the proliferation of differentiated histiocytes (Fig. 27.7). These generally have abundant acidophilic cytoplasm and ovoid or kidney-shaped nuclei. Nuclear chromatin is finely distributed, and the prominence of nucleoli is variable. The cytoplasm may be vacuolated and is rarely foamy. The cells may have phagocytized inclusions or hemosiderin (47). Letterer-Siwe disease bears a definite resemblance to the well-differentiated form of reticulum cell sarcoma. The possibility of a relation between Letterer-Siwe disease and other less differentiated histiocytic proliferative disorders is suggested by the occasional report of illness that begins as Letterer-Siwe disease and terminates in monocytic leukemia (7, 73, 83).

Hand-Schüller-Christian disease and eosinophilic granuloma of bone will be considered in subsequent portions of this chapter, and their similarities to and differences from Letterer-Siwe disease will be discussed.

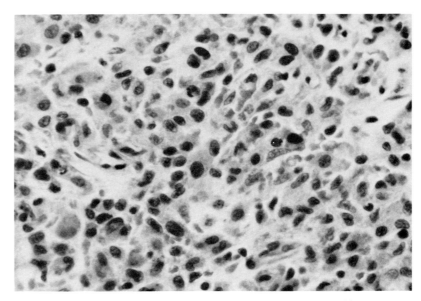

Figure 27.7 Moderately differentiated histiocytes infiltrating the spleen of a patient with Letterer-Siwe disease. (From M. J. Cline and D. W. Golde, *Am. J. Med.* 55:49, 1973. Reprinted by permission of authors and publisher.)

Histiocytic Medullary Reticulosis

The term *histiocytic medullary reticulosis* was originally used by Robb-Smith in 1938 (149) and further amplified by Scott and Robb-Smith the following year (167). These authors classified malignant lymphomas on the basis of anatomic sites within the lymph node and predominant cell type. They observed four patients whom they considered to have a unique form of the lymphoma with focal proliferation of histiocytes within the medullary portion of the lymph node, hence the rather cumbersome name of histiocytic medullary reticulosis. They, as well as subsequent authors, believed that this was a distinctive disorder differentiated from monocytic leukemia on the basis of absence of peripheral blood involvement and prominent erythrophagocytosis by the histiocytes.

In fact, neither of these features is unique to those cases classified as histiocytic medullary reticulosis. Blood and bone marrow involvement in patients with otherwise typical features of histiocytic medullary reticulosis has been described (31), and erythrophagocytosis may be a feature of both reticulum cell sarcoma and monocytic leukemia. It is likely that histiocytic medullary reticulosis is merely a variant of the well-differentiated form of reticulum cell sarcoma. Nevertheless, the cytological and clinical features are sufficiently distinctive to merit separate discussion.

Cytological Features   In the bone marrow, lymph nodes, and scattered throughout the parenchymal organs are large reticulum cells 30 to 50 microns in the long axis containing one, two, or three eccentric nuclei and a few nucleoli. These cells resemble moderately well-differentiated macrophages with a high proliferative capacity and well-developed phagocytic activity. They most closely resemble the immature macrophage (Fig. 27.1). Erythrophagocytosis is generally prominent (Figs. 27.8 and 27.9), and preparations stained with Prussian blue reveal extensive hemosiderosis. When stained with oil red O, droplets may be demonstrated within the cytoplasm of histiocytes. By electron microscopy the nuclei are large, often indented, and contain evenly dispersed chromatin. The abundant cytoplasm has irregular pseudopodal extensions and contains a variety of vacuoles, vesicles, and inclusions (119, 197, 198).

Clinical Features   Histiocytic medullary reticulosis is a rapidly progressive and fatal disease with a median survival time of less than 6 months, rarely lasting more than 15 months after appearance of symptoms (67, 75, 180, 197). No sex predilection has been noted, and the disease has been observed from young adult life to age seventy.

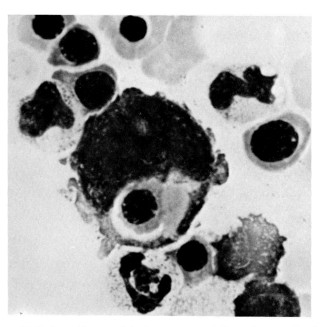

Figure 27.8 A malignant histiocyte containing phagocytized normoblasts from the bone marrow of a patient with histiocytic medullary reticulosis (moderately differentiated malignant histiocytosis). (From M. J. Cline and D. W. Golde, *Am. J. Med.* 55:49, 1973. Reprinted by permission of authors and publisher.)

Occurrence before age twenty is rare, however, and familial occurrence has been infrequently observed (17).

Prominent clinical features of this disease include hepatosplenomegaly, lymphadenopathy, anemia, fever, and pancytopenia. Phagocytosis of blood elements by his-

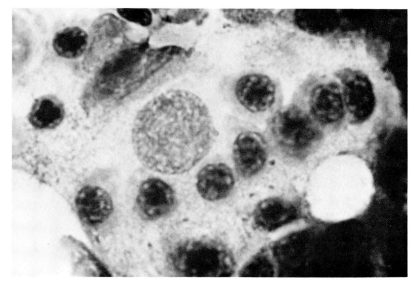

Figure 27.9 A malignant histiocyte that has phagocytized normoblasts.

tiocytes may contribute to the anemia, to leukopenia (see Fig. 25.7), to thrombocytopenia, or to pancytopenia (30, 116, 130, 168, 198). Rarely, abnormal cells circulate in the blood and the clinical picture may resemble acute leukemia (28, 31, 67). Even more unusual is histiocytic proliferation within the bowel wall producing symptomatology including that of protein-losing enteropathy (31, 119). In all, over 50 cases of histiocytic medullary reticulosis have been reported (31, 67, 75, 115, 197).

In general, treatment of this condition has been unsatisfactory and only transient responses to corticosteroids and cytotoxic agents have been reported.

Leukemic Reticuloendotheliosis

In 1923 Ewald described an unusual form of chronic leukemia whose principal features were the presence of circulating mononuclear cells with many cytoplasmic projections (hairy cells) and a very large spleen in the absence of significant lymphadenopathy (57). The disease is extremely rare, accounting for less than 2 percent of all leukemias. Onset is generally insidious, occurring after age fifty and more commonly in males than in females. Repeated infections are frequent, as are anemia and lymphocytopenia. The white count may be elevated, but in about half the patients leukopenia is present. The massive splenomegaly may be associated with splenic infarcts, perisplenitis, and splenic rupture.

It is difficult to know how to classify this disease. Despite numerous clinical, cytological, and histochemical studies, the origin of the malignant cells is unknown (21, 72, 87, 125, 154, 165). Recent studies suggest a relation of the malignant cells to the reticular cells of the lymph nodes, spleen, and bone marrow (178). The malignant cells are PAS positive and acid phosphatase positive, but lack detectable peroxidase or alkaline phosphatase activity or sudanophilia.

Malignant Histiocytic Diseases with Well-differentiated Cells

Hand-Schüller-Christian Disease

Hand-Schüller-Christian disease is a rare histiocytic disorder of childhood that in the classic form consists in the triad of defects of membranous bone, diabetes insipidus, and exophthalmos. It is unusual, however, for all three abnormalities to be expressed in the same patient.

Over the years there has been considerable debate over whether Hand-Schüller-Christian disease represents a chronic and differentiated form of Letterer-Siwe disease or is a distinct disease entity (111).

History In 1921 Hand wrote a paper entitled "Defects of Membranous Bones, Exophthalmos and Polyuria in Childhood: Is It Dyspituitarism?" (77) in which he reviewed the histories of two of his own patients and the four patients of Drs. Kay (94), Christian (29) and Schüller (166). One of Hand's patients, first described in 1893, was thought to have had tuberculosis (76). In 1928 Rowland wrote a now classic description that provided a firm histologic basis for the clinical syndrome (153). He initiated an era of investigation of Hand-Schüller-Christian disease as a possible metabolic storage disease. However, by 1938 the old concept that this was a primary disorder of lipid metabolism was discarded, and Hand-Schüller-Christian disease was classified among the xanthomatoses with normal levels of serum lipids and cholesterol (177). This classification was supported by later conclusions that this disorder was *not* the result of a metabolic defect leading to lipid or carbohydrate storage.

The next phase in the history of Hand-Schüller-Christian disease arrived when this disorder came to be regarded as a disease variant intermediate in severity and degree of cellular differentiation between Letterer-Siwe disease and eosinophilic granuloma of bone. Hand-Schüller-Christian disease came to be referred to as chronic disseminated histiocytosis-X (108).

In the last and current phase of the history of this interesting disorder, it is again regarded as a separate nosologic entity with multiple localized areas of histiocytic proliferation, distinct from Letterer-Siwe disease (111).

Cytological Features Histologically, Hand-Schüller-Christian disease is characterized by the focal accumulation within bone and sometimes within skin and lungs of masses of tissue macrophages, some of which have a foamy appearance (Fig. 27.10). These lesions may have a variable admixture of lymphocytes, plasma cells, neutrophils, and eosinophils. Eosinophilic infiltration is not usually outstanding.

Clinical Manifestations Although the great majority of cases have their onset before age four, occasional reports document the onset of illness in early adult life (7). Males predominate over females in most series of cases (7, 27, 181). The classic triad of diabetes insipidus, exophthalmos, and skull lesions in a young child occurs relatively rarely in Hand-Schüller-Christian disease, perhaps in one patient in ten (7). The major clinical features resulting from histiocytic proliferation are listed in Table 27.3.

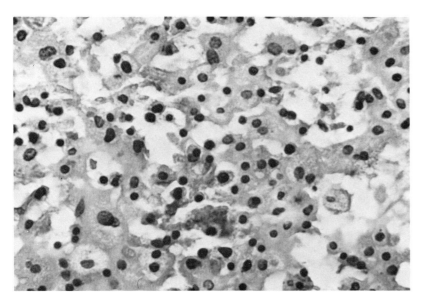

Figure 27.10 Histiocytes from a bone lesion of a patient with Hand-Schüller-Christian disease. Some cells have a foamy appearance. Hematoxylin and eosin stain. (From M. J. Cline and D. W. Golde, *Am. J. Med.* 55:49, 1973. Reprinted by permission of authors and publisher.)

Defects of bone. Radiologically, the common sites of proliferation of tumor cells include the calvaria, petrous and mastoid bones, mandible, and sinuses. Less frequently, the ribs, pelvis, and long bones are involved. The sella is only rarely destroyed. This pattern of distribution of lesions is similar to that of eosinophilic granuloma (43). Soft tissues other than the lungs are only rarely involved (7).

The bone defects may be single or multiple and vary in size from barely perceptible to large, irregular, geographic defects. Soft tissue nodules are sometimes palpable in the

Table 27.3 Sites of neoplastic cell proliferation in Hand-Schüller-Christian disease, and percentage of patients in which these clinical features are found.

Characteristic	Percent
Defect in membranous bone	50
Hypothalamic infiltration + diabetes insipidus	50
Orbital infiltration + exophthalmos	30
Otitis media	40
Skin infiltration	30
Gum infiltration	30
Lung infiltration	30

skin overlying bony defects. Both tables of the skull are usually involved; lesions may extend epidurally, but rarely involve the brain itself.

Diabetes insipidus. In large series of patients with Hand-Schüller-Christian disease about half have diabetes insipidus. Usually the onset of this manifestation is insidious, with gradual increase in polyuria and fluid requirement. The presumed mechanism is involvement of the pituitary stalk or hypothalamus. Growth hormone deficiency may be associated (22).

Exophthalmos. Exophthalmos occurs in about one-third of patients. It may be uni- or bilateral and results from orbital infiltration with typical proliferative cells. Destruction of orbital bones may take place.

Otitis media. In one series, chronic otitis media was the most common complaint of children with Hand-Schüller-Christian disease (7). Otitis media is often accompanied by radiological changes in mastoid bone or the petrous portion of the temporal bone. An early sign is clouding of the mastoid air cell; later, destructive foci are evident.

Skin lesions. Skin involvement occurs in about one-third of patients. They are initially diagnosed as having seborrheic dermatitis because of the erythematous and scaling nature of the rash. Eczema is another common early diagnosis. The skin may be involved by isolated granulomatous nodules or may show diffuse histiocytic infiltration with atrophy of the epithelium and hyperkeratosis.

Jaw and gum lesions. Lesions of the jaw often begin in the tooth-bearing areas of the mandible in the region of the apexes of the teeth. Uni- or multicystic destruction of bone is associated with localized erosion of the lamina dura of adjacent teeth. Destruction of bone produces a "teeth in air" appearance radiologically and eventually results in extrusion of affected teeth.

Ulcerative lesions of the gums occur in about one-third of patients and are not usually associated with underlying mandibular lesions.

Pulmonary involvement. When pulmonary involvement is present, it is usually restricted to the central and perihilar areas of the lung, with the periphery of the lung being clear. Although readily apparent radiologically, lung involvement only rarely gives rise to serious symptoms. However, extensive interstitial fibrosis with cor pulmonale has been described in some patients (144). Lesions may be solitary nodules or diffuse miliary infiltrates.

Other manifestations. Lymphadenopathy and hepatosplenomegaly rarely are prominent manifestations of Hand-Schüller-Christian disease (66, 111). Other organs, such as the thyroid, may be infiltrated and enlarged (7,

161). Occurrence of disease early in childhood may be associated with moderate to severe stunting of growth.

Course and Prognosis   The course of Hand-Schüller-Christian disease is extremely variable. In general, the disease is chronic, often waxing and waning in severity. In at least one-third—and probably over one-half—of patients the disease eventually "burns out" and the lesions slowly heal and resolve. In a small fraction of patients (probably less than 15 percent) the disease is fatal within months or a few years as a consequence of complications such as infection or, rarely, pulmonary insufficiency (7, 111). Anemia is said to be a poor prognostic sign in this disease.

The disease rarely, if ever, makes the transition to a more fulminant type of histiocytic proliferation. The clinical pattern is reflected in the changes in tissue histology. During an active phase of disease, rapidly developing lesions resemble inflammatory histiocytosis with a variable degree of eosinophilic infiltration. With a more chronic illness, the histiocytes become lipid-laden and fibrosis appears. Ultimately the lesions are densely fibrotic.

Local lesions are often responsive to X-irradiation, and generalized disease may respond to corticosteroids or cytolytic agents (8, 111).

Uni- and Multifocal Eosinophilic Granuloma of Bone

History   In 1940 Otani and Ehrlich (137) and Lichtenstein and Jaffe (109) drew attention to a group of patients with solitary eosinophilic granuloma of bone "simulating primary neoplasm." An example of one of the first patients described was an eleven-year-old boy with an isolated rib lesion, which was treated with local irradiation and excision. The patient did well postoperatively.

In 1942 Green and Farber published an important article discussing the nature of solitary eosinophilic granuloma of bone (74). They introduced the concept that this disease entity was part of a spectrum of Letterer-Siwe disease and Hand-Schüller-Christian disease. As we have seen, this concept has not gained universal acceptance.

Cytological Features   The basic histologic picture of eosinophilic granuloma of bone is of a mixture of eosinophils and histiocytes in variable proportions (Fig. 27.11). The histiocytes often contain ingested cells and cell debris. The eosinophils generally are typically mature cells. Mitotic figures are rare. Healing lesions show fibrotic appearance.

Clinical Manifestations and Prognosis   Eosinophilic granuloma of bone may be unifocal, as well as multifocal. It is a disease of childhood, with most patients presenting

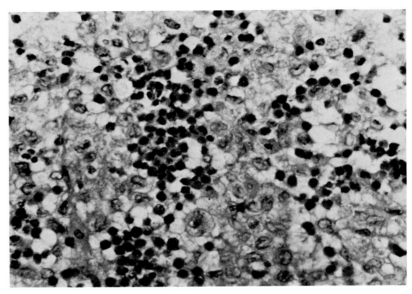

Figure 27.11   Histiocytes and eosinophils (small dark cells) in a lesion of eosinophilic granuloma of bone. Hematoxylin and eosin stain. (From M. J. Cline and D. W. Golde, *Am. J. Med.* 55:49, 1973. Reprinted by permission of authors and publisher.)

before the age of ten years. However, cases with onset well into adult life are not rare (111). In most series there is a predominance of males over females.

Presentation of disease is usually with bone pain; the head, ribs, femur, and pelvis are the most common sites of involvement. Systemic manifestations are rare with unifocal disease. With multifocal disease there is clear overlap in symptomatology with Hand-Schüller-Christian disease, and the two entities may be difficult to separate on either clinical or pathological grounds.

Unifocal eosinophilic granuloma is almost invariably benign and responds readily to excision or to radiation therapy.

Extraosseous Eosinophilic Granulomas and Focal Histiocytosis

A body of literature has accumulated documenting the appearance of "eosinophilic granulomata" in various organs. Whether such granulomatas bear any relation to similar granulomata in bone or whether they are malignant in nature is unknown. Probably the most common site of such disease is in the gastrointestinal tract, including stomach and large and small bowel (19, 157, 160, 179). These granulomas may be either focal or diffuse; the former are often polypoid. These lesions for the most part are benign, although perforation has been observed (111).

Eosinophilic granuloma of the lung is also well described (6, 42, 81, 96, 99, 106). It is unlikely, however, that all the descriptions are concerned with a single disease entity. It is more likely that histiocytic and eosinophilic accumulation occurs in response to a multiplicity of stimuli. In some instances diffuse fibrosis takes place in association with eosinophilic granulomata.

Numerous reports in the literature have described eosinophilic granulomas of the mucous membrane and skin in patients with and without bone lesions (5, 95, 103, 118).

In addition to mixed eosinophilic and histiocytic granulomas, localized histiocytic tumors have been recognized (49, 93). These are usually benign.

Multicentric Reticulohistiocytosis

Multicentric reticulohistiocytosis is a rare systemic disease of unknown etiology whose major manifestation is the gradual development of nodules in the skin, subcutaneous tissues, synovia, and at times in the bone and periosteum. These nodules are composed of multinucleate giant cells and histiocytes with a ground-glass appearance of the cytoplasm (11). Lesions result in a destructive arthritis and disfigurement of the facies.

These nodules are quite easily distinguished histologically from those of rheumatoid arthritis, a disease which may occasionally be mistaken for multicentric reticulohistiocytosis on clinical grounds. A variety of terms has been used to describe the disease syndrome of multifocal reticulohistiocytosis (3, 188). Histochemical studies indicate that the giant cells and histiocytes contain neutral fats, phospholipids, iron granules, and PAS-reactive material (11). The disease on the whole is benign, although patients may die during the acute early stages.

It is uncertain whether this rare disease entity reflects histiocytic proliferation in response to an unknown inciting agent or is neoplastic in nature.

Summary and Opinion

In the author's opinion unifocal and multifocal eosinophilic granuloma of bone and Hand-Schüller-Christian disease are variants of the same basic disease process, manifested as localized or widespread lesions. These entities are distinctly less "malignant" than Letterer-Siwe disease and reticulum cell sarcoma, and bear no definite relation to them. Their cytological hallmark is the differentiated histiocyte. Letterer-Siwe disease is clinically and cytologically similar to a childhood variant of differentiated reticulum cell sarcoma with progressive and generalized proliferation of immature and moderately differentiated histiocytes, whereas uni- and multifocal eosinophilic granulomas of bone behave like "reactive" histiocytic lesions.

Several points emerge from the foregoing discussion of malignant histiocytic diseases.

(a) Cells of the monocyte-histiocyte series may become malignant; that is, they may undergo a transformation that permits unrestrained proliferation. This concept is supported by recent observations of malignant transformation of animal macrophages induced by an oncogenic DNA virus.

(b) Malignant cells of the monocyte-macrophage series may show a variable degree of differentiation—from relatively undifferentiated monoblasts at the one extreme to well-differentiated functional histiocytes at the other extreme.

(c) Neoplastic diseases of the histiocytic cells also embrace a wide spectrum—from disorders in which there is extensive proliferation of poorly differentiated cells (for example, acute monocytic leukemia) to disorders in which there is limited and circumscribed proliferation of well-differentiated cells. Clearly there will be overlap among these diseases, depending on how "tightly" or "loosely" the neoplastic clone is regulated in its differentiation.

(d) It is convenient to catalog these diseases on the basis of cellular differentiation:

(1) Disease with little cellular differentiation, including acute monocytic leukemia and undifferentiated reticulum cell sarcoma;

(2) Disease with a moderate degree of histiocytic differentiation, including chronic monocytic leukemia, well-differentiated reticulum cell sarcoma, Letterer-Siwe disease, and histiocytic medullary reticulosis;

(3) Disease with well-differentiated histiocytes, including Hand-Schüller-Christian disease, unifocal and multifocal eosinophilic granuloma of bone, and localized histiocytoma.

Although there is little dispute about the malignant nature of the disorders in groups (1) and (2), it is not certain that the entities listed in group (3) are indeed neoplastic. The clinically chronic disorders characterized by proliferation of well-differentiated histiocytes may represent a reactive response to an unidentified antigen or parasite. In this regard they may be viewed as having more in common with sarcoidosis, for example, than with a true malignancy.

We are now entering an era in which it is possible to evaluate malignant histiocytic disorders by several methods: standard morphology, histochemistry, and functional and proliferative assessment of isolated cells. By combining these approaches it should be possible to classify the histiocytic disorder in a given patient in a manner that reflects the biological properties of the proliferating cell. Such an approach has more to recommend it than the present attempts to force complex and varying constellations of clinical findings into rigid disease categories with uninformative and unpronounceable names.

Chapter 27 References

1. Abt, A. F., and Denenholz, E. J. Letterer-Siwe's disease. Splenohepatomegaly associated with widespread hyperplasia of nonlipoid-storing macrophages; discussion of the so-called reticulo-endothelioses, *Am. J. Dis. Child.* 51:499, 1936.

2. Ackerman, L. V., and Spjut, H. J. Tumors of bone and cartilage, *in* Atlas of Tumor Pathology, sect. II, fasc. 4, Armed Forces Inst. of Pathol., Washington, D.C., 1962.

3. Albert, J., Bruce W., Allen, A. C., and Blank, H. Lipoid dermato-arthritis. Reticulohistiocytoma of the skin and joints, *Am. J. Med.* 28:661, 1960.

4. Allen, D. H., Berg, O. C., and Rosenblatt, W. Lymphosarcoma of the kidney. A case report and description of roentgen findings, *Radiology* 55:731, 1950.

5. Altman, J., and Winklemann, R. K. Xanthomatous cutaneous lesions of Histiocytosis X, *Arch. Dermatol.* 87:164, 1963.

6. Auld, D. Pathology of eosinophilic granuloma of the lung, *Arch. Pathol.* 63:113, 1957.

7. Avery, M. E., McAfee, J. G., and Guild, H. G. The course and prognosis of reticuloendotheliosis (eosinophilic granuloma, Schüller-Christian disease and Letterer-Siwe disease). A study of forty cases, *Am. J. Med.* 22:636, 1957.

8. Avioli, L. V., Lasersohn, J. T., and Lopresti, J. M. Histiocytosis X (Schüller-Christian disease): a clinicopathological survey, review of ten patients and the results of prednisone therapy, *Medicine* 42:119, 1963.

9. Barnes, J. M. The enzymes of lymphocytes and polymorphonuclear leucocytes, *Br. J. Exp. Pathol.* 21:264, 1940.

10. Baron, M. G., and Whitehouse, W. M. Primary lymphosarcoma of the lung, *Am. J. Roentgenol.* 85:294, 1961.

11. Barrow, M. V., and Holubar, K. Multicentric reticulohistiocytosis, *Medicine* 48:287, 1969.

12. Barth, R. F., Vergara, G. G., Khurana, S. K., et al. Rapidly fatal familial histiocytosis associated with eosinophilia and primary immunological deficiency, *Lancet* ii:503, 1972.

13. Basset, F., Nezelof, C., Mallet, R., et al. Nouvelle mise en évidence, par la microscopie électronique, de particules d'allure virale dans une seconde forme clinique de l'histiocytose X, le granulome éosinophile de l'os, *C. R. Acad. Sci. (Paris)* 261:5719, 1965.

14. Beier, F. R., Thatcher, L. G., and Lahey, M. E. Treatment of reticuloendotheliosis with vinblastine sulfate, *J. Pediatr.* 63:1087, 1963.

15. Belding, H., Dalad, A. G., and Parker, F. Histiocytic and monocytic leukemia. A clinical, hematological and pathological differentiation, *Cancer* 8:237, 1955.

16. Bingham, C. T., and Quarrier, S. S. Reticulum cell sarcoma. Report of a case with pronounced cutaneous manifestations, *Arch. Dermatol.* 41:722, 1940.

17. Boake, W. C., Card, W. H., and Kimmey, J. F. Histiocytic medullary reticulosis concurrence in father and son, *Arch. Intern. Med.* 116:245, 1965.

18. Bodel, P. T., and Atkins, E. Release of endogenous pyrogen by human monocytes, *N. Engl. J. Med.* 276:1002, 1967.

19. Booher, R. J., and Grant, R. N. Eosinophilic granuloma of the stomach and small intestine, *Surgery* 30:388, 1951.

20. Borella, L. Reticulum cell sarcoma in children, *Cancer* 17:26, 1964.

21. Bouroncle, B. A., Wiseman, B. K., and Doan, C. A. Leukemic reticuloendotheliosis, *Blood* 13:609, 1958.

22. Braunstein, G. D., and Kohler, P. O. Pituitary function in Hand-Schüller-Christian disease, *N. Engl. J. Med.* 286:1225, 1972.

23. Briggs, R. S., Perillie, P. E., and Finch, S. C. Lysozyme in bone marrow and peripheral blood cells, *J. Histochem.* 14:167, 1966.

24. Broun, G. O. Chronic erythromonocytic leukemia, *Am. J. Med.* 47:785, 1969.

25. Cancilla, P. A., Lahey, M. E., and Carnes, W. H. Cutaneous lesions of Letterer-Siwe disease. Electron microscopic study, *Cancer* 20:1986, 1967.

26. Catovsky, D., Galton, D. A. G., and Griffin, C. The significance of lysozyme estimations in acute myeloid and chronic monocytic leukemia, *Br. J. Haematol.* 21:565, 1971.

27. Chester, W., and Kugel, V. H. Lipoidgranulomatosis (type, Hand-Schüller-Christian). Report of a case, *Arch. Pathol.* 14:595, 1932.

28. Chih-Fei, Y., et al. Histiocytic medullary reticulosis, *Chin. Med. J.* 80:466, 1960.

29. Christian, H. A. Defects in membraneous bones, exophthalmos and diabetes insipidus; an unusual syndrome of dyspituitarism, *Med. Clin. North Am.* 3:849, 1920.

30. Civin, H., Gotshalk, H. C., and Okazaki, K. Histiocytic medullary reticulosis. Report of two cases, *Arch. Intern. Med.* 94:375, 1954.

31. Clark, B. S., and Dawson, P. J. Histiocytic medullary reticulosis presenting with a leukemic blood picture, *Am. J. Med.* 47:314, 1969.

32. Cline, M. J., and Golde, D. W. Review and re-evaluation of the histiocytic disorders, *Am. J. Med.* 55:49, 1973.

33. Cline, M. J., and Metcalf, D. Cellular differentiation in a murine myelomonocytic leukemia, *Blood* 39:771, 1972.

34. Cline, M. J., and Moore, M. A. S. Embryonic origin of the mouse macrophage, *Blood* 39:842, 1972.

35. Cline, M. J., and Sumner, M. A. Bone marrow macrophage precursors. I. Some functional characteristics of the early cells of the mouse macrophage series, *Blood* 40:62, 1972.

36. Clough, P. W. Monocytic leukemia, *Bull. Johns Hopkins Hosp.* 51:148, 1932.

37. Cohen, D. M., Mitchell, C. B., and Alexander, J. W. Letterer-Siwe disease in a newborn, *Arch. Pathol.* 81:347, 1966.

38. Cohn, Z. A. The structure and function of monocytes and macrophages, *Adv. Immunol.* 9:163, 1968.

39. Coles, W. C., and Schulz, M. D. Bone involvement in malignant lymphoma, *Radiology* 50:458, 1948.

40. Cooper, M. D., Peterson, R. D. A., Gabrielsen, E., and Good, R. A. Lymphoid malignancy and develop-

ment, differentiation and function of the lymphoreticular system, *Cancer Res.* 26:1165, 1966.

41. Cooper, M. D., Peterson, R. D. A., South, M. A., and Good, R. A. The functions of the thymus system and the bursa system in the chicken, *J. Exp. Med.* 123:75, 1966.

42. Cruthirds, T. P., and Johnson, H. R. Solitary primary eosinophilic granuloma of lung, *J.A.M.A.* 196:295, 1966.

43. Dargeon, H. W. K. Reticuloendothelioses in Childhood; A Clinical Survey, Charles C Thomas, Springfield, Ill., 1966.

44. Deeb, P. H., and Stilson, W. L. Roentgenologic manifestations of lymphosarcoma of the small bowel, *Radiology* 63:235, 1954.

45. Diamandopoulos, G. Th., and Smith, E. B. Phagocytosis in reticulum cell sarcoma, *Cancer* 17:329, 1964.

46. Doan, C. A., and Wiseman, B. K. The monocyte, monocytosis, and monocytic leukosis: a clinical and pathological study, *Ann. Intern. Med.* 8:383, 1934.

47. Doede, K. G., and Rappaport, H. Long-term survival of patients with acute differentiated histiocytosis (Letterer-Siwe disease), *Cancer* 20:1782, 1967.

48. Downey, H. Monocytic leucemia and leucemic reticuloendotheliosis, *in* H. Downey (ed.), Handbook of Hematology, vol. 2, p. 1273, Paul B. Hoeber, New York, 1938.

49. Dubilier, L. D., Bryant, L. R., and Danielson, G. K. Histiocytoma (fibrous xanthoma) of the lung, *Am. J. Surg.* 115:420, 1968.

50. Eckert, H., and Smith, J. P. Malignant lymphoma of the testis, *Br. Med. J.* 2:891, 1963.

51. Editorial. A new lymphoma syndrome, *Lancet* i:139, 1973.

52. Eidelman, S., Parkins, R. A., and Rubin, C. E. Abdominal lymphoma presenting as malabsorption. A clinico-pathologic study of nine cases in Israel and a review of the literature, *Medicine* 45:111, 1966.

53. Engelbreth-Holm, J., Teilum, G., and Christensen, E. Eosinophil granuloma of bone—Schüller-Christian disease, *Acta Med. Scand.* 118:292, 1944.

54. Ereaux, L. P., and Schopflocher, P.

Histiocytosis X in an infant, *Cutis* 3:223, 1967.

55. Esterly, N. B., and Swick, H. M. Cutaneous Letterer-Siwe disease, *Am. J. Dis. Child.* 117:236, 1969.

56. Evans, T. S. Monocytic leukemia. (General review of the subject), *Medicine* 21:421, 1942.

57. Ewald, O. Die leukämische Reticuloendotheliose, *Dtsch. Arch. Klin. Med.* 142:222, 1923.

58. Falk, W., and Gellei, B. The familial occurrence of Letterer-Siwe disease, *Acta Paediatr.* 46:471, 1957.

59. Farber, S. The nature of "solitary or eosinophilic granuloma" of bone, *Am. J. Pathol.* 17:625, 1941.

60. Farrar, G. E., Jr., and Cameron, J. D. Monocytic leukemia with data on the individuality and development of the monocyte, *Am. J. Med. Sci.* 184:763, 1932.

61. Federman, J., Goldstein, M. E., and Weingarten, B. Malignant lymphoma of over fifteen years' duration masquerading as ulcerative colitis, *Am. J. Roentgenol.* 89:771, 1963.

62. Fink, M. E., and Finch, S. C. Serum muramidase and granulocyte turnover, *Clin. Res.* 14:316, 1966.

63. Forkner, C. E. Clinical and pathologic differentiation of the acute leukemias with special reference to acute monocytic leukemia, *Arch. Intern. Med.* 53:1, 1934.

64. Francis, K. C., Higinbotham, N. L., and Coley, B. L. Primary reticulum cell sarcoma of bone. Report of 44 cases, *Surg. Gynecol. Obstet.* 99:142, 1954.

65. Frei, P. C., Benacerraf, B., and Thorbecke, G. J. Phagocytosis of the antigen, a crucial step in the induction of the primary response, *Proc. Natl. Acad. Sci. U.S.A.* 53:20, 1965.

66. Freund, M., and Ripps, M. L. Hand-Schüller-Christian disease. A case in which lymphadenopathy was a predominant feature, *Am. J. Dis. Child.* 61:759, 1941.

67. Friedman, R. M., and Steigbigel, N. H. Histiocytic medullary reticulosis, *Am. J. Med.* 38:130, 1965.

68. Gall, E. A., and Mallory, T. B. Malignant lymphoma. A clinico-pathologic survey of 618 cases, *Am. J. Pathol.* 18:381, 1942.

69. Garvey, J. S., and Campbell, D. H.

The retention of S³⁵-labelled bovine serum albumin in normal and immunized rabbit liver tissue, *J. Exp. Med.* 105:361, 1957.

70. Ghadially, F. N., and Skinnider, L. F. Ultrastructure of hairy cell leukemia, *Cancer* 29:444, 1972.

71. Gore, I. Proliferative disorders of blood, *in* O. Saphir (ed.), A Text on Systemic Pathology, vol. 1, p. 792, Grune & Stratton, New York, 1958.

72. Gosselin, G. R., Hanlon, D. G., and Pease, G. L. Leukaemic reticuloendotheliosis, *Can. Med. Assoc. J.* 74:886, 1956.

73. Gray, J. D., and Taylor, S. Acute systemic reticulo-endotheliosis terminating as a monocytic leukaemia, *Cancer* 6:333, 1953.

74. Green, W. T., and Farber, S. "Eosinophilic or solitary granuloma" of bone, *J. Bone Joint Surg.* 24:499, 1942.

75. Greenberg, E., Cohen, D. M., Pease, G. L., and Kyle, R. A. Histiocytic medullary reticulosis, *Mayo Clin. Proc.* 37:271, 1962.

76. Hand, A., Jr. General tuberculosis, *Trans. Pathol. Soc. Phila.* 16:282, 1893.

77. Hand, A. Defects of membranous bones, exophthalmos and polyuria in childhood: is it dyspituitarism?, *Am. J. Med. Sci.* 162:509, 1921.

78. Hayhoe, F. G. J., Quaglino, D., and Doll, R. The cytology and cytochemistry of acute leukaemias, Med. Res. Council Spec. Rept., Ser. 304, London, 1964.

79. Herbut, P. A., and Miller, F. R. Histopathology of monocytic leukemia, *Am. J. Pathol.* 23:93, 1947.

80. Hertz, C. G., and Hambrick, G. W. Congenital Letterer-Siwe disease. A case treated with vincristine and corticosteroids, *Am. J. Dis. Child.* 116:553, 1968.

81. Hoffman, L., Cohn, J. E., and Gaensler, E. A. Respiratory abnormalities in eosinophilic granuloma of the lung. Long-term study of five cases, *N. Engl. J. Med.* 267:577, 1962.

82. Hoogstraten, B., Owens, A. H., Lenhard, R. E., et al. Combination chemotherapy in lymphosarcoma and reticulum cell sarcoma, *Blood* 33:370, 1969.

83. Imamura, M., Sakamoto, S., and Hanazono, H. Malignant histiocy-

tosis: a case of generalized histiocytosis with infiltration of Langerhans' granule-containing histiocytes, *Cancer* 28:467, 1971.

84. Inai, S., et al. Studies on serum lysozyme, *Med. J. Osaka Univ.* 9:33, 1958.

85. Jackson, H., Jr., Parker, F., Jr., and Brues, A. M. Malignant lymphoma of the tonsils, *Am. J. Med. Sci.* 191:1, 1936.

86. Jaffe, H. L., and Lichtenstein, L. Eosinophilic granuloma of bone: condition affecting one, several, or many bones, but apparently limited to skeleton, and representing mildest clinical expression of peculiar inflammatory histiocytosis also underlying Letterer-Siwe disease and Schüller-Christian disease, *Arch. Pathol.* 37:99, 1944.

87. James, G. W. III, and Goodwin, A. R. Leukemic reticuloendotheliosis: clinical and hematologic manifestations, *Trans. Am. Clin. Climatol. Assoc.* 75:175, 1963.

88. Johnson, D. E., Griep, J. A., and Baehner, R. L. Histiocytic leukemia following lifelong infection and thrombocytopenia: histologic, metabolic and bactericidal studies, *J. Pediatr.* 82:664, 1973.

89. Jollès, P., Sternberg, M., and Mathé, G. The relationship between serum lysozyme levels and the blood leukocytes, *Isr. J. Med. Sci.* 1:445, 1965.

90. Jones, B., Welton, W. A., and Gilbert, E. F. Congenital Letterer-Siwe disease—report of three cases, *Cutis* 3:750, 1967.

91. Jordan, H. E. Hemoblastic leukemia. Study of a case, *Arch. Pathol.* 23:653, 1937.

92. Kaplan, H. S., and Rosenberg, S. A. Cure of Hodgkin's disease and other malignant lymphomas, *Postgrad. Med.* 43:146, 1968.

93. Kauffman, S. L., and Stout, A. P. Histiocytic tumors (fibrous xanthoma and histiocytoma) in children, *Cancer* 14:469, 1961.

94. Kay, T. W. Acquired hydrocephalus with atrophic bone changes, exophthalmos, and polyuria (with presentation of the patient), *Pa. Med. J.* 9:520, 1905-1906.

95. Kierland, R. B., Epstein, J. G., and Weber, W. E. Eosinophilic granuloma of skin and mucous membrane. Association with diabetes in-

sipidus, *Arch. Dermatol.* 75:45, 1957.

96. Knudson, R. J., Badger, T. L., and Gaensler, E. A. Eosinophilic granuloma of the lung, *Med. Thorac.* 23:248, 1966.

97. Kostich, N. D., and Rappaport, H. Diagnostic significance of the histologic changes in the liver and spleen in leukemia and malignant lymphoma, *Cancer* 18:1214, 1965.

98. Kress, M. B., and Brantigan, O. C. Primary lymphosarcoma of the lung, *Ann. Intern. Med.* 55:582, 1961.

99. Lackey, R. W., Leaver, F. Y., and Farinacci, C. J. Eosinophilic granuloma of the lung, *Radiology* 59:504, 1952.

100. Lahey, M. E. Prognosis in reticuloendotheliosis in children, *J. Pediatr.* 60:664, 1962.

101. Lehrer, R. I., and Cline, M. J. Leukocyte myeloperoxidase deficiency and disseminated candidiasis: the role of myeloperoxidase in resistance to *Candida* infection, *J. Clin. Invest.* 48:1478, 1969.

102. Letterer, E. Aleukämische Reticulose (ein Beitrag zu den proliferativen Erkrankungen des Retikuloendothelialapparates), *Frankfurt. Z. Pathol.* 30:377, 1924.

103. Lever, W. F., and Leeper, R. W. Eosinophilic granuloma of the skin. Report of cases representing the two different diseases described as eosinophilic granuloma, *Arch. Dermatol. Syph.* 62:85, 1950.

104. Levine, M., Schwartz, S., Allen, A., and Narcisco, F. V. Lymphosarcoma and periureteral fibrosis, *Radiology* 82:90, 1964.

105. Levitt, M., Marsh, J., DeConti, R., et al. Combination sequential chemotherapy in advanced reticulum cell sarcoma, *Cancer* 29:630, 1972.

106. Lewis, J. G. Eosinophilic granuloma and its variants with special reference to lung involvement. A report of 12 patients, *Q. J. Med.* 33:337, 1964.

107. Lichtenstein, L. Histiocytosis X. Integration of eosinophilic granuloma of bone, "Letterer-Siwe disease," and "Schüller-Christian disease" as related manifestations of a single nosologic entity, *Arch. Pathol.* 56:84, 1953.

108. Lichtenstein, L. Histiocytosis X (eosinophilic granuloma of bone, Let-

terer-Siwe disease, and Schüller-Christian disease). Further observations of pathological and clinical importance, *J. Bone Joint Surg.* 46A:76, 1964.

109. Lichtenstein, L., and Jaffe, H. L. Eosinophilic granuloma of bone. With report of a case, *Am. J. Pathol.* 16:595, 1940.

110. Lichtman, M. A., and Weed, R. I. Peripheral cytoplasmic characteristics of leukocytes in monocytic leukemia: relationship to clinical manifestations, *Blood* 40:52, 1972.

111. Lieberman, P. H., Jones, C. R., Dargeon, H. W. K., and Begg, C. F. A reappraisal of eosinophilic granuloma of bone, Hand-Schüller-Christian syndrome and Letterer-Siwe syndrome, *Medicine* 48:375, 1969.

112. Lightwood, R., and Tizard, J. P. M. Recovery from acute infantile nonlipoid reticulo-endotheliosis (? Letterer-Siwe disease), *Acta Paediatr.* 100:453, 1954 (suppl.).

113. Litwack, G. Photometric determination of lysozyme activity, *Proc. Soc. Exp. Biol. Med.* 89:401, 1955.

114. Lowenbraun, S., DeVita, V. T., and Serpick, A. Combination chemotherapy with nitrogen mustard, vincristine, procarbazine and prednisone in lymphosarcoma and reticulum cell sarcoma, *Cancer* 25:1018, 1970.

115. Lutman, G. B., and Senhauser, D. A. Histiocytic medullary reticulosis: report of a case with autopsy findings, *South. Med. J.* 59:1345, 1966.

116. Lynch, E. C., and Alfrey, C. P., Jr. Histiocytic medullary reticulosis. Hemolytic anemia due to erythrophagocytosis by histiocytes, *Ann. Intern. Med.* 63:666, 1965.

117. McGavran, M. H., and Spady, H. A. Eosinophilic granuloma of bone. A study of twenty-eight cases, *J. Bone Joint Surg.* 42A:979, 1960.

118. McKay, D. G., Street, R. B., Jr., Benirschke, K., and Duncan, C. J. Eosinophilic granuloma of the vulva, *Surg. Gynecol. Obstet.* 96:437, 1953.

119. Marshall, A. H. E. Histiocytic medullary reticulosis, *J. Pathol. Bacteriol.* 71:61, 1956.

120. Mathé, G., Schwarzenberg, L., Mery, A. M., Cattan, A., Schneider, M., Amiel, J. L., Schlumberger, J.

R., Poisson, J., and Wajcner, G. Extensive histological and cytological survey of patients with acute leukaemia in "complete remission," *Br. Med. J.* 1:640, 1966.

121. Meacham, G. C., and Weisberger, A. S. Early atypical manifestations of leukemia, *Ann. Intern. Med.* 41:780, 1954.

122. Melamed, M. R. The cytological presentation of malignant lymphomas and related diseases in effusions, *Cancer* 16:413, 1963.

123. Metcalf, D. Transformation of granulocytes to macrophages in bone marrow colonies in vitro, *J. Cell Physiol.* 77:277, 1971.

124. Mikal, S. Primary lymphoma of the thyroid gland, *Surgery* 55:233, 1964.

125. Mitus, W. J., Mednicoff, I. B., Wittels, B., and Dameshek, W. Neoplastic lymphoid reticulum cells in the peripheral blood; a histochemical study, *Blood* 17:206, 1961.

126. Morris, R. C., Ueki, I., Sebastian, A., and Morris, E. Lysozymuria in acidification defects of the proximal nephron, *Clin. Res.* 15:142, 1967.

127. Morris, R. C., Jr., and Fudenberg, H. H. Impaired renal acidification in patients with hypergammaglobulinemia, *Medicine* 46:57, 1969.

128. Moxley, J. H. III, DeVita, V. T., Brace, K., and Frei, E. III. Intensive combination chemotherapy and X-irradiation in Hodgkin's disease, *Cancer Res.* 27:1258, 1967.

129. Myer, K., Gellhorn, A., Prudden, J. F., Lehman, W. L., and Steinberg, A. Lysozyme activity in ulcerative alimentary disease. II. Lysozyme activity in chronic ulcerative colitis, *Am. J. Med.* 5:469, 1948.

130. Natelson, E. A., Lynch, E. C., Hettig, R. A., et al. Histiocytic medullary reticulosis. The role of phagocytosis in pancytopenia, *Arch. Intern. Med.* 122:223, 1968.

131. Nies, B. A., Bodey, G. P., Thomas, L. B., Brecher, G., and Freireich, J. The persistence of extramedullary leukemic infiltrates during bone marrow remission of acute leukemia, *Blood* 26:133, 1965.

132. Ohara, K., Fried, J., Dowling, M. D., Jr., et al. Studies of cellular proliferation in human leukemia. VII.

Cytokinetic behavior of neoplastic cells in a patient with reticulum cell sarcoma in a leukemic phase, *Cancer* 28:862, 1971.

133. Ohta, H., and Nagase, H. Serial estimation of serum, urine and leukocyte muramidase (lysozyme) in monocytic leukemia, *Acta Haematol.* 46:257, 1971.

134. Osgood, E. E. Monocytic leukemia. Report of six cases and review of one hundred and twenty-seven cases, *Arch. Intern. Med.* 59:931, 1937.

135. Osserman, E. F., and Lawlor, D. P. Serum and urinary lysozyme (muramidase) in monocytic and monomyelocytic leukemia, *J. Exp. Med.* 124:921, 1966.

136. Otani, S. A discussion on eosinophilic granuloma of bone, Letterer-Siwe disease and Schüller-Christian disease, *J. Mount Sinai Hosp.* 24:1079, 1957.

137. Otani, S., and Ehrlich, J. C. Solitary granuloma of bone simulating primary neoplasm, *Am. J. Pathol.* 16:479, 1940.

138. Perillie, P. E., Kaplan, S. S., Lefkowitz, E., Rogaway, W., and Finch, S. C. Studies of muramidase (lysozyme) in leukemia, *J.A.M.A.* 203:317, 1968.

139. Pollock, J. J., Chipman, D. M., and Sharon, N. The active site of lysozyme: some properties of subsites *E* and *F*, *Biochem. Biophys. Res. Commun.* 28:779, 1967.

140. Pretlow, T. G. II. Chronic monocytic dyscrasia culminating in acute leukemia, *Am. J. Med.* 46:130, 1969.

141. Prockop, D. J., and Davidson, W. D. A. A study of urinary and serum lysozyme in patients with renal disease, *N. Engl. J. Med.* 270:269, 1964.

142. Prudden, J. F., Lane, N., and Meyer, K. Lysozyme content of granulation tissue, *Proc. Soc. Exp. Biol. Med.* 72:38, 1949.

143. Pruzanski, W., and Platts, M. E. Serum and urinary proteins, lysozyme (muramidase) and renal dysfunction in mono- and myelomonocytic leukemia, *J. Clin. Invest.* 49:1694, 1970.

144. Pugh, D. G. Reticulosis, in Roentgenographic Diagnosis of Diseases of Bones, p. 475, Williams &

Wilkins Co., Baltimore, 1954.

145. Rappaport, H. Tumors of the hematopoietic system, in Atlas of Tumor Pathology, sect. III, Fasc. 8, p. 63, Armed Forces Inst. of Pathol., Washington, D.C., 1966.

146. Reid, M. J., and Gottlieb, B. Congenital histiocytosis X, *Calif. Med.* 111:275, 1969.

147. Reilly, C. J., Han, T., Stutzman, L., Slack, N. H., and Webster, J. Reticulum cell sarcoma. A review of radiotherapeutic experience, *Cancer* 29:1314, 1972.

148. Reshcad, H., and Schilling-Torgau, V. Ueber eine neue Leukämie durch echte Uebergangsformen (Splenozytenleukämie) und ihre Bedeutung für die Selbstandigkeit, *Munch. Med. Wochenschr.* 60:1981, 1913.

149. Robb-Smith, A. H. T. Reticulosis and reticulosarcoma: a histological classification, *J. Pathol. Bacteriol.* 47:457, 1938.

150. Rosai, J., and Dorfman, R. F. Sinus histiocytosis with massive lymphadenopathy, *Arch. Pathol.* 87:63, 1969.

151. Rosenberg, S. A., Diamond, H. D., Dargeon, H. W., and Craver, L. F. Lymphosarcoma in childhood, *N. Engl. J. Med.* 259:505, 1958.

152. Rosenberg, S. A., Diamond, H. D., Jaslowitz, B., and Craver, L. F. Lymphosarcoma: a review of 1269 cases, *Medicine* 40:31, 1961.

153. Rowland, R. S. Xanthomatosis and the reticuloendothelial system. Correlation of an unidentified group of cases described as defects in membraneous bones, exophthalmos and diabetes insipidus (Christian's syndrome), *Arch. Intern. Med.* 42:611, 1928.

154. Rubin, A. D., Douglas, S. D., Chessin, L. N., Glade, P. R., and Dameshek, W. Chronic reticulolymphocytic leukemia. Reclassification of "leukemic reticuloendotheliosis" through functional characterization of the circulating mononuclear cells, *Am. J. Med.* 47:149, 1969.

155. Rupley, J. A., and Gates, V. Studies on the enzymic activity of lysozyme. II. The hydrolysis and transfer reactions of N-acetylglucosamine oligosaccharides, *Proc. Natl. Acad. Sci. U.S.A.* 57:496, 1967.

156. Sachs, L. In vitro control of growth and development of hematopoietic cell clones, *in* A. S. Gordon (ed.), Regulation of Hematopoiesis, p. 217, Appelton-Century-Crofts, New York, 1970.

157. Salmon, P. R., and Paully, J. W. Eosinophilic granuloma of the gastrointestinal tract, *Gut* 8:8, 1967.

158. Salmon, S. E., Cline, M. J., Schultz, J., and Lehrer, R. I. Myeloperoxidase deficiency: immunologic study of a genetic leukocyte defect, *N. Engl. J. Med.* 282:250, 1970.

159. Salton, M. R. J., and Ghuysen, J. M. The structure of *di-* and *tetra*-saccharides released from cell walls by lysozyme and streptomyces F_1 enzyme and the β $(1 \rightarrow 4)$ N-acetyl-hexosaminidase activity of these enzymes, *Biochim. Biophys. Acta* 36:552, 1959.

160. Samter, T. G., Alstott, D. F., and Kurlander, G. J. Inflammatory fibroid polyps of the gastrointestinal tract. A report of 3 cases, 2 occurring in children, *Am. J. Clin. Pathol.* 45:420, 1966.

161. Schafer, E. L. Nonlipid reticulo-endotheliosis: Letterer-Siwe's disease. A report of three cases, *Am. J. Pathol.* 25:49, 1949.

162. Schaumburg, H. H., Plank, C., and Adams, R. The reticulum cell sarcoma–microglioma group of brain tumours, *Brain* 95:199, 1972.

163. Schnitzer, B., and Kass, L. Leukemic phase of reticulum cell sarcoma (histiocytic lymphoma), *Cancer* 31:547, 1973.

164. Schoek, V. W., Peterson, R. D. A., and Good, R. A. Familial occurrence of Letterer-Siwe disease, *Pediatrics* 32:1055, 1963.

165. Schrek, R., and Donnelly, W. J. "Hairy" cells in blood in lymphoreticular neoplastic disease and "flagellated" cells of normal lymph nodes, *Blood* 27:199, 1966.

166. Schüller, A. Über eigenartige Schädeldefekte im Jugendalter, *Fortschr. Roentgenstr.* 23:12, 1915–1916.

167. Scott, R. B., and Robb-Smith, A. H. T. Histiocytic medullary reticulosis, *Lancet* ii:194, 1939.

168. Seligman, B. R., Rosner, F., Lee, S. L., et al. Histiocytic medullary reticulosis. Fatal hemorrhage due to massive platelet phagocytosis, *Arch. Intern. Med.* 129:109, 1972.

169. Sherrick, D. W., Hodgson, J. R., and Dockerty, M. B. The roentgenologic diagnosis of primary gastric lymphoma, *Radiology* 84:925, 1965.

170. Shoji, H., and Miller, T. R. Primary reticulum cell sarcoma of bone, *Cancer* 28:1234, 1971.

171. Sinn, C. M., and Dick, F. W. Monocytic leukemia, *Am. J. Med.* 20:588, 1956.

172. Siwe, S. A. Die Reticuloendotheliose—ein neues Krankheitsbild unter den Hepatosplenomegalien, *Z. Kinderheilkd.* 55:212, 1933.

173. Siwe, S. A. The reticulo-endothelioses in children, *Adv. Pediatr.* 4:117, 1949.

174. Skarin, A. T., Matsuo, Y., and Moloney, W. C. Muramidase in myeloproliferative disorders terminating in acute leukemia, *Cancer* 29:1336, 1972.

175. Spellberg, M. A., and Zivin, S. Lymphosarcoma of the gastrointestinal tract. With a report of twenty-one cases, *Arch. Intern. Med.* 83:135, 1949.

176. Steinman, R. M., and Cohn, Z. A. Identification of a novel cell type in peripheral lymphoid organs of mice, *J. Exp. Med.* 137:1142, 1973.

177. Thannhauser, S. J., and Magendantz, H. The different clinical groups of xanthomatous diseases; a clinical physiological study of 22 cases, *Ann. Intern. Med.* 11:1662, 1938.

178. Trubowitz, S., Masek, B., and Frasca, J. M. Leukemic reticuloendotheliosis, *Blood* 38:288, 1971.

179. Ureles, A. L., Alschibaja, T., Lodico, D., and Stabins, S. J. Idiopathic eosinophilic infiltration of the gastrointestinal tract, diffuse and circumscribed. A proposed classification and review of the literature, with two additional cases, *Am. J. Med.* 30:899, 1961.

180. Vaithianathan, T., Fishkin, S., and Gruhn, J. G. Histiocytic medullary reticulosis, *Am. J. Clin. Pathol.* 47:160, 1967.

181. Van Creveld, S. The lipoidoses, *in* S. Z. Levine (ed.), Advances in Pediatrics, vol. 6, p. 190, Yearbook Publishers, Chicago, 1953.

182. van Furth, R., and Diesselhoff-Den Dulk, M. M. C. The kinetics of promonocytes and monocytes in the bone marrow, *J. Exp. Med.* 132:813, 1970.

183. Vieta, J. O., Friedell, H. L., and Craver, L. F. Survey of Hodgkin's disease and lymphosarcoma in bone, *Radiology* 39:1, 1942.

184. Wainwright, C. W., and Duff, G. L. Monocytic leukemia, *Bull. Johns Hopkins Hosp.* 58:267, 1936.

185. Wallgren, A. Systemic reticuloendothelial granuloma. Nonlipoid reticuloendotheliosis and Schüller-Christian disease, *Am. J. Dis. Child.* 60:471, 1940.

186. Watkins, C. H., and Hall, B. E. Monocytic leukemia of the Naegeli and Schilling types, *Am. J. Clin. Pathol.* 10:387, 1940.

187. Weber, F. P. Lipoid rheumatism, *Br. J. Dermatol. Syph.* 60:106, 1948.

188. Weber, F. P. Reticulohistiocytosis, *Br. Med. J.* 3:103, 1957.

189. Wechsler, L., and Zahavi, J. The latent period of acute leukemia. Report of a case of unusual duration, *Isr. J. Med. Sci.* 2:355, 1966.

190. Welborn, J. K., Ponka, J. L., and Rebuck, J. W. Lymphoma of the stomach. A diagnostic and therapeutic problem, *Arch. Surg.* 90:480, 1965.

191. Welch, J. W., Chesky, V. E., and Hellwig, C. A. Malignant lymphoma of the thyroid, *Surg. Gynecol. Obstet.* 106:70, 1958.

192. West, W. O. Primary lymphosarcoma of prostate gland, *Arch. Intern. Med.* 109:469, 1962.

193. Wiernik, P. H., and Serpick, A. A. Clinical significance of serum and urinary muramidase activity in leukemia and other hematologic malignancies, *Am. J. Med.* 46:330, 1969.

194. Wintrobe, M. M. Clinical Hematology, 6th ed., Lea & Febiger, Philadelphia, 1967.

195. Woolner, L. B., McConahey, W. M., Beahrs, O. H., and Black, B. M. Primary malignant lymphoma of the thyroid. Review of forty-six cases, *Am. J. Surg.* 111:502, 1966.

196. Yam, L. T., Castoldi, G. L., Garvey, M. B., and Mitus, W. J. Functional cytogenetic and cytochemical study of the leukemic reticulum cells, *Blood* 32:90, 1968.

197. Zak, F. G., and Rubin, E. Histiocytic medullary reticulosis, *Am. J. Med.* 31:813, 1961.

198. Zawadzki, Z. A., Pena, C. E., and Fisher, E. R. Histiocytic medullary reticulosis. Case report with electron microscopic study, *Acta Haematol.* 42:50, 1969.

199. Zussman, W. V. Monocytic leukemic glossitis. Report of a case, *Oral Surg.* 21:205, 1966.

Additional References

Index

Additional References

The bibliography that follows is supplementary to the references listed at the close of each chapter. These are articles that have appeared in the past year or two; while not cited in the text, they are pertinent to the material contained therein.

Chapter 1

Bretz, U., and Baggiolini, M. Biochemical and morphological characterization of azurophil and specific granules of human neutrophil polymorphonuclear leukocytes, *J. Cell Biol.* 63:251, 1974.

Murata, F., and Spicer, S. S. Morphologic and cytochemical studies of rabbit heterophilic leukocytes. Evidence for tertiary granules, *Lab. Invest.* 29:65, 1973.

Olsson, I., and Venge, P. Cationic proteins of human granulocytes. II. Separation of the cationic proteins of granules of leukemic myeloid cells, *Blood* 44:235, 1974.

Spitznagel, J. K., Dalldorf, F. G., Leffell, M. S., et al. Character of azurophil and specific granules purified from human polymorphonuclear leukocytes, *Lab. Invest.* 30:774, 1974.

West, B. C., Rosenthal, A. S., Gelb, N. A., and Kimball, H. R. Separation and characterization of human neutrophil granules, *Am. J. Pathol.* 77:41, 1974.

Chapter 2

Cerny, J. Stimulation of bone marrow haemopoietic stem cells by a factor from activated T cells, *Nature* 249:63, 1974.

Cline, M. J., Craddock, C. G., Gale, R. P., Golde, D. W., and Lehrer, R. I. Granulocytes in human disease, *Ann. Intern. Med.* 81:801, 1974.

Cline, M. J., and Golde, D. W. Production of colony stimulating factor by human lymphocytes, *Nature* 248:703, 1974.

Golde D. W., and Cline, M. J. Medical progress: regulation of granulopoiesis, *N. Engl. J. Med.,* 291:1388, 1974.

Lind, D. E., Bradley, M. L., Gunz, F. W., et al. The non-equivalence of mouse and human marrow culture in the assay of granulopoietic stimulatory factors, *J. Cell. Physiol.* 83:35, 1974.

Moore, M. A. S., Spitzer, G., Metcalf, D., et al. Monocyte production of colony stimulating factor in familial cyclic neutropenia, *Br. J. Haematol.* 27:47, 1974.

Petersen, B. H., Meyer, T., and Tjernshaugen, H. Kinetics of rat bone marrow cells cultured in diffusion chambers: effect of heterologous implantation and irradiation of the host, *Scand. J. Haematol.* 13:39, 1974.

Schroder, J., Tiilikainen, A., and de la Chapelle, A. Fetal leukocytes in the maternal circulation after delivery. I. Cytological aspects, *Transplantation* 17:346, 1974.

Vincent, P. C., Chanana, A. D., Cronkite, E. P., et al. The intravascular survival of neutrophils labeled in vivo, *Blood* 43:371, 1974.

Chapter 3

Bryant, R. E., and Sutcliffe, M. C. The effect of 3',5'-adenosine monophosphate on granulocyte adhesion, *J. Clin. Invest.* 54:1241, 1974.

DeChatelet, L. R., McCall, C. E., McPhail, L. C., et al. Superoxide dismutase activity in leukocytes, *J. Clin. Invest.* 53:1197, 1974.

DePierre, J. W., and Karnovsky, M. L. Ecto-enzymes of the guinea pig polymorphonuclear leukocyte. I. Evidence for an ecto-adenosine monophosphatase, -adenosine triphosphatase, and -*p*-nitrophenyl phosphatase, *J. Biol. Chem.* 249:7111, 1974.

DePierre, J. W., and Karnovsky, M. L. Ecto-enzymes of the guinea pig polymorphonuclear leukocyte. II. Properties and suitability as markers for the plasma membrane, *J. Biol. Chem.* 249:7121, 1974.

Salin, M. L., and McCord, J. M. Superoxide dismutases in polymorphonuclear leukocytes, *J. Clin. Invest.* 54:1005, 1974.

Scott, R. B., and Cooper, L. W. Leucocyte glycogen response in inflammatory exudates, *Br. J. Haematol.* 26:485, 1974.

Chapter 4

Bryant, R. E., and Sutcliffe, M. C. The effect of 3',5'-adenosine monophosphate on granulocyte adhesion, *J. Clin. Invest.*, 54:1241, 1974.

Gamow, E., and Barnes, F. S. Chemotactic responses of human polymorphonuclear leukocytes to cyclic GMP and other compounds, *Exp. Cell Res.* 87:1, 1974.

Giordano, G. F., and Lichtman, M. A. The role of sulfhydryl groups in human neutrophil adhesion, movement and particle ingestion, *J. Cell. Physiol.* 82:387, 1973.

Ignarro, L. J., and George, W. J. Mediation of immunologic discharge of lysosomal enzymes from human neutrophils by guanosine 3′,5′-monophosphate, *J. Exp. Med.* 140:225, 1974.

Keller, H. U., Hess, M. W., and Cottier, H. Physiology of chemotaxis and random motility, *Semin. Hematol.* 12:47, 1975.

Stossel, T. P. Medical progress. Phagocytosis, *N. Engl. J. Med.* 290:717, 1974.

Tatsumi, N., Shibata, N., Okamura, Y., et al. Actin and myosin A from leucocytes, *Biochim. Biophys. Acta* 305:433, 1973.

Weiss, J., Franson, R. C., Beckerdite, S., et al. Partial characterization and purification of rabbit granulocyte factor that increases permeability of *Escherichia coli*, *J. Clin. Invest.* 55:33, 1975.

Wilkinson, P. C. Surface and cell membrane activities of leukocyte chemotactic factors, *Nature* 251:58, 1974.

Chapter 5

Bell, D. A., Thiem, P. A., Vaughan, J. H., et al. Studies with human leukocyte lysosomes. Evidence for antilysosome antibodies in lupus erythematosis and for the presence of lysosomal antigen in inflammatory diseases, *J. Clin. Invest.* 55:256, 1975.

Lalezari, P., and Radel, E. Neutrophil-specific antigens: immunology and clinical significance, *Semin. Hematol.* 11:281, 1974.

Chapter 6

Cohn, D. A., Athanassiades, T. J., and Speirs, R. S. Inflammatory cell responses to antigen in thymus deprived mice: reduced eosinophils and mononuclear cells, *J. Reticuloendothel. Soc.* 15:199, 1974.

Kay, N. E., Nelson, D. A., and Gottlieb, A. J. Eosinophilic Pelger-Huët anomaly with myeloproliferative disorder, *Am. J. Clin. Pathol.* 60:663, 1973.

Mahmoud, A. F., Kellermeyer, R. W., and

Warren, K. S. Production of monospecific rabbit antihuman eosinophil serums and demonstration of a blocking phenomenon, *N. Engl. J. Med.* 290:417, 1974.

Presentey, B. Partial and severe peroxidase and phospholipid deficiency in eosinophils. Cytochemical and generic considerations, *Acta Haematol.* 44:345, 1970.

Tchernitchin, A., Roorijck, J., Tchernitchin, X., et al. Dramatic early increase in uterine eosinophils after oestrogen administration, *Nature* 248:142, 1974.

Wasserman, S. I., Goetzl, E. J., Ellman, L., and Austen, K. F. Tumor-associated eosinophilotactic factor, *N. Engl. J. Med.* 290:420, 1974.

Chapter 7

Kulzycki, A., Jr., Isersky, C., and Metzger, H. The interaction of IgE with rat basophilic leukemia cells. I. Evidence for specific binding of IgE, *J. Exp. Med.* 139:600, 1974.

Chapter 8

Boggs, D. R. Transfusion of neutrophils as prevention or treatment of infection in patients with neutropenia, *N. Engl. J. Med.* 290:1055, 1974.

Boxer, L. A., Hedley-Whyte, E. T., and Stossel, T. P. Neutrophil actin dysfunction and abnormal neutrophil behavior, *N. Engl. J. Med.* 291:1093, 1974.

Craddock, P. R., Yawata, Y., Van Santen, L., Gilberstadt, S., Silvis, S., and Jacob, H. S. Acquired phagocyte dysfunction; a complication of the hypophosphatemia of parenteral hyperalimentation, *N. Engl. J. Med.* 290:1403, 1974.

Dale, D. C., Fauci, A. S., and Wolff, S. M. Alternate-day prednisone; leukocyte kinetics and susceptibility to infections, *N. Engl. J. Med.* 291:1154, 1974.

MacGregor, R. R., Spagnuolo, P. J., and Lentnek, A. L. Inhibition of granulocyte adherence by ethanol, prednisone, and aspirin, measured with an assay system, *N. Engl. J. Med.* 291:642, 1974.

Miller, M. E. Pathology of chemotaxis and random mobility, *Semin. Hematol.* 12:59, 1975.

Tan, J. S., Strauss, R. G., Akabutu, J., et al. Persistent neutrophil dysfunction in an adult. Combined defect in chemotaxis, phagocytosis and intracellular killing, *Am. J. Med.* 57:251, 1974.

Chapter 9

Boggs, D. R. Medical progress: transfusion of neutrophils as prevention or treatment of infection in patients with neutropenia, *N. Engl. J. Med.* 290:1055, 1974.

Dale, D. C. Transplantation of allogeneic bone marrow in canine cyclic neutropenia, *Science* 183:83, 1974.

Hansen, N. E., Andersen, V., and Karle, H. Plasma lysozyme in drug-induced and spontaneous cyclic neutropenia, *Br. J. Haematol.* 25:485, 1973.

Herring, W. B., Smith, L. G., Walker, R. I., et al. Hereditary neutrophilia, *Am. J. Med.* 56:729, 1974.

Kjeldsberg, C. R., and Swanson, J. Platelet satellitism, *Blood* 43:831, 1974.

Weiden, P. L., Robinett, B., Graham, T. C., et al. Canine cyclic neutropenia. A stem cell defect, *J. Clin. Invest.* 53:950, 1974.

Chapter 10

Gilbert, H. S. The spectrum of myeloproliferative disorders, *Med. Clin. North Am.* 57:355, 1973.

Rosenoff, S. H., Canellos, G. P., O'Connell, M., et al. Mediastinal adenopathy in granulocytic leukemia, *Arch. Intern. Med.* 134:135, 1974.

Rowley, J. D. A new consistent chromosomal abnormality in chronic myelogenous leukaemia identified by quinacrine fluorescence and Giemsa staining, *Nature* 243:290, 1973.

Vallejos, C. S., Trujillo, J. M., Cork, A., et al. Blastic crisis in chronic granulocytic leukemia: experience in 39 patients, *Cancer* 34:1806, 1974.

Chapter 11

Brandt, L., Levan, G., Mitelman, F., et al. Trisomy G-21 in adult myelomonocytic leukaemia. An abnormality common to granulocytic and monocytic cells, *Scand. J. Haematol.* 12:117, 1974.

Gallagher, R. E., and Gallo, R. C. Type C RNA tumor virus isolated from cultured human acute myelogenous leukemia cells, *Science* 187:350, 1975.

Gutterman, J. U., Rodriguez, V., Mavligit, G., et al. Chemoimmunotherapy of adult acute leukemia: prolongation of remission in myeloblastic leukemia with B.C.G., *Lancet* ii:7894, 1974.

Rosman, M., Lee, M. H., Creasey, W. A., et al. Mechanisms of resistance to 6-thiopurines in human leukemia, *Cancer Res.* 34:1952, 1974.

Seeber, S., Käding, J., Brucksch, K. P., et al. Defective rRNA synthesis in human leukaemic blast cells? *Nature* 248:673, 1974.

Trujillo, J. M., Cork, A., Hart, J. S., et al. Clinical implications of aneuploid cytogenetic profiles in adult acute leukemia, *Cancer* 33:824, 1974.

Chapter 12

Trainin, N. Thymic hormones and the immune response, *Physiol. Rev.* 54:272, 1974.

Chapter 14

Ahern, T., Sampson, J., and Kay, J. E. Initiation of protein synthesis during lymphocyte stimulation, *Nature* 248:519, 1974.

Krishnaraj, R., and Talwar, G. P. Role of cyclic AMP in mitogen induced transformation of human peripheral leukocytes, *J. Immunol.* 111:1010, 1973.

Lesniak, M. A., Gorden, P., Roth, J., et al. Binding of ^{125}I-human growth hormone to specific receptors in human cultured lymphocytes, *J. Biol. Chem.* 249:1661, 1974.

Torelli, U., and Torelli, G. Poly(A)-containing RNA molecules in electrophoretically separated fractions of rapidly labeled nuclear RNA from unstimulated and PHA-stimulated human lymphocytes, *Acta Haematol.* 51:140, 1974.

Werthamer, S., Samuels, A. J., and Amaral, L. Identification and partial purification of "transcortin"-like protein within human lymphocytes, *J. Biol. Chem.* 248:6398, 1973.

Chapter 15

Choi, T. K., Sleight, D. R., and Nisonoff, A. General method for isolation and recovery of B cells bearing specific receptors, *J. Exp. Med.* 139:761, 1974.

Lawrence, D. A., Weigle, W. O., and Spiegelberg, H. L. Immunoglobulins cytophilic for human lymphocytes, monocytes, and neutrophils, *J. Clin. Invest.* 55:368, 1975.

Menzoian, J. O., Glasgow, A. H., Nimberg, R. D., et al. Regulation of T lymphocyte function by immunoregulatory alphaglobulin (IRA), *J. Immunol.* 113:266, 1974.

Stocker, J. W., Marchalonis, J. J., and Harris, A. W. Inhibition of a T-cell-dependent immune response in vitro by thymoma cell immunoglobulin, *J. Exp. Med.* 139:785, 1974.

Strosberg, A. D., Collins, J. J., Black, P., et al. Transformation by simian virus 40 of spleen cells from a hyperimmune rabbit: demonstration of production of specific antibody to the immunizing antigen, *Proc. Natl. Acad. Sci. U.S.A.* 71:263, 1974.

Chapter 16

Chapuis, R. S., and Koshland, M. E. Mechanism of IgM polymerization (J chain/J stoichiometry), *Proc. Natl. Acad. Sci. U.S.A.* 71:657, 1974.

DeCoteau, W. E. The role of secretory IgA in defense of the distal lung, *Ann. N.Y. Acad. Sci.* 221:214, 1974.

Ishizaka, K. Dean's lecture. Immunoglobulin E and reaginic hypersensitivity, *Johns Hopkins Med. J.* 135:67, 1974.

Mendez, E., Prelli, F., Fragione, B., et al. Characterization of a disulfide bridge linking the J chain to the α chain of polymeric immunoglobulin A, *Biochem. Biophys. Res. Commun.* 55:1291, 1973.

Mestecky, J., Schrohenloher, R. E., Kulhavy, R., et al. Site of J chain attachment to human polymeric IgA, *Proc. Natl. Acad. Sci. U.S.A.* 71:544, 1974.

Poger, M. E., and Lamm, M. E. Localization of free and bound secretory component in human intestinal epithelial cells. A model for the assembly of secretory IgA, *J. Exp. Med.* 139:629, 1974.

Schechter, I. Biologically and chemically pure mRNA coding for a mouse immunoglobulin L-chain prepared with the aid of antibodies and immobilized oligothymidine, *Proc. Natl. Acad. Sci. U.S.A.* 70:2256, 1973.

Chapter 17

Ascher, M. S., Schneider, W. J., Valentine, F. T., et al. *In vitro* properties of leukocyte dialysates containing transfer factor, *Proc. Natl. Acad. Sci. U.S.A.* 71:1173, 1974.

Barth, R. F., and Gillespie, G. Y. The use of technetium-99m as a radioisotopic label to assess cell-mediated immunity *in vitro, Cell. Immunol.* 10:38, 1974.

Gallin, J. I., and Kirkpatrick, C. H. Chemotactic activity in dialyzable transfer factor, *Proc. Natl. Acad. Sci. U.S.A.* 71:498, 1974.

Kirkpatrick, C. H., and Gallin, J. I. Treatment of infectious and neoplastic diseases with transfer factor, *Oncology* 29:46, 1974.

Rosenfeld, S., and Dressler, D. Transfer factor: a subcellular component that transmits information for specific immune responses, *Proc. Natl. Acad. Sci. U.S.A.* 71:2473, 1974.

Weisbart, R. H., Bluestone, R., Goldberg, L., et al. Migration enhancement factor: a new lymphokine, *Proc. Natl. Acad. Sci. U.S.A.* 71:875, 1974.

Chapter 18

Biggar, W. D., and Park, B. H. Variability in immunologic reconstitution following bone marrow transplantation, *Clin. Immunol. Immunopathol.* 2:501, 1974.

Buckley, R. H., and Fiscus, S. A. Serum IgD and IgE concentrations in immunodeficiency diseases, *J. Clin. Invest.* 55:157, 1975.

Geha, R. S., Schneeberger, E., Merler, E., and Rosen, F. S. Heterogeneity of "acquired" or common variable agammaglobulinemia, *N. Engl. J. Med.* 291:1, 1974.

Scott, C. R., Chen, S-H., and Giblett, E. R. Detection of the carrier state in combined immunodeficiency disease associated with adenosine deaminase deficiency, *J. Clin. Invest.* 53:1194, 1974.

Wu, L. Y. F., Lawton, A. R., and Cooper, M. D. Differentiation capacity of cultured B lymphocytes from immunodeficient patients, *J. Clin. Invest.* 52:3180, 1973.

Chapter 19

Catovsky, D., Pettit, J. E., Galetto, J., et al. The B-lymphocyte nature of the hairy cell of leukaemic reticuloendotheliosis, *Br. J. Haematol.* 26:29, 1974.

Catovsky, D., Pettit, J. E., Galton, D. A. G., et al. Leukaemic reticuloendotheliosis ("hairy" cell leukaemia): a distinct clinico-pathological entity, *Br. J. Haematol.* 26:9, 1974.

Cohen, H. J. Human lymphocyte surface immunoglobulin capping. Normal characteristics and anomalous behavior of chronic lymphocytic leukemic lymphocytes, *J. Clin. Invest.* 55:84, 1975.

Schnitzer, B., and Kass, L. Hairy-cell leukemia. A clinicopathologic and ultrastructural study, *Am. J. Clin. Pathol.* 61:176, 1974.

Shevach, E., Edelson, R., Frank, M., et al. A human leukemia cell with both B and T cell surface receptors, *Proc. Natl. Acad. Sci. U.S.A.* 71:863, 1974.

Chapter 20

Arend, W. P., and Adamson, J. W. Non-secretory myeloma. Immunofluorescent demonstration of paraprotein within bone marrow plasma cells, *Cancer* 33:721, 1974.

Cohen, H. J., and Lefer, L. G. Intranuclear inclusions in Bence Jones lambda plasma cell myeloma, *Blood* 45:131, 1975.

Isobe, T., and Osserman, E. F. Plasma cell dyscrasia associated with the production of incomplete (? deleted) IgGλ molecules, gamma heavy chains, and free lambda chains containing carbohydrate: description of the first case, *Blood* 43:505, 1974.

Mundy, G. R., Raisz, L. G., Cooper, R. A., Schechter, G. P., and Salmon, S. E. Evidence for the secretion of an osteoclast stimulating factor in myeloma, *N. Engl. J. Med.* 291:1041, 1974.

Salmon, S. E. Expansion of the growth fraction in multiple myeloma with alkylating agents, *Blood* 45:119, 1975.

Chapter 21

Aur, R. J. A., Simone, J. V., Hustu, H. O., et al. Cessation of therapy during complete remission of childhood acute lymphocytic leukemia, *N. Engl. J. Med.* 291:1230, 1974.

Fefer, A., Einstein, A. B., Thomas, E. D., Buckner, C. D., Clift, R. A., Glucksberg, H., Neiman, P. E., and Storb, R. Bone-marrow transplantation for hematologic neoplasia in 16 patients with identical twins, *N. Engl. J. Med.*, 290:1389, 1974.

Haghbin, M., Tan, C. C., Clarkson, B. D., et al. Intensive chemotherapy in children with acute lymphoblastic leukemia (L-2 protocol), *Cancer* 33:1491, 1974.

Moore, M. A. S., Spitzer, G., Williams, N., et al. Agar culture studies in 127 cases of untreated acute leukemia: the prognostic value of reclassification of leukemia according to in vitro growth characteristics, *Blood* 44:1, 1974.

Pattengale, P. L., Smith, R. W., and Perlin, E. Atypical lymphocytes in acute infectious mononucleosis; identification by multiple T and B lymphocyte markers, *N. Engl. J. Med.* 291:1145, 1974.

Simone, J. Acute lymphocytic leukemia in childhood, *Semin. Hematol.* 11:25, 1974.

Chapter 22

Abt, A. B., Kirschner, R. H., Belliveau, R. E., et al. Hepatic pathology associated with Hodgkin's disease *Cancer* 33:1564, 1974.

Goldsmith, M. A., and Carter, S. K. Combination chemotherapy of advanced Hodgkin's disease. A review, *Cancer* 33:1, 1974.

Jaffe, E. S., Shevach, E. M., Frank, M. M., et al. Nodular lymphoma—evidence for origin from follicular B lymphocytes, *N. Engl. J. Med.* 290:813, 1974.

Levine, G. D., and Dorfman, R. F. Nodular lymphoma: an ultrastructural study of its relationship to germinal centers and a correlation of light and electron microscopic findings, *Cancer* 35:148, 1975.

Long, J. C., Aisenberg, A. C., and Zamecnik, P. C. An antigen in Hodgkin's disease tissue cultures: radioiodine-labeled antibody studies, *Proc. Natl. Acad. Sci. U.S.A.* 71:2605, 1974.

Lukes, R. J., and Tindle, B. H. Immunoblastic lymphadenopathy: a hyperimmune entity resembling Hodgkin's disease, *N. Engl. J. Med.* 292:1, 1975.

Shipley, W. U., Piro, A. J., and Hellman, S. Radiation therapy of Hodgkin's disease: significance of splenic involvement, *Cancer* 34:223, 1974.

Chapter 23

Meuret, G., Bammert, J., and Hoffman, G. Kinetics of human monocytopoiesis, *Blood* 44:801, 1974.

Meuret, G., Bremer, C., Bammert, J., et al. Oscillation of blood monocyte counts in healthy individuals, *Cell Tissue Kinet.* 7:223, 1974.

Nichols, B. A., and Bainton, D. F. Differentiation of human monocytes in bone marrow and blood, *Lab. Invest.* 29:27, 1973.

Reaven, E. P., and Axline, S. G. Subplasmalemmal microfilaments and microtubules in resting and phagocytizing cultivated macrophages, *J. Cell Biol.* 59:12, 1973.

Weiss, L. A scanning electron microscopic study of the spleen, *Blood* 43:665, 1974.

Chapter 24

Ackerman, N. R., and Beebe, J. R. Release of lysosomal enzymes by alveolar mononuclear cells, *Nature* 247:475, 1974.

Cohen, A. B. Interrelationships between the human alveolar macrophage and alpha-1-antitrypsin, *J. Exp. Med.* 52:2793, 1973.

Gemsa, D., Wood, C. H., Fudenberg, H. H., et al. Stimulation of heme oxygenase in macrophages and liver by endotoxin, *J. Clin. Invest.* 53:647, 1974.

Gordon, S., Todd, J., and Cohn, Z. A. In vitro synthesis and secretion of lysozyme by mononuclear phagocytes, *J. Exp. Med.* 139:1228, 1974.

Olsen, G. N., Harris, J. O., Castle, J. R., et al. Alpha-1-antitrypsin content in the serum, alveolar macrophages, and alveolar lavage fluid of smoking and nonsmoking normal subjects, *J. Clin. Invest.* 55:427, 1975.

Sandler, J. A., Clyman, R. I., Manganiello, V. C., et al. The effect of serotonin (5-hydroxytryptamine) and derivatives on guanosine 3′,5′-monophosphate in human monocytes, *J. Clin. Invest.* 55:431, 1975.

Chapter 25

Anderson, S. E., and Remington, J. S. Effect of normal and activated human macrophages on *Toxoplasma gondii*, *J. Exp. Med.* 139:1154, 1974.

Bast, R. C., Jr., Cleveland, R. P., Littman, B. H., et al. Acquired cellular immunity: extracellular killing of *Listeria monocytogenes* by a product of immunologically activated macrophages, *Cell. Immunol.* 10:248, 1974.

Lehrer, R. I. The fungicidal mechanisms of human monocytes. I. Evidence for myeloperoxidase-linked and myeloperoxidase-independent candidacidal mechanisms, *J. Clin. Invest.* 55:330, 1975.

Rinehart, J. J., Sagone, A. L., Balcerzak, S. P., et al. Effects of corticosteroid therapy on human monocyte function, *N. Engl. J. Med.* 292:236, 1975.

Willenborg, D. O., and Prendergast, R. A. The effect of sea star coelomocyte extract on cell-mediated resistance to *Listeria monocytogenes* in mice, *J. Exp. Med.* 139:820, 1974.

Chapter 26

McClure, P. D., Strachan, P., and Saunders, E. F. Hypofibrinogenemia and thrombocytopenia in familial hemophagocytic reticulosis, *J. Pediatr.* 85:67, 1974.

Twomey, J. J., and Gyorkey, F. The monocyte disorder with herpes zoster, *J. Lab. Clin. Med.* 83:768, 1974.

Chapter 27

DeVita, V. T., et al. Advanced diffuse histiocytic lymphoma, a potentially curable disease, *Lancet* i:248, 1975.

Glick, A. D., and Horn, R. G. Identification of promonocytes and monocytoid precursors in acute leukaemia of adults: ultrastructural and cytochemical observations, *Br. J. Haematol.* 26:395, 1974.

Shaw, M. T., and Nordquist, R. E. "Pure" monocytic or histiomonocytic leukemia: a revised concept, *Cancer* 35:208, 1975.

Warnke, R. A., Kim, H., and Dorfman, R. F. Malignant histiocytosis (histiocytic medullary reticulosis)—I. Clinicopathologic study of 29 cases, *Cancer* 35:215, 1975.

Index